Water-Soluble Vitamins							Minerals						
Vitamin C (mg)	Thiamin (mg)	Riboflavin (mg)	Niacin (mg NE)	Vitamin B6 (mg)	Folate (µg)	Vitamin B12 (µg)	Calcium (mg)	Phosphorus (mg)	Magnesium (mg)	Iron (mg)	Zinc (mg)	Iodine (µg)	Selenium (µg)
30	0.3	0.4	5	0.3	25	0.3	400	300	40	6	5	40	10
35	0.4	0.5	6	0.6	35	0.5	600	500	60	10	5	50	15
40	0.7	0.8	9	1.0	50	0.7	800	800	80	10	10	70	20
45	0.9	1.1	12	1.1	75	1.0	800	800	120	10	10	90	20
45	1.0	1.2	13	1.4	100	1.4	800	800	170	10	10	120	30
50	1.3	1.5	17	1.7	150	2.0	1,200	1,200	270	12	15	150	40
60	1.5	1.8	20	2.0	200	2.0	1,200	1,200	400	12	15	150	50
60	1.5	1.7	19	2.0	200	2.0	1,200	1,200	350	10	15	150	70
60	1.5	1.7	19	2.0	200	2.0	800	800	350	10	15	150	70
60	1.2	1.4	15	2.0	200	2.0	800	800	350	10	15	150	70
50	1.1	1.3	15	1.4	150	2.0	1,200	1,200	280	15	12	150	45
60	1.1	1.3	15	1.5	180	2.0	1,200	1,200	300	15	12	150	50
60	1.1	1.3	15	1.6	180	2.0	1,200	1,200	280	15	12	150	55
60	1.1	1.3	15	1.6	180	2.0	800	800	280	15	12	150	55
60	1.0	1.2	13	1.6	180	2.0	800	800	280	10	12	150	55
70	1.5	1.6	17	2.2	400	2.2	1,200	1,200	320	30	15	175	65
95	1.6	1.8	20	2.1	280	2.6	1,200	1,200	355	15	19	200	75
90	1.6	1.7	20	2.1	260	2.6	1,200	1,200	340	15	16	200	75

Retinol equivalents. 1 retinol equivalent = 1 µg retinol or 6 µg β-carotene.

[c]α-Tocopherol equivalents. 1 mg d-α tocopherol = 1 α-TE.

[d]As cholecalciferol. 10 µg cholecalciferol = 400 IU of vitamin D.

[f]1 NE (niacin equivalent) is equal to 1 mg of niacin or 60 mg of dietary tryptophan.

ESTIMATED SAFE AND ADEQUATE DAILY DIETARY INTAKES OF SELECTED VITAMINS AND MINERALS[a]

Category	Age (years)	Vitamins	
		Biotin (µg)	Pantothenic Acid (mg)
Infants	0-0.5	10	2
	0.5-1	15	3
Children and adolescents	1-3	20	3
	4-6	25	3-1
	7-10	30	4-5
	11 +	30-100	4-7
Adults		30-100	4-7

Category	Age (years)	Trace Elements[b]				
		Copper (mg)	Manganese (mg)	Fluoride (µg)	Chromium (µg)	Molybdenum (mg)
Infants	0-0.5	0.4-0.6	0.3-0.6	0.1-0.5	10-40	15-30
	0.5-1	0.6-0.7	0.6-1.0	0.2-1.0	20-60	20-40
Children and adolescents	1-3	0.7-1.0	1.0-1.5	0.5-1.5	20-80	25-50
	4-6	1.0-1.5	1.5-2.0	1.0-2.5	30-120	30-75
	7-10	1.0-2.0	2.0-3.0	1.5-2.5	50-200	50-150
	11 +	1.5-2.5	2.0-5.0	1.5-2.5	50-200	75-250
Adults		1.5-3.0	2.0-5.0	1.5-4.0	50-200	75-250

* Because there is less information on which to base allowances, these figures are not given in the main table of RDA and are provided here in the form of ranges of recommended intakes.

* Since the toxic levels for many trace elements may be only several times usual intakes, the upper levels for the trace elements given in this table should not be habitually exceeded.

Essentials of Nutrition and Diet Therapy

Sue Rodwell Williams, Ph.D., M.P.H., R.D.

President, SRW Productions, Inc. and
Clinical Nutrition Consultant, Davis, California;
Formerly Metabolic Nutritionist, Kaiser-Permanente Northern
California Regional Newborn Screening and Metabolic
Program, Kaiser-Permanente Medical Center, Oakland, and
Field Faculty, M.P.H.-Dietetic Internship Program and
Coordinated Undergraduate Program in Dietetics,
University of California, Berkeley, California

Sixth Edition

with 110 illustrations

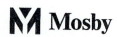

St. Louis Baltimore Boston Chicago London Madrid Philadelphia Sydney Toronto

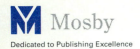
Mosby

Dedicated to Publishing Excellence

Editor-in-Chief: James M. Smith
Editor: Vicki Malinee
Developmental Editors: Loren M. Stevenson, Terry Eynon
Project Manager: Peggy Fagen
Designer: Jeanne Wolfgeher
Design Manager: Betty Schulz
Manufacturing Supervisor: Theresa Fuchs
Cover art: "Melon by the Mountain," WRK, Inc.

Printed in the United States of America
Composition/color separation by The Clarinda Company
Printing/binding by Von Hoffmann Press, Inc.

Mosby–Year Book, Inc.
11830 Westline Industrial Drive
St. Louis, Missouri 63146

International Standard Book Number 0-8016-7923-0

94 95 96 97 98 / 9 8 7 6 5 4 3 2 1

To My Students
whose "whys" and "hows" and "so whats"
keep my feet to the fire of knowledge
and make the learning process exciting
and ever new to me

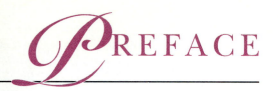

PREFACE

Through five previous editions, this compact "little" book has served the needs of students and teachers in the health sciences in many colleges and universities and has provided a sound but simple reference for busy practitioners. In truth, in all its editions, it has captured and distilled the essence of my larger, more comprehensive textbook, *Nutrition and Diet Therapy*, to lay a faithful foundation for further study and practice.

In this new sixth edition I have adhered to these same fundamental goals. But as in the previous completely reformatted edition, here I have rewritten much of the material to reflect a rapidly developing science and society. Thus its expanded current material and its organization continue to meet the more comprehensive needs of beginning students in the allied health professions today. All the while, it retains its sound, simple, substantive content, thoroughly updated and realistically applied to meet human health needs in our rapidly changing world.

New to this Edition

As indicated, this book is in essence an abridgement of my larger text. It follows a similar format and style to facilitate learning and lay a beginning foundation for sound clinical practice. To achieve these goals in this current edition, I have made a number of changes:

New Chapters. Several new chapters apply the expanding science of nutrition to changing health care needs and developing technologic tools for its clinical practice and management. I have included two new chapters to help meet current practice needs: Chapter 18, Feeding Methods: Enteral and Parenteral Nutrition, to update and expand information about these rapidly developing means of special nutrition support; and Chapter 24, Nutrition and AIDS, to provide current coverage of the special nutritional needs of the rapidly growing number of HIV-infected and AIDS patients worldwide.

New Chapter Order and Coordination. Several chapters have been repositioned or combined to aid learning and reflect current science and practice.

Chapter 2, Digestion, Absorption, and Metabolism, has been repositioned before the chapters on the macronutrients—carbohydrates, fats, and proteins—at the request of teachers and students using this beginning text, to provide basic knowledge of the body systems involved.

Chapter 6, Energy Balance and Weight Management, combines two topics previously treated in separate chapters for a better understanding of their basic relationship in practice.

Chapter 13, Nutrition for Adults: Early, Middle, and Later Years, provides a more balanced and comprehensive view of the varying needs of adults at different age periods, rather than the previous limited focus mainly on the aged, to better reflect the current health care emphasis on health maintenance and disease prevention.

Chapter 19, Gastrointestinal Diseases, has been expanded to include increased current knowledge and changes in nutritional management of problems of the gastrointestinal tract and its accessory organs. For example, new knowledge has changed the treatment of peptic ulcer disease; discovery of the cystic fibrosis gene and its biochemical mechanism effect on pancreatic secretions has changed treatment of the resulting pancreatic insufficiency and malabsorption; and advancing knowledge of viruses causing liver disease has led to new vaccines and reinforced nutritional care of the various stages of the disease, including advanced cirrhosis and encephalopathy.

Chapter 20, Diseases of the Heart, Blood Vessels, and Lungs, has been rewritten and renamed to reflect the coordinated functions of each component of the overall circulatory system and newly discovered unique actions of system sections, such as the role of the arterial vessels' inner endothelial lining in controlling hypertension.

Chapter 26, Nutrition Support in Disabling Disease and Rehabilitation, has been rewritten and expanded to include late-breaking news of current discoveries, treatment, and rehabilitative care in the fields of *musculoskeletal problems* such as rheumatoid arthritis and osteoarthritis; *neuromuscular injury and disease* from the growing problem of neurologic injuries or from developmental disabilities of childhood (cerebral palsy, epilepsy, spina bifida, Down's syndrome); and *progressive neurologic disorders* of middle and older adulthood (Parkinson's and Huntington's diseases, Guillain-Barré syndrome, amyotrophic lateral sclerosis or Lou Gehrig disease, multiple sclerosis, myasthenia gravis, Alzheimer's disease). In each case I have focused on life-changing effects and the role of nutritional support.

New Illustrations and Design.   A new four-color design, incorporating numerous color illustrations, greatly enhances the overall visual appeal and provides learning support. These added graphs, charts, and photographs portray concepts introduced and help students grasp the clinical problems encountered in patient care.

Enhanced Readability and Student Interest.   A large amount of the text has been rewritten to incorporate new material. The writing style is designed to capture student interest and present comprehensive subject matter in a sound and simple manner. Many new advances in basic and clinical science are explained and applied. Issues of student interest and public-professional controversy are discussed. The many examples used open up meaning and understanding. Topics of current relevance clarify questions and concerns.

Learning Aids Within the Text

This new edition continues to use many learning aids throughout the text.

Chapter Openers.   To alert students to the topic of each chapter and draw them into its study, each chapter opens with an illustration, and brief focusing paragraphs on the Chapter topic.

Chapter Outlines.   The major sections are listed at the beginning of each chapter and indicated by special type for ease in reading comprehension.

Key Terms.   Key terms important to the student's understanding and application of the material in patient care are presented in three steps. They are first identified by boldface type in the body of the text. Some are particularly pertinent to the discussion and defined on the right-hand side of each right page. And finally, all are collected in a comprehensive glossary for easy reference at the end of the book. This three-level approach to vocabulary development greatly improves the overall study and use of the text.

Chapter Summaries.   To help the student pull the chapter material together again as a whole, each chap-

ter concludes with a summary of the key concepts presented and their significance or application. The student can then return to any part of the material for repeated study and clarification as needed.

Review Questions for Testing Comprehension.   To help the student understand key parts of the chapter or apply it to patient problems, questions are given after each chapter text for review and analysis of the material presented.

Chapter References.   To provide immediate access to all references cited in the chapter text, a full list of these key references is given at the end of each chapter, rather than collected at the end of the book as in the previous edition.

Further Reading.   In addition to referenced material in the text, an annotated list of suggestions for further reading for added interest and study is provided at the end of each chapter. These selections extend or apply the material in the text according to student needs or areas of special interest. The annotations themselves improve the student's ability to use them by identifying pertinent parts of that reference.

Issues and Answers.   A special feature of each chapter is a concluding brief article on nutrition-related issues or controversies based on the text discussion. These interesting and motivating studies help the student to see the importance of scientific thinking and develop sound judgment and openness to different points of view.

Case Studies.   In many chapters realistic case studies lead the student to apply the text material to related patient care problems. Each case is accompanied by questions for case analysis. These cases also help alert the student to applications of nutritional therapy for similar patient care needs in their own clinical assignments.

Diet Guides.   A variety of diet guidelines are highlighted in the clinical chapters in Part Three.

Appendixes.   The revised Appendixes include a number of materials for use as reference tools and guidelines in learning and practice. Food value tables include nutrient and energy references for a variety of basic foods.

Index.   The index extends the basic text cross-referencing and provides a quick reference to the book's content.

Supplementary Materials

Several supplements enhance the teaching-learning process. Further information on these helpful packages may be obtained from your publisher's representative.

Instructor's Manual.   Prepared by Joanne Spaide, University of Northern Iowa, this valuable tool features suggested course syllabuses; chapter reviews; behavioral objectives; key terms; chapter outlines with teaching notes on controversial topics; nutrition in the news; additional resources, including slides, films, and filmstrips; transparency masters; and an extensive test-item band of approximately 1500 questions.

Computerized Test Bank.   Qualified adopters of the text receive a computerized test bank package compatible with the IBM, Macintosh, Apple IIc, or Apple IIe computers. This software provides a unique combination of user-friendly aids and enables the instructor to select, edit, delete, or add questions and construct and print tests and answer keys. The Gradebook segment features computerized record-keeping, with class, test, or individual grade analysis displayed as bar charts. The Proctor segment allows instructors to set up student tutorials, using items from the test bank or specially written tests.

Overhead Transparency Acetates.   Illustrations of important, hard-to-understand concepts are available as transparency acetates. These useful tools facilitate learning of key concepts discussed in the text and are available to qualified adopters of the text.

Self-Study Guide.   This concise little companion continues to serve as a general learning aid during initial courses, as well as a tool for review of the text for professional examinations or for practitioners needing to update knowledge. It includes many items to support learning of each chapter's content: (1) chapter focus; (2) summary-review quiz; (3) discussion questions to stimulate thinking; (4) true-false and multiple choice test items to test comprehension; (5) numerous guides for individual and group projects that involve experiments, case studies, and situational problems that apply learning; and (6) inquiry questions that relate an "Issues and Answers" article to current health care problems.

Mosby Diet Simple 2.0 Software.   This interactive nutrient analysis software includes a unique food list with more than 2250 items, selected activities, and food exchange lists. The program allows students to input food intake and physical activities to determine total kcalories consumed and expended over a certain period of time.

Personal Approach.   My person-centered approach in past editions remains in this new text. It is enhanced by (1) a personal writing style that reflects my own convictions and commitments about student learning and patient care; (2) extensive use of ever-expanding personal files and materials gathered from current research, my own clinical practice, teaching, and biochemical-metabolic work; and (3) practical applications of scientific knowledge in realistic *human* terms to find personal solutions to individual problems.

Acknowledgments

Many persons have helped me in this book project, and I am grateful for their contributions. To these persons I give my thanks: my editor-in-chief Jim Smith, whose demands for scientific integrity strengthen my own convictions and guide my work; the editorial staff, especially Vicki Malinee, Loren Stevenson, and Terry Eynon, for their constant skill and support; the project managers in Book Production Editing for their constant push toward perfection; the reviewers for their valuable time and suggestions:

Betty Helgerson, M.A.
Northeast Iowa Community College

Jane M. Krump, M.S.
North Dakota State College of Science

Carol Satterberg, R.N., M.N.
Highline Community College

Marie L. Smith, M.Ed., M.S.
SUNY-Morrisville

Linda H. Youngstrom, M.S.
Delaware County Community College

I also thank my own staff for all their personal skills and support, especially to Jim Williams and Mary Herbert, whose computer savvy, research skills, and personal support keep me and my system going; my many students, interns, colleagues, clients, and patients, all of whom have taught me much; and my family, who never cease to support all my efforts and who always share in whatever I am able to achieve.

Sue Rodwell Williams
Davis, California

CONTENTS IN BRIEF

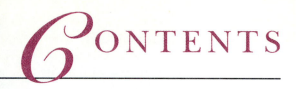

CONTENTS

PART

1

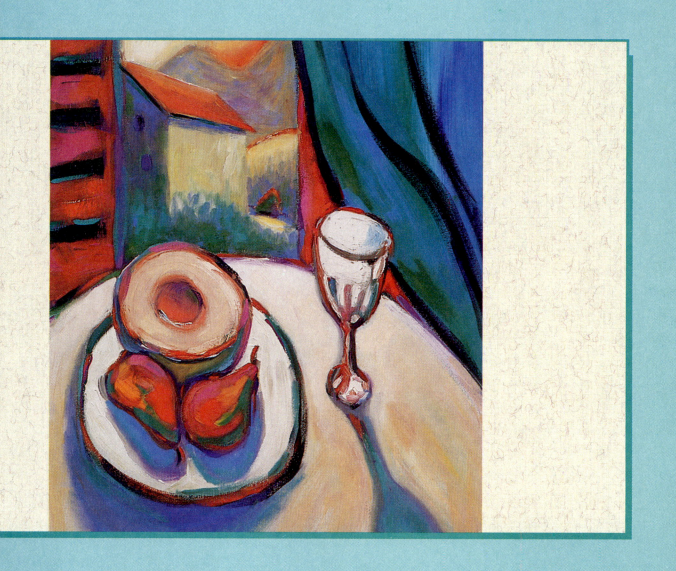

*I*ntroduction to Human Nutrition

CHAPTER 1

Nutrition and Health

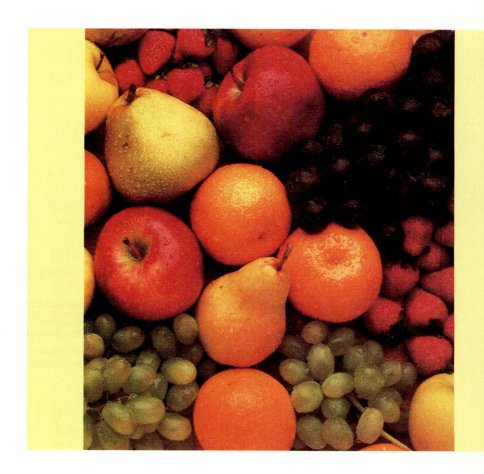

This chapter introduces the study of nutrition in health and health care. Whatever the basis of your present interest, a sound base of nutrition knowledge and skills is fundamental.

Current knowledge of nutrition and its basic science foundations reflect our rapidly changing world in terms of a changing food supply, expanding population, and phenomenal scientific knowledge. Nutrition is rapidly emerging as a vital component in personal health care and in our national nutrition and health policies to meet human need.

A primary means of promoting health and preventing disease for all people rests on a wholesome food supply and the sound nutrition it pro-

vides. In this first chapter we introduce this person-centered approach to nutrition and health care, an important focus throughout your study.

Nutrition and Human Health

The Science of Nutrition

For the most part, knowledge about nutrition builds on two fundamental areas of science. First, the physical sciences of biochemistry and physiology help us to see how nutrition relates to our physical health and well-being. Second, behavioral sciences help us to better understand how nutrition is interwoven with our unique nature as human beings. Throughout our study here, you will see both of these areas of learning at work in our lives.

Basic principles of biochemistry show us that human organisms are marvelously complex groupings of chemical compounds constantly at work in an array of reactions designed to sustain life. Nutrients, the basic currency of nutrition, are chemical compounds or elements. The integrating work of human physiology brings the beauty of order out of a seeming internal chaos of individually functioning cells and organs, blending them into a total functioning whole. Physiologists call this highly sensitive level of internal control **homeostasis.**

However, if we were defined only by our physical components, we would not be fully human. We learn human aspects of being and nutrition from the behavioral sciences, which are rooted in our earliest awareness of psychosocial beginnings and life experiences. Attitudes toward food and eating patterns develop throughout our lifespan from the acculturating influences of family, group, ethnic group, community, nation, even our world. How we perceive ourselves and our food, what we choose to eat, why we eat what we do and in what manner, all become integral parts of human nutrition.

Food and Nutrients

The word **nutrition** refers to nourishment that sustains life. The science and art of human nutrition both focus on nourishing human life. They do this in many ways. From the moment of conception until death, the body needs energy to carry out vital functions such as breathing. In addition, people need energy to support physical activity. They must constantly replenish these energy needs with food to sustain physical life. But food also nourishes the human spirit. We all have our particular "soul foods," "comfort foods," or special "warm fuzzies" for the human spirit.

Nutrition is thus defined as the food people eat and how it nourishes their bodies. **Nutritional science** com

prises the body of scientific knowledge governing the nutritional requirements of humans for maintenance, growth, activity, and reproduction. **Dietetics** is the health profession having primary responsibility for the practical application of nutritional science to persons and groups of persons in various states of health and disease. The **registered dietitian (RD),** especially the **clinical nutrition specialist,** is the nutrition authority on the health care team. The RD, in collaboration with the physician and nurse, carries the major responsibility for nutritional care of patients and clients. The **public health nutritionist** is responsible for nutritional care of groups of people in the community, especially those high-risk groups who require assessment of need and community programs to meet these needs.

Functions of Food and Nutrients

The respective functions of food and nutrients in human nutrition need to be distinguished. First of all, dispense with the myth that any particular food or food combination is required by the body for health. The human race has subsisted for centuries with wide varieties of foods, depending on what was available to eat and what the culture designated as human food. Various foods serve as important vehicles for taking nutrients into the body and bringing human pleasure and comfort. Instead, it is these specific chemical compounds or elements—the **nutrients**—in a wide *variety* of foods that the body requires. Approximately 40 essential nutrients are known; others are probably yet to be discovered. Known essential nutrients include **macronutrients**—carbohydrates, fats, and proteins—whose constituent substances supply energy and build tissue, and **micronutrients,** vitamins and minerals that the body uses in much smaller amounts to regulate and control body processes. Water is the overall vital nutrient sustaining all life processes. The term **metabolism** refers to the sum of these chemical processes in the body that sustain life and health. The first part of this text will cover your study of these important nutrients.

Nutrient Interrelationships

An important nutritional metabolic fact will emerge increasingly in your study of nutrition, the fundamental principle of *nutrient interaction.* The principle states that:

1. Individual nutrients have many specific metabolic functions, including primary and supporting roles, and
2. No nutrient ever works alone

The human body is a fascinating whole made up of many parts and processes. Intimate metabolic relationships exist among all the basic nutrients and their **metabolites.** This key principle of nutrient interaction will be demonstrated more clearly in the following chapters. Remember, we may separate nutrients for study purposes, but they do not exist that way in the body. Nutrients are always interacting as a dynamic whole to produce and maintain the human body, providing energy, building and rebuilding tissue, and regulating metabolic processes.

Energy Sources

The energy-yielding macronutrients—carbohydrates, fats, and proteins—provide primary and alternate sources of energy.

Carbohydrates

Dietary carbohydrates, starches and sugars, provide the body's primary source of fuel for heat and energy. Carbohydrates also maintain a backup source of quick energy known as *glycogen*, sometimes called "animal starch" because its structure is similar to that of plant starch. Each gram of carbohydrate consumed yields **4 kilocalories** (kcalories or kcal). This number is called the "fuel factor" for carbohydrates. A well-balanced diet for a healthy person should supply approximately 50% to 60% of the total kcalories from carbohydrates. The majority of these kcalories should be derived from complex carbohydrate foods, the starches, rather than from simple carbohydrate foods, the sugars.

Fats

Dietary fats from animal and plant sources provide the body's alternate or storage form of heat and energy. Fats are a more concentrated fuel, yielding 9 kcalories for each gram consumed. The fuel factor of fats is therefore 9. Fats should supply no more than 25% to 30% of the total kcalories of a healthy person's well-balanced diet. The majority of these kcalories, approximately two thirds, should consist of vegetable oil products (unsaturated fats) rather than animal food products (saturated fats).

Proteins

The body may draw on dietary or tissue protein to obtain needed energy when the fuel supply from carbohydrates and fats is insufficient. Protein yields 4 kcalories per gram, making its fuel factor 4. Quality protein should provide approximately 15% to 29% of the total kcalories of a healthy person's well-balanced diet. Thus,

---

clinical nutrition specialist • Specialty practice of a registered dietitian with an advanced degree in nutritional science and training in clinical nutrition.

dietetics • Management of diet and the use of food; the science concerned with the nutritional planning and preparation of foods.

homeostasis • State of relative dynamic equilibrium within the body's internal environment; a balance achieved through the operation of various interrelated physiologic mechanisms.

kilocalorie • The general term *calorie* refers to a unit of heat measure and is used alone to designate the *small calorie*. The calorie used in nutritional science and the study of metabolism is the *large calorie*, 1000 calories, or kilocalorie, to be more accurate and avoid use of very large numbers in calculations.

macronutrients • The three large energy-yielding nutrients: carbohydrates, fats, and proteins.

metabolism • Sum of all the various biochemical and physiologic processes by which the body grows and maintains itself (anabolism) and breaks down and reshapes tissue (catabolism), transforming energy to do its work. Products of these various reactions are called *metabolites*.

metabolites • Any substance produced by metabolism or by a metabolic process.

micronutrients • The two classes of small non-energy-yielding elements and compounds: minerals and vitamins, essential in very small amounts for regulation and control functions in cell metabolism and building certain body structures.

nutrients • Substances in food that are essential for energy, growth, normal functioning of the body, and maintenance of life.

nutrition • The sum of the processes involved in taking in food nutrients, assimilating and using them to maintain body tissue and provide energy; a foundation for life and health.

nutritional science • The body of scientific knowledge, developed through controlled research, that relates to the processes involved in nutrition—national, international, community, and clinical.

public health nutritionist • A professional nutritionist, accredited by academic degree course of university and special graduate study (MPH, DrPH) in schools of public health accredited by the American Association of Public Health, responsible for nutrition components of public health programs in varied community settings—county, state, national, international.

registered dietitian (RD) • A professional dietitian, accredited by academic degree course of university and graduate study (MS, PhD), clinical and administration training, and having passed required registration examinations administered by the American Dietetic Association.

although protein's primary function is tissue building, some may be available for energy as needed.

Tissue Building

Protein is the primary nutrient used in tissue building; minerals, vitamins, and fatty acids also play a role.

Proteins

The primary function of protein is tissue building. Dietary protein foods provide **amino acids,** the building units necessary for constructing and repairing body tissues. This is a constant, dynamic process of modeling and remodeling according to need that ensures growth and maintenance of a strong body structure and vital substances for tissue functioning.

Minerals

Two of the major minerals, calcium and phosphorus, help build and maintain bone tissue. Iron helps build hemoglobin, a red blood cell's vital oxygen carrier.

Vitamins

As just one example, vitamin C helps develop the cementing intercellular ground substance necessary to build strong tissue and prevent bleeding in the tissues.

Metabolic Regulation and Control

All of the multiple biochemical processes that comprise body metabolism, which are required to provide energy and build tissue, must be controlled in exquisite detail to maintain a smooth-running, balanced operation. Otherwise, there would be chaos within the body system and death would eventually result. Life and health result from a dynamic balance, a state of *homeostasis,* among all of the body parts and processes. Vitamins and minerals are nutrients that play a vital role in metabolic regulation and control; water provides the necessary fluid environment.

Vitamins

Many vitamins function as coenzyme factors, or components of cell enzyme systems, to govern chemical reactions in cell metabolism. This is true, for example, of most B-complex vitamins.

Minerals

Many minerals also serve as coenzyme factors in cell metabolism. An interesting structural example is that of the trace element cobalt, a central constituent of vitamin B_{12} (cobalamin), which functions with this vitamin to combat pernicious anemia.

Other Nutrients

Water and dietary fiber also function as regulatory agents. In fact, water is *the* fundamental agent for life itself, providing the essential solution base for all metabolic processes. Dietary fiber helps regulate the passage of food through the gastrointestinal tract and influences absorption of various nutrients.

Levels of Nutritional Status

Individual nutritional status will vary depending on a person's living situation, available food supply, and health. You will be concerned with these varying levels as you assess your own nutritional status or that of others.

Ideal Nutrition

Evidence of sound positive nutrition includes a well-developed body, ideal weight for body composition (ratio of muscle mass to fat) and height, and good muscle development and tone. The skin is smooth and clear, the hair glossy, the eyes clear and bright. Posture is good; facial expression is alert. Appetite, digestion, and elimination are normal. Detailed characteristics of good and poor states of nutrition are given in Table 1-1. Begin to think about these signs as you get into your nutrition study and look for them as you become a more skilled observer. Well-nourished persons are much more likely to be alert, both mentally and physically. They are meeting not only their day-to-day needs but also maintaining essential nutrient reserves for resisting infectious diseases and generally extending their years of normal functioning.

Borderline Nutrition

As the descriptive label indicates, persons with only a borderline nutritional status may manage to meet their minimum day-to-day nutritional needs. However, they lack nutritional reserves to meet any added physiologic or metabolic demand resulting from injury or illness, sustain fetal development during pregnancy or attain proper growth in childhood. A state of borderline nutrition may exist in persons with poor eating habits or those who are living in stressed environments on low incomes. Dietary surveys have shown that approximately one third of the U.S. population is living on diets below the optimal level. This does not necessarily mean that these Americans are undernourished; some persons can maintain general health on somewhat less than the optimal amounts of various nutrients. On the average, however, persons who do not get enough of these nutrients have greater risk of physical illness than persons who are well nourished. The human body has great capacity to adapt to lowered nutritional states, but it can only sustain a given amount of physiologic stress before signs of malnutrition appear.

Malnutrition

Signs of malnutrition appear when nutritional reserves are depleted and nutrient and energy intake is insuffi-

TABLE 1-1

Clinical Signs of Nutritional Status

Features	Good	Poor
General appearance	Alert, responsive	Listless, apathetic, cachexic
Hair	Shiny, lustrous, healthy scalp	Stringy, dull, brittle, dry, depigmented
Neck glands	No enlargement	Thyroid enlarged
Skin, face, neck	Smooth, slightly moist, good color, reddish pink mucous membranes	Greasy, discolored, scaly
Eyes	Bright, clear, no fatigue circles	Dryness, signs of infection, increased vascularity, glassiness, thickened conjunctivae
Lips	Good color, moist	Dry, scaly, swollen, angular lesions (stomatitis)
Tongue	Good pink color, surface papillae present, no lesions	Papillary atrophy, smooth appearance, swollen, red, beefy (glossitis)
Gums	Good pink color, no swelling or bleeding, firm	Marginal redness or swelling, receding, spongy
Teeth	Straight, no crowding, well-shaped jaw, clean, no discoloration	Unfilled cavities, absent teeth, worn surfaces, mottled, malpositioned
Skin, general	Smooth, slightly moist, good color	Rough, dry, scaly, pale, pigmented, irritated; petechiae, bruises
Abdomen	Flat	Swollen
Legs, feet	No tenderness, weakness, swelling, good color	Edema, tender calf, tingling, weakness
Skeleton	No malformations	Bowlegs, knock-knees, chest deformity at diaphragm, beaded ribs, prominent scapulas
Weight	Normal for height, age, body build	Overweight or underweight
Posture	Erect, arms and legs straight, abdomen in, chest out	Sagging shoulders, sunken chest, humped back
Muscles	Well-developed, firm	Flaccid, poor tone, undeveloped, tender
Nervous control	Good attention span for age, does not cry easily, not irritable or restless	Inattentive, irritable
Gastrointestinal function	Good appetite and digestion, normal, regular elimination	Anorexia, indigestion, constipation or diarrhea
General vitality	Endurance, energetic, sleeps well at night, vigorous	Easily fatigued, no energy, falls asleep in school, looks tired, apathetic

cient to meet day-to-day needs or added metabolic stress. A large number of malnourished people live in high-risk conditions of poverty. These conditions influence the health of all persons involved, but especially the lives of the most vulnerable ones—infants, children, pregnant women, and elderly adults. Infant mortality rates continue at a high level, especially among Black and other minority populations.[1] Prenatal care for many women who are young, poor, and uneducated is not of even minimally acceptable quality.[2] One out of four young children in the United States lives in poverty and suffers from stunted growth and deficiency diseases such as anemia. These children also have lowered resistance to infection and disease, impaired learning ability, apathy, and reduced activity levels.[3] Low socioeconomic status and malnutrition are positively related in the increasing American population of older adults.[4,5] Many studies also document widespread hunger and malnutrition among the poor, especially among the growing number of homeless persons.[6-8]

We also find malnutrition in our hospitals and long-term care facilities. For example, hypermetabolic disease or prolonged illness, especially among older persons with chronic conditions, places added stress. In these situations, the person's daily nutrient and energy intake is often insufficient to meet needs. Nutrition as-

sessment procedures fundamental to appropriate clinical care are described in Chapter 16.

Overnutrition

Some persons may be in a state of overnutrition that gradually results in degrees of overweight and obesity from excess energy intake over time. In a sense, overnutrition can be viewed as another form of malnutrition, especially when excess caloric intake produces gross harmful body weight and fatness—morbid obesity. Childhood and adolescent obesity may set the stage for continuing adult obesity, increasing the risk for chronic disease. Harmful overnutrition also occurs in persons who use excessive "megadoses" of nutrient supplements that, over time, produce damaging tissue effects.

---

amino acid • An acid containing the essential element nitrogen (in the chemical group $-NH_2$). Amino acids are the structural units of protein and the basic building blocks of the body.

anemia • Blood condition characterized by decreased number of circulating red blood cells, hemoglobin, or both.

Nutrition and National Health Problems
Diet, Nutrition, and Chronic Disease

Over the past few years, a series of reports to the American people and national health policy makers have related specific dietary factors to leading U.S. health threats and chronic disease problems: coronary heart disease, high blood pressure, stroke, some types of cancer, diabetes, and obesity.

Nutrition and Health

In 1988, *The Surgeon General's Report on Nutrition and Health* was issued in response to the increasing concerns of scientists, health professionals, and the American public about the effects of typical American dietary patterns on the incidence of chronic diseases that are leading causes of death and disability in this country.[9] Based on the weight of evidence presented and the magnitude of health problems involved, recommendation was made for dietary changes to reduce use of foods high in fats and salt and to increase foods high in complex carbohydrates and fiber.

Diet and Health

In 1989, the Diet and Health Committee of the Food and Nutrition Board, National Research Council, issued their extensive research report, *Diet and Health: Implication for Reducing Chronic Disease Risk*.[10] On the basis of systematic evaluation of scientific evidence relating dietary components, foods, food groups, and dietary patterns to health maintenance and reduction of chronic disease risk, the 19-member interdisciplinary committee proposed dietary guidelines in line with those of the Surgeon General, specifically, reducing total fat intake to 30% or less of the total kcalories, with associated reductions in saturated fats and cholesterol.

Healthy People 2000

In 1990, the U.S. Department of Health and Human Services, Public Health Services, issued a report applying the recommendations indicated above in a system of specific objectives to reach these national health goals by the year 2000.[11-12] Targeted are particularly vulnerable groups in our population who suffer from poor diets, malnutrition, and poor health: older Americans with chronic disease and disability, infants and young children (one in four live in poverty), and the increasing numbers of homeless people.

Nutritional Guides for Health Promotion

During the years since the early 1900s, a number of food and nutrient guides have been developed to meet nutrition and health needs of Americans. Although not always apparent in these guides, some underlying assumptions about food, nutrition, and health have directed their design and reflected not only developing nutritional science but also social, political, and economic events of the times. They have addressed nutritional needs during wars and emergencies as well as in economic depressions. With our changing modern health problems, the focus of these guides has shifted from preventing primary deficiency diseases of insufficient nutritional intake to controlling chronic diseases of affluence and excess.

In general, these nutritional guides may be classified into three groups: nutrient and energy standards, food guides, and dietary guidelines; each serves different needs. They are reviewed briefly here for reference and guidance in your study.

Nutrient Standards: The Recommended Dietary Allowances (RDAs)
United States Standards

Most of the developed countries of the world have set up standards for intake of major nutrients by healthy persons categorized by age and sex. They serve as guidelines for maintaining healthy populations. These standards are not intended to indicate individual requirements or therapeutic needs. Rather they serve as a reference based on current scientific knowledge for intake levels of the essential nutrients judged to be adequate for meeting the known nutritional needs of most healthy population groups. In the United States these nutrient and energy standards are called the **Recommended Dietary Allowances (RDAs).** Such standards are similar in different countries, but may vary somewhat according to their purpose and use.

Development of the RDAs

The first RDA standards grew out of a national nutrition conference for defense held in 1941 during World War II.[12] A summary background for the nutrient and energy recommendations, based on developing nutritional science, was first published in 1943 as a guide for nutrition workers in planning and obtaining food supplies for national defense and in determining general population needs for good nutrition. Since this first edition of the RDAs, a new edition has been published about every 4 years, with revisions of the standards based on expanding current scientific research. The current tenth edition, issued in 1989, is the work of the present Dietary Allowances Subcommittee of the Food and Nutrition Board, National Research Council, National Academy of Sciences.[13] The Academy has numerous councils and is supported by the National Institutes of Health. (See U.S. RDA tables inside book covers.)

Other Standards

Canadian and British standards are similar to U.S. standards. (See Appendix L for the current Canadian stan-

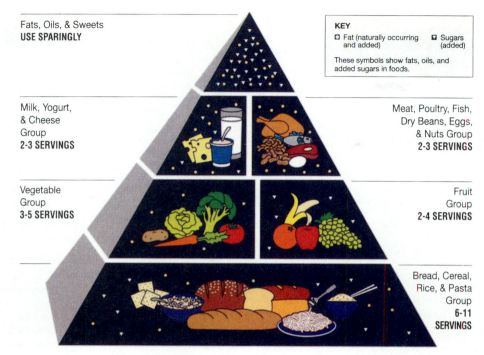

FIG. 1-1   Eating right pyramid. A guide to daily food choices. *(Adapted from the US Department of Agriculture, 1992.)*

dards for comparison.) In less developed countries where such factors as quality of protein foods available must be considered, workers look to standards such as those set by the Food and Agriculture Organization (FAO) of the World Health Organization (WHO). All of these standards provide nutrient and energy guidelines to help health workers in a variety of population groups promote good health through sound nutrition.

Food Group Guides

To interpret and apply sound nutrient standards, health workers need practical food guides to use in nutrition education and food planning for individuals and families. Two such food guides, very different in nature and serving different needs, are the *Basic Four Food Groups Guide* and the *Food Exchange Lists*.

Basic Four Food Groups Guide

Probably the most familiar food group guide is the long-used but limited tool issued by the U.S. Department of Agriculture (USDA), reflecting in its origin agricultural commodity concerns as well as nutritional ones: the Basic Four Food Groups Guide. Over the years, the USDA has issued a succession of basic food guides, each reflecting needs and concerns of the time.

In 1991, the U.S. Department of Agriculture issued a revised edition, reflecting current national goals for increasing carbohydrate intake to supply the bulk of the energy needs with the fruit, vegetable, and starch/bread groups; the revision also recommended limiting fat intake by modifying the milk, meat, and fat groups.[14] This new approach, titled *The Guide to Daily Food Choices*, is summarized in Table 1-2 (p. 10). A subsequent graphic form, *The Food Guide Pyramid* (Fig. 1-1), was issued the following year to illustrate the relative amounts of each food group in the daily diet. This revised basic food groups guide continues in its modified form. It is designed to represent a total diet and not just a foundation, to fill a need for simple guidance.[15]

The Exchange Lists Food Guide

This guide was introduced in 1950 by the American Diabetes Association and the American Dietetic Association as a meal planning tool for managing the diet of persons with diabetes. Organized quite differently from the USDA guide, *The Exchange Lists Food Guide* was based on the unique concept of food exchanges, with foods grouped on the basis of equivalent food values. Soon it became apparent that this guide was also a use-

Recommended Dietary Allowances (RDAs) • Recommended daily allowances of nutrients and energy intake for population groups according to age and sex, with defined weight and height. The RDAs are established and reviewed periodically by a representative group of nutritional scientists, in response to current research. These standards vary very little among the developed countries.

TABLE 1-2
The Guide to Daily Food Choices—a Summary

Food group	Servings	Major contributions	Foods and serving sizes*
Bread, cereals, rice, pasta	6-11	Starch Thiamin Riboflavin† Iron Niacin Folate Magnesium‡ Fiber‡ Zinc	1 slice of bread 1 oz ready-to-eat cereal ½-¾ cup cooked cereal, rice, pasta
Vegetables	3-5	Vitamin A Vitamin C Folate Magnesium Fiber	½ cup raw or cooked vegetables 1 cup raw leafy vegetables
Fruits	2-4	Vitamin C Fiber	¼ cup dried fruit ½ cup cooked fruit ¾ cup juice 1 whole piece of fruit 1 melon wedge
Milk, yogurt, cheese	2 (adult§) 3 (children, teens, young adults, pregnant or lactating women)	Calcium Riboflavin Protein Potassium Zinc	1 cup milk 1½ oz cheese 2 oz processed cheese 1 cup yogurt 2 cups cottage cheese 1 cup custard/pudding 1½ cups ice cream
Meat, poultry, fish, dry beans, eggs, nuts	2-3	Protein Niacin Iron Vitamin B_6 Zinc Thiamin Vitamin B_{12}‖	2-3 oz cooked meat, poultry, fish 1-1½ cups cooked dry beans 4 tbsp peanut butter 2 eggs ½-1 cup nuts
Fats, oils, sweets	Foods from this group should not replace any from the other groups. Amounts consumed should be determined by individual energy needs.		

From the U.S. Department of Agriculture, revised edition of former *Basic Four Food Groups Guide,* 1985.
*May be reduced for child servings.
†If enriched.
‡Whole grains especially.
§≥25 years of age.
‖Only in animal food choices.

ful short-method tool for calculating and planning any diet, such as those for weight reduction, in which control of the energy nutrients—carbohydrate, fat, and protein—as well as kcalories, for both total and nutrient distribution, was the goal.

Since foods in each group in the exchange system are equal to one another in the portions indicated, group items could be freely exchanged within individual groups, thus maintaining consistent food values and kcalories. At the same time, this freedom of exchange within single groups allowed a great variety of foods and food combinations to be used in planning meals and snacks. This food exchange group guide has been widely used as a nutrition tool for meal planning, education, and counseling.

In 1986, a major revision of the exchange lists was published to meet current nutrition and medical research and national dietary guidelines for health promotion and reduction of chronic disease risk factors.[16] The basic six food groups have been completely reorganized and their list order changed to emphasize use for health: (1) starch/bread, (2) meat, with subgroups of lean, medium-fat, and high-fat items and tips for reducing portion size and fat, (3) vegetables, (4) fruits, (5) milk, with subgroups for reducing fat, and (6) fat, with subgroups for unsaturated and saturated food sources (see Appendix K). Three expanded lists were added: free foods and seasonings, combination foods, and foods for occasional use. In all groups, values for dietary fiber and sodium have been identified and food sources flagged. A new edition has been issued that is specifically revised and designed for weight management.[18]

Health Promotion Guidelines

In recent years, several general dietary guidelines for health promotion have been issued in the United States that reflect the growing health concerns of government, professional groups, and the public. Though not quantifying food use as do the food groups guides, above, they call attention to proposed food habit changes to reduce chronic disease risks and enhance health. The guidelines have proved useful in nutrition education and counseling.

U.S. Dietary Guidelines

These basic health guidelines have developed from public and professional concern about chronic health problems in an aging population and a changing food environment. The U.S. Departments of Agriculture and Health and Human Services issued the current third edition in 1990, *Nutrition and Your Health: Dietary Guidelines for Americans,* based on extensive study by expert advisory committees and supplying extensive supporting references for each guideline.[19] The statements emphasize health promotion through risk reduction and

---

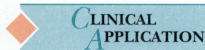

CLINICAL APPLICATION

Nutrition and Your Health: Dietary Guidelines for Americans

Eat a variety of foods

About 40 different known nutrients, and probably additional as yet unknown factors, are needed to maintain health. No single food can supply all the essential nutrients in the amounts needed. Thus the greater the variety of foods used, the less likely a person is to develop either a deficiency or an excess of any single nutrient. One way to ensure variety, and with it a balanced diet, is to select foods each day from all the major food groups.

Maintain ideal weight

Excessive fatness is associated with some chronic disorders such as hypertension and diabetes, which in turn relate to heart disease. The "ideal" body weight, however, must be determined individually, for many factors are involved, such as body composition, body metabolism, genetics, and physical activity.

Avoid too much fat, saturated fat, and cholesterol

Americans as a population have traditionally consumed a high-fat diet. In some persons, excess fat leads to high levels of blood fats and cholesterol carried in lipoprotein compounds. Elevated serum levels of these fats and cholesterol are associated with a higher risk of coronary heart disease. Thus it is wise to cut down on fats in general, using them only in moderation.

Eat foods with adequate starch and fiber

Complex carbohydrate foods (starches) are better fuel sources for energy than are simple carbohydrates (sugars) and fats. Starches also contain many essential nutrients and kcalories needed for energy. With increased use of processed and refined foods, the modern American diet is relatively low in dietary fiber. Increasing the use of less-refined complex carbohydrates will help increase dietary fiber. Evidence exists that certain types of dietary fiber may help control chronic bowel diseases, contribute to improved blood glucose management for persons with diabetes mellitus, and bind dietary lipids such as cholesterol. Starches, especially forms with more dietary fiber, may therefore be sustained for some of the fats and sugars as energy sources.

Avoid too much sugar

The major health hazard from eating too much sugar is tooth decay (dental caries). Contrary to popular opinion, however, too much sugar does not in itself cause diabetes. It can only contribute to poor control of diabetes in persons who have inherited the disease. Most Americans consume a relatively large amount of sugar, much of it coming from processed food products. Again, moderation is the key.

Avoid too much sodium

Excessive sodium is not healthy for anyone, especially persons with high blood pressure. In general, since many processed food products contain considerable sodium or salt and since most Americans eat more sodium than they need, it is wise to limit the use of these products, especially "salty" ones, and reduce added salt in food preparation. These practices will lower individual salt tastes, which are learned habits and not biologic necessities. Ample sodium is found as a natural mineral in foods to meet usual needs.

If you drink alcohol, do so in moderation

Alcoholic beverages tend to be high in kcalories and low in other nutrients. Limited food intake may accompany large alcohol intake. Also, heavy drinking contributes to chronic liver disease and some neurologic disorders, as well as some throat and neck cancers. Thus moderation is the key, if alcohol is used at all. ◆

relate current scientific thinking to America's leading health problems. They have been actively supported by the American Dietetic Association and continue to serve as useful general guides for a concerned public. Although no guidelines can guarantee health or well-being, and although people differ widely in their food needs, these seven general statements can lead people to evaluate their food habits and move toward general improvements. Good food habits based on moderation and variety help build sound healthy bodies (see box, p. 11). Shortly after the initial publication of the general U.S. Dietary Goals, two similar, but more specific sets of dietary guidelines were issued applying these general goals to two major U.S. health problems, heart disease and cancer. These disease prevention guidelines are summarized below.

Dietary Guidelines for Heart Disease Prevention

Following the general dietary guidelines just discussed, the Nutrition Committee of the American Heart Association (AHA) published a report in 1982 outlining basic modifications in the American diet that, based on current research, would help reduce identified risk factors contributing to the development of coronary heart disease.[20] These guidelines represented an effort to quantify more specifically the general principles of the U.S. dietary goals. The AHA Nutrition Committee agreed that at that time, although all the answers were certainly not in, a wise approach would be to at least moderate our excesses in kcalories, fat, cholesterol, and sodium, replacing reduced fat kcalories with increased carbohydrate sources. It was called a "prudent diet" and the name has remained. Its six basic statements define these prudent dietary changes:

1. *Total energy intake.* Adjust dietary kcalorie value sufficiently to maintain ideal body weight.
2. *Fats.* Reduce the total dietary fat kcalories to no more than 30% to 35% of the total kcalories. Of these total fat kcalories, saturated fat should contribute 10% or less, monounsaturated 15%, and polyunsaturated 10%.
3. *Carbohydrates.* Replace reduced fat with increased carbohydrates to provide 50% to 55% of the total kcalories. Of these total carbohydrate kcalories, complex carbohydrates (starches) should contribute the majority of 30% to 35%, with simple carbohydrates (sugars) limited to 10%.
4. *Proteins.* Use protein in moderation, about 12% to 20% of the diet's total kcalories, with less use of animal protein which carries more fat.
5. *Cholesterol.* Limit dietary cholesterol to 300 mg or less per day, which is about half to a third of the usual American diet. Since cholesterol occurs only in animal food sources, mainly with fat tissues, this means fewer egg yolks, well-trimmed leaner meat in small portions, limited use of organ meats or processed meats, and use of nonfat dairy products.

6. *Sodium.* Limit the use of salt and salty foods. A reasonable limit of 2 to 3 g of sodium a day can be achieved by using salt only lightly in cooking, adding none at the table, and avoiding highly salted processed foods.

The American Heart Association provides a number of leaflets and booklets based on the prudent diet guidelines for use in diet counseling and meal planning. These principles have also been incorporated into a wide variety of "light cooking" recipe books, as well as appearing on restaurant menus.

Dietary Guidelines for Cancer Prevention

In 1982 the Committee on Diet, Nutrition and Cancer of the National Cancer Institute, National Institutes of Health, published its initial report containing what it termed "interim" guidelines for reducing cancer risks.[21] The report was based on available data indicating potential health benefits with no known health risks from these diet principles. You will note several similar guidelines here to those for heart disease prevention, especially in relation to fat, fiber-rich foods, and alcohol use:

1. *Fats.* Reduce fat intake from its present level (approximately 40%) to 30% of the diet's total kcalories, and avoid obesity.
2. *Dietary fiber.* Include fruits, vegetables, and whole-grain cereals in the daily diet.
3. *Preserved food.* Limit use of food preserved by salt-curing (including salt pickling), smoking, or nitrite-curing.
4. *Contaminated food.* Avoid contamination of foods with carcinogens from any known source. Identify mutagens in food and test for their carcinogenicity.
5. *Alcohol.* Use alcoholic beverages in moderation, if at all.

All of these guidelines apply to consumers, except number 4, which is directed to the food industry. In the 1985 revision, the American Cancer Society updated these guidelines by directing them specifically to consumers and health care professionals. They eliminated number 4 and added two descriptive guidelines about vegetables and fruits following the statement on dietary fiber:

1. Include foods rich in vitamins A and C in your daily diet.
2. Include **cruciferous** vegetables in your diet.

A number of pamphlets are available for using these guidelines in nutrition education and counseling.

Personal Assessment of Food Patterns
Personal Perceptions of Food

Traditionally, each person develops food habits and ways of eating from birth that are influenced by factors such as ethnic background, cultural patterns, family habits, socioeconomic status, health, available food,

Personal Perceptions and Analysis of Food Patterns

TO PROBE FURTHER

What are your own personal perceptions of your eating patterns? What are your food habits, attitudes, and values? To find some answers, check yourself for a few days, using some of the procedures discussed here.

First, keep a detailed record of everything you eat and drink for 2 week days and 1 weekend day. Make it as complete as possible. Keep a small pocket pad with you and jot down what you eat or drink throughout the day and evening, while your memory is still clear on details. Include any factors influencing your choices: what was it, how much, how prepared or brand name, where and what time, alone or with someone, how you were feeling at the time. Just this brief recording process alone is a good start, because it may tell you some things about your eating habits that you were not aware of. Remember, you are going to analyze this record, so make it as readable, accurate, and detailed as possible.

Second, using the Basic Four Food Groups Guide to Daily Food Choices (Table 1-2), list the foods you ate or drank under their respective food groupings. Then compare what you ate with the amounts listed and estimate how closely your choices fulfilled the recommended daily food choices. Also, estimate your diet's shortcomings.

Third, list the foods you ate in their respective food groups, referring to the Food Exchange Lists (see Appendix K) to integrate your choices with the energy-yielding macronutrients: carbohydrates, proteins, and fats. Total the amount of each nutrient you consumed. Pay particular attention to the total amount of fat (g) and kcalories. How close is your total amount to the recommended 30% of kcalories per day in the national diet and health objectives? How close is your total RDA for kcalories?

Fourth, compare your eating patterns with the national Dietary Guidelines for Americans (see the box on p. 11). Are there any statements that your eating patterns do not fit? Can you change your eating habits so they more closely adhere to the guidelines?

Fifth, classify yourself according to (1) Fairweather's study of personal perceptions of food attitudes and behaviors (see p. 13), and (2) the eating patterns described by Bailey and Goldberg (see p. 14).

Now that you have considered your food habits and patterns, how do you view your eating habits? Are there any food behaviors that you may want to modify to promote health? Which food behaviors enhance your health?

---

and personal likes and dislikes. However, today increasing ethnic diversity has influenced food patterns and brought a greater intermingling variety of foods and ideas about food. How people perceive themselves in relation to food and food patterns plays an important role in developing their own attitudes toward food and personal eating behavior.

In a recent study of these subjective personal perceptions of food, Fairweather[22] used a system of ranking objects or statements, asking each subject to place them in a significant personal order. Statements ranked by the subjects covered 13 topics related to eating: time—when one should eat; preparation—cooked vs raw; vegetarianism; "bad" or "junk" food; changes in nutrition—traditional vs new; health; organic food; the experience of eating; quantity of food and food as fuel; taste; cost; allergies and reactions; and the food industry. The results identified four interesting and distinctive perceptions of food among contemporary people:

1. *The gregarious gourmet*—eats many types of foods, values the taste, and savors the social experience.
2. *The virtuous vegetarian*—actively seeks the "right" foods and values foods that are nonmeat, unprocessed, and natural.
3. *The traditional meat eater*—also actively seeks the "right" foods, but prefers traditional foods; neither health nor sociability is at issue.
4. *The selective connoisseur*—health conscious, selec

tive in choice of food, enjoys taste and sociability, but emphasizes that food is a needed fuel.

A simple way to get a basic idea of the general nutritional value of your own food habits is to apply both of the food guides discussed here. First, keep a record of everything you eat and drink for a few days, noting the time, place, activity, and persons with you, if any. Sometimes these factors are a revelation, because we eat by habit, usually according to where we are and what we are doing, not because of any serious thought or plan. Second, evaluate everything you had to eat or drink each day. (1) Check the revised basic food groups shown in Table 1-2 to get a rough estimate of your use of representative foods in each group. (2) Check the food exchange lists provided in Appendix K to determine the energy-yielding values of the macronutrients involved in your food choices (see the box above).

---

cruciferous • Bearing a cross; botanical term for plants belonging to the botanical family *Cruciferae* or *Brassicaceae*, the mustard family, so-called because of cross-like, four-petaled flowers; name given to certain vegetables of this family, such as broccoli, cabbage, brussels sprouts, and cauliflower.

This method of food records and food groupings has even been useful in larger studies of population groups to provide meaningful information about the quality of food habits. Bailey and Goldberg[23] used a similar approach to identify particular patterns of eating behavior in relation to food intake and weight concerns of college women. The students found by their analysis of their food records that meal frequency generally follows characteristic patterns and that eating habits generally fall into one of four basic types.

1. *Regular eaters*—those who eat regular meals and snacks, have a morning snack instead of a full breakfast, and are unconcerned with weight.
2. *Morning eaters*—those who eat breakfast and morning snacks, have less dinner and evening snacks, and have little concern about weight.
3. *Concerned eaters*—those who eat breakfast and dinner and less lunch and snacks, and are strongly concerned with being overweight.
4. *Lunch avoiders*—those who eat breakfast, dinner, and an evening snack, seldom have lunch or afternoon snacks, and consider themselves underweight.

The simple approach of analyzing food records by basic food groups and food exchange lists can be helpful for increased awareness of personal food patterns or related concerns such as weight management.

Nutritional Analysis by Nutrients and Energy Values

A more comprehensive nutritional analysis of food intake records for a wide range of macronutrients and their subgroupings, as well as micronutrient and energy values, can be easily accomplished by using a number of computer programs. In this age of computers, colleges usually have computer equipment available in a computer laboratory or individual students may have their own. If computer equipment is not available, a limited analysis can be done by hand using standard food value reference tables (see Appendix A). Currently, there is general concern about dietary fat in relation to risk of heart disease, so an analysis that focuses on total fat and cholesterol would prove useful in making changes in food habits.

To Sum Up

Over the past few years, the role of nutrition in human health has been changing in response to our changing society. The scientific base of nutrition is expanding in both its physical and its behavioral foundations. Health goals and objectives have become more person-centered, with a focus on health promotion.

Health status in general has a fundamental nutritional base. To meet these needs, nutritional standards (RDAs) have been developed on the basis of current scientific research, as have a number of general and specific food guides and dietary guidelines, for the purpose of disease prevention.

QUESTIONS FOR REVIEW

1. Describe the science of nutrition in terms of its major basic science foundations. What contributions does each make toward understanding human nutrition?
2. Why is the concept of change fundamental in the science of nutrition?
3. Define the terms *nutrition* and *dietetics*. Identify personal roles of professional practitioners in the field of human nutrition.
4. Compare the four general levels of individual nutritional status, and describe factors or situations that would contribute to each condition.
5. Compare the three major types of nutritional guides in terms of their nature and use. Give illustrations of each type, and describe what you see as strengths and weaknesses in each case.
6. Keep a 1-day food record of everything you eat or drink, noting nature of the food, method of preparation, and portion consumed. Analyze your food record—by computer if available—in terms of nutrient and kcalorie intake in comparison with the RDAs and the prudent AHA dietary guidelines. Do you see ways of improving your diet?

REFERENCES

1. Yankauer A: What infant mortality tells us, *Am J Pub Health* 80(6):653, 1990.
2. Hansell MJ: Sociodemographic factors and the quality of prenatal care, *Am J Pub Health* 81(8):1023, 1991.
3. Splett PL, Story M: Child nutrition: objectives for the decade, *J Am Diet Assoc* 91(6):665, 1991.
4. White JV and others: Consensus of the Nutrition Screening Initiative: risk factors and indicators of poor nutritional status in older Americans, *J Am Diet Assoc* 91(7):783, 1991.
5. White JV and others: Nutrition Screening Initiative: development and implementation of the public awareness checklist and screening tools, *J Am Diet Assoc* 92(2):163, 1992.
6. Luder E and others: Health and nutrition survey in a group of urban homeless adults, *J Am Diet Assoc* 90(10):1387, 1990.
7. Carrillo TE and others: Soup kitchen meals: an observation and nutrient analysis, *J Am Diet Assoc* 90(7):989, 1990.
8. ADA Reports: Position of the American Dietetic Association: domestic hunger and inadequate access to food, *J Am Diet Assoc* 90(10):1437, 1990.
9. US Department Health and Human Services, Public Health Service: *The surgeon general's report on nutrition and health,* PHS Pub No 88-50210, Washington, DC, 1988, US Government Printing Office.

10. Food and Nutrition Board, Committee on Diet and Health, National Academy of Sciences—National Re search Council: *Diet and health: implications for reducing chronic disease risk,* Washington, DC, 1989, National Academy Press.

11. US Department of Health and Human Services, Public Health Service: *Healthy people 2000: national health promotion and disease prevention objectives,* Washington, DC, 1990, US Government Printing Office.

12. American Dietetic Association: Healthy people 2000: nutrition objectives, *J Am Diet Assoc* 91(12):1515, 1991.

13. Food and Nutrition Board, National Research Council: *Recommended dietary allowances,* ed 10, Washington, DC, 1989, National Academy Press.

14. US Department of Agriculture: *Guide to daily food choices,* Washington, DC, 1991, US Government Printing Office.

15. US Department of Agriculture: Eating right food pyramind, Washington, DC, 1992, US Government Printing Office.

16. American Dietetic Association, American Diabetes Association: *Exchange lists for meal planning,* Chicago, 1986, American Dietetic Association.

17. Franz MJ and others: Exchange lists: revised 1986, *J Am Diet Assoc* 87(1):28, 1987.

18. American Dietetic Association: *Exchange lists for weight management,* Chicago, 1989, American Dietetic Association.

19. US Department of Agriculture, US Department of Health and Human Services: *Nutrition and your health: dietary guidelines for Americans,* ed 3, Home and Garden Bulletin No 232, November, 1990.

20. American Heart Association Nutrition Committee: Ratio-nale of the diet-heart statement of the American Heart Association, *Arteriosclerosis* 4:177, 1982.

21. Committee on Diet, Nutrition, and Cancer: *Diet, nutrition, and cancer,* Washington, DC, 1982, National Academy Press.

22. Fairweather JR: Subjective perceptions of food, *J NZ Diet Assoc* 45:19, 1991.

23. Bailey S, Goldberg JP: Eating patterns and weight concerns of college women, *J Am Diet Assoc* 89(1): 1989.

FURTHER READING

Danford DE, Stephenson MG: Healthy people 2000: development of nutrition objectives, *J Am Diet Assoc* 91(12):1517, 1991.
Report: Healthy people 2000: nutrition objectives, *J Am Diet Assoc* 91(12):1515, 1991.

These key reports list the specific nutrition objectives among the current national health objectives and describes how they were developed and what the implications are for their application in practice.

Hinton AW and others: ADA Reports: Position of the American Dietetic Association: domestic hunger and inadequate access to food, *J Am Diet Assoc* 90(10):1437, 1990.

This professional position paper describes the extent of the problem of hunger in America and and its resulting malnutrition, especially among families living in poverty, the homeless, and vulnerable groups such as pregnant women, infants, children, and elderly persons. The report includes a five-point program with the goal of achieving food security for all persons.

Positive Health Promotion, Not Negative Blame

Some critics of the current health promotion/self-care movement sabotage some people's efforts to maintain health by blaming them when they become ill. This is a misplaced accusation. It apparently started when the public and practitioners alike, alarmed by the soaring costs of health care, sought ways in which individuals could reduce their chances of becoming ill. The result is the growing field of preventive health.

Many preventive health care practitioners are sensitive, skilled professionals who have used various methods of sharing their knowledge and skills with the public:

- Identification of risks
- Patient education regarding special illnesses
- Medical self-care
- Alternatives to traditional medical care
- Promotion of "wellness" as a state of mind or attitude

Their task has not been easy, since (1) their recommendations are often taken over and redefined or changed by business opportunists; (2) there are no guarantees that every recommendation will achieve the same results (for example, everyone who jogs 10 miles a day does not escape heart disease); (3) our culture stresses "antihealth" habits (for example, high-sodium/high-fat convenience foods, a high level of alcohol use, and overeating are promoted by the media); and (4) health activists are viewed as attempting to impose their personal value systems on others.

However, recommendations of some of these practitioners are not based on solid research and tend to yield inconsistent results. Because these "opinions" almost always involve the personal habits of the client, the "wellness" promoter is in effect telling people that it's their own fault if they're sick—they don't eat the right foods, they aren't keeping their weight at the correct level, they smoke/drink too much, they even *think* too much. In doing so they may be confusing the issue in several cases:

- Is it really the 16-year-old's fault that he eats too much when in his lifetime he's seen over 300,000 television commercials, most of which advertise readily available food?
- Is it the fault of the working woman that she relies on high-sodium/high-fat convenience foods to feed her family?
- Is the low-income patient with no recreation available other than meal preparation totally at fault for his obesity?
- What about the countless patients with chronic diseases who did not receive preventive health information from their physicians for decades before seeing a wellness practitioner? Are they responsible for their heart attacks or liver disease?

Physicians and other health professionals who have improved their own health because of wellness practices can contribute to the wellness of their patients without conducting a crusade against them. They can teach those same health-promoting ideas nonjudgmentally, rather than concentrating *only* on the "challenge" or threat of illness.

When the "victim" role is reinforced, circumstances that created vulnerability to poor health in the first place are perpetuated and legitimized. Further attempts to help are often turned down. To avoid this type of situation, the health practitioner should:

Examine personal value systems. Is my own work designed to point a finger at the victim or truly help the client help himself?

Consider every aspect of the client. Is it really within my client's power to control food intake at home? What social, financial, or other factors may be limiting choice of foods or activities other than eating? How can these be addressed?

Be realistic. If current research is not conclusive, should I avoid presenting recommendations as being "failure proof"?

Practitioners may benefit in their health promotion activities by determining which persons may be open to such approaches and which may not. Researchers have used a health-promoting lifestyle profile to investigate patterns of health behavior and the effects of efforts to change these behaviors. They identified six areas involved in these behaviors that need to be considered in working with each client: (1) degree of health responsibility, (2) capacity for self-fulfillment, (3) exercise capacity and amount, (4) nutritional status and problems, (5) interpersonal support, and (6) capacity for coping with stress. As a result of these studies, a useful checklist of positive health behaviors was constructed. Items concerned with nutrition focused on meal patterns and food choices.

Current trends in health promotion indicate that health and nutrition education efforts have increased dramatically over the past decade and resulted in behavioral change. Substantial evidence supports the fact that these health promotion activities can alter public health behaviors, preventing disease by reducing risks for health problems.

REFERENCES

American Medical Association, Council on Scientific Affairs: Education for health: a role for physicians and the efficacy of health education, *JAMA* 263:1816, 1990.

Walker SN, Sechrist KR, Pender NJ: The health-promoting lifestyle: development and psychometric characteristics, *Nurs Res* 36:76, 1987.

*C*HAPTER 2

Digestion, Absorption, and Metabolism

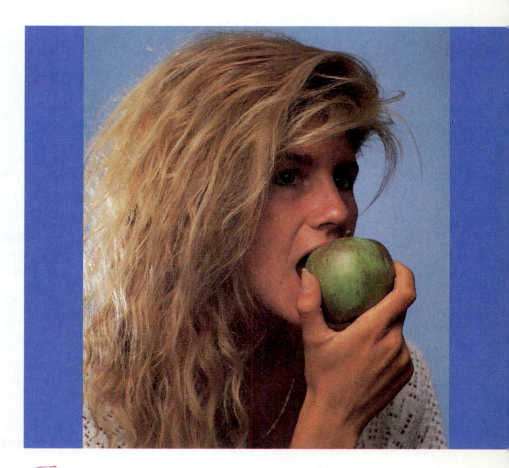

*I*n this chapter, at the beginning of your study of the three macronutrients—carbohydrates, fats, and protein—we will look first at the integrated overall body systems that handle them. Once the body receives the foods we eat, unique structures and functions transform them for our use.

The overall physiologic and biochemical process involved has three integrated parts: digestion, absorption, and metabolism. We begin with a look at the gastrointestinal tract and then follow the path of the nutrients to the cells. We see how each part of the system makes its own special contribution to the whole integrated operation.

The Human Body as a Dynamic Whole
The Concepts of Change and Balance

Through a successive interrelated system of balanced change, the foods we eat must be transformed into simpler substances and then into other, still simpler, substances that our cells can use to sustain life. All these many changes prepare food for use by the body. Together they constitute the overall digestion-absorption-metabolism process.

The Concept of Wholeness
Body Integrity

The parts of this overall process of change do not exist separately. Rather they comprise one continuous *whole.* Look carefully at the respective components of the gastrointestinal tract and their relative position in this overall body system (Fig. 2-1). In your review here, follow the fate of food components as they travel *together* through the successive parts of the gastrointestinal tract and into the body cells. This fundamental body system has indeed rightly been called "the portal to nutrient utilization."[1]

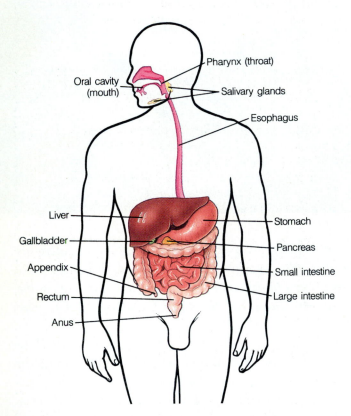

FIG. 2-1   The gastrointestinal system. Through the successive parts of the system, multiple activities of digestion liberate and reform food nutrients for our use.

Reasons for Human Life Systems

Why is this intricate complex of activities so necessary to human life? Two reasons are apparent: (1) *Food* as it naturally occurs and as we eat it is not a single component but a mixture of chemical substances, or nutrients. If these substances are to release their stored energy and building materials for use, they must be separated into their respective components so that the body may handle each one as a separate unit. (2) *Nutrients* released from the food may still remain unavailable to the body, and some additional means of changing their forms must follow. The intermediate units must be broken down, simplified, regrouped, and rerouted. This complex chemical work must take place because the human being, whose life is developed and sustained in a dynamic internal chemical environment, is the most highly organized and intricately balanced of all organisms. Essentially, this high level of internal bodily control and balance is called **homeostasis**, which is achieved through the effectiveness and beauty of the body's homeostatic mechanisms.[2] This view of the human body as an integrated physiochemical organism is basic to an understanding of human nutrition, both in health and in disease.

Basic Principles of Digestion

Digestion initially prepares the food for the body's use. Two basic types of action are involved—muscular and chemical.

Gastrointestinal Motility: Muscles and Movement

Food is prepared for chemical digestion by initial break down with specific enzymes, which takes place through a number of neuromuscular, self-regulating processes. These actions work together to move the food mass along the alimentary tract at the best rate for digestion and absorption of nutrients.

Types of Muscles

Organized muscle layers of the gastrointestinal wall, shown in Fig. 2-2, provide the necessary motility for digestion. From the outside surface inward the layers are (1) the **serosa,** (2) a *longitudinal muscle layer,* (3) a *circular muscle layer,* (4) the *submucosa,* and (5) the **mucosa.** Embedded in the deeper layers of the mucosa is a thin layer of smooth muscle fibers called the *muscularis mucosae.* The interaction of these smooth muscle layers make possible four necessary types of movement (Fig. 2-3, p. 20):

1. *Longitudinal muscles.* The long, smooth muscles, arranged in fiber bundles that extend lengthwise along the gastrointestinal tract, help propel the food mass along the tract.
2. *Circular contractile muscles.* In the circular muscle layer, smooth muscle fibers extend around the gut.

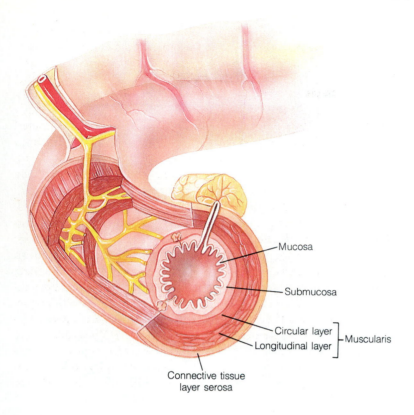

FIG. 2-2 Muscle layers of the intestinal wall.

Mucosa

Submucosa

Circular layer
Longitudinal layer }Muscularis

Connective tissue
layer serosa

They form rhythmic contractile rings that cause sweeping waves along the digestive tract and push the food mass forward. These regularly occurring propulsive movements are called **peristalsis.**

3. *Sphincter muscles.* More defined circular muscles occur at strategic points to provide muscle sphincters that act as valves—pyloric, ileocecal, and anal—to prevent reflux and control movement of food mass in its forward passage.

4. *Mucosal muscles.* The embedded, thin layer of smooth muscle produces *local constrictive contractions* that occur every few centimeters. They mix and chop the food mass as it moves along the tract, effectively churning the mass and mixing it with secretions to form a semiliquid **chyme** ready for digestion and absorption.

Thus, in summary, the interaction of the gastrointestinal muscle produces two basic types of action:

• General muscle tone or tonic contraction that ensures continuous passage and valve control

• Periodic, rhythmic contractions that mix and propel the food mass

As a result, these alternating muscular contractions and relaxations force the contents forward and facilitate specific digestion and absorption.

Nervous System Control

Throughout the gastrointestinal tract, specific nerves regulate these muscular actions. An interrelated network of nerves within the gastrointestinal wall, called the **intramural nerve plexus** (Fig. 2-4, p. 20), extends from the esophagus to the anus. This network of nerve fibers controls muscle tone of the gastrointestinal wall, regulates the rate and intensity of muscle contractions, and coordinates the various movements.[3]

chyme • Semifluid food mass in gastrointestinal tract following gastric digestion.

digestion • The process of breaking down food to release its nutrients for absorption and transport to the cells for use in body functions.

homeostasis • State of relative dynamic equilibrium within the body's internal environment; a balance achieved through the operation of various interrelated physiologic mechanisms.

intramural nerve plexus • Network of nerves in the walls of the intestine that make up the enteric nervous system controlling muscle action and secretions for digestion and absorption.

mucosa • The mucous membrane comprising the inner surface layer of gastrointestinal tract tissues, providing extensive nutrient absorption and transport functions.

peristalsis • A wave-like progression of alternate contraction and relaxation of the muscle fibers of the gastrointestinal tract.

serosa • Outer surface layer of the intestines interfacing with the blood vessels of the portal system going to the liver.

Gastrointestinal Secretions

Food is digested chemically by the combined action of a number of secretions. Generally these secretions are of four types:

1. *Enzymes.* Specific kind and quantity split designated chemical bonds within the structure of specific nutrient compounds, freeing their component parts.
2. *Hydrochloric acid and buffer ions.* These agents produce the necessary pH for the activity of given enzymes.
3. *Mucus.* This agent lubricates and protects the inside wall tissues of the gastrointestinal tract and facilitates food mass passage.
4. *Water and electrolytes.* These agents provide a balanced solution base in sufficient volumes to circulate the organic substances released.

Special cells in the mucosal tissue of the gastrointestinal tract, or in adjacent accessory organs, especially the pancreas, produce these secretions. The secretory action of these cells or glands is stimulated by the intake of food, by the sensory nerve network, or by hormones specific for certain nutrients.

Mouth and Esophagus: Preparation and Delivery

Up to this point, we have generally viewed the gastrointestinal tract in terms of integrated muscular/secretory functions that govern its operation as a whole.

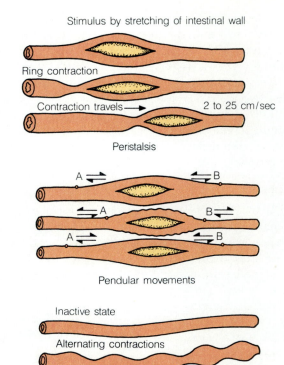

FIG. 2-3 Types of movement produced by muscles of the intestine: peristaltic waves from contraction of deep circular muscle, pendular movements from small local muscles, and segmentation rings formed by alternate contraction and relaxation of circular muscle.

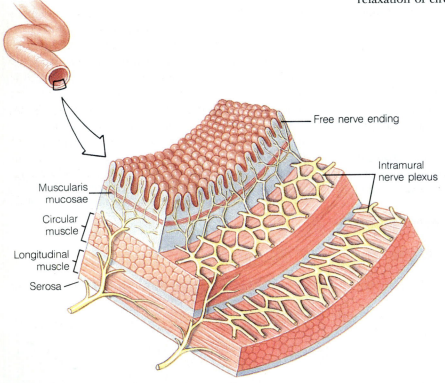

FIG. 2-4 Innervation of the intestine by intramural nerve plexus.

Here we begin to follow this operation through its successive parts to see what happens when we eat food. Actually, eating starts a remarkable physiologic event. It prepares food for entry into a complex system that radically changes its form and finally nourishes the body with its contents. Each step requires motility and secretions. In this first step, highly synchronized actions prepare food in the mouth, control the intricate act of swallowing, and deliver the food to the stomach by way of the esophagus.

Mastication

Initial biting and chewing begin to break food down into smaller particles. The teeth and other oral structures are particularly suited for this function. The incisors cut; the molars grind. Tremendous force is supplied by the jaw muscles: 55 lb of muscular pressure is applied through the incisors, 200 lb through the molars. Mastication allows an enlarged surface area of food to receive constant enzyme action. Also, the fineness of the food particles eases the continued passage of material through the gastrointestinal tract.

Swallowing

The process of swallowing involves both the mouth and the pharynx. Swallowing is extremely rapid, taking less than 1 second. It can be initiated voluntarily, but once started it proceeds as an involuntary reflex. Coordination of this reflex flows from the "swallowing center" area in the brain stem.[4] The mixed **bolus** of food particles then passes immediately down the esophagus largely by perstaltic waves controlled by nerve reflexes. Muscles at the base of the tongue aid the process of swallowing and gravity aids the movement of food down the esophagus in the upright position.

Entry into the Stomach

At the point of entry into the stomach, the *gastroesophageal constrictor muscle* relaxes to allow food to enter. Then it contracts again to prevent regurgitation or reflux of the now acidic stomach contents up into the esophagus. When regurgitation does occur, through failure of this mechanism, the person feels it as "heartburn." Two clinical problems may hinder normal food passage at this point: (1) *cardiospasm*, caused by failure of the constrictor muscle to relax properly, or (2) *hiatal hernia*, caused by protrusion of the upper part of the stomach into the thorax through an abnormal opening of the diaphragm.

Chemical or Secretory Digestion

In the mouth, three pairs of salivary glands—*parotid*, *submaxillary*, and *sublingual*—secrete serous material containing *salivary amylase*. This is an enzyme specific for starches. Mucus is also secreted to lubricate and bind the food particles. Stimuli such as sight, smell,

TABLE 2-1

Comparative pH Values and Approximate Daily Volumes of Gastrointestinal Secretions

Secretion	pH	Daily volume (ml)
Salivary	6.0-7.4	1000
Gastric	1.0-3.5	1500
Pancreatic	8.0-8.3	1000
Small intestinal	7.5-8.0	1800
Brunner's gland	8.0-8.9	200
Bile	7.5-7.8	1000
Large intestinal	7.5-8.0	200
TOTAL		6700

Adapted from Guyton AC: *Textbook of medical physiology*, ed 8, Philadelphia, 1991, Saunders.

taste, and touch—even thoughts of likes and dislikes in food—greatly influence these secretions. The normal daily secretion of saliva ranges between 800 and 1500 ml, with a pH range approximately neutral at 6.0 to 7.4, as shown in Table 2-1. Food remains in the mouth only a short time, so starch digestion here is brief and is terminated by the acid medium of the stomach.

Stomach: Storage and Initial Digestive Processes

Motility

The major parts of the stomach are shown in Fig. 2-5. Muscles in the stomach wall provide three basic motor functions: storage, mixing, and controlled emptying. As the food mass enters the stomach, it lies against the stomach walls, which can stretch outward to store as much as 1 L. Local tonic muscle waves gradually increase their kneading and mixing action as the mass of food and secretions moves on toward the pyloric valve at the distal end of the stomach. Here waves of peristaltic contractions reduce the mass to a semifluid chyme. Finally, with each wave, small amounts of chyme are forced through the pyloric valve. This sphincter muscle constricts and periodically relaxes, then constricts again to control the emptying of the stomach contents into the duodenum. This control releases the acid chyme slowly enough to be buffered by the alkaline intestinal secretions. The kcaloric density of a meal, in addition to its particular volume and composition, influences the rate of stomach emptying.[1]

Chemical or Secretory Digestion
Types of Secretion

Stomach secretions contain three basic types of materials: acid, mucus, and enzymes.

bolus · Rounded mass of food formed in the mouth and ready to be swallowed.

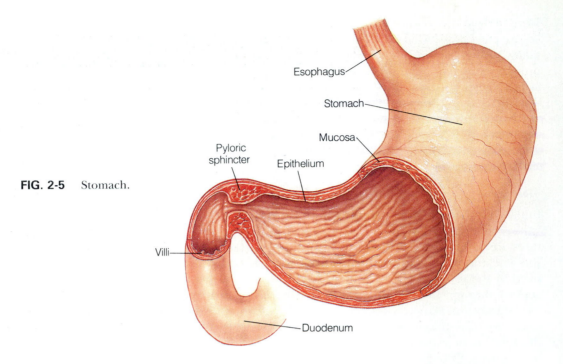

FIG. 2-5   Stomach.

1. *Acid*. Hydrochloric acid is produced to prepare certain enzymes and materials for digestion and absorption by creating the necessary degree of acidity for given enzymes to work.
2. *Mucus*. Special mucous secretions protect the stomach lining from the eroding effect of the acid. This **mucus** also binds and mixes the food mass and helps move it along.
3. *Enzymes*. The main enzyme in the stomach is *pepsin*, which begins the breakdown of protein. It is first secreted in the inactive form *pepsinogen,* which is then activated by the hydrochloric acid present. A small amount of *gastric lipase (tributyrinase)* is present and works on emulsified fats such as butterfat. This is a relatively minor activity, however. In childhood, an enzyme called *rennin* (not to be confused with the vital lifelong renal enzyme *renin*) is also present in gastric secretions to aid in the coagulation of milk. Rennin is absent in adults.

Control of Secretions

Stimuli for these gastric secretions come from two sources:
1. **Nerve stimulus** is produced in response to the senses, ingested food, and emotions. For example, anger and hostility increase secretions. Fear and depression decrease secretions and inhibit blood flow and motility.
2. **Hormonal stimulus** is produced in response to the entrance of food into the stomach. Certain stimulants, especially caffeine, alcohol, and meat extracts, cause the release of a local gastrointestinal hormone **gastrin** from mucosal cells in the antrum, which in

turn stimulates the secretion of more hydrochloric acid. When the pH reaches 2.0, a feedback mechanism stops further secretion of the hormone to prevent excess acid formation. Another local gastrointestinal hormone, **enterogastrone,** is produced by glands in the duodenal mucosa. Enterogastrone counteracts excessive gastric activity by inhibiting acid secretion, pepsin secretion, and gastric motility.

Small Intestine: Major Digestion and Absorption

Motility

Intestinal Muscle Layers

Note the exquisite structural arrangement of the intestinal wall shown in Fig. 2-2. Finely coordinated intestinal motility is achieved by the three basic layers of muscle: (1) the thin layer of smooth muscle embedded in the mucosa, the *muscularis mucosae,* with fibers extending up into the villi, (2) the circular muscle layer, and (3) the longitudinal muscle next to the outer serosa.

Types of Intestinal Muscle Actions

Under the control of the nerve plexus, wall-stretch pressure from food, or hormonal stimuli, these muscles produce several different types of movement to aid digestion:
1. *Segmentation contractions* of circular muscle rings progressively chop the food into successive boluses, mixing food and secretions.
2. *Longitudinal rotation* of the long muscle running

TABLE 2-2

Summary of Digestive Processes

Nutrient	Mouth	Stomach	Small intestine
Carbohydrate	Starch $\xrightarrow{\alpha\text{-amylase}}$ Dextrins		Pancreas
			(Disaccharides)
			Starch $\xrightarrow{\text{Amylase}}$ Maltose and sucrose
			Intestine
			(Monosaccharides)
			Lactose $\xrightarrow{\text{Lactase}}$ Glucose and galactose
			Sucrose $\xrightarrow{\text{Sucrase}}$ Glucose and fructose
			Maltose $\xrightarrow{\text{Maltase}}$ Glucose and glucose
Protein		Protein $\xrightarrow{\text{Pepsin HCl}}$ Polypeptides	Pancreas
			Proteins, Polypeptides $\xrightarrow{\text{Trypsin}}$ Dipeptides
			Proteins, Polypeptides $\xrightarrow{\text{Chymotrypsin}}$ Dipeptides
			Polypeptides, Dipeptides $\xrightarrow{\text{Carboxypeptidase}}$ Amino acids
			Intestine
			Polypeptides, Dipeptides $\xrightarrow{\text{Aminopeptidase}}$ Amino acids
			Dipeptides $\xrightarrow{\text{Dipeptidase}}$ Amino acids
Fat		Tributyrin $\xrightarrow{\text{Tributyrinase}}$ Glycerol	Pancreas
		(butterfat) Fatty acids	Fats $\xrightarrow{\text{Lipase}}$ Glycerol
			Glycerides (di-, mono-)
			Fatty acids
			Intestine
			Fats $\xrightarrow{\text{Lipase}}$ Glycerol
			Glycerides (di-, mono-)
			Fatty acids
			Liver and gallbladder
			Fats $\xrightarrow{\text{Bile}}$ Emulsified fat

the length of the intestine rolls the slowly moving food mass in a spiral motion, mixing it and exposing new surfaces for absorption.

3. *Pendular movements* of small local muscle contractions sweep back and forth and stir the chyme at the mucosal surface.

4. *Peristalsis* produced by waves of contracting deep circular muscle propels the food mass slowly forward. The intensity of the wave may be increased by food intake or by the presence of irritants which in some cases causes long, sweeping waves over the entire intestine.

5. *Villi motions* constantly sweep the mucosal surface with alternating contractions and extensions of mucosal muscle fibers. This action agitates the mucosal surface, stirring and mixing chyme in contact with the intestinal wall and exposing additional nutrient material for absorption.

Chemical or Secretory Digestion
Major Role of Small Intestine

More than any other part of the entire gastrointestinal tract, the small intestine carries the major burden of chemical digestion. Thus this area secretes a large number of enzymes, each specific for some member of the macronutrients—carbohydrates, fats, and proteins. These specific enzymes are secreted from both the intestinal glands and the pancreas. (See Table 2-2.)

Types of Secretions

Four basic types of digestive secretions complete this final process of chemical breakdown in the small intestine:

1. *Enzymes.* A number of specific enzymes (see Table 2-2), act on specific nutrients to cause a final breakdown of the nutrient materials in food to forms the body can absorb and use.

2. *Mucus.* Intestinal glands located immediately inside the duodenum secrete large quantities of mucus. This secretion protects the mucosa from irri-

enterogastrone • A duodenal peptide hormone that inhibits gastric hydrochloric acid secretion and motility.

gastrin • Hormone secreted by mucosal cells in the antrum of the stomach that stimulates the parietal cells to produce hydrochloric acid. Gastrin is released into the stomach in response to stimulants, especially coffee, alcohol, and meat extracts. When the gastric pH reaches 2.0 to 3.0, a feedback mechanism cuts off gastrin secretion and prevents excess acid formation.

mucus • Viscid fluid secreted by mucous membranes and glands, consisting mainly of mucin (a glycoprotein), inorganic salts, and water. Mucus serves to lubricate and protect the gastrointestinal mucosa and to help move the food mass along the digestive tract.

Absorption Aids: Bile Circulation and Pumping Mechanisms

The body has a remarkable capacity for developing mechanisms to maintain its metabolic balances. Two such mechanisms are the enterohepatic circulation of bile and the pumping mechanisms for absorbing nutrients.

TO PROBE FURTHER

Enterohepatic circulation of bile

The efficiency of the enterohepatic circulation of bile salts between the small intestine and the liver demonstrates the body's amazing ability to conserve materials needed for its basic functions. These built-in conservation systems are re ferred to as *homeostatic mechanisms* because they maintain their own balance. They are specifically designed to sustain life in a relatively stable state of equilibrium among the multitude of interdependent elements and subsystems that make up the human organism.

For example, of the 20 to 30 g of bile acids circulated daily in the body to aid in the digestion and absorption of fats, only about 0.8 g is lost in the feces. Therefore, only this small amount needs to be replaced daily by newly synthesized bile. After its tasks in digestion and absorption of fat—emulsifying and transporting—are completed, the bile is separated from its fat complex, returned to the liver, and recirculated again and again.

Pumping mechanisms for absorbing nutrients

Various nutrients cross absorbing membranes by biologic devices called "pumps." The use of the word *pump* for this type of absorbing mechanism may be confusing at first. But it is a helpful term when you think about it.

Remember that what makes a pump pump is the *threat of vacuum,* a situation that cannot exist in biologic organisms. A pump pulls material from one place to another by the exercise of negative pressure.

The pump is able to "suck" material from one place to another because the new site *cannot endure the absence of material.*

It is from this characteristic of nature that biochemists and physiologists have adapted the name *pump.* The empty site's absolute necessity for something to fill its space provides the impetus to move molecules across membranes. A biochemical "pumping mechanism" is one that works by pulling a fresh molecule in to fill a place that has been emptied by the removal of a molecule that was formerly present.

tation and digestion by the highly acid gastric juices at this point. Additional mucous cells on the intestinal surface continue to secrete mucus when touched by the moving food mass. This secretion lubricates and protects the tissues.

3. *Hormone.* In response to the presence of acid in the entering food mass, mucosal cells in the upper part of the small intestine produce the local gastrointestinal peptide hormone **secretin.** In turn, secretin then stimulates the pancreas to send alkaline pancreatic juices into the duodenum to buffer the entering gastric acid chyme. The unprotected intestinal mucosa alone at this

point could not withstand this high degree of acidity.

4. *Bile.* Another important aid to digestion and absorption in the small intestine is bile, an emulsifying agent for fats (see the box above). A large volume of bile is produced in the liver as a dilute watery solution. It is then concentrated and stored by the gallbladder. When fat enters the duodenum, the local gastrointestinal peptide hormone **cholecystokinin** is secreted by glands in the intestinal mucosa and stimulates the gallbladder to contract and release the needed bile. The bile-conserving *enterohepatic circulation of bile* (Fig. 2-6), between the liver, gallbladder, and gastrointestinal tract, serves the needs of all organs involved.

Factors Influencing Secretions

Here in the small intestine, as well as in other sections of the system, many factors influence various secretions. These factors include controls by hormones and nerve plexus, stimulated by physical contact with the food materials and by emotions. These influencing factors are summarized in Fig. 2-7.

Absorption
End Products of Digestion

After digestion of the food nutrients is complete, the simplified end products are ready for **absorption,** aided by a number of transport mechanisms. The end prod-

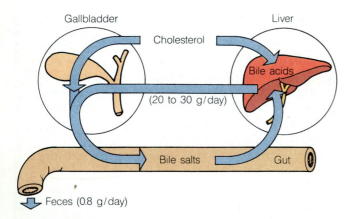

FIG. 2-6   Enterohepatic circulation of bile salts.

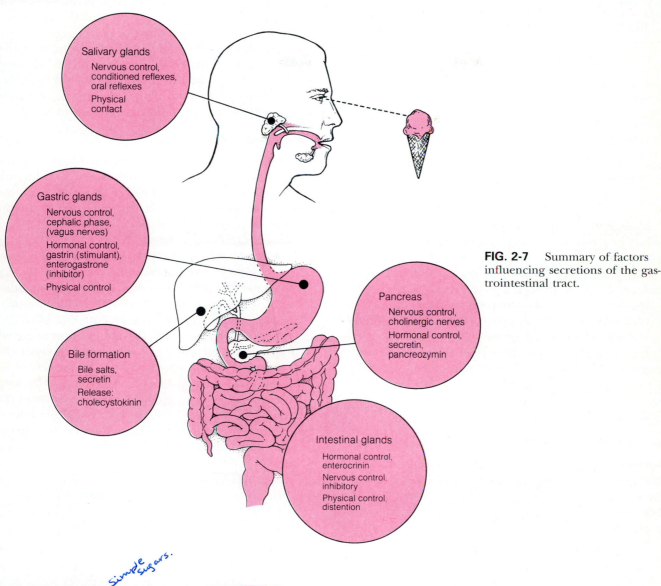

Salivary glands

Nervous control, conditioned reflexes, oral reflexes

Physical contact

Gastric glands

Nervous control, cephalic phase, (vagus nerves)

Hormonal control, gastrin (stimulant), enterogastrone (inhibitor)

Physical control

Bile formation

Bile salts, secretin

Release: cholecystokinin

Pancreas

Nervous control, cholinergic nerves

Hormonal control, secretin, pancreozymin

Intestinal glands

Hormonal control, enterocrinin

Nervous control, inhibitory

Physical control, distention

FIG. 2-7 Summary of factors influencing secretions of the gastrointestinal tract.

ucts include the *monosaccharides* glucose, fructose, and galactose from carbohydrates; *fatty acids* and *glycerides* from fats; and *amino acids* from proteins. In some cases, incompletely digested nutrients, such as lactose in the absence of lactase, remain in the intestine and cause problems for sensitive persons. (See Issues and Answers, p. 33). Some small peptides may be absorbed intact and finally broken down to amino acids within the mucosal absorptive cells. Vitamins and minerals are also liberated. Finally, with a water base for solution and transport plus necessary electrolytes, the total fluid food mass is now prepared for absorption as part of the large gastrointestinal circulation (Table 2-3, p. 26).

Surface Structures

Viewed from the outside, the intestine appears smooth, but the inner mucosal surface lining is quite different. Note carefully in Fig. 2-8 the three types of convolutions and projections that greatly enhance the absorbing surface area:

absorption • Transport of digested nutrients into body circulation to cells.

cholecystokinin (CCK) • A peptide hormone secreted by the mucosa of the duodenum in response to the presence of fat. The cholecystokinin causes the gallbladder to contract. This contraction propels bile into the duodenum, where it is needed to emulsify the fat. The fat is thus prepared for digestion and absorption.

secretin • Hormone produced in the mucous membrane of the duodenum in response to the entrance of the acid contents of the stomach into the duodenum. Secretin in turn stimulates the flow of pancreatic juice, providing needed enzymes and the proper alkalinity for their action.

Daily Absorption Volume in Gastrointestinal System

	Intake (L)	Intestinal absorption (L)	Elimination (L)
Food ingested	1.5		
Gastrointestinal secretions	8.5		
TOTAL	10.0		
Fluid absorbed in small intestine		9.5	
Fluid absorbed in large intestine		0.4	
TOTAL		9.9	
Feces			0.1

Mucosal folds. Large mucosal folds, similar to hills and valleys in a mountain range, can easily be seen by the naked eye.

Villi. Finger-like projections on these folds, called **villi,** can be seen through a simple microscope.

Microvilli. Extremely small projections on each villus, can be seen only with an electron microscope. The array of **microvilli** covering the edge of each villus is called the *brush border* because it looks like bristles on a brush. Each villus has an ample network of blood capillaries as well as a central lymph vessel called a *lacteal* because the fat substances it absorbs have a creamy, milk-like appearance at this point.

Absorbing Surface Area

The three structures of the small intestine—mucosal folds, villi, and microvilli—increase the inner absorbing surface area some 600 times over that of the outside serosa.[6] These special structures, plus the contracted length of the live organ—630 to 660 cm (21 to 22 ft)—produce a tremendously large absorbing surface. This inner surface of the small intestine, if stretched out flat, would be as large or larger than half a basketball court! All three of these mucosal structures serve as a unit for the absorption of nutrients. Although the intestine is popularly known as the lowly "gut," it is actually one of the most highly developed, exquisitely fashioned, specialized tissues in the human body.

Mechanisms of Absorption

Absorption of the finely dispersed water-based nutrient solution is accomplished through the wall of the small intestine by means of a number of transport processes, depending on the nature of the nutrient and the prevailing fluid pressure gradient.

1. *Passive diffusion and osmosis.* When no opposing pressure exists, molecules small enough to pass through the capillary membranes diffuse easily into the capillaries of the villi in the direction of pressure flow, in quantities that depend on their concentration or electrochemical chemical gradient (Fig. 2-9).

2. *Facilitated diffusion.* Even though the pressure gradient is favorably flowing from greater to lesser concentration, which characterized the process of diffusion, some particular molecules may be too large to go through the membrane pores easily and may require assistance. In such cases, a specific integral membrane protein facilitates passage by carrying the particular nutrient molecules across the membrane.

3. *Energy-dependent active transport.* Nutrient molecules must cross the intestinal epithelial membrane to feed hungry tissue cells even when the fluid flow pressures are against them. Such "active" work re-

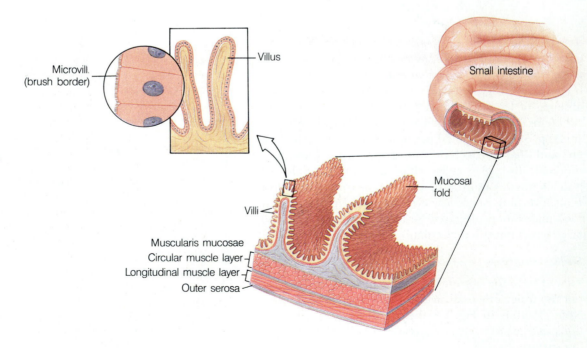

FIG. 2-8 Intestinal wall. Note the arrangement of muscle layers and the structures of the mucosa that increase the surface area for absorption—mucosal folds, villi, and microvilli.

Microvill. (brush border)

Villus

Small intestine

Mucosal fold

Villi

Muscularis mucosae

Circular muscle layer

Longitudinal muscle layer

Outer serosa

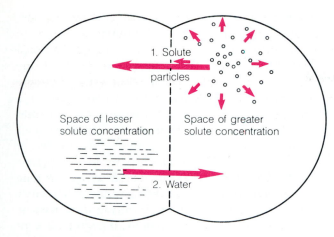

FIG. 2-9 Movement of molecules, water, and solutes by osmosis and diffusion.

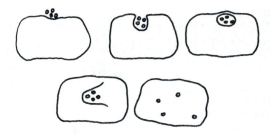

FIG. 2-10 Pinocytosis—engulfing of large molecules by the cell.

quires extra energy supplied by the cell's metabolism and a "pumping" mechanism (see box, p. 24). A special membrane protein carrier, often coupled with the active transport of sodium, assists the process. The active sodium-coupled transport of glucose is an example of this action. A remarkable enzyme, *sodium- and potassium-dependent adenosine triphosphatase (Na$^+$-, K$^+$-, ATPase)*, which is present in the cell membrane, supplies the energy for this interesting pumping action.

4. *Engulfing pinocytosis.* At times, fluid and nutrient molecules use still another means of reaching the tissue circulation outposts in the villi. In these instances, when the particular particle touches the absorbing cell membrane, the membrane dips inward around the fluid and nutrient material, surrounding it to form a *vacuole,* and then engulfs it. The materials are then conveyed through the cell cytoplasm and discharged into circulation. Occasionally, smaller whole proteins, as well as neutral fat droplets, may be absorbed by pinocytosis (Fig. 2-10).

Routes of Absorption

After their absorption by these various processes, the nutrients from carbohydrates and proteins, being water soluble, enter the portal bloodstream directly and travel to the liver and other body tissues. Only fat, which is not water soluble, is unique in its route. Fats are carried in a bile complex into the cells of the intestinal wall, enzyme-processed to human lipid compounds, converted to a complex with protein as a carrier, and packaged as lipoproteins. These packages of fat flow into the lymph; empty into the **cisterna chyli,** the major central abdominal collecting vessel of the body's lymphatic system; travel upward into the chest through the thoracic duct; and finally flow into the venous blood at the left subclavian vein. Then these initial lipoproteins, called chylomicrons from the large fat

load just absorbed, are rapidly cleared from the blood by the special fat enzyme lipoprotein lipase. Exceptions to this route of fat absorption are the medium-chain and short-chain fatty acids, which are more water soluble and hence absorbed directly into blood circulation. However, most of the fats in the human diet are made of long-chain fatty acids, are not water soluble, and must travel the lacteal lymphatic route described.

Large Intestine: Final Absorption and Waste Elimination

Absorption of water is the main task remaining for the large intestine. The actual capacity of the colon for water absorption is great; the net maximum is approximately 5 to 6 L.[1] In daily function, however the large intestine absorbs most of the 1 to 2 L it receives from the ileum. Related nutrient factors, such as electrolytes, minerals, vitamins, amino acids, intestinal bacteria, and nondigestible residue, are also involved.

cisterna chyli • Cistern or receptacle of the chyle; a dilated sac at the origin of the thoracic duct, which is the common truck that receives all the lymphatic vessels. The cisterna chyli lies in the abdomen between the second lumbar vertebra and the aorta. It receives the lymph from the intestinal trunk, the right and left lumbar lymphatic trunks, and two descending lymphatic trunks. The chyle, after passing through the cisterna chyli, is carried upward into the chest through the thoracic duct and empties into the venous blood at the point where the left subclavian vein joins the left internal jugular vein.

microvilli • Minute vascular structures protruding from the surface of villi covering the inner surface of the small intestine, forming a "brush border" that facilitates absorption of nutrients.

villi • Small protrusions from the surface of a membrane; finger-like projections covering mucosal surfaces of the small intestine.

Water Absorption

Within a 24-hour period about 500 ml of the remaining food mass leaves the *ileum,* the last portion of the small intestine, and enters the *cecum,* the pouch at the start of the large intestine. Here the *ileocecal valve* controls passage of the semiliquid chyme. Normally the valve remains closed, but each peristaltic wave relaxes the valve and squirts a small amount of chyme into the cecum. This mechanism holds the food mass in the small intestine long enough to ensure digestion and absorption of vital nutrients.

The watery chyme continues to move slowly through the large intestine, aided by mucous secretion from mucosal glands and muscle contractions. The major portion of the water in the chyme, 350 to 400 ml, is absorbed in the first half of the **colon.** Only about 100 to 150 ml remains to form the feces.

This food residue mass now begins to slow its passage. A meal, having traveled the 630 to 660 cm (21 to 22 ft) of the small intestine, usually starts to enter the cecum about 4 hours after it is consumed. About 8 hours later it reaches the sigmoid colon, having traveled about 90 cm (3 ft) through the large intestine. In the sigmoid colon the residue descends still more slowly toward the anus, where the remainder is finally eliminated as feces. As much as 25% of a meal may remain in the rectum for up to 72 hours.

Mineral Absorption

Electrolytes, mainly sodium, are transported into the bloodstream from the colon. Intestinal absorption is a major balance control point for many of the minerals, and much of the dietary intake remains unabsorbed for elimination in the feces. For example, 20% to 70% of calcium and 80% to 85% of iron ingested are eliminated. The bioavailability of nutrients, especially minerals and vitamins, is largely reflected by their relative overall absorption from the diet during their passage through the gastrointestinal system.[7] This is an important aspect of nutrient balance and dietary evaluation.

Vitamin Absorption and Bacterial Action

Intestinal absorption also serves as a balance control point for some of the vitamins, determining how much the body will keep and how much it will excrete.[8] In addition, bacteria in the colon are closely associated with a number of vitamins. For example, colon bacteria synthesize vitamin K and some of the B-complex vitamins, which are then absorbed from the colon to help meet daily needs. At birth the colon is sterile, but in-

---

CLINICAL APPLICATION   *Digestion's Sometimes Embarrassing Effects*

A common complaint of many persons after eating a meal or certain foods is the discomfort, and sometimes embarrassment, of "gas." This gas is a normal byproduct of digestion, but when it becomes painful or apparent to others it may become a physical and social problem.

The gastrointestinal tract normally holds about 3 oz of gas, moving along with the food mass and silently absorbed into the bloodstream. Sometimes extra gas collects in the stomach or intestine, creating an embarrassing, though usually harmless, situation.

Stomach gas

Gas in the stomach results from uncomfortable air bubbles trapped there. It occurs when a person eats too fast, drinks through a straw, or otherwise takes in extra air while eating. Burping relieves it. But these tips may help to avoid this social slip:
• Avoid carbonated beverages
• Don't gulp

• Chew with your mouth closed
• Don't drink from a can or through a straw
• Don't eat when you're nervous

Intestinal gas

The passing of gas from the intestine is usually a social embarrassment. This gas is formed in the colon, where bacteria attack nondigested items, causing them to decompose and produce gas. Carbohydrates release hydrogen, carbon dioxide, and, in people with certain types of bacteria in the gut, *methane.* All three of these products are odorless (though noisy) gases. Protein produces *hydrogen sulfide* and such volatile amines as *indole* and *skatole,* which add a distinctive aroma to the expelled air. However, these suggestions may help control the problem:
• Cut down on simple carbohydrates— sugars. Especially observe milk's effect because *lactose intolerance* may be the real culprit. Substitute cultured dairy

products such as yogurt or drink milk treated with a lactase product such as LactAid or Lactrace.
• Eliminate all known food offenders. These vary among individuals, but beans, onions, cabbage, and high fiber wheat are among the most common.

Once relief is achieved, you may add more complex carbohydrates and high-fiber foods to the diet—slowly. Once small amounts are tolerated, somewhat greater amounts can be tried. If there is still no relief, a medical examination may be needed to rule out or treat an overactive gastrointestinal tract.

REFERENCES

Brand JC, Holt S: Relative effectiveness of milks with reduced amounts of lactose in alleviating milk intolerance, *Am J Clin Nutr* 54:148, 1991.

Martini MC, Savaiano DA: Reduced intolerance symptoms from lactose consumed during a meal, *Am J Clin Nutr* 47:57, 1988. ◆

TABLE 2-4

Intestinal Absorption of Some Major Nutrients

Nutrient	Form	Means of absorption	Control agent or required cofactor	Route
Carbohydrate	Monosaccharides (glucose and galactose)	Competitive	—	Blood
		Selective	—	
		Active transport via sodium pump	Sodium	
Protein	Amino acids	Selective	—	Blood
	Some dipeptides	Carrier transport systems	Pyridoxine (pyridoxal phosphate)	Blood
	Whole protein (rare)	Pinocytosis	—	Lymph
Fat	Fatty acids	Fatty acid-bile complex (micelles)	Bile	
	Glycerides (mono-, di-)		—	Lymph
	Few triglycerides (neutral fat)	Pinocytosis	—	Lymph
Vitamins	B$_{12}$	Carrier transport	Intrinsic factor (IF)	Blood
	A	Bile complex	Bile	Blood
	K	Bile complex	Bile	From large intestine to blood
Minerals	Sodium	Active transport via sodium pump	—	Blood
	Calcium	Active transport	Vitamin D	Blood
	Iron	Active transport	Ferritin mechanism	Blood (as transferritin)
Water	Water	Osmosis	—	Blood, lymph, interstitial fluid

testinal bacterial flora quickly become well established. The adult colon contains large numbers of bacteria; the predominant species is *Escherichia coli*. Great masses of the bacteria are passed in the stool.

Other Bacterial Action

Intestinal bacteria also affect the color and odor of the stool. The brown color is due to bile pigments formed by the colon bacteria from **bilirubin**. Thus in conditions that hinder bile flow, the feces may become clay colored or white. The characteristic odor results from *amines*, especially *indole* and *skatole*, which are formed by bacterial enzymes from amino acids.

Intestinal gas, or flatus, contains hydrogen sulfide or methane produced by the bacteria. Gas formation, a common complaint, is often caused not so much by specific foods as by the state of the body that receives them (see the box). Many foods have been labeled "gas formers" but in reality these effects are highly variable from one person to another and such classifications have little or no scientific basis.

Dietary Fiber

Since humans have no microorganisms or enzymes to break down dietary fiber, this residue from plant carbohydrate remains after nutrient digestion and absorption (see Chapter 3). However, pectin, one of the soluble fibers, is degraded in the large intestine. Undigested fiber contributes important bulk to the diet and helps form the feces. Fully formed and ready for elimination, normal feces contain about 75% water and 25% solids. The solids include fiber, bacteria, inorganic matter such as minerals, a small amount of fat and its derivatives, some mucus, and sloughed off mucosal cells.

Some major features of nutrient absorption are summarized in Table 2-4.

Metabolism

The various absorbed nutrients, including water and electrolytes, are carried to the cells to produce many substances the body needs to sustain life. Cell metabolism encompasses the total continuous complex of chemical changes that determine the final use of the individual nutrients.

---

bilirubin • A reddish bile pigment resulting from the degradation of heme by reticuleodothelial cells in the liver; a high level in the blood produces the yellow skin symptomatic of jaundice.

colon • The large intestine extending from the cecum to the rectum.

Carbohydrate Metabolism
Sources of Blood Glucose

Both carbohydrate and noncarbohydrate substances provide sources of blood glucose:

1. *Carbohydrate sources.* Three carbohydrate sources provide blood glucose: (1) dietary starches and sugars, (2) glycogen stored in liver and muscle tissue (the hydrolysis of glycogen to form glucose is called **glycogenolysis** or simply **glycolysis**), and (3) products of intermediary carbohydrate metabolism, such as lactic acid and pyruvic acid.
2. *Noncarbohydrate sources.* Both protein and fat provide additional indirect sources of glucose. Certain amino acids from protein are called *glucogenic amino acids* because they form glucose after they are broken down. About 58% of the protein in a mixed diet is composed of glucogenic amino acids. Thus more than half of dietary protein may ultimately be used for energy if sufficient carbohydrate and fat are not available for fuel. After the breakdown of fat into fatty acids and *glycerol*, the small glycerol portion (about 10% of the fat) can be converted to glycogen in the liver and made available for glucose formation. The production of glucose from protein, fat, and intermediary carbohydrate metabolites is called **gluconeogenesis.**

Uses of Blood Glucose

Three uses of glucose serve to regulate the blood sugar within a normal range of 70 to 120 mg/dL (3.9 to 6.6 mmol/L):

1. *Energy production.* The primary function of glucose is to supply energy to meet the body's constant demand. A vast array of interacting metabolic pathways employing many specific successive cell enzymes accomplish this task in a highly efficient manner.
2. *Energy storage.* Two storage forms may be used for glucose: (a) *glycogen*—glucose may be converted to glycogen and stored in limited amounts in the liver and muscle tissue. Only a small supply of glycogen is present at any one time and it turns over rapidly. (b) *Fat*—after energy demands have been fulfilled, any excess glucose is converted to fat and stored as adipose tissue.
3. *Glucose products.* Small amounts of glucose are used in the production of various carbohydrate compounds, which have significant roles in overall body metabolism. Examples include DNA and RNA, galactose, and certain amino acids.

These sources and uses of glucose act as checks and balances to maintain normal blood sugar levels by adding sugar to the blood or removing it as needed.

Hormonal Controls

A number of hormones directly and indirectly influence the metabolism of glucose and regulate the blood sugar level.

Blood sugar–lowering hormone. Only one hormone, *insulin,* acts to lower blood sugar. It is produced by special beta cells in the pancreas. These cells are scattered in cell clusters forming "islands" in the pancreas, thus are called *islets of Langerhans,* named for the scientist Paul Langerhans (1847-1888), who, as a young German medical student, first discovered and studied them. Insulin regulates blood sugar through several actions: (1) *glycogenesis* stimulates the conversion of glucose to glycogen in the liver for constant energy reserve; (2) *lipoprotein* stimulates conversion of glucose to fat for storage in adipose tissue; and (3) *cell permeability* to glucose is increased, allowing it to pass into the cells for oxidation to supply needed energy.

Blood sugar–raising hormones.   A number of hormones effectively raise blood sugar levels:

- *Glucagon*, produced by pancreatic islet alpha cells, acts opposite to insulin, increasing breakdown of liver glycogen to glucose and maintaining blood glucose during fasting sleep hours.
- *Somatostatin*, produced in the pancreatic delta cells and in the hypothalamus, suppresses insulin and glucagon and acts as a general modulator of related metabolic activities.
- *Steroid hormones*, originating from the adrenal cortex, release glucose-forming carbon units from protein and act as insulin antagonists.
- *Epinephrine*, originating from the adrenal medulla, stimulates the breakdown of liver glycogen and a quick release of immediate glucose.
- *Growth hormone* (GH) and *adrenocorticotropic hormone* (ACTH), released from the anterior pituitary gland, act as insulin antagonists.
- *Thyroxine*, originating from the thyroid gland, influences the rate of insulin breakdown, increases glucose absorption from the intestine, and liberates epinephrine.

Lipid Metabolism
Fat Synthesis and Breakdown

Two organ tissues, the liver and adipose tissue, form an overall balanced axis of fat metabolism. Both function in fat synthesis and breakdown. The fatty acids released from fat are used by body cells as concentrated fuel to produce energy.

Lipoproteins

These lipid-protein complexes provide the major transport form of fat in the blood circulation. An excess amount in the blood produces a clinical condition called *hyperlipoproteinemia*. Lipoproteins are produced in the intestinal wall after initial absorption of dietary fat and in the liver for constant recirculation to and from cells.

Hormonal Controls

Since fat and carbohydrate metabolism are closely interrelated, the same hormones are involved:

- *GH, ACTH,* and *thyroid-stimulating hormone (TSH),* all from the pituitary gland, increase the release of free fatty acids from stored body fat by imposing energy demands.
- *Cortisone* and *hydrocortisone,* from the adrenal gland, cause release of free fatty acids.
- *Epinephrine* and *norepinephrine* stimulate breakdown of fat.
- *Insulin,* from the pancreas, promotes fat synthesis, whereas glucagon has the opposite effect of breaking fat tissue to release free fatty acids.
- *Thyroxine,* from the thyroid gland, stimulates fat tissue release of free fatty acids and also lowers blood cholesterol levels.

Protein Metabolism

Anabolism or Tissue Building

Protein metabolism centers on the essential balance between anabolism (tissue building) and catabolism (tissue breakdown). The process of anabolism builds protein tissue through the synthesis of new protein. This build-up is specifically governed by a definite pattern—a specific "blueprint" provided by DNA in the cell nucleus—that requires specific amino acids. Specific selection and supply of amino acids are necessary. Control agents include specific cell enzymes and coenzymes. Also, specific hormones—growth hormone, gonadotropins, and thyroxine—control or stimulate the building of tissue protein.

Catabolism or Tissue Breakdown

Amino acids released by tissue breakdown, if not reused in new tissue synthesis, are further broken down and used for other purposes. Two main parts of these amino acids result: the nitrogen-containing group and the remaining nonnitrogen residue.

1. *Nitrogen group.* The nitrogen portion is first split off of the amino acid, a process called **deamination.** The nitrogen is converted to ammonia and excreted in the urine or retained for use in making other nitrogen compounds.
2. *Nonnitrogen residue.* The nonnitrogen residues are called **keto acids.** They may be used to form either carbohydrates or fats. They may also be reanimated to form a new amino acid.
3. *Control agents.* As in the case of tissue building, cell enzymes and coenzymes as well as hormones influence tissue catabolism. In health, there is a dynamic equilibrium between the two processes of anabolism and catabolism to sustain growth and maintain sound tissue.

Metabolic Interrelationships

Each of the chemical processes of overall body metabolism is purposeful and all are interdependent. They are designed to fill two essential needs: to produce energy and to grow and maintain healthy tissue. The controlling agents in the cells for all of these intricately balanced processes to proceed in an orderly fashion are the cell enzymes, their coenzymes (many of which involve key vitamins and minerals), and special hormones. Overall human metabolism is an exciting biochemical process designed to develop, sustain, and protect our most precious possession—life itself.

To Sum Up

Nutrients are converted into usable forms via digestion and absorption. Metabolism is the means by which the body uses these nutrients to produce energy, build and rebuild body tissues, and maintain normal body functions.

Digestion consists of two basic activities: muscular and chemical. Muscular activity is responsible for food's mechanical breakdown by such means as mastication and movement of food along the gastrointestinal tract by such motions as peristalsis. Chemical activity involves enzymatic action that degrades food into smaller and smaller components for absorption.

Absorption involves the passage of food's nutrients from the gut into the blood stream across the intestinal wall. It occurs mainly in the small intestine via a number of efficient mechanisms.

Cell metabolism handles the absorbed nutrients. This metabolic work is accomplished by a large number of biochemical reactions that result in energy and

---

deamination • Removal of amino group (NH_2) from amino acid.

gluconeogenesis • Production of glucose from keto acid carbon skeleton from deaminated amino acids and the glycerol portion of fatty acids.

glycogenolysis • Specific term for conversion of glycogen into glucose in the liver; chemical process of enzymatic hydrolysis or breakdown by which this conversion is accomplished.

glycolysis • Initial energy production enzyme pathway outside the mitochondria, by which six-carbon glucose is changed to active three-carbon fragments of acetyl CoA, the fuel ready for final energy production in the mitochondria to the high-energy phosphate bond compound adenosine triphosphate (ATP).

keto acid • Amino acid residue after deamination. The glycogenic keto acids are used to form carbohydrates. The ketogenic keto acids are used to form fats.

maintain a dynamic balance between tissue breakdown and rebuilding.

QUESTIONS FOR REVIEW

1. Describe five types of movement involved in the motility necessary for digestive processes.
2. Identify digestive enzymes and any cofactors secreted by the following glands or organs: salivary, mucosal, intestinal, pancreatic, liver. What activity do they perform on fats, proteins, and carbohydrates? What stimulates their release? What inhibits their activity?
3. Describe four mechanisms of nutrient absorption from the small intestine. Describe the routes taken by the breakdown products of fats, proteins, and carbohydrates after absorption. Why must fat follow a different initial route?
4. Describe in detail two major activities that occur in the large intestine.

REFERENCES

1. Wilson PC, Greens HL: The gastrointestinal tract: portal to nutrient utilization. In Shils ME, Young VR, editors: *Modern nutrition in health and disease,* ed 7, Philadelphia, 1988, Lea & Febiger.
2. Guyton AC: *Textbook of medical physiology,* ed 8, Philadelphia, 1991, WB Saunders.
3. Furness JB, Bornstein JC: The enteric nervous system and its extrinsic connections. In Yamada T editor: *Textbook of gastroenterology,* vol 1, New York, 1991, JB Lippincott.
4. Weisbrodt NW: Swallowing. In Johnson LR, editor: *Gastrointestinal physiology,* ed 4, St Louis, 1991, Mosby.
5. Taylor IL, Mannon P: Gastrointestinal hormones. In Yamada T, editor: *Textbook of gastroenterology,* vol 1, New York, 1991, JB Lippincott.
6. Caspary WF: Physiology and pathophysiology of intestinal absorbtion, *Am J Clin Nutr* 55(suppl):299, 1992.
7. Castro GA: Digestion and absorption. In Johnson LR, editor: *Gastrointestinal physiology,* ed 4, St Louis, 1991, Mosby.
8. Sauberlich HE: Vitamins—how much is for keeps? *Nutr Today* 22(1):20, Jan/Feb 1987.

FURTHER READING

Eastwood MA, Morris ER: Physical properties of dietary fiber that influence physiological function: a model for polymers along the gastrointestinal tract, *Am J Clin Nutr* 55:436, 1992.

This article reviews the varying physical characteristics of different dietary fibers and the diverse actions of each as it becomes part of the gastrointestinal functions. It also examines differences in action that are influenced by related situations along the gastrointestinal tract. How these varying fiber actions may be modified by processing and cooking is described.

Shamburek RD, Farrar JT: Disorders of the digestive system in the elderly, *N Engl J Med* 322:438, 1990.

In this excellent review the authors discuss the anatomic and physiologic changes that aging may bring and relate them in a systematic manner to all parts of the gastrointestinal tract, their altered functions, and related problems.

Lactose Intolerance: Common Problem Worldwide

Picture this: a natural disaster strikes a poor nation, leaving thousands homeless and with very little food. CARE, UNICEF, and other international organizations work quickly to collect and ship foodstuffs to the area. Yet the people find it difficult to be grateful: since the shipments began, they have found themselves not only without shelter but also in distress—gastrointestinal distress.

One of the most common foodstuffs shipped to improverished areas is milk. And one of the most common problems throughout the world is *lactose intolerance*—a condition that results in abdominal cramps, nausea, bloating, or diarrhea when milk is consumed. The problem stems from a deficiency of *lactase,* a digestive enzyme found in the microvilli of the small intestine that hydrolyzes milk sugar (lactose) into its component monosaccharides, glucose and galactose, for absorption.

All mammals are born with sufficient amounts of lactase to accommodate the very high lactose levels in "mother's milk." In animal species the amount of enzyme activity drops off significantly shortly after birth. In most human beings this drop occurs after age 5.

Only a few among the human species of the world do not experience this significant childhood drop in the enzyme lactase. These are mostly Northern Europeans, a few African cattle-raisers, and residents of the northwestern sector of India who manage to digest lactose very easily throughout adulthood. The remaining majority of the world's population experience symptoms on drinking as little as a half pint of milk.

Most lactose-intolerant persons can digest cultured or fermented milk products such as buttermilk, yogurt, or cheese very well, and can use these products as a primary source of calcium. But the problem of supplying these items in disaster areas is difficult or unacceptable. Even cheese is too expensive an item to be used frequently to satisfy calcium needs of American school children through school breakfast and lunch programs. The nutritional benefits of lactose-rich foods may become crucial in offsetting deficiency signs among those in dire need.

Continuing study seems to cloud the calcium relationship issue further. Sensitive tests used to measure the subjects' calcium absorption and lactase status have indicated that calcium may be absorbed better in lactase-deficient persons than in lactase-sufficient ones. Also, it seems that the presence or absence of lactose in the intestinal food mix when the calcium was ingested had no effect on its absorption. So what do we tell persons who are lactase-deficient about supplementing their dietary intake of calcium? They have several options, all of which may have drawbacks: (1) use low-lactose milk treated with lactase products, such as Lactaid or Latrase; (2) use cultured or fermented forms of milk such as yogurt or buttermilk; (3) drink small amounts of milk at a time and only with meals; and (4) use lactose supplements in tablet form with meals.

To cloud the issue still further, there is a question concerning the validity of peoples' subjective responses and symptoms about milk tolerance. In some studies of adults who claimed to be lactose-intolerant, only about a third were proved through testing to be truly lactose-intolerant.

Nonetheless, the option of substituting cultured milk products or lactase-treated milk is a possible solution. The low-lactose milks are sweeter than regular milk but have proved to be both acceptable and more effective at reducing symptoms than the alternate product, sweet acidophilus milk. Processing of the low-lactose product involves incubation with yeast lactose, which increases the cost only 2 to 3 cents per liter, keeping it inexpensive enough to be considered for mass distribution. If it continues to demonstrate its effectiveness and safety, those involved with food assistance programs may find low-lactose milk to be the means of overcoming an enzymatic barrier to optimal nutrition throughout the world.

REFERENCES

Brand JC, Holt S: Relative effectiveness of milks with reduced amounts of lactose in alleviating milk intolerance, *Am J Clin Nutr* 54:148, 1991.

Editorial: Mankind, calcium, and milk, *Gastroenterology* 92:260, 1987.

Rosado JL, Allen LH, Solomans NW: Milk consumption, symptom response, and lactose digestion in milk intolerance, *Am J Clin Nutr* 45:1457, 1987.

CHAPTER 3

Carbohydrates

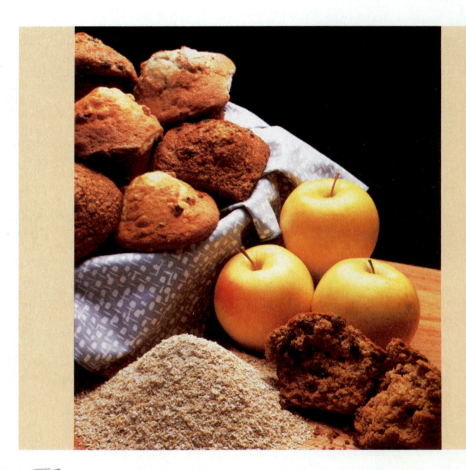

Here we begin a three-chapter sequence on the macronutrients, car-bohydrates, fats, and proteins. Among all the nutrients, these three share a unique capacity, the ability to yield energy.

Carbohydrates have long been of prime importance in the human diet, because they provide the primary source of energy for the body. Over the ages they have nurtured cultures throughout the world, providing the major energy source to sustain work and human development.

In this chapter we look first at the nature of this major macronutri-ent and its function as the basic body fuel.

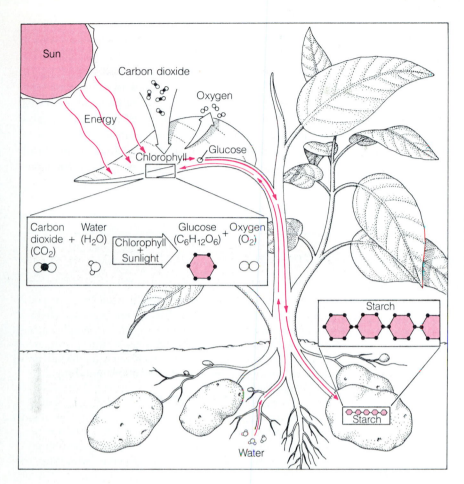

FIG. 3-1 Photosynthesis. In the presence of sunlight and the green leaf pigment chlorophyll, green plants use the raw materials water and carbon dioxide to produce glucose and starch by capturing the sun's energy and transforming it into chemical energy in the food products stored in roots, stems, and leaves and returning oxygen to the atmosphere.

The Nature of Carbohydrates

Basic Fuels: Starches and Sugars

The basic fuel forms of carbohydrates are starches and sugars that occur naturally in our foods. Energy on the planet Earth comes ultimately from the sun and its tremendous nuclear reactions. In the presence of this life-giving sunlight, plants use their internal process of **photosynthesis** to transform the sun's energy into the stored plant fuel form of carbohydrates, as shown in Fig. 3-1. In this important process, plants use carbon dioxide from the air and water from the soil—along with the plant pigment *chlorophyll* in their green leaves, which serves as a chemical catalyst—to manufacture starches and sugars. Because the human body can rapidly break down these starches and sugars to yield body energy, carbohydrates are called "quick energy" foods. They provide our major source of energy.

Dietary Importance

There are practical reasons for the large quantities of carbohydrates in diets all over the world. First, carbohydrates are widely available, because they are easily grown in such plants as grains, vegetables, and fruits. In some countries, carbohydrate foods make up almost the entire diet of the people. In the American diet, about half of the total kilocalories is in the form of carbohydrates. Second, carbohydrates are relatively low in cost. And third, they may be stored easily. Compared with other types of foods, carbohydrate foods can be kept in dry storage for relatively long periods without spoilage. Modern processing and packaging further extend the shelf life of carbohydrate products almost indefinitely.

Classification of Carbohydrates

The term **carbohydrate** comes from its chemical nature. It is composed of the elements carbon, hydrogen,

---

carbohydrate • Compound of carbon, hydrogen, and oxygen; starches, sugars, cellulose, and gums made and stored in plants; major energy source in the human diet.

photosynthesis • Process by which plants containing chlorophyll are able to manufacture carbohydrate by combining CO_2 from air and water from soil. Sunlight is used as energy; chlorophyll is a catalyst.

$6\ CO_2 + 6\ H_2O + Energy \rightarrow Chlorophyll \rightarrow C_6H_{12}O_6 + 6\ O_2$

and oxygen, with the hydrogen/oxygen ratio usually that of water—CH_2O. Carbohydrates are classified according to the number of basic sugar, or *saccharide*, units making up their structure.

Monosaccharides

The simplest form of carbohydrate is the **monosaccharide,** often called a simple (single) sugar. The three main monosaccharides important in human nutrition are glucose, fructose, and galactose.

Glucose

A moderately sweet sugar, glucose is found naturally preformed in only a few foods, such as corn syrup. It is mainly created in the body from starch digestion. In human metabolism, all other types of sugar are converted into glucose. Glucose, sometimes called by its older name *dextrose* in some hospital intravenous solutions, is the form in which sugar circulates in the bloodstream. Blood sugar levels normally range from about 3.9 to 6.1 mmol/L (70 to 110 mg/dl). The term *hyper-*

CLINICAL APPLICATION

How Much Fat Are You Eating?

Recent controversy has developed concerning *hypoglycemia*, the condition of low blood sugar. Is it fact or fiction? Probably some of both. The lay public associates hypoglycemia with an excessive amount of sugar in the diet and at various times has attributed a number of symptoms to this condition, ranging from hunger and headaches to depression and crime. On the other hand, members of the medical community have fueled the problem with statements about "nonhypoglycemia" as a "nondisease."

Clinically, hypoglycemia is usually defined as a blood glucose level of 40 md/dl or lower after consumption of a meal or a glucose load. Clinicians and consumers alike agree on some of the symptoms—for example, nervousness, anxiety, hunger, palpitations, and headaches. But they disagree about causes of the problem, methods of diagnosis, and treatment.

Cause

While consumers have generally named excess dietary sugar as the culprit, clinicians have specifically identified two types of hypoglycemia and their known causes:

- **Reactive hypoglycemia** occurs after a meal and most frequently affects persons who have recently had abdominal surgery or who have diabetes.
- **Fasting hypoglycemia** occurs after extended periods of inadequate food intake or from poor eating habits. It may also be caused by several drugs: (1) alcohol, which blocks glucose production by the liver, (2) hypoglycemic

medications used to treat diabetes, and (3) salicylate in aspirin. More serious conditions that may cause this effect include tumors of the pancreas that stimulate excessive insulin secretion and adrenal insufficiency, a rare condition that prevents the adrenal glands from responding to certain body needs, especially under stress. Unrelieved general stress, whatever the cause, increases metabolic demands on the body and can contribute to hypoglycemia.

Diagnosis

Normal blood glucose levels range from about 3.9 to 6.1 mmol/L (70 to 110 mg/dl). The traditional basis for a medical diagnosis of hypoglycemia has been the oral glucose tolerance test. The patient drinks a beverage containing 75 to 100 g of glucose, and the blood glucose levels are measured at half-hour intervals for up to 5 hours. But this very test situation is unrealistic and induces the abnormal response itself. So, more recently, physicians have used blood tests at the time the person exhibits the characteristic symptoms to obtain a more realistic measure.

Treatment

In general, the lay public believes that hypoglycemia should be treated with a very low-carbohydrate, high-protein diet. However, a very low-carbohydrate diet will make it difficult for the body to obtain sufficient amounts of glucose to achieve and maintain normal blood sugar levels. It is evident now from current carbohydrate research that a diet

of frequent small meals, rich in complex carbohydrates and a good dietary fiber content, with fewer simple carbohydrates and sugars, will maintain a more stable blood sugar level while preventing periods of low blood sugar.

Sound approaches

The simple procedure for home blood glucose monitoring developed for persons with diabetes can be used by persons with hypoglycemic symptoms to test their own blood sugar levels at the time they exhibit symptoms. They should keep a record of results which will provide an accurate profile of the blood glucose levels in the free home environment. This procedure can provide a therapeutic tool for use in counseling and teaching. If the record shows no documented hypoglycemic periods, a sensitive counselor can help the person gain more insight into the problem, exploring other reasons for the symptoms. On the other hand, if the record documents actual hypoglycemia, further diagnostic evaluation is required. This technique is simple, accurate, and effective for persons being evaluated for reactive or postprandial hypoglycemia.

REFERENCES

Andreani D and others: *Hypoglycemia*, Serono Symposia Publications, vol 38, New York, 1987, Raven Press.

Guyton AC: *Textbook of medical physiology,* Philadelphia, 1991, WB Saunders.

Woodley M, Whelan A, editors: *Manual of medical therapeutics,* ed 27, Boston, 1992, Little, Brown & Co. ◆

TABLE 3-1

Summary of Physiologic and Nutritional Significance of Selected Monosaccharides

	Source	Significance
Hexoses		
D-Glucose	Fruit juices; hydrolysis of starch, cane sugar, maltose, and lactose	Body "sugar"; blood and tissue fluids; cell fuel
D-Fructose	Fruit, juices, honey; hydrolysis of sucrose from cane sugar	Changed to glucose in the liver and intestine to serve as basic body fuel
D-Galactose	Hydrolysis of lactose (milk sugar)	Changed to glucose in the liver; cell fuel; synthesized in mammary gland to make lactose of milk; constituent of glycolipids and glycoproteins

glycemia refers to an elevated blood glucose level. *Hypoglycemia* results from blood glucose levels below the normal range. In recent years, public controversy has developed concerning the condition of hypoglycemia (see box). Glucose is the ultimate common refined body fuel that is oxidized in the cells to give energy.

Fructose

The sweetest of the simple sugars, fructose is found in fruits and other substances, such as honey. In the United States, fructose intake has greatly increased since it was introduced in 1970 as a high-fructose corn syrup used in food processing.[1] In human metabolism, fructose is converted to glucose to be burned for energy.

Galactose

The simple sugar galactose is not found free in foods but is produced in human digestion from lactose (milk sugar) and is then changed to glucose for energy. This reaction is reversible, and during lactation glucose may be reconverted to galactose for use in milk production.

The general physiologic and nutritional importance of these major monosaccharides (called *hexoses* from their basic 6-carbon structure) is summarized in Table 3-1.

Disaccharides

The **disaccharides** are simple (double) sugars composed of two monosaccharides linked together. The three main disaccharides of physiologic importance are sucrose, lactose, and maltose. Their respective monosaccharide components follow:

> Sucrose = glucose + fructose
> Lactose = glucose + galactose
> Maltose = glucose + glucose

Notice that glucose is a major component in each of these disaccharides.

Sucrose

Sucrose is the common "table sugar" made commercially from sugar cane and sugar beets. It is the most prevalent disaccharide. With the increasing use of processed foods, sucrose contributes some 30% to 40% of the total kilocalories in the American diet (see Issues and Answers, p. 47). Sucrose can be found in all forms of common sugar, molasses, and in some fruits and vegetables, such as pineapple and carrots.

Lactose

The sugar in milk is called *lactose* because of its source. It is formed in the body from glucose to supply the needed sugar component of milk during lactation. It is the least sweet of the disaccharides, about one sixth as sweet as sucrose. When milk sours, as in the initial stages of cheese making, the lactose changes its form and separates out the liquid whey from the solid curd. The curd is then processed for cheese. Thus, although milk has a relatively high carbohydrate content in the form of lactose, one of its main products—cheese—has very little or none.

Maltose

Maltose occurs in commercial malt products of starch breakdown and in germinating cereal grains. As such, it is a negligible *dietary* carbohydrate. But it is a highly significant *metabolic* carbohydrate as an intermediate product of starch digestion.

The general physiologic and nutritional significance of the disaccharides is sumarized in Table 3-2.

Polysaccharides

The much more complex carbohydrates are called **polysaccharides,** because they are made up of *many*

---

disaccharides • Class of compound sugars composed of two molecules of monosaccharide. The three most common are sucrose, lactose, and maltose.

monosaccharide • Simple single sugar; a carbohydrate containing a single saccharide (sugar) unit.

polysaccharides • Class of complex carbohydrates composed of many monosaccharide units. Common members are starch, dextrins, dietary fiber, and glycogen.

TABLE 3-2

Summary of Physiologic and Nutritional Significance of Selected Disaccharides

	Source	Significance
Maltose	Starch digestion by amylase, commercial hydrolysis; malt and germinating cereals	Hydrolyzed to D-glucose; basic body fuel and metabolite; fermentable
Sucrose	Cane and beet sugar, sorghum cane, carrots, pineapple	Hydrolyzed to glucose and fructose; body fuel
Lactose	Milk	Hydrolyzed to glucose and galactose; body fuel; constituent for milk production during lactation

single sugar (saccharide) units. The most important polysaccharide in human nutrition is starch. Other forms are glycogen and dextrins. The nondigestible forms of dietary fiber, cellulose and other noncellulose polysaccharides, provide important bulk in the diet.

Starch

In human nutrition, starch is by far the most significant polysaccharide. It is a relatively large complex compound made up of many coiled or branching chains of simple sugar (glucose) units. It yields only glucose on digestion. The cooking of starch not only improves its flavor, but also softens and ruptures the starch cells, which makes digestion easier. Starch mixtures thicken when cooked, because the portion that encases the starch granules has a gel-like quality that thickens the mixture in the same way that pectin causes jelly to set.

Starch is also by far the most important source of dietary carbohydrate worldwide. It is recognized as a significant factor in human nutrition and health. For example, standards of U.S. dietary guidelines, as outlined in Chapter 1, recommend that about 50% to 55% of the total kilocalorie value of the diet come from carbohydrates, with a greater portion of that allowance coming from complex carbohydrate starch foods.[2] In many other countries, where starch is the staple food material, it makes up an even greater portion of the diet. The major food sources of starch include cereal grains, legumes, potatoes, and other vegetables.

Glycogen

The animal storage compound comparable to starch in plants is **glycogen.** It is formed during cell metabolism and stored in relatively small amounts in the liver and muscle tissues. These stores help sustain normal blood glucose levels during fasting periods, such as sleep hours, and provide immediate fuel for muscle action, especially during athletic activity.[3] Sometimes athletes practice pregame "glycogen loading" to provide added fuel stores for use during athletic events (see Chapter 14). Dietary carbohydrate is essential to maintain these needed glycogen stores and prevent the symptoms of low carbohydrate intake—fatigue, dehydration, and en-

ergy loss—as well as other undesirable metabolic effects, such as *ketoacidosis* (see Chapter 21) and excessive protein breakdown. The Food and Nutrition Board of the National Research Council recommends a carbohydrate intake of at least 100 g/day to prevent these symptoms.[2] Most diets provide well over 200 g/day, with the average diet containing 300 g or more.

Dextrins

Dextrins are polysaccharide compounds formed as intermediate products in the breakdown of starch. This starch breakdown occurs constantly in the process of digestion.

Starch + water →	soluble starch + maltose
Soluble starch + water →	dextrins + maltose
Dextrins + water →	maltose
Maltose + water →	glucose + glucose

Oligosaccharides

These carbohydrates are small portions of partially digested starch, ranging in size from about 3 to 10 monosaccharides. They form either naturally through the process of digestion or commercially through acid hydrolysis. **Oligosaccharides** are irregular in form and, when digested, yield their few constitutent monosaccharides. These small sugars are used extensively in special formulas for infants or persons with gastrointestinal problems, because they are designed for easier digestion. These smaller sugars are also used in sports drinks—for example, Exceed (Ross)—in which they may contribute about 47.5% of the total glucose in the solution (see Chapter 14).

Some naturally occurring oligosaccharides are constructed with bonds that cannot be broken by human enzymes, so they are indigestible.[4] For example, two of these—stachyose and **raffinose**—are found in legumes, such as beans, peas, and soybeans. These small sugars provide a feast for bacterial flora in the intestines, producing a large amount of gas that can bring discomfort and embarrassment.

Dietary Fiber

Based on current research, dietary fiber may be classed into three major groups according to structure and

TABLE 3-3

Summary of Dietary Fiber Classes

Dietary fiber class	Plant parts	Functions
Cellulose	Main cell wall constituent	Insoluble; holds water, functions as laxative, reduces elevated colonic intraluminal pressure; binds minerals
Noncellulose polysaccharides		
Hemicellulose	Secretions, cell wall material	Mostly insoluble; holds water, increases stool bulk, reduces colonic pressure; binds bile acids
Pectins	Intracellular cement material	Soluble; binds cholesterol and bile acids
Gums	Special cell secretions	Soluble; binds cholesterol and bile acids; slows gastric emptying; provides fermentable material for colonic bacteria with production of volatile fatty acids and gas
Mucilages	Cell secretions	Soluble; slows gastric emptying time; fermentable substrate for colonic bacteria; binds bile acids
Algal substances	Algae, seaweeds	Soluble; slows gastric emptying time; fermentable substrate; binds bile acids
Noncarbohydrate		
Lignin	Woody part of plants	Insoluble; antioxidant; binds bile acids and metals

TABLE 3-4

Summary of Soluble and Insoluble Fibers in Total Dietary Fiber

Insoluble	Soluble
Cellulose	Gums
Most hemicelluloses	Mucilages
Lignin	Algal polysaccharides
	Most pectins

properties, with one of these groups having five different members.[1]

Cellulose

This **dietary fiber** is the chief constituent of the framework of plants. Humans cannot digest cellulose, because they lack the necessary digestive enzymes. Therefore it remains in the digestive tract and contributes important bulk to the diet. This bulk helps move the food mass along and stimulates *peristalsis* (see Chapter 5). Cellulose makes up the principal structural material in plant cell walls and provides most of the substance labeled "crude fiber" (see box, p. 40). The main food sources are stems and leaves of vegetables, seed and grain coverings, skins, and hulls. 20-25s

Noncellulose Polysaccharides

The noncellulose fiber carbohydrates include hemicellulose, pectins, gums, mucilages, and algal substances. They absorb water and slow gastric emptying time. All of them, except hemicellulose, are gumlike water-soluble substances that aid in binding cholesterol and controlling its absorption. They also prevent colon pressure by providing bulk for normal intestinal muscle action.

Lignin

This substance is the only noncarbohydrate type of dietary fiber. It is a large compound that forms the woody part of plants. In the intestine it combines with bile acids to form insoluble compounds, thus preventing their absorption. They contribute the memorable sandy texture of pears and lima beans.

A summary of these dietary fiber classes is given in Table 3-3. Compare the classes with their solubility groupings in Table 3-4. Some main food sources of the various types of dietary fiber are indicated in Table 3-5 (p. 40). Also, in the food exchange lists (Appendix K), the high-fiber foods in each food group are indicated. Comparisons of the fiber content of some selected foods are given in Table 3-6 (p. 41).

dietary fiber • Nondigestible form of carbohydrate that is of nutritional importance in gastrointestinal disease such as diverticulosis and in reducing serum lipid and glucose levels related to chronic conditions such as heart disease and diabetes.

glycogen • A polysaccharide, that is, a large compound of many saccharide (i.e., sugar) units. It is the main body storage form of carbohydrate, largely stored (with relatively rapid turnover) in the liver, with lesser amounts stored in muscle tissue.

oligosaccharides • Intermediate products of polysaccharide carbohydrate breakdown that contain a small number (from 4 to 10) of single sugar units of the monosaccharide glucose.

raffinose • A colorless crystalline trisaccharide component of legumes, composed of galactose and sucrose connected by bonds that human enzymes cannot break, thus it remains whole in the intestines and produces gas as bacteria attack it.

TABLE 3-5

Selected Food Sources of Various Classes of Dietary Fiber

Dietary fiber class	Grains	Fruits	Vegetables
Cellulose	Bran Whole wheat Whole rye	Apples Pears	Beans, peas Cabbage family Root vegetables Tomatoes, fresh
Noncellulose polysaccharides			
Hemicellulose	Bran Cereals Whole grains		
Pectins		Apples Citrus fruits Berries, especially strawberries	Green beans Carrots
Gums	Oatmeal	Food products thickener, stabilizer	Dried beans, other legumes Vegetable gums used in food processing
Mucilages		Food products thickener, stabilizer	
Algal substances		Food products thickener, stabilizer	
Noncarbohydrate			
Lignins	Whole wheat Whole rye	Strawberries Peaches Pears Plums	Mature vegetables

TO PROBE FURTHER

Much of the confusion concerning fiber in the diet has centered on semantics. No term has seemed fully acceptable to cover all the different types of fiber or the various meanings involved. The older word *roughage* and the current general term *fiber* denote a rough abrasive material of the physical nature observed in plant cellulose, a woody type of material. However, a number of the indigestible materials in food have a soft amorphous gel-like character, more soluble in physical nature and hence having different properties and functions.

This difference in physical properties adds to the problem nutritionists and clinicians have had in determining a more precise nutritional and clinical significance for fiber in the diet and in defining the variety of food substances involved. Further problems have surrounded methods of accurately analyzing and measuring these substances in the variety of food sources in which they occur.

The general term *fiber* was initially applied to a variety of indigestible carbohydrate and noncarbohydrate substances for which specific hydrolytic enzymes are lacking in the human digestive system. Confusion has resulted mainly from the erroneous interchange of the two terms *dietary fiber* and *crude fiber*.

Dietary fiber refers to the total amount of naturally occurring material in foods, mostly plants, that is not digested. This includes (1) plant dietary fiber from such foods as whole grains, legumes, vegetables, fruits, seeds, and nuts, (2) undigested animal tissue polysaccharides, (3) undigested pharmaceutical products, and (4) undigested biosynthetic polysaccharides. Refined diets in Western countries usually contain little fiber in the energy foods—starches, sugars, and fats. Diets in rural communities of other developing countries contain much more fiber. Research suggests that these higher-fiber diets protect against a wide variety of Western diseases.

Crude fiber is the material remaining after vigorous treatment of the food sources with acid and alkaline agents in the laboratory. These were the initial results given in most food value tables. These strong laboratory processes remove a good portion of the total dietary fiber, which cannot withstand such treatment. Because the proportion of total dietary fiber and crude fiber varies widely among specific foods, depending on the fiber composition of a particular food, the fiber values given in earlier food value tables have had limited usefulness. However, as new laboratory procedures are developed, better information is being provided. Thus the term *crude fiber* is of little value in current usage.

The current term of choice, although not perfect, is *dietary fiber*. It refers to the indigestible residues of plant foods: (1) cellulose, (2) noncellulose polysaccharides, including hemicellulose, pectins, gums, mucilages, and algal substances, and (3) the single noncarbohydrate member, lignin. All resist digestion by any human digestive enzymes, but all are valuable in nutrition and related disease.

REFERENCES

Marlett JA: Content and composition of dietary fiber in 117 frequently consumed foods, *J Am Diet Assoc* 92(2):175, 1992.
Slavin JL: Dietary fiber: classification, chemical analysis, and food sources, *J Am Diet Assoc* 87(9):1164, Sept 1987.
Slavin JL: Dietary fiber: mechanism or magic on disease prevention, *Nutr Today* 25(6):6, 1990.

TABLE 3-6

Dietary Fiber and Kcalorie Values for Selected Foods

Foods	Serving	Dietary fiber (g)	
Breads and cereals			
All Bran	½ cup	8.5	70
Bran (100%)	½ cup	8.4	75
Bran Buds	⅓ cup	7.9	75
Corn Bran	⅔ cup	5.4	100
Bran Chex	⅔ cup	4.6	90
Cracklin' Oat Bran	⅓ cup	4.3	110
Bran Flakes	¾ cup	4.0	90
Air-popped popcorn	1 cup	2.5	25
Oatmeal	1 cup	2.2	144
Grapenuts	¼ cup	1.4	100
Whole-wheat bread	1 slice	1.4	60
Legumes, cooked			
Kidney beans	½ cup	7.3	110
Lima beans	½ cup	4.5	130
Vegetables, cooked			
Green peas	½ cup	3.6	55
Corn	½ cup	2.9	70
Parsnip	½ cup	2.7	50
Potato, with skin	1 medium	2.5	95
Brussels sprouts	½ cup	2.3	30
Carrots	½ cup	2.3	25
Broccoli	½ cup	2.2	20
Beans, green	½ cup	1.6	15
Tomato, chopped	½ cup	1.5	17
Cabbage, red and white	½ cup	1.4	15
Kale	½ cup	1.4	20
Cauliflower	½ cup	1.1	15
Lettuce, fresh	1 cup	0.8	7
Fruits			
Apple	1 medium	3.5	80
Raisins	¼ cup	3.1	110
Prunes, dried	3	3.0	60
Strawberries	1 cup	3.0	45
Orange	1 medium	2.6	60
Banana	1 medium	2.4	105
Blueberries	½ cup	2.0	40
Dates, dried	3	1.9	70
Peach	1 medium	1.9	35
Apricot, fresh	3 medium	1.8	50
Grapefruit	½ cup	1.6	40
Apricot, dried	5 halves	1.4	40
Cherries	10	1.2	50
Pineapple	½ cup	1.1	40

From Lanza E, Butrum RR: A critical review of food fiber analysis and data, *J Am Diet Assoc* 86:732, 1986.

Physiologic Effects

In general, dietary fiber produces various effects on the food mix consumed and its fate in the body. Most of these effects are caused by its physiologic properties:

- **Water absorption.** Dietary fiber's capacity to absorb water contributes to its bulk-forming laxative effect, thus influencing the transit time of the food mass through the digestive tract and the consequent absorption of the various nutrients.
- **Binding effect.** Such fibers as the noncellulose substances influence blood lipid levels through a binding effect, a capacity to bind cholesterol and bile salts

TABLE 3-7

Relationship Between Fiber and Various Health Problems

Problem	Effect of fiber	Possible mode of action	Future research needs
Diabetes mellitus	Reduces fasting blood sugar levels Reduces glycosuria Reduces insulin requirements Increases insulin sensitivity	Slows carbohydrate absorption by: Delaying gastric emptying time Forming gels with pectin or guar gum in the intestine, thus impeding carbohydrate absorption "Protecting" carbohydrates from enzymatic activity with a fibrous coat Allowing "protected" carbohydrates to escape into large colon where they are digested by bacteria	Influence of short-chain fatty acid production or metabolism of glucose and fats in the liver Exact mechanisms by which fiber influences glucose metabolism
	Inhibits postprandial (after meals) hyperglycemia	Alters gut hormones (for example, glucagon) to enhance glucose metabolism in the liver	
Obesity	Increases satiety rate	Prolongs chewing and swallowing movements	Cause of increased satiety rate reported by subjects
	Reduces nutrient bioavailability	Increases fecal fat content	Effect of nutrient binding on nutritional status
	Reduces energy density	Inhibits absorption of carbohydrates in high-fiber foods	Studies based on food composition and kcaloric density instead of fiber content alone
		Decreases transit time	Effects of different types of fiber on gastric, small intestine, and colonic emptying time
	Alters hormonal response	Alters action of insulin, gut glucagon, and other intestinal hormones	
	Alters thermogenesis		
Coronary heart disease	Inhibits recirculation of bile acids	Alters bacterial metabolism of bile acids	Influence of fiber on cholesterol content of specific lipoprotein fractions (see Chapter 20)
		Alters bacterial flora, resulting in a change in metabolic activity	Influence on production of short-chain fatty acids
		Forms gels that bind bile acids	Role of dietary fiber as an independent variable in reducing risk of heart disease
		Alters the function of pancreatic and intestinal enzymes	
	Reduces triglyceride and cholesterol levels*	Reduces insulin levels†	Relationship between lipoprotein turnover and glucose turnover/ sensitivity to insulin
		Binds cholesterol, preventing absorption	Effect of higher concentration of bile salts on colon function
		Slows fat absorption by forming gel matrices in the intestine	
Colon cancer	Reduces incidence of disease‡	Bile acids or their bacterial metabolites may affect the structure of the colon, its cell turnover rate, and function	Testing of current hypotheses regarding the effects of dietary factors on the structure of the colon and cell turnover rate
Other gastrointestinal disorders	Reduces pressure from within the intestinal lumen	Decreases transit time	
Diverticular disease Constipation Hiatal hernia Hemorrhoids	Increases diameter of the intestinal lumen, thus allowing intestinal tract to contract more, propelling contents more rapidly and inhibiting segmentation§	Increases water absorption resulting in a larger, softer stool	

*This effect is based on epidemiologic studies, usually observed in combination with reduced fat intake.

†Insulin is required for fat synthesis.

‡Preventive effect of fiber is assumed from epidemiologic studies that associate low-fiber, high-fat diets with an *increased* incidence of disease.

§Segmentation increases pressure and weakness along the walls of the intestinal tract.

and prevent their absorption. However, excessive dietary fiber can have the undesirable effect of binding such minerals as iron, zinc, or calcium, thus preventing needed absorption.[6]

- **Colon bacteria effect.** The colon bacteria effect on fermentation substrates for bacterial action produces volatile fatty acids and gas.[7]

Current research concerning various clinical applications has centered largely on diabetes mellitus, coronary heart disease, colon cancer, and other intestinal problems, such as diverticulosis.[7-9] Some of these clinical associations between dietary fiber and various health problems are summarized in Table 3-7.

Dietary Fiber Recommendation

Sufficient evidence now exists to suggest that Americans should increase their intake of dietary fiber by consuming more whole grain products, fruits, and vegetables, and that fiber supplements are not appropriate for healthy persons. Recent studies indicate that the average dietary fiber intake of American adults is only 11 g/day, when a recommendation of about 20 to 25 g/day appears wise.[2] This goal can easily be achieved through generous use of whole grains, legumes, vegetables, fruits, seeds, and nuts. Indiscriminate use of bran is not justified. While more analysis of the various types of dietary fiber is still needed, Marlett has provided dietary fiber values for a number of foods by food groups.[5]

Functions of Carbohydrates

Energy

As indicated, the primary function of carbohydrate in nutrition is to provide fuel for energy production. Fat is also a fuel, but the body needs only a small amount of dietary fat, mainly to supply the essential fatty acids. To function properly, however, the body tissues require a daily dietary supply of carbohydrate sufficient to provide 50% to 55% of the total kilocalories.

The amount of carbohydrate in the body, though relatively small, is important to maintain energy reserves. For example, in an adult male about 300 to 350 g is "stored" in the liver and muscle tissues as glycogen, and about 10 g is present in circulating blood glucose (Table 3-8). This total amount of available glycogen and glucose provides energy sufficient for only about half a day of moderate activity. Thus carbohydrate foods must be eaten regularly and at moderately frequent intervals to meet the constant energy demands of the body.

Special Functions of Carbohydrates in Body Tissues

As part of their general function as the body's main energy source, carbohydrates serve special functions in many body tissues.

TABLE 3-8

Postabsorptive Carbohydrate Storage in Normal Adult Man (70 kg [154 lb])

	Glycogen (g)	Glucose (g)
Liver (weight 1800 g)	72	
Muscles (mass weight 35 kg [77 lb])	245	
Extracellular fluids (10 L)		10
Component totals	317	10
TOTAL STORAGE	327	

Glycogen Reserves

As indicated, the liver and muscle glycogen reserves provide a constant interchange with the body's overall energy balance system. Thus these reserves protect cells from depressed metabolic function and injury.

Protein-sparing Action

channels excess protein

Carbohydrate helps regulate protein metabolism. The presence of sufficient carbohydrate for energy demands of the body prevents the channeling of too much protein for this purpose. This protein-sparing action of carbohydrate allows the major portion of protein to be used for its basic structural purpose of tissue building.

Antiketogenic Effect

Carbohydrate also relates to fat metabolism. The amount of carbohydrate present in the diet determines how much fat will be broken down, thus affecting the formation and disposal rates of *ketones*. Ketones are intermediate products of fat metabolism, which normally are produced at a low level during fat oxidation. However, in such extreme conditions as starvation and uncontrolled diabetes, as well as the unwise use of very low-carbohydrate diets, carbohydrate is inadequate or unavailable for energy needs, so too much fat is oxidized. Ketones accumulate, and the result is *ketoacidosis* (see Chapter 21). Sufficient carbohydrate prevents this damaging excess of ketones.

Heart Action

Heart action is a life-sustaining muscular exercise. Although fatty acids are the preferred regular fuel for the heart muscle, the glycogen reserve in cardiac muscle is an important emergency source of contractile energy. In a damaged heart, poor glycogen stores or low carbohydrate intake may cause cardiac symptoms and angina.

Central Nervous System Function

A constant supply of carbohydrate is necessary for the proper functioning of the central nervous system (CNS). The CNS regulatory center, the brain, contains no stored supply of glucose and is therefore especially dependent on a minute-to-minute supply of glucose from the blood. Sustained and profound hypoglycemic shock may cause irreversible brain damage. In all nerve tissue, carbohydrate is indispensable for functional integrity.

Although a more detailed and integrated discussion of digestion, absorption, and metabolism of the macronutrients is given in Chapter 2, a brief summary of these aspects for each individual macronutrient is presented at the end of each introductory macronutrient chapter, to set the scene for the larger picture that follows. Here we provide that summary outline for carbohydrates.

Digestion-Absorption-Metabolism Summary

Digestion

Most carbohydrate foods, starches and sugars, cannot immediately be used by the cells to make energy available. They must first be changed into the refined fuel for which the cell is designed—*glucose.* The process by which these vital changes are made is *digestion.* The digestion of carbohydrate foods proceeds through the successive parts of the gastrointestinal tract, accomplished by two types of actions: (1) mechanical or muscle functions that render the food mass into smaller particles, and (2) chemical processes in which specific enzymes break down food nutrients into smaller usable metabolic products.

Mouth

Mastication breaks food into fine particles and mixes it with the salivary secretions. During this process, a salivary amylase (ptyalin) is secreted by the parotid gland. It acts on starch to begin its breakdown into dextrins and maltose.

Stomach

Successive wavelike contractions of the muscle fibers of the stomach wall continue the mechanical digestive process. This action is called *peristalsis.* It further mixes food particles with gastric secretions to allow chemical digestion to take place more readily. The gastric secretion contains no specific enzyme for the breakdown of carbohydrate. The hydrochloric acid in the stomach stops the action of salivary amylase. But before the food mixes completely with the acid gastric secretion, as much as 20% to 30% of the starch may have been changed to maltose. Muscle actions continue to bring the food mass to the lower part of the stomach. Here the food mass is now a thick creamy *chyme,* ready for its controlled emptying through the *pyloric valve* into the duodenum, the first portion of the small intestine.

Small Intestine

Peristalsis continues to aid digestion in the small intestine by mixing and moving the chyme along the **lumen**

in the length of the tube. Chemical digestion of carbohydrate is completed in the small intestine by specific enzymes from two sources: the pancreas and intestine.

Pancreatic Secretions

Secretions from the pancreas enter the duodenum through the common bile duct. They contain pancreatic amylase, which continues the breakdown of starch to maltose.

Intestinal Secretions

Intestinal secretions contain three disaccharidases—**sucrase, lactase,** and **maltase.** These enzymes act on their respective disaccharides to render the monosaccharides—glucose, galactose, and fructose—ready for absorption. These specific disaccharidases are integral proteins of the brush border of the small intestine that break down the disaccharides as absorption takes place. The digestive products, the monosaccharides, are then immediately absorbed into the portal blood circulation.

A summary of the major aspects of carbohydrate digestion through these successive parts of the gastrointestinal tract is given in Table 3-9.

Absorption

The refined fuel glucose is now ready to be carried to the individual cells to be "burned" or stored to produce energy. The process by which the body carries this basic end product of carbohydrate digestion to the cells throughout the body is called *absorption* or *transport.* The major glucose absorption mechanism is an active transport "pumping" system requiring sodium as a carrier substance.

Absorbing Structures

The absorbing surface area of the small intestine is uniquely enhanced by its three basic structures—mucosal folds, villi, and microvilli—which are described in detail in Chapter 2. Together, these structures provide

TABLE 3-9		
Summary of Carbohydrate Digestion		
	Enzyme	Action
Mouth	Salivary amylase: ptyalin	Starch→dextrins→maltose
Stomach	None	Starch hydrolysis continued briefly
Small intestine	Pancreatic amylase: amylopsin	Starch→dextrins→maltose
	Intestinal disaccharidases:	
	Sucrase	Sucrose→glucose + fructose
	Lactase	Lactose→glucose + galactose
	Maltase	Maltose→glucose + glucose

a greatly increased absorbing surface that allows 90% of the digested food material to be absorbed in the small intestine. Only water absorption remains for the large intestine.

Route of Absorption

By way of the capillaries of the villi, the simple sugars enter **portal** circulation and are transported to the liver. Here fructose and galactose are converted to glucose, which is either used immediately for fuel or converted to glycogen for brief storage. Then glycogen constantly reconverts to glucose as needed by the body.

Metabolism

Definition

The general term **metabolism** refers to the sum of the various chemical processes in a living organism by which energy is made available for the functioning of the entire organism. It includes all the processes by which basic structures are built and maintained, function, and then break down to be rebuilt. Products of specific metabolic processes are called **metabolites.**

Cell Metabolism of Carbohydrate Products

Cells are the functional units of life in the human body. In cell nutrition the most important end product of carbohydrate digestion is glucose, because the other two monosaccharides—fructose and galactose—are eventually converted to glucose. The liver is the major site of the intricate machinery that handles glucose. However, energy metabolism occurs in all cells. In these individual cells, glucose is burned to produce energy through a series of chemical reactions involving specific cell enzymes. The final energy produced is then available to the cell to do its work. Extra glucose not immediately needed for energy may also be changed to fat and stored as a reserve fuel. Details of these interactive metabolic activities among the nutrients are discussed in Chapter 2.

Metabolic Concept of Unity

Here and in following discussions of other nutrients, a central significant scientific principle emerges—*unity of the human organism.* The human body is a whole made up of many parts and processes that possess unequaled specificity and flexibility. Intimate metabolic relationships exist among all the basic nutrients and metabolites. Thus it is impossible to understand any one of the body's many metabolic processes without viewing it in relationship to the whole.

Therefore, in all your study and work with patients and clients, remember this important fact: **All nutrients do their best work in partnership with other nutrients.** From this fundamental fact you can draw two practical conclusions: (1) the emphasis in health teaching and nutrition education should be on achieving a sound balanced nutritional basis for any dietary program, and

(2) some deficiency states may be *iatrogenic* (induced by medical treatment), may have their origin in a fad, or may be caused by long-term, overzealous emphasis on one particular nutrient to the exclusion of other equally essential ones.

To Sum Up

Carbohydrate supplies most of the world's population with its primary source of energy. A product of photosynthesis, it is widely distributed in nature and its food products are easy to store and generally low in cost.

There are two basic types of carbohydrates: simple and complex. *Simple carbohydrates* consist of single- and double-sugar units (monosaccharides and disaccharides), which are easily digested and provide quick energy. *Complex carbohydrates,* or polysaccharides, are less easily prepared for use. Though they vary somewhat in their effect on blood sugar, they generally provide energy more slowly and prevent large fluctuations in blood glucose levels.

In addition to providing general body energy, carbohydrates maintain liver, heart, brain, and nerve tissue function. They also prevent the breakdown of both fats and proteins for energy, which results in excessive production of toxic metabolic byproducts. *Dietary fiber,* a complex carbohydrate that forms the indigestible part of plants, also affects the digestion and absorption of foods in ways that have proved beneficial to good health.

---

lactase • Enzyme that splits the disaccharide lactose into its two monosaccharides, glucose and galactose.

lumen • The cavity or channel within a tube or tubular organ, such as the intestines.

maltase • Enzyme that breaks down the disaccharide maltose into two units of glucose, a monosaccharide.

metabolism • Sum of all the various biochemical and physiologic processes by which the body grows and maintains itself (anabolism) and breaks down and reshapes tissue (catabolism), transforming energy to do its work. Products of these various reactions are called *metabolites.*

metabolite • Any substance produced by metabolism or by a metabolic process.

portal • An entryway, usually referring to the portal circulation of blood through the liver. Blood is brought into the liver by the portal vein and out by the hepatic vein.

sucrase • Enzyme splitting the disaccharide sucrose into its two monosaccharides of glucose and fructose.

QUESTIONS FOR REVIEW

1. Refer to the RDA table to determine the daily caloric need of a 25-year-old woman who is 5 ft 4 in tall and weighs 125 lbs. How many kilocalories should be provided by carbohydrate in her diet? How much fiber is recommended?

2. Give a general description of the clinical effects of fiber in each of the following disease states: diverticular disease, hyperlipidemia, diabetes mellitus, and colon cancer.

3. Your client, Mr. Brown, wants desperately to lose 20 lbs before meeting his future in-laws next month. He purchased a month's worth of liquid protein and takes multivitamins daily. He seems adamant about not eating any starches or sweets. Based on your readings, how would you explain the effects of a very low-carbohydrate diet on carbohydrate functions, so that he will know why carbohydrates are important even in a weight-loss program?

REFERENCES

1. Food and Nutrition Board, National Academy of Sciences—National Research Council: *Recommended dietary allowances*, ed 10, Washington, DC, 1989, National Academy Press.

2. Food and Nutrition Board, Committee on Diet and Health, National Academy of Sciences—National Research Council: *Diet and health: implications for reducing chronic disease risk*, Washington, DC, 1989, National Academy Press.

3. Sherman WM and others: Carbohydrate feedings 1 hour before exercise improves cycling performance, *Am J Clin Nutr* 54:866, 1991.

4. Olsen WA, Lloyd ML: Carbohydrate assimilation. In Yamada T, editor: *Textbook in gastroenterology*, vol 1, New York, 1991, JB Lippincott.

5. Marlett JA: Content and composition of dietary fiber in 117 frequently consumed foods, *J Am Diet Assoc* 92(2):175, 1992.

6. Wisker E and others: Calcium, magnesium, zinc, and iron balances in young women: effects of a low-phytate barley-fiber concentrate, *Am J Clin Nutr* 54:553, 1991.

7. Kashtan H and others: Colonic fermentation and markers of colorectal cancer risk, *Am J Clin Nutr* 55:723, 1992.

8. Anderson JW and others: Metabolic effects of high-carbohydrate, high-fiber diets for insulin-dependent diabetic individuals, *Am J Clin Nutr* 54:936, 1991.

9. Dietzen CD, Pemberton JH: Diverticulitis. In Yamada T, editor: *Textbook of gastroenterology*, vol 2, New York, 1991, JB Lippincott.

FURTHER READING

Endres J: Acceptance and consumption of crystalline fructose menu items by institutionalized elderly persons, *J Am Diet Assoc* 90(3):431, 1990.

This brief report describes the use of crystalline fructose, along with other nutrient-dense foods, in the menus of elderly, diabetic persons in long-term care facilities to add energy, satisfy the taste for sweet foods, and at the same time maintain stable blood sugar levels.

Marlett JA: Content and composition of dietary fiber in 117 frequently consumed foods, *J Am Diet Assoc* 92(2):175, 1992. Slavin JL: Dietary fiber: mechanism of magic on disease prevention? *Nutr Today* 25(6):6, 1990.

These two articles provide helpful material for understanding the role of dietary fiber in relation to health problems and may be used as a resource for planning personal diets with increased dietary fiber.

The Sugar Phobia Syndrome

The Puritan ethic that "pleasure is evil" has probably done as much as has the lack of accurate nutrition information in the popular media to promote Americans' general fear of sweets in their diet. But like so many other things in our lives, sugar itself is not "bad." Rather, it is *excess* sugar and the health implications of overconsumption that is the real problem.

Actually, carbohydrate-rich foods have provided people with one of their primary sources of nutrients—and pleasure—since the beginning of time. Because of our inborn taste for sweets, the simpler the carbohydrates, the greater the pleasure they often provide. Nonetheless, as some persons protest and as any good Puritan can tell you, "If it's good tasting, it must be bad for you," because pleasure is to be avoided at all costs.

Although this premise is highly conjectural, it is becoming obvious that Americans have developed a fear of carbohydrates, especially in one of its simplest forms—sugar. This fear is greatly manifest in the American obsession with weight control and the use of sugar substitutes. Popular media usually advise dieters to eliminate excess kilocalories by avoiding starches, especially sugar. This advice is based on the belief that sugar not only contributes a large number of kilocalories to the average diet, but also is responsible for such ills as heart disease, diabetes, hypoglycemia, hyperactivity in children, and dental caries. Only in the case of dental caries is the evidence indisputable. Much of the belief in other areas is based on limited evidence and requires both clarification and qualified application.

Kilocalories

Approximately 20% of the total kilocaloric intake of the average American diet is provided by sugar, often through pies, cakes, ice cream, and other rich desserts high in fat. Because fat provides more than twice the number of kilocalories per serving as sugar, the dieter should be concerned with reducing this nutrient as well. In fact, the intelligent dieter should be concerned with reducing overall *excessive* kilocaloric intake.

Heart disease

Sucrose has been associated with elevated levels of cholesterol, low-density lipoproteins (LDLs), and plasma triglycerides, especially in carbohydrate-sensitive persons. The same association has been made with fructose, a nutritive sweetener currently being promoted as an alternate to sugar (sucrose), because it is 1.5 times sweeter and less is therefore required to achieve the desired taste level. Of course, if high sugar use replaces factors in the diet, such as fiber and other nutrients that are believed to be associated with reducing heart disease risk, it may contribute significantly to an *increased* risk for heart disease.

Diabetes mellitus

Sugar and other simple carbohydrates can contribute to elevated blood glucose levels in persons with diabetes. But contrary to popular opinion, sugar is *not* a cause of diabetes. It is only one of many variables, such as total kilocaloric intake or stress, that can raise blood sugar levels.

Hypoglycemia

Sugar intake initially brings hyperglycemia, which in turn triggers the release of insulin. The insulin output, which may exceed the need, then reduces the blood sugar level, and in some sensitive individuals these levels may become abnormally low. The popular press has often recommended a very low-carbohydrate, high-protein diet to counteract this effect, while condemning the use of sugar entirely. However, current research indicates that a diet low in simple sugars, whatever their form, and more liberal in complex carbohydrates and dietary fiber is effective in raising the blood glucose to a normal level, even in persons with diabetes.

Attention deficit hyperactivity disorder

Practitioners have observed changes in the behavior of some children consuming high-sugar diets and have noted greater activity, ease of stimulation, and other signs suggesting an association between sugar intake and an attention deficit disorder, or hyperactivity. But a number of problems have clouded the issue, including the absence of reliable methods for measuring a child's behavior; the possibility of environmental factors, such as stress, contributing to the changed behavior; and the lack of conclusive controlled studies relating sugar intake to a decreased attention span and hyperactivity.

Dental caries

Dental caries is the one health problem that has been proved to be "caused" by sugar. However, the effect of sugar has been waning because of the widespread practice of fluoridation, which together with better dental care has greatly reduced the incidence of caries.

Despite sugar's questionable contribution to major health problems, the "fear of sugar" has led the public to increase its demand for alternative sweeteners (see Chapter 21). These agents include both nonnutritive sweeteners, such as saccharin, and nutritive sweeteners, such as aspartame (made from two amino acids, phenylalanine and aspartic acid), and other sugars (for example, lactose or fructose) in smaller amounts. But our history of the use of such alternative sweeteners is rather dismal. For example, although consuming enough saccharin, and now aspartame, to replace 150 kilocalories worth of sugar every day, Americans still have failed to make a dent either in the total amount of sugar they consume—as much as 63 kg (140 lb) per person per year—or in the average body weight of the population.

The Sugar Phobia Syndrome—cont'd

There are two possible explanations for the failure of artificial sweeteners to work as sugar substitutes:

Physiologic response differences. Artificial sweeteners do not replace the desire for sugar, because they do not trigger the same physiologic responses mediated by neurotransmitters in the brain and induced by sugar to produce satiety. Although for many persons the level of natural sweetness provided by vegetables, fruits, and milk often satisfies the need for a sweet taste, the average user of nonnutritive sweeteners may find that the desire for "something sweet" is even greater than that of the average sugar user.

Increased fat intake. Often users of artificial sweeteners try to achieve satiety by increasing their intake of fats, thereby sabotaging their weight loss efforts.

To complicate matters even further, a number of studies indicate that individuals who consume average or even above average amounts of sugar tend to be thinner, not because of the sugar, but because they lead much more active lives. It has been suggested that persons use sugar as a means of satisfying short-term energy needs, because of its kilocaloric content and ease of digestion. For example, a group of South African sugar cane cutters who manually move up to 7 tons of cane every day and consume approximately 27% of their 6000 kilocalorie/day diet in the form of sugar are neither obese nor diabetic and maintain serum cholesterol levels that average 100 mg/dl *less* than those of most healthy Americans.

Even though there is growing evidence indicating that sugar may not be as "bad" as some people seem to believe, sugar eaters may benefit from a little pseudo-Puritanical advice: too much of *anything* can be harmful. The *excessive* sugar users may well consider these objective facts:

Sugar is purely a fuel supplying energy to the body. It lacks other nutrients essential for growth and health maintenance. Thus if it replaces significant amounts of other foods in the diet, the result may be malnutrition and obesity.

Sugar is cariogenic, and although fluoride and good dental care do reduce the incidence of dental caries, controlled intake of sugar is recommended as another preventive measure.

Excessive sugar can elevate blood lipid levels in susceptible persons and contribute to elevated blood glucose levels in persons with diabetes.

The use of artificial sweeteners may help prevent some of these health problems, but it is wise to temper their use in the light of current knowledge.

Artificial sweeteners cannot satisfy the need for satiety or the physiologic experience of a sweet taste. In fact, they may even increase the desire for "real" sweets.

Excessive amounts of sugar substitutes also can cause problems, such as diarrhea in the case of sorbitol. Saccharin, although approved for use by the general public, is still considered a weak carcinogen. Aspartame—approved for widespread use in soft drinks—enjoys a large consumer market, but because it is made from two amino acids—phenylalanine and aspartic acid—it cannot be used freely by those with phenylketonuria (PKU).

Summing up, consumers should become aware of the benefits of *moderate* sugar use, as well as the hazards of *excessive* amounts of sugar and its substitutes. We can then make intelligent decisions about their use.

REFERENCES

American Dietetic Association: Position paper: appropriate use of nutritive and nonnutritive sweeteners, *J Am Diet Assoc* 87:1698, 1987.

Chen LA, Parham ES: College students' use of high-intensity sweeteners is not consistently associated with sugar consumption, *J Am Diet Assoc* 90(2):686, 1991.

Pivonka EEA, Grunewald KK: Aspartame- or sugar-sweetened beverages: effects of mood in young women, *J Am Diet Assoc* 90(2):250, 1990.

Rodin J: Comparative effects of fructose, aspartame, glucose, and water preloads on calorie and macronutrient intake, *Am J Clin Nutr* 51:428, 1990.

CHAPTER 4

Fats

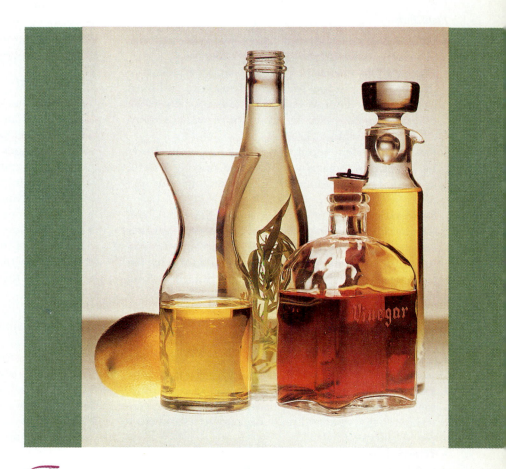

Fat—the second of our energy-yielding macronutrients—has for the most part had negative reporting for the past few years, because of its association with a number of current health problems. This is especially true with heart disease problems. But the real culprit, as with many things, is the excess *fat we eat. Fat itself is an essential nutrient.*

Traditionally fat has held a prominent place in the American diet. However, spurred by our justified health concerns, our attitudes and habits regarding fat have begun to change.

Our goal here is to help achieve some balance in our food habits and our attitudes toward fat and health. Based on the information provided about the nature of fat and its role in nutrition, we will see why we need a moderate amount of fat for energy and overall health.

Fats in Nutrition and Health

Health Needs for Fat

We need some fat in our food and in our bodies to keep us healthy. This need is indicated by the number of functions fat performs in nutrition, both in our diets and in our overall body metabolism.

Food Fats

The fat in our food provides energy, essential nutrients, and satiety, as the following list explains:

- **Fuel source for energy.** Food fats supply a basic continuing source of fuel for the body to store and burn as needed for energy. Food fat yields 9 kcal/g when oxidized in the body, in comparison with carbohydrate, which yields 4 kcal/g.
- **Essential nutrient supply.** Food fats supply the essential fatty acids, especially **linoleic acid,** and cholesterol as needed to supplement the body's endogenous supply.
- **Food satiety.** Fats in the diet supply flavor to food, which contributes to a feeling of satisfaction that lasts longer than does the feeling of satisfaction after eating carbohydrates. This satiety is enhanced by the fuller texture and body that fat contributes to food mixtures and the slower gastric emptying time it brings.

Body Fats

Fat in our body tissues serves a number of vital functions that are essential to health and life itself:

- **Energy.** A major function of fat in nutrition is to supply an efficient fuel to all tissues, although the central nervous system and brain depend on a steady supply of glucose.
- **Thermal insulation.** The layer of fat directly underneath the skin controls body temperature within the range necessary for life.
- **Vital organ protection.** A weblike padding of **adipose** fat surrounds vital organs, such as the kidneys, protecting them from mechanical shock and providing a structure to support them.
- **Nerve impulse transmission.** Fat layers surrounding nerve fibers provide electrical insulation and transmit nerve impulses.
- **Tissue membrane structure.** Fat serves as a vital constituent of the cell membrane structure, helping transport nutrient materials and metabolites across cell membranes.
- **Cell metabolism.** Combinations of fat and protein,

known as **lipoproteins,** carry fat in the blood to all cells.
- **Essential precursor substances.** Fat supplies necessary components, such as fatty acids and cholesterol, for the synthesis of many materials required for metabolic functions and tissue integrity.

Health Problems with Fat

From these lists, it is evident that fat is an essential nutrient. But if fat is as vital to human health as indicated, what is the problem about fat in the diet? As with so many things, and certainly with fat, the old maxim still holds true: you need what you need, but you don't need more than you need. Specifically, health problems with fat focus on two main issues: too much dietary fat, reflected in too much body fat, and too much of the dietary fat coming from animal food sources.

Amount of Fat

Too much fat in the diet provides excessive kilocalories, more than required for immediate energy needs. The excess is stored as excess adipose tissue, thereby increasing body weight. How much fat is in your own diet? You might try figuring it out for a day (see box, p. 51). This increased body weight—more precisely, an increased proportion of body fat making up the total body composition—has been associated with such health problems as diabetes, hypertension, and heart disease. Look for the specific relationships between increased body weight and these health problems in later chapters on these topics.

Kind of Fat

Current research has shown a clear relation between a diet containing excess saturated fat and cholesterol, which come from animal sources, to *atherosclerosis,* a blood vessel disease characterized by fatty plaques on interior vessel walls that can eventually fill the vessel and cut off blood circulation (see Chapter 20). This disease process contributes to heart attacks and strokes (see Issues and Answers, pp. 60-61).

The Physical and Chemical Nature of Lipids

Physical Characteristics

Fats include such substances as fat, oil, and related compounds that are greasy to the touch and insoluble in water. Some basic food forms of fat are easily seen as fat: butter, cream, exterior meat fat, bacon, oil, mayonnaise, and salad dressings. Other food forms of fat are more hidden: egg yolk, internal tissue fat of meats, olives, avocados, nuts, and seeds.

Chemical Nature

The chemical class name for fats and fat-related compounds is **lipids.** By chemical definition these are all organic compounds, consisting mainly of a chain of the basic element carbon as a "backbone," with attached hydrogen and oxygen atoms and other radicals. They all have in common a relation to the **fatty acids.** Thus the same basic chemical elements that make up carbohydrates—carbon, hydrogen, and oxygen—also make up the fatty acids and their related fats. But in general the two nutrients differ in two main ways: fats are more complex in structure, and their common structural units are the fatty acids. Fatty acids are also refined fuel forms that some cells, such as those constituting the heart muscle, prefer over glucose. In our discussion here, we look first at the basic structural units, the fatty acids, and their unique characteristics of saturation, essentiality, and chain length. Then we focus on the nature of the fats, known as triglycerides, that the fatty acids build.

Basic Lipids: Fatty Acids and Triglycerides

Saturation of Fatty Acids

The state of **saturation** or unsaturation gives fats their varying textural characteristics. Saturated fats are harder, less saturated ones are softer, and unsaturated ones are usually liquid oils. This differing state results from the ratio of hydrogen to carbon in the structures of the respective fatty acids that make up a particular fat. If a given fatty acid is filled with as much hydrogen as it can take, the fatty acid is said to be completely *saturated* with hydrogen. If, however, the fatty acid has less hydrogen, it is obviously less saturated. Three terms designate the varying degree of saturation:

- **Saturated.** Food fats composed of saturated fatty acids are called *saturated fats*. These fats are of animal origin.
- **Monounsaturated.** Food fats composed mainly of fatty acids, with one less hydrogen atom creating one double bond, are called *monounsaturated fats*. These fats are mostly from plant sources—for example, olive oil.
- **Polyunsaturated.** Food fats composed mainly of un-

saturated fatty acids, with two or more places unfilled with hydrogen creating double bonds, are called *polyunsaturated fats*. These fats are from plant sources. Notable exceptions are coconut oil, palm oil, and cocoa butter, which are saturated.

Essential Fatty Acids

The terms *essential* and *nonessential* are applied to nutrients according to their relative necessity in the diet. The nutrient is essential if the body cannot manufacture it and therefore must obtain it from the diet, because a failure to do so would result in a specific disease. If fat makes up only 10% or less of the diet's daily kilocalories, the body cannot obtain adequate amounts of the essential fatty acids. Three fatty acids—linoleic, linolenic, and arachidonic—are the only ones known

adipose • Fat present in cells of adipose (fatty) tissue.

fatty acid • The structural components of fats.

linoleic acid • The ultimate essential fatty acid for humans.

lipids • Chemical group name for fats and fat-related compounds such as cholesterol, lipoproteins, and phospholipids; general group name for organic substances of a fatty nature, including fats, oils, waxes, and related compounds.

organic • Carbon-based chemical compounds.

saturated • To cause to unite with the greatest possible amount of another substance through solution, chemical combination, or the like. A saturated fat, for example, is one in which the component fatty acids are filled with hydrogen atoms. A fatty acid is said to be saturated if all available chemical bonds of its carbon chain are filled with hydrogen. If one bond remains unfilled, it is a monounsaturated fatty acid. If two or more bonds remain unfilled, it is a polyunsaturated fatty acid. Fats of animal sources are more saturated. Fats of plant sources are unsaturated.

to be essential for the complete nutrition of humans. Actually only linoleic acid is a *true* **essential fatty acid (EFA),** because the other two may be naturally synthesized from it. These fatty acids—linoleic acid, along with linolenic and arachidonic acids—serve important body functions:

- **Membrane structure.** Linoleic acid strengthens cell membranes, helping prevent a harmful increase in skin and membrane permeability. A linoleic acid deficiency leads to a breakdown in skin integrity, resulting in a characteristic eczema and skin lesions. A similar effect also occurs in other tissue membranes throughout the body.
- **Cholesterol transport.** Like other fatty acids, linoleic acid combines with cholesterol to form cholesterol esters for transport in the blood.
- **Serum cholesterol.** As do other unsaturated fatty acids, linoleic acid helps lower serum cholesterol levels. It plays a key role in both the transport and metabolism of cholesterol.
- **Blood clotting.** With its closely associated metabolic products arachidonic acid and linolenic acid, linoleic acid helps prolong blood clotting time and increase fibrinolytic activity.
- **Local hormonelike effects.** Linoleic acid is a major metabolic precursor of a group of physiologically and pharmacologically active compounds known as *pros-*

taglandins, prostacyclins, thromboxanes, and *leukotrienes,* which are called **eicosanoids** because of their structure (see box below). These eicosanoid compounds have extensive local hormonelike effects.[1] They are synthesized in the body from arachidonic acid, which is derived from essential linoleic acid. The synthesis of these highly active important compounds is diagrammed in Fig. 4-1, which also shows some of their significant physiologic functions and sites.

Prostaglandins

Of these groups of *eicosanoid* compounds related to the omega-3 long-chain fatty acids, perhaps the most familiar is the group of **prostaglandins** because of their extensive functions. They were first discovered by Swedish investigators in their study of reproductive physiology, identified initially in human semen, and named prostaglandins because they were thought to originate in the prostate gland. They are now known to exist in virtually all body tissues, acting as local hormones to direct and coordinate important biologic functions. For example, they have been shown to be powerful modulators of vascular smooth muscle tone and platelet aggregation and hence have a significant relationship to cardiovascular disease.[2]

Omega-3 Fatty Acids: Health or Hype?

TO PROBE FURTHER

Often with new nutrition research findings comes a heavy dose of hype and a new diet fad. This is especially true when the research holds promise for combating heart disease and its dreaded fatty arteries, as well as other chronic health problems. Such is the case with the *omega-3* fatty acids and their rich presence in fatty fish.

But if you can get past the commercial hype and maintain perspective, you'll find some remarkable scientific data accumulating. Scientific interest was first sparked by earlier observations among Greenland Eskimos, who eat a diet rich in fish oils but have a low incidence of heart disease. These fish oils contain high levels of the class of long-chain polyunsaturated fatty acids called *omega-3* fatty acids. (Omega [ω] is the last letter in the Greek alphabet, used by scientists for naming fatty acid classes by the structure of their carbon chain, counting from the end of the chain.) There is an especially high level of one of these omega-3 fatty acids in fish oils, **eicosapentaenoic acid (EPA)** (from Greek *eicosa-,* twenty; *penta-,* five). The name designates its structure, abbreviated 20:5ω3, meaning a long-chain polyunsaturated fatty acid of 20 carbons with 5 double bonds (unsaturated points), the first double bond located at carbon 3 counting from the omega end of the carbon chain.

Accumulating evidence supports the potential nutritional and clinical relevance of these omega-3 fatty acids. The National Institutes of Health (NIH) is studying both synthesis and comparative effects of these fatty acids. The human body obtains omega-3 EPA mainly from fatty fish in the diet but can synthesize it from linolenic acid. The other two essential fatty acids, linoleic and arachidonic, are omega-6 fatty acids, closely related in their metabolic pathways and functions. In fact, the two precursor essential fatty acids, linolenic (omega-3) and linoleic (omega-6) acids, compete for the same metabolic enzyme systems in the body in producing their *eicosanoid* substances. The optimal dietary balance of omega-3 and omega-6 fatty acids and their metabolic balance effects is under study. These highly active local hormone substances have very significant physiologic effects in helping to modulate and balance cardiovascular functions, as well as in supporting normal growth and development.

REFERENCES

Anderson PA, Sprecher HW: Omega-3 fatty acids in nutrition and health, *Diet Curr* 14(2):7, 1987.
Simopoulos AP: Omega-3 fatty acids in health and disease and in growth and development, *Am J Clin Nutr* 54:438, 1991.

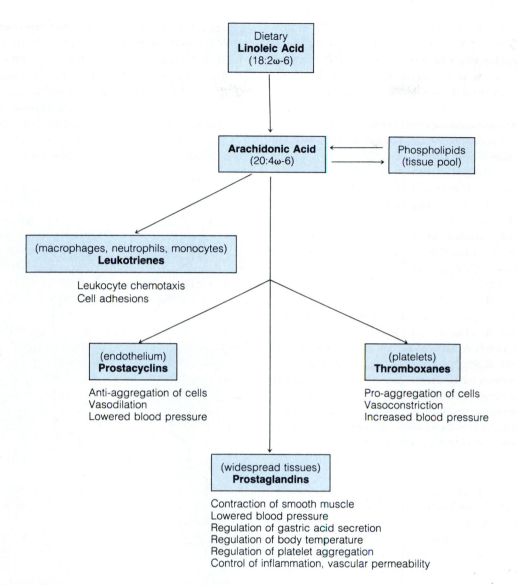

FIG. 4-1   Spectrum of food fats according to degree of saturation of component fatty acid.

Chain Length of Fatty Acids

Another characteristic of fatty acids, important in their absorption, is the length of the carbon chain composing their structure. The long-chain fatty acids are more difficult to absorb and require a helping carrier. The short- and medium-chain fatty acids are more soluble in water and hence easier to absorb directly into the blood stream. In intestinal malabsorption disease, when the absorbing mucosal surface is inflamed or infected, short- or medium-chain fat products are preferred. A commercial product called MCT (medium-chain triglycerides) is an oil made of short- and medium-chain fatty acids that can be used in the diet just as any ordinary vegetable oil.

eicosanoids • Long chain fatty acids composed of 20 carbon atoms.

essential fatty acid • A fatty acid required in the diet because the body cannot synthesize it.

prostaglandins • Group of naturally occurring substances, first discovered in semen, derived from long-chain fatty acids that have multiple local hormonelike actions, including regulation of gastric acid secretion, platelet aggregation, body temperature, and tissue inflammation.

Triglycerides

Basic structure

The chemical name for fat is **triglyceride.** The name indicates its basic chemical structure: three fatty acids attached to a **glycerol** base. Thus fats are **glycerides** composed of glycerol and fatty acids. When glycerol is combined with one fatty acid it is called a *monoglyceride,* with two fatty acids a *diglyceride,* and with three fatty acids a *triglyceride.* Whether in food or in the body, fatty acids combine with glycerol to form glycerides. Most natural fats, whether from animal or plant sources, are triglycerides. These fats, the triglycerides, occur in body cells as oily droplets. They circulate in water-based blood serum encased in a covering of water-soluble protein. These fat-protein complexes are called *lipoproteins.* They serve multiple functions throughout the body.

Nature of Food Fats

Food fats, as well as body fats, are composed of saturated and unsaturated fatty acids. If the food fat is made up mainly of saturated fatty acids, it is called a saturated fat. Foods from animal sources—such as meat, milk, and eggs—contain saturated fats. Conversely, food from plant sources, such as the vegetable oils, are unsaturated fats. A general saturated-unsaturated spectrum of food fats is shown in Fig. 4-2. The animal food fats on the saturated end of the spectrum are solid; those toward the center become somewhat less saturated and are softer. The plant fats on the unsaturated end are free-flowing oils that do not solidify even at low temperatures. Exceptions are coconut oil, palm oil, and cocoa butter, which are saturated fats. These saturated plant fats are used extensively in commercial products, because they are usually cheaper oils. Therefore it is important to read product labels carefully. The new food labels on processed foods indicate these distinctions in fat composition. This distinction in saturation, as shown in Fig. 4-2, is helpful in explaining to persons on modified fat diets the correct choices of food fats.

Cis and Trans Unsaturated Fatty Acid Products

The unsaturated oils can be hardened commercially into such products as margarine and shortening by in-jection of hydrogen gas to saturate them, a process called **hydrogenation.** Recently, health professionals have been concerned about the increasing number of hydrogenated food products being made from the *cis* and *trans* forms of unsaturated fatty acids. First, compare this difference in the structure of the commonly occurring monounsaturated fatty acid, oleic acid, with its one unsaturated double bond occurring in the middle of its chain of 18 carbon atoms.

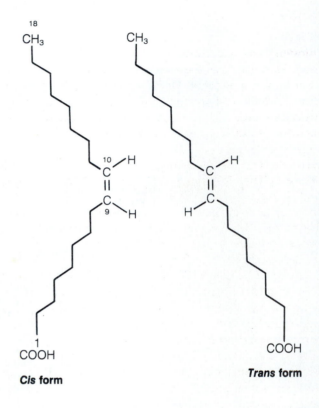

Cis form   **Trans form**

When double bonds occur naturally in food fats, the fatty acid chains usually bend at those points so that the remaining parts of the structure are on the same side of the bond. In this case the form is called *cis* (same side). All fatty acids in naturally occurring fats are in the *cis* form. However, when vegetable oils are partially hydrogenated to make food products, the normal bend is changed so that the remaining parts are on opposite

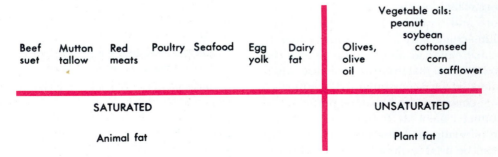

Beef suet	Mutton tallow	Red meats	Poultry	Seafood	Egg yolk	Dairy fat	Olives, olive oil	Vegetable oils: peanut soybean cottonseed corn safflower
		SATURATED						UNSATURATED
		Animal fat						Plant fat

FIG. 4-2 Synthesis, sites, and functions of eicosanoids.

sides of the bond. In this case the form is called *trans* (opposite side). Commercially hydrogenated fats in margarine and many other products are in the *trans* form. With the increasing use of these products, especially margarine, there is some debate about possible effects of the accumulating *trans* form in the body.[3,4] Some of these observed effects include elevation of serum lipid levels, inhibition of essential fatty acid metabolism, and modification of membrane properties.

Visible and Hidden Food Fat

As indicated, food fats are sometimes called "visible" or "hidden" fats according to how obvious they are in food. In most cases the food fat is quite evident, such as in butter, margarine, oil, salad dressing, bacon, and cream, which account for about 40% of the fat in the American diet. However, less obvious hidden fats in such foods as meat, milk (unless it is a nonfat form), eggs (only in the yolk; the white is pure protein), nuts, seeds, olives, and avocados contribute more to our fat intake. A large part of this fat comes from our relatively high consumption of meats. Even when all the fat is trimmed off a cut of meat, its lean portion still contains 4% to 12% hidden fat. Higher grades of meat, both prime and choice, have considerable "marbling"—tiny fat deposits within the muscle tissue. This is especially true of beef, a major meat on the American market. Thus the meat and milk food groups together contribute about half the fat in the American diet. Thus, considering all sources, about 45% of the total kilocalories come from fat—an excessive amount.

Yet even with increasing health concerns about their fat intake, Americans still seem ambivalent. They cut down in some areas, but at the same time purchase larger amounts of red meats with considerable non-separable fat, such as ground beef and hamburgers. This conflicting pattern of meat fat consumption, termed "meat fat madness" by one research team, suggests that such contradictory choices are made by an ill-informed public.[5] But the meat industry, challenged by health-conscious consumers, has been developing leaner breeds through genetic engineering, the so-called Lite or Ultra label for meat containing 25% less fat, and promoting leaner cuts in smaller portions for low-fat cooking.[6] In addition, fast-food restaurants have begun to develop leaner menu items.[7]

Special Fat-Related Compound: Cholesterol
Structure

Although **cholesterol** is often discussed in connection with dietary fat, it is not a fat (triglyceride) itself. Many people confuse cholesterol with saturated fat. It is a fat-related compound that is quite different from triglycerides in structure. Generally, cholesterol travels in the bloodstream attached to long-chain fatty acids, forming cholesterol **esters.**

Functions

Cholesterol is a vital substance in human metabolism. It belongs to a family of substances called **steroids,** or sterols, and is a precursor to all steroid hormones. A cholesterol compound in the skin, *7-dehydrocholesterol,* is irradiated by sunlight's ultraviolet rays and activated in the body to produce vitamin D hormone. It is also essential in the formation of bile acids, which emulsify fats for enzymatic digestion and then serve as a carrier for fat absorption. Cholesterol is widely distributed in all cells of the body and is found in large amounts in brain and nerve tissue. It is an essential component of cell membranes. It is small wonder therefore that a constant supply of so vital a material for body processes would be made in body tissues, mainly in the liver. If a person consumed *no* cholesterol at all, the body would still synthesize a needed supply.

---

cholesterol • A fat-related compound, a sterol ($C_{27}H_{45}OH$). It is a normal constituent of bile and a principal constituent of gallstones. In body metabolism cholesterol is important as a precursor of various steroid hormones, such as sex hormones and adrenal corticoids. Cholesterol is synthesized by the liver. It is widely distributed in nature, especially in animal tissue such as glandular meats and egg yolk.

ester • A compound produced by the reaction between an acid and an alcohol with elimination of a molecule of water. This process is called esterification. For example, a triglyceride is a glycerol ester. Cholesterol esters are formed in the mucosal cells by combination with fatty acids, largely linoleic acid.

glyceride • Group name for fats; any of a group of esters obtained from glycerol by the replacement of one, two, or three hydroxyl (OH) groups with a fatty acid. Monoglycerides contain one fatty acid; diglycerides contain two fatty acids; triglycerides contain three fatty acids. Glycerides are the principal constituent of adipose tissue and are found in animal and vegetable fats and oils.

glycerol • A colorless, odorless, syrupy, sweet liquid; a constituent of fats usually obtained by the hydrolysis of fats. Chemically glycerol is an alcohol; it is esterified with fatty acids to produce fats.

hydrogenation • Process of hardening liquid vegetable oils by injecting hydrogen gas to produce margarines and shortenings.

steroids • Group name for lipid-based sterols, including hormones, bile acids, and cholesterol.

triglyceride • Chemical name for fat, indicating structure; attachment of three fatty acids to a glycerol base. A neutral fat, synthesized from carbohydrate and stored in adipose tissue, it releases free fatty acids into the blood when hydrolyzed by enzymes.

Food Sources

Cholesterol occurs naturally in all animal foods. There is none in plant foods. Its main food sources are egg yolks and organ meats, such as liver and kidneys. In fact, cholesterol occurs *only* in animal fats and tissues, *not* in plant fats or tissues. Therefore vegetable oils do not contain cholesterol. Plant oils may vary in degree of saturation, but *none* of them contain cholesterol.

Health Concerns

Cholesterol has been increasingly implicated in vascular disease as a large risk factor in the development of *atherosclerosis,* the underlying pathology in coronary heart disease, in which cholesterol-containing fatty plaques build up on blood vessel walls. If this plaque forms a blood clot and narrows the major arteries serving the heart muscle, a heart attack is triggered. If this process initiates a clot that finally lodges in an artery in the brain, it causes a stroke. Current research has confirmed the association of this process with elevated serum cholesterol levels (see Chapter 20). Thus government health officials and health professionals have recommended that Americans reduce their dietary cholesterol to no more than 300 mg/day, from a high of about twice that amount.[8-10] The various U.S. dietary guidelines (see Chapter 1) likewise recommend that Americans reduce their dietary cholesterol intake to about 300 mg/day, along with maintaining an appropriate level of physical exercise and body weight.[11] An increase in soluble types of dietary fiber—described in the previous chapter—is also recommended, because these fibers bind bile acids and dietary cholesterol, which helps in eliminating excess cholesterol from the body.

Special Compound Lipids: Lipoproteins

Function

The lipoproteins are important combinations of fat with protein and other fat-related components that are highly significant in human nutrition. Chemically they are not true compound lipids but are *complexes* (noncovalent structures) of lipids and covering protein, which—together with **apoproteins**—serve as the major vehicle for fat transport in the bloodstream (see Chapter 20).

Fat Transport

Fat is insoluble in water. This simple characteristic poses a problem in carrying fat to cells in a water-based circulatory system. The body has solved this problem through the development of the **lipoproteins,** packages of fat wrapped in water-soluble protein. These plasma lipoproteins contain fatty acids, triglycerides, cholesterol, **phospholipids,** and traces of other materials, such as fat-soluble vitamins and steroid hormones. The high or low density of the lipoprotein is determined by its relative loads of fat and protein. The higher the protein ratio, the higher the density.

Thus the lipoproteins are classified according to density and by relative fat and cholesterol loads as follows:

1. **Chylomicrons.** These are formed in the intestinal wall after a meal and carry the large fat load from the meal just consumed to liver cells for initial conversion to other transport lipoproteins.
2. **Very low-density lipoproteins (VLDLs).** These are formed in the chylomicrons in the continuing process of lipid transport and metabolism and deliver endogenous triglycerides to tissue cells.
3. **Intermediate low-density lipoproteins (ILDLs).** These are formed from VLDLs and continue the delivery of endogenous triglycerides to tissue cells.
4. **Low-density lipoproteins (LDLs).** These are formed from VLDLs and ILDLs and carry cholesterol to the peripheral tissue cells.
5. **High-density lipoproteins (HDLs).** These are formed in cell metabolism and carry cholesterol from the cells to the liver for breakdown and elimination from the body.

The lipoproteins are closely associated with lipid disorders and vascular disease, so look for details of their structures and functions in Chapter 20.

Digestion-Absorption-Metabolism Summary

Digestion

The basic fat fuel—various animal and plant fats (triglycerides) that naturally occur in foods—is taken into the body with the diet. Then the task is to change these basic fuel fats into a refined fuel form of fat that the cells can burn for energy. This key refined fuel is the individual *fatty acid*. The body accomplishes this task through the process of fat digestion.

Mouth

No major chemical fat breakdown takes place in the mouth. In this first portion of the gastrointestinal tract, the main action is mechanical as fat is broken up into smaller particles through chewing and moistened for passage into the stomach with the general food mass.

Stomach

Little if any chemical fat digestion takes place in the stomach. General peristalsis continues the mechanical mixing of fats with the stomach contents. No significant amount of enzymes specific for fats is present in the gastric secretions except a gastric **lipase** (tributyrinase), which acts on emulsified butterfat. As the main gastric enzymes act on other specific nutrients in the food mix, fat is separated from them and made readily accessible to its own specific chemical breakdown in the small intestine.

TABLE 4-1		
Summary of Fat Digestion		
Organ	**Enzyme**	**Activity**
Mouth	None	Mechanical, mastication
Stomach	No major enzyme	Mechanical separation of fats as protein and starch digested out
	Small amount of gastric lipase tributyrinase	Tributyrin (butterfat) to fatty acids and glycerol
Small intestine	Gallbladder bile salts (emulsifier)	Emulsifies fats
	Pancreatic lipase (steapsin)	Triglycerides to diglycerides and monoglycerides in turn, then fatty acids and glycerol

Small Intestine

Not until fat reaches the small intestine do the chemical changes necessary for fat digestion occur. Digestive agents from three major sources are present: the biliary tract—consisting of the liver and gallbladder—which contributes a preparation agent, and the pancreas and small intestine itself, which both release specific enzymes.

1. **Bile from the liver and gallbladder.** The presence of fats in the duodenum stimulates the secretion of cholecystokinin, a local hormone from glands in the intestinal walls. In turn, cholecystokinin causes contraction of the gallbladder, relaxation of the sphincter muscle, and subsequent secretion of **bile** into the intestine via the common bile duct. The liver produces a large amount of dilute bile, then the gallbladder concentrates and stores it, ready for use with fat as needed. Its function is that of an **emulsifier.** The process of *emulsification* is not a chemical digestive action itself, but it is an important first preparation step for the chemical digestion of fat through its specific enzymes. This preparation process accomplishes two important tasks: (1) it breaks the fat into small particles, or globules, which greatly enlarges the total surface area available for action of the enzyme, and (2) it lowers the surface tension of the finely dispersed and suspended fat globules, which allows the enzymes to penetrate more easily. This process is similar to the wetting action of detergents. The bile also provides an alkaline medium for the action of the fat enzyme lipase.

2. **Enzymes from the pancreas.** Pancreatic juice contains an enzyme for fat and one for cholesterol. First, *pancreatic lipase,* a powerful fat enzyme, breaks off one fatty acid at a time from the glycerol base of fats. One fatty acid plus a diglyceride, then another fatty acid plus a monoglyceride, are produced in turn. Each successive step of this breakdown occurs with increasing difficulty. In fact, separation of the final fatty acid from the remaining monoglyceride is such a slow process that less than one third of the total fat present actually breaks down completely. The final products of fat digestion to be absorbed are fatty acids, diglycerides, monoglycerides, and

glycerol. Some remaining fat may pass into the large intestine for fecal elimination. Second, the enzyme *cholesterol enterase* acts on free cholesterol to form cholesterol esters by combining free cholesterol and fatty acids in preparation for absorption.

3. **Enzyme from the small intestine.** The small intestine secretes an enzyme in the intestinal juice called *leci*

---

apoprotein • A separate protein compound that attaches to its specific receptor site on a particular lipoprotein and activates certain functions, such as synthesis of a related enzyme. An example is apoprotein C II, an apoprotein of HDL and VLDL that functions to activate the enzyme lipoprotein lipase.

bile • A fluid secreted by the liver and transported to the gallbladder for concentration and storage. It is released into the duodenum upon entry of fat to facilitate enzymatic fat digestion by acting as an emulsifying agent.

cholecystokinin (CCK) • A peptide hormone secreted by the duodenal mucosa in the presence of fat. The cholecystokinin causes the gallbladder to contract. This contraction propels bile into the duodenum, where it is needed to emulsify the fat. The fat is thus prepared for digestion and absorption.

emulsifier • An agent that breaks down large fat globules to smaller, uniformly distributed particles. This action is accomplished in the intestine chiefly by the bile acids, which lower surface tension of the fat particles. Emulsification greatly increases the surface area of fat, facilitating contact with fat-digesting enzymes.

lipase • Group of fat enzymes that cut the ester linkages between the fatty acids and glycerol of triglycerides (fats).

lipoprotein • Noncovalent complexes of fat with protein. The lipoproteins function as major carriers of lipids in the plasma, since most of the plasma fat is associated with them. Such a combination makes possible the transport of fatty substances in a water medium such as plasma.

phospholipid • Any of a class of fat-related substances that contain phosphorus, fatty acids, and a nitrogenous base. The phospholipids are essential elements in every cell.

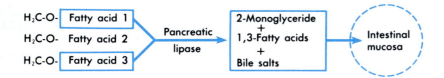

FIG. 4-3 Micellar complex of fats with bile salts for transport of fats into intestinal mucosa.

thinase. As its name indicates, it acts on lecithin, a *phospholipid,* to break it down into its components for absorption.

A summary of fat digestion in the successive parts of the gastrointestinal tract is given in Table 4-1.

Absorption

The task of fat absorption is not easy. The problem is that fats are not soluble in water and blood is basically water. Hence fat always requires some type of solvent carrier. To accomplish this task of transporting fat from the small intestine into the bloodstream, the body has three basic stages of operation.

Stage I: Initial fat absorption. In the small intestine, bile combines with products of fat digestion in a **micellar bile-fat complex.** This unique carrier system, shown in Fig. 4-3, takes fat digestion products along its initial passage into the intestinal wall.

Stage II: Absorption within the intestinal wall. Once inside the wall of the small intestine, the bile separates from the fat complex and returns in the *enterohepatic circulation* to accomplish its task over and over again. Two important actions on the fat digestion products occur inside the intestinal wall: (1) *enteric lipase action:* an enteric lipase within the cells of the intestinal wall completes the digestion of the remaining glycerides, and (2) *triglyceride synthesis:* with the resulting fatty acids and glycerol, new human triglycerides are formed as body fats, ready now for final absorption and circulation.

Stage III: Final fat absorption and transport. These newly formed human fats—triglycerides—and other fat materials present are combined with a small amount of protein covering to form lipoproteins called **chylomicrons.** These packages of fat, in a milk-like liquid called *chyle,* cross the cell membrane intact into the lymphatic system and then into the portal blood. Here a final fat-clearing enzyme, *lipoprotein lipase,* helps clear the large meal load of dietary fat from circulation. In the liver the fat is converted to other lipoproteins for transport to the body cells for energy and other structural functions.

Fig. 4-4 illustrates the general process of lipid absorption through its three stages.

Metabolism

In the body cells, fatty acids are "burned" as concentrated fuel to produce energy. These derived units of

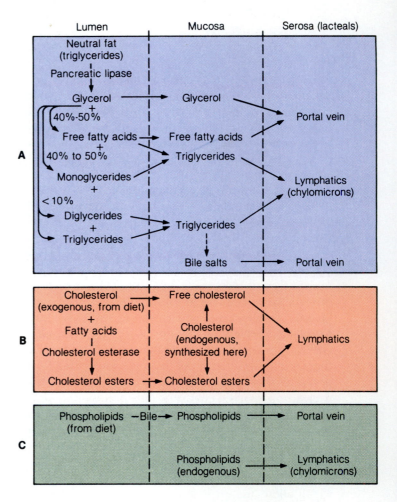

FIG. 4-4 Absorption of fat, cholesterol, and phospholipids.

fat have about twice the energy value of glucose products. As seen in the broad picture of metabolism discussed in Chapter 2, cell metabolism of fat is closely interrelated with that of the other nutrients.

To Sum Up

Fat is an essential nutrient that, in addition to supplying the highest density of energy among the energy nutrients, insulates the body against low temperatures and protects vital organs from damage. It also aids in the transmission of nerve impulses, production of metabolic precursors, formation of cell membrane structure, and transport of other molecules, such as protein.

Fats are composed of glycerol and attached fatty acids of varying lengths and degreees of saturation. Essential fatty acids are long-chain unsaturated fatty acids that cannot be manufactured by the body. The major one is linoleic acid. Its functions include improving skin integrity, lowering serum cholesterol levels, prolonging blood clotting time, and developing a group of special substances called *ecosanoids*—including *prostaglandins*—that are involved in many tissue activities, such as the maintenance of the smooth muscle tone of blood vessels and platelet aggregations.

The type and amount of dietary fat can affect health. Large amounts of saturated fat and cholesterol increase the risk for cardiovascular disease and other general health problems. Too small an amount of fat can result in a deficiency of the essential fatty acid, linoleic acid. Americans get about 40% to 45% of their total kilocalories from fat; the U.S. Dietary Guidelines recommends about 30%. When fat provides 10% or less of total kilocalories, deficiency symptoms occur.

QUESTIONS FOR REVIEW

1. Two persons with strong family histories of cardiovascular disease are concerned about preventing heart problems. Both reduce their cholesterol intake and avoid butter. The first person replaces butter with stick margarine made from corn oil, the second with corn oil itself. Which person might have more success with avoiding heart disease? Identify and describe two characteristics of a dietary lipid component that may affect this rate of success.
2. A woman runner concerned about her health dropped her total fat intake to an amount supplying about 10% of her total kilocaloric intake. What health problems would you expect her to encounter?

REFERENCES

1. Simopoulos AP: Omega-3 fatty acids in health and disease and in growth and development, *Am J Clin Nutr* 54:438, 1991.
2. Knapp HR and others: In vivo indexes of platelet and vascular function during fish-oil administration in patients with arteriosclerosis, *N Engl J Med* 314:937, 1986.
3. Mensink RP, Katan MB: Effect of *trans* fatty acids on high-density and low-density lipoprotein cholesterol levels in healthy subjects, *N Engl J Med* 323:439, 1990.
4. Kris-Etherton PM: The effects of *trans*-fatty acids on high-density and low-density lipoprotein cholesterol levels, *Nutr Today* 25(5):6, 1990.
5. Ratje WL, Ho EE: Meat fat madness: conflicting patterns of meat fat consumption and their public health implications, *J Am Diet Assoc* 87(10):1357, 1987.
6. Report: Genetic engineering produces low-fat Ultra Beef, *Food Engineering* 59:48, 1987.
7. Shields JE, Young E: Fat in fast foods—evolving changes, *Nutr Today* 25(2):32, 1990.
8. US Department of Health and Human Services, Public Health Service: *Healthy people 2000: national health promotion and disease prevention objectives*, Pub No 91-50212, Washington, DC, 1990, US Government Printing Office.
9. Food and Nutrition Board, Committee on Diet and Health, National Academy of Sciences-National Research Council: *Diet and health: implications for reducing chronic disease risk*, Washington, DC, 1989, National Academy Press.
10. O'Keefe CE and others: Physician perspectives on cholesterol and heart disease, *J Am Diet Assoc* 91(2):189, 1991.
11. Wood PD and others: The effects on lipoproteins of a prudent weight-reducing diet, with or without exercise, in overweight men and women, *N Engl J Med* 325(7):461, 1991.

FURTHER READING

Key JO, Rocchini AP: A family focus program to lower blood cholesterol, *J Am Diet Assoc* 91(9):1113, 1991.

This article describes ways to help people change food behavior relating to dietary cholesterol within the family with practical knowledge and family support, especially in families with a high risk for heart disease.

Shields JE, Young E: Fat in fast foods—evolving changes, *Nutr Today* 25(2):32, 1990.

Because fast food is such a regular part of American food habits and traditionally has centered around high-fat foods, these authors have provided needed information on changes the industry is trying to make to reduce the fat in their food items.

Skinner JD: Changes in students' dietary behavior during a college nutrition course, *J Nutr Educ* 23(2):72, 1991.

This author describes ways in which college students in an introductory nutrition course made positive changes in their food habits, especially in reducing their fat intake.

chylomicrons • Initial lipoproteins, carrying a large fat load, formed in the intestinal wall after a meal for absorption of the food fats into circulation.

micellar bile-fat complex • A combination of bile and fat in which the bile emulsifies fat into very minute globules or particles that can be absorbed easily into the small intestine wall in preparation for the final stage of absorption into circulation to the cells.

The Dietary Fat and Cholesterol Controversy

Over the past two decades, despite overwhelming evidence linking fat and cholesterol to heart disease, questions about the nature and extent of this relationship still seem to arise. What have we learned? Has learning led to actions? What issues remain? How are they being resolved?

Background

Controversy first arose when individual studies led to the first official concern about Americans' habit of consuming rich foods. Justly alarmed by the increasing extent of major disease in the population, a Senate Committee on Nutrition and Health issued a plan for attacking the leading cause of death—coronary heart disease. Its approach was direct and apparently simple: it would advise millions of Americans to reduce their dietary intake of fats, saturated fats, and cholesterol. These early recommendations were based on research showing that people who eat large amounts of fat, as Americans do, tend to develop heart disease more often than people who follow leaner diets. This sounds reasonable. But it is not as simple as it sounds. Americans seem to love their fat, and a great many food industries with vested interests would like to whet these appetites.

We soon learned that getting Americans to reduce their fat intake was not easy then, nor is it any easier now, for several reasons:

1. *Taste and texture.* Fats make food more tasteful and give a pleasing texture. This is a taste cultivated over the past few years by our marketplace and is probably why some 40% to 45% of the kilocalories of the American diet were then made up of fats.
2. *Prevalence in the diet.* Meat, milk, eggs, and cheese provide about half of the fat Americans consume. Because these products are so prevalent in the diet, the task of reducing animal fat components—such as saturated fats and cholesterol—is *very* challenging, to say the least.

   Further, the task of making *any* dietary recommendations for Americans is always complicated by the nature of our society.
3. *Heterogenous population.* The U.S. population is such a heterogenous group—with wide variety of food preferences dictated by culture, religion, food availability, and personal likes and dislikes—that change is extremely difficult.
4. *Population size.* The U.S. population is so large—with persons who require a wide range of dietary fat, depending on individual health and energy needs—that making any standard to cover personal requirements is also difficult.

Obviously any recommendation that attempts to be specific about amounts of nutrients or types of food to eat would be difficult to make. Yet specifics were apparent in these initial guidelines:

- *Total fat.* Reduce total fat consumption to 30% of energy intake.
- *Saturated fat.* Reduce saturated fat consumption to about 10% of the total energy intake. Balance that with polyunsaturated and monounsaturated fats, which should account for about 10% of the energy intake.
- *Cholesterol.* Reduce cholesterol consumption to about 10% of the energy intake.

These initial guidelines also recommended that Americans cut their meat consumption to meet these recommendations. Obviously, this conflicted with the interests of meat-producing and meat-marketing industries.

During the following years, health officials and professional groups began to recognize that dietary guidelines must provide for a three-way balance among the following:

- The individual's *need* for fat
- The effects of *excess* dietary fat
- The public's *need* for education and guidance in preventive health

Apparently, these suggestions were taken to heart. Through two revisions our current national dietary guidelines have emerged, in essence advising Americans to eat a variety of foods, maintain an appropriate weight, and limit intake of total fat, saturated fat, and cholesterol. These early recommendations strengthened our preventive care approach to health maintenance and vascular disease. These goals are now embodied not only in the current dietary guidelines, but also in official reports, such as the National Research Council's *Diet and Health: Implications for Reducing Chronic Disease Risk* and the U.S. Department of Health and Human Services's specific directions in *Healthy People 2000: National Health Promotion and Disease Prevention Objectives.* A part of this pattern was the establishment of the National Cholesterol Education Program by the Heart, Lung, and Blood Institute of the National Institutes of Health, based on the strong findings of the large Lipid Clinics Coronary Primary Prevention Trials. A panel of experts brought together by the Institute, working with more than 20 health agencies, outlined for physicians important steps of cholesterol monitoring and diet as the primary attack on heart disease. In addition, the Bogalusa Heart Study, a longitudinal study now in its sixteenth year of monitoring the health and life-style of children growing into adulthood in this Louisiana town, continues to reinforce the fact that the artery changes underlying heart disease begin early in life in genetically predisposed individuals and are enhanced by elevated serum cholesterol levels. This investigator and other cardiologists indicate that preventive cardiology should start early in life, especially with children at high risk, instilling principles of a "prudent" diet to control for excess fat, cholesterol, and energy intake, along with the value of exercise and an active life-style.

The Dietary Fat and Cholesterol Controversy—cont'd

Current issues

The current debate focuses on three basic questions:

1. Why do the large number of studies that show a definite decline in heart disease with lowering cholesterol fail to show a similar reduction in deaths from heart disease?
2. How should we deal with children's diets in the light of the demonstrated diet-cholesterol link?
3. And what do we do about drug alternatives in this age of scarce health care dollars?

The question of heart disease mortality

Multifactorial disease. The question about results of the cholesterol campaign in terms of fewer deaths from heart disease appears to be part of the reality that heart disease is multifactorial, with numerous factors other than just cholesterol contributing to its development. These well-known factors include life-style behaviors, such as lack of exercise, smoking, the consumption of excessive high-kilocaloric food, and obesity; predisposing disease factors, such as hypertension and diabetes; and the important genetic factor. There is a difficulty in untangling these many intertwined factors. It also shows how difficult it is in a free-living population to know precisely what people eat and the limitations of the dietary history method. One large, ongoing study of coronary artery disease risk development in young adults reports that early data show a general difference between the recommended intakes of total fat, saturated fat, and cholesterol and the actual dietary intakes of young adults, regardless of age and educational level. It seems that we still have a long way to go toward improving our food habits.

Data analysis. Another possible answer and resolution of the mortality issue may lie in the method used to analyze the large amount of data collected. For the most part, each of the many experimental and clinical studies have been analyzed separately. Now an Oxford University statistician indicates that the new technique of meta-analysis, or overview of all the accumulative data, would vastly add to the power of the analysis.

The question of children and cholesterol

An important question concerns what to do about screening and proposing dietary intervention for children. Long-standing studies show that fatty streaks of the arterial disease process begin in childhood, as indicated by autopsies of young Americans killed in the Korean War, who showed a high frequency of advanced lesions. Also, an ongoing study that tracks children through adulthood has indicated a correlation between a childhood elevated blood cholesterol level and continued serum elevation in adulthood. But other investigators believe that childhood screening, family conflicts, the potential labeling, and as well as the cost of universal screening, exceed its benefits. Officially, the National Cholesterol Education Program has endorsed a specific cholesterol monitoring program limited to children over 2 years of age whose genetic predisposition is evidenced by parents who have premature coronary heart disease. Most families and practitioners express approval of this approach. A good plan with children's diets, expressed by one wise nutritionist, may well be one that gradually reduces fat intake while maintaining a normal eating environment and avoiding strained relationships involving food. One of the easiest ways of focusing on the positive aspects of such a diet is to increase the child's intake of fruits, vegetables, and low-fat whole-grain products—such as cereals and breads—in snacks and at meals, as well as to moderate the amounts of low-fat meats and nonfat milk.

The question of drug alternatives

A final question involves the alternative therapy if diet therapy fails—the use of drugs. Several drugs have proved useful in clinical studies for their cholesterol-lowering effect. But the magnitude of the cost involved for a significant number of our population would be enormous. Estimates for such drug therapy have ranged from $329 to $1744 per patient per year, depending on the drug chosen and its dose. These figures are based on wholesale drug costs. It is clear that future recommendations for these drugs must include a careful assessment of their cost-effectiveness.

As you can see, there are no easy answers. But there are real proposals that are bringing some solutions. In the meantime, perhaps more of us can examine our own lifestyles and turn our basic food habits in the lower fat direction.

REFERENCES

Dalen JE: Detection and treatment of elevated blood cholesterol: what have we learned? *Arch Intern Med* 151:25, 1991.

Palca J: Getting to the heart of the cholesterol debate, *Science* 247:1170, 1990.

Schucker B and others: Change in cholesterol awareness and action: results from the National Physician and Public Surveys, *Arch Intern Med* 151:666, 1991.

Van Horn LV and others: Diet, body size, and plasma lipids-lipoproteins in young adults: differences by race and sex, *Am J Epidemiol* 133(1):9, 1991.

Webber LS and others: Tracking of serum lipids and lipoproteins from childhood to adulthood: the Bogalusa Heart Study, *Am J Epidemiol* 133(9):884, 1991.

Wilson DKW, Lewis NM: Weight-for-height measurements and saturated fatty acid intake are predictors of serum cholesterol level in children, *J Am Diet Assoc* 92(2):192, 1992.

CHAPTER 5

Proteins

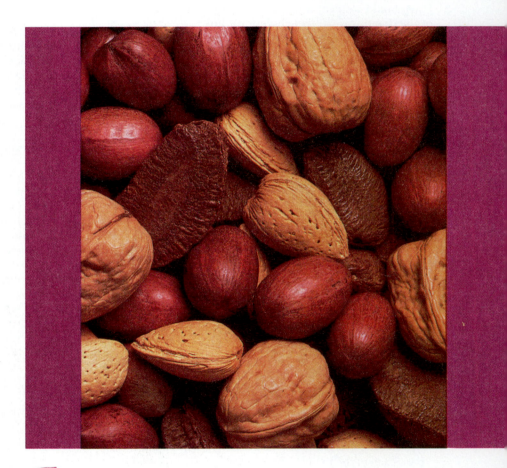

In this chapter, which completes our introductory sequence on the macronutrients, we look at protein. It is quite different from its partners, carbohydrates and fats. Although protein also yields energy as needed, its main job is building and rebuilding body tissue. It is the body's major provider of nitrogen, the essential element for all living beings.

Here, then, we focus primarily on the body's builder. We see how protein accomplishes this unique task through its marvelous building units, the amino acids.

Physical and Chemical Nature of Proteins

General Definition

When Dutch chemist Johann Mulder (1802-1880) first classified protein in 1838 as a prime substance of all life forms, he could scarcely guess how far-reaching his work would become. From Mulder's early grasp of what he was seeing, protein has become recognized as the essential life-substance of all living matter.[1] Today we know as fact his early insight.

In many ways, proteins act to shape our lives. They act as structural units to build our bodies. As enzymes, they change our food into nutrients our cells can use. As antibodies, they shield us from disease. As peptide hormones, they send messages that coordinate continuous body activity, and much more. They guide our growth during childhood and then maintain our bodies throughout adulthood. They ensure our nutritional well-being. They make us the unique individuals that we are.

Chemical Nature

The proteins we eat do none of this wonderful work as proteins. Their specific structural chemical units—*amino acids* released at initial digestion—provide the living, working currency of our body cells. These unique units are composed of the basic elements carbon, hydrogen, and oxygen and the special element of all living matter—nitrogen. So it is with these basic units of life-substance that we begin this chapter.

The Nature of Amino Acids

The story of protein must begin with its unique building materials, the amino acids. A major life-sustaining task of the human body is the constant building and rebuilding of all its body tissues. The name of these building units, the amino acids, indicates that they have a dual nature. The word *amino* refers to base (alkaline) substance, so we at once confront a paradox. How can a chemical material be both a base and an acid at the same time, and why is this important here? Consider the significance of this fact as you first examine the structure of amino acids.

General Pattern and Specific Structure

A general fundamental pattern holds for all amino acids. It is the unique side group radical (R) attached to the common baseline pattern that makes each of the amino acids that constitute protein different. Amino acids are made of the same three elements—carbon, hydrogen, and oxygen—that make up carbohydrates and fats. But amino acids and their proteins have an additional important element—*nitrogen*—as the base (alkaline—NH_2) portion of their structure. There are some 22 amino acids, all of which are important in the body's metabolism. They all have the same basic core pattern, but each is unique because it has a specific different side group attached.

This dual chemical structure of amino acids, combining both acid (**carboxyl** group—COOH) and base (amino) factors, gives them a unique **amphoteric** nature. As a result, an amino acid in solution can behave either as an acid or a base, depending on the pH of the solution. This means that amino acids have a **buffer** capacity, which is an important clinical characteristic.

Essential Amino Acids

Nine of the amino acids are vital in our diets and have been termed **essential amino acids.** Note these nine amino acids carefully in Table 5-1 (p. 64). They are significant in our diets, because they are the only ones that we cannot make. Over the years of human development, we have apparently lost the ability to synthesize these nine amino acids, so we must get them in our foods. Thus the label "essential" means that they are *dietary* essentials. The remaining amino acids—some 13 of them, which we can synthesize in our own bodies—are then labeled "nonessential" amino acids. Actually, this is a poor choice of label in the sense that all 22 of the amino acids are necessary for building the various body tissue proteins. However, the concept of *dietary* essentiality for these so-designated nine amino acids is important to remember in assessing food protein quality and protein-controlled diets, such as vegetarian food patterns.

---

amino acid • An acid containing the essential element nitrogen (in the chemical group $-NH_2$). Amino acids are the structural units of protein and are the basic building blocks of the body.

amphoteric • Having opposite characteristics; capable of acting either as an acid or a base, combining with both acids and bases.

buffer • Mixture of acidic and alkaline components that, when added to a solution, is able to protect the solution against wide variations in its pH, even when strong acids and bases are added to it. If an acid is added, the alkaline partner reacts to counteract the acidic effect. If a base is added, the acid partner reacts to counteract the alkalizing effect. A solution to which a buffer has been added is called a buffered solution.

carboxyl (COOH) • The monovalent radical, -COOH, occurring in those organic acids termed carboxylic acids.

essential amino acid • Any one of nine amino acids that the body cannot synthesize at all or in sufficient amounts to meet body needs, so it must be supplied by the diet and is hence a *dietary* essential. These nine specific amino acids are histidine, isoleucine, leucine, lysine, methionine, phenylalanine, threonine, tryptophan, and valine.

TABLE 5-1

Amino Acids Required in Human Nutrition, Grouped According to Nutritional (Dietary) Essentiality

Essential amino acids	Semiessential amino acid*	Nonessential amino acids
Histidine	Arginine	Alanine
Isoleucine		Aspargine
Leucine		Aspartic acid
Lysine		Cystine (cysteine)
Methionine		Glutamic acid
Phyenylalanine		Glutamine
Threonine		Glycine
Tryptophan		Hydroxylysine
Valine		Hydroxyproline
		Proline
		Serine
		Tyrosine

*Considered semiessential because the rate of synthesis in the body is inadequate to support growth; therefore essential for children.

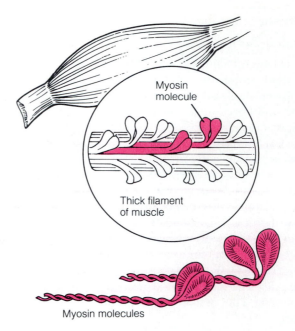

FIG. 5-1 Myosin is a globulin in muscle that, in combination with actin, forms actomyosin, the fundamental contractile unit of muscle active with ATP.

The Building of Proteins

The building units, amino acids, are used by the body to construct specific tissue proteins. This process is made possible by the nature of amino acids, which enables them to form peptide linkages and arrange themselves into peptide chains.

Tissue Protein Structure

Peptide Bond

The dual chemical nature of amino acids—the presence of a base (amino—NH_2) group containing nitrogen on one end and an acid (carboxyl—COOH) group on the other—enables them to join in the characteristic chain structure of proteins. The end amino group of one amino acid joins the end carboxyl group of another amino acid beside it. This characteristic joining of specific amino acids in a specific sequence to make a specific protein is called a **peptide bond.** Long chains of amino acids linked in this manner form proteins and are called *polypeptides*. These peptides may vary in chain length from relatively short chains of 3 to 15 amino acids, called *oligopeptides,* to medium-sized polypeptides, such as insulin, with chains of either 21 or 30 amino acids.

Large Complex Proteins

Larger still are complex proteins of several hundred amino acids that require special techniques to study, such as x-ray crystallography. Scientists can now view polypeptides in the exciting four-dimensional technique of nuclear magnetic resonance (NMR) spectroscopy, allowing them to examine closely much bigger complex proteins.[2] This new view enables researchers to learn how long protein chains fold and twist in space,

helping them understand how enzymes and other proteins work and aiding them in new drug design.

To make a compact structure, the long polypeptide chains coil or fold back on themselves in a spiral shape called a **helix** or in a "pleated sheet" arrangement. They are held together in some instances by additional strengthening cross-links of sulfur and hydrogen bonds.

Types of Proteins

The proteins illustrate a huge diversity of compounds produced by specific amino acid linkages. As a result, according to their varied specific structures, tissue proteins perform many vital roles in body structure and metabolism. Consider several examples here.

Myosin

This fibrous type of protein in muscle fiber, shown in Fig. 5-1, is composed of 153 amino acid long chains that coil and unfold on contraction and relaxation. Shaped into long rods, these fibers end in two-headed bundles so that they can change their shape and bend, making it possible to tighten and contract muscles and then relax them.

Collagen

This structural protein, shown in Fig. 5-2, is made up of three separate polypeptide chains wound around each other to produce a triple helix. Thus strengthened, the collagen is shaped into long rods and bundled into stiff fibers, because its job is to strengthen

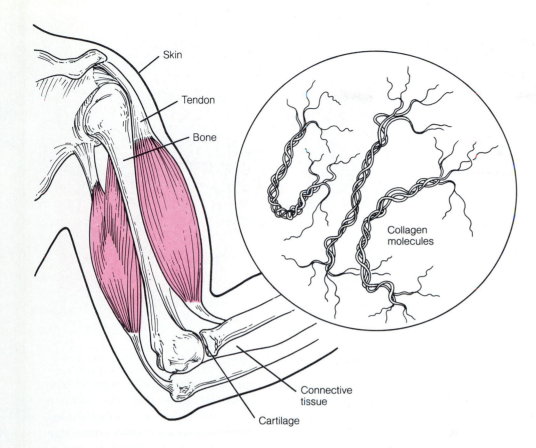

FIG. 5-2   Tissues that contain collagen, the basic structural material forming connective tissue throughout the body.

bone, cartilage, skin, and other body structures to maintain their form.

Hemoglobin

This globular type protein, shown in Fig. 5-3 (p. 66), is made up of four globin polypeptide chains in a molecule of hemoglobin. Each chain has several hundred amino acids, conjugated with the nonprotein portion—an oxygen-carrying pigment *heme*—which attaches to iron. The globin, in a compact globular shape, wraps around the heme and forms protective pockets to secure the iron and facilitate its exposure to oxygen as it travels in circulating red blood cells.

Albumin

This major plasma protein is made up of similar compact globular shaping. It consists of a single polypeptide chain of 584 amino acids, twisted and coiled into helixes held together by 17 disulfide bridges.[3]

Other examples of tissue proteins shaped for special structural or metabolic roles in the body include antibodies of the immune system, such as gammaglobulin; the blood protein fibrinogen; some regulating hormones, such as insulin, thyroxin, and the gastrointestinal peptides; and all of the enzymes.

Complete and Incomplete Food Proteins

A common way of designating the quality of protein foods is whether they are complete or incomplete in terms of the amounts of essential amino acids that they contain.

Complete Protein Foods

Foods called complete protein foods are those which contain all the essential amino acids in sufficient quantity and ratio to meet the body's needs. These proteins are of animal origin: eggs, milk, cheese, and meat. Another protein of animal origin, gelatin, does not qualify because it lacks three essential amino acids—tryptophan, valine, and isoleucine—and has only small amounts of leucine.

---

peptide bond • The characteristic joining of amino acids to form proteins. Such a chain of amino acids is termed a peptide. Depending on its size, it may be a dipeptide fragment of protein digestion or a large polypeptide.

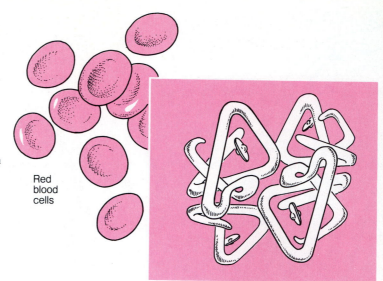

FIG. 5-3   Hemoglobin is an oxygen-carrying protein of red blood cells.

Red blood cells

Hemoglobin molecule

Incomplete Protein Foods

Foods called **incomplete protein foods** are those deficient in one or more of the essential amino acids. These proteins are mostly of plant origin: grains, legumes, nuts, and seeds. In a mixed diet, however, animal and plant proteins complement one another. Even a mixture of plant proteins alone may provide an adequate, balanced ratio of amino acids if planned carefully, especially if some form of soy protein is included.[4] The value of *variety* in the diet is therefore evident.

Thus, in the last analysis, the most significant measure of the protein quality of the diet depends on the total food mix consumed; how well the amino acid patterns of the various diet components, both complete and incomplete food proteins, complement one another; and how efficiently the protein is used at given levels of intake. A sound diet is the best way to obtain needed protein, eliminating any need for amino acid supplements (see box, p. 67).

Functions of Protein

Growth and Tissue-Building Maintenance

The primary function of dietary protein is to supply building material for growth and maintenance of body tissue. It does this by furnishing amino acids in appropriate amounts and types for efficient synthesis of specific cellular tissue proteins. Nitrogen, with its key position in amino acids and hence in building body tissues, is *the* vital element in our body's structure. Without it, we—and life on our planet as we know it—would not exist. Unlike carbohydrates and fats, which contain no nitrogen, protein is about 16% nitrogen. Protein also supplies amino acids for other essential nitrogen-containing substances, such as enzymes and hormones.

Specific Physiologic Roles

All amino acids supplied by dietary protein participate in growth and tissue maintenance. But some also perform other important physiologic and metabolic roles. For example, *methionine* is an agent in the formation of choline, which is a precursor of acetylcholine, one of the major neurotransmitters in the brain. In addition, methionine is not only the precursor of the nonessential amino acid cystine, but also of the lesser known ones **carnitine** and **taurine,** which are now known to have widespread metabolic functions (see box, p. 68). *Tryptophan* is the precursor of the B vitamin niacin and of the neurotransmitter serotonin. *Phenylalanine* is the precursor of the nonessential amino acid tyrosine, leading to formation of the hormones thyroxine and epinephrine. In addition, protein antibodies provide essential components of the body's immune system, and plasma proteins guard water balance.

Available Energy

Protein also contributes to the body's overall energy metabolism. This occurs as needed in the fasting state or during extended physical effort, such as marathon running, but not in the fed state. After the removal of the nitrogen-containing portion of the constituent amino acid, the amino acid residue—its carbon "skeleton" called a *keto*-acid—may be converted either to glucose or to fat. On the average, 58% of the total dietary protein may become available when needed to be burned for energy. Thus sufficient amounts of nonprotein kilocalories from carbohydrate are always needed to spare protein for its primary building purpose and to prevent unnecessary protein breakdown in the process of providing energy.

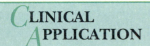

CLINICAL APPLICATION   *Amino Acids on the Grocery Shelf*

Be aware of persons shopping for amino acids and taking them singly or as multiple supplements for a number of supposed improvements in health and fitness or as remedies for health problems. Such persons buy tryptophan for insomnia, lysine and arginine for herpes, even glutamine for gluttony, and multiple combinations for athletic prowess or chronic illness. But these and other such health claims have repeatedly been refuted.

Two groups of persons most vulnerable to such claims are athletes and elderly persons. In the first group, athletes and their coaches are always searching for that "competitive edge" and often turn to various substances to advance it. The belief that protein is a major energy source and builds muscle strength leads to the use of amino acid supplements in an effort to attain this result. But carbohydrate and fat—not protein—are fuel substrates in muscle tissue, and excess protein only places excess metabolic burden on the body. It is exercise, not protein, that increases and strengthens muscles. In the second group, older adults seek to avoid health problems or relieve the pain and stress of the chronic illnesses of aging. The belief that amino acids will provide such magic elixirs is ill advised. They are both an expensive burden for many older adults on fixed incomes and an ineffective source of needed protein, the latter of which is better found in an improved diet containing all the nutrients that work best together.

In the case of one essential amino acid—tryptophan—touted among food faddists as a "natural" agent to relieve depression and insomnia, the megadose toxic levels of use—about 3000 mg every night—had severe, even deadly, consequences for a number of persons. When a significant number of such cases were reported, including 19 deaths, the Food and Drug Administration recalled all products containing tryptophan nationwide. The products may now be off the shelves of health food stores and pharmacies, but the lesson of such abuses remains.

This health fad of "amino acid shopping" is probably only partially based on new research redefining our ideas about "essential" and "nonessential" amino acids. More likely, it is taking advantage of the public's ignorance about the function of amino acids. Even if each individual amino acid is found to have a specific physiologic effect, they must *all* be present in specific amounts to build and maintain body proteins.

Thus persons concerned about their amino acid intake and seeking some supplement to enhance it should be cautioned as follows:

- They probably already get at least twice as much protein as they need, including all the essential amino acids, if their diet is based on typical American fare.
- Research on the effect of each amino acid refutes claims in most cases and warns of possible severe effects, even death, of toxic megadose abuse, as was the case with tryptophan.
- They can get all the currently known essential amino acids from a diet that includes even small amounts of animal products or that mixes vegetable proteins to complement their amino acid content.

In the final analysis, such individuals need to be reminded, as researchers and practitioners alike state: "Sound diet is still the best way to maintain health."

REFERENCES

Hertzman PA and others: Association of the eosinophilia-myalgia syndrome with the ingestion of tryptophan, *N Engl J Med* 322:869, 1990.

Kessler DA: The Food and Drug Administration and its problems, *N Engl J Med* 326:70, 1992.

Philen RM and others: Survey of advertising for nutritional supplements in health and bodybuilding magazines, *JAMA* 268(8):1009, 1992.

Shocket ID, Golar K: L-Tryptophan use and the eosinophilia-myalgia syndrome, *Nutr Rev* 48(8):313, 1990. ◆

Digestion-Absorption-Metabolism Summary

After the source of basic body-building materials—the food protein—is secured, it must be changed into the needed ready-to-use building units—the amino acids. This work is done through the successive parts of the gastrointestinal tract by the mechanical and chemical processes of digestion.

Mouth

In the mouth, only mechanical breaking up of the protein foods by chewing occurs. Here the food particles are mixed with saliva and passed on as a semisolid mass into the stomach.

carnitine • A naturally occurring amino acid ($C_{17}H_{15}NO_3$) formed from methionine and lysine, required for transport of long-chain fatty acids across the mitochondrial membrane, where they are oxidized as fuel substrate for metabolic energy.

incomplete protein food • A protein food having a ratio of amino acids different from that of the average body protein and therefore less valuable for nutrition than complete protein food.

taurine • A sulfur-containing amino acid, $NH_2(CH_2)_2SO_2OH$, formed from the essential amino acid methionine. It is found in various body tissues, such as lungs and muscles, and in bile and breast milk.

Recently Rediscovered Amino Acids

Sometimes little-known nutrients that have really been around for some time spark renewed interest and are "rediscovered" as their metabolic and clinical importance becomes more evident. Such is the case with two more recently rediscovered nutrients usually classed as amino acids—taurine and carnitine. Taurine was first isolated in 1872 and carnitine in 1905, but only now are their extensive metabolic activities and nutritional needs being recognized by modern research.

TO PROBE FURTHER

Taurine

Taurine is a sulfur-containing amino acid [NH$_2$(CH$_2$)$_2$ SO$_3$H] formed from methionine. The new interest in taurine has stemmed largely from increased awareness of its need in infant formulas to make them nutritionally similar to human milk. It is one of the most abundant free amino acids in human milk and was first added to infant formulas in 1984 to meet the body's need for amino acids. Taurine is also the most abundant free amino acid in the body's total intracellular fluid.

Dietary sources of taurine are largely animal protein foods. It is virtually absent in plant foods and hence in strict vegetarian diets. Its now known list of wide metabolic credits is receiving well-deserved attention, and continued research is ongoing. Its functions, for example, relate to bile acid synthesis, regulation of heart beat, control of brain neurons and central nervous system activity, maintenance of membrane stability, and integrity of retinal and vision function. Perhaps its key functional word is *stability*.

Carnitine

Carnitine (C$_7$H$_{15}$NO$_3$) is formed from methionine and lysine, with vitamins C, and B$_6$, niacin, and iron acting as necessary nutrient cofactors with the cell enzymes in its synthesis. Thus the nutritional status of the individual greatly influences the capacity of the liver and kidney, major synthesis sites, to make carnitine.

Renewed research and clinical interest in carnitine have increased with the advent of total parenteral nutrition (TPN) technology and advanced knowledge of genetic disease. Carnitine deficiences have been observed in persons with related genetic metabolic disorders and hypermetabolic disease and trauma patients who are receiving TPN. These deficiencies have been corrected by carnitine supplementation. Its major metabolic role is associated with the transport of long-chain fatty acids across the mitochondria membranes, thus stimulating the oxidation of these fuel substrates for metabolic energy. Continuing research is revealing broader functions in forming complex esters with many of the *acyl compounds,* metabolic intermediary products from fats and carbohydrates. An accumulation of such metabolites in cells can inhibit cell enzyme functions and become toxic, creating a secondary carnitine deficiency. Carnitine supplements have been effective, for example, in such conditions as ischemic heart disease, drug reactions, and a number of inborn errors of metabolism, including organic acidemias. Carnitine converts many of the acyl compounds to less toxic forms and removes them from the cell.

As with taurine, dietary sources of carnitine are largely limited to animal protein foods. It is absent from plant proteins, hence from strict vegetarian diets. Actually, the only carnitine in such vegan diets would be from the soy-based Indonesian food *tempeh* and only then from the mold used in the fermentation process. Infants receiving soy formula, then, would need a supplement, so carnitine is now being added to such products. Current studies indicate that oral carnitine is about 55% to 85% bioavailable from normal Western diets.

As a result of carnitine's metabolic functions, it has now become an important metabolic tool in conditions often requiring carnitine supplementation: (1) diseases of the liver and kidney, the major sites of carnitine synthesis, (2) major chronic illnesses or extensive injuries complicated by malnutrition and requiring TPN, (3) genetic metabolic disease affecting fatty acid metabolism and producing organic acidemias, and (4) deficiencies in premature infants with immature enzyme systems. Its current clinical nutrition and medical attention is obviously well-deserved.

REFERENCES

Borum PR: Carnitine—who needs it? *Nutr Today* 21(6):4, 1986.

Desai TK and others: Taurine deficiency after intensive chemotherapy and/or radiation, *Am J Clin Nutr* 55:708, 1992.

Lombard KA and others: Carnitine status of lactoovovegetarians and of vegetarian adults and children, *Am J Clin Nutr* 50:301, 1989.

Picone TA: Taurine update: metabolism and function, *Nutr Today* 22(4):16, 1987.

Rebouche CJ, Chenard CA: Metabolic fate of dietary carnitine in human adults: identification and quantification of urinary and fecal metabolites, *Am Inst Nutr* 121:539, 1991.

Wang W-Y, Liaw K-Y: Effect of a taurine-supplemented diet on conjugated bile acids in biliary surgical patients, *J Parenter Enteral Nutr* 15(3):294, 1991.

Stomach

Because proteins are such large complex structures, a series of enzymes is necessary to finally break them down to produce the amino acids. These chemical changes, through a system of enzymes, begin in the stomach. In fact, the stomach's chief digestive function in relation to all foods is the initial partial enzymatic breakdown of protein. Three agents in the gastric secretions help with this task: pepsin, hydrochloric acid, and rennin.

1. **Pepsin.** The main gastric enzyme, specific for proteins, is **pepsin.** It is first produced as an inactive **proenzyme (zymogen),** *pepsinogen,* by a single layer of cells (the chief cells) in the mucosa of the stom-

TABLE 5-2
Summary of Protein Digestion

Organ	Enzyme			Digestive action
	Inactive precursor	Activator	Active enzyme	
Mouth			None	Mechanical only
Stomach (acid)	Pepsinogen	Hydrochloric acid	Pepsin	Protein→polypeptides
			Rennin (infants) (calcium necessary for activity)	Casein→coagulated curd
Intestine (alkaline)				
Pancreas	Trypsinogen	Enterokinase	Trypsin	Protein, polypeptides→polypeptides, dipeptides
	Chymotrypsinogen	Active trypsin	Chymotrypsin	Protein, polypeptides→polypeptides, dipeptides
			Carboxypeptidase	Polypeptides→simpler peptides, dipeptides, amino acids
Intestine			Aminopeptidase	Polypeptides→peptides, dipeptides, amino acids
			Dipeptidase	Dipeptides→amino acids

ach wall. Pepsinogen then requires hydrochloric acid to be transformed into the enzyme pepsin. The active pepsin then begins splitting the peptide linkages between the protein's amino acids, changing the large polypeptides into successively smaller peptides. If the protein were held in the stomach longer, pepsin could continue the breakdown until individual amino acids resulted. However, with normal gastric emptying time, only the beginning stage is completed by the action of pepsin.

2. **Hydrochloric acid.** Gastric hydrochloride is an important catalyst in gastric protein digestion. It provides the acid medium necessary to convert pepsinogen to pepsin. Clinical problems result from lack of the normal secretion of hydrochloric acid.

3. **Rennin.** This gastric enzyme (not to be confused with the renal enzyme *renin*) is present only in infancy and childhood and disappears in adulthood. It is especially important in the infant's digestion of milk. Rennin and calcium act on the casein of milk to produce a curd. By coagulating milk, rennin prevents too rapid a passage of food from the child's stomach.

Small Intestine

Protein digestion begins in the acid medium of the stomach and is completed in the alkaline medium of the small intestine. A number of enzymes, from secretions of both the pancreas and the intestine, take part in protein digestion:

1. **Pancreatic secretions.** Three enzymes produced by the pancreas continue breaking down proteins to simpler and simpler substances:
    - **Trypsin** is secreted first as inactive trypsinogen and is then activated by the hormone enterokinase, which is produced by glands in the duodenal wall.

The active enzyme trypsin then acts on protein and large polypeptide fragments carried over from the stomach, producing smaller polypeptides and dipeptides.
- **Chymotrypsin** is produced by special cells in the pancreas as inactive chymotrypsinogen and then activated by the trypsin already present. Chymotrypsin continues the same protein-splitting action of trypsin.
- **Carboxypeptidase,** as its name indicates, attacks the carboxyl end (acid—COOH) of the peptide chain. It in turn produces smaller peptides and some free amino acids.

carboxypeptidase • A protein enzyme that splits off the chemical group *carboxyl* (-COOH) at the end of peptide chains, acting on the peptide bond of the terminal amino acid having a free-end carboxyl group.

chymotrypsin • One of the protein-splitting and milk-curdling pancreatic enzymes, activated in the intestine from precursor chymotrypsinogen. It breaks peptide linkages of the amino acids phenylalanine and tyrosine.

pepsin • The main gastric enzyme specific for proteins. Pepsin begins breaking large protein molecules into shorter chain polypeptides, proteoses, and peptones. Gastric hydrochloric acid is necessary to activate pepsin.

proenzyme • An inactive precursor converted to the active enzyme by the action of an acid, another enzyme, or other means. Also called zymogen.

trypsin • A protein-splitting enzyme formed in the intestine by action of enterokinase on the inactive precursor trypsinogen.

2. **Intestinal secretions.** Glands in the intestinal wall produce two more protein-splitting enzymes in the peptidase group:
   - **Aminopeptidase** releases amino acids one at a time from the nitrogen-containing amino end (base—NH_2) of the peptide chain. Through this cleavage, it produces smaller short-chain peptides and free amino acids.
   - **Dipeptidase,** final enzyme in this protein-splitting system, breaks the remaining dipeptides into their two, now free, amino acids.

Through this total system of protein-splitting enzymes, the large complex proteins are broken down into progressively smaller peptide chains and finally into free amino acids, now ready for absorption by the intestinal mucosa. A summary of these steps in protein digestion is given in Table 5-2.

Absorption

The construction sites in the body for building necessary specific tissue proteins are in the *cells.* Each cell, depending on its particular nature and function, has a specific job to do. Thus its proteins must be specifically structured.

Absorption of Amino Acids

The end products of protein digestion are the amino acids. They are water-soluble, so their absorption directly into the water-based bloodstream poses no problem. These building units are rapidly absorbed from the small intestine into the portal blood system through the fine network of villus capillaries, by means of competitive active transport.

1. **Active transport system.** Most of the amino acid absorption takes place in the first section of the small intestine, the duodenum. An energy-dependent active transport, using pyridoxine (vitamin B_6) as a carrier, absorbs the amino acids into the blood circulation, delivering them into the cells for eventual metabolism.
2. **Competition for absorption.** When we eat a mixed diet containing a variety of different amino acids, the amino acids compete with each other for absorption. The amino acid present in the largest quantity retards the absorption of the others. In plasma, circulating amino acids also compete for entry receptor sites for transport across cell membranes into the cell.

Absorption of Peptides and Whole Proteins

A few larger fragments of short-chain peptides or smaller intact proteins are absorbed as such and then by **hydrolysis** within the absorbing cells yield their amino acids. These whole protein molecules may play a part in the development of immunity and sensitivity. For example, antibodies in the mother's colostrum, the premilk breast secretion, are passed on to her nursing infant.

Metabolism

In human nutrition the amino acids are the "metabolic currency" of protein. It is with the fate of these vital compounds that the metabolism of protein is ultimately concerned. Protein's fascinating array of complex metabolic activities are intricately interwoven with those of carbohydrates and fats. Here we will look briefly at the fundamental metabolic concept of protein and nitrogen balance. This will provide a base for relating the tissue-building processes of **anabolism** with those of the breaking-down processes of **catabolism** to maintain these important protein balances.

The Concept of Balance

Many interdependent checks and balances exist throughout the body to keep it in its fine working order. There is a constant ebb and flow of materials, a building up and breaking down of parts, and a depositing and taking up of components. The body has built-in controls that operate as finely tuned coordinated responses to meet any situation that tends to disturb its normal condition or function. This resulting state of dynamic equilibrium is called **homeostasis,** and the various mechanisms designed to preserve it are called *homeostatic mechanisms.* This highly sensitive balance between body parts and functions is life-sustaining. As more and more is learned about human nutrition and physiology, older ideas of a rigid body structure are giving way to this important concept of *dynamic equilibrium*—balance amid constant change. All body constituents are in a constant state of flux, although some tissues are more actively engaged than are others. This dynamic concept can be seen in all metabolism. It is especially striking in protein metabolism.

Protein Balance

Overall protein balance involves concepts of protein turnover, compartments, amino acid pool, and nitrogen balance.

1. **Protein turnover.** For a number of years the use of radioactive isotopes has clearly demonstrated that the body's protein tissues are continuously being broken down into amino acids and then resynthesized into tissue proteins. When "labeled" amino acids are fed, they can be traced—that is, rapidly incorporated into various body tissue proteins. The rate of this protein turnover varies in different tissues. It is highest in the intestinal mucosa, liver, pancreas, kidney, and plasma. It is lower in muscle, brain, and skin. It is much slower in structural tissues, such as collagen and bone.
2. **Protein compartments.** Body protein exists in a balance between two compartments—tissue protein

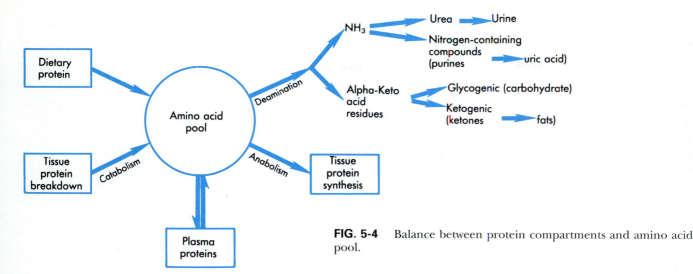

FIG. 5-4 Balance between protein compartments and amino acid pool.

and plasma protein. These stores are further balanced with dietary protein intake. Protein from one compartment may be drawn to supply need in the other. For example, during fasting, resources from the body protein stores may be used for tissue synthesis. But even when the intake of protein and other nutrients is adequate, the tissue proteins are still being constantly broken down, reshaped, and reformed according to body need. Such a dynamic state is necessary to life and growth because the body is an open system. It must sustain a dynamic balance not only within its own internal environment, but also with its larger and extended external environment.

The body's state of stability then is the result of tissue **protein balance** between the rates of protein breakdown (catabolism) and protein synthesis (anabolism). In periods of growth the synthesis rate is higher so that new tissue can be formed. In conditions of starvation, wasting disease, and more gradually as aging continues in elderly persons, tissue breakdown exceeds that of synthesis, and the body gradually deteriorates.

3. **Metabolic amino acid pool.** Amino acids derived from tissue breakdown and amino acids from dietary protein digestion and absorption both contribute to a common collective metabolic "pool" of amino acids throughout the body available for use (Fig. 5-4). A balance of amino acids is thus maintained to supply the body's constant needs. Shifts in balances between tissue breakdown and dietary protein intake ensure a balanced mixture of amino acids. From this reserve pool, specific amino acids are supplied to synthesize specific body proteins.

4. **Nitrogen balance.** Another useful reference for indicating a person's state of protein balance is **nitrogen balance.** Total nitrogen balance involves all

aminopeptidase • Protein-splitting enzyme that cuts the peptide bond (linkage) at the amino end of amino acids, splitting off the amino group -NH_2.

anabolism • Metabolic process by which body tissues are built.

catabolism • The breaking-down phase of metabolism, the opposite of anabolism. Catabolism includes all the processes in which complex substances are progressively broken down into simpler ones. Catabolism usually involves the release of energy. Together, anabolism and catabolism constitute metabolism, which is the coordinated operation of anabolic and catabolic processes into a dynamic balance of energy and substance.

dipeptidase • Final enzyme in the protein-splitting series that cleaves the one remaining amino acid bond in dipeptides.

homeostasis • State of relative dynamic equilibrium within the body's internal environment; a balance achieved through the operation of various interrelated physiologic mechanisms.

hydrolysis • Process by which a chemical compound is split into other simpler compounds by taking up the elements of water, as in the manufacture of infant formulas to produce easier-to-digest derivatives of the main protein casein in the cow's milk base. This process occurs naturally in digestion.

nitrogen balance • The metabolic balance between nitrogen intake in dietary protein and output in urinary nitrogen compounds such as urea and creatinine. For every 6.25 g dietary protein consumed, 1 g nitrogen is excreted.

protein balance • Body tissue protein balance between building up tissue (anabolism) and breaking down tissue (catabolism) to maintain healthy body growth and maintenance.

sources of nitrogen in the body—protein nitrogen, as well as nonprotein nitrogen present in other compounds, such as urea, uric acid, ammonia, and other body tissues and fluids. It is the net result of nitrogen gains and losses in all the body protein. A person is in a harmful state of negative nitrogen balance when the loss of body protein exceeds the input of food protein, as occurs in such conditions as long-term illness, a hypermetabolic wasting disease, or starvation.

Protein Requirements

It is clear that protein is an essential nutrient. But just how much and what kind do we actually need? We know that some people get far less than they need. On a worldwide basis, protein-energy malnutrition is a major health concern, especially in underdeveloped countries. In contrast, however, protein deficiency is not a problem in America and most other Western societies. Actually most persons in America eat two or three times as much protein as they really need, largely due to the extensive role of meat and dairy products in cultural food habits. For example, U.S. surveys indicate that foods of animal origin contribute about two thirds of the daily protein intake, with some 48% from meat, 17% from daily products, and 4% from eggs.[5] But such excess protein intake often creates other problems. First, excessive intake of animal protein foods—which carry animal fat—can contribute to obesity and vascular health problems. Second, the excessive nitrogen load can place accumulative burden on the kidneys for nitrogen excretion. Clinicians have begun to raise questions about the long-term effects of habitual excess protein intake on the human kidney, which was designed in earlier ages to handle a different supply of protein.

Factors Influencing Protein Requirements
Tissue Growth

The primary purpose of protein in the diet is to supply amino acids in the quantity and quality necessary for growth and maintenance of tissue. Thus any period of growth increases the need for protein. Growth-related factors include age, body size, and general physical state. Also, special periods of rapid growth—such as the growth of the fetus and maternal tissue during pregnancy—require added protein.

Diet

Other factors include the nature of the protein in the diet and its ratio or pattern of amino acids. There must be sufficient nonprotein foods in the diet to have a protein-sparing effect, so that the total amount of protein will not be diminished for energy requirements. Also, the digestibility and absorption of the protein is affected by the cooking of the food, and time intervals between eating protein foods lowers the competition for absorption sites and enzymes.

Illness or Disease

Any illness or disease will usually increase the requirement for protein. Diseases accompanied by fever usually increase the need for protein, because of the increase in basal metabolic rate and the general breaking down of tissue. Traumatic injury requires extensive tissue rebuilding. Postsurgical states require protein for wound healing and to replenish losses.[6] Extensive tissue destruction, as occurs with burns, requires considerable increase in protein intake for the healing process.

Measurement of Protein Requirements

It is evident, then, that two basic measures of protein requirement must be considered: quantity and quality.

Protein Quantity

The quantity of protein needed is the basis for establishing the total protein requirement. Actually, the human body *requires* somewhat less than the nutrient standards state, because the standard *allows* for a safety margin to cover the variety of needs in a given population. Thus the U.S. standards are stated in terms of recommended dietary *allowances,* not as set *requirements.* The current RDA standard for adults has been generally set at 0.8 g/kg (2.2 lb) of body weight.[5] This amounts to about 56 g/day for a man weighing 70 kg (154 lb) and 44 g/day for a woman weighing 55 kg (120 lb). Increased protein is indicated during pregnancy and lactation. The needs of infants and children vary according to age and growth patterns.

Protein Quality

Because the value of a protein depends on its content of essential amino acids, in the final analysis the measure of protein need must be based on its amino acid quality. Guidelines for protein needs, based on nitrogen balance studies determining specific amino acid requirements, have been developed (Table 5-3).

Comparative Quality of Food Proteins

The nutritive value of a food protein is often expressed in terms of its *chemical score*, a value derived from its amino acid composition. Using the amino acid pattern of a high-quality protein food—such as egg—and giving it a value of 100, other foods are compared according to their ratios of essential amino acids. Of these necessary amino acids, the one showing the greatest dietary deficit is called the **limiting amino acid** because when it is used up in making a specific protein, it limits the ability of the body to make more of that protein.

TABLE 5-3

Estimates of Amino Acid Requirements

Amino acid	Requirements, mg/kg per day, by age-group			
	Infants, age 3-4 mo	Children, age ~ 2 yr	Children, age 10-12 yr	Adults
Histidine	28	?	?	8-12
Isoleucine	70	31	28	10
Leucine	161	73	42	14
Lysine	103	64	44	12
Methionine plus cystine	58	27	22	13
Phenylalanine plus tyrosine	125	69	22	14
Threonine	87	37	28	7
Tryptophan	17	12.5	3.3	3.5
Valine	93	38	25	10
Total without histidine	714	352	214	84

From the Food and Nutrition Board, National Academy of Sciences—National Research Council: *Recommended dietary allowances,* ed 10, Washington, DC, 1989, National Academy Press.

TABLE 5-4

Comparative Protein Quality of Selected Foods According to Chemical (Amino Acid) Score, Biologic Value (BV), Net Protein Utilization (NPU), and Protein Efficiency Ratio (PER)

Food	Chemical score	BV	NPU	PER
Egg	100	100	94	3.92
Cow's milk	95	93	82	3.09
Fish	71	76	—	3.55
Beef	69	74	67	2.30
Unpolished rice	67	86	59	—
Peanuts	65	55	55	1.65
Oats	57	65	—	2.19
Polished rice	57	64	57	2.18
Whole wheat	53	65	49	1.53
Corn	49	72	36	—
Soybeans	47	73	61	2.32
Sesame seeds	42	62	53	1.77
Peas	37	64	55	1.57

Data adapted from Food and Nutrition Board, National Academy of Sciences—National Research Council: *Recommended dietary allowances,* ed 10, Washington, DC, 1989, National Academy Press.

Other measures also determine aspects of protein quality:

1. **Biologic value (BV)** based on nitrogen balance
2. **Net protein utilization (NPU)** based on biologic value and degree of digestibility
3. **Protein efficiency ratio (PER)** based on weight gain of a growing test animal divided by its protein intake

A comparison of the scores of various protein foods with their nutritive values based on these measures is shown in Table 5-4. A sound diet is the best way to obtain needed protein. There is no need for amino acid supplements. They are both costly and inefficient (see box, p. 68).

Vegetarian Diets: Complementary Food Proteins

Protein requirements in various vegetarian diets may be met by applying the principle of combining complementary plant proteins, complete and incomplete protein foods, to achieve the necessary balance of essential amino acids.[7,8] There are three basic types of vegetarian diets: (1) lactoovovegetarian (including dairy foods and eggs), (2) lactovegetarian (including dairy foods), and (3) pure vegan (no animal protein). Each must be planned carefully to secure needed essential amino acids (see Issues and Answers, p. 75). Guidelines for vegetable protein combinations and interesting recipes for preparing these foods are now widely available because of increased public interest. A favorite of many remains *Laurel's Kitchen.*[9] In general, in relation to animal protein sources, larger amounts of vegetable protein foods must be consumed to obtain comparable amounts of complete protein.

To Sum Up

Proteins build tissue, perform various physiologic roles, and provide energy. Amino acids are the structural components of proteins. There are 22 in total, 9 of which the body cannot synthesize in adequate amounts. These 9 are called essential amino acids (EAAs). Food proteins are considered "complete" when they contain all 9 EAAs in appropriate amounts. Animal proteins are complete. Vegetable proteins are incomplete but can be mixed with complete proteins or with each other to provide all 9 EAAs for the day.

Amino acids participate in protein building (anabolism) or breakdown (catabolism). Both processes are dictated by genetic information and hormonal influences. *Anabolism* occurs when specific amino acids required for each protein are present. If one is missing, the protein is not formed—the law of "all or none." *Catabolism* occurs when the body tissues are broken down. The amino acid splits into its nitrogen group, which helps to form amino acids or other nitrogen compounds, and its nonnitrogen residue, which can form carbohydrates for energy or fat storage. In the unfed

limiting amino acid • The amino acid in foods occurring in the smallest amount, thus limiting its availability for tissue structure.

state, proteins are broken down for energy. Thus dietary carbohydrates have a protein-sparing effect.

Protein requirements are influenced by growth needs and rate of protein synthesis, food protein quality, and dietary carbohydrate and fat levels. Clinical factors affecting protein needs include fever, disease, surgery, or other trauma to body tissues.

QUESTIONS FOR REVIEW

1. What is the difference between *essential* and *nonessential* amino acids? List the names of the essential amino acids.
2. Explain the term "protein-sparing effect." Which nutrients have this effect?
3. List and describe factors that affect dietary protein needs.
4. Calculate your own protein intake for a day and compare it with your general need according to the RDA allowances.
5. A vegetarian couple decides to raise their 2-year-old daughter on a strict vegan diet. As expected, the child does not often finish meals and snacks of fruits and whole-grain biscuits. Eventually, they notice that she is falling behind in her growth rate and becoming thin. What food patterns would you expect in this family? What dietary factor may be involved in the child's poor growth? What advice would you offer these parents to improve their child's nutritional status? Plan 1 day's meals for this family, indicating amounts that would meet the child's dietary protein need, while still adhering to a typical vegan meal pattern.

REFERENCES

1. Munro HN: Historical introduction: the origin and growth of our present concepts of protein metabolism. In Munro HN, Allison JB, editors: *Mammalian protein metabolism,* vol 1, New York, 1964, Academic Press.
2. Pool R: Seeing protein in 4-D: nuclear magnetic resonance spectroscopy in protein structure analysis, *Science* 249(476):364, 1990.
3. Doweiko JP, Nompleggi DJ: Role of albumin in human physiology and pathophysiology, *J Parenter Enteral Nutr* 15(2):207, 1991.
4. Young VR: Soy protein in relation to human protein and amino acid nutrition, *J Am Diet Assoc* 91(7):828, 1991.
5. Food and Nutrition Board, National Academy of Sciences—National Research Council: *Recommended dietary allowances,* ed 10, Washington, DC, 1989, National Academy Press.
6. Hammarqvist F and others: Alpha-ketoglutarate preserves protein synthesis and free glutamine in skeletal muscle after surgery, *Surgery* 109(1):28, 1991.
7. Resnicow K and others: Diet and serum lipids in vegan vegetarians: a model for risk reduction, *J Am Diet Assoc* 91(4):447, 1991.
8. Dwyer JT: Nutritional consequences of vegetarianism, *Annu Rev Nutr* 11:61, 1991.
9. Robertson L and others: *The new Laurel's kitchen,* Berkeley, Calif, 1986, Ten Speed Press.

FURTHER READING

Resnicow K and others: Diet and serum lipids in vegan vegetarians: a model for risk reduction, *J Am Diet Assoc* 91(4):447, 1991.

This study clearly shows how a strict vegan diet—which is very low in saturated fat and dietary cholesterol—can not only provide adequate balanced protein intake, but also help children and adults maintain desirable serum lipid levels.

Young VR: Soy protein in relation to human protein and amino acid nutrition, *J Am Diet Assoc* 91(7):828, 1991.

This review of the many uses of soy protein products in the diets of infants, children, adolescents, and adults provides helpful information about the important role of these plant protein sources in the diet. In each case these diets replaced much of the excess animal protein foods usually consumed, thereby lowering serum lipid values, and also retained an essentially equivalent dietary protein value.

Vegetarian Food Patterns: Harm or Health?

At least 7 million Americans have become vegetarians, replacing meats as a main entree item with legumes, grains, and vegetables. Their meals follow a variety of patterns. Some groups call themselves "true" vegetarians, because they allow no animal products in their diets. But their highly restrictive "dietary laws" have caused serious malnutrition problems. These problems are found among the following persons:

Zen macrobiotics, who eat only brown rice and herb tea to achieve a perfect balance of yin and yang in order to fend off disease

Vegans—who rely on fruits, vegetables, nuts, and seeds—and use no source of animal protein, fortified foods, or nutritional supplements

Fruitarians, who eat only fresh and dried fruits, nuts, honey, and sometimes olive oil

Other vegetarian diets, however, as well as a strict vegan diet—if well planned—can be very nutritious. These alternate forms of "animal-product" vegetarianism include the following:

Lactovegetarians, who allow milk, cheese, yogurt, and other milk products as the only animal protein in their diets

Ovovegetarians, who use eggs as their only source of animal protein

Lactoovovegetarians, who permit fish as their only animal product

Pescovegetarians, who allow only poultry

"Red-meat abstainers," who eat any animal product except red meat and consider themselves to be vegetarians, too

Reasons people give for becoming vegetarian are as varied as these diets:

Religion. Religious communities, such as the Seventh-Day Adventists, use vegetarianism as a means of self-discipline, as well as promoting good health. Other vegetarians may or may not be religious but feel it is "sinful" to kill a living animal for food.

Ecology. Approximately half of the world's grain output is used to feed livestock. Some vegetarians feel it could be better used to feed people so that less land would be used to meet the world's protein needs. Some also feel that using less land would result in a reduction in the use of pesticides now used to ensure large crops.

Economics. Beans, grains, and vegetables are cheaper than meat. Some vegetarians are concerned not only with saving money for themselves, but also with finding a way to meet food shortages in poor nations throughout the world.

Health. Another common reason for selecting vegetarianism is to achieve good health. By avoiding animal products, vegetarians manage to reduce their intake of cholesterol and saturated fats, thus perhaps gaining some protection against heart disease.

Does a vegetarian diet offer other important nutrients besides protein?

Yes. Vegetarians can meet the recommended dietary allowance (RDA) for most major nutrients without taking supplements. However, a few key nutrients create problems if the vegetarian is not careful:

- **Vitamin B$_{12}$.** This vitamin is found only in animal products. People who follow veganism or the macrobiotic diets are at the greatest risk for a deficiency. Vegans may be at special risk because they take in a large amount of folacin, another B vitamin that can mask signs of B$_{12}$ deficiency. A deficiency can be avoided, however, by including fortified foods or taking a B$_{12}$ supplement, along with sufficient complete protein from complementary amino acids to ensure synthesis of the intrinsic factor (a mucoprotein) necessary for B$_{12}$ absorption.
- **Vitamin A.** Vegetarians tend to get more provitamin A, carotene, than they need. This usually isn't a problem, unless they are also taking supplements that include vitamin A. One study shows that 85% of vegetarians take supplements. These may include as much as 10 times the RDA for vitamin A! As a fat-soluble vitamin, vitamin A can build up in body tissues and reach toxic levels. The result could be anorexia, irritability, dry skin, and hair loss.
- **Iron.** Grains and legumes have iron, but much of it is poorly absorbed from the gut. Absorption can be enhanced, however, by including a good source of vitamin C in the same meal.

Can vegetarian women get enough protein for a successful pregnancy?

Yes, though including animal products—as in lactoovovegetarianism—may become essential to meet extra nutritional needs. Supplements are also recommended for such hard-to-get nutrients as iron.

Is the vegetarian diet safe for children?

Children manage to grow and develop fairly well on a vegetarian diet that includes the nonmeat animal proteins milk, cheese, and eggs. They tend to be a little shorter than average, but this may be the result of other genetic or environmental factors. Vegetarian children also tend to be mildly anemic, probably because of the poor availability of iron from grains and legumes. Again, including a source of vitamin C with meals may be helpful. The vegan diet, unless it is carefully planned and monitored, and all levels of macrobiotic diets are too poor in required nutrients to sustain childhood growth needs.

Can you lose weight on a vegetarian diet?

Yes, definitely. Eliminating meats automatically removes a major source of fat in the diet. Because fats provide more

Vegetarian Food Patterns: Harm or Health?—cont'd

than twice the number of kilocalories per gram than carbohydrates or protein, the vegetarian diet is usually much lower in kilocalories than the "meat-and-potatoes" diet. In fact, some vegetarians—especially pregnant women, children, and athletes—have to be careful to get *enough* kilocalories.

Thus the well-planned vegetarian diet can be nutritious.

If used wisely, especially in its lactoovo forms, it can offer many advantages in terms of health, economy, and ecology.

REFERENCES

Dwyer JT: Nutritional consequences of vegetarianism, *Annu Rev Nutr* 11:61, 1991.

Havala S, Dwyer JT: Position of the American Dietetic Association: vegetarian diets—technical support paper, *J Am Diet Assoc* 88(3):352, 1988.

Resnicow K and others: Diet and serum lipids in vegan vegetarians: a model for risk reduction, *J Am Diet Assoc* 91(4):447, 1991.

Young VR: Soy protein in relation to human protein and amino acid nutrition, *J Am Diet Assoc* 91(7):828, 1991.

CHAPTER 6

Energy Balance and Weight Management

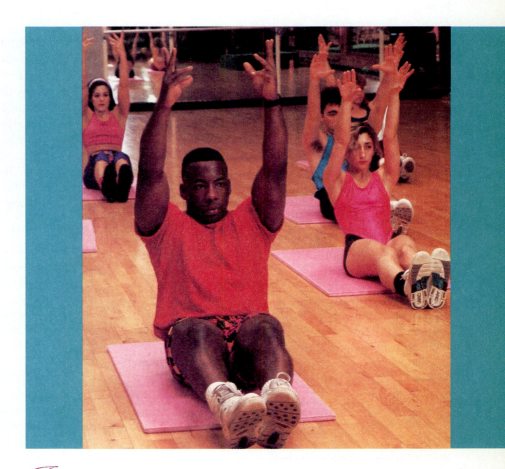

In a previous chapter, we reviewed the overall digestion-absorption-metabolism continuum in our bodies for handling the three energy nutrients. In this chapter we consider the relationship between body energy balance and body weight, problems of overweight and underweight, and their effects on health.

We will find, however, that this balance is not a simple matter. We are not all alike, and our energy needs vary in different circumstances and different body types. Each of us is unique, and sometimes our varying body weights reflect this fact. This individual view of weight patterns is difficult for many modern societies to accept, and the social norm of thinness creates undue pressure for many whose natural weight cannot conform.

Here we will seek an improved goal of weight management based on sound nutrition, health, and physical fitness. This approach is important for all persons, but especially for those with health risks related to excess body weight.

The Human Energy System

Energy Cycle and Transformation

Forms of Human Energy

It is clear that in our physical world **energy,** like matter, is neither created nor destroyed. When we speak of energy "production," what we really mean is that it is being *transformed*. Energy is being changed in form and cycled throughout a system. In the human body the various metabolic processes convert stored chemical energy in our food to other forms of energy for the body's work. In our bodies, energy is available in four basic forms for life processes: *chemical, electrical, mechanical,* and *thermal*. Our ultimate source of power is the sun with its vast reservoir of nuclear reactions (Fig. 6-1). Then through the process of photosynthesis, as shown in the previous chapter on carbohydrates (see Fig. 3-1), using water and carbon dioxide as raw materials, plants transform the sun's energy into food storage forms of chemical energy. In the body these stored food fuels are converted to the basic energy unit glucose, which together with fatty acids is metabolized to release its energy to be transformed and cycled through body systems. Water and carbon dioxide, the initial materials used by the plants, are retrieved as end products of this process of oxidation in the body. And so the cycle goes on and on.

Transformation of Energy

Through the many processes of metabolism, after stored chemical energy in food is taken into the body, it is converted further to chemical energy in other metabolic products to do the body's work. This chemical energy is then changed still further to other forms of energy as this work is performed. For example, chemical energy is changed to electrical energy in brain and nerve activity. It is changed to mechanical energy in muscle contraction. It is changed to thermal energy in the regulation of body temperature. It is changed to still other types of chemical energy in the synthesis of new compounds. In all these work activities of the body, heat is given off to the surrounding atmosphere and larger biosphere.

In human *metabolism,* as in any energy system, energy is always present as either *free energy* or *potential energy*.

Free energy is the energy involved at any given moment in the performance of a task. It is unbound and in motion. Potential energy is the energy that is stored or bound in the various chemical compounds, available for conversion to free energy as needed for work. For example, energy stored in sugar is potential energy. When we eat it and it is metabolized, free energy is released and body work results. As work is done, energy in the form of heat is released.

Energy Balance: Input and Output

Whether the energy system is electrical, mechanical, thermal, or chemical, in the course of the many reactions that compose its operation, free energy is decreased and the reservoir of potential energy is secondarily diminished. Therefore the system must be constantly refueled from some outside source. In the human energy system this basic input of fuel is our food.

The energy demands of the body require a constant supply of available energy. These energy needs support the body's total basic metabolic needs, as well as the additional physical activity requirements. In the human energy system this physical energy output is evident in our activities. But energy output to an even larger degree is also going on internally at all times to meet our basal or resting energy needs.

Energy Control in Human Metabolism

In the human body the energy produced in its many chemical reactions, if "exploded" all at once, would be destructive. There must be some mechanism therefore by which energy is controlled in the human system, so that it may support life and not destroy it. Several basic means of control, chemical bonding and controlled reaction rates, accomplish this task.

Chemical Bonding

The main mechanism controlling energy in the human system is **cheminal bonding.** The chemical bonds that hold elements of compounds together consist of energy. As long as the compound remains constant, energy is being exerted to maintain it. When the compound is taken into the body and broken into its parts, this energy is released and available for body work. Three basic types of chemical bonds transfer energy in the body:

- **Covalent bonds.** These are regular bonds, based on relative **valence** of constituent elements, that link the elements of a chemical compound together—for example, those which hold carbon atoms together in the core of an organic compound.
- **Hydrogen bonds.** Weaker than covalent bonds, these bonds are nonetheless significant because they can be formed in large numbers. Also, the very fact that they are less strong and can be broken easily makes them important because they can be transferred or

passed readily from one substance to another to help form still another substance.

- **High-energy phosphate bonds.** A main example of these high-energy phosphate bonds at work is the compound **adenosine triphosphate (ATP),** which is the unique compound the human body uses to store energy for its cell work. Like storage batteries for electrical energy, these bonds become the controlling force for ongoing energy needs.

Controlled Reaction Rates

The many chemical reactions that make up the body's energy system must also have controls. Some of the reactions that break down proteins—for example, if left to themselves (as in sterile decomposition)—would span several years. Such reactions must be accelerated, or else getting the needed energy from a meal would take years. At the same time, they must be regulated so that too fast a reaction will not produce a burst of energy in a single "explosion." Control agents regulating these cell activities are the enzymes, coenzymes, and hormones.

1. **Enzymes.** Many specific **enzymes** in every cell control specific cell reactions. All enzymes are protein compounds. They are produced in the cells under control of specific genes. One specific gene controls the making of one specific enzyme, and there are thousands of enzymes in each cell. Each enzyme

adenosine triphosphate (ATP) • The high-energy compound formed in the cell called the "energy currency" of the cell because of the binding of energy in its high-energy phosphate bonds for release for cell work as these bonds are split. A compound of adenosine (a nucleotide containing adenine and ribose) that has three phosphoric acid groups. ATP is a high-energy phosphate compound important in energy exchange for cellular activity. The splitting off of the terminal phosphate bond (PO_4) of ATP to produce adenosine diphosphate (ADP) releases bound energy and transfers it to free energy available for body work. The reforming of ATP in cell oxidation again stores energy in high-energy phosphate bonds for use as needed. They may be charged and discharged according to conditions in the cell.

chemical bonding • Process of linking the radicals, chemical elements, or groups of a chemical compound.

energy • The capacity of a system for doing work; available power. Energy is manifest in various forms—motion, position, light, heat, and sound. Energy is interchangeable among these various forms and is constantly being transformed and transferred among them.

enzyme • Various complex proteins produced by living cells that act independently of these cells. Enzymes are capable of producing certain chemical changes in other substances without themselves being changed in the process. Their action is therefore that of a catalyst. Digestive enzymes of the gastrointestinal secretions act on food substances to break them down into simpler compounds and greatly accelerate the speed of these chemical reactions. An enzyme is usually named according to the substance (substrate) on which it acts, with the common suffix *-ase;* for example, sucrase is the specific enzyme for sucrose and breaks it down to glucose and fructose.

valence • Power of an element or a radical to combine with or to replace other elements or radicals. Atoms of various elements combine in definite proportions. The valence number of an element is the number of atoms of hydrogen with which one atom of the element can combine.

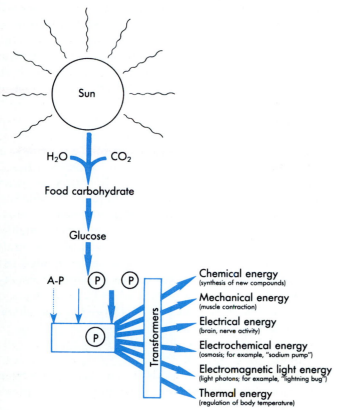

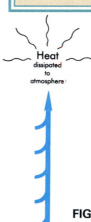

FIG. 6-1 Transformation of energy from its primary source (the sun) to various forms for biologic work by means of metabolic processes ("transformers").

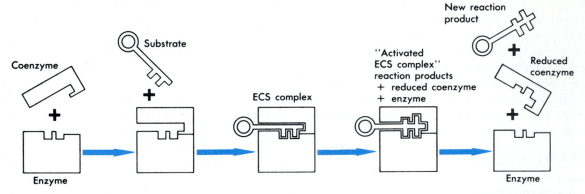

FIG. 6-2　Lock and key concept of the action of enzyme, coenzyme, and substrate to produce a new reaction product.

works on its own particular substance, which is called its **substrate.** The enzyme and its substrate lock together to produce a new reaction product, and the original enzyme remains unchanged, ready to do its specific work over and over again (Fig. 6-2).

2. **Coenzymes.** Many reactions require a partner to assist the enzyme in completing the reaction. These coenzyme factors in many instances involve several of the vitamins, especially the B-complex vitamins and some of the minerals. It may be helpful to think of the coenzyme as another substrate, because in receiving the material transferred, the coenzyme is changed or reduced.

3. **Hormones.** In energy metabolism **hormones** act as messengers to trigger or control enzyme action. For example, the rate of oxidative reactions in the tissues—the body's metabolic rate—is controlled by the *thyroid-stimulating hormone (TSH)* from the anterior pituitary gland. Another familiar example is the controlling action of insulin from the pancreas islet cells on the rate of glucose utilization in the tissues. Steroid hormones also have the capacity to regulate the cell's ability to synthesize enzymes.

Types of Metabolic Reactions

The two types of reaction constantly going on in energy metabolism are anabolism and catabolism. Each requires energy. The processes of *anabolism* synthesize new and more complex substances. The processes of *catabolism* break down more complex substances to simpler ones. These processes release free energy, but the work also uses up some free energy. Therefore there is a constant energy deficit, which must be supplied by food.

Sources of Stored Energy

When food is not available, as in periods of fasting or starvation, the body must draw on its own stores for energy:

1. **Glycogen.** Only a 12- to 48-hour reserve of glyco-

gen exists in liver and muscle and is quickly depleted.

2. **Muscle mass.** Storage of energy as protein exists in limited amounts in muscle mass, but in greater volume than glycogen stores.

3. **Adipose fat tissue.** Although fat storage may be larger, the supply varies from person to person and from circumstance to circumstance.

Measurement of Energy Balance
Kilocalorie

Because the body performs work only as energy is released by chemical reactions, and because all work takes the form of heat production, energy may be measured in terms of heat equivalents. Such a heat measure is the **calorie.** To avoid using large numbers the professional nutritionist and biochemist use the term **kilocalorie** (1000 calories), abbreviated kcalorie or kcal. This is the amount of heat required to raise 1 kg of water 1° C.

Joule (J)

The international (SI) unit of energy measurement is the **joule.** It expresses the amount expended when 1 kg of a substance is moved 1 meter by a force of 1 newton. It was named for James Prescott Joule (1818-1889), an English physicist who discovered the first law of thermodynamics and invented an electromagnetic engine. The conversion factor for changing kilocalories (kcal) to kilojoules (kJ) is 4.184—one kilocalorie equals 4.184 kilojoules. Because the conversion product of energy values of diets in kilojoules renders large numbers, a simpler term is the megajoule (MJ)—one megajoule equals 239 kilocalories.

Food Energy Measure

The energy in various foods is generally measured in two basic ways: calorimetry and computing the approximate composition.

Calorimetry

The caloric values of various foods expressed in food value tables have usually been determined by direct calorimetry.[1] In this process a metal container called a *bomb calorimeter* is used. The name comes from its long tubular shape. A weighed amount of food is placed inside, and the instrument is immersed in water. The food is then ignited by an electric spark in the presence of oxygen and burned. The increase in the temperature of the surrounding water indicates the number of kilocalories given off by the oxidation of the food. Remember when you use food value tables, however, that these values represent averages of a number of samples of the given food tested. The value of a particular serving of that food varies around that figure.

Approximate Composition

An alternate method of measuring food energy is by computing the approximate nutrient composition of a given food using values in food value tables or data bases. These values are based on the average kilocalorie value of each of the three energy-yielding macronutrients. These values are known as their respective **fuel factors:** 1 g of carbohydrate yields 4 kcal, 1 g of fat yields 9 kcal, and 1 g of protein yields 4 kcal. In comparison, 1 g of beverage alcohol yields 7 kcal.

Total Energy Requirements

The total energy expended by an individual supports three essential energy uses: (1) basal metabolic needs (basal energy expenditures [BEE] or resting energy expenditures [REE]), (2) food intake effect, and (3) physical activities.

Basal Metabolic Needs

Basal Metabolic Rate (BMR)

The sum of all internal chemical activities that maintain the body at rest comprise its basal metabolism. The **basal metabolic rate (BMR),** frequently referred to as **resting metabolic rate (RMR),** is a measure of the energy required by these activities of resting tissue. Certain small but vitally active tissues—brain, liver, gastrointestinal tract, heart, and kidneys—together make up less than 5% of the total body weight, yet they contribute about 60% of the total basal metabolic processes. This resting metabolic rate is the largest component of energy expenditure in humans, constituting about 60% to 70% of the daily energy expenditure of individuals, and is influenced by the state of fitness and the pretesting environment.[2,3]

Measuring BMR

Direct and indirect methods of measuring BMR are used:

1. **Direct calorimetry.** In direct methods, a chamber

---

basal metabolic rate (BMR) • Amount of energy required to maintain the resting body's internal activities after an overnight fast. See also **resting metabolic rate (RMR).**

calorie • A unit of heat energy. The calorie used in the study of metabolism is the large calorie, or *kilocalorie,* defined as the amount of heat required to raise the temperature of 1 kg of water 1° Celsius (centigrade).

calorimentry • Measurement of amounts of heat absorbed or given out. *Direct method:* measurement of amount of heat produced by a subject enclosed in a small chamber. *Indirect method:* measurement of amount of heat produced by a subject by the quantity of nitrogen and carbon dioxide eliminated.

fuel factor • The kilocalorie value (energy potential) of food nutrients; that is, the number of kilocalories that 1 g of the nutrient yields when oxidized. The kilocalorie fuel factor for carbohydrate is 4; for protein, 4; and for fat, 9. The basic figures are used in computing diets and energy values of foods. (For example, 10 g of fat yields 90 kcal.)

hormones • Various internally secreted substances from the endocrine organs, which are conveyed by the blood to another organ or tissue on which they act to stimulate increased functional activity or secretion. This tissue or substance is called its target organ or substance.

joule • The international (SI) unit of energy and heat, defined as the work done by the force of 1 newton acting over the distance of 1 meter. A newton (named for Sir Isaac Newton, 1643-1727, English mathematician, physicist, and astronomer) is the international unit of force, defined as the amount of force that, when applied in a vacuum to a body having a mass of 1 kg, accelerates it at the rate of 1 meter per second. These are examples of the exactness with which terms and values used by the world's scientific community must be defined, as illustrated in the *Système International d'Unités (SI).*

kilocalorie • The general term *calorie* refers to a unit of heat measure and is used alone to designate the *small calorie.* The calorie used in nutritional science and the study of metabolism is the *large calorie,* 1000 calories, or kilocalorie, to be more accurate and avoid use of very large numbers in calculations.

resting metabolic rate (RMR) • Amount of energy required to maintain the resting body's internal activities when in a normal environment temperature. Because of small differences in measuring techniques, RMR may be slightly different from the same person's **basal metabolic rate (BMR).** In practice, however, RMR and BMR measurments may be used interchangeably.

substrate • The specific organic substance on which a particular enzyme acts to produce new metabolic products.

large enough for a person to enter is used, and the body's heat production at rest is measured. This instrument is large and costly and is therefore limited to research studies.[1,4]

2. **Indirect calorimetry.** In this indirect method a smaller portable instrument, sometimes called a *metabolator,* can be brought to the side of the bed or chair on a cart. The person breathes into the instrument through a mouthpiece and the exchanges of gases in respiration, the *respiratory quotient* (CO_2/O_2), is measured while the subject is at rest. The metabolic rate is calculated with a high degree of accuracy from the rate of oxygen utilization, because more than 95% of the energy expended by the body is derived from metabolic reactions with oxygen.[1] Energy (BMR) measured in this manner is equivalent to the heat released by the body.

3. **Indirect laboratory tests.** Because the thyroid hormone regulates BMR, thyroid function tests are used in clinical practice to serve as indirect measures of BMR. These tests include measures of serum protein-bound iodine (PBI), and serum thyroxin levels, both triiodothyronine (T_3) and thyroxin (T_4), as well as the radioactive iodine uptake test. The free thyroxine index (FTI) is an overall measure based on the product of T_3 and T_4. These two compounds are produced in the final two stages of thyroid hormone synthesis. This product ($T_3 \times T_4$) reflects the relative functioning of the thyroid gland and the amount of hormone activity influencing the BMR.

Factors Influencing BMR

The four main factors influencing BMR are lean body mass, growth, fever and disease, and cold climate.

1. **Lean body mass.** Lean body mass is the major factor influencing BMR, because of its greater level of metabolic activity than that of less active tissues, such as fat and bones. Differences, for example, in metabolic requirements for women are primarily related to their generally lower amount of lean muscle mass in comparison with men.

2. **Growth.** Growth during childhood and pregnancy, as well as milk production during lactation, requires anabolic work under the influence of growth hormone.

3. **Fever and disease.** Fever increases BMR about 7% for each 0.83° C (1° F) rise. In addition, diseases involving increased cell activity—such as cancer, certain anemias, cardiac failure, hypertension, and respiratory problems, such as occur with emphysema—usually increase BMR. Conversely, the abnormal states of starvation and malnutrition lower BMR, because the lean body mass is diminished.

4. **Cold climate.** BMR rises in response to lower temperatures as a compensatory mechanism to main body temperature.

Food Intake Effect

Food ingestion stimulates metabolism and requires energy to meet the multiple activities of digestion, absorption, and transport of nutrients. This overall metabolic stimulation is called the **thermic effect of food (TEF).** About 10% to 15% of the body's total energy needs are used in activities related to metabolizing food.

Physical Activity Needs

Exercise involved in work and recreation or in physical training and competition accounts for wide individual variations in energy requirements (see Chapter 14). The effects of various activities on energy metabolism have been measured by the oxygen consumption method of indirect calorimetry. Some of these representative kilocalorie expenditures in various types of work and recreation are given in Table 6-1. The feelings of fatigue after periods of study are not caused by vast cerebral activity but by the various amounts of muscle tension or moving about involved. Heightened emotional states alone do not increase the metabolic activity, but they may bring additional energy needs because they involve increased muscle tension, restlessness, and agitated movements.

Total Energy Expenditure Requirements

In summary, then, the basic components of energy expenditure required during weight maintenance are (1) *resting metabolic rate (RMR),* the energy demands of the basal metabolic activity—about 70% of the total, (2) the *thermic effect of food (TEF)*—about 10% of the total, and (3) the variable requirements of *physical activity.*[5] To these factors another factor called *adaptive thermogenesis* is sometimes added. This is defined as the change in resting metabolic rate associated with adaptation to environmental stress, such as changes in dietary intake, area temperature, and emotional state.

Obesity, in the traditional sense, represents an energy imbalance resulting from an excess of energy input (fuel from food) over energy output (energy requirement or expenditure). However, investigators are increasingly recognizing a genetic-based low resting metabolic rate characteristic of an inherited obesity disorder—perhaps better termed, they suggest, *essential obesity*—approached and understood much like essential hypertension, for example.[5] On the other end of the weight disorder continuum, extreme weight loss—such as anorexia nervosa—results from a deficit of energy input under energy output or requirement (see Issues and Answers, p. 99).

Where do you stand in your own energy balance? Try estimating your own energy requirement using the

TABLE 6-1

Energy Expenditure/Hour During Various Activities*

Light activities (120-150 kcal/hr)	Light to moderate activities (150-300 kcal/hr)	Moderate activities (300-400 kcal/hr)	Heavy activities (420-600 kcal/hr)
Personal care	**Domestic work**	**Yard Work**	**Yard work**
Dressing	Ironing	Digging	Chopping wood
Shaving	Making beds	Mowing lawn (not motorized)	Digging holes
Washing	Sweeping floors	Pulling weeds	Shoveling snow
	Washing clothes		
Sitting		**Walking**	**Walking**
	Yard work		
Peeling potatoes		3½ to 4 mph on level surface	5 mph
Playing cards	Light gardening	Up and down small hills	Up stairs
Playing piano	Mowing lawn (power mower)		Up hills
Rocking		**Recreation**	Climbing
Sewing	**Light work**		
Typing		Badminton	**Recreation**
Writing	Auto repair	Ballet exercises	
	Painting	Calisthenics	Bicycling 11 to 12 mph or up and
Standing or	Shoe repair	Canoeing 4 mph	down hills
slowly moving	Store clerk	Dancing (waltz, square)	Cross-country skiing
around	Washing car	Golf (no cart)	Jogging 5 mph
		Ping-Pong	Swimming
Billiards	**Walking**	Tennis (doubles)	Tennis (singles)
		Volleyball	Waterskiing
	2 to 3 mph on level surface or down stairs		
	Recreation		
	Archery		
	Bicycling 5½ mph on level surface		
	Bowling		
	Canoeing 2½ to 3 mph		

*Energy expenditure depends on the physical fitness (that is, amount of lean body mass) of the individual and continuing of exercise. Note that some of these activities can be used as aerobic activities to promote cardiovascular fitness.

steps indicated here (see box, p. 84). Compare your estimate with your general energy needs as indicated in the RDA standards.

Body Composition: Fatness and Leanness

Body Weight vs Body Fat

Sometimes the common terms *obesity* and *overweight* are used without the necessary attention to *body composition*. It is helpful to consider first the distinct meanings and concepts embodied in each of these terms.

Obesity

As it is used in the traditional medical model, the word **obesity** is a clinical term for excess body weight, defining it in the sense of a disease. It is generally applied to a person who is 20% to 30% or more above a so-called standard weight, usually displayed in weight-height tables. These Metropolitan tables were constructed a number of years ago from information obtained from life insurance holders, largely white

middle-aged males, hardly representative of our current diverse and aging U.S. population. Thus they tell us little about particular individuals. The problem lies in defining the word *standard*. This term is usually defined in reference to average weight according to height and frame. But even this is not much help, because an average person does not really exist. Every person is individual, a unique and complex human being, and *normal* values in healthy persons vary over a relatively wide range. Age plays a large role in this variance.

obesity • Fatness; an excessive accumulation of fat in the body.

thermic effect of food • Body heat produced by food; amount of energy required to digest and absorb food and transport nutrients to the cells. This basic preparatory work accounts for about 10% of the day's total energy (kcalories) requirement.

CLINICAL APPLICATION   *Evaluate Your Own Daily Energy Requirements*

Your total energy output (in kcal) per day is the sum of your body's three uses of energy:
1. Resting metabolic rate
2. Thermic effect of food
3. Physical activity

1. Resting metabolic rate (RMR):

Use general formula: Women: 0.9 kcal/kg/hr
                                       Men: 1.0 kcal/kg/hr
Convert weight (lb) to kg: 1 kg = 2.2 lb
Multiply by formula:

RMR (kcal) = 1 (or 0.9) × kg weight × 24 (hours in day)

2. Thermic effect of food intake (TEF):

The thermic effect of food is the energy the body uses in the processes of digestion and absorption. It averages 10% of the energy in the food.

Record your food intake for one day (24 hours) and calculate approximate energy value (kcal), using either Table of Food Values in Appendix A or a simple computer program.

Find energy cost of thermic effect of food (TEF):

TEF (kcal) = 10% of total kcal in food consumed

3. Physical activity:

Estimate your general average level of physical activity.

The energy used by physical activity can be approximated as a percentage of your RMR and varies with the degree of physical activity. Use this list to select your activity level:

Average Activity Level	Energy Cost: % of RMR
Sedentary	20%
Very light	30%
Moderate	40%
Heavy	50%

Find the energy cost of your activity level:

Physical activity energy cost (kcal) = RMR × your activity %

For example, if you are sedentary (mostly sitting): RMR x 20%

4. Calculate your total energy output:

Total energy output (kcal) = RMR + TEF + physical activity

Example 1:

A woman who weighs 130 lbs (59 kg), who eats an average of 1800 kcal per day, and who has started and maintains a regular physical exercise program.

RMR	= 0.9 × 59 × 24 =	1274 kcal
TEF	= 1800 × 10% =	180 kcal
Activity = RMR × 40% =		510 kcal
Total energy output	=	**1964 kcal**

Result: This woman will lose weight. Her energy output is around 150 kcal per day greater than her food intake. Because 1 lb of body weight equals approximately 3500 kcal, she will lose about 1 lb every 20 to 30 days with the above eating and exercise routine.

Example 2:

A man who weighs 180 lbs (82 kg), who eats an average of 2700 kcal per day, and who has a sedentary lifestyle.

RMR	= 1 × 82 × 24 =	1968 kcal
TEF	= 2700 × 10% =	270 kcal
Activity = RMR × 20% =		394 kcal
Total energy output	=	**2632 kcal**

Result: This man will tend to gain weight slowly over time. What would your clinical advice be to him? ◆

Body Weight vs Body Fat

We often use the term *overweight* as a synonym for obesity. But the two terms are not interchangeable, and the distinction is important. For example, a football player in peak condition can be markedly "overweight" according to standard weight-height charts. That is, he can weigh considerably more than the "average" man of the same height, but much of his greater weight is not fat at all. In clinical usage, the term *overweight* refers to persons with body weight in excess of the weight-height standard but below the 20% excess designated as obesity. In relation to health, however, the term *over-fat* would be a more correct designation, because it refers to the percentage of excess body fat in the overall total body composition. As a result of this understanding, experts in the field of nutrition have now defined *obesity* in relation to severe obesity and its implications for health as "an excess of body *fat* frequently resulting in a significant impairment of health."[6]

Body Composition

What is critical, then, in determining a reasonable body weight is **body composition.** In relation to our concern about body weight and health, we need to know what the body composition is and how much of the body weight comes from fat and how much is from lean body mass. It is much more precise to talk in terms of *fatness* and *leanness* than overweight. When speaking of weight, we need to ask for whom, under what circumstances, and by what measures. We need to consider individual body composition and use some practical means of determining it as a guideline for planning individual care. On the basis of metabolic activity—hence energy (kilocalories) demand—and comparative size, the four-compartment model of body composition is divided into lean body mass, body fat, body water, and mineral mass—mainly bone. In this basic model, based on laboratory studies with adults, approximately 50% of the body weight is contributed by water, 25% by fat, 20% by lean body mass, and 5% by mineral mass.[7]

1. **Lean body mass (LBM).** This major body component of active fat-free cell mass largely determines the basal metabolic rate and energy and nutrient need. It changes through the life cycle and in adulthood accounts for some 30% to 65% of the total body weight. In any person it accounts for almost all of the energy requirement. When persons lose weight from changes in their diet, the loss reflects changes not only in body fat, but also in LBM. Physical activity and exercise are essential for developing and maintaining the relative LBM size.

2. **Body fat.** Gross body fat varies widely with individual degrees of fatness or leanness. These differences reflect the number and size of fat cells, the **adipocytes,** that make up the adipose tissue. In an adult man, for example, fat accounts for a range of 14% to 28% of total body weight. In a woman, it is somewhat larger, about 15% to 29% of body weight. These amounts vary with age, climate, exercise, and fitness. About half the body fat is in the subcutaneous fat layers as insulation, thus providing a useful measure—the triceps skinfold—for estimating body fat in relation to LBM (see Chapter 16).

3. **Body water.** The body water content varies with relative leanness or fatness and with age, hydration, and health status. Generally it makes up about 50% to 65% of body weight. Lean persons have a somewhat larger proportion of body water than do fat persons, because lean muscle tissue contains more water than does any other body tissue except blood.

4. **Bone.** The remaining mineral mass, largely in the skeletal structure, accounts for only about 4% to 6% of the total body weight. The major mineral component is calcium, as you would expect, which makes up about 75% of the body mineral mass in bone and other body cells and fluids.

In free-living populations, however, individuals vary widely around these body composition proportions. A number of factors influence these variances[7]:

- **Gender.** Women have more fat tissue, and men have more muscle mass.
- **Age.** Younger adults have more lean body mass and less fat than do older adults.
- **Physical exercise.** Persons physically fit from daily work and other physical activities have less fat and more relative lean body mass than do those leading sedentary lives.
- **Race.** Black women have more mineral mass than do white women.
- **Climate.** Those in cold climates have somewhat more subcutaneous fat than those in hot tropical areas to protect body temperature.
- **Weight extremes.** Obese persons have excess fat in relation to lean body mass.

Measuring Body Composition

Various indirect methods of measuring body composition have been developed. These include such classic means as water displacement (weighing under water) and measuring radioactive body emissions. Newer methods include ultrasonics, light absorption and reflection, electrical conductivity and resistance, radioactive absorption, and other research techniques.[8] In clinical practice, related estimates are made from various measurements of body circumferences and skinfold thicknesses (see Chapter 16).

Standard Weight-for-Height Measurements

Two basic approaches have been used to evaluate body weight, although each has flaws. These are (1) a general guide and (2) standard weight tables.

General Guide

A general rule of thumb in common speech and practice has been passed along for some years:

1. For men, begin with 106 lb (47.7 kg) for the first 5 ft (150 cm), then add 6 lb/in (2.7 kg/2.5 cm), plus or minus 10 lb (4.5 kg).
2. For women, begin with 100 lb (45 kg) for the first 5 ft (150 cm), then add 5 lb/in (2.25 kg/2.5 cm), plus or minus 10 lb (4.5 kg).

This calculation may have been helpful initially for individuals of average height, but not for short or tall height extremes. In addition, for many persons—especially women—unrealistically low figures are produced by this method, and it has been largely discarded.

Weight-Height Tables

Most of the standard U.S. tables, as indicated, are based on the Metropolitan Life Insurance Company's so-called ideal weight-for-height charts, derived from life expectancy data gathered by the company since the 1930s. (These tables are printed inside the back book cover for reference.) But there are problems with this information base for today's total diverse population.

---

adipocyte • A fat cell. All cell names end in the suffix *-cyte,* with the type of cell indicated by the root word to which it is added.

body composition • The relative sizes of the four basic body compartments that make up the total body: lean body mass (muscle mass), fat, water, and bone.

TABLE 6-2

Good Body Weights-for-Height for Adults, Expressed in Pounds (for Height, in Feet-Inches) and Kilograms (for Height, in Centimeters) and Related to BMI*

Height (ft-in)†	19-34 years Average weight (lb)	19-34 years Range (lb)	35 years + Average weight (lb)	35 years + Range (lb)	Centimeters	19-34 years Average weight (kg)	19-34 years Range (kg)	35 years + Average weight (kg)	35 years + Range (kg)
5′0″	112	97-128	123	108-138	152	51	44-58	55	49-62
5′1″	116	101-132	127	111-143	155	53	46-60	58	50-65
5′2″	120	104-137	131	115-148	157	54	47-62	59	52-67
5′3″	124	107-141	135	119-152	160	56	49-64	61	54-69
5′4″	128	111-146	140	122-157	163	58	51-66	64	56-72
5′5″	132	114-150	144	126-162	165	60	52-68	65	57-74
5′6″	136	118-155	148	130-167	168	62	54-71	68	59-76
5′7″	140	121-160	153	134-172	170	64	55-72	69	61-78
5′8″	144	125-164	158	138-178	173	66	57-75	72	63-81
5′9″	149	129-169	162	142-183	175	67	58-77	74	64-83
5′10″	153	132-174	167	146-188	178	70	60-79	76	67-86
5′11″	157	136-179	172	151-194	180	71	62-81	78	68-88
6′0″	162	140-184	177	155-199	183	74	64-84	80	70-90
6′1″	166	144-189	182	159-205	185	75	65-86	82	72-92
6′2″	171	148-195	187	164-210	188	78	67-88	85	74-95
6′3″	176	152-200	192	168-216	191	80	69-91	88	77-99
6′4″	180	156-205	197	173-222	193	82	71-93	89	78-101
6′5″	185	160-211	202	177-228	196	85	73-96	92	81-104
6′6″	190	164-216	208	182-234	198	86	75-98	94	82-106
					BMI (kg/m²)	22	19-25	24	21-27

Data adapted from US Department of Agriculture, US Department of Health and Human Services: Nutrition and your health: dietary guidelines for Americans, ed 3, Washington, DC, 1990, US Government Printing Office; and from Bray GA: Pathophysiology of obesity. *Am J Clin Nutr* 55:448S, 1992.

*Without clothes.

†Without shoes.

Also, investigators have found that health risks are as great—if not greater—in the thin, low-weight range as for the obese group. For example, data from the long-standing Framingham study have shown that within each age-group, extremely thin—as well as extremely fat—persons have higher mortality rates.[9] The message seems to be that persons should strive to be neither excessively overweight nor excessively underweight and that the multitude of health problems attributed to moderate amounts of overweight are unfounded.

National Research Council Tables and Body Mass Index

Other more recent height-weight tables have been developed that are more realistic for practitioners. They are based on the National Research Council data on weight and health and the dietary guidelines.[10,11] These guides, shown in Table 6-2, relate height and adult age ranges to good ranges of body weight, as well as to body mass index (BMI).[12] The BMI can be calculated as follows:

$$BMI = weight\ (kg) \div height\ (meters)^2$$

The metric conversion factors involved are (1) 1 kg equals 2.2 lb, and (2) 1 meter (m) equals 39.37 in. The desired health maintenance BMI range for adults is 20 to 25 kg/m². Health risks associated with obesity begin at about 30 kg/m². Values above 40 kg/m² indicate severe obesity.

Individual Variation

"Ideal" Weight vs Good Individual Body Weight

The basic problem with the idea of "ideal" weight, as we have seen, is that it really doesn't exist. A person's ideal body weight depends on many different factors, including age, body shape, metabolic rate, genetic makeup, gender, physical activity, among many others. Persons need varying amounts of weight and can carry different amounts of weight in good health.

Necessity of Body Fat

Some body fat is necessary to survival. This has been demonstrated in times of human starvation. Such victims die of fat loss, not protein depletion. For mere survival, men require 3% body fat and women require 12%. However, we need to do more than just stay alive. For the human race to continue, we need to be able to work and reproduce. The additional body fat carried by women has evolved to enable them to bear children. Especially for reproductive capacity, women require about 20% body fat. Menstruation—**menarche**—begins when the female body reaches a certain size or, more precisely, when the young girl's body fat reaches this critical proportion of body weight, somewhere near 20%. Approximately this amount is needed for ovulation and thus for eventual pregnancy. Most women gain body fat during pregnancy. This fat storage is important for lactation, because the production of breast milk requires energy. Usually the lactation process then brings a gradual loss of these body fat stores. Dieting during pregnancy in an attempt to avoid storing this needed body fat is extremely dangerous and leads to a low-birth-weight baby at risk for developmental difficulties.

Health Obesity, and Social Images

Obesity and Health

Many common beliefs about the relation of obesity and health conflict with data available from scientific studies.

Common Beliefs

Common folk knowledge holds that being fat is "bad for you." Also, traditional medical opinion has contended for many years that obesity is an illness and contributes to a wide number of health problems, including hyperlipidemia, carbohydrate intolerance, surgical risk, anesthesia risk, pulmonary and renal problems, pregnancy complications, diabetes, and hypertension.

Conflicting Data

Often in such broad statements the distinction is not made between moderate overweight states and massive or morbid variances. Both extremes of fatness and thinness pose medical problems. The major issue relates to the effect of degrees of general overweight in the population and requires closer study. For example, recent studies of the Framingham data show clear health risks in *extreme* obesity, but unless a person is at least 30% *overfat*, the relationship of weight to mortality is questionable.[13]

Specific Health Implications

These data, however, might obscure important health implications of obesity. A recent National Institutes of Health (NIH) consensus development conference of experts identified adverse effects of obesity on health in three main areas[6]:

1. **Hypertension, hypercholesterolemia, and diabetes.** Experts agree that evidence indicates a strong association between obesity and the three health problems of essential hypertension, elevated serum cholesterol levels, and non–insulin-dependent diabetes mellitus (NIDDM), although the association varies directly with the extent of the obesity and is reversible with weight reduction.[14,15] BMI values at or above 27.8 for men and 27.3 for women (the 85th percentile level), especially for young adults aged 20

to 44, carry the greatest risk. There is a genetic factor in each of these chronic conditions. Thus early intervention in developing health habits in diet and exercise to maintain optimal weight, especially for children in families at high risk, is important.

2. **Coronary heart disease (CHD).** Although the evidence was not as strong, the NIH panel agreed that sufficient long-term data from the classic Framingham study shows association of degree of obesity with CHD, independent of other risk factors.[16] In any event, the primary conditions of hypertension, elevated blood cholesterol, and NIDDM are strong risk factors for CHD, thus linking obesity indirectly to CHD.

3. **Cancer.** Evidence indicates strong associations between some types of cancer with dietary fat and obesity.[17] These data show that obese men, regardless of smoking habits, had a higher mortality from cancer of the colon, rectum, and prostate. Obese women had a higher mortality from cancer of the breast (postmenopausal), uterus (including cervix and endometrium), and ovaries, as well as the gallbladder and biliary passages.

Social Images: Fear of Fatness and Eating Disorders

The Thinness Model

A model of thinness, especially directed toward women, pervades American society. Fueled by capital investment in New York City's Madison Avenue advertising, successful use of an exaggerated image of thinness has been the drive for marketing many products. The "ideal" woman has been remade in the eyes of America. The gaunt, almost cadaverous models adorning the covers of many glamor magazines seem to mock most women's attempts to feel good about themselves and their bodies. In many instances, these social pressures have created a fear of fatness that leads to a persistent pursuit of the abnormal thin ideal marketed constantly in the media.[18] These fears of fatness develop early among young girls. A recent survey of weight-related behaviors among fourth-grade 9-year-old children indicated that 60.3% of the girls wanted to be thinner, but about the same number of boys (67.2%) wanted only to be taller.[19] In another survey of middle-class children aged 9 to 18 in a senior high school and its two feeder middle-class schools, the fear of fatness has already begun to cause disordered eating, restraint, and binging in young girls—up to 46% of 9-year-olds and up to 81% of 10-year-olds.[20]

---

menarche • The beginning of first menstruation with the onset of puberty.

Evolutionary Conflict and Social Pressure

This extreme degree of thinness now popular in America, however, goes against evolutionary body wisdom. It took the human species thousands of centuries to evolve the greater fat-carrying capacity of women for reproductive purposes. The largely futile and often dangerous attempts to lower body weight drastically have damaged the self-image of many women and men alike. Strong prejudice exists against obese persons, regardless of their age, gender, race, or socioeconomic status. But some people, try as they might, simply cannot and do not lose weight, or they live "yo-yo" lives of perpetual ups and downs of weight—an even greater threat to their physical and emotional health.[21,22] They do not and cannot conform to the social norms, no matter how hard they try, and are somehow blamed for their condition. Many people see fat people as (1) *gluttonous*—they eat more than they should, (2) *lazy*—if they wanted to, they could lose weight, (3) *neurotic*—they have an oral fixation caused by arrested development during childhood, or (4) *unhappy*—they eat because they are depressed. Many studies of comparative behavior have shown no evidence for any of these stereotyped beliefs about overweight persons.

Eating Disorders

Unfortunately, in some extreme cases, this obesssion with thinness has led to serious distortion of body image and eating disorders.

1. **Anorexia nervosa,** a form of self-induced starvation, has reached alarming proportions among adolescent girls. They become terrified of gaining weight and refuse to eat, even though they may be hungry. They often perceive themselves to be "fat," "gross," and "ugly," even though they are severely underweight or emaciated. This condition can become life-threatening, inducing malnutrition and requiring hospitalization (see Issues and Answers, p. 99). A small percentage of these young victims eventually die from this disorder.
2. **Bulimia nervosa,** a gorging-purging syndrome, also creates both emotional and physical problems. It is increasingly common among young women. Some estimate that as many as 20% of college women engage in bulimic behavior. In a sense, a bulimic person is a "failed anorectic" one. Unable to go without eating, these persons engage in the practice of gorging themselves with large amounts of food and subsequently purging themselves, usually by induced vomiting.

The Problem of Weight Management

How does a person go about losing excess weight, or more correctly, excess fat? Simple, you say—just reverse the process by which it was gained. Everybody knows that on the energy balance sheet, when energy taken in does not equal energy expended, the difference is reflected in weight either stored or lost. And 3500 kcal is the equivalent of 0.45 kg (1 lb) of body fat. That is part of the answer, but it is not altogether quite that simple, as you shall see.

Individual Variances
Energy Balance Factors

Keeping a weight balance score in such arithmetic terms is not that easy. First, it's difficult to know *precisely* how many kilocalories are in the food you are eating. Second, it's even more difficult to know how many kilocalories you are burning up. This depends on your basal metabolic activity, the resting metabolic rate and thermic effect of food, body size, amount of lean body mass, age, gender, and physical activity, among other things.

Metabolic Efficiency

Some persons have proclaimed for years, "It's not fair! She can eat twice as much as I can and never gains an ounce." The medical rejoiner has been, until recently, "She gets more exercise than you do." That may be true in some cases, but not all. Recent work indicates that some people do metabolize food more easily than others, whereas in others a low metabolic rate—especially a low thermic effect of food (see p. 82)—contributes to their overweight state.[23]

Extreme Approaches

For such lazy, weak-willed, and morally inferior creatures, as some deride them, overweight persons endure rather incredible experiences in their constant struggle to lose weight, including some of the following.

Fad Diets

A constant array of various "diet books" flood the American market. They usually sell briefly and then fade away, largely because their "quick fix" does not work. Moreover, nutritional science finds itself caught in the "diet wars" because there are no magic, simple answers to a far more complex problem. Most of the fad diets fail on two counts: (1) they are based on scientific inaccuracies and misinformation; hence they are often nutritionally inadequate, and (2) they do not address the basic behavioral problem involved in life-long food and exercise habit change, actually a new life-style, required to maintain a healthy weight for a given individual once it is achieved. For some persons the degree of kilocaloric restriction required places impossible demands and they find themselves caught in the **chronic dieting syndrome,** with its harmful physical and psychologic effects.[22] To conform to society's thinness values, they are often consigned to a lifetime battle against biologic mechanisms that operate within their bodies to return them to their natural, or metabolic set-point, weight—a high price for false hope.[24] They often become caught up in our burgeoning U.S. diet industry, where it is estimated that in 1995 $51 billion will be spent on a wide range of weight loss diets, products, and services.[25]

Fasting

This drastic approach takes many forms, from literal fasting to use of very-low-calorie diets of special formulas. Effects may be those of semi-starvation: acidosis, postural hypotension, increase in urinary loss of important electrolytes, increase in serum uric acid, constipation, and a decrease in basal metabolic rate (BMR). In past use of such extreme practices, there has been sufficient loss of heart muscle to cause death.[26] And, at best, more recent programs have failed in the critical period after initial weight loss to help persons maintain the new weight when refeeding began.[27,28]

Special Clothing and Body Wraps

Special "sauna suits" are claimed to help weight loss in specific spots of the body or to help clear up so-called "cellulite" tissue. To the scientific community, "spot reduction" is a fabrication, as is "cellulite," which is a word coined some years ago in Europe by a "beauty operator" and has no factual basis. This mummylike wrapping is endured by some persons in an attempt to reduce body size. What small weight loss may result is usually caused by temporary water loss. The only way to lose weight is to metabolize more kilocalories than are consumed.

Drugs

The amphetamines, commonly called "speed," were once popular in the treatment of obesity. They are no longer used because of their danger to health. An over-the-counter drug available now is *phenylpropanolamine (PPD)* (Dexatrim), a stimulant similar to amphetamine. However, the disordered metabolism of severe obesity and its high risk in chronic disease has renewed medical interest in drug research for its treatment. Initial studies are producing several experimental agents that act on hunger-satiety brain centers, **serotonin** neurotransmitters, or hormonal metabolism regulators.[29]

Surgery

Surgical intervention is usually reserved for medical treatment of severely obese persons after more traditional methods have failed. They include earlier procedures such as intestinal bypass, which resulted in serious side effects and is no longer used. Current procedures focus on gastric bypass, including several forms of gastroplasty (Fig. 6-3), but these surgeries are not without problems and require skilled team management, including nutritional care.[30,31]

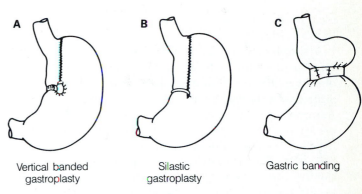

Vertical banded gastroplasty / Silastic gastroplasty / Gastric banding

FIG. 6-3 Simple gastric-restriction procedures for treatment of obesity in order of frequency in current practice: **A,** Vertical banded gastroplasty—50%. **B,** Silastic ring gastroplasty—5%. **C,** Gastric banding—4%. More complex procedures that bypass part of the digestive tract are reserved for treating severe massive obesity. (*Adapted from Grace DM: Gastric restriction procedures for treating severe obesity.* Am J Clin Nutr 55:556S, 1992 and Mason EE and others: *Perioperative risks and safety of surgery for severe obesity,* Am J Clin Nutr *55:573S, 1992.*)

A more limited type of cosmetic surgery, developed in the 1980s and still in current vogue, is a form of local fat removal, lipectomy, commonly called *liposuction.* It is used to remove fat deposits under the skin in places of cosmetic or figure concern, such as the hip and thigh areas. A thin tube is inserted through a small incision in the skin and a desired amount of the fat deposit is suctioned away. However, this procedure is quite painful and carries risks of infection, large disfiguring skin depressions, or blood clots that lead to dangerous circulatory problems and possible kidney failure. Any sur-

---

anorexia nervosa • Extreme psychophysiologic aversion to food, resulting in life-threatening weight loss. A psychiatric eating disorder caused by a morbid fear of fatness, in which the person's distorted body image is reflected as fat when the body is actually malnourished and extremely thin from self-starvation.

bulimia nervosa • A psychiatric eating disorder related to the person's fear of fatness, in which cycles of gorging on large quantities of food are followed by self-induced vomiting and use of diuretics and laxatives to maintain a "normal" body weight.

chronic dieting syndrome • A compulsive eating disorder, commonly referred to as **compulsive overeating**. It includes binge eating episodes, but without the purging behavior of persons with bulimia nervosa. This is an emotional, reactive eating pattern occurring in response to stress or anxiety and used to soothe painful feelings.

serotonin • A neurotransmitter in the brain that effectively suppresses appetite and heavy eating.

gical procedure carries risk and may cause other problems as side effects.

A simpler, noninvasive, less costly procedure developed in the mid-1980s as an alternative to surgery for obesity is the insertion of a gastric balloon.[32] However, gastrointestinal problems caused the Food and Drug Administration to recall it from the market. Researchers are now developing new polymers for its restructuring that are better tolerated and simpler to remove, before it is returned to the market for treating severe obesity. In this procedure, a small cylindric sac is inserted into the stomach through a tube, then inflated and the tube removed. The free-floating balloon, about the shape and size of a small juice can, remains to give a feeling of fullness and reduce food intake. It is not a permanent fixture and can be removed at intervals and replaced as needed.

Types and Causes of Obesity

Theories about the cause of obesity have varied in recent years. The prior simplistic terms *exogenous* (external cause) and *endogenous* (internal cause) are too vague to be useful and have been discarded. Rapidly developing research, however, is providing better knowledge of the types and causes of various obesities, which is gradually dispelling some of the long-standing social myths and prejudices about obesity. We are beginning to understand that there are different forms of obesity, which vary in extent, body distribution, and underlying genetic-metabolic factors.[33] This knowledge provides a more realistic individual approach to care. Four basic factors may be identified: genetic-metabolic, psychologic, social, and physiologic.

Genetic-metabolic Factors

There is increasing evidence that familial tendencies probably influence a person's chances of becoming fat more than any other basic factor. A genetic base may regulate differences in body fat, including gender variances. Only recently, studies have confirmed that gene-controlled low resting metabolic rate (RMR) is a contributor to obesity, not a result, and that adaptive thermic effect of food (TEF) has genetic influences.[5,23,33] It has been shown that the semistarvation of rigorous dieting reduces the RMR even further as an adaptive response to the dietary restriction. Further validation studies on the metabolic set-point for adipocyte or total body fat that predisposes an individual for a particular natural weight level are continuing.[33]

Family studies covering several generations, as well as studies of identical and fraternal twins reared apart and of adopted children, also indicate a strong heritability factor in obesity. Although the family and environment influence food habits and attitudes, in the adoption studies the children reflect weight patterns of their biologic parents, not of their adoptive parents.[34,35] In addition, current ongoing studies of the heart disease-lipid link in three generations of a large Midwestern family suggest a genetic basis for obesity through the metabolic role of the human lipoprotein lipase (LPL) gene, the molecular biology of which has been understood only since 1986.[36] Investigators indicate that a possible defect in the LPL gene contributes to obesity, because of the central role of LPL in breaking down fats to be either stored or used as fuel. These results further reinforce that there is a genetic link to obesity, as indicated by many other studies in both animals and humans. In the model of other genetic diseases, eventual distinction is made between obesities that arise from genetic-metabolic defects and those which result from overeating. An increasing number of researchers and clinicians in the field are concluding that we are dealing with different obesities with different causes and characteristics, indicating different approaches to treatment.[33,37] In fact a recent survey of physicians and scientists involved in obesity research in North America, Europe, and the United Kingdom indicated that genetic factors were considered important areas of study overall.[38] Of course, overweight is not *strictly* a genetic condition, but in some persons this factor may well relate to food habits learned over time, as other factors discussed here indicate.

Psychologic Factors

The public perceives fat persons as having less control over their appetites and as being more responsive to external cues than to internal ones. That is, some believe obese persons eat (1) when it's mealtime by the clock or when they're surrounded by tasty foods, instead of when they're really hungry, (2) when they're unhappy, or (3) because as children they associated food with maternal love. It is true that reactive eating from stress or anxiety contributes to obesity.[39] However, these factors cannot be applied to *all* fat persons as a group. They have no more tendency to these actions and feelings than anyone else. But there is no question about the role that psychology must play in any weight management program. Our cultural ideal thin body type and social discrimination against obese persons have created psychologic problems in many individuals that must be addressed. Psychosocial support—in the form of a counselor, a support group, friends, or family—is critical for a successful weight management program.[40]

Social Factors

The class values placed on the obese state by different social groups also influence its frequency. As a person moves upward in social class, there is a tendency to be more highly motivated to maintain a moderate or normal body weight. In lower socioeconomic status groups, obesity is more common and considered normal. In higher-level groups, greater social value is usually placed on the nonobese state. The length of exposure to these values and their pressure on individuals in any social class determine reaction to them. Other social and environmental factors associated with obesity include cultural and family food patterns, job environments and recreational eating that encourage use of kilocalorie-dense foods, the social role of eating, the sedentary patterns of recreation and employment, and television viewing time with its inactivity and constant snacking.

Physiologic Factors

Normal physiology during the growth years contributes to the accumulation of fat tissue deposits. There are critical periods during growth for the development of obesity, such as early childhood and early stages of puberty. Early and middle adulthood are other potential periods, because of reduced physical activity with no adjustment of caloric intake. For women other times may be during pregnancy and after menopause, resulting from hormonal changes. For men a critical period is early to middle adulthood, generally due to decreasing activity with no change in food habits formed during adolescence, when the body has high energy needs. Both men and women tend to gain weight after age 50 because of the lower resting metabolic rate (RMR), decreased physical exercise, and failure to adjust food habits accordingly.

A significant physiologic factor in obesity is fat cell increase. Normally, the full genetic complement of fat cells is reached by puberty and then remains constant.[33] After puberty, these fat cells may increase in mass within limits, rarely exceeding about 1.5 µg, but not usually in number. However, if overeating continues after the fat cells have reached their maximal capacity, cell proliferation is triggered again. Once this increased cell number has occurred, it cannot be reversed. In extreme obesity, for example, the number of fat cells may increase from a norm of about 30 billion to approximately 120 billion, each one of which is also increased in size. The only means of weight reduction then is to diminish individual cell size. Once the body has added fat cells to accommodate extra fuel storage, these cells remain and store varying amounts of fat. A similar harmful pattern of increased fat storage occurs in individuals whose natural metabolic setpoint for body weight is higher than cultural ideals of thinness when they respond to unrealistic weight goals and constant diets. Hunger and frustration are inevitable, and rebound overeating follows in a repeated cycling of weight loss and regain in the chronic dieting syndrome.

Increased fat cell formation also affects body fat distribution. A form of localized fat cell increase occurs in women over the lower body areas of thighs and hips,

called *gynecoid*—or lower body—obesity. This form of obesity is benign and unrelated to the metabolic complications of obesity. However, a second type of central abdominal fat deposit—called *android,* because it is the usual pattern of adult male fat distribution—is a typical pattern that also occurs in women and is associated with metabolic complications, such as non–insulin-dependent diabetes mellitus (NIDDM) in males and females.

The Health Model: A Positive Personal Approach

General Components

Healthful, successful, and lasting weight management occurs through combined wisdom from nutritional and behavioral research. A well-balanced, individually tailored food plan, together with a gradually increased exercise program and supportive behavioral change measures, can be effective and personally rewarding. In health care practice the general approach to weight management is based on underlying sound nutrition and energy balance and the client's personal situational needs. It focuses on two main aspects: (1) motivation and support and (2) a personalized program.

Motivation and Support

The degree of personal motivation is a prime factor. Through initial interviews, the nutrition counselor—usually a specially trained registered dietitian (RD)—seeks to determine individual needs, attitudes toward food and weight, and the meaning food has for the client. Recognition is given to emotional factors involved, and support is provided by the nutritionist—together with the nurse and the physician—to meet the client's particular needs.

Personal Program

To be successful, a weight-management program must meet personal needs and goals. Such a program has some form of the following parts:

1. **Food behaviors.** Note the quantity of food served and eaten. Use moderate to small portions, attractively served. Take time to eat *slowly* and savor the food taste and texture. Reduce hidden factors added in food preparation, mainly fat. Increase fiber content. Use a variety of food choices from a basic food guide, which serves as a focus for sound realistic nutrition education. Emphasize whole primary foods and a minimum of processed foods. Plan a fairly even food distribution throughout the day.
2. **Exercise behaviors.** Plan a regular daily exercise schedule. Start with walking, building to a brisk aerobic pace, for about a half hour a day. Aerobic exercise benefits a person in a weight-management program because it (1) lowers the body-weight set-

point, (2) suppresses appetite, (3) reduces body fat, (4) increases basal metabolic rate, (5) increases energy expenditure, and (6) retains and builds LBM levels. Thus gradually increase the time of the exercise period to 45 to 60 minutes, and add other activities that can have aerobic value, such as swimming, or develop a set of body exercises, including stretching, body and muscle development, aerobic periods, and a cool-down period. Set occasional goals and keep a record of progress. Use variety in your program and enjoy it.

3. **Stress-reduction exercises.** Practice progressive muscle relaxation and stress-reduction exercises (see Chapter 15). Learn an appropriate pattern as a guide, using imagery as a mental focusing devise, or use tapes or environmental recordings if they are helpful. Select a suitable time and stay with it for daily practice. Start with a brief 10-minute period and increase as desired.

4. **Personal interest area.** Develop some creative interest area for intellectual stimulation, personal enjoyment, and fulfillment. Explore various community groups or resources to support such activities.

5. **Follow-up program.** A follow-up schedule of appointments with the nutrition counselor is then outlined, and its values are discussed with the client. On subsequent visits, progress can be reviewed, problems discussed, and solutions to them mutually explored. Continuing support can be provided. Practical suggestions for dealing with such things as realistic goals, food and exercise behaviors, meals at home and away from home, and any other special situations can be discussed. This follow-up support helps the client anticipate needs, reinforce new learnings, avoid pitfalls, sustain motivation, and deal positively with periods of frustration.

Behavioral Aspects

Behavioral change in respect to food and exercise is an important component of long-term weight management. It requires family, individual, or group support. Experienced and sensitive practitioners in health care settings recognize increasingly the need to provide ongoing training and support for the obese client, both individually and in peer support groups, to modify undesirable food behaviors and lack of physical activity that may have contributed to the obesity, if long-range success is to be achieved. Food behavior particularly is rooted in many human experiences and associations and environmental situations. These experiences often produce addictive forms of eating responses. Behavior-oriented therapies are designed to help the person change food, eating, and exercise patterns that contribute to the excessive fat and weight. These strategies help to increase insight, awareness, and understanding of present behaviors; to motivate toward positive

change; and to recondition behaviors into new ones to meet personal goals. When the person changes associations with the undesirable habit patterns, he or she can then plan a means of constructive action. Supportive behavioral change activities are directed toward (1) management of eating behavior—the when, what, why, where, how, and how much, and (2) promotion of physical activity and increased energy output, providing a better total energy balance, as well as an added means of reducing stress.

Principles of a Sound Food Plan

On the basis of careful interviewing, body composition measures, and evaluation of available laboratory data, the nutritionist makes a comprehensive assessment of nutritional and health status, food and physical activity habits and behaviors, and living situation. Details for such full assessment are described in Chapter 16. Then, on the basis of this individual assessment, personal needs and goals can be established with the client. An appropriate food plan is developed together to meet normal nutritional needs and any necessary therapeutic modification for health problems that are present. Such a personal plan has several basic parts.

Energy Balance

The energy intake level (kilocalories) is adjusted to meet individual weight-management needs. A moderate normal eating pattern is outlined. This gradual process is best for long-term success and health. On the average, for women, a sound plan for energy needs is based on about 1200 to 1500 kcal/day. For larger women and for men, a plan of about 1500 to 1800 kcal/day would meet gradual weight adjustment energy needs. It may be helpful to some persons to determine what their basal and activity needs are as a basis for understanding their overall energy expenditure factors (Table 6-3). Examples of several weight-management guides, using the exchange system food value listings, are given in Table 6-4 for general focus on a regular meal pattern. The exchange food lists are given in Appendix K.

Nutrient Balance

Basic energy nutrients are outlined to achieve the following nutrient balance:

1. **Carbohydrate.** About 50% to 55% of total kilocalories, with emphasis on complex forms, such as starches with fiber, and moderation of sugars

2. **Protein.** Approximately 20% of total kilocalories, with emphasis on lean food choices and small portions to curtail fat

3. **Fat.** About 25% to 30% of total kilocalories, with emphasis on plant fats, scant use, and alternate seasonings

TABLE 6-3

General Approximations for Daily Adult Basal and Activity Needs

Basal energy needs (avg. 1 kcal/kg/hr)	Male (70 kg) kcal 70 × 24 = 1680	Female (58 kg) kcal 58 × 24 = 1392
Activity energy needs		
Very sedentary + 20% basal	1680 + 336 = 2016	1392 + 278 = 1670
Sedentary +30% basal	1680 + 504 = 2184	1392 + 418 = 1810
Moderately active +40% basal	1680 + 672 = 2352	1392 + 557 = 1949
Very active + 50% basal	1680 + 840 = 2520	1392 + 696 = 2088

TABLE 6-4

Weight Reduction Food Plans Using the Exchange System of Dietary Control* (Total Kilocalorie Distribution: 50% Carbohydrate, 20% Protein, 30% Fat)

Food Exchange Groups	1200 kcal	1500 kcal	1800 kcal
Total number exchanges/day			
Milk (nonfat)	2	2	2
Vegetable	3	4	4
Fruit	3	4	4
Bread	5	7	9
Meat	4	5	7
Fat	4	5	5
Meal pattern of food exchanges			
Breakfast			
Fruit	1	1	1
Meat		1	1
Bread	1	2	2
Fat	1	1	1
Milk	½	½	½
Lunch/supper			
Meat	1	1	2
Vegetable	1	2	2
Bread	2	2	3
Fat	1	2	2
Fruit	1	1	1
Milk	½	½	½
Dinner			
Meat	2	2	3
Vegetable	2	2	2
Bread	1	2	3
Fat	2	2	2
Fruit		1	1
Milk	½	½	½
Snack (afternoon or evening)			
Milk	½	½	½
Meat	1	1	1
Bread	1	1	1
Fruit	1	1	1

*See food exchange lists, Appendix K.

In general, this nutrient balance approximates the recommendations of the U.S. Dietary Guidelines for Healthy Americans. Review these guidelines in Chapter 1. They are helpful as a good basic nutrition education tool.

Distribution Balance

Spread food fairly evenly through the day to meet energy needs. Consider any daily "problem times" and plan simple snacks to meet such needs.

Food Guide

Use some type of general food reference lists from which the client can make a variety of food choices to fulfill the basic food plan. The food exchange system provides such a guide (see box, p. 94). This system provides a good general reference guide for comparative food values and portions, variety in food choices, and basic meal planning. Food items can easily be combined into desired dishes. To control fat in food preparation, use alternate seasonings, such as herbs and spices, onion and garlic, lemon juice, vinegar, wine, fat-free broth, mustard, and other condiments.

Personal Needs

Individual Adaptations

Throughout the planning, remember to focus on the individual client and personal needs. If the plan is unrealistic, whatever its form or basis, it will not be followed. Some persons find it helpful to keep a daily journal, which can include notes of food intake, environmental food cues, feelings, physical symptoms, and any stress factors related to food behavior. It may also include notes about other activities, such as physical exercise or stress-reduction practice. A periodic review of such notes may help in making general observations, determining problem areas, monitoring progress, and gaining insights for setting personal goals to achieve desired health and fitness behavior changes. Essential parts of all programs are nutrition counseling and education—especially in reducing total fat, ongoing support for behavioral change, and increased physical activity.

Currently in the United States, there is a healthy growing awareness among health professionals, their clients, and the public in general that the modern phenomenon of constant restrictive "dieting" and the U.S. diet industry is counterproductive and harmful in the long run to many persons, especially to overweight women whose natural body weight levels do not conform to society's thinness model.[21,41,42] As a result, health professionals are developing alternative ap-

Food Guide: The Exchange System of Dietary Management

TO PROBE FURTHER

The exchange system of dietary management, developed by two professional organizations—the American Dietetic Association and the American Diabetes Association—is based on the concept of nutritional equivalency. Thus its basic food lists are simple groupings of common foods according to their generally equivalent nutritional values. This system may be used for any situation requiring a balance of the energy nutrient foods—carbohydrates, fats, and proteins.

The foods are divided into six basic groups (with subgroups), called the "exchange lists." Each food item within a group or subgroup contains about the same food value as other food items in that group, allowing for exchange within groups, and thereby providing for variety in food choices, as well as food value control. Hence the term *food exchanges* is sometimes used to refer to food choices or servings.

The total number of "exchanges" per day depends on individual nutritional needs, based on normal nutritional standards. Although the composition of foods within each exchange group varies somewhat, the following energy and nutrient values are used for simplicity. The full listings of foods in each exchange group is given in Appendix K. Note how these food listings may be used as a reference, along with current nutrient values on food product labels, for controlling a particular nutrient, such as grams of fat consumed each day.

Exchange Lists

Food Groups	Carbohydrate (g)	Protein (g)	Fat (g)	Kilocalories
Starch or bread	15	3	trace	80
Meat				
Lean	—	7	3	55
Medium-fat	—	7	5	75
High-fat	—	7	8	100
Vegetable	5	2	—	25
Fruit	15	—	—	60
Milk				
Skimmed	12	8	trace	90
Low-fat	12	8	5	120
Whole	12	8	8	150
Fat	—	—	5	45

From Franz MJ and others: Exchange lists: revised 1986, *J Am Diet Assoc* 87(1):28, 1987.

---

proaches, based on a health and fitness model, for persons who benefit from a more supportive gradual plan with emphasis on exercise and small gradual diet changes focused first on fat. Such health and fitness models provide needed help with positive behavioral changes through ongoing supportive counseling and peer group support.

Preventive Approach

In the last analysis, it seems that the most constructive work in weight management is aimed at *prevention*. Early nutrition education, positive food and fitness behavior, and habit formation in the family—with support and guidance for young parents and children before an obese condition develops—will help prevent many problems in later adulthood.

The Problem of Underweight

We have discussed at length the major problem of excess weight. But conversely, what about the state of less-than-adequate weight? Excluding the self-imposed eating disorders of anorexia nervosa and bulimia nervosa, what dangers lie in being generally underweight? What are some of its causes and approaches to treatment?

Definition

Extremes of underweight, just as in overweight, bring or accompany serious health problems. Although general underweight is a less common problem in the American population than is overweight, it does occur in a small percentage—estimated at somewhat less than 10%—among persons who have trouble gaining and maintaining weight.[41] Such persons seem to lack control over how much they eat at a meal and reach a full feeling with less food than do persons of normal weight. The underweight condition may be associated with poverty, poor living conditions, or long-term disease. A person with more than 10% below the average weight for height and age is considered underweight; 20% or more is cause for concern. Serious problems may result in these persons, especially young children who may suffer long-term growth retardation or failure to thrive. Resistance to infection is lowered, general health is poor, malnutrition develops, and strength is reduced.

General Causes

In general, underweight is associated with conditions that cause basic malnutrition, such as the following:

- **Wasting disease.** Long-term hypermetabolic disease, such as cancer or short- or long-term infection and fever, place metabolic demands on the body that drain the body's resources.
- **Poor food intake.** Diminished food intake results from physiologic causes suggested before or from other situations, such as (1) psychologic factors that cause a person to refuse to eat, (2) loss of appetite or imbalance in the brain's hunger-satiety centers, or (3) personal poverty and limited food supply.
- **Malabsorption.** Poor nutrient absorption results from (1) prolonged diarrhea, (2) gastrointestinal disease, or (3) abuse of laxatives.
- **Hormonal imbalance.** Hyperthyroidism or other abnormalities may increase the needs of the body.
- **Energy imbalance.** Greatly increased physical activity without a corresponding increase in food brings an energy balance deficit.
- **Poor living situation.** An unhealthful home environment or no home at all results in irregular and inadequate meals, or in some persons, an indifferent or defeated attitude toward food.

Nutritional Care

Underweight persons require special nutritional care to rebuild their body tissues and nutrient stores and regain their health. Any food plan needs to be adapted for each person's unique situation, whether it involves personal or economic needs, living situation, or underlying disease. The dietary goal, according to each person's tolerance, is to increase energy and nutrient intake in a diet that is (1) high-calorie, at least 50% above standard needs, (2) high-protein, to rebuild tissue, (3) high-carbohydrate, to provide a primary energy source in easily digested form, (4) moderate-fat, to add kilocalories but not exceed toleration limits, and (5) a good source of all the vitamins and minerals, including individual supplements when deficiencies require them. Good food of wide variety, well-prepared and seasoned and attractively presented, helps revive lagging appetites and increases the desire to eat. Frequent small nourishing meals and snacks spread through the day, including favorite foods, stimulate interest in eating and increase optimal use of foods and their nutrients. To achieve the desired increase in kilocalories, use (1) food seasonings, such as margarine or butter, sauces, and dressings, and (2) a food supplement such as Ensure (Ross) to add kilocalories and key nutrients.

A basic aim is to help build the best food habits possible, within any limitations that may exist, so that the improved nutritional status and weight can be maintained once it is regained. This rehabilitation process requires much creative counseling with each individual and family, with attention to the underlying socioeconomic or disease conditions. Practical personal guides and ongoing support are needed to counteract root causes of the malnutrition. In some extreme cases, tube feeding or total parenteral nutrition (TPN) may be necessary (see Chapter 18).

To Sum Up

Energy is that force or power that enables the body to maintain its life-sustaining metabolic work, as well as all its physical work and activity. The energy provided by food is measured in *kilocalories* or *joules*. Body energy cycles among various basic forms, such as chemical, electric, mechanical, and thermal. *Metabolism* is the body's way of changing the chemical energy of food into these cycling forms of body energy according to body needs. When food is not available, the body draws on its own stores to meet energy needs: glycogen from carbohydrate stores, fatty acids from fat tissue, and amino acids from lean body mass.

Total energy needs are based on basal (maintenance) and nonbasal (exercise) requirements. The *basal metabolic rate (BMR)*—or the currently used term *resting metabolic rate (RMR)*, the amount of energy required to maintain the body at rest after a 12-hour fast—and the added total effect of food (TEF) comprise the body's metabolic energy needs, with variable needs for work and other physical activities. The four main compartments of body composition are lean body mass, body fat, body water, and mineral mass. Body composition is measured by a number of methods developed for research, population surveys, and clinical practice.

Body weight has traditionally been used as an indicator of obesity, which raises the risk of health problems. But it is the *composition* of the weight, lean vs fat tissue, that is the most important aspect. Weight-management programs have traditionally been designed for obese persons. However, a growing modern obsession with thinness has created new weight-management problems—the development of the *chronic dieting syndrome,* which leads to ever-increasing cycles of dieting and regaining and decreasing self-esteem, as well as fostering eating disorders that result in semi-starvation.

In general, the health and fitness model of weight management is based on personal motivation and support for the individual. Aspects of such a program include changing food attitudes and behaviors, increasing physical activity, learning and practicing relaxation techniques, and developing personal interests. Behavioral strategies, with counselor and group support, help the individual examine the effect of life situations on eating habits and change those situations that encourage overeating. According to individual needs, sound weight management is based on adjusted energy level, mainly in decreasing fat and increasing exercise, that allows for (1) gradual small-to-moderate rates of loss, or in some instances a more healthful holding pattern that recognizes individual natural weight levels, (2) sound nutrition, and (3) support for food and exercise behavior changes. The ideal plan begins with prevention, stressing positive food habits and physical fitness from early childhood to help prevent major problems later in life.

The opposite problem of underweight also brings food problems. It results from physiologic, psychosocial, economic, or disease causes. A nutrient and energy-rich diet supplied through multiple small meals is needed, with ongoing counseling to help with the underlying causes and rehabilitation process.

QUESTIONS FOR REVIEW

1. What does the term *fuel factor* mean? What is this comparative factor for each of the energy-yielding nutrients?
2. Define *resting metabolic rate.* What factors influence this rate? Which body tissues contribute most of the body's basal metabolic needs and what approximate percentage of the total energy expenditure do these internal basal metabolic activities require?
3. What factors influence nonbasal energy needs?
4. Calculate your own energy balance for 1 day based on your energy input (food) and your energy output (RMR + TEF + physical activity). (See box, p. 84.)
5. Describe three major eating disorders associated with America's growing obsession with thinness. What social factors contribute to this obsession? Compare these with the factors that contribute to the growing tendency of overweight.
6. Discuss the safety of five popular means of trying to lose weight.
7. Describe four basic types of causes of obesity.
8. Describe five components of the "health model" for weight management. How does it differ from the traditional medical model?
9. What are the basic principles of a sound food-exercise plan for weight-management programs?
10. List some ways of increasing energy intake for an underweight person.

REFERENCES

1. Guyton AC: *Textbook of medical physiology,* ed 8, Philadelphia, 1991, WB Saunders.
2. Poehlman ET and others: The impact of exercise and diet restriction on daily energy expenditure, *Sports Med* 11:78, 1991.
3. Berke EM and others: Resting metabolic rate and the influence of the pretesting environment, *Am J Clin Nutr* 55:626, 1992.
4. Hill JO and others: Nutrient balance in humans: effects of diet composition, *Am J Clin Nutr* 54:10, 1991.
5. Ravussin E, Bogardus C: A brief overview of human energy metabolism and its relationship to essential obesity, *Am J Clin Nutr* 55:242S, 1992.
6. Burton BT, Foster WR: Health implications of obesity: an NIH consensus development conference, *J Am Diet Assoc* 85(9):1117, 1985.
7. Heymsfield SB, Waki M: Body composition in humans: advances in the development of multicompartment chemical models, *Nutr Rev* 49(4):97, 1991.
8. Jenson MD: Research techniques for body composition assessment, *J Am Diet Assoc* 92(4):454, 1992.
9. Kannel WB, Gordon T: Physiological and medical concomitants of obesity: the Framingham study. In Bray GA, editor: *Obesity in America,* Department of Health, Education, and Welfare, Pub No (NIH) 79-359, Washington, DC, 1979, US Government Printing Office.
10. Food and Nutrition Board, Committee on Diet and Health, National Academy of Science—National Research Council: *Diet and health: implications for reducing chronic disease risk,* Washington, DC, 1989, National Academy Press.
11. US Department of Agriculture, US Department of Health and Human Services: *Nutrition and your health: dietary guidelines for Americans,* Home and Garden Bulletin No 232, ed 3, Washington, DC, 1990, US Government Printing Office.
12. Bray GA: Pathophysiology of obesity, *Am J Clin Nutr* 55:488S, 1992.
13. Lissner L and others: Variability of body weight and health outcomes in the Framingham population, *N Engl J Med* 324:1839, 1991.
14. Dustan HP: Obesity and hypertension, *Diabetes Care* 14(6):488, 1991.
15. Haffner SM and others: Greater influence of central distribution of adipose tissue on incidence of non-insulin-dependent diabetes in women than in men, *Am J Clin Nutr* 53:1312, 1991.
16. Hubert HB and others: Obesity as an independent risk factor for cardiovascular disease: a 26-year follow-up of participants in the Framingham Heart Study, *Circulation* 67:968, 1993.
17. Wynder EL: Primary prevention of cancer: planning and policy considerations, *J Natl Cancer Inst* 83(7):475, 1991.
18. Czajka-Narins DM, Perham ES: Fear of fat: attitudes toward obesity, *Nutr Today* 25(1):26, 1990.
19. Gustafson-Larson AM, Terry RD: Weight-related behaviors and concerns of fourth-grade children, *J Am Diet Assoc* 92(7):818, 1992.
20. Mellin LM and others: Prevalence of distorted eating: a survey of middle-class children, *J Am Diet Assoc* 92(7):851, 1992.

21. Berdanier CD, McIntosh MK: Weight loss–weight regain: a vicious cycle, *Nutr Today* 20(5):6, 1991.

22. Grodner M: "Forever dieting": chronic dieting syndrome, *J Nutr Educ* 24(4):207, 1992.

23. Nelson KM and others: Effect of weight reduction on resting energy expenditure, substrate utilization, and the thermic effect of food in moderately obese women, *Am J Clin Nutr* 55:924, 1992.

24. Wooley SC, Garner DM: Obesity treatment: the high cost of false hope, *J Am Diet Assoc* 91(10):1248, 1991.

25. Begley CE: Government should strengthen regulation in the weight loss industry, *J Am Diet Assoc* 91(10):1255, 1991.

26. Report: Survey of very-low-calorie weight reduction diets, *Arch Intern Med* 143(7):1423, 1983.

27. Legislative highlights: ADA testifies on very-low-calorie diets before the Subcommittee on Regulation, Business Opportunities, and Energy, *J Am Diet Assoc* 90(5):722, 1990.

28. Position of the American Dietetic Association: Very-low-calorie weight loss diets, *J Am Diet Assoc* 90(5):722, 1990.

29. Bray GA: Drug treatment for obesity, *Am J Clin Nutr* 55:538S, 1992.

30. Forse A and others: Morbid obesity: weighing treatment options—surgical intervention, *Nutr Today* 24(5):10, 1989.

31. Kral JG: Overview of surgical techniques for treating obesity, *Am J Clin Nutr* 55:552S, 1992.

32. Morrow SR, Mona IK: Effect of gastric balloons on nutrient intake and weight loss in obese subjects, *J Am Diet Assoc* 90(5):717, 1990.

33. Willard MD: Obesity: types and treatments, *Am Fam Physician* 43(6):2099, 1991.

34. Stunkard AJ and others: An adoption study of human obesity, *N Engl J Med* 314:193, 1986.

35. Berdanier CR: You are what you inherit, *Nutr Today* 21(5):18, 1986.

36. Goldsmith MF: Heart disease researchers tailor new theories—now maybe it's genes that make people fat, *JAMA* 263(1):17, 1990.

37. Bouchard C: Heredity and the path to overweight and obesity, *Med Sci Sports Exerc* 23(3):285, 1991.

38. Bray GA and others: A survey of the opinions of dietary experts on the causes and treatment of obesity, *Am J Clin Nutr* 55:151S, 1992.

39. Ganley RM: Emotions and eating: a review of the literature, *Int J Eating Disord* 8:343, 1989.

40. Hart J and others: The importance of family support in a behavior modification weight loss program, *J Am Diet Assoc* 90(9):1270, 1990.

41. Goodrick GK, Foreyt JP: Why treatments for obesity don't last, *J Am Diet Assoc* 91(10):1243, 1991.

42. Foreyt JP, Goodrick GK: Weight management without dieting, *Nutr Today* 28(2):4, 1993.

43. Underweight people bear a heavy burden, too, *Tufts University Diet and Nutrition Letter* 6(3):7, 1988.

FURTHER READING

American Dietetic Association: *The healthy weight: a practical food guide*, Chicago, 1992, The Association.

This new food guide from the ADA explains why popular diets often fail and provides a plan for a healthy weight.

Czajka-Narins DM, Parham ES: Fear of fat: attitudes toward obesity, *Nutr Today* 25(1):26, 1990

Wooley SC, Garner DM: Obesity treatment: the high cost of false hope, *J Am Diet Assoc* 91(10):1248, 1991.

These authors, nutritionists and clinical psychologists, give us sensitive views of the psychologic burden many naturally overweight persons bear from the social stigma and false presumptions attached to obesity in America and the many failing attempts to conform to the impossible thin ideal.

Berdanier CD, McIntosh MK: Weight loss–weight regain: a vicious cycle, *Nutr Today* 26(5):6, 1991.

Foreyt JP, Goodrick GK: *Living without dieting*, Houston, 1992, Harrison House.

Foreyt JP, Goodrick GK: Weight management without dieting, *Nutr Today* 28(2):4, 1993.

Perri MG and others: *Improving the long-term management of obesity: theory, research, and clinical guidelines*, New York, 1992, John Wiley & Sons.

These authors are all involved in the frontiers of research and practice in the evolving directions of a positive health and fitness approach to realistic weight management without the repeated dieting cycles. They provide ample background and guidelines for developing such a program.

CASE STUDY

The Obese Patient with Hypertension

Rosanna Giovanni is a 45-year-old woman, mother of three children, first seen in the clinic 6 months ago for a routine checkup. At that time she weighed 90 kg (200 lb) and had a blood pressure reading of 152/88 mm Hg. She is 155 cm (5 ft 2 in) tall. At the initial visit she had no serious complaints other than a bad cold. Her physician warned her that her blood pressure was somewhat elevated and scheduled a return visit for another reading the following week. After two more readings of 160/95 and 155/89 mm Hg consecutively, Mrs. Giovanni was told that she had hypertension. No medication was prescribed. However, she was referred to the nutritionist to begin weight-management and sodium-control programs.

During the assessment interview the clinic nutritionist discovered that Mrs. Giovanni ate two meals at home and one at work. Breakfast usually consisted of scraps of food left on plates by her school-age children. Lunch was a hot meal with dessert purchased in the cafeteria of the hospital where she worked part-time as an admissions clerk. Dinner was almost always an Italian-style meal, often including pasta with rich sauces and cheese or filled with meat, plus a variety of vegetables and salads. Desserts, usually made from scratch, were served with every dinner.

Mrs. Giovanni was very interested in gradually losing some weight to avoid taking antihypertensive medication, if possible. However, she was apprehensive about the possibility of having to give up her favorite foods to do so. The nutritionist reassured her. With Mrs. Giovanni, the nutritionist helped with a food preparation plan to reduce fat and salt by using a number of alternative seasonings in the family recipes. Then she arranged for Mrs. Giovanni to join one of the clinic's peer support groups where she could learn some stress-reduction exercises and new ways of looking at food.

Three months later Mrs. Giovanni had lost 8 kg (18 lbs). She reported feeling much better and said her family was very supportive of her efforts. As a result of new cooking methods, her overweight husband had finally started to lose weight as well. She continued to lose an average of 0.7 kg (1.4 lb) per week for another month, but suddenly she gained 2.5 kg (5 lb) in a 2-week period. At a nutrition interview conducted shortly after that time, she revealed that her husband had recently been hospitalized with a stroke. Apparently he also had hypertension but had refused to see a physician for many years. The effects of the stroke were very mild; however, Mrs. Giovanni continued to worry about her husband's health. She began to eat desserts with lunch again and kept nuts, candies, and other snack foods at home for "nibbling." The nutritionist provided personal support in the office and suggested adding exercise to the routine as a good form of stress management and weight control. Mrs. Giovanni resisted the idea at first, saying that she could not fit it into her current schedule of caring for three children and her husband and working part-time at the hospital. However, after bringing the subject up in her weight-management group meeting, she gained positive feedback and practical ideas for fitting some aerobic activities into her busy schedule.

During the next 3 months, Mrs. Giovanni resumed her previous weight-loss pattern and began to feel better. The exercise routine had also helped her to look better and to feel better about herself. She informed the nutritionist that, aside from her appearance, she is most proud of the effect of her healthful diet program on her family. Her children have reduced their junk food intake, and her husband has even begun exercising with her almost every day.

Questions For Analysis

1. How do you think Mrs. Giovanni's life-style, meal pattern, food habits, and food preparation methods influenced her weight status?
2. What is hypertension? What role does weight management play in controlling it? Why did Mrs. Giovanni's physician recommend nondrug methods of control through diet?
3. In developing a meal plan with Mrs. Giovanni, what advice would you offer to help her retain the cultural flavor of her meals while reducing her kilocalorie intake?
4. What are some ways that Mrs. Giovanni may strengthen her behavioral changes toward food and exercise? What other behavioral approaches may be useful?
5. What is aerobic exercise? Why is it effective for a weight-management program?
6. What practical suggestions would you offer to Mrs. Giovanni for helping her incorporate exercise time into her busy routine? Why?

"Bean lean, slender as the night, narrow as an arrow, pencil thin, get the point?" So reads the clever advertising copy of a well-known New York fashion house, one of many such Madison Avenue reflections of our American culture's obsession with thinness, especially for women. Many of these women are paying a heavy price in physical and psychologic illness from eating disorders.

America's developing thinness drive

This obsessive cultural drive for thinness is, in fact, a comparatively recent social phenomenon in the American experience. At the beginning of the 1900s, the skinny woman would have been seen as awkward, unsightly, perhaps piteously at risk for disease, and certainly not a standard of beauty. Even in the 1950s, Marilyn Monroe's hourglass figure would have been considered overweight by today's standards. Then in the 1960s, the fashion world discovered a model named "Twiggy" from her small, straight-as-a-stick, little-girl figure. The thinner form became the ideal, and fashions were developed based on her thin type of body shape. But Twiggy was *naturally* thin, and many naturally moderate-weight women could reach that ideal only by becoming *unnaturally* thin through constant dieting. Thus the trend to be acceptable by reshaping the body through weight loss and restrained eating became entrenched, fueled by a growing diet industry, the profits of which made its purveyors willing partners. This trend strengthened through the 1970s and 1980s. Now in the 1990s, the model form is somewhat more "athletic" in appearance but still thin, so women must add workouts to dieting to meet society's ideals. The notion is perpetuated that personal worth and self-esteem derive from how we look rather than who we are.

General nature and extent of thinness pressure and disordered eating

The drive for thinness is now appearing even in very young girls early in their initial grade school social experiences. In one recent survey among nine-year-olds in the fourth grade, for example, a majority of the girls were already saying that they wanted to be thinner and were beginning to restrict normal eating of foods they labeled as "bad." By the high school years, the pressure to be thin intensifies. Adolescents learn early, even before puberty and its rapid growth effects, that thinness in women and athletic leanness and muscle development in men are major cultural criteria for determining attractiveness and social acceptability. Unfortunately, however, many soon learn that it is difficult to meet these standards because genetic inheritance plays a major role in determining body size and shape. They also find themselves in a double bind with the inactivity and snacking that attends watching television. Dieting may appear an attractive tool to offset these effects and reshape their bodies, including such practices

as fasting, low-energy–deficit diets, heavy workouts, purging behavior such as induced vomiting, and the use of laxatives, diuretics, and diet pills. An increasing number of girls and boys, especially those in wrestling and body-building activity, practice such on and off cycles of dieting and purging to accomplish this body reshaping. Students are waving red flags for eating problems, such as preoccupation with food and body weight, inappropriate body image, and reluctance to eat.

Researchers studying eating disorders tell us that the percentage of persons with eating problems is increasing and that this is a true increase and not just a factor of increased reporting. Most scientific evidence indicates that both biologic and psychosocial factors are involved, especially impaired family communication patterns. Eating moderately to maintain a natural weight level is perfectly healthful and promotes wellness of mind and body. For some individuals, however, who are sensitive to family and social pressures about acceptably thin body weight and labels of "good" and "bad" food, dieting begins to serve other purposes of achieving acceptance and a sense of self-worth. This pattern of chronic restrictive dieting has been strongly related to the development of eating disorders, in which feelings about self and body image are projected to food. Eating, then, becomes fueled by emotional rather than actual physiologic needs. Two forms of such eating disorders, *anorexia nervosa* and *bulimia nervosa,* have been recognized by the American Psychiatric Association (APA) and described in its current guide for mental health professionals, the *Diagnostic and Statistical Manual for Mental Disorders,* third edition, revised *(DSM III-R).* A third eating disorder now being described for the fourth edition is the problem of compulsive overeating related to the *chronic dieting syndrome.* Each has distinctive characteristics, based on the APA's diagnostic criteria and symptoms.

Anorexia nervosa

The eating disorder anorexia nervosa—"appetite loss from nervous disease"—is actually misnamed. It is starvation with excessive weight loss, self-imposed at great physical and psychologic cost. Through their distorted body image, those with anorexia nervosa do not see themselves as underweight and emaciated but as always fat, and they continue to restrict their eating in ritualistic ways. Anorexia nervosa affects about 1% of young women, but its dangerous path can lead to sudden death from severe hypoglycemia and cardiac arrest. Significant deficits of bone mass occur as a frequent and often early complication of anorexia nervosa in adolescence, so that osteoporosis and bone fractures have become a "new morbidity" for dieting adolescent girls.

Diagnostic criteria. *DSM III-R* describes the following states as diagnostic for anorexia nervosa:
1. Refusal to eat sufficient food to maintain body weight over a minimal normal weight for age and height—for example, weight loss leading to maintenance of body weight 15% below that expected, or failure to make expected weight gain during a pe-

riod of growth, leading to body weight 15% below that expected

2. Intense fear of gaining weight or becoming fat, even though underweight
3. Disturbance in the way in which one's body weight, size, or shape is experienced—for example, the person claims to "feel fat" even when emaciated, believes that one area of the body is "too fat" even when obviously underweight
4. In females, absence of at least three consecutive menstrual cycles when otherwise expected to occur

Bulimia nervosa

Bulimia, literally "ox-hunger," is descriptive of the massive amounts of food sometimes consumed and has been called the binge and purge syndrome. Because the person is eating, though in a disorderly manner, a fairly normal weight level is usually maintained and the underlying problem is a guilt-ridden secret. Control is lost when eating, and extremely large amounts of food are consumed. Then in response the individual attempts to purge the body from the effects of the large amount of food by self-induced vomiting, fasting, excessive exercise, or the use of laxatives, diuretics, or diet pills. The emotional and physical cost of maintaining such disordered behavior is great.

Diagnostic criteria. The *DSM III-R* describes specific behavioral criteria for bulimia nervosa and the psychologic and physical effects:
1. Recurrent episodes of binge eating—rapid consumption of a large amount of food in a single, relatively short time
2. A feeling of loss of control over eating behavior during the binges
3. Regular self-induced vomiting, use of laxatives or diuretics, strict dieting or fasting, or vigorous exercise to prevent weight gain
4. Minimal average of two binge eating episodes a week for at least 3 months
5. Persistent overconcern with body shape and weight

Compulsive overeating

This newly developed third eating disorder, commonly referred to as compulsive overeating, includes binge eating episodes without the purging behavior of persons with bulimia nervosa. This reactive type of eating occurs in response to stress or anxiety as an emotional eating pattern to soothe or relieve painful feelings. The binges may be triggered in part by physiologic factors. Dietary restriction and failure to achieve satiety precede binges and probably help drive them in a cyclic pattern.

The chronic dieting syndrome fueled by our cultural drive for thinness contributes to this compulsive eating disorder. Persons who attempt to reach these unrealistic, and for them unnatural, weight goals are "forever dieting" and inevitably experience hunger and frustration. Rebound eating, or binging, usually occurs, followed by more attempts to lose weight, creating the characteristic weight cycling with its physiologic effects compounding the psychologic problem. With each successive weight loss, the resting metabolic rate (RMR) drops more quickly; thus the weight comes off with greater difficulty. Evidence now suggests that lean body mass lost with such dieting cycles may not be recovered with each regain in weight, thus altering body composition. Even if the final weight achieved is in a so-called normal range, the increased percentage of body fat can cause abnormalities, creating the "metabolically obese" individual of normal weight.

Treatment approaches

Eating disorders take a high toll in both physical and psychologic health of many adolescent girls and young women and require individualized care. First, the best chances for success in improving their condition lies with team care by a sensitive, experienced group of health professionals, including a physician, clinical psychologist, clinical nutritionist, and nurse. Outpatient care may provide needed care for less serious cases of bulimia nervosa, but often for life-threatening anorexia nervosa, more intense inpatient care is essential. Second, with an individualized approach, especially for bulimia nervosa, a "stepped-care" program at five levels of intervention may provide appropriate options. At least five levels may be used: (1) some form of self-help with written material, (2) nutrition and diet education and counseling—individual or group, (3) antidepressant drug therapy in combination with counseling and support, (4) individual outpatient psychologic treatment, including cognitive behavior therapy, and (5) period of day patient or inpatient care, with follow-up outpatient care.

These are serious health matters. How long are we willing to pay this heavy price for distorted societal images of personal worth based on how we look instead of who we are? Change in any area is difficult, but it rests on a foundation of awareness and knowledge of the problem. Then changes in attitude can come. Only then will we see a weakening of America's drive for thinness and its feeding of serious eating disorders. Certainly we need to seek more ethical practices in our own work, as well as reforms in the diet industry. More realistic individualized approaches to help persons with weight and health will follow and will help to reduce the risks for serious eating disorders.

REFERENCES

Czajka-Narins DM, Parham ES: Fear of fat: attitudes toward obesity, *Nutr Today* 25(1):26, 1990.

Fairburn CG, Peveler RC: Bulimia nervosa and a stepped care approach to management, *Gut* 31:1220, 1990.

Grodner M: *The psychology of eating disorders*, Nutri-News, 1991, Mosby–Year Book.

Grodner M: "Forever dieting": chronic dieting syndrome, *J Nutr Educ* 24(4):207, 1992.

Lustig A: Weight loss programs: failing to meet ethical standards? *J Am Diet Assoc* 91(10):1252, 1991.

Willard MD: Obesity: types and treatments, *Am Fam Physician* 43(6):2099, 1991.

Wooley SC: Obesity treatment: the high cost of false hope, *J Am Diet Assoc* 91(10):1248, 1991.

Vitamins

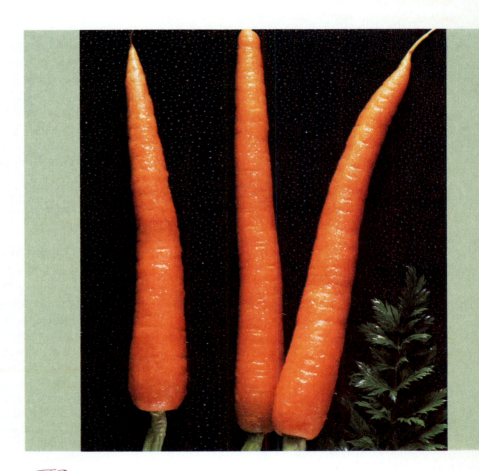

Here we begin a two-chapter sequence on the non–energy-yielding micronutrients: the vitamins and minerals. First we look at the vitamins.

Probably no other group of nutritional elements has so captured the interest of scientists, health professionals, and the general public as has the vitamin group. Attitudes toward vitamins have varied widely, running the gamut from wise functional use to wild flagrant abuse.

In this chapter we will review both fat- and water-soluble vitamins. We will focus on why we need them and how we may obtain them.

The Study of Vitamins

General Nature and Classification

During the five decades of vitamin discovery in the first half of the 1900s, the remarkable nature of these vital agents became more and more apparent. Three key characteristics were evident: (1) they were not metabolized to yield energy as were the energy nutrients carbohydrate, fat, and sometimes protein; (2) they were vital to life; and (3) often not a single substance but a group of related substances turned out to have the particular metabolic activity. The name *vitamin* developed during initial research years when one of the early scientists working with a nitrogen-containing chemical substance called an **amine** thought that this was the common nature of these vital agents. So he named his discovery *vitamine* (vital amine). Later the final *e* was dropped when other similarly vital substances turned out to be a variety of organic compounds. The name vitamin has been retained to designate compounds of this class of essential substances. At first letter names were given to individual vitamins discovered. But as the number of them increased rapidly, this practice created confusion. So in recent years more specific names based on structure or function have developed. Today these scientific names are preferred and commonly used.

Definition of a Vitamin

As the vitamins were discovered one by one and the list of them grew, two basic characteristics clearly emerged to define a compound as a vitamin:

1. It must be a vital organic dietary substance that is not an energy-producing carbohydrate, fat, or protein, and is usually necessary in only very small quantities to perform a particular metabolic function or to prevent an associated deficiency disease.

2. It cannot be manufactured by the body and therefore must be supplied in food.

Classification

Vitamins are usually grouped and distinguished according to their solubility in either fat or water.

Fat Soluble

The fat-soluble vitamins are A, D, E, and K. They are closely associated with lipids in their fate in the body. They can be stored, and their functions are generally related to structural activities.

Water Soluble

The water-soluble vitamins are C and the B-complex family. These have fewer problems in absorption and transport. They cannot be stored except in the general tissue saturation sense. The B vitamins function mainly as coenzyme factors in cell metabolism. Vitamin C is a vital structural agent.

Current Concepts and Key Questions

To clarify current concepts concerning each known vitamin, consider these key questions as basis for your study:

Nature: What is the vitamin's general structural nature?

Absorption and transport: How does the body handle this particular vitamin?

Function: What does this vitamin do? This is perhaps the most significant question.

Requirement and sources: How much of this vitamin do we need and where can we obtain it?

Here, then, we will briefly review each of the vitamins in turn—four fat-soluble (A, D, E, K) and nine water-soluble (C and B vitamins). In each case we will identify the specific chemical name, a more common usage now, and review answers to the key questions above. In some cases, a group of similar substances have the vitamin activity, not just the single substance bearing the specific name.

FAT-SOLUBLE VITAMINS

Vitamin A

Chemical and Physical Nature

Vitamin A is a generic term for a group of compounds having similar biologic activity. These compounds include **retinol, retinal,** and retinoic acid. The term *retinoids* refers to both the natural forms of retinol and its synthetic copies. Chemically, retinol is a primary alcohol of high molecular weight ($C_{20}H_{29}OH$). Because it has a specific function in the retina of the eye and is an alcohol, vitamin A has been given the specific chemical name *retinol*. It is soluble in fat and in ordinary fat solvents. Because it is insoluble in water, it is fairly stable in cooking.

Forms

1. *Preformed vitamin A: retinol.* This is the natural form of vitamin A, found only in animal food sources and usually associated with fats. Vitamin A compounds are deposited primarily in the liver but also in small amounts in the kidneys, lungs, and fat tissue. In this form, its dietary sources are mainly the fat portion of dairy products, egg yolk, and storage organs such as liver.

2. *Provitamin A: beta-carotene.* This is the original substance, the provitamin A behind the animal sources of vitamin A itself, in plants that animals have eaten and converted to the vitamin. This original plant source is beta-carotene ($C_{40}H_{56}$), which is found in plant pigments. It is called carotene because one of its main

sources is the yellow pigment of carrots. Beta-carotene is significant in human nutrition and is the common precursor of vitamin A. It supplies about two thirds of the vitamin A necessary in human nutrition.

Absorption and Storage
Substances That Aid Absorption

Vitamin A enters the body as the preformed vitamin A from animal sources and as the precursor carotene from plant sources. Several substances aid in the absorption of vitamin A and carotene by the body.

Bile salts. With fat and other fat-related compounds, bile transports vitamin A in micelles, minute fat globules formed in the small intestine after initial digestion and then carried into the intestinal wall for further preparation. Clinical conditions affecting the biliary system, such as obstruction of the bile ducts, infectious hepatitis, and liver cirrhosis, hinder vitamin A absorption.

Pancreatic lipase. This fat-splitting enzyme is necessary for initial hydrolysis in the upper small intestine of fat emulsions or oil solutions of the vitamin. Water-based preparations of retinol are available for use in conditions where secretion or absorption of pancreatic lipase is curtailed, such as in cystic fibrosis or pancreatitis.[1]

Dietary fat. Some fat in the food mix, simultaneously absorbed, stimulates bile release for effective absorption of vitamin A.

Carotene Conversion

In the intestinal wall during absorption some of the carotene is converted to vitamin A. The remainder is absorbed and transported as such, dissolved in the fat part of lipoproteins.

Transport and Storage

The route of absorption of both vitamin A and carotene parallels that of fat. In the intestinal mucosa all the retinol, from both natural preformed animal sources and from plant carotene conversion, is incorporated into the chylomicrons. In this form it enters the blood stream via the lymphatic system and is carried to the liver for storage and distribution to the cells. The liver, by far the most efficient storage organ for vitamin A, contains about 90% of the body's total quantity. This amount is sufficient to supply the body's needs for about 6 to 12 months, and some persons have been known to store as much as a 4-year supply. These stores are reduced, however, during infectious disease, especially in childhood infections such as measles. For example, among malnourished nonimmunized children in many parts of the world, measles has become a lead-

ing killer disease and is now designated by the WHO Expanded Program on Immunization as a target for both vitamin A supplementation and immunization.[2,3] Age is also a factor in absorption. For example, in the newborn, especially the premature infant, absorption is poor. With advancing age, elderly persons may experience increasing difficulties with absorption.[4] In addition, chronic use of mineral oil as a laxative hinders vitamin A absorption.

Functions of Vitamin A

Vitamin A's role in visual adaptation to light and dark has been well established. It also has a number of more generalized functions that influence vision, the health of body coverings and linings (epithelial tissue), the process of growth, antioxidant capacity, and reproductive functions.

Vision

The eye's ability to adapt to changes in light depends on a light-sensitive pigment—rhodopsin, commonly known as visual purple—in the rods of the retina (Fig. 7-1). Rhodopsin is composed of the vitamin A substance retinal and the protein opsin (Fig. 7-2). When the body is deficient in vitamin A, the normal rhodopsin cannot be made and the rods and cones of the retina become increasingly sensitive to light changes, causing **night blindness.** This condition can usually be cured in about 30 minutes by an injection of vitamin A (retinol), which is readily converted into retinal and then into rhodopsin.

Epithelial Tissue

Vitamin A is necessary to build and maintain healthy epithelial tissue, which provides our primary barrier to

---

amine • An organic compound containing nitrogen. There are many different amine organic compounds.

night blindness • Inability to see well at night in diminished light, resulting from lack of required vitamin A.

retinal • Organic compound that is the aldehyde form of retinol, derived by the enzymatic splitting of absorbed carotene. It performs vitamin A activity. In the retina of the eye, retinal combines with opsins to form visual pigments. In the rods it combines with scotopsin to form rhodopsin (visual purple). In the cones it combines with photopsin to form the three pigments responsible for color vision.

retinol • Chemical name for vitamin A derived from its function relating to the retina of the eye and light-dark adaptation. Daily RDA standards are stated in retinol equivalents (RE) to account for sources of the preformed vitamin A and its precursor provitamin A, beta-carotene.

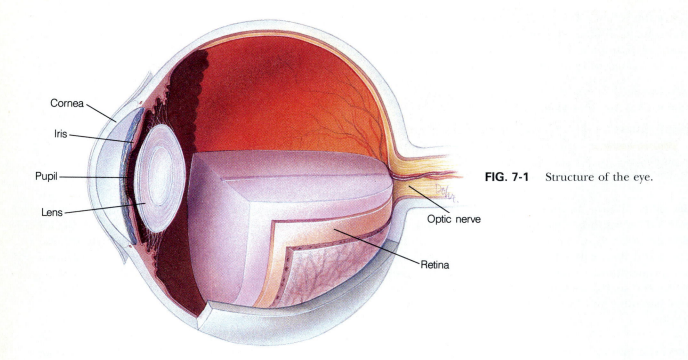

FIG. 7-1   Structure of the eye.

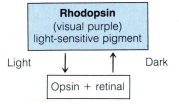

FIG. 7-2   The vision cycle: light-dark adaptation role of vitamin A.

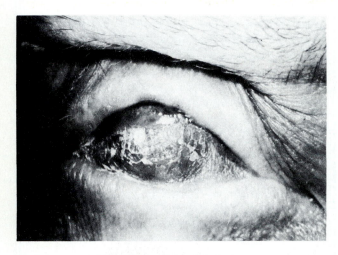

FIG. 7-3   Xerophthalmia.

infections. The epithelium includes not only the outer skin but also the inner mucous membranes. This function of vitamin A is the basis for current study of retinoids and carotene in relation to cancers of epithelial origin (see Issues and Answers, p. 132).

Without vitamin A, the epithelial cells become dry and flat. They gradually harden to form keratin, a process called **keratinization.** Keratin is a protein that forms dry, scalelike tissue, normal in the case of nails and hair but abnormal in the case of skin and mucosale membranes. When the body is deficient in vitamin A, many such abnormal epithelial tissue changes may occur.

1. *Eye.* The cornea dries and hardens, a condition called xerophthalmia (Fig. 7-3). In extreme deficiency the process may progress to blindness. This progressive blindness resulting from vitamin A deficiency is a serious public health problem; it affects the health and sight of a staggering number of persons in many parts of the world.[5] The tear ducts dry, robbing the eye of its cleansing and lubricating means, and infection follows easily.

2. *Respiratory tract.* Ciliated epithelium in the nasal passages dries and the cilia are lost, thus removing a barrier to entry of infection. The salivary glands dry, and the mouth becomes dry and cracked, open to invading organisms.

3. *Gastrointestinal tract.* Mucosal membrane secretions decrease so that tissues dry and slough off, affecting digestion and absorption.

4. *Genitourinary tract.* As epithelial tissue breaks down, problems such as urinary tract infections, calculi, and vaginal infections increase.

5. *Skin.* As skin becomes dry and scaly, small pustules

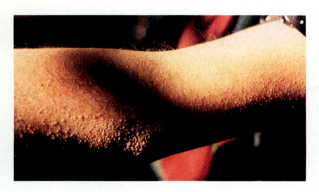

FIG. 7-4   Follicular hyperkeratosis caused by vitamin A deficiency. *(From files of Therapeutic Notes, Parke, Davis & Co, Detroit, Mich; courtesy Dr. Orson D. Bird.)*

or hardened, pigmented, papular eruptions appear around hair follicles, a condition called *follicular hyperkeratosis* (Fig. 7-4).

6. *Tooth formation.* Specific epithelial cells surrounding tooth buds in fetal gum tissue that normally become specialized cup-shaped organs called *ameloblasts* may not develop properly. These little organs form the enamel of the developing tooth.

Growth

Vitamin A is essential for the growth of bones and soft tissues. This effect is probably caused by the vitamin's influence on protein synthesis, mitosis (cell division), or stability of cell membranes. Growth and maintenance of bone require constant remodeling of the bone tissue according to growth and repair needs. To accomplish this constant reshaping and balance task, continuous growth of new bone and removal of old bone must occur. Vitamin A participates in the important job of tunneling out old bone to make way for new bone; the tunnels are filled in to accommodate growth needs, all the while maintaining the precise pattern set in the initial embryonic cartilage model.

Antioxidant Capacity

The provitamin A, beta-carotene, has been shown to have **antioxidant** capacity, raising interest in its ability to protect persons as they grow older from cell damage caused by free radicals.[6] The free radicals are parts of compounds that are by-products of normal metabolism in cells, or they may be created by environmental exposure to sunlight, tobacco smoke, car exhaust fumes, ozone, or x rays. In any case, free radicals damage the DNA, cell membranes, and cell compounds, or kill the cell outright. These accumulative effects advance the aging process of cell deterioration. Antioxidant substances help to neutralize free radicals in the cell, protecting those persons susceptible to such oxidative stress.

Reproduction

The retinoids, except for retinoic acid, are necessary to support normal sexual maturation during adolescence and function of the adult reproductive system.[7] Vitamin A deficiency causes glandular degeneration and sterility.

Vitamin A Requirement
Influencing Factors

A number of variables modify vitamin A needs. Although the vitamin is generally ample in most diets, many factors may alter need in a given individual: (1) the amount stored in the liver, (2) the form in which it is taken (carotene or vitamin A), (3) illness, and (4) gastrointestinal or hepatic defects. Vitamin A deficiency may occur due to: (1) inadequate dietary intake, (2) poor absorption due to lack of bile or defective absorbing surface, and (3) inadequate conversion of carotene because of liver or intestinal disease.

Units of Measure

To cover such variables, the RDA standard recommends a margin of safety above minimal needs. Traditionally, vitamin A has been measured in international units (IU). Currently, the RDA uses the measure of **retinol equivalents (RE)**. These RDA standards are printed inside this book's covers for quick reference, with footnotes giving the weight equivalents for retinol and beta-carotene. The RE provides a more accurate measure because it accounts for individual absorption and conversion variances. All other countries and international agencies have also adopted the RE measure.

Hypervitaminosis A

Because the liver can store large amounts of vitamin A, and many persons take additional megadose supplements, it is clearly possible to consume a potentially toxic quantity. Hypervitaminosis A is manifested by joint pain, thickening of long bones, loss of hair, and jaundice. Excess vitamin A may also cause liver injury with resulting portal hypertension and ascites.

---

antioxidant • A substance that inhibits oxidation of polyunsaturated fatty acids and formation of free radicals in the cells.

keratinization • The process of creating the protein *keratin*, which is the principal constituent of skin, hair, nails, horny tissues, and the organizing matrix of the enamel of the teeth. It is a very insoluble protein.

retinol equivalent (RE) • Unit of measure for dietary sources of vitamin A, both preformed vitamin, retinol, and the precursor provitamin, beta-carotene. 1 RE = 1 μg retinol or 6 μg beta-carotene.

TABLE 7-1

Food Sources of Vitamin A (RDA for Adults: Women, 800 μg RE; Men, 1000 μg RE)

	Quantity	Vitamin A (μg RE)
Bread, cereal, rice, pasta		
This food group is not an important source of vitamin A.		
Vegetables		
Asparagus	½ cup	196
Beet greens	½ cup	1110
Bok choy cabbage	½ cup	790
Broccoli (fresh)	1 med stalk	1350
Broccoli (frozen)	½ cup (chopped)	721
Brussels sprouts	½ cup (4 sprouts)	121
Carrots (raw)	½ cup (1 med)	2379
Collard greens	½ cup	2223
Corn	1 sm cob	93
Dandelion greens	½ cup	1843
Green beans	½ cup	102
Green peas	½ cup	144
Kale	½ cup	1369
Lima beans	½ cup	60
Mustard greens	½ cup	1218
Pumpkin (canned)	½ cup	2352
Romaine lettuce	½ cup (chopped)	157
Spinach	½ cup	2187
Summer squash	½ cup	123
Sweet potato (baked, in skin)	1 med	2769
Tomato (cooked)	½ cup	325
Winter squash	½ cup	1021
Fruits		
Apricot (dried)	4 halves	490
Apricot (fresh)	3 med	867
Avocado	1 med	189
Banana	1 med	69
Cantaloupe	¼ med	1386
Grapefruit (pink)	½ med	162
Orange juice	½ cup	75
Papaya	1 cup (cubes)	735
Peach	1 med	399
Prunes (dried)	4 prunes	207
Tangerine	1 med	108
Watermelon	1 wedge (4 × 8 in)	753
Meat, poultry, fish, dry beans, eggs, nuts		
Clams (canned)	3 oz	144
Egg, whole	1 large	78
Liver, beef	3.5 oz	10,831
Liver, chicken	3.5 oz	4912
Salmon, pink (raw)	3 oz	30
Milk, dairy products		
Cheddar cheese	1 oz	90
Milk, lowfat 2% (fortified)	8 fl oz	150
Milk, skim (fortified)	8 fl oz	150
Milk, whole (unfortified)	8 fl oz	101
Ricotta cheese, whole milk	½ cup	182
Swiss cheese	1 oz	72
Yogurt, whole	8 fl oz	84
Fats, oils, sugar		
Butter	1 tbsp	138
Margarine	1 tbsp	141

Food Sources of Vitamin A

There are few animal sources of natural preformed vitamin A: liver, kidney, cream, butter, and egg yolk. Our main dietary sources are the yellow and green vegetable and fruit sources of carotene. In addition, commercial products such as margarine are fortified with vitamin A. The vitamin A values of selected foods are given in Table 7-1.

Vitamin D

Chemical and Physical Nature

Early investigators wrongly classed this substance as a vitamin. But it is now clear that it is really a prohormone of a sterol type and in its active form is viewed as a hormone. The precursor base in human skin is the lipid cholesterol material **7-dehydrocholesterol.** Thus all forms of these compounds with vitamin D activity are soluble in fat but not in water. They are heat stable and are not easily oxidized.

Forms

Two compounds with vitamin D activity are involved in nutrition: *ergocalciferol (vitamin D_2)* and *cholecalciferol (vitamin D_3).* Vitamin D_2 is formed by irradiating ergosterol (provitamin D_2), which is found in ergot (a fungus growth on rye and other cereal grains) and yeast. The much more significant product in human nutrition is D_3, **cholecalciferol,** which is formed by irradiating 7-dehydrocholesterol (provitamin D_3) in the skin. D_3 occurs also in fish liver oils.

Absorption, Transport, and Storage

Absorption

The absorption of dietary vitamin D_3 occurs in the small intestine with the aid of bile. It mixes with the intestinal bile-fat complex and is absorbed in these fat packets. Malabsorption diseases such as celiac syndrome, colitis, and Crohn disease hinder vitamin D absorption.

Active Hormone Synthesis

The synthesis of the active hormonal form of *1,25-dihydroxycholecalciferol [1,25 $(OH)_2$ D_3]* is accomplished by the combined action of skin, liver, and kidneys, an overall process now called the vitamin D endocrine system.

Skin.   In the skin, 7-dehydrocholesterol, the precursor cholesterol compound, is irradiated by the sun's ultraviolet rays to produce vitamin D_3. The amount of D_3 produced by this irradiation in the skin depends on a number of variables, including length and intensity of sunlight exposure and color of the skin (see box, p. 107). For example, heavily pigmented skin can prevent up to 95% of ultraviolet radiation from reaching the deeper layer of the skin for adequate synthesis of the

Sunlight—or the Milky Way?

Sunlight and milk, that is, fortified milk, are the primary sources of vitamin D. But can we rely on them to supply our needs?

Sunlight, we have long held, is the least constant of the two because of the number of factors that can affect its absorption and ability to transform cholesterol into provitamin D_3, a precursor to vitamin D. However, we are now learning, after U.S. milk fortification regulations have been in place since the early 1930s, that we can't always count on milk either. First, a look at sunlight as a source.

Season of the year

Ultraviolet exposure varies by season, depending on the type of activity (especially indoor versus outdoor) of the individual and the type of clothing worn. Studies of older persons with hip fractures show high correlation with very little exposure to sunshine.

Body composition

It has also been shown that gross obesity, which reduces the person's mobility and often confines them indoors, decreases exposure to ultraviolet light, even to the point of increasing the risk of a vitamin D deficiency.

Second, consider milk as an alternate source. We have looked to milk as the most reliable source of vitamin D, especially for persons at risk for deficiency problems (for example, postmenopausal women, especially those who spend much of their time indoors, and infants). However,

TO PROBE FURTHER

as we have known, the milk must be fortified with vitamin D, 10 µg (400 IU)/quart by U.S. regulations, to provide necessary amounts with a reasonable intake.

However, we now find that we can't always rely on the fortification process either. Recent news of an outbreak of vitamin D toxicity from drinking milk traced to a single dairy raises questions about just how reliable milk really is as a consistent source of vitamin D. Not so reliable, subsequent investigations proved through sampling milk and infant formulas in five adjacent states. Labels on these random products showed the required amount of fortification, but actual analysis indicated a wide range of added vitamin D from toxic levels to none.

So now we answer our initial question with "both." We need to benefit from both sunlight and milk, but in controlled amounts. Just as we have learned that too little or too much sunlight can do harm, we are now learning the same thing about milk fortification. Vigilant monitoring and enforcement of regulations is necessary if fortification of milk and other foods is to remain a reliable source of vitamin D.

REFERENCES

DeLuca HF: The vitamin D story: a collaborative effort of basic science and clinical medicine, *FASEB J* 2:224, March 1, 1988.

Holick MF and others: The vitamin D content of fortified milk and infant formula, *N Engl J Med* 326(18):1178, April 30, 1992.

Jacobus CH and others: Hypervitaminosis D associated with drinking milk, *N Engl J Med* 326(18):1173, April 30, 1992.

steroid hormone. Also, persons who lack exposure to sunlight—house-bound elderly persons or those living in crowded city areas with high air pollution rates—would fail to receive adequate skin irradiation.

Liver. After synthesis in the skin, vitamin D_3 is transported by its special globulin protein carrier to the liver. Here a special liver enzyme converts D_3 to **25-hydroxycholecalciferol, [25(OH)D_3]**, the intermediate product. This intermediate product is then transported by the same serum protein carrier to the kidney for final activation.

Kidneys. In the kidney a special renal enzyme, 1-alpha-hydroxylase, forms the physiologically active vitamin D hormone, *1-alpha,25-dihydroxycholecalciferol [1α,25(OH)$_2$D$_3$].*[7,8] In general usage, the chemical name of the active vitamin D hormone is **calcitriol.**

Functions of Vitamin D Hormone

Vitamin D in the body is predominantly associated with calcium and phosphorus metabolism. It influences the

calcitriol • Activated hormone form of vitamin D [1,25(OH)$_2$D$_3$]—1,25-dihydroxycholecalciferol.

cholecalciferol • Chemical name for vitamin D in its inactive dietary form (D_3). When the inactive cholecalciferol is consumed or its counterpart cholesterol compound is developed in the skin, its first stage of activation occurs in the liver and then is completed in the kidney to the active vitamin D hormone form *calcitriol,* 1,25-dihydroxycholecalciferol, or shorter form 1,25 (OH)$_2$D$_3$.

7-dehydrocholesterol • A precursor cholesterol compound in the skin that is irradiated by sunlight to produce an initial stage in the process of forming activated vitamin D hormone.

25-hydroxycholecalciferol [25,(OH)D_3] • Initial product formed in the liver in the process of developing the active vitamin D hormone.

absorption of these minerals and their deposit in bone tissue.

Calcium and Phosphorus Absorption and Bone Mineralization

In balance with the parathyroid hormone, the vitamin D endocrine system based in the kidneys stimulates the active transport of calcium and phosphorus in the small intestine and promotes normal bone mineralization. First, vitamin D stimulates calcium and phosphorus absorption in the intestine and their deposit in bone tissue. Second, balanced with this action, parathyroid hormone stimulates calcium withdrawal from the bone and excretion of phosphorus in the urine to help maintain the normal calcium-phosphorus balance in the blood. A third hormone participates in this triad of regulatory agents in calcium metabolism. This is calcitonin, a polypeptide secreted by connective tissue cells in the thyroid gland.

Role in Bone Disease

When the body does not have enough vitamin D, it cannot build normal bones. In children this vitamin D deficiency disease is call *rickets*. In the growing child the condition is characterized by malformation of skeletal tissue (Fig. 7-5). In adults the disease is called *osteomalacia*. It occurs mostly in women of childbearing age who get little exposure to sunlight or have poor diets, or who have frequent pregnancies, each followed by periods of lactation. The wide use of vitamin D–fortified foods, especially milk, has nearly eliminated common

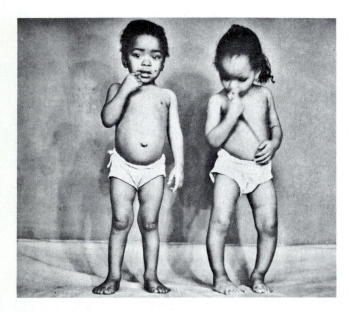

FIG. 7-5   Rachitic children. Note the knock-knees on the child on the left and the bowlegs on the child on the right. *(From files of Therapeutic Notes, Parke, Davis & Co, Detroit, Mich; courtesy Dr. Orson D. Bird.)*

vitamin D deficiency rickets in developed countries, but it does occur, most frequently in infants 6 to 18 months of age. Cases recently reported in the United States occurred among breast-fed infants who were not receiving the recommended vitamin D supplements.[9] In other parts of the world, rickets remains a public health problem. It occurs more often in northern countries with limited winter sunlight or in dark-skinned races whose skin pigmentation inhibits passage of the sun's ultraviolet rays.

In addition, because of the active regulatory role of vitamin D as a balancing hormone, it has been used to treat a bone disease secondary to kidney failure, renal **osteodystrophy,** which is characterized by defective bone formation. Vitamin D also contributes to the treatment of **osteoporosis,** a bone loss disease common in older women that leads to fractures.

Basic Cell Processes

Beyond this role in bone and mineral metabolism, evidence is growing that the vitamin D hormone system is involved in widespread basic cell processes with targets in a number of organ tissues, such as brain, kidney, liver, skin, and reproductive tissue; hormone-secreting glands; and certain cells of the immune system. Investigators suggest that these expanded metabolic activities probably relate to an active hormonal role in controlling basic cell functions such as cell reproduction and spread, as well as cell differentiation. This ongoing work may lead to possible use of the vitamin D analogs in treatment of some types of leukemias and the persistent skin disorder psoriasis.[7]

Vitamin D Toxicity

Toxic amounts of vitamin D build up in the body easily because vitamin D is stored in adipose tissue and is released slowly. Toxic intakes of vitamin D may result from self-administered large doses of the vitamin supplement or from unknowing intake of large amounts in fortified foods such as milk. In the United States milk has been fortified with vitamin D since the 1930s, which has had the result of largely eradicating common rickets. The U.S. federal regulations specify that each quart of milk contain 10 μg (400 IU). However, experience has shown that vitamin D has to be used cautiously and carefully. Adults taking continued megadoses of 1500 μg (60,000 IU) have shown signs of severe intoxication.[10]

Yet even today cases of intoxication occur, usually from excessively fortified food. For example, a recent U.S. outbreak of vitamin D intoxication was traced to a single local dairy's sporadic addition of excessive vitamin D to milk, ranging from 19.87 to 5814 μg (795 to 232,565 IU)/quart during the fortification process.[11] Symptoms included failure to thrive and calcium deposits in soft tissue of the kidney nephrons in a 15-month-old child and progressive weakness, bone pain, and hypercalcemia in adults. A follow-up investigation of fortified milk and infant formula from supermarkets in five Eastern states showed similar irregularities in fortification from their labeled content of vitamin D addition of 10 μg (400 IU)/quart.[12] In fact, the actual vitamin D amounts ranged from no detectable amount to 12.9 μg (515 IU)/quart in the milk samples and from 17.9 to 40.2 μg (715 to 1608 IU)/quart in the infant formulas. Infant feeding poses special problems. Excess intake is possible in infant feeding practices where fortified milk, fortified cereal, plus variable vitamin supplements are used. The infant needs only 10 μg (400 IU) daily, whereas the amount in all of these items can easily total 100 μg (4000 IU).

Vitamin D Requirement

Influencing Factors

Difficulties exist in setting requirements for vitamin D. Variables arise from numerous sources: a limited number of food sources available, lack of knowledge of precise body needs, and differing degrees of skin synthesis by irradiation. Needs vary between winter and summer in northern climates. Also, a person's way of living and working determines the degree of sunlight exposure and thus influences individual need. Persons living and working indoors need more than someone who works outside all day. Elderly people or invalids who do not go out-of-doors may need supplementary vitamin D.[13] Growth demands in childhood and in pregnancy and lactation necessitate increased intake.

RDA Standard

The RDA standard is 10 μg of cholecalciferol (400 IU) daily for children and for women during pregnancy and lactation. The daily allowance for persons from 6 months to 24 years of age is the same—10 μg (400 IU), and for all adults 25 years of age and older it is 5 μg (200 IU). Questions are raised about the adequacy of this allowance for older adults above age 65, especially elderly homebound persons for whom there is as yet no consensus of need.[13,14]

Food Sources of Vitamin D

Few natural food sources of vitamin D exist. The two basic substances with vitamin D activity, D_2 and D_3, occur only in yeast and fish liver oils. The main food sources are those to which crystalline vitamin D has been added. Milk, because it is commonly used, has proved to be the most practical carrier. However, such food must be fortified accurately and consistently and the products monitored regularly by public health officials to avoid toxic excesses. It is now a widespread commercial practice to standardize the added vitamin content of milk at 10 μg (400 IU)/quart. But, as we have learned from recent toxic outbreaks and follow-up

TABLE 7-2
Food Sources of Vitamin D (RDA for Adults: 5 μg)

	Quantity	Vitamin D (μg)
Bread, cereal, rice, pasta		
Corn flakes	1 cup (1 oz)/28 g	1.00
Granola	¼ cup (1 oz)/28 g	1.23
Raisin bran	½ cup (1 oz)/28 g	1.23
Vegetables		
This food group is not an important source of vitamin D.		
Fruits		
This food group is not an important source of vitamin D.		
Meat, poultry, fish, dry beans, nuts		
This food group is not an important source of vitamin D.		
Eggs		
Egg, whole	1 large/50 g	0.68
Egg yolk	Yolk of 1 large egg/17 g	0.68
Milk, dairy products		
Cheddar cheese	1 oz/28 g	0.08
Cream cheese	1 oz/28 g	0.05
Evaporated milk (vitamin D fortified)	½ cup (4 fl oz)/126 g	2.50
Milk, whole or nonfat (vitamin D fortified)	1 qt/960 g	10.00
Milk, whole or nonfat (vitamin D fortified)	1 cup (8 fl oz)/240 g	2.50
Fats, oils, sugar		
Margarine	1 tbsp	1.50

investigations, this is not always a reliable addition.[11,12] Milk is also a good carrier for the vitamin because it contains calcium and phosphorus as well. Margarines are also fortified with 37.5 μg (1500 IU)/lb to serve as butter substitutes. A summary of food sources of vitamin D is given in Table 7-2.

Vitamin E

Chemical and Physical Nature

Vitamin E was discovered in connection with studies concerning the reproductive responses of rats and was identified as an alcohol. Because of this rat reproduc-

osteodystrophy • Defective bone formation.

osteoporosis • Abnormal thinning of bone, producing a porous, fragile, latticelike bone tissue of enlarged spaces, prone to fracture or deformity.

tive function and its chemical nature as an alcohol, it was named **tocopherol** from the Greek word *tokos* meaning "childbirth." Since then, tocopherol has come to be commonly known as the antisterility vitamin, but this effect has been demonstrated only in rats and not in humans, despite all advertising claims for its contribution to sexual powers.

Forms

Vitamin E is the generic name for a group of compounds with similar physiologic activity. One of these, alpha-tocopherol, is the most significant in human nutrition. It is a pale yellow oil, stable to acids and heat and insoluble in water. It oxidizes very slowly, which gives it an important role as an antioxidant with widespread clinical application.

Absorption, Transport, and Storage

Vitamin E is absorbed with the aid of bile. With other lipids in the chylomicrons, it is transported out of the intestinal wall into body circulation in the blood plasma lipoproteins. Accumulated intake is stored in the liver and mainly in fat tissue. In adipose tissue, vitamin E is held mainly in bulk liquid droplets, and mobilization of alpha-tocopherol from these droplets is slow.[15]

Functions of Vitamin E
Antioxidant

Vitamin E acts as nature's most potent fat-soluble antioxidant. The polyunsaturated fatty acids in the structural lipid membranes of cells are particularly vulnerable to oxidative breakdown by free radicals in the cell. The tocopherols can interrupt this oxidation process, protecting the cell membrane fatty acids from the oxidative damage.

Selenium Relationship

Even with adequate vitamin E intake, some damaging cell peroxides may be formed, so a second line of defense is needed to destroy them before they can damage the cell membrane. The agent providing this added defense is a selenium-containing enzyme. Thus the trace element selenium spares vitamin E by reducing the vitamin's requirement. Similarly, in this partnership role, vitamin E helps reduce the selenium requirements.

Vitamin E Deficiency

When adequate vitamin E is not available, the cells are more vulnerable to oxidative attack and damage. For example, if vitamin E is deficient, the lipid membranes of red blood cells are exposed to oxidation of their structural polyunsaturated fatty acids. The membranes are broken, the contents lost, and the cells destroyed. The continued loss of red blood cells leads to anemia.

This vitamin E deficiency disease is thus called **hemolytic anemia.** Premature infants are especially vulnerable because they missed the last month or two of fetal life, when vitamin E stores are normally built up.

In older children and adults, vitamin E deficiency presents a different set of symptoms, sometimes called neurologic syndrome of vitamin E deficiency. These symptoms are associated with functions of the nervous system. The main nerves involved are (1) spinal cord fibers that affect physical activity such as walking, and (2) the retina of the eye, which affects vision. This group of neurologic problems has just been recognized recently, since medical advances have enabled children, such as those with cystic fibrosis and pancreatic insufficiency, to live longer with chronic defective absorption of fats and fat-soluble vitamins.[15] The loss of the pancreatic fat-digesting enzyme lipase and its associated emulsifying agent bile leads to a chronic fatty diarrhea and inability to absorb fat and fat-soluble nutrients such as vitamin E. This vitamin E deficiency disrupts the making of **myelin,** the protective fat covering for the long axons of nerve cells that help pass messages along to muscles they serve. In children and adults this neurologic disorder, the lack of vitamin E, causes pigment degeneration of the retina's rods and cones. These light-sensitive cell membranes are rich in polyunsaturated fatty acids, and vitamin E is critical for preventing oxidation damage.[16]

Vitamin E Requirement
RDA Standard

The requirements for vitamin E vary with the amount of polyunsaturated fatty acids in the diet. The RDA standard for adults in alpha-tocopherol equivalents (α-TE) is 10 mg for men and 8 mg for women. Needs during childhood growth years range from 3 to 10 mg. These stated allowances are based on an estimate of a diet composed of 80% α-TE and 20% other tocopherols with varying potencies.[17]

Special Clinical Needs

Since vitamin E protects cellular and subcellular membranes and hence tissue health, it is an important nutrient in the diets of pregnant and lactating women, and especially for newborn infants. Two medical problems found in infants, particularly premature ones, have responded positively to vitamin E therapy: (1) retrolental fibroplasia, a condition causing severely limited vision or complete blindness from the effect of excess oxygen therapy following birth; and (2) hemolytic anemia, a condition in which fragile erythrocyte membranes break down because of high cell peroxide levels and the induced deficiency of vitamin E. Also, older persons may require more vitamin E. It has been proved effective for those suffering circulatory distur-

TABLE 7-3

Food Sources of Vitamin E as alpha-Tocopherol (RDA for Adults: Women, 8 mg; Men, 10 mg)

	Quantity	Vitamin E (mg α-TE)
Bread, cereal, rice, pasta		
This food group is not an important source of vitamin E.		
Vegetables		
Asparagus (raw)	4 spears/58 g	1.15
Avocado (raw)	1 med/173 g	2.32
Brussels sprouts (boiled)	½ cup (4 sprouts)/78 g	0.66
Cabbage, green (raw)	½ cup shredded/35 g	0.58
Carrot (raw)	1 med/72 g	0.32
Lettuce, iceberg (raw)	¼ head/135 g	0.54
Spinach (raw)	½ cup chopped/28 g	0.53
Sweet potato (raw)	1 med/130 g	5.93
Fruits		
Apple (raw, with skin)	1 med/138 g	0.81
Apricot (canned)	4 halves/90 g	0.80
Banana (raw)	1 med/114 g	0.31
Mango (raw)	1 med/207 g	2.32
Pear (raw)	1 med/166 g	0.83
Meat, poultry, fish, dry beans, eggs		
This food group is not an important source of vitamin E.		
Nuts		
Almonds (dried)	1 oz (24 nuts)/28 g	6.72
Hazelnuts (dried)	1 oz/28 g	6.70
Peanut butter	1 tbsp/16 g	3.00
Peanuts (dried)	1 oz/28 g	2.56
Walnuts (dried)	1 oz (14 halves)/28 g	0.73
Milk, dairy products		
This food group is not an important source of vitamin E.		
Fats, oils, sugar		
Corn oil	1 tbsp/14 g	1.90
Cottonseed oil	1 tbsp/14 g	4.80
Olive oil	1 tbsp/14 g	1.60
Palm oil	1 tbsp/14 g	2.60
Peanut oil	1 tbsp/14 g	1.60
Safflower oil	1 tbsp/14 g	4.60
Soybean oil	1 tbsp/14 g	1.50

bances such as pain in the legs (intermittent claudication) after walking has begun. This therapy helps reduce the arterial blockage causing the pain.

Vitamin E is the only one of the fat-soluble vitamins for which no toxic effect in humans is known. Its use as a supplement has shown no harmful effects. Regular vitamin E replacement therapy is needed for the chronic pancreatic insufficiency and malabsorption conditions described. Current interest in ongoing research concerning vitamin E and its antioxidant role in decreasing free radical damage to cells has led researchers and clinicians to recommend use of moderate supplements of 200 to 300 mg α-TE/day for many middle-age and older adults.[18]

Food Sources of Vitamin E

The richest dietary sources of vitamin E are the vegetable oils. Curiously enough, these are also the richest sources of polyunsaturated fatty acids, which vitamin E protects from oxidation. Other food sources include nuts, certain vegetables and fruits, and only small amounts in cereals, dairy products, and meats. A summary of main food sources is given in Table 7-3.

Vitamin K

Chemical and Physical Nature

The studies of a biochemist at the University of Copenhagen working with a hemorrhagic disease in chicks that were fed a fat-free diet led to the discovery of vitamin K. He found that the absent factor responsible was a fat-soluble blood-clotting vitamin. Because of its blood clotting function, he called it *koagulationsvitamin,* or vitamin K, from this Swedish word for its physiologic action. Later he succeeded in isolating and identifying the compound from alfalfa, for which he received the Nobel Prize in physiology and medicine. This major form of the vitamin found in plants has been named **phylloquinone** for its chemical structure. This is our dietary form of vitamin K; its name is generally used as the vitamin's basic chemical name. **Menaquinone** (K_2) is synthesized by intestinal bacterial flora and contributes about half our daily supply. **Menadione** (K_3) is the

hemolytic anemia • An anemia (reduced number of red blood cells) caused by breakdown of red blood cells and loss of their hemoglobin.

menadione • The parent compound of vitamin K in the body; also called *vitamin K₂*

menaquinone • Form of vitamin K synthesized by intestinal bacteria; also called *vitamin K₂.*

myelin • High lipid-to-protein substance forming a fatty sheath to insulate and protect neuron axons and facilitate their neuromuscular impulses.

phylloquinone • A fat-soluble vitamin of the K group, $C_3H_{46}O_2$, found in green plants or prepared synthetically.

tocopherol • Chemical name for vitamin E. It was so named by early investigators because their initial work with rats indicated a reproductive function, which did not turn out to be the case with humans. In humans it functions as a strong antioxidant to preserve structural membranes, such as cell walls.

parent compound in the body; a water-soluble synthetic copy is used widely in animal feeds but is no longer used in clinical medicine.[19]

Forms

As with most of the vitamins, several forms of vitamin K comprise a group of substances with similar biologic activity in blood clotting. There are three main forms of vitamin K:

1. K_1, which is the major form found in plants
2. K_2, which is synthesized by intestinal bacteria, so vitamin K is not required directly in the diet
3. K_3, a water-soluble analog, which does not require bile for absorption and goes directly into the portal blood system

Absorption, Transport, and Storage

K_1 and K_2 require bile for absorption as with other fat-related products. They are packaged in the intestinal chylomicrons and travel via the abdominal lacteals into the lymphatic system and then into the portal blood for transport to the liver. In the liver, vitamin K is stored in small amounts, though its concentration there declines rapidly. It is excreted in considerable quantity after administration of therapeutic doses.

Function of Vitamin K

The one basic function of vitamin K is to catalyze the synthesis of blood-clotting factors in the liver. Vitamin K produces the active form of several precursors, mainly **prothrombin** (factor II), which combines with calcium (factor IV) to help produce the clotting effect. In the absence of functioning liver tissue, vitamin K cannot act. When liver damage has caused decreased blood levels of prothrombin, and this problem in turn has led to hemorrhage, vitamin K is ineffective as a therapeutic agent. Several clinical problems relate to vitamin K.

Neonatology

The sterile intestinal tract of the newborn can supply no vitamin K during the first few days of life until normal bacterial flora develop. During this immediate postnatal period, therefore, hemorrhagic disease of the newborn can occur. To prevent this result, a prophylactic dose of vitamin K is usually given to the infant soon after birth.

Malabsorption Disease

Any defect in fat absorption will cause a failure in vitamin K absorption, resulting in prolonged blood clotting time. For example, patients with bile duct obstruction are usually given vitamin K before surgery. Also, after a cholecystectomy, which hinders normal bile release, vitamin K, which requires bile and fat for normal absorption, is not readily absorbed.

Drug Therapy

Several drug-nutrient interactions involve vitamin K. An anticlotting drug such as bishydroxycoumarin (dicumarol) acts as an **antimetabolite,** thus inhibiting the action of vitamin K. When a drug of this nature is used for treating conditions such as blood clots in the lung or blood vessels, vitamin K may be used as a balancing "antidote" to the drug in the management of blood clotting time. Also, in extended use of antibiotics, the intestinal bacterial flora is diminished, thus reducing one of the body's main sources of vitamin K.

Vitamin K Requirement

In past years, it has been difficult to determine a specific dietary level for vitamin K for several reasons: (1) part of the body's apparent need is supplied by bacterial synthesis; (2) our body reserves are small and turn over rapidly; and (3) instruments for measuring such small amounts were just developing. Also, we lacked reliable food source information. Now, however, with increasing knowledge and advances in laboratory equipment for measuring small amounts, a more specific RDA has recently been established.[17] Thus, based on an approximate need in adults of 1 μg/kg body weight per day, the current RDA for men is stated as 80 μg/day, and for women, it is 65 μg/day. The average daily intake of vitamin K by surveyed individuals in the United States seems to be adequate.[17] Therefore, no additional amount is stated for pregnancy and lactation or for older adults. However, older adults who have chronic diseases, are on drug therapy, or are consuming poor diets may need more. Newborns require a vitamin K injection shortly after birth. The RDA standard during the first 6 months of life is 5 μg/day, and during the second 6 months of the first year it is 10 μg/day. Persons who are taking antibiotics, who are being fed by tube or total parenteral nutrition (TPN) by vein for long periods, or who have biliary obstruction or chronic malabsorption disease require monitoring and therapeutic supplementation as indicated.[17]

A deficiency of vitamin K is unlikely except in the clinical conditions indicated. An adequate amount is usually ensured because intestinal bacteria usually synthesize an added supply and the amount needed is apparently quite small.[20] Toxicity from vitamin K, even

---

antimetabolite • A substance bearing a close structural resemblance to one required for normal physiologic functioning and exerting its effect by interfering with the utilization of the essential metabolite.

prothrombin • Blood-clotting factor (number II) synthesized in the liver from glutamic acid and CO_2, catalyzed by vitamin K.

TABLE 7-4

Food Sources of Vitamin K (RDA for Adults: Women, 65 μg; Men, 80 μg)

	Quantity	Vitamin K (μg)		Quantity	Vitamin K (μg)
Bread, cereal, rice, pasta			**Fruits**		
Oats (dry)	100 g	63	This food group is not an important source of vitamin K.		
Wheat bran	100 g	83			
Whole wheat flour	100 g	30	**Meat, poultry, fish, dry beans, eggs, nuts**		
			Beef liver	100 g	104
Vegetables			Chicken liver	100 g	80
			Pork liver	100 g	88
Broccoli (raw)	100 g	132			
Cabbage (raw)	100 g	149	**Milk, dairy products**		
Cauliflower (raw)	100 g	191	This food group is not an important source of vitamin K.		
Lentils (dry)	100 g	223			
Lettuce, iceberg (raw)	100 g	112	**Fats, oils, sugar**		
Spinach (raw)	100 g	266			
Turnip greens (raw)	100 g	650	Corn oil	100 g	60
			Soybean oil	100 g	540

TABLE 7-5

Summary of Fat-Soluble Vitamins

Vitamin	Physiologic functions	Results of deficiency	Requirement	Food sources
Vitamin A				
Provitamin: beta-carotene Vitamin: retinol	Production of rhodopsin and other light-receptor pigments Formation and maintenance of epithelial tissue Growth Reproduction Toxic in large amounts	Poor dark adaptation, night blindness, xerosis, xerophthalmia Keratinization of epithelium Growth failure Reproductive failure	Adult male: 1000 μg or RE (5000 IU) Adult female: 800 μg or RE (4000 IU) Pregnancy: 1000 μg or RE (5000 IU) Lactation 1200 μg or RE (6000 IU) Children: 400 μg or RE (2000 IU) to 800 or RE (4000 IU)	Liver, cream, butter, whole milk, egg yolk Green and yellow vegetables, yellow fruits Fortified margarine
Vitamin D				
Provitamins: ergosterol (plants); 7-dehydrocholesterol (skin) Vitamins: D$_2$ (ergocholecalciferol) and D$_3$ (cholecalciferol)	Calcitriol a major hormone regulator of bone mineral (calcium and phosphorus) metabolism Calcium and phosphorus absorption Toxic in large amounts	Faulty bone growth; rickets, osteomalacia	Adult: 5-10 μg cholecalciferol (200-400 IU) Pregnancy and lactation: 10-12.5 μg (400-500 IU) depending on age Children: 10 μg (400 IU)	Fortified milk Fortified margarine Fish oils Sunlight on skin
Vitamin E				
Tocopherols	Antioxidant Hemopoiesis Related to action of selenium	Anemia in premature infants	Adult: 8-10 mg α-TE Pregnancy and lactation: 10-11 mg α-TE Children: 3-10 mg α-TE	Vegetable oils
Vitamin K				
K$_1$ (phylloquinone) K$_2$ (menaquinone) Analog: K$_3$ (menadione)	Activates blood-clotting factors (for example, prothrombin) by alpha-carboxylating glutamic acid residues Toxicity can be induced by water-soluble analogs	Hemorrhagic disease of the newborn Defective blood clotting Deficiency symptoms are produced by coumarin anticoagulants and by antibiotic therapy	Adult: 70-140 μg Children: 15-100 μg Infants: 12-20 μg	Cheese, egg yolk, liver Green leafy vegetables Synthesized by intestinal bacteria

with large amounts taken over extended periods, has not been observed.

Food Sources of Vitamin K

Dietary vitamin K, phylloquinone, is present to some degree in most vegetables (Table 7-4). It is found especially in green leafy vegetables and liver.

WATER-SOLUBLE VITAMINS

Vitamin C

Chemical and Physical Nature

The recognition of vitamin C is associated with the history of an unrelenting search for the cause of the ancient hemorrhagic disease **scurvy.** Early observations, mostly among British sailors and explorers, led to the American discovery of an acid in lemon juice that prevented or cured scurvy. The specific chemical name of vitamin C is ascorbic acid, given to this substance because of its antiscorbutic, or antiscurvy, properties. The structure of vitamin C is similar to that of glucose, its metabolic precursor in most animals, but humans lack a specific enzyme needed to change glucose to ascorbic acid. Thus, human scurvy can be called a disease of distant genetic origin, an inherited metabolic defect.

Vitamin C is an unstable, easily oxidized acid. It can be destroyed by oxygen, alkalis, and high temperatures. Thus, cook vitamin C foods in as little water as possible for brief periods and keep covered. Do not cut vegetables into small pieces until time of use, to curtail cut surface exposure to the air. Keep juices tightly closed.

Absorption, Transport, and Storage

Vitamin C is easily absorbed from the small intestine. But this absorption is hindered by a lack of hydrochloric acid or by bleeding from the gastrointestinal tract. Vitamin C is not stored in single tissue deposits as is vitamin A. Rather it is more generally distributed throughout the body tissues, maintaining a tissue saturation level. Any excess is excreted in the urine. The tissue levels relate to intake, and the size of the total body pool adjusts to maintain balances. The total amount in adults varies from about 4 g to as little as 0.3 g. Tissue levels diminish slowly, so with no intake deficiency symptoms would not appear for approximately 3 months. This explains why generally healthy people in more isolated living situations can survive the winter without eating many fresh fruits and vegetables. Sufficient vitamin C for early infancy needs is present in breast milk if the mother has a good lactation diet. Cow's milk, however, contains very little vitamin C; remember that these animals have the enzymes to make their own vitamin C from glucose. Because of this, human infant formulas made from cow's milk are supplemented with ascorbic acid.

Functions of Vitamin C

General Antioxidant Capacity

In general, along with vitamins A and E, vitamin C is an antioxidant. This means that vitamin C also takes up free oxygen in the cells resulting from cell metabolism. This action prevents oxygen from feeding hungry oxygen-free radicals that also result from normal metabolism in cells but damage or destroy cells if they are not defused.[21,22]

Intercellular Cement Substance

We require vitamin C to build and maintain body tissues in general, including bone matrix, cartilage, dentin, collagen, and connective tissue. When vitamin C is absent, the important ground substance does not develop into collagen. When the vitamin is given, formation of cartilaginous tissue follows quickly. **Collagen** is a protein substance that exists in many body tissues, such as the white fibers of connective tissue. Blood vessel tissue particularly is weakened without the cementing substance from vitamin C's metabolic action that helps provide firm capillary walls. Thus vitamin C deficiency is characterized by fragile capillaries, easily ruptured by blood pressure or trauma, resulting in diffuse tissue bleeding. Deficiency signs include easy bruising, pinpoint hemorrhages of the skin, bone and joint hemorrhages, easy bone fracture, poor wound healing, and soft bleeding gums, a condition called gingivitis.

General Body Metabolism

The concentration of vitamin C is greater in the more metabolically active tissue such as the adrenal glands, brain, kidney, liver, pancreas, thymus, and spleen than in less active tissues. More vitamin C is also present in a child's actively multiplying tissue than in adult tissue. Vitamin C helps in the formation of hemoglobin and the development of red blood cells in two ways: (1) it aids in the absorption of iron, and (2) it influences the removal of iron from ferritin, the protein-iron-phosphorus complex in which iron is stored, so that more iron is made available to tissues producing the hemoglobin.[23]

Vitamin C also participates in other tissues in numerous processes that have clinical implications. For example, in addition to its role in collagen formation, vitamin C is needed for the synthesis of carnitine, an amino acid that transports long-chain fatty acids into cell mitochondria where they are used to produce energy. Also, vitamin C is necessary for synthesis of many peptide hormones, the hormone norepinephrine, and many receptors for the neurotransmitter acetylcholine.[23]

Clinical Problems and Normal Growth

Some basic clinical problems, as well as normal growth, require additional vitamin C.

TABLE 7-6

Food Sources of Vitamin C (RDA for Adults: 60 mg)

	Quantity	Vitamin C (mg)		Quantity	Vitamin C (mg)
Bread, cereal, rice, pasta			**Fruits—cont'd**		
This food group is not an important source of vitamin C.			Orange juice (fresh)	8 fl oz	124
			Orange, navel	1 med	80
Vegetables			Papaya (raw)	1 med	188
Asparagus (boiled)	½ cup (6 spears)	18	Pineapple (raw)	½ cup	12
Avocado (raw)	1 med	14	Raspberries (raw)	½ cup	15
Broccoli (raw)	½ cup	41	Strawberries (raw)	½ cup	44
Brussels sprouts (boiled)	½ cup (4 sprouts)	48	Tangerine (raw)	1 med	26
Cauliflower (raw)	½ cup, pieces	38			
Green pepper (raw)	½ cup, chopped	64	**Meat, poultry, fish, dry beans, eggs, nuts**		
Kale (boiled)	½ cup	27	Beef liver (fried)	3.6 oz	23
Potato (baked, with skin)	1 med	26	Ham, lean (canned; vitamin C added)	3.5 oz	27
Sweet potato (baked)	1 med	28	Lentils (boiled)	1 cup	3
Tomato (raw)	1 med	22	Soybeans (boiled)	1 cup	3
Fruits			**Milk, dairy products**		
Cantaloupe (raw)	½ cup, pieces	34	Milk, skim	8 fl oz	2
Grapefruit, white	½ med	39	Milk, whole	8 fl oz	4
Kiwi (raw)	1 med	75	**Fats, oils, sugar**		
Lemon	1 med	31	This food group is not an important source of vitamin C.		
Lemon juice (fresh)	8 fl oz	112			

Wound healing. The significant role of vitamin C in cementing the ground substance of supportive tissue makes it an important agent in wound healing. This creates added demands for vitamin C in traumatic injury or surgery, especially where extensive tissue regeneration is involved.

Fevers and infections. Infectious processes deplete tissue stores of vitamin C. Optimal tissue stores help maintain resistance to infection. Just how large an amount may be required to maintain this protection is not known. Fevers also deplete tissue stores of vitamin C as they accompany the infectious processes and produce a catabolic effect.

Growth periods. Additional vitamin C is required during the growth periods of infancy and childhood. It is also needed during pregnancy to supply demands for rapid fetal growth and development of maternal tissues.

Stress and body defense. Body stress from injury, fracture, general illness, or shock calls on vitamin C tissue saturation. A large amount of vitamin C is present in the adrenal glands, which play a primary role in the stress response pattern (see Chapter 15).

Vitamin C Requirement

Difficulties in establishing requirements for vitamin C involve questions about individual tissue needs and whether minimum or optimum intakes are desired. From numerous studies, estimates of a desired body pool size of vitamin C in healthy adults average 1500 mg, which an intake of about 45 mg/day will maintain. The RDA standard for adults is 60 mg/day for an optimal margin to cover variances in tissue demand.[17] Cigarette smokers require about twice as much. Additional amounts are added for pregnancy and lactation needs. Gradual increases during childhood support growth needs.

Although pharmacologic doses of 1 g or more daily have been reported to reduce frequency and severity of symptoms of the common cold and other respiratory problems, controlled trials have not supported this claim. Thus such amounts are not recommended for

collagen • The protein substance of the white fibers (collagenous fibers) of skin, tendon, bone, cartilage, and all other connective tissue; it is converted into gelatin by boiling.

scurvy • A hemorrhagic disease caused by lack of vitamin C. Diffuse tissue bleeding occurs, limbs and joints are painful and swollen, bones thicken because of subperiosteal hemorrhage, ecchymoses (large irregular discolored skin areas resulting from tissue hemorrhages) form, bones fracture easily, wounds do not heal well, gums are swollen and bleeding, and teeth loosen.

TABLE 7-7

Summary of Vitamin C (Ascorbic Acid)

Physiologic functions	Clinical applications	Requirement	Food sources
Antioxidation Collagen biosynthesis General metabolism 　Makes iron available for hemo- 　　globin synthesis 　Influences conversion of folic 　　acid to folinic acid 　Oxidation-reduction of the amino 　　acids, phenylalanine and ty- 　　rosine	Scurvy (deficiency) Wound healing, tissue formation Fevers and infections Stress reactions Growth	60 mg Vegetables, such as tomatoes, cab- 　bage, potatoes, chili peppers, and 　broccoli	Fresh fruits, especially citrus

the entire population. Nonetheless, many persons do habitually ingest this dose daily without developing any toxic effects. On the other hand, others have experienced adverse effects. Because the risk is unknown, routine use of such large doses is not recommended.[17]

Food Sources of Vitamin C

Vitamin C can be oxidized easily. Thus the handling, preparation, cooking, and processing of any food source of the vitamin should be considered in evaluating that food's contribution of the vitamin to the diet. Well-known sources include citrus fruit and tomatoes. Less regarded but good additional sources include white potatoes, sweet potatoes, cabbage, broccoli, and other green and yellow vegetables and fruits. A summary of food sources of vitamin C is given in Table 7-6.

A summary of vitamin C and its role in the body is given in Table 7-7. Some guidelines for vitamin supplementation are provided in the *Clinical Application* on p. 117.

B Vitamins

Deficiency Disease and Vitamin Discoveries

The story of the B vitamins is a compelling one. It tells of persons dying of a puzzling, age-old disease for which there was no cure. It was eventually learned that common, everyday food held the answer. The paralyzing disease was **beriberi,** which had plagued the Orient for centuries and caused persons in many places to search for its solution (Fig. 7-6). Early observations and studies provided important clues, but application of the "vitamine" connection to the creeping human sickness was needed. This was finally achieved when an American chemist, R.R. Williams, and his associates with the Philippine Bureau of Science used extracts of rice polishings and cured the epidemic infantile beriberi, a paralysis named by the repeated native words, "I can't, I can't," describing its crippling effects. The food factor

was named water-soluble B because it was thought to be a single vitamin. Now we know it consists of a large group of individual B vitamins, all water soluble but each having unique metabolic functions in human health. The original letter-naming scheme has long since become meaningless and we are now accustomed to calling the B vitamins by their familiar specific chemical names.

Vital Coenzyme Role

The B vitamins, originally believed to be important only in preventing the deficiency diseases that led to their discovery, have now been identified in relation to many important metabolic functions. As vital control agents, they serve in many specific reactions as **coenzyme** part-

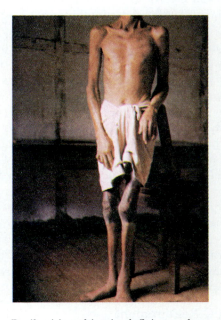

FIG. 7-6   Beriberi is a thiamin deficiency characterized by extreme weakness, paralysis, anemia, and wasting away (for example, decreased metabolic function in the liver).

Toddler Feeding Made Simple

In 1954 researchers found out that large doses, 10 to 1000 times the RDA, of specific nutrients helped alleviate symptoms in certain genetic disorders. Later the public got the idea that this would be helpful for healthy people, too. So they began using nutrients as drugs.

A similarity does exist. Both nutrients and drugs are used by the body in specific amounts to control or improve a physiologic condition or illness, to prevent a disease, or to relieve symptoms. But the similarity ends there for many people. They know that too much of any drug can be harmful, but they fail to apply this wise logic to nutrients, too. As a result, some persons have had to learn the hard way.

Some bad results

Toxic effects of vitamin megadoses. Physicians may prescribe large doses of water-soluble vitamins, believing them safe because they are not stored in the body. However, they have recently discovered the potential toxicity of at least one such vitamin—pyridoxine (B_6). Gynecologists have been prescribing this vitamin at levels that were 1000 to 2700 times its RDA to help patients relieve the discomfort of edema during their menstrual cycle. The patients eventually developed unstable gaits, with such numbness in the hands that they were unable to walk or carry out their usual duties at work. To make matters worse, the prescription did nothing to relieve their discomfort.

"Artificially induced" deficiency symptoms. These occur when blood levels of one nutrient rise above normal, resulting in an increased need for other nutrients with which it interacts. Deficiencies also occur when large doses are suddenly removed, creating a rebound effect. This effect has been seen in infants born to mothers who took megadoses of vitamin C during pregnancy, yet developed scurvy after birth when their high nutrient supply was cut off.

Wise warnings

The megavitamin lesson is not easily taught. Megadose salespersons frequently have more time, money, and better selling techniques with which they can misinform the public. Nonetheless, for your client's welfare, you will still want to apprise them of the following considerations:

Vitamins, like drugs, can be harmful in large amounts. The only time megadoses are helpful is when the body already has a severe deficiency or is unable to absorb or metabolize the nutrient efficiently.

All nutrients work in harmony to promote good health. Adding large amounts of one only makes the body believe that it isn't getting enough of the others and increases the risk of developing deficiency symptoms.

Supplements should not be taken without first analyzing nutrient levels currently in the diet. This helps avoid problems of excess, which may increase with an accumulative effect over time.

Food remains the best source of nutrients. Most food items provide a wide variety of nutrients in every bite, as opposed to the dozen or so found in a vitamin bottle. By itself a vitamin can actually do very little. Its action is catalytic and so it requires a substrate to work on. These necessary substrates are the energy nutrients carbohydrate, protein, fat and their metabolites. With careful selection of a variety of foods and wise storage, meal-planning, and preparation, most people can still secure an ample amount of essential nutrients. Food provides these necessities and a great deal of pleasure as well.

A last word on balance

Remember that as more is known about the pharmacologic effects of some vitamins, special use of them in larger prescribed therapeutic doses will occur. For example, niacin is already being used as a drug in medical care of cardiovascular disease to effectively lower elevated blood cholesterol levels. And some physicians have suggested increased use of vitamin E to decrease free radical cell damage, as well as more vitamin B_6 to counter the large loss induced by the drug theophylline, which is used to treat respiratory problems such as asthma. But such therapeutic use is not to be equated with nutritional needs or effects. As with any drug, pharmacologic use follows regular testing and approval procedures for designated medical therapy.

REFERENCES

Berman MK and others: Vitamin B-6 in premenstrual syndrome, *J Am Diet Assoc* 90(6):859, 1990.

Horwitt MK: Data supporting supplementation of humans with vitamin E, *J Nutr* 121:424, 1991.

Ubbink JB and others: Relationship between vitamin B-6 status and elevated pyridoxal kinase levels induced by theophylline therapy in humans, *J Nutr* 120:1359, 1990. ◆

---

ners with key cell enzymes in energy metabolism and tissue building.

Here we will review briefly the eight basic vitamins in this group of water-soluble compounds. First we will look at the three classic deficiency disease factors—thiamin, riboflavin, and niacin. Then we will explore more recently discovered coenzyme factors—pyridoxine, pantothenic acid, and biotin. Finally, we will examine the important blood-forming factors—folic acid and cobalamin.

beriberi • A disease of the peripheral nerves caused by a deficiency of thiamin (vitamin B_1). It is characterized by pain (neuritis) and paralysis of the extremities, cardiovascular changes, and edema. Beriberi is common in the Orient, where diets consist largely of milled rice with little protein.

coenzyme factors • A major metabolic role of the micronutrients, vitamins and minerals, as essential partners with cell enzymes in a variety of reactions in both energy and protein metabolism.

Thiamin

The search of many persons for the cause of beriberi led eventually to a successful conclusion with the identification of thiamin as the control agent involved. Its basic nature and metabolic function were then clarified in the early 1930s.

Chemical and Physical Nature

Thiamin is a water-soluble, fairly stable vitamin. However, it is destroyed by alkalis. Its name comes from its chemical ringlike structure. One of its major parts is a thiazole ring: *thi*(o + vit)*amin.*

Absorption and Storage

Thiamin is absorbed more readily in the acid medium of the first section of the small intestine, the duodenum. In the lower duodenum the acidity of the food mass is buffered by the alkaline intestinal secretions. Thiamin is not stored in large quantities in the tissues. The tissue content is highly relevant to increased metabolic demand, as in fever, increased muscular activity, pregnancy, and lactation. The tissue stores also depend on the adequacy of the diet and on its general composition. For example, carbohydrate increases the need for thiamin, whereas fat and protein spare thiamin. Any unused thiamin is constantly excreted in the urine.

Function of Thiamin

Basic Coenzyme Role

The main function of thiamin as a metabolic control agent relates to energy metabolism. When actively combined with phosphorus as the coenzyme **thiamin pyrophosphate (TPP),** thiamin serves as a coenzyme in key reactions that produce energy from glucose or that convert glucose to fat for tissue energy storage. Thus the symptoms of beriberi—muscle weakness, gastrointestinal disturbances, and neuritis—can be traced to problems related to these basic energy functions of thiamin.

Clinical Problems

Inadequate thiamin to provide the key energizing coenzyme factor in the cells produces broad clinical effects in the following systems.

Gastrointestinal system. Various symptoms such as anorexia, indigestion, constipation, gastric atony, and deficient hydrochloric acid secretion may result from thiamin deficiency. When the cells of the smooth muscles and the secretory glands do not receive sufficient energy from glucose, they cannot do their work in digestion to provide still more glucose. A vicious cycle ensues as the deficiency continues.

Nervous system. The central nervous system depends on glucose to do its work. Without sufficient thiamin to help provide this constant fuel, neuronal activity is impaired, alertness and reflex responses are diminished, and general apathy and fatigue result. If the deficiency continues, lipogenesis is hindered and damage or degeneration of myelin sheaths—lipid tissue covering the nerve fibers—follows. This causes increasing nerve irritation, pain, and prickly or deadening sensations. Paralysis results if the process continues unchecked, as in the classic thiamin deficiency disease beriberi.

Cardiovascular system. With continuing thiamin deficiency, the heart muscle weakens and cardiac failure results. Also, smooth muscle of the vascular system may become involved, causing dilation of the peripheral blood vessels. As a result of cardiac failure, edema appears in the lower legs.

Musculoskeletal system. A chronic painful musculoskeletal condition called primary fibromyalgia results from inadequate amounts of TPP in muscle tissue. The widespread muscle pain responds to TPP therapy, as indicated by measuring the activity of a key related enzyme, transketolase, in red blood cells. This is a common test for individual thiamin status.

Thiamin Requirement
RDA Standard

The thiamin requirement in human nutrition is stated in terms of carbohydrate and energy needs, as expressed in kcaloric intake. On this basis, the current RDAs for adults are 0.5 mg/1000 kcal daily, with a minimum of 1 mg/day, even for those consuming less than 2000 kcal daily. An increase of 0.4 mg/day is needed for pregnancy, and an added 0.5 mg/day is needed for lactation. The allowance for children and teenagers is the same as for adults. For infants the need is 0.4 mg/1000 kcal, the same as that recommended by the American Academy of Pediatrics.[17] Since excess thiamin is easily cleared by the kidneys, there is no evidence of toxicity from oral doses.

Special Needs

Several important conditions influence thiamin requirements.

Alcoholism. Thiamin is most important in nutritional therapy for persons with alcoholism. Both a primary (lack of adequate diet) and a conditioned (effect of alcohol itself) malnutrition may develop and bring serious neurologic disorders.

Other disease. Fevers and infections increase cellular energy requirements. Persons with chronic illness, especially older adults, require particular attention to prevent deficiencies.

TABLE 7-8

Food Sources of Thiamin (RDA for Adults: Women, 1.0 mg; Men, 1.4 mg)

	Quantity	Thiamin (mg)		Quantity	Thiamin (mg)
Bread, cereal, rice, pasta			**Meat, poultry, fish, dry beans, eggs, nuts**		
Bran flakes	1 cup	0.46	Beef liver (fried)	3.5 oz	0.21
Bread, whole wheat	1 slice	0.10	Black-eyed peas (boiled)	1 cup	0.35
Corn muffin	1 muffin	0.10	Cashews (roasted)	1 oz	0.12
Egg noodles, enriched	1 cup	0.20	Chicken, light and dark (roasted, without skin)	3.5 oz	0.07
Pasta, enriched	1 cup	0.23	Chicken liver (simmered)	3.5 oz	0.18
Rice, enriched	1 cup	0.23	Ham (canned)	3.5 oz	0.88
Wheat flakes	1 cup	0.40	Kidney beans (boiled)	1 cup	0.28
			Lentils (boiled)	1 cup	0.34
Vegetables			Lima beans (boiled)	1 cup	0.30
Asparagus (boiled)	½ cup (6 spears)	0.09	Navy beans (boiled)	1 cup	0.37
Avocado (raw)	1 med	0.19	Peanuts (roasted)	1 oz	0.12
Brussels sprouts (boiled)	½ cup (4 sprouts)	0.08	Pecans (dried)	1 oz	0.24
Corn, yellow (boiled)	½ cup	0.18	Pinto beans (boiled)	1 cup	0.32
Green peas (boiled)	½ cup	0.21	Sirloin steak (broiled)	3.5 oz	0.13
Potato (baked, with skin)	1 med	0.22	Soybeans (boiled)	1 cup	0.27
			Top round (broiled)	3.5 oz	0.12
Fruits			Tuna (baked)	3 oz	0.24
Figs (dried)	10 figs	0.13			
Orange juice (fresh)	8 fl oz	0.22	**Milk, dairy products**		
Orange, navel (raw)	1 med	0.13	Milk, skim	8 fl oz	0.09
Raisins, seedless	⅔ cup	0.16	Milk, whole	8 fl oz	0.09
			Fats, oils, sugar		
			This food group is not an important source of thiamin.		

Normal growth and development. About a 50% increase in thiamin requirement accompanies pregnancy and lactation, demanded by the rapid fetal growth, the increased metabolic rate during pregnancy, and the production of milk. Continuing growth during infancy, childhood, and adolescence requires attention to thiamin needs. At any point in the life cycle, the larger the body and its tissue volume is, the greater are cellular energy requirements and thus thiamin needs.

Food Sources of Thiamin

Although thiamin is widespread in almost all plant and animal tissues commonly used as food, the content is usually small. Deficiency of thiamin is a distinct possibility when kcalories are markedly curtailed, as in alcoholism, and when persons are following some highly inadequate special diet. Good food sources include lean pork, beef, liver, whole and enriched grains, and legumes. Table 7-8 provides some comparative food sources of thiamin.

Riboflavin

Discovery

As early as 1897 a London chemist first observed in milk whey a water-soluble pigment with peculiar yellow-green fluorescence. But it was not until 1932 that riboflavin was actually discovered by researchers in Germany. The vitamin was given the chemical group name flavins from the Latin word for yellow. Later, because the vitamin was found also to contain a sugar named ribose, the name riboflavin was officially adopted.

Chemical and Physical Nature

Riboflavin is a yellow-green fluorescent pigment that forms yellowish brown, needlelike crystals. It is water soluble and relatively stable to heat but easily destroyed by light and irradiation.

Absorption and Storage

Absorption of riboflavin occurs readily in the upper section of the small intestine, assisted by combination with phosphorus in the intestinal mucosa. Studies indicate that long-term laxative use of some bulk fiber supplements such as psyllium gum, especially when taken with

---

thiamin pyrophosphate (TPP) • Activating coenzyme form of thiamin that plays a key role in carbohydrate metabolism.

milk or near meals, can hinder riboflavin absorption and contribute to its deficiency in body metabolism.[26] Storage is limited, although small amounts are found in liver and kidney. Day-to-day tissue turnover needs must be supplied in the diet.

Functions of Riboflavin

Basic Coenzyme Role

The cell enzymes of which riboflavin is an important part are called flavoproteins. Riboflavin enzymes operate at vital reaction points in the process of energy metabolism and in deamination. This is the key reaction that removes the nitrogen-containing amino group from certain amino acids. Thus riboflavin acts as a control agent in both energy production and tissue building.

Clinical Problems

Problems associated with riboflavin deficiency include the following two conditions.

Ariboflavinosis. A deficiency of riboflavin, or **ariboflavinosis,** brings a combination of symptoms, which centers on tissue inflammation and breakdown and poor wound healing. Even minor injuries easily become aggravated and do not heal easily. The lips become swollen, cracking easily, and characteristic cracks develop at the corners of the mouth, a condition called cheilosis. Cracks and irritation develop at nasal angles. The tongue becomes swollen and reddened, a condition called **glossitis** (Fig. 7-7). Extra blood vessels develop in the cornea, creating corneal vascularization, and the eyes burn, itch, and tear. A scaly, greasy skin condition, seborrheic dermatitis, may develop, especially in skin folds. Since nutritional deficiencies are usually multiple rather than single, riboflavin deficiencies seldom occur alone. They are especially likely to occur in conjunction with deficiencies of other B vitamins.

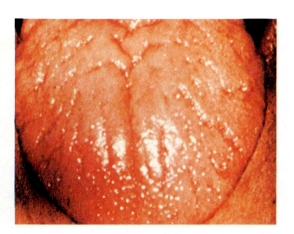

FIG. 7-7 Glossitis.

Deficiency in newborns. Because riboflavin is light sensitive, newborn infants with elevated blood levels of bilirubin treated with phototherapy have shown signs of riboflavin deficiencies even when supplements were provided.

Riboflavin Requirement

Influencing Factors

The body's riboflavin requirement is related to total energy needs, level of exercise, body size, metabolic rate, and rate of growth—all of which are related to protein intake.

RDA Standard

For practical purposes the general RDA standard for riboflavin is based on 0.6 mg/1000 kcal for all ages.[17]

Risk Groups

Persons in certain risk groups or clinical situations may require increased riboflavin. These include persons living in poverty or following bizarre food habits. It also applies to those with gastrointestinal disease or chronic illness where poor appetite and malabsorption exist. In addition, at risk are people who have poor wound healing, and those persons in growth periods such as in childhood, pregnancy, and lactation.

Food Sources of Riboflavin

The most important source of riboflavin is milk. There are several flavins in milk. The most abundant one, initially named lactoflavin, has been renamed specifically riboflavin, to distinguish it from the others.[27] Each quart of milk contains 2 mg of riboflavin, which is more than the daily requirement. Other good sources are organ meats such as liver, kidney, and heart, whole or enriched grains, and vegetables. Since riboflavin is water soluble and is destroyed by light, considerable loss can occur in open, excess-water cooking. Table 7-9 gives some food sources of riboflavin.

Niacin

The age-old disease related to niacin (nicotinic acid) is *pellagra* (Fig. 7-8). It is characterized by a typical dermatitis and often has fatal effects on the nervous system.[28] Pellagra was first observed in eighteenth century Europe, where it was endemic in populations subsisting largely on corn. Later the American physician Goldberger, who made his now classic observations while studying the problem in the Southern states, found further clues among children in an orphanage. He noticed that, although the majority of the children had pellagra to some degree, a few of them did not. He discovered that the few who were free of pellagra were sneaking into the pantries at night and eating the orphanage's limited supply of milk and meat. His in-

TABLE 7-9
Food Sources of Riboflavin (RDA for Adults: Women, 1.2 mg; Men, 1.6 mg)

	Quantity	Riboflavin (mg)		Quantity	Riboflavin (mg)
Bread, cereal, rice, pasta			**Meat, poultry, fish, dry beans, eggs, nuts—cont'd**		
Bran flakes	1 cup	0.40	Chicken liver (simmered)	3.5 oz	1.76
Bread, whole wheat	1 slice	0.05	Clams (baked)	3 oz (9 small)	0.36
English muffin, plain	1 muffin	0.18	Egg, fresh	1 large	0.18
Noodles, enriched	1 cup	0.18	Ground beef, regular (broiled)	3.5 oz	0.19
Spaghetti, enriched	1 cup	0.11	Ham loin, lean (broiled)	3.5 oz	0.31
Wheat flakes	1 cup	0.42	Kidney beans (boiled)	1 cup	0.10
			Lentils (boiled)	1 cup	0.18
Vegetables			Lima beans (boiled)	1 cup	0.10
Asparagus (boiled)	½ cup (6 spears)	0.11	Mackerel (baked)	3 oz	0.35
Avocado (raw)	1 med	0.21	Rainbow trout (baked)	3 oz	0.19
Mushrooms (boiled)	½ cup pieces	0.23	Sirloin steak (broiled)	3.5 oz	0.30
Spinach (boiled)	½ cup	0.21	Soybeans (boiled)	1 cup	0.49
Sweet potato (baked)	1 med	0.15	Top round (broiled)	3.5 oz	0.27
Fruits			**Milk, dairy products**		
Blueberries (raw)	1 cup	0.07	Brie cheese	1 oz	0.15
Figs (dried)	10 figs	0.17	Buttermilk	8 fl oz	0.38
Pear (raw)	1 med	0.07	Cheddar cheese	1 oz	0.11
Prunes (dried)	10 prunes	0.14	Cottage cheese, creamed	1 cup	0.34
Raspberries (raw)	1 cup	0.11	Cottage cheese, 2% fat	1 cup	0.42
			Milk, skim	8 fl oz	0.34
Meat, poultry, fish, dry beans, eggs, nuts			Milk, whole	8 fl oz	0.39
Almonds (oil roasted)	1 oz	0.28	Ricotta cheese, whole milk	1 cup	0.48
Beef liver (fried)	3.5 oz	4.14	Yogurt, whole	8 fl oz	0.32
Chicken, dark (roasted, without skin)	3.5 oz	0.23	**Fats, oils, sugar**		
Chicken, light (roasted, without skin)	3.5 oz	0.12	This food group is not an important source of riboflavin.		

vestigation established the relation of the disease to a certain food factor. But it was not until 1937 that University of Wisconsin scientist Elvehjem definitely associated niacin with pellagra by using it to cure a related disease—black tongue in dogs. Correlation between human pellagra and niacin deficiency was then rapidly secured.[28]

Chemical and Physical Nature

Further study of niacin and pellagra made clear a close connection of niacin to the essential amino acid tryptophan.

Precursor Role of Tryptophan

Curious observations were made by early investigators that raised puzzling questions. Why was pellagra rare in some population groups whose diets were actually low in niacin, whereas the disease was common in other groups whose diets were higher in niacin? And why did milk, which is low in niacin, cure or prevent pellagra? Furthermore, why was pellagra so common in groups subsisting on diets high in corn? In 1945, scientists at the University of Wisconsin finally made the key discovery—tryptophan can be used by the body to make niacin; it is a **precursor** of niacin. Milk prevents pellagra because it is high in tryptophan. Almost exclusive use of corn contributes to pellagra because it is low in tryptophan. And some populations with diets low in niacin may never have pellagra because they happen also to be consuming adequate amounts of tryptophan.

ariboflavinosis • Group of clinical manifestations of riboflavin deficiency.

glossitis • Swollen, reddened tongue; riboflavin deficiency symptom.

precursor • Something that precedes; in biology, a substance from which another substance is derived.

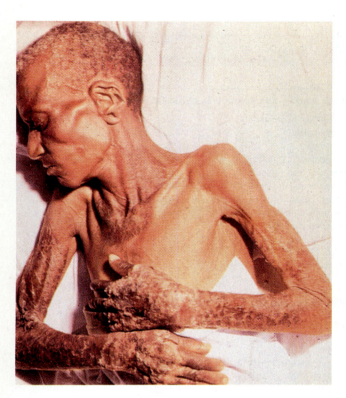

FIG. 7-8   Pellagra.

Niacin Equivalent

This tryptophan-niacin relationship led to the development of the unit of measure called **niacin equivalent (NE)**. In persons with average physiologic needs, approximately 60 mg of tryptophan produces 1 mg of niacin, the amount designated as a niacin equivalent. Dietary requirements are now given in terms of total milligrams of niacin equivalents.

Forms

Two forms of niacin exist. Niacin (nicotinic acid) is easily converted to its amide form, nicotinamide, which is water soluble, stable to acid and heat, and forms a white powder when crystallized.

Functions of Niacin
Basic Coenzyme Role

Niacin is a partner with riboflavin in the cellular coenzyme systems that convert proteins, and the small amount of glycerol from fats, to glucose and then oxidize glucose to release energy.

Drug Therapy

High doses of nicotinic acid act as vasodilators and cause skin flushing, gastrointestinal distress, and itching. Such a dosage has been effective in lowering serum cholesterol.

Clinical Problems

Generally niacin deficiency appears as weakness, anorexia, indigestion, and various skin eruptions. More specific symptoms involve the skin and nervous system. Skin areas exposed to sunlight develop a dark, scaly dermatitis. If deficiency continues, the central nervous system becomes involved, and confusion, apathy, disorientation, and neuritis occur.

Niacin Requirement
Influencing Factors

Factors such as age and growth periods, pregnancy and lactation, illness, tissue trauma, body size, and physical activity affect the niacin requirement.

RDA Standard

The current RDAs for adults of all ages are 6.6 mg/1000 kcal and not less than 13 NE at intakes of less than 2000 kcal. These recommendations allow for the contribution of tryptophan, in terms of niacin equivalents, from the dietary protein sources.[17]

Food Sources of Niacin

Meat is a major source of niacin. Good sources include peanuts, dried beans, and peas. Enrichment makes good sources of all grains. Otherwise corn and rice are poor food sources of niacin because they are low in tryptophan. Table 7-10 gives some comparative food sources of niacin.

Pyridoxine
Chemical and Physical Nature

The chemical structure of pyridoxine, a pyridine ring, accounts for its specific name. It is water soluble, heat stable, but sensitive to light and alkalis.

Forms

Vitamin B_6 is a generic term for a group of vitamins with a similar function. Three forms occur in nature—pyridoxine, pyridoxal, and pyridoxamine. In the body all three forms are equally active as precursors of the potent pyridoxine coenzyme pyridoxal phosphate (B_6PO_4), PLP.

Absorption and Storage

Pyridoxine is easily absorbed in the upper portion of the small intestine. It is "stored" in the tissue saturation sense and found throughout the body, evidence of its many essential metabolic activities.

Functions of Pyridoxine
Coenzyme in Protein Metabolism

In its active phosphate form (PLP), pyridoxine is a coenzyme in many types of amino acid reactions:
1. *Neurotransmitters.* Converts glutamic acid to gamma-

TABLE 7-10

Food Sources of Niacin (RDA for Adults: Women, 13 mg NE; Men, 18 mg NE)

	Quantity	Niacin (mg)		Quantity	Niacin (mg)
Bread, cereal, rice, pasta			**Fruits—cont'd**		
Bread, whole wheat	1 slice	1.0	Mango (raw)	1 med	1.2
Corn meal, yellow, enriched	1 cup	4.8	Raspberries (raw)	1 cup	1.1
Cream of wheat (regular, cooked)	¾ cup	1.1			
Oatmeal (cooked)	¾ cup (⅓ cup dry)	0.2	**Meat, poultry, fish, dry beans, eggs, nuts**		
Rice, white, enriched (cooked)	½ cup	1.1	Beef liver (fried)	3.5 oz	14.4
Wheat flour, all-purpose, enriched	1 cup	4.8	Chicken liver (simmered)	3.5 oz	4.6
			Ground beef, regular (broiled)	3.5 oz	6.8
Vegetables			Ham, cured, regular	3.5 oz	4.8
Asparagus (boiled)	½ cup (6 spears)	0.9	Peanut butter	1 tbsp	2.2
Avocado (raw)	1 med	3.3	Peanuts (dry roasted)	1 oz	3.8
Broccoli (raw)	½ cup chopped	0.3	Salmon (baked)	3 oz	5.7
Carrot (raw)	1 med	0.7	Sirloin steak (lean, broiled)	3.5 oz	4.3
Corn, yellow (boiled)	½ cup	1.3	Swordfish (baked)	3 oz	10.0
Mushrooms (raw)	½ cup pieces	1.4	Top round, lean (broiled)	3.5 oz	6.0
Peas, green (boiled)	½ cup	1.8			
Potato (baked, with skin)	1 med	3.3	**Milk, dairy products**		
Tomato (boiled)	½ cup	0.9	Milk, skim	8 fl oz	0.2
Tomato juice	6 fl oz	1.2	Milk, whole	8 fl oz	0.2
Fruits			**Fats, oils, sugar**		
Banana (raw)	1 med	0.8	This food group is not an important source of niacin.		
Figs (dried)	10 figs	1.3			

aminobutyric acid (GABA), a substance found in the gray matter of the brain, and converts the essential amino acid tryptophan to serotonin, a potent regulatory substance in brain activity.

2. *New amino acids.* Transfers nitrogen from amino acids to form new ones and releases carbon residues for energy.
3. *Sulfur transfer.* Moves sulfur from an essential sulfur-containing amino acid (methionine) to form other sulfur compounds.
4. *Niacin.* Controls formation of niacin from tryptophan.
5. *Hemoglobin.* Incorporates amino acids into heme, the essential nonprotein core of hemoglobin.
6. *Amino acid transport.* Actively transports amino acids from the intestine into circulation and across cell walls into the cells.

Coenzyme in Carbohydrate and Fat Metabolism

PLP provides metabolites for energy-producing fuel. It also converts the essential fatty acid, linoleic acid, to another fatty acid, arachidonic acid.

Clinical Problems

It is evident from this sample list of metabolic activities that pyridoxine holds a key to a number of clinical problems.

Anemia. A hypochromic type of anemia relates to the role of pyridoxine in heme formation. It can occur even in the presence of a high serum iron level. Such deficiency of pyridoxine has been demonstrated by a special test and the anemia cured by supplying the deficient vitamin.

Central nervous system problems. Through its role in the formation of the two regulatory compounds in brain activity, serotonin and GABA, pyridoxine controls related neurologic conditions. In infants deprived of the vitamin, as was the case when a batch of formula was mistakenly autoclaved at high temperature, there is increased irritability progressing to convulsions. Immediate supplementation with the vitamin restores function.

Physiologic demands in pregnancy. Pyridoxine deficiencies during pregnancy have been demonstrated

---

niacin equivalent (NE) • A measure of the total dietary sources of niacin equivalent to 1 mg of niacin. Thus an NE is 1 mg of niacin or 60 mg of tryptophan.

by special tests and subsequently alleviated by supplementation. Fetal growth creates greater maternal metabolic needs and increases pyridoxine requirement.

Oral contraceptive use. Women taking estrogen-progesterone oral contraceptives require additional pyridoxine. An abnormal state of tryptophan metabolism contributes to the increased need.

Drug therapy. The drug isoniazid (isonicotinic acid hydrazide, or INH), used as a chemotherapeutic agent for tuberculosis, is an antagonist to pyridoxine. Also, it inhibits the conversion of glutamic acid, the only amino acid the brain metabolizes, and causes a side effect of neuritis. Treatment with large doses of pyridoxine, 50 to 100 mg/day, prevents this effect.

Pyridoxine Requirement
RDA Standard

A deficiency of pyridoxine is unlikely because the amounts present in the general diet are large relative to the requirement. Since pyridoxine is involved in amino acid metabolism, the need varies with dietary protein intake. The RDA standard is 2 mg/day for men and 1.6 mg/day for women with additions for pregnancy and lactation. Amounts for infants and children are shown in the RDA tables inside the book covers.

Toxic Effects

Acute toxicity of pyridoxine is rare.[30] However, when pyridoxine is taken in larger amounts, up to 5 g/day, for long periods of time, as in therapy for premenstrual syndrome (PMS), it causes lack of muscular coordination and in some cases severe nerve damage. Symptoms disappear when the large supplement is discontinued.

Food Sources of Pyridoxine

Pyridoxine is widespread in foods, but many sources provide only very small amounts. Good sources include grains, seeds, liver and kidney, and other meats. Table 7-11 gives some comparative food sources of pyridoxine.

Pantothenic Acid
Discovery

Pantothenic acid was isolated and synthesized between 1938 and 1940. Because it occurs in all forms of living things and is an acid, it was named **pantothenic acid.** True to its name, it is widespread in nature and in body functions. Intestinal bacteria synthesize considerable amounts. This source, together with its widespread natural occurrence, makes deficiencies unlikely.

TABLE 7-11
Food Sources of Pyridoxine (Vitamin B₄) (RDA for Adults: Women, 1.6 mg; Men, 2.0 mg)

	Quantity	Pyridoxine (mg)		Quantity	Pyridoxine (mg)
Bread, cereal, rice, pasta			**Meat, poultry, fish, dry beans, eggs, nuts—cont'd**		
Wheat germ (toasted)	¼ cup (1 oz)	0.28	Ham (canned)	3.5 oz	0.48
			Kidney beans (boiled)	1 cup	0.21
Vegetables			Lentils (boiled)	1 cup	0.35
Avocado (raw)	1 med	0.48	Lima beans (boiled)	1 cup	0.30
Asparagus (boiled)	1 med	0.13	Navy beans (boiled)	1 cup	0.30
Broccoli (boiled)	½ cup	0.15	Peanut butter (chunk style)	1 tbsp	0.14
Carrot (raw)	1 med	0.11	Peanut butter (creamy)	1 tbsp	0.06
Potato (baked, with skin)	1 med	0.70	Peanuts (roasted)	1 oz	0.07
			Pinto beans (boiled)	1 cup	0.27
Fruits			Sirloin steak (broiled)	3.5 oz	0.45
Apple (raw, with skin)	1 med	0.07	Soybeans (boiled)	1 cup	0.40
Banana (raw)	1 med	0.66	Swordfish (baked)	3 oz	0.32
Figs (dried)	10 figs	0.42	Top round (broiled)	3.5 oz	0.61
Grape juice (bottled)	8 fl oz	0.16	Walnuts (dried)	1 oz	0.18
Meat, poultry, fish, dry beans, eggs, nuts			**Milk, dairy products**		
Beef liver (fried)	3.5 oz	0.27	Milk, skim	8 fl oz	0.10
Cashews (roasted)	1 oz	0.07	Milk, whole	8 fl oz	0.10
Chicken light meat (roasted, without skin)	3.5 oz	0.60			
Chicken liver (simmered)	3.5 oz	0.68	**Fats, oils, sugar**		
Ground beef, regular (broiled)	3.5 oz	0.27	This food group is not an important source of pyridoxine.		

TABLE 7-12

Food Sources of Pantothenic Acid (RDA for Adults: 4-7 mg)

	Quantity	Pantothenic acid (mg)		Quantity	Pantothenic acid (mg)
Bread, cereal, rice, pasta			**Meat, poultry, fish, dry beans, eggs, nuts—cont'd**		
All-bran	⅓ cup (1 oz)	0.49	Cashews (roasted)	1 oz (16 med nuts)	0.34
Bagel	1 bagel	0.20	Chicken, dark meat (roasted, without skin)	3.5 oz	1.21
Bread, whole wheat	1 slice	0.18			
English muffin, plain	1 muffin	0.29	Chicken, light meat (roasted, without skin)	3.5 oz	0.97
Oatmeal, regular (quick)	¾ cup (1 oz)	0.35			
Shredded wheat	1 oz	0.24	Chicken liver (simmered)	3.5 oz	5.41
Soybean flour (defatted)	½ cup	1.00	Egg, fresh	1 large	0.85
Wheat germ (toasted)	¼ cup (1 oz)	0.39	Egg yolk, fresh	Yolk of 1 large egg	0.76
			Garbanzo beans (boiled)	½ cup	0.24
Vegetables			Ground beef, regular (broiled)	3.5 oz	0.38
Avocado (raw)	1 med	1.68	Ham, cured, regular	3.5 oz	0.50
Broccoli (raw)	½ cup, chopped	0.24	Lentils (boiled)	½ cup	0.83
Corn, yellow (boiled)	½ cup	0.72	Lima beans (boiled)	½ cup	0.36
Potato (baked, with skin)	1 med	1.12	Peanut butter (chunk style)	2 tbsp	0.31
Squash, winter, all varieties, (baked)	½ cup	0.36	Peanuts (roasted)	1 oz	0.39
			Pinto beans (boiled)	½ cup	0.26
Sweet potato (boiled)	½ cup, mashed	0.87	Salmon (smoked)	3 oz	0.74
Tomato (boiled)	½ cup	0.35	Sirloin steak (broiled)	3.5 oz	0.35
			Top round (broiled)	3.5 oz	0.48
Fruits			Turkey, light meat (roasted, without skin)	3.5 oz	0.63
Apricots (raw)	3 med	0.25			
Banana (raw)	1 med	0.30			
Figs (dried)	10 figs	0.81	**Milk, dairy products**		
Orange juice (fresh)	8 fl oz	0.47	American cheese, processed	1 oz	0.14
Orange, navel (raw)	1 med	0.35	Blue cheese	1 oz	0.49
Papaya (raw)	1 med	0.86	Cheddar cheese	1 oz	0.12
Pomegranate (raw)	1 med	0.92	Milk, skim	8 fl oz	0.81
			Milk, whole	8 fl oz	0.76
Meat, poultry, fish, dry beans, eggs, nuts			Yogurt, whole	8 fl oz	0.88
Almonds (dried)	1 oz (24 nuts)	0.13			
Beef liver (fried)	3.5 oz	5.92	**Fats, oils, sugar**		
Black beans (boiled)	½ cup	0.24	This food group is not an important source of pantothenic acid.		
Black-eyed peas (boiled)	½ cup	0.35			

Chemical and Physical Nature

Pantothenic acid is a white crystalline compound. It is readily absorbed in the intestine and combines with phosphorus to form the active coenzyme A. It is in this key controlling compound of coenzyme A that pantothenic acid has such widespread metabolic presence and use throughout the body. There is no known toxicity or a natural deficiency.

Functions of Pantothenic Acid

In its one basic role as an essential constituent of the body's key activating agent acetylcoenzyme A (acetyl-CoA), pantothenic acid is vital to metabolic reactions involving carbohydrate, fat, and protein metabolism.

Pantothenic Acid Requirement

Since deficiency is unknown, a requirement for pantothenic acid has not been stated. The RDA's estimated safe and adequate range for adults is 4 to 7 mg. The daily intake in an average American diet ranges from about 5 to 10 mg.[17] Thus a deficiency is unlikely with the widespread occurrence of the vitamin in food sources.

Food Sources of Pantothenic Acid

Sources of pantothenic acid are equally as widespread as its occurrence in body tissue. Rich sources include metabolically active tissue such as liver and kidney. Egg

> **pantothenic acid** • A B vitamin found widely distributed in nature and occurring throughout the body tissues. Pantothenic acid is an essential constituent of coenzyme A, which has extensive metabolic responsibility as an activating agent of a number of compounds in many tissues.

yolk and milk contribute more. Table 7-12 shows some food sources of pantothenic acid.

Biotin

General Nature of Biotin

The minute traces of biotin in the body perform multiple metabolic tasks. Its potency is great and natural deficiency is unknown. But some cases of induced deficiency have occurred in patients on long-term TPN, and several inborn errors of biotin metabolism have been defined according to the specific enzyme that is lacking.[31,32] There is no known toxicity.

Functions of Biotin

Biotin functions as a partner with acetyl-CoA in reactions that transfer carbon dioxide from one compound and fix it onto another. Examples of this combination of cofactors at work include: (1) initial steps in synthesis of some fatty acids, (2) conversion reactions involved in synthesis of some amino acids, and (3) carbon dioxide fixation in forming purines.

Biotin Requirements

Since the amount needed for metabolism is so small, the human requirement for biotin has not yet been established in specific terms. The RDA adult estimate is 30 to 100 µg/day. Intestinal bacteria synthesis contributes to the body's supply of biotin, but the amount is uncertain.[17]

Food Sources of Biotin

Biotin is widely distributed in natural foods, but its bioavailability is highly variable in different foods. For example, the biotin of corn and soy meals is completely available, whereas that of wheat is almost unavailable. Excellent food sources include egg yolk, liver, kidney, and other animal tissues, as well as tomatoes among the vegetables, and yeast. Fruit and meat are poor sources. The biotin in general U.S. diets ranges from about 30 to 45 µg/day.

Folate

Discovery

Folate is the generic name for a group of substances that have similar nutritional properties and chemical structures. One of these substances was first extracted from dark green, leafy vegetables such as spinach and thus initially given the name folic acid, or folacin, from the Latin word *folium*, meaning "leaf." The reduced form of folic acid is folinic acid. Folic acid was then identified and isolated in laboratory studies of anemias and growth factors in animals. In 1945 folic acid was obtained from liver and finally synthesized. The term *folate* is the the salt form of folic acid, and both terms are often used interchangeably for the vitamin.

Chemical and Physical Nature

Folic acid forms yellow crystals and is a conjugated substance made up of three acids: (1) pteroic acid, (2) para-aminobenzoic acid (PABA), and (3) glutamic acid (an amino acid). The chemical name for folic acid, from its structure, is pteroylglutamate (PGA).

PABA is sometimes touted in nutrition supplement claims as a separate essential factor in human nutrition. It is not. Its only role in human nutrition is that of a component of the vitamin folic acid. Animal and human cells are capable neither of synthesizing PABA nor of attaching it to the rest of the vitamin molecule. Only plants and certain bacteria can do this. Thus dietary folic acid, preformed by plants, is the essential substance in human nutrition, and the major source of this folic acid is green leafy vegetables.

Functions of Folate
Basic Coenzyme Role

Folates function as necessary coenzyme agents in the important task of attaching single carbons to many metabolic compounds. Several key compounds are examples:

1. *Purines.* Nitrogen-containing compounds essential to all living cells, involved in cell division and in the transmission of inherited traits
2. *Thymine.* Essential compound forming a key part of deoxyribonucleic acid (DNA), the important material in the cell nucleus that controls and transmits genetic characteristics
3. *Hemoglobin.* Heme, the iron-containing nonprotein portion of hemoglobin

Clinical Problems

Some clinical problems associated with folate follow:

Anemia. A nutritional **megaloblastic anemia** occurs in simple folate deficiency. Since tissue growth requires additional folate, this folate deficiency anemia is a special risk in pregnant women, growing infants, and young children.

Sprue. Folate is an effective agent in the treatment of **sprue,** a gastrointestinal disease characterized by intestinal lesions, malabsorption defects, diarrhea, macrocytic anemia, and general malnutrition. The vitamin corrects both the blood-forming and the gastrointestinal defects of the disease.

Chemotherapy. The drug amethopterin (Methotrexate), currently used in cancer chemotherapy, acts as a folate antagonist to reduce the tumor growth. The effect of this action is to prevent synthesis of DNA and purines.

Growth and stress. Increased folate is needed during periods of rapid growth, especially during fetal development.

Folate Requirement

Average American and Canadian diets contribute about 0.3 µg/kg body weight of folate and provide approximately 90% of the adult population with sufficient absorbable folate to meet daily needs and maintain adequate storage.[17] On this basis the current RDA for folate is 200 µg for men and 180 µg for women. Based on a 50% food folate absorption, the RDA for folate is 400 µg/day for women during pregnancy to meet increased needs for fetal and maternal tissue growth. Increases are also indicated for lactation. The varying needs of infants, children, and adolescents are indicated in the summary RDA tables inside the book covers.

This current RDA for folate is about 50% lower than the amounts previously recommended. This reduction has raised some concern that the new allowance may not provide adequate safety for specific population groups at risk, such as pregnant women, adolescents, and older adults, especially those with the added burdens of low socioeconomic status.[33,34]

Food Sources of Folate

Folate is widely distributed in foods. Good sources include green leafy vegetables, liver, legumes, and a few fruits. Table 7-13 gives a summary of food sources of folate. However, household preparation plus food processing and storage may destroy as much as 50% of the folate. Since there is potential for toxicity from the increased intake of folate, excessive supplemental use is not recommended.[17]

Cobalamin

Discovery

The discovery of cobalamin (vitamin B_{12}) was associated with the search for the specific agent responsible for control of **pernicious anemia.** At first the disease was thought to be related to a deficiency of folate. However, although folate helped the initial red blood cell regeneration, it was not permanently effective and did not control the nerve problems associated with the disease. When folate was found to be lacking in full effectiveness, the search continued for the remaining piece of the disease puzzle.

In 1948 two groups of workers, one in America and one in England, crystallized a red compound from liver, which they then numbered B_{12}. In the same year

TABLE 7-13

Food Sources of Folate (RDA for Adults: Women, 180 µg; Men, 200 µg)

	Quantity	Folate (µg)
Bread, cereal, rice, pasta		
Bread, whole wheat	1 slice	14
Wheat germ (toasted)	¼ cup (1 oz)	100
Vegetables		
Asparagus (boiled)	½ cup (6 spears)	88
Avocado (raw)	1 med	113
Peas, green (boiled)	1 cup	51
Spinach (boiled)	1 cup	262
Fruits		
Banana (raw)	1 med	22
Figs (dried)	10 figs	14
Orange (raw)	1 med	47
Strawberries (raw)	1 cup	26
Meat, poultry, fish, dry beans, eggs, nuts		
Beef liver (fried)	3.5 oz	220
Black beans (boiled)	1 cup	256
Black-eyed peas (boiled)	1 cup	358
Chicken liver (simmered)	3.5 oz	770
Chick-peas (boiled)	1 cup	282
Egg, whole	1 large	32
Green beans (boiled)	1 cup	42
Kidney beans (boiled)	1 cup	229
Lima beans, baby (boiled)	1 cup	273
Navy beans (boiled)	1 cup	255
Peanut butter	1 tbsp	13
Peanuts (dry roasted)	1 oz	41
Pinto beans (boiled)	1 cup	794
Milk, dairy products		
Milk, whole	8 fl oz	12
Yogurt, whole	8 fl oz	17
Fats, oils, sugar		
This food group is not an important source of folate.		

megaloblastic anemia • Anemia resulting from faulty production of abnormally large immature red blood cells, caused by a deficiency of vitamin B_{12} and folate.

pernicious anemia • A chronic macrocytic anemia occurring most commonly after age 40. It is caused by absence of the intrinsic factor normally present in the gastric juices and necessary for the absorption of cobalamin (B_{12}) and controlled by intramuscular injections of vitamin B_{12}.

it was clearly shown that this new vitamin could control both the blood-forming defect and the neurologic involvement in pernicious anemia. Soon afterward, the working groups of scientists were able to produce the vitamin through a process of bacterial fermentation. This process remains the main source of commercial supply today. The scientists named their vitamin discovery cobalamin because of its unique structure with a single brilliant red atom of the trace element cobalt at its center.

Chemical and Physical Nature

Cobalamin is a complex red crystalline compound of high molecular weight, with a single cobalt atom at its core. It occurs as a protein complex in foods, so its food sources are mainly of animal origin. The ultimate source, however, may be designated as the synthesizing bacteria in the intestinal tract of herbivorous animals. Some synthesis is done by human intestinal bacteria.

Absorption, Transport, and Storage

Absorption

Intestinal absorption takes place in the ileum. Cobalamin is first split from its protein complex by the gastric hydrochloric acid and then bound to a specific glycoprotein called intrinsic factor, secreted by the gastric mucosal cells. This cobalamin–intrinsic factor complex then moves into the intestine, where it is absorbed by special receptors in the ileal mucosa.

Storage

Cobalamin is stored in active body tissues. Organs holding the greatest amounts are the liver, kidney, heart, muscle, pancreas, testes, brain, blood, spleen, and bone marrow. These amounts are very minute, but the body holds them tenaciously and the stores are only slowly depleted. For example, a typical postgastrectomy anemia does not become apparent until 3 to 5 years after removal of the organ and subsequent loss of its secretions.

Functions of Cobalamin

Basic Coenzyme Role

As an essential coenzyme factor, cobalamin is closely related to amino acid metabolism and the formation of the heme portion of hemoglobin. Its requirement increases as protein intake increases.

Clinical Problems

Special needs for cobalamin occur in several problems related to blood forming.

Pernicious anemia.   In the absence of the intrinsic factor, the specific component of gastric secretion required for cobalamin absorption, pernicious anemia develops. The vitamin is then not available for its key role in heme formation, and adequate hemoglobin cannot be synthesized.

Conversely, however, folate is not the primary agent for treating pernicious anemia. As indicated, although folate results in blood cell regeneration in persons with pernicious anemia, its effect is not permanent, nor does it control the degenerative neurologic problems. This is the critical distinction between cobalamin and folate in the diagnosis and treatment of this anemia. Therefore, the American Medical Association and the U.S.

TABLE 7-14

Food Sources of Vitamin B_{12} (RDA for Adults: 2 µg)

	Quantity	Vitamin B_{12} (µg)		Quantity	Vitamin B_{12} (µg)
Bread, cereal, rice, pasta			**Meat, poultry, fish, dry beans, eggs, nuts—cont'd**		
This food group is not an important source of vitamin B_{12}.			Mackerel (baked)	3 oz	16.18
			Oysters (steamed)	3 oz (12 med)	32.63
Vegetables			Salmon (baked)	3 oz	4.93
This food group is not an important source of vitamin B_{12}.			Sirloin steak (lean, broiled)	3.5 oz	2.86
			Swordfish (baked)	3 oz	1.72
Fruits			Top round, lean (broiled)	3.5 oz	2.48
This food group is not an important source of vitamin B_{12}.			**Milk, dairy products**		
			Cheddar cheese	3.5 oz	0.83
Meat, poultry, fish, dry beans, eggs, nuts			Milk, skim	8 fl oz	0.83
Beef liver (fried)	3.5 oz	111.80	Milk, whole	8 fl oz	0.87
Chicken liver (simmered)	3.5 oz	19.39	Swiss cheese	3.5 oz	1.86
Chicken, white meat (roasted)	3.5 oz	0.34	Yogurt, whole	8 fl oz	0.84
Clams (steamed)	3 oz (9 small)	84.05			
Egg, fresh	1 large	0.77	**Fats, oils, sugar**		
Ground beef, regular (broiled)	3.5 oz	2.93	This food group is not an important source of vitamin B_{12}.		
Ham, cured, regular	3.5 oz	0.80			

Food and Drug Administration have recommended that no more than 0.4 mg of folate be included in multivitamin preparations, as this amount would suffice for common needs and not mask the development of pernicious anemia or prevent its diagnosis.

A person with defective cobalamin absorption, and hence pernicious anemia, can be given from 15 to 30 μg/day of cobalamin in intramuscular injections during a relapse and can be maintained afterward by an injection of about 30 μg every 30 days. This treatment controls both the blood-forming disorder and the degenerative effects on the nervous system.

Megaloblastic anemia. Since cobalamin shares close metabolic relations with folate, a megaloblastic anemia develops when either of the vitamins is deficient. Cobalamin indirectly affects blood formation by providing an activated form of folate.

TABLE 7-15

Summary of B-Complex Vitamins

Vitamin	Coenzyme: physiologic function	Clinical applications	Requirement	Food sources
Thiamin	Carbohydrate metabolism Thiamin pyrophosphate (TPP): oxidative decarboxylation	Beriberi (deficiency) Neuropathy Wernicke-Korsakoff syndrome (alcoholism) Depressed muscular and secretory symptoms	0.5 mg/1000 kcal	Pork, beef, liver, whole or enriched grains, legumes
Riboflavin	General metabolism Flavin adenine dinucleotide (FAD) Flavin mononucleotide (FMN)	Cheilosis, glossitis, seborrheic dermatitis	0.6 mg/1000 kcal	Milk, liver, enriched cereals
Niacin (nicotinic acid, nicotinamide)	General metabolism Nicotinamide adenine dinucleotide (NAD) Nicotinamide adenine dinucleotide phosphate (NADP)	Pellagra (deficiency) Weakness, anorexia Scaly dermatitis Neuritis	6.6 NE/1000 kcal	Meat, peanuts, enriched grains (protein foods containing tryptophan)
Vitamin B_4 (pyridoxine, pyridoxal, pyridoxamine)	General metabolism Pyridoxal phosphate (PLP): transamination and decarboxylation	Reduced serum levels associated with pregnancy and use of oral contraceptives Antagonized by isoniazid, penicillamine, and other drugs	2 mg (men) 1.6 mg (women)	Wheat, corn, meat, liver
Pantothenic acid	General metabolism CoA (coenzyme A): acetylation	Many roles through acyl-transfer reactions (for example, lipogenesis, amino acid activation, and formation of cholesterol, steroid hormones, heme)	4 to 7 mg	Liver, egg, milk
Biotin	General metabolism N-Carboxybiotinyl lysine: CO_2 transfer reactions	Deficiency induced by avidin (a protein in raw egg white) and by antibiotics Synthesis of some fatty acids and amino acids	30 to 100 μg	Egg yolk, liver Synthesized by intestinal microorganisms
Folate (folic acid, folacin)	General metabolism Single carbon transfer reactions (for example, purine nucleotide, thymine, heme synthesis)	Megaloblastic anemia	200 μg (men) 180 μg (women)	Liver, green leafy vegetables
Cobalamin	General metabolism Methylcobalamin: methylation reactions (for example, synthesis of amino acids, heme)	Pernicious anemia induced by lack of intrinsic factor Megaloblastic anemia Methylmalonic aciduria Homocystinuria Peripheral neuropathy (strict vegetarian diet)	2 μg	Liver, meat, milk, egg, cheese

Sprue. Like folate, cobalamin is effective in the treatment of the intestinal syndrome of **sprue.** However, it is most effective when used in conjunction with folate, because its role is indirect activation of folic acid.

Cobalamin Requirement

The amount of dietary cobalamin needed for normal human metabolism is very small. Reported minimum needs have been from 0.6 to 1.2 µg/day, with a range upward to approximately 2.8 µg to allow for individual variances. The ordinary diet easily provides this much and more. For example, one cup of milk, one egg, and 4 oz meat provide 2.4 mg. The RDA standard recommends an intake of 3 µg/day for adults. This amount allows a safety margin to cover variances in individual need, absorption, and body stores.

Food Sources of Cobalamin

Cobalamin is supplied by animal foods. The richest sources are liver and kidney, lean meat, milk, egg, and cheese. Natural dietary deficiency is rare. It has been observed only in some groups of strict vegetarians, who displayed symptoms of nervous disorders, sore mouth and tongue, neuritis, and amenorrhea. Table 7-14 gives food sources of cobalamin.

A summary of the water-soluble B vitamins is given in Table 7-15.

To Sum Up

A vitamin is an organic, noncalorigenic food substance that is required in small amounts for certain metabolic functions and cannot be manufactured by the body. Vitamins may be fat or water soluble, and their solubility affects their absorption and mode of transport to target tissues.

The fat-soluble vitamins are A, D, E, and K. Their metabolic tasks are mainly structural in nature, and their fate in the body is associated with lipids. The possibility of toxicity is enhanced for fat-soluble vitamins because the body can store them. Such toxicity is no longer rare because of the current popularity of vitamin supplements.

The remaining vitamins are water soluble: ascorbic acid (C) and the B complex. These vitamins share three characteristics: (1) synthesis by plants and thus dietary supply by plant foods or animal foods (except vitamin B_{12}); (2) no stable "storage" form and thus must be provided regularly in the diet (except vitamin B_{12}); and (3) function as a coenzyme factor in cell metabolism (ex-

cept vitamin C). Toxicity levels are usually not associated with water-soluble vitamins because excess is easily excreted in the urine. However, two vitamins have shown toxic effects when taken in megadoses (that is, in gram amounts): pyridoxine (B_6), which can result in severe nerve damage, and ascorbic acid (C), which has been associated with gastrointestinal disturbances, renal calculi, and lowered resistance to infection. All water-soluble vitamins, especially vitamin C, are easily oxidized and care must be taken in food storage and preparation practices.

QUESTIONS FOR REVIEW

1. List and describe three health problems caused by a vitamin A deficiency. Give three possible causes of a deficiency.
2. How do the absorption and storage of a vitamin affect its potential deficiency or toxicity? Give several examples to illustrate.
3. Describe the function of the vitamin D hormone calcitriol. Who is at risk for developing a deficiency? Why?
4. List three conditions that increase the risk for vitamin K deficiency. How do these deficiencies develop?
5. What three characteristics are shared by most water-soluble vitamins? Identify an exception to each and explain the reason.
6. Define the term *coenzyme factor* as applied to the role of vitamins, especially water-soluble vitamins. Give several examples to illustrate.
7. Which water-soluble vitamins are potentially toxic? Why? What signs of toxicity have been observed for each?
8. Which B vitamins play significant roles in blood formation? Describe their roles and interactions.

REFERENCES

1. Johnson EJ and others: Evaluation of vitamin A absorption by using oil-soluble and water-miscible vitamin A preparations in normal adults and in patients with gastrointestinal disease, *Am J Clin Nutr* 55:857, 1992.
2. Hussey GD, Klein M: A randomized controlled trial of vitamin A in children with severe measles, *N Engl J Med* 323:160, 1990.
3. Report: Vitamin A administration reduces mortality and morbidity from severe measles in populations nonendemic for hypervitaminosis A, *Nutr Rev* 49(3):89, 1991.
4. Report: Processing of dietary retinoids is slowed in the elderly, *Nutr Rev* 49(4):116, 1991.
5. Mele L and others: Nutritional and household risk factors for xerophthalmia in Aceh, Indonesia: a case-control study, *Am J Clin Nutr* 53:1460, 1991.
6. Willett WC: Vitamin A and lung cancer, *Nutr Rev* 48(5):201, 1990.
7. DeLuca HF: The vitamin D story: a collaborative effort of basic science and clinical medicine, *FASEB J* 2:224, 1988.
8. Glorieux FH: Rickets: the continuing challenge, *N Engl J Med* 325(26):1875, 1991.

sprue • Alternate term for adult celiac disease, a malabsorption syndrome.

9. Bhowmick SK, Retting KR: Rickets caused by vitamin D deficiency in breast-fed infants in the southern United States, *Am J Dis Child* 145:127, 1991.

10. Haynes PC Jr: Agents affecting calcification: calcium, parathyroid hormone, calcitonin, vitamin D, and other compounds. In Gilman AG and others, eds: *Goodman and Gilman's the pharmacological basis of therapeutics*, ed 8, New York, 1990, Pergamon Press.

11. Jacobus CH and others: Hypervitaminosis D from drinking milk, *N Engl J Med* 326(18):1173, 1992.

12. Holick MF and others: The vitamin D content of fortified milk and infant formula, *N Engl J Med* 326(18):1178, 1992.

13. Gloth FM and others: Is the recommended daily allowance for vitamin D too low for the home-bound elderly? *J Am Geriatr Soc* 39(2):137, 1991.

14. Zheng JJ, Rosenberg JH: What is the nutritional status of the elderly? *Geriatrics* 44:57, 1989.

15. Bjorneboe A and others: Absorption, transport, and distribution of vitamin E, *J Nutr* 120:233, 1990.

16. Howard LJ: The neurologic syndrome of vitamin E deficiency: laboratory and electrophysiologic assessment, *Nutr Rev* 48(4):169, 1990.

17. Food and Nutrition Board, National Academy of Science-National Research Council: *Recommended dietary allowances*, ed 10, Washington, DC, 1989, National Academy Press.

18. Horwitt MK: Data supporting supplementation of humans with vitamin E, *J Nutr* 121:424, 1991.

19. Suttie JW: Vitamin K and human nutrition, *J Am Diet Assoc* 92(5):585, 1992.

20. Booth C, Dugdale A: Vitamin K, the neglected vitamin: a review of its requirements and role, *Aust J Nutr Diet* 47:115, 1990.

21. Niki E: Action of ascorbic acid as a scavenger of active and stable oxygen radicals, *Am J Clin Nutr* 54(suppl):1119S, 1991.

22. Frei B: Ascorbic acid protects lipids in human plasma and low-density lipoproteins against oxidative damage, *Am J Clin Nutr* 54(suppl):1113S, 1991.

23. Block G and others: Vitamin C—a new look, *Ann Intern Med* 114(10):1991.

24. McCormick DB: Thiamin. In Shils ME, Young VR, eds: *Modern nutrition in health and disease*, ed 7, Philadelphia, 1988, Lea & Febiger.

25. Eisinger J, Ayavou T: Transketolase stimulation in fibromyalgia, *J Am Coll Nutr* 9(1):56, 1990.

26. Roe DA and others: Effect of fiber supplements on the apparent absorption of pharmacologic doses of riboflavin, *J Am Diet Assoc* 88(2):211, 1988.

27. Roughead Z, McCormick DB: Qualitative and quantitative assessment of flavins in cow's milk, *J Nutr* 120:382, 1990.

28. McCormick DB: Niacin. In Shils ME, Young VR, eds: *Modern nutrition in health and disease*, ed 7, Philadelphia, 1988, Lea & Febiger.

29. Report: Assessment of niacin status in humans, *Nutr Rev* 48(8):318, 1990.

30. Leklem JE: Vitamin B_6: a status report, *J Nutr* 120:1503, 1990.

31. McCormick DB: Biotin. In Shils ME, Young VR, eds: *Modern nutrition in health and disease*, ed 7, Philadelphia, 1988, Lea & Febiger.

32. Mack DM and others: Effects of biotin deficiency on fatty acid composition: evidence for abnormalities in humans, *J Nutr* 118:342, 1988.

33. Tsui JC, Nordstrom JW: Folate status of adolescents: effects of folic acid supplementation, *J Am Diet Assoc* 90(11):1551, 1990.

34. Bailey LB: Evaluation of a new recommended dietary allowances for folate, *J Am Diet Assoc* 92(4):463, 1992.

FURTHER READING

Gloth FM and others: Is the recommended daily allowance for vitamin D too low for the homebound elderly? *J Am Geriatr Soc* 39(2):137, 1991.

On the basis of limited exposure to sunlight accompanied by chronic conditions and limited mobility in their study of elderly nursing home residents, these authors answer their question with a definitive "yes."

Horwitt MK: Data supporting supplementation of humans with vitamin E, *J Nutr* 121:424, 1991.

The author, an eminent nutrition scientist, presents a timely review of current vitamin E research that underscores its antioxidant function and identifies older adults and persons with chronic disease as those who may need physiologic supplementation.

Suttie JW: Vitamin K and human nutrition, *J Am Diet Assoc* 92(5):585, 1992.

This leader in vitamin K research provides current information about the recently discovered role of vitamin K in bone growth, as well as the status of food analysis to produce needed food value tables.

Merkel JM and others: Vitamin and mineral supplement use by women with school-age children, *J Am Diet Assoc* 90(3):462, 1990.

Read MA and others: Relationship of vitamin/mineral supplementation to certein psychologic factors, *J Am Diet Assoc* 91(11):1429, 1991.

These two articles provide some interesting answers to the question of why persons choose to use vitamin and mineral supplements, ranging from the insurance approach to concern about illness.

Guidelines for Vitamin Supplementation

"Charlatan!" cry the conservative health workers at anyone who suggests a need for vitamin supplements.

"Fuddy-duddy!" reply the self-proclaimed nutrition experts who prescribe megadoses of everything from A through zinc to cure anything that ails you.

Who's right? Probably someone who suggests something between these two extremist views. The RDAs are based on the average needs of a healthy population, not on specific individual needs, which can vary widely. But extremists may take these two concepts too far. Extreme traditionalists try to apply these standards rigidly to every individual. "Pill-pushers" recommend megadoses of everything to cover all the bases and increase their profits.

Biochemical individuality is a real concept. It cannot be overlooked when assessing an individual's nutritional needs. Since it is influenced by health status, personal habits, age, and other factors, the assessment process should consider at least the following conditions.

Pregnancy and lactation. The RDA takes into account increased nutrient requirements for these situations. But individual food preferences and food availability may make meeting these increased nutrient needs by diet alone difficult. Supplements then become a more reasonable way of ensuring an adequate intake to meet the increased nutrient demands.

Oral contraceptive use. The use of oral contraceptives lowers serum levels of several B vitamins, including vitamin B_6 (pyridoxine) and niacin, as well as vitamin C. If nutrient intake levels are marginal, some supplements may be necessary. Of course, it is more important to encourage the client to improve her diet or assist her in obtaining nutritious foods.

Aging. The aging process may increase the need for some nutrients because of decreased food intake and impaired nutrient metabolism. Marginal or so-called subclinical deficiencies of ascorbic acid, thiamin, riboflavin, and pyridoxine are seen in the elderly, even among individuals using supplements. This suggests that current RDA standards may be too low to meet their particular needs.

Restricted diets. Persons who are eternally dieting may find it difficult to meet many of the nutrient standards if they take in less than 1200 kcal/day. Strict diets are not recommended anyway. In any event, carefully assess anyone on a weight-reduction regimen.

Exercise. Persons involved in physical exercise programs have been shown to require increased riboflavin to maintain normal tissue levels. Most people who exercise consume adequate amounts of food to compensate for this possible deficit. But the combination of restricting kcalories and exercising accentuates this need even more and may indicate the need for a B-complex supplement, especially in women who do not tolerate milk (the major source of riboflavin) well.

Smoking. This unhealthful, addictive habit reduces ascorbic acid levels by as much as 30%. If dietary intake is marginal, a small supplement (for example, 100 mg/day) may help compensate for the reduction. Of course, stopping the harmful habit helps even more.

Alcohol. Chronic or abusive use of alcohol impedes absorption and utilization of the B-complex vitamins, especially thiamin, and even destroys folate. Supplements of multivitamins rich in B-complex vitamins, as well as ascorbic acid, help. However, a change in alcohol consumption must accompany nutritional therapy to prevent recurrence of deficiency signs.

Caffeine. Taken in large quantities, caffeine flushes water-soluble vitamins from the body faster than usual. Small supplements of B-complex and ascorbic acid may help. Reduced caffeine intake helps even more.

Disease. In a state of disease, malnutrition, debilitation, or hypermetabolic demand, each patient must of course be carefully assessed to determine just what degree of overall nutrient supplementation and diet modification may be indicated for clinical purposes. These needs are particularly evident in long-term illness.

Once all these conditions are carefully evaluated, a wise nutrition program can be developed. In many situations, supplementation can be avoided by a change in personal habits. Best of all, people in general are better served by changing personal habits. They are able to maintain good health while avoiding artificially induced deficiencies and expensive health food store bills.

REFERENCES

Chen MF and others: Effect of ascorbic acid on plasma alcohol clearance, *J Am Coll Nutr* 9(3):185, 1990.

Schectman G and others: Ascorbic acid requirements for smokers: analysis of a population survey, *Am J Clin Nutr* 53:1466, 1991.

White-O'Connor B and others: Dietary habits, weight history, and vitamin supplement use in elderly osteoarthritis patients, *J Am Diet Assoc* 89(3):378, 1989.

CHAPTER 8

Minerals

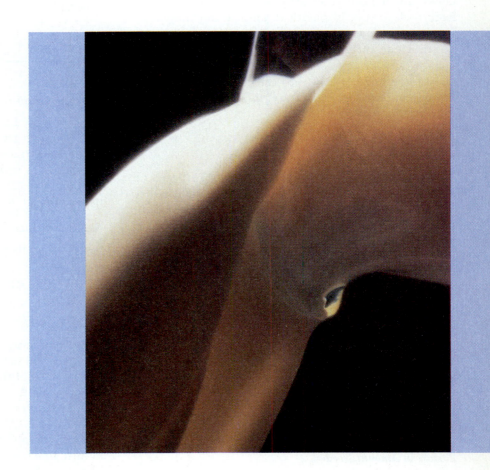

In this chapter we look at the remaining micronutrients, the minerals. They may seem simple in comparison to the complex organic vitamin compounds, but they fulfill a variety of metabolic functions.

Elements for which the requirement is greater than 100 mg/day are called major minerals, not because they are more important, but just because there are more of them in the body. Those needed in much smaller amounts are called trace elements, of which a few in minute amounts are called ultratrace elements.

Here we review each of these groups of minerals. As with the vita-

mins, we focus on why we need them and how we may obtain them.

Minerals in Human Nutrition
Our Cycle of Minerals

Here on our planet Earth we live within a vast slow-motion cycle of minerals essential to our existence as humans. Over eons of time, shifting oceans and mountains have deposited an array of elements that move from rock to soil, to plants, to animals and humans.[1] Until recent times our access to some of these elements in sufficient measure for health has depended on luck—where we happened to live. But over time, with more knowledge of how they can be processed, transported, and used in agriculture, there has come better distribution.

Metabolic Roles
Variety of Functions

Minerals are inorganic elements widely distributed in nature. They have vital roles in human metabolism that are as varied as are the minerals themselves. These substances, which appear so inert in comparison with the complex organic vitamin compounds, fulfill an impressive variety of metabolic functions: building, activating, regulating, transmitting, and controlling. For example, ionized sodium and potassium exercise all-important control over shifts in body water. Dynamic calcium and phosphorus provide structure for the body's framework. Oxygen-hungry iron gives a core to heme in hemoglobin. Brilliant red cobalt is the atom at the core of cobalamin (vitamin B_{12}). Iodine is the necessary constituent of the thyroid hormones, which in turn control the rate of body metabolism. Far from being static and inert, minerals are active participants, helping to control many of the metabolic processes in the body.

Variety in Amount Needed

Minerals also differ from vitamins in another way. Vitamins, as you saw in the previous chapter, all require very small amounts of their complex organic compounds to do their metabolic jobs. Minerals, however, require varying amounts, from the relatively large amounts of the major minerals to the exceedingly small amounts of the trace elements. For example, the major mineral calcium forms a relatively large amount of body weight—about 2%. Most of this is in skeletal tissue. Thus an adult weighing 150 lb has about 3 lb of calcium in the body. On the other hand, the trace element iron is present in very small amounts. This same adult has only about 3 g (about 1/10 oz) of iron in the body, mostly in the hemoglobin of red blood cells.

TABLE 8-1
Major Minerals and Trace Elements in Human Nutrition

Major minerals (required intake over 100 mg/day)	Trace elements	
	Essential (required intake under 100 mg/day)	Essentiality unclear
Calcium (Ca)	Iron (Fe)	Silicon (Si)
Phosphorus (P)	Iodine (I)	Vanadium (V)
Magnesium (Mg)	Zinc (Zn)	Nickel (Ni)
Sodium (Na)	Copper (Cu)	Tin (Sn)
Potassium (K)	Manganese (Mn)	Cadmium (Cd)
Chloride (Cl)	Chromium (Cr)	Arsenic (As)
Sulfur (S)	Cobalt (Co)	Aluminum (Al)
	Selenium (Se)	Boron (B)
	Molybdenum (Mo)	
	Fluoride (F)	

Classification

In your study here you will find these important mineral elements grouped in three main sections, one major and two trace. These commonly used divisions are based on (1) how much of the mineral is required by the body and (2) how much we know at this point about its essentiality, in cases of some of the trace elements.

Major Minerals

Seven minerals present in the body in large amounts are called the major minerals. These include calcium, magnesium, sodium, potassium, phosphorus, sulfur, and chloride.

Trace Elements

The remaining minerals are present in smaller amounts and are called trace elements. The essential nature of 10 of these has been determined. For the remaining eight, their precise functioning is as yet not entirely clear.

In Table 8-1, as a study guide, you will find a listing of the minerals in each group. We briefly review each in turn, looking at (1) balance controls maintaining the body's needed amount, (2) physiologic function, (3) associated clinical problems, (4) the body's requirement, and (5) food sources.

MAJOR MINERALS
Calcium

Of all the minerals in the body, calcium by far occurs in the largest amount. The total amount of body calcium is in constant balance with food sources from the outside as well as with tissue calcium within the body among its various parts. A number of dynamic balance mechanisms are constantly at work to maintain these levels within normal ranges. The balance concept, therefore, can be applied at three basic levels: (1) the intake-absorption-output balance, (2) the bone-blood balance, and (3) the calcium-phosphorus blood serum balance.

Intake-Absorption-Output Balance
Calcium Intake

The average adult American diet contains about 700 to 1200 mg of calcium. Most of this comes from dairy products and some from green leafy vegetables and grains. However, the absorption of minerals in general is less efficient than that of the vitamins and macronutrients. Not all of the food intake of minerals is necessarily available. The term **bioavailability** refers to the degree to which the body uses a particular nutrient, such as calcium in this case, which depends on many factors that influence its absorption-excretion balance or its balance in body tissues.[2] This is one of the basic facts that makes the setting of precise requirements for minerals difficult. Stated requirements for many of these elements are given as estimated ranges of need rather than as precise figures.

Absorption of Calcium

Only about 10% to 30% of the calcium in an average diet is absorbed. Most food calcium occurs in complexes with other dietary components. These complexes must be broken down and the calcium released in a soluble form before it can be absorbed. Absorption takes place in the small intestine, chiefly in the first section, the duodenum, where the gastric acidity is still effective rather than being buffered as the food mass moves along.

Factors Increasing Calcium Absorption

The following factors increase calcium absorption:

Vitamin D hormone.   An optimum amount of this control agent is necessary for calcium absorption. This agent controls the synthesis of a calcium-binding protein carrier in the duodenum that transports the mineral into the mucosal cells amd blood circulation.[3]

Body need.   During periods of greater body demand, such as growth or depletion states, more calcium is absorbed. Physiologic states in the life cycle—growth, pregnancy and lactation, and old age—have a strong influence on the amount of absorption needed to meet body requirements. In elderly persons in general and in postmenopausal women in particular, the ability to absorb calcium is reduced.[4]

Dietary protein and carbohydrate.   A greater percentage of calcium is absorbed when the diet is high in protein. However, this larger amount absorbed results in increased renal excretion, with a negative cal-

cium balance following. Thus, in essence, high-protein diets only induce increased calcium requirements to maintain calcium balance. Lactose enhances calcium absorption through the action of the lactobacilli, which produce lactic acid and lower intestinal pH. However, this effect is not always consistent.[5]

Acidity.   Lower pH (increased acidity) favors solubility of calcium and consequently its absorption.

Factors Decreasing Calcium Absorption

The following factors decrease calcium absorption:

Vitamin D deficiency.   Vitamin D hormone, along with parathyroid hormone, is essential for calcium absorption.

Dietary fat.   Excess dietary fat or poor absorption of fats results in an excess of fat in the intestine. This fat combines with calcium to form insoluble soaps. These insoluble soaps are excreted, with consequent loss of the incorporated calcium.

Fiber and other binding agents.   An excess of dietary fiber binds calcium and hinders its absorption. Other binding agents include oxalic acid, which combines with calcium to produce calcium oxalate, and phytic acid, which forms calcium phytate. Oxalic acid is a constituent of green leafy vegetables, but the amount of oxalates in them varies, making some of them better sources of calcium than others. Phytic acid is found in the outer hull of many cereal grains, especially wheat.

Alkalinity.   Calcium is insoluble in an alkaline medium and consequently is poorly absorbed.

Calcium Output

The overall body calcium balance is maintained first, therefore, at the point of absorption. A large unabsorbed amount—some 70% to 90% varying according to body need—remains to be eliminated in the feces. A small amount of calcium may be excreted in the urine, about 200 mg/day, to maintain normal levels in the body fluids.

Bone-Blood Balance
Calcium in the Bones

In a healthy state the body maintains a constant turnover of the calcium in the bone tissue, which is the ma-

bioavailability • Amount of a nutrient ingested in food that is absorbed and thus available to the body for metabolic use.

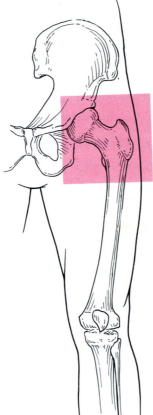

FIG. 8-1
Bone and cartilage development.

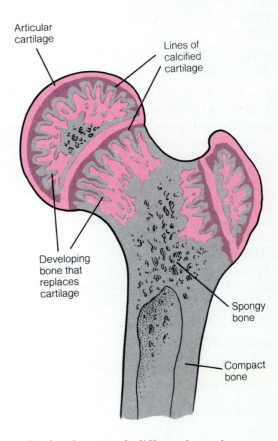

jor site of calcium storage. Calcium in the bones and teeth is about 99% of that in the entire body. However, this is not a static storage. Bone tissue is constantly being built and reshaped according to various body needs and stresses (Fig. 8-1). As much as 700 mg calcium enters and leaves the bones each day. And all the while the body maintains a dynamic equilibrium. But in certain conditions or disease, withdrawals may exceed deposits and a state of calcium imbalance occurs. For example, conditions such as immobility from a body cast or diseases such as osteoporosis would cause excess bone calcium withdrawals.

Calcium in the Blood

The remaining small amount of calcium not in bone tissue—about 1%—circulates in the blood and other body fluids. Despite its small amount, however, this serum calcium plays a vital role in controlling body functions. Calcium in the blood occurs in two main forms.

Bound calcium. About half the calcium in the blood is bound in the plasma proteins, hence is not free or diffusible, that is, able to move about or to enter into other activities.

Free ionized calcium. Free particles of calcium, carrying electrical charges and hence in an active ionized form, move freely about and diffuse through membranes to control a number of body functions. These functions include blood clotting, transmission of nerve impulses, muscle contraction and relaxation, membrane permeability, and enzyme activation. This is a good illustration of a small amount of a nutrient doing a great deal of metabolic work because it is in an activated form.

Calcium-Phosphorus Serum Balance

A final level of calcium balance is that which calcium maintains with phosphorus in the blood serum. Amounts of these two minerals in the blood are normally maintained in a definite relationship because of their relative solubility. This relationship is called the *calcium-phosphorus serum balance*. This serum balance is the solubility product of calcium times phosphorus, expressed in milligrams per deciliter of each mineral. Normal serum levels are 10 mg/dl of calcium in children and adults, and 4 mg/dl of phosphorus in adults and 5 mg/dl in children. Thus the normal serum calcium-phosphorus solubility products are $10 \times 4 = 40$ for adults and $10 \times 5 = 50$ for children. Any situation that causes an increase in the serum phosphorus level would cause a resulting decrease in the serum calcium level to hold the calcium-phosphorus solubility product constant. In such a case the decreased serum calcium may bring on signs of tetany from lack of neuromuscular controls. To help maintain the normal serum calcium-phosphorus balance, the ideal dietary calcium-phosphorus balance is 1.0:1.5 for children and women during pregnancy and lactation. Other adults require a 1:1 dietary balance, meaning equal amounts of dietary calcium and phosphorus, for ideal absorption and utilization.

Control Agents For Calcium Balance

Two main control agents work together to maintain these vital levels of calcium balance in the body: parathyroid hormone and vitamin D hormone *(calcitriol)*. The cooperative action of these two factors is a good example of the **synergistic** behavior of metabolic controls. Consider the interdependent relationship of these agents.

Parathyroid hormone. The parathyroid glands, lying adjacent to the thyroid glands, are particularly sensitive to changes in the circulating blood level of free ionized calcium. When this level drops, the parathyroid gland releases its hormone, which then acts in three ways to restore the normal blood calcium level: (1) it stimulates intestinal mucosa to absorb more calcium; (2) it withdraws more calcium rapidly from the bone **compartment,** and (3) it causes kidneys to excrete more phosphate. These combined activities then restore calcium and phosphorus to their correct balance in the blood.

Vitamin D hormone. In general, along with parathyroid hormone, vitamin D hormone controls absorption of calcium. However, still with parathyroid hormone, it also affects the deposit of calcium and phosphorus in bone tissue. Thus these two agents balance each other, with vitamin D hormone acting more to control calcium absorption and bone deposit and parathyroid acting more to control calcium withdrawal from bone and kidney excretion of its partner serum phosphorus.

A third hormonal agent, **calcitonin,** is also involved in calcium balance. Produced by special C cells in the thyroid gland, it prevents abnormal rises in serum calcium by modulating release of bone calcium. Thus its action counterbalances that of parathyroid hormone to help regulate serum calcium at normal levels in balance with bone calcium.

The overall balance relationship of the various factors involved in calcium metabolism is illustrated in Fig. 8-2.

Physiologic Functions of Calcium
Bone Formation

The physiologic function of 99% of the body calcium is to build and maintain skeletal tissue. This is done by special types of cells that are in constant balance between depositing and withdrawing bone calcium.

Tooth Formation

Special tooth-forming organs in the gums deposit calcium to form teeth. The mineral exchange continues as in bone. This exchange in dental tissue occurs mainly in the dentin and cementum. Very little deposit occurs in the enamel once the tooth is formed.

General Metabolic Functions

The remaining 1% of the body's calcium performs a number of vital physiologic functions.

Blood clotting. In the blood clotting process, serum calcium ions are required for cross-linking of fibrin, giving stability to the fibrin threads.

Nerve transmission. Normal transmission of nerve impulses along axons requires calcium. A current of calcium ions triggers the flow of signals from one nerve cell to another and on to the waiting target muscles.

Muscle contraction and relaxation. Ionized serum calcium helps initiate contraction of muscle fibers and control of contraction following. This catalyzing action of calcium ions on the muscle protein filaments allows the sliding contraction between them to occur (see Chapter 14). This action of calcium is particularly vital in the constant contraction-relaxation cycle of the heart muscle.

Cell membrane permeability. Ionized calcium controls the passage of fluids and solutes through cell membranes by affecting membrane permeability. It influences the integrity of the intercellular cement substance.

Enzyme activation. Calcium ions are important activators of specific cell enzymes, especially ones that release energy for muscle contraction. They play a similar role with other enzymes, including lipase, which di-

---

calcitonin • A polypeptide hormone secreted by the thyroid gland in response to hypercalcemia, which acts to lower both calcium and phosphate in the blood.

compartment • The collective quantity of material of a given type in the body. The four body compartments are *lean body mass* (muscle), *bone, fat,* and *water.*

synergism • The joint action of separate agents in which the total effect of their combined action is greater than the sum of their separate actions. (Adjective: synergistic.)

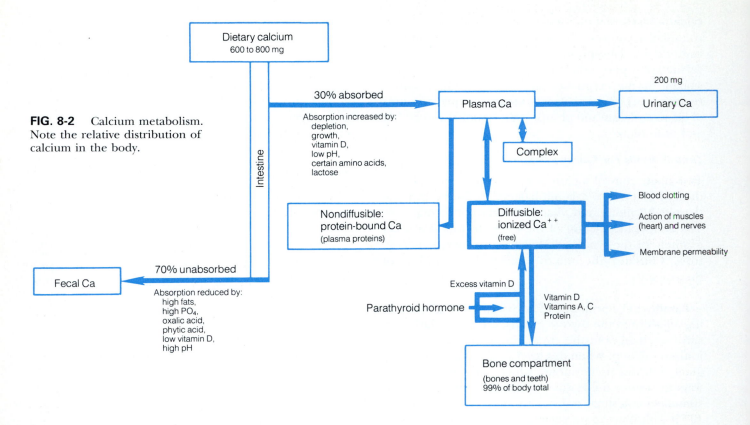

FIG. 8-2 Calcium metabolism. Note the relative distribution of calcium in the body.

gests fat, and with some members of the protein-splitting enzyme system.

Clinical Problems

A number of clinical problems may develop from imbalances that interfere with the various physiologic and metabolic functions of calcium.

Tetany

A decrease in ionized serum calcium causes tetany, a state marked by severe, intermittent spastic contractions of the muscle and by muscular pain.

Rickets

A deficiency of vitamin D hormone causes rickets. When there is inadequate exposure to sunlight or deficient dietary intake of vitamin D, proper bone formation cannot take place.

Osteoporosis

The usual form of osteoporosis, which is characterized by bone mineral loss, occurs mainly in older persons, especially in postmenopausal women. In affected women the most rapid rate of loss occurs in the first 5 years after menopause. There is a negative calcium balance of about 40 to 120 mg/day, indicating loss from both the outer bone layer—*cortex*—and the small developing needlelike projections of bone—*trabeculae*—into the central marrow forming the calcium-anchoring network of bone matrix.[6] Afterward the rate of bone

loss is about 1% a year. In most patients it is not corrected by increased calcium alone but is often improved by exercise coupled with supplements.[7] Current approaches to stimulate new bone growth involve hormonal therapy with both vitamin D hormone and estrogen. An idiopathic osteoporosis occurring in young adults does not respond to calcium therapy.

Resorptive Hypercalciuria and Renal Calculi

Two conditions can tilt the usually fine-tuned calcium deposition-mobilization balance maintained by the controlling hormones. When this normal balance is disturbed, resorption of calcium from bone and subsequent increased urinary calcium excretion occurs. A main factor leading to such a condition is prolonged immobilization. Such an imbalance may occur, for example, from a full body cast after orthopedic surgery or a spinal cord injury, or with a body brace following a back injury. In such cases, normal muscle tension on bones that is necessary for calcium balance is lessened, and the risk of renal stones from increased urinary calcium is increased.

Calcium Requirement

Recognizing that peak bone mass is attained by about age 25, the RDA standard has been raised for young adults. An intake of 1200 mg/day for both sexes from ages 11 to 24 is made to cover the important accelerated growth years of adolescence and early adulthood.[8] A conservative estimate of a 40% absorption rate is as-

TABLE 8-2
Food Sources of Calcium (RDAs for Adults: 800 mg)

	Quantity	Calcium (mg)
Bread, cereal, rice, pasta		
Bran muffin, homemade	1 muffin	54
Bread, whole wheat	1 slice	18
Corn muffin, from mix	1 muffin	96
Cream of wheat (cooked)	¾ cup	38
Pasta, enriched (cooked)	1 cup	16
Rice, enriched	1 cup	21
Wheat flakes	1 cup	43
Vegetables		
Artichoke (boiled)	1 med	47
Asparagus (boiled)	½ cup (6 spears)	22
Avocado (raw)	1 med	19
Broccoli (raw)	½ cup	21
Brussels sprouts (boiled)	½ cup (4 sprouts)	28
Carrots (raw)	1 med	19
Collards (boiled)	1 cup	148
Corn, yellow (boiled)	½ cup	2
Kale (chopped)	½ cup	47
Peas, green (boiled)	½ cup	19
Potato (baked, with skin)	1 med	115
Tomato (raw)	1 med	8
Fruits		
Apricots (raw)	3 med	15
Banana (raw)	1 med	7
Cantaloupe (raw)	½ cup	8
Figs (dried)	10 figs	269
Orange juice (fresh)	8 fl oz	27
Orange, navel (raw)	1 med	56
Papaya (raw)	1 med	72
Raspberries (raw)	½ cup	14
Strawberries (raw)	½ cup	11
Tangerine (raw)	1 med	12
Meat, poultry, fish, dry beans, eggs, nuts		
Almonds (roasted)	1 oz	148
Beef liver (fried)	3.5 oz	11
Cashews (roasted)	1 oz	13
Chicken, dark (roasted, without skin)	3.5 oz	179
Chicken, light (roasted, without skin)	3.5 oz	216
Egg, whole	1 large	90
Ham (canned)	3.5 oz	6
Kidney beans (boiled)	1 cup	50
Lentils (boiled)	1 cup	37
Lima beans (boiled)	1 cup	32
Peanuts (roasted)	1 oz	15
Soybeans (boiled)	1 cup	175
Milk, dairy products		
Milk, skim	8 fl oz	302
Milk, whole	8 fl oz	290
Yogurt, whole	8 fl oz	355
Fats, oils		
This food group is not an important source of calcium.		
Sugar		
Brown sugar	1 cup	123
Molasses, barbados	1 tbsp	49

sumed. The previous allowance for older adults is continued at 800 mg/day. An allowance of 1200 mg/day is made for pregnancy and lactation, irrespective of age. The standard for formula-fed infants is 400 mg/day for the first 6 months and 600 mg/day for the remainder of the first year. For children ages 1 to 10, the standard is 800 mg/day. Higher intakes with supplementation may lead to problems such as constipation, urinary stones, or interference with absorption of other essential minerals, so supplementation beyond these RDAs is not recommended.

Food Sources of Calcium

Dairy products provide the bulk of dietary calcium. One quart of milk contains about 1 g of calcium. Cheese is also a major source. Other sources, including eggs, green leafy vegetables, broccoli, legumes, nuts, and whole grains, contribute smaller amounts. Table 8-2 provides some comparative food sources of calcium.

Phosphorus

Phosphorus makes up about 1% of total body weight. It is closely associated with calcium in human nutrition and has been called its metabolic twin. However, it has some unique characteristics and functions of its own.

Absorption-Excretion Balance
Absorption

The same factors that control calcium absorption also regulate phosphorus. Free phosphate is absorbed in the jejunum of the small intestine in relation to calcium and is also regulated by active vitamin D hormone, although the hormonal effect is greater on calcium absorption than on phosphorus.[9] Equal amounts of calcium and phosphorus should exist in the diet in an optimal ratio. Since phosphate occurs in food as a phosphate compound, mainly with calcium, the first step for its absorption is its splitting off as the free mineral. Factors similar to those which influence calcium absorption also affect phosphorus absorption. For example, an excess of calcium or other binding material, such as aluminum or iron, inhibits phosphorus absorption.

Excretion

The kidneys provide the main excretion route for regulation of the serum phosphorus level. Usually, 85% to 95% of plasma phosphate is filtered at the renal glomeruli and largely reabsorbed at the tubules, along

> **osteoporosis** • Abnormal thinning of bone, producing a porous, fragile, latticelike bone tissue of enlarged spaces that is prone to fracture or deformity.

with calcium, under the influence of vitamin D hormone. But when increased phosphate excretion is needed to maintain the normal serum calcium-phosphate balance, parathyroid hormone acts to override the effect of vitamin D hormone. The amount of phosphorus excreted in the urine of a person ingesting an average diet is 0.6 to 1.8 g/day.

Bone-Blood-Cell Balance
Bone

From 80% to 90% of the body's phosphorus is in the skeleton, including the teeth, compounded with calcium. This bone compartment of phosphorus is in constant interchange with the rest of the body's phosphorus, which is circulating in the blood and other body fluids.

Blood

The serum phosphorus level normally ranges from 3 to 4.5 mg/dl in adults and somewhat higher, 4 to 7 mg/dl, in children. The higher range in growth years is a significant clue to its role in cell metabolism.

Cells

In its active phosphate form phosphorus plays a major role in the structure and function of all living cells. Here it works with proteins, lipids, and carbohydrates to produce energy, build and repair tissues, and to act as a buffer.

Hormonal Controls

Since calcium and phosphorus work closely together, phosphorus balance is under the direct control of the same two hormones controlling calcium—vitamin D hormone and parathyroid hormone. A deficiency or depletion of phosphate occurs from dietary lack, diminished absorption from the intestine, or excessive wasting through the kidney.

Physiologic Functions of Phosphorus
Bone and Tooth Formation

From 80% to 90% of the body phosphorus helps make bones and teeth. As a component of calcium phosphate, it is constantly being deposited and reabsorbed in the process of bone formation.

General Metabolic Activities

Far out of proportion to the relatively small remaining amount, the rest of the phosphorus is intimately involved in overall human metabolism in every living cell. It has several vital roles.

Absorption of glucose and glycerol. Phosphorus combines with glucose and glycerol to assist in their intestinal absorption. It also promotes renal tubular reabsorption of glucose to return this sugar to the blood.

Transport of fatty acids. Phospholipids provide a form of fat transport.

Energy metabolism. Phosphorus-containing compounds, for example, adenosine triphosphate (ATP), are key cell substances in energy metabolism.

Buffer system. The phosphate buffer system of phosphoric acid and phosphate helps control acid-base balance in the blood.

Physiologic Changes

Situations involving physiologic and clinical changes in serum phosphorus level include the following:

Recovery from diabetic acidosis. Active carbohydrate absorption and metabolism use much phosphorus, depositing it with glycogen and causing temporary hypophosphatemia.

Growth. Growing children usually have higher serum phosphate levels, resulting from high levels of growth hormone.

Hypophosphatemia. Low serum phosphorus levels occur in intestinal diseases such as sprue and celiac disease, which hinder absorption; in bone disease such as rickets or osteomalacia, which upset the calcium-phosphorus serum balance; and in primary hyperparathyroidism, in which the excess secretion of parathyroid hormone causes excess renal tubular excretion of phosphorus. Symptoms of hypophosphatemia include muscle weakness, because the cells are deprived of phosphorus essential for energy metabolism.

Hyperphosphatemia. Both renal insufficiency and hypoparathyroidism cause excess accumulation of serum phosphate. As a result, the calcium side of the serum calcium-phosphorus balance is low, causing tetany.

Phosphorus Requirement
Dietary Ratio

During growth, pregnancy, and lactation the balance of dietary phosphorus to calcium should ideally be 1:1. In ordinary adult life the intake of phosphorus is about 1.5 times that of calcium. In general, since these two minerals are found in the same food sources, if calcium needs are met, adequate phosphorus will be ensured.

RDA Standard

The current RDA standard for phosphorus is 800 mg for children 1 to 10 years of age, 1200 mg for ages 11 to 24, and 800 mg for all adults beyond the age of 24. For formula-fed infants from birth to 6 months of age the standard is 300 mg/day, and for infants ages 6 to 12 months, 500 mg/day.

TABLE 8-3
Food Sources of Phosphorus (RDAs for Adults: 800 mg)

	Quantity	Phosphorus (mg)		Quantity	Phosphorus (mg)
Bread, cereal, rice, pasta			**Meat, poultry, fish, dry beans, eggs, nuts—cont'd**		
Bran flakes	¾ cup	158	Chicken, dark (roasted, without skin)	3.5 oz.	179
Bran muffin, homemade	1 muffin	111	Chicken, light (roasted, without skin)	3.5 oz	216
Bread, whole wheat	1 slice	65	Chick-peas (boiled)	1 cup	275
Cream of wheat (cooked)	¾ cup	31	Clams, canned	3 oz	287
English muffin, plain	1 muffin	64	Cod (baked)	3 oz	117
Oatmeal (cooked)	¾ cup	133	Crab, Alaska king (steamed)	3 oz	238
Pasta, enriched (cooked)	1 cup	70	Egg, whole	1 large	90
Rice, enriched (cooked)	1 cup	57	Ground beef, regular (broiled)	3.5 oz	170
Wheat flakes	1 cup	98	Halibut (baked)	3 oz	242
			Ham, canned (lean)	3.5 oz	224
Vegetables			Lentils (boiled)	1 cup	356
Artichoke (boiled)	1 med	72	Lobster (steamed)	3 oz	157
Avocado (raw)	1 med	73	Oysters (steamed)	3 oz (12 med)	236
Brussels sprouts (boiled)	½ cup (4 sprouts)	44	Peanut butter, creamy	1 tbsp	60
Carrots (raw)	1 med	32	Peanuts (roasted)	1 oz	100
Corn, yellow (boiled)	½ cup	84	Pinto beans (boiled)	1 cup	273
Peas, green (boiled)	½ cup	94	Sirloin steak, lean (broiled)	3.5 oz	244
Potato (baked, with skin)	1 med	115	Sole (baked)	3.5 oz	344
Spinach (boiled)	½ cup	50	Soybeans (boiled)	1 cup	421
Sweet potato (baked)	1 med	62	Trout, rainbow (baked)	3 oz	272
			Tuna, light, canned in water	3 oz	158
Fruits			Walnuts, dried	1 oz	132
Figs (dried)	10 figs	128			
Kiwi fruit (raw)	1 med	31	**Milk, dairy products**		
Orange juice (fresh)	8 fl oz	42	Cheddar cheese	1 cup	145
Orange, navel (raw)	1 med	27	Cottage cheese, creamed	1 cup	277
Raisins, seedless	⅔ cup	97	Milk, skim	8 fl oz	247
			Milk, whole	8 fl oz	227
Meat, poultry, fish, dry beans, eggs, nuts			Swiss cheese	1 oz	171
Almonds (roasted)	1 oz (22 nuts)	156	Yogurt, whole	8 fl oz	215
Bacon (fried)	3 med	64			
Beef liver (fried)	3.5 oz	461	**Fats, oils, sugar**		
Beef top round, lean (broiled)	3.5 oz	246	This food group is not an important source of phosphorus.		
Black-eyed peas (boiled)	1 cup	266			

Food Sources of Phosphorus

Milk and milk products are the most significant sources of phosphorus as they are for calcium. However, because phophorus plays such a large role in cell metabolism, it is also found in lean meats. Table 8-3 provides a list of food sources of phosphorus.

Sodium

Sodium is one of the most plentiful minerals in the body. About 120 mg (4 oz) is in the body of an adult, with one third in the skeleton as inorganic bound material. The remaining two thirds is free ionized sodium, the major electrolyte in body fluids outside the cells.

Absorption-Excretion Balance
Absorption

Sodium intake is readily absorbed from the intestine. Normally only about 5% remains for elimination in the feces. Larger amounts are lost in abnormal states such as diarrhea.

Excretion

The major route of excretion is through the kidney, under the powerful hormonal control of **aldosterone,** the sodium-conserving hormone from the adrenal glands.

> **aldosterone** • Potent hormone of the cortex of the adrenal glands, which acts on the distal renal tubule to cause reabsorption of sodium in an ion exchange with potassium. The aldosterone mechanism is essentially a sodium-conserving mechanism but indirectly also conserves water since water absorption follows the sodium reabsorption.

Physiologic Functions of Sodium

Water Balance

Ionized sodium is the major guardian of body water outside of cells. Variations in its body fluid concentrations largely determine the distribution of water by *osmosis* from one body area to another.

Acid-Base Balance

In association with chloride and bicarbonate ions, ionized sodium helps regulate acid-base balance.

Cell Permeability

The sodium pump in all cell membranes helps exchange sodium and potassium and other cellular materials. A major substance carried into cells by this active transport system is glucose.

Muscle Action

Sodium ions play a large part in transmitting electrochemical impulses along nerve and muscle membranes and help maintain normal muscle action. Potassium and sodium ions balance the response of nerves to stimulation, the travel of nerve impulses to muscles, and the resulting contraction of the muscle fibers.

Sodium Requirement

RDA Standard

The body can function on a rather wide range of dietary sodium by mechanisms designed to conserve or excrete the mineral. Thus there is no specific stated requirement. However, the RDAs do include a table of estimated minimum requirements of the three minerals—sodium, chloride, and potassium—that are major electrolytes in body fluid balance. This RDA standard estimates a minimum sodium requirement for healthy persons over age 18 to be about 500 mg/day to cover wide variations in individual patterns of physical activity and climate, which influence relative losses in perspiration.[8] Thus a safe and adequate sodium intake for

TABLE 8-4

Food Sources of Sodium (Estimated Safe and Adequate Daily Intakes for Adults: 1100-3300 mg)

	Quantity	Sodium (mg)		Quantity	Sodium (mg)
Bread, cereal, rice, pasta			**Meat, poultry, fish, dry beans, eggs, nuts—cont'd**		
Bran flakes	¾ cup	264	Egg, whole	1 large	69
Bran muffin, homemade	1 muffin	168	Ground beef, regular (broiled)	3.5 oz	83
Bread, whole wheat	1 slice	159	Halibut (baked)	3 oz	59
Corn flakes	1 cup	310	Ham, canned (lean)	3.5 oz	1255
Wheat flakes	1 cup	270	Lentils (boiled)	1 cup	4
			Lobster (steamed)	3 oz	323
Vegetables			Mackerel (baked)	3 oz	71
Artichoke (boiled)	1 med	79	Oysters (steamed)	3 oz (12 med)	190
Broccoli (boiled)	½ cup	12	Peanut butter, creamy (unsalted)	1 tbsp	3
Brussels sprouts (boiled)	½ cup	17	Peanut butter, creamy (with salt)	1 tbsp	131
Carrot (raw)	1 med	25	Shrimp (steamed)	3 oz (15 large)	190
Potato (baked, with skin)	1 med	16	Sirloin steak, lean (broiled)	3.5 oz	66
Spinach (boiled)	½ cup	63	Soybeans (boiled)	1 cup	1
Tomato (raw)	1 med	10	Tuna, light, canned in water (with salt)	3 oz	303
Fruits			**Milk, dairy products**		
This food group is not an important source of sodium.			Cheddar cheese	1 oz	176
			Cottage cheese, creamed	1 cup	850
Meat, poultry, fish, dry beans, eggs, nuts			Milk, skim	8 fl oz	126
			Milk, whole	8 fl oz	119
Almonds (roasted, unsalted)	1 oz (22 nuts)	3	Swiss cheese	1 oz	74
Bacon (broiled/fried)	3 med pieces	303	Yogurt, whole	8 fl oz	105
Beef liver (fried)	3.5 oz	106			
Beef top round, lean (broiled)	3.5 oz	61	**Fats, oils, sugar**		
Black-eyed peas (boiled)	1 cup	6	Butter (salted)	1 tbsp	123
Chicken, dark (roasted, without skin)	3.5 oz	93	Butter (unsalted)	1 tbsp	2
			Margarine, stick, corn oil (salted)	1 tbsp	132
Chicken, light (roasted, without skin)	3.5 oz	77	Margarine, stick, corn oil (unsalted)	1 tbsp	3
			Molasses, black	1 tbsp	19
Clams (steamed)	3 oz (9 small)	95	Sugar, brown	1 cup	44
Crab, blue (steamed)	3 oz	237			

adults has been set at approximately 1100 to 3300 mg/day.

General Dietary Intake

Sodium in the average American diet, mainly in processed foods, usually far exceeds the RDA estimate of adequate intake, even excluding the added amount in table salt. There is about 4 g sodium in the average 10 g of table salt consumed daily. A wiser adult intake of about 2 g sodium would equal about 5 g (1 tsp) of salt.

Food Sources of Sodium

The main dietary source of sodium is common salt used in cooking, seasoning, and processing of foods. Natural food sources include milk, meat, eggs, and certain vegetables such as carrots, beets, leafy greens, and celery. Some comparative food sources of sodium are provided in Table 8-4.

Potassium

Potassium is about twice as plentiful as sodium in the body. An adult body contains about 270 mg (9 oz, 4000 mEq). By far the greater portion is found inside the cells, since potassium is the major guardian of the body water inside cells. However, the relatively small amount in fluid outside cells has a significant effect on muscle activity, especially heart muscle.

Absorption-Excretion Balance

Absorption

Dietary potassium is easily absorbed in the small intestine. Potassium also circulates in the gastrointestinal secretions, and is reabsorbed in the digestive process. However, diseases such as prolonged diarrhea cause dangerous losses.

Excretion

Urinary excretion is the principal route of potassium loss. There is excess loss with some diuretic drugs. Since maintenance of serum potassium within the narrow normal range is vital to heart muscle action and electrolyte balance, the kidneys guard potassium carefully. However, they cannot guard potassium as effectively as sodium. In the renal aldosterone mechanism for sodium conservation, potassium is lost in exchange for sodium. The normal obligatory loss is about 160 mg/day.

Physiologic Functions of Potassium

Water and Acid-Base Balance

As the major guardian of cell water, potassium inside the cells balances with sodium outside the cells to maintain normal osmotic pressures and water balance to protect cellular fluid. Potassium also works with sodium and hydrogen to maintain acid-base balance.

Muscle Activity

Potassium plays a significant role in the activity of skeletal and cardiac muscle. Together with sodium and calcium, potassium regulates neuromuscular stimulation, transmission of electrochemical impulses, and contraction of muscle fibers. This effect is particularly notable in the action of the heart muscle. Even small variations in serum potassium concentration are reflected in electrocardiographic (ECG) changes. Variations in serum levels or low serum potassium may cause muscle irritability and paralysis. The heart may even develop a gallop rhythm and finally cardiac arrest.

Carbohydrate Metabolism

When blood glucose is converted to glycogen for storage, 0.36 mmol of potassium is stored for each 1 g glycogen. When a patient in diabetic acidosis is treated with insulin and glucose, rapid glycogen production draws potassium from the serum. Serious hypokalemia can result unless adequate potassium replacement accompanies treatment.

Protein Synthesis

Potassium is required for the storage of nitrogen in muscle protein and general cell protein. When tissue is broken down, potassium is lost together with the nitrogen. Amino acid replacement includes potassium to ensure nitrogen retention.

Potassium Requirement

As with sodium, no specific dietary requirement is given for potassium. However, based on balance studies of the amount needed to replace losses and maintain normal body stores and plasma levels, the RDA standard estimates a minimum safe daily intake for adults of approximately 1600 to 2000 mg.[8] In light of considerable evidence that dietary potassium has a beneficial effect on hypertension, in its report *Diet and health: implications for reducing chronic disease risk*, the National Research Council has recommended an increase in potassium by eating more fruits and vegetables.[10] The RDA has stated a safe and adequate range of daily potassium intake for adults of 1875 to 5625 mg. The usual diet contains from 2000 to 4000 mg/day, which is ample for common need.

Food Sources of Potassium

Potassium is widely distributed in natural foods, since it is an essential constituent of all living cells. Legumes, whole grains, fruits such as oranges and bananas, leafy green vegetables, broccoli, potatoes, and meats supply considerable amounts. People who eat large amounts of fruits and vegetables have a high potassium intake of about 8 to 11 g/day, well above the minimum safe level of 2 g/day. Table 8-5 gives some comparative food sources of potassium.

TABLE 8-5

Food Sources of Potassium (Estimated Safe and Adequate Daily Intake for Adults: 1875-5625 mg)

	Quantity	Potassium (mg)		Quantity	Potassium (mg)
Bread, cereal, rice, pasta			**Meat, poultry, fish, dry beans, eggs, nuts—cont'd**		
Bran flakes	¾ cup	184	Beef top round, lean (broiled)	3.5 oz	442
Bran muffin, homemade	1 muffin	99	Black-eyed peas (boiled)	1 cup	476
Bread, whole wheat	1 slice	44	Chicken, dark (roasted, without skin)	3.5 oz	240
Oatmeal (cooked)	¾ cup	99	Chicken, light (roasted, without skin)	3.5 oz	247
Pasta, enriched (cooked)	1 cup	85	Clams (steamed)	3 oz (9 small)	534
Rice, white, enriched	1 cup	57	Crab, blue (steamed)	3 oz	275
Wheat flakes	1 cup	110	Egg, whole	1 large	65
Wheat germ, toasted	¼ cup (1 oz)	268	Ground beef, regular (broiled)	3.5 oz	292
			Halibut (baked)	3 oz	490
Vegetables			Ham, canned (lean)	3.5 oz	364
Artichoke (boiled)	1 med	316	Lentils (boiled)	1 cup	731
Asparagus (boiled)	½ cup (6 spears)	279	Lima beans (boiled)	1 cup	955
Avocado (raw)	1 med	1097	Lobster (steamed)	3 oz	299
Broccoli (raw)	½ cup, chopped	143	Mackerel (baked)	3 oz	341
Brussels sprouts (boiled)	½ cup (4 sprouts)	247	Oysters (steamed)	3 oz (12 med)	389
Carrot (raw)	1 med	233	Peanut butter, creamy	1 tbsp	110
Corn, yellow (boiled)	½ cup	204	Peanuts (dry roasted)	1 oz	184
Mushrooms (boiled)	½ cup, pieces	277	Pinto beans (boiled)	1 cup	800
Potato (baked, with skin)	1 med	844	Salmon (baked)	3 oz	319
Spinach (boiled)	½ cup	419	Sirloin steak, lean (broiled)	3.5 oz	403
Sweet potato (baked)	1 med	397	Soybeans (boiled)	1 cup	886
Tomato (raw)	1 med	254	Trout, rainbow (baked)	3 oz	539
			Tuna, light, canned in water (with salt)	3 oz	267
Fruits					
Apple (raw, with skin)	1 med	159	**Milk, dairy products**		
Banana	1 med	451	Cottage cheese, creamed	1 cup	177
Cantaloupe	1 cup, pieces	494	Milk, skim	8 fl oz	406
Dates (dried)	10 dates	541	Milk, whole	8 fl oz	368
Figs (dried)	10 figs	1332	Yogurt, whole	8 fl oz	351
Orange juice (fresh)	8 fl oz	486			
Orange, navel	1 med	250	**Fats, oils**		
Prunes (dried)	10 prunes	626	This food group is not an important source of potassium.		
Prune juice (canned)	8 fl oz	706			
Raisins, seedless	⅔ cup	751	**Sugar**		
			Molasses, black	1 tbsp	585
Meat, poultry, fish, dry beans, eggs, nuts			Sugar, brown	1 cup	499
Almonds (dry roasted)	1 oz (22 nuts)	219			
Beef liver (fried)	3.5 oz	364			

Other Major Minerals

Three additional minerals are assigned to the major minerals group because of the extent of their occurrence in the body. These are magnesium, chloride, and sulfur.

Magnesium

Magnesium has widespread metabolic functions and is present in all body cells. An adult body contains about 25 g of magnesium, or a little less than an ounce. About 70% of this small but vital amount is combined with calcium and phosphorus in the bone. The remaining 30% is distributed in various tissues and body fluids, where it has widespread metabolic use in all cells as a control agent. It acts as an enzyme activator for energy production and building tissue protein. It also aids in normal muscle action. The RDA standard is 350 mg/day for men and 300 mg for women. Magnesium is relatively widespread in nature and thus in unprocessed foods. For example, large concentrations of magnesium occur in unmilled grains, but more than 80% is lost by removal of the germ and outer layers.[8] Its main food sources include nuts, soybeans, cocoa, seafood, whole grains, dried beans and peas, and green vegetables. Most fruits, except bananas, are relatively poor sources, as are milk, meat, and fish. Thus, on the whole, diets rich in vegetables and unrefined grains are much higher in magnesium than are diets made up mostly

TABLE 8-6

Food Sources of Magnesium (RDAs for Adult Women, 300 mg; for Adult Men, 350 mg)

	Quantity	Magnesium (mg)		Quantity	Magnesium (mg)
Bread, cereal, rice, pasta			**Meat, poultry, fish, dry beans, eggs, nuts—cont'd**		
Bran flakes	¾ cup	68	Crab, blue (steamed)	3 oz	28
Bran muffin, homemade	1 muffin	35	Egg, whole	1 large	6
Bread, whole wheat	1 slice	23	Ground beef, regular (broiled)	3.5 oz	20
Oatmeal (cooked)	¾ cup	42	Halibut (baked)	3 oz	91
Pasta, enriched (cooked)	1 cup	28	Ham, canned (lean)	3.5 oz	17
Wheat flakes	1 cup	31	Lentils (boiled)	1 cup	71
			Lobster (steamed)	3 oz	30
Vegetables			Mackerel (baked)	3 oz	83
Artichoke (boiled)	1 med	47	Oysters (steamed)	3 oz (12 med)	92
Avocado (raw)	1 med	70	Peanut butter, creamy	1 tbsp	28
Corn, yellow (boiled)	½ cup	26	Peanuts (roasted)	1 oz	49
Okra (boiled)	½ cup	46	Pinto beans (boiled)	1 cup	95
Peas, green (boiled)	½ cup	31	Sirloin steak, lean (broiled)	3.5 oz	32
Potato (baked, with skin)	1 med	55	Soybeans (boiled)	1 cup	148
Spinach (boiled)	½ cup	79	Trout, rainbow (baked)	3 oz	33
Sweet potato (baked)	1 med	23	Tuna, light, canned in water	3 oz	25
			Walnuts, dried	1 oz	57
Fruits					
Figs (dried)	10 figs	111	**Milk, dairy products**		
Kiwi (raw)	1 med	23	Cheddar cheese	1 oz	8
Orange juice (fresh)	8 fl oz	27	Cottage cheese, creamed	1 cup	11
Raisins, seedless	⅔ cup	33	Milk, skim	8 fl oz	28
			Milk, whole	8 fl oz	33
Meat, poultry, fish, dry beans, eggs, nuts			Swiss cheese	1 oz	10
Almonds (roasted)	1 oz (22 nuts)	86	Yogurt, whole	8 fl oz	26
Beef liver (fried)	3.5 oz	23			
Beef top round, lean (broiled)	3.5 oz	31	**Fats, oils, sugar**		
Black-eyed peas (boiled)	1 cup	91	This food group is not an important source of magnesium.		
Chicken, dark (roasted, without skin)	3.5 oz	23			
Chicken, light (roasted, without skin)	3.5 oz	27			
Chick-peas (boiled)	1 cup	78			
Cod (baked)	3 oz	36			

of refined foods, meat, and dairy products.[8] Table 8-6 gives some comparative food sources of magnesium.

Chloride

Chloride accounts for about 3% of the body's total mineral content, mainly as a part of the fluid outside of cells, where it helps control water and acid-base balances. Spinal fluid has the highest concentration. A relatively large amount of ionized chloride is found in the gastrointestinal secretions, especially as a component of gastric hydrochloric acid (HCl).

Sulfur

Sulfur is present in all body cells, usually as a constituent of cell protein. Elemental sulfur occurs in sulfate compounds with sodium, potassium, and magnesium. Organic forms occur mainly with other protein compounds: (1) sulfur-containing amino acids, such as me-thionine and cystine, (2) glycoproteins in cartilage, tendons, and bone matrix, (3) detoxification products formed in part by bacterial activity in the intestine, (4) other organic compounds such as heparin, insulin, coenzyme A, lipoic acid, thiamin, and biotin, and (5) keratin in hair and nails.

The major minerals are summarized in Table 8-7.

TRACE ELEMENTS: THE CONCEPT OF ESSENTIALITY

By the simplest definition, an essential element is one required for existence; conversely, its absence brings death. For major elements that occur in relatively large amounts in the body, as we have seen, such determinations can be made easily because the quantity present is sufficiently available for study. However, for things that occur in very small amounts, this determination of

TABLE 8-7

Summary of Major Minerals (Required Intake Over 100 mg/day)

Mineral	Metabolism	Physiologic functions	Clinical applications	Requirements	Food sources
Calcium (Ca)	Absorption according to body need; requires Ca-binding protein and regulated by vitamin D, parathyroid hormone, and calcitonin; absorption favored by protein, lactose, acidity Excretion chiefly in feces: 70%-90% of amount ingested Deposition-mobilization is bone tissue constant, regulated by vitamin D and parathyroid hormone	Constituent of bones and teeth Participates in blood clotting, nerve transmission, muscle action, cell membrane permeability, enzyme activation	Tetany (decrease in serum Ca) Rickets, osteomalacia Osteoporosis Resorptive hypercalcinuria, renal calculi Hyperthyroidism and hypothyroidism	Adults: 800 mg Pregnancy and lactation: 1200 mg Infants: 400-600 mg Children: 800-1200 mg	Milk, cheese Green, leafy vegetables Whole grains Egg yolk Legumes, nuts
Phosphorus (P)	Absorption with Ca aided by vitamin D and parathyroid hormone as for calcium; hindered by binding agents Excretion chiefly by kidney according to serum level, regulated by parathyroid hormone Deposition-mobilization in bone compartment constant	Constituent of bones and teeth, ATP, phosphorylated intermediary metabolites Participates in absorption of glucose and glycerol, transport of fatty acids, energy metabolism, and buffer system	Growth Recovery from diabetic acidosis Hypophosphatemia: bone disease, malabsorption syndromes, primary hyperparathyroidism Hyperphosphatemia: renal insufficiency, hypothyroidism, tetany	Adults: 800 mg Pregnancy and lactation: 1200 mg Infants: 300-500 mg Children: 800-1200 mg	Milk, cheese Meat, egg yolk Whole grains Legumes, nuts
Magnesium (Mg)	Absorption according to intake load; hindered by excess fat, phosphate, calcium, protein Excretion (regulated by kidney)	Constituent of bones and teeth Coenzyme in general metabolism, smooth muscle action, neuromuscular irritability Cation in intracellular fluid	Low serum level following gastrointestinal losses Tremor, spasm in deficiency induced by malnutrition, alcoholism	Adults: 280-350 mg Pregnancy and lactation: 290-355 mg Infants: 40-60 mg Children: 80-170 mg	Milk, cheese Meat, seafood Whole grains Legumes, nuts
Sodium (Na)	Readily absorbed Excretion chiefly by kidney, controlled by aldosterone	Major cation in extracellular fluid, water balance, acid-base balance Cell membrane permeability, absorption of glucose Normal muscle irritability	Losses in gastrointestinal disorders, diarrhea Fluid-electrolyte and acid-base balance problems Muscle action	Adults: 500 mg Infants: 120-200 mg Children: 225-500 mg	Salt (NaCl) Sodium compounds in baking and processing Milk, cheese Meat, eggs Carrots, beets, spinach, celery
Potassium (K)	Readily absorbed Secreted and resorbed in gastrointestinal circulation Excretion chiefly by kidney, regulated by aldosterone	Major cation in intracellular fluid, water balance, acid-base balance Normal muscle irritability Glycogen formation Protein synthesis	Losses in gastrointestinal disorders, diarrhea Fluid-electrolyte, acid-base balance problems Muscle action, especially heart action Losses in tissue catabolism	Adults: 2000 mg Infants: 500-700 mg Children: 1000-2000 mg	Fruits Vegetables Legumes, nuts Whole grains Meat

TABLE 8-7

Summary of Major Minerals (Required Intake Over 100 mg/day)—cont'd

Mineral	Metabolism	Physiologic functions	Clinical applications	Requirements	Food sources
Potassuim (K)—cont'd			Treatment of diabetic acidosis: rapid glycogen production reduces serum potassium level Losses with diuretic therapy		
Chloride (Cl)	Readily absorbed Excretion controlled by kidney	Major anion in extracellular fluid, water balance, acid-base balance, chloride-bicarbonate shift Gastric hydrochloride—digestion	Losses in gastrointestinal disorders, vomiting, diarrhea, tube drainage Hypochloremic alkalosis	Adults: 750 mg Infants: 180-300 mg Children: 350-750 mg	Salt (NaCl)
Sulfur (S)	Elemental form absorbed as such; split from amino acid sources (methionine and cystine) in digestion and absorbed into portal circulation Excreted by kidney in relation to protein intake and tissue catabolism	Essential constituent of protein structure Enzyme activity and energy metabolism through free sulfhydryl group (—SH) Detoxification reactions	Cystine renal calculi Cystinuria	Diet adequate in protein contains adequate sulfur	Meat, eggs Milk, cheese Legumes, nuts

essentiality is not easy to make. For example, of the 54 known chemical elements in the major part of the periodic table, 27 have been determined to be essential to human life and function. By far most living matter as we know it is made up of five fundamental elements: hydrogen (H), carbon (C), nitrogen (N), oxygen (O), and sulfur (S). We know these elements well because their concentrations are relatively large, hence more easily studied, and their requirements for human function can be stated in multiples of grams per gram of body weight. This is a recognizable quantity with which we can be comfortable. We have means for analysis of such quantities and can easily see that these are essential elements. Also, the major minerals you have just reviewed here occur in respectable amounts in the body, so their essentiality has been more easily studied and determined.

A much larger number of elements—microelements or trace elements—occur in biologic matter in such very small amounts that measurement and analysis are exceedingly difficult. So in many cases we know little about them and understand even less. It is much harder to determine the essentiality of these trace elements because we apparently require so little of them. In general, trace elements have been defined as those having a required intake of less than 100 mg/day. Yet some of them exist in fairly large amounts in our diet and our environment.

Essential Function

Despite difficulties in determining the essentiality of these very small amounts of trace elements in our bodies, Mertz, a leading researcher and authority in trace element metabolism, has indicated that essentiality can be determined on the basis of function and effect of deficiency.[11]

Basic Functions of Trace Elements

An element is essential when a deficiency causes an impairment of function and when supplementation with that substance, but not with others, prevents or cures this impairment. Studies in this field have identified the two basic functions of trace elements in terms of *catalytic* and *structural* components of larger molecules.

Deficiency and Requirement

Because these small amounts of trace elements are not easily measured, specific needs have been stated only for the following: (1) iron (Fe), because it has a long history, (2) zinc (Zn), because it occurs in higher concentration than some of the others, (3) iodine (I), because it has only one specific known function, and (4) selenium (Se), because of its recently recognized partnership with vitamin E as an antioxidant agent. Thus far the RDA standard only estimates requirements for the others in terms of a general range of need.

TABLE 8-8

Summary of Trace Elements (Required Intake Less Than 100 mg/day)

Element	Metabolism	Physiologic functions	Clinical applications	Requirements	Food sources
Iron (Fe)	Absorption controls bio-availability; favored by body need, acidity, and reduction agents such as vitamins; hindered by binding agents, reduced gastric HCl, infection, gastrointestinal losses Transported as transferrin, stored as ferritin or hemosiderin Excreted in sloughed cells, bleeding	Hemoglobin synthesis, oxygen transport Cell oxidation, heme enzymes	Anemia (hypochromic, microcytic) Excess: hemosiderosis, hemochromatosis Growth and pregnancy needs	Adults: men—10 mg, women—15 mg Pregnancy and lactation: 30 and 15 mg, respectively Infants: 6-10 mg Children: 10-12 mg	Liver, meats, eggs Whole grains Enriched breads and cereals Dark green vegetables Legumes, nuts (Iron cookware)
Iodine (I)	Absorbed as iodides, taken up by thyroid gland under control of thyroid-stimulating hormone (TSH) Excretion by kidney	Synthesis of thyroxin, which regulates cell metabolism, basal metabolic rate (BMR)	Endemic colloid goiter, cretinism Hypothyroidism and hyperthyroidism	Adults: 150 μg Infants: 40-50 μg Children: 70-150 μg	Iodized salt Seafood
Zinc (Zn)	Absorbed with zinc-binding ligand (ZBL) from pancreas Transported in blood by albumin; stored in many sites Excretion largely intestinal	Essential coenzyme constituent: carbonic anhydrase, carboxypeptidase, lactic dehydrogenase	Growth: hypogonadism Sensory impairment: taste and smell Wound healing Malabsorption disease	Adults: 12-15 mg Infants: 5 mg Children: 10-15 mg	Widely distributed Seafood, oysters Liver, meat Milk, cheese, eggs Whole grains
Copper (Cu)	Absorbed with copper-binding protein metallothionein Transported in blood by histidine and albumin Stored in many tissues	Associated with iron in enzyme systems, hemoglobin synthesis Metalloprotein enzyme constituent	Hypocupremia: nephrosis and malabsorption Wilson's disease, excess copper storage	Adults: 1.5-3 mg Infants: 0.4-0.7 mg Children: 0.7-2.5 mg	Widely distributed Liver, meat Seafood Whole grains Legumes, nuts (Copper cookware)
Manganese (Mn)	Absorbed poorly Excretion mainly by intestine	Enzyme component in general metabolism	Low serum levels in diabetes, protein-energy malnutrition Inhalation toxicity	Adults: 2-5 mg Infants: 0.3-1.0 μg Children: 1-5 μg	Cereals, whole grains Legumes, soybeans Leafy vegetables
Chromium (Cr)	Absorbed in association with zinc Excretion mainly by kidney	Associated with glucose metabolism; improves faulty glucose uptake by tissues; glucose tolerance factor	Potentiates action of insulin in persons with diabetes Lowers serum cholesterol, LDL-cholesterol* Increases HDL*	Adults: 50-200 μg Infants: 10-60 μg Children: 2-200 μg	Cereals Whole grains Brewer's yeast Animal protein
Cobalt (Co)	Absorbed as component of food source, vitamin B$_{12}$ Elemental form shares transport with iron Stored in liver	Constituent of vitamin B$_{12}$, functions with vitamin	Deficiency associated only with deficiency of vitamin B$_{12}$	Unknown, evidently minute	Vitamin B$_{12}$ source
Selenium (Se)	Absorption depends on solubility of compound form Excreted mainly by kidney	Constituent of enzyme glutathione peroxidase Synergistic antioxidant with vitamin E Structural component of teeth	Marginal deficiency when soil content is low Deficiency secondary to parenteral nutrition (TPN), malnutrition Toxicity observed in livestock	Adults: 55-70 μg Infants: 10-15 μg Children: 20-50 μg	Varies with soil content Seafood Legumes Whole grains Low-fat meats and dairy products Vegetables

*LDL = low density lipoprotein; HDL = high density lipoprotein.

TABLE 8-8

Summary of Trace Elements (Required Intake Less Than 100 mg/day)—cont'd

Element	Metabolism	Physiologic functions	Clinical applications	Requirements	Food sources
Molybdenum (Mo)	Readily absorbed Excreted rapidly by kidney Small amount excreted in bile	Constituent of oxidase enzymes, xanthine oxidase	Deficiency unknown in humans	Adults: 75-250 μg Infants: 15-30 μg Children: 25-250 μg	Legumes Whole grains Milk Organ meats Leafy vegetables
Fluoride (F)	Absorption in small intestine; little known of bioavailability Excreted by kidney—80%	Accumulates in bones and teeth, increasing hardness	Dental caries inhibited Osteoporosis: may help control Excess: dental fluorosis	Adults: 1.5-4 mg Infants: 0.1-0.5 mg Children: 0.5-2.5 mg	Fish Fish products Tea Foods cooked in fluoridated water Drinking water

Essential Trace Elements: Definite and Probable

On the basis of current knowledge, these small trace elements may be classed in two groups: those which are definitely essential and those which are probably essential.

Definitely Essential Elements

Ten trace elements have been assigned essential roles in human nutrition based on defined function and need determined from research. This group includes iron (Fe), iodine (I), zinc (Zn), copper (Cu), manganese (Mn), chromium (Cr), cobalt (Co), selenium (Se), molybdenum (Mo), and fluoride (F).

Probably Essential Elements

All the remaining eight trace elements are probably essential, but a more complete understanding awaits the development of better means of analysis and tests for function. These elements include silicon (Si), vanadium (V), nickel (Ni), tin (Sn), cadmium (Cd), arsenic (As), aluminum (Al), and boron (B).

We look first at iron and iodine because of their long history and clearly defined specific function. Then in turn we briefly review the remainder. These essential elements are summarized in Table 8-8.

Iron

Forms of Iron in the Body

The human body contains only about 45 mg iron/kg body weight. This iron is distributed in four forms that point to its basic metabolic function.

Transport Iron

A trace of iron, 0.05 to 0.18 mg/dl, is in plasma bound to its transport carrier protein *transferrin*.

Hemoglobin

Most of the body's iron, about 70%, occurs in red blood cells as a vital constituent of the heme portion of **hemoglobin.** Another 5% is a part of the muscle oxygen–carrying hemoglobin *myoglobin*.

Storage Iron

About 20% of the body iron is stored as the protein-iron compound **ferritin,** mainly in liver, spleen, and bone marrow. Excess iron is stored in the body as **hemosiderin,** interchanging with ferritin as needed.

Cellular Tissue Iron

The remaining 5% of body iron is distributed throughout all cells as a major component of oxidative enzyme systems for the production of energy.

Absorption-Transport-Storage-Excretion Balance

In the body, iron follows a unique system of interrelated absorption, transport, storage, and excretion. Optimal levels of body iron are not maintained by urinary excretion as is the case with most plasma constituents. Rather, the mechanisms of iron control lie in the absorption-transport-storage complex.

---

ferritin • Protein-iron compound in which iron is stored in tissues; the storage form of iron in the body.

hemoglobin • Oxygen-carrying pigment in red blood cells; a conjugated protein containing four heme groups combined with iron and four long polypeptide chains forming the protein globin, named for its ball-like form; made by the developing red blood cells in bone marrow. Hemoglobin carries oxygen in the blood to body cells.

hemosiderin • Insoluble iron oxide-protein compound in which iron is stored in the liver if the amount of iron in the blood exceeds the storage capacity of ferritin, for example, during rapid destruction of red blood cells (malaria, hemolytic anemia).

Absorption

The main control of the body's iron balance is at the point of intestinal absorption. Dietary iron enters the body in two forms: **heme** and **nonheme** (Table 8-9). By far the larger portion is nonheme—all plant sources plus 60% of animal sources. But it is absorbed at a much slower rate than the smaller heme portion, because nonheme iron is tightly bound in its food sources to organic molecules in the form of ferric iron (Fe^{+++}). In the acidic medium of the stomach, it must be disassociated and reduced to the more soluble ferrous iron (Fe^{++}).[12] This is a source of nutritional concern because of nonheme's greater quantity in the diet.

Control of iron distribution and transfer in the absorbing cell involves several receiving substances. Iron is never allowed to travel about the body unescorted. First the iron, all now in ferric form, is bound by an initial intracellular molecule (ICM). This ICM first leaves a portion to serve needs of the absorbing cell's mitochondria, then delivers specific proportions to its regular receptors and carriers: (1) apoferritin (*apo-*, meaning derived or separated from something), the cell's special protein receptor with which iron combines to form the immediate holding compound, epithelial ferritin, and (2) apotransferrin, the blood's special protein receptor with which iron combines to form its circulating carrier compound, serum transferrin.

The amount of ferritin already present in the intestinal mucosa determines the amount of ingested iron that is absorbed or rejected. When all available apoferritin has been bound to iron to form ferritin, any additional iron that arrives at the binding site is rejected, returned to the lumen of the intestine, and passed on for excretion in the feces. In all, only 10% to 30% of the ingested iron is absorbed, mostly in the duodenum. The remaining 70% to 90% is eliminated.

The following factors favor absorption:
1. *Body need.* In deficiency states or in periods of extra demand, as in growth or pregnancy, mucosal ferritin is lower and more iron is absorbed. When tissue reserves are ample or saturated, iron is rejected and excreted.
2. *Acidity and reduction agents.* Vitamin C (ascorbic acid) aids iron absorption by its reducing action and effect on acidity. Other metabolic reducing agents have similar effects, as does gastric hydrochloric acid, which provides the optimal acid medium for preparing iron for use.
3. *Calcium.* An adequate amount of calcium helps bind and remove agents such as phosphate and phytate, which would combine with iron and prevent its absorption.

The following factors hinder absorption:
1. *Binding agents.* Materials such as phosphate, phytate, and oxalate bind iron and remove it from the body. Tea and coffee have also been shown to inhibit nonheme iron absorption.
2. *Reduced gastric acid secretion.* Surgical removal of stomach tissue (gastrectomy) reduces the number of cells that secrete hydrochloric acid, thus reducing the necessary acid medium for iron reduction.
3. *Infection.* Severe infection hinders iron absorption.
4. *Gastrointestinal disease.* Malabsorption or any disturbance that causes diarrhea or *steatorrhea* (fatty diarrhea) hinders iron absorption.

Thus the bioavailability of iron essentially depends on its absorption, which in turn depends on a number of influencing factors in the body. This is a unique and precarious arrangement.

Transport

As we have seen in the mucosal cells of the duodenum and proximal jejunum, iron is oxidized and bound with the plasma transferrin for transport to body cells. Normally, only about 20% to 35% of the iron-binding capacity of transferrin is filled. The remaining capacity forms an unsaturated plasma reserve for handling variances in iron intake.

Storage

Bound to plasma transferrin, iron is delivered to its storage sites in bone marrow and to some extent in the liver. Here it is transferred to apoferritin again to form ferritin for storage and use as needed in synthesizing hemoglobin for red blood cells. This binding with apoferritin provides a stable, exchangeable storage form for the body needs. A second, less soluble storage compound, hemosiderin, provides reserve storage in the liver. From these storage compounds, iron is mobilized for hemoglobin synthesis as needed. In the average adult, 20 to 25 mg/day of iron is used in hemoglobin synthesis. However, the body avidly conserves the iron in hemoglobin, recycling the iron when red cells are destroyed after their average life span of about 120 days. These interrelationships of body iron absorption-

TABLE 8-9

Characteristics of Heme and Nonheme Portions of Dietary Iron

	Dietary Iron	
	Heme (smallest portion)	**Nonheme (largest portion)**
Food sources	None in plant sources; 40% of iron in animal sources	All plant sources of iron; 60% of iron in animal sources
Absorption rate	Rapid; transported and absorbed intact	Slow; tightly bound in organic molecules

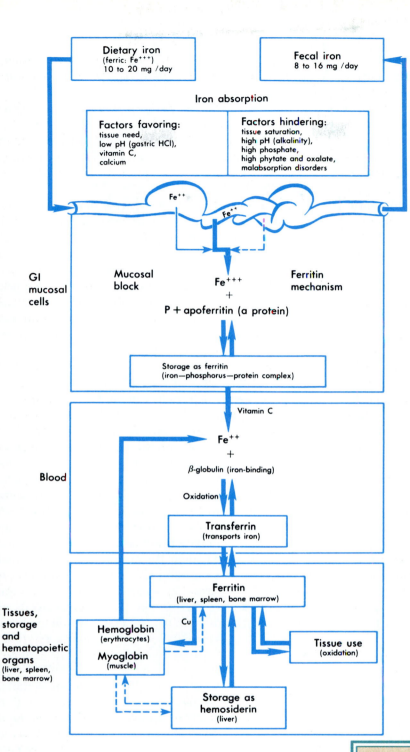

FIG. 8-3 Summary of iron metabolism, showing its absorption, transport, main use in hemoglobin formation, and its storage forms (ferritin and hemosiderin).

transport-storage mechanisms are diagrammed in Fig. 8-3 for review.

Excretion

Because the main regulatory mechanism controlling iron levels in the body occurs at the point of absorption, only minute amounts are lost by renal excretion. Essentially none is in the urine, as is the case with other circulating minerals. Rather, the small amounts of iron excreted normally come from the sloughing off of skin tissue, gastrointestinal cells, and normal gastrointestinal and menstrual blood loss. Unusual blood loss such

heme iron • Dietary iron from animal sources, from the heme portion of hemoglobin in red blood cells. Heme iron is more easily absorbed and transported in the body than nonheme iron from plant sources, but it supplies the smaller portion of the body's total dietary iron intake.

nonheme iron • The larger portion of dietary iron, including all the plant food sources and 60% of the animal food sources, which lacks the more easily absorbed and bioavailable heme iron in the remaining 40% of the animal food sources that contain hemoglobin residues of iron containing heme.

as that from heavy menstrual flow, childbirth, surgery, acute and chronic hemorrhage, gastrointestinal disease, or parasitic infestation may bring severe iron loss.

Physiologic Functions of Iron

Oxygen Transport

Iron is "pocketed" within the heme molecule, which is the fundamental nonprotein part of hemoglobin in the red blood cells. As such, iron functions as a major transporter of vital oxygen to the cells for respiration and metabolism. Iron is also a constituent of the similar compound myoglobin in muscle tissue.

Cellular Oxidation

Although in smaller amounts, iron also functions in the cells as a vital component of enzyme systems for oxidation of glucose to produce energy.

Growth Needs

During growth, demands for positive iron balance is imperative. At birth, the infant has a small 4- to 6-month supply of iron stored in the liver from fetal development. Breast-fed infants obtain some iron in breast milk. However, since cow's milk does not supply iron, iron is added to commercial formulas. Supplementary iron-rich and fortified foods are added to the diet at about 4 to 6 months of age. In this way the classic milk anemia of young children is prevented. Iron is also needed for continued growth and to build up reserves for the physiologic stress of adolescence, especially the onset of menses in girls. The woman's need for iron is increased greatly during pregnancy to maintain the increased number of red blood cells in an expanded circulating blood volume and to supply the iron needed for storage in the developing fetal liver. Finally, normal blood loss during delivery reduces iron stores further.

Clinical Problems

Because of the unique physiologic controls of the body's iron content, clinical abnormalities may result from either a deficiency or an excess of iron.

Iron Deficiency

Surprisingly iron deficiency occurs in both developed and underdeveloped countries for two main reasons: (1) the modest dietary supply is not readily absorbed; and (2) the body holds to its iron, and it is excreted not through the urine but rather through a number of avenues of potential loss. Iron deficiency then results in a hypochromic microcytic anemia. This deficiency may result from several causes[13]:

1. *Nutritional anemia:* An inadequate dietary supply of iron and other nutrients needed for hemoglobin and red blood cell production
2. *Hemorrhagic anemia:* Excessive blood iron loss
3. *Postgastrectomy anemia:* Lack of gastric hydrochloric acid necessary to liberate iron for absorption
4. *Malabsorption anemia:* The presence of iron-binding agents that prevent its absorption or mucosal lesions that affect the absorbing surface
5. *Chronic disease anemia:* Abnormalities in the recycling of iron from hemoglobin of old blood cells that frequently accompany infections, inflammatory disorders, or connective tissue diseases such as arthritis.

The World Problem of Iron-Deficiency Anemia

Nutritional anemias, of which iron deficiency is the greatest, constitute the second most prevalent nutritional deficiency in the world, second only to protein-energy malnutrition. Iron-deficiency anemia in particular respects neither social class nor geographic situation. General iron balance in many places is often precarious. Vulnerable life cycle periods include infancy and early childhood, adolescence, the reproductive years of women from menses to menopause, pregnancy, and older adulthood.

Iron Requirement

Iron stores vary widely, being about 300 mg in women and 1000 mg in men. Iron losses in healthy men average about 1 mg/day; in women the loss is about 1.5 mg/day. The addition for women is based on usual menstrual losses averaged over the month. Considering the iron balance studies, usual U.S. surveys of intake from the general food supply, and the need to maintain adequate iron reserves, the current RDAs are set at 15 mg/day for women and 10 mg/day for men. The needs of postmenopausal women are about the same as the standard for men. During pregnancy, the total allowance increases to 30 mg/day, but no addition is necessary during lactation because the menses are usually absent during this period. The growth needs of children are indicated in the RDA table inside the book covers.

Iron Toxicity

Iron toxicity has not been observed in the general population from dietary sources, except for ingestion of "home brews" made in iron vessels.[8] However, there are some 2000 cases of iron poisoning every year in the United States, second only to aspirin poisoning, that occur among small children who pick up and eat the bright-colored adult iron dose tablets carelessly left within their reach. The only other cause of iron overload is the genetic disease hemochromatosis.

Food Sources of Iron

Iron is widespread among foods in the U.S. food supply, especially in meats (particularly in organ meats such as liver), eggs, vegetables, and cereals (fortified cereal products). This fortification of grain products such as flour, breads, and cereals has at times been controversial among some nutritionists and policy makers. Nonetheless, it has helped to reduce our incidence of

TABLE 8-10

Food Sources of Iron (RDAs for Adult Women, 15 mg; for Adult Men, 10 mg)

	Quantity	Iron (mg)		Quantity	Iron (mg)
Bread, cereal, rice, pasta			**Meat, poultry, fish, dry beans, eggs, nuts—cont'd**		
Bran flakes	¾ cup	4.50	Chick-peas (boiled)	1 cup	4.74
Bran muffin, homemade	1 muffin	1.26	Clams (steamed)	3 oz (9 small)	23.76
Bread, whole wheat	1 slice	0.86	Crab, blue (steamed)	3 oz	0.77
Cream of wheat, regular (cooked)	¾ cup	7.70	Egg, whole	1 large	1.04
Oatmeal (cooked)	¾ cup	1.19	Ground beef, regular (broiled)	3.5 oz	2.44
Pasta, enriched (cooked)	1 cup	2.40	Halibut (baked)	3 oz	0.91
Rice, white, enriched (cooked)	1 cup	1.80	Ham, canned (lean)	3.5 oz	0.94
Wheat flakes	1 cup	4.45	Lentils (boiled)	1 cup	6.59
			Lima beans (boiled)	1 cup	4.50
Vegetables			Mackerel (baked)	3 oz	1.33
Artichoke (boiled)	1 med	1.62	Oysters (steamed)	3 oz (12 med)	11.39
Avocado (raw)	1 med	2.04	Pinto beans (boiled)	1 cup	4.47
Broccoli (boiled)	½ cup	0.89	Shrimp (steamed)	3 oz (15 large)	2.62
Brussels sprouts (boiled)	½ cup	0.94	Sirloin steak, lean (broiled)	3.5 oz	3.36
Peas, green (boiled)	½ cup	1.24	Sole (baked)	3.5 oz	1.40
Potato (baked, with skin)	1 med	2.75	Soybeans (boiled)	1 cup	8.84
Spinach (boiled)	½ cup	3.21	Trout, rainbow (baked)	3 oz	2.07
			Tuna, light, canned in water	3 oz	2.72
Fruits					
Dates (dried)	10 dates	0.96	**Milk, dairy products**		
Figs (dried)	10 figs	4.18	Cheddar cheese	1 oz	0.19
Prune juice (canned)	8 fl oz	3.03	Cottage cheese, creamed	1 cup	0.29
Prunes (dried)	10 prunes	2.08	Milk, skim	8 fl oz	0.10
Raisins, seedless	⅔ cup	2.08	Milk, whole	8 fl oz	0.12
			Yogurt, whole	8 fl oz	0.11
Meat, poultry, fish, dry beans, eggs, nuts					
Almonds (roasted)	1 oz (22 nuts)	1.08	**Fats, oils**		
Beef liver (fried)	3.5 oz	6.28	This food group is not an important source of iron.		
Beef top round, lean (broiled)	3.5 oz	2.88			
Black-eyed peas (boiled)	1 cup	4.29	**Sugar**		
Cashews (roasted)	1 oz	1.70	Molasses, black	1 tbsp	3.20
Chicken, dark (roasted, without skin)	3.5 oz	1.33	Sugar, brown	1 cup	4.90
Chicken, light (roasted, without skin)	3.5 oz	1.06			

childhood iron-deficiency anemia. Table 8-10 gives some comparative food sources of iron.

Iodine

Iodine shares with iron a longer history of study than that of other trace minerals. Thus its function and requirement are clearly defined. The basic function of iodine is to participate in the synthesis of the hormone *thyroxine* by the thyroid gland.

The body of the average adult contains a small amount of the trace element iodine, from 20 to 50 mg. Approximately 50% of this is in the muscles, 20% in the thyroid glands, 10% in the skin, and 6% in the skeleton. The remaining 14% is scattered in other endocrine tissue, in the central nervous system, and in plasma transport. By far, the greatest iodine tissue concentration is in the thyroid glands, where its one function is to participate in the synthesis of thyroxine.

Absorption-Excretion Balance

Absorption

Dietary iodine is absorbed in the small intestine in the form of iodides. These are loosely bound with proteins and carried by the blood to the thyroid gland. About one third of this iodide is selectively absorbed by the thyroid cells and removed from circulation.

Excretion

The remaining two thirds of the iodide is usually excreted in the urine within 2 to 3 days after ingestion.

Hormonal Control

A pituitary hormone, thyroid-stimulating hormone (THS), stimulates the uptake of iodine by the thyroid cells in direct feedback response to the plasma levels of the hormone. This normal physiologic feedback mechanism maintains a healthy circular balance between supply and demand. This is a characteristic pattern for governing all the hormones from the several endocrine glands that are controlled by the pituitary master gland.

Physiologic Function of Iodine
Thyroid Hormone Synthesis

Iodine participates in the synthesis of thyroid hormone as its only known function in human metabolism. The hormone thyroxine in turn stimulates cell oxidation and regulates basal metabolic rate (BMR), apparently by increasing oxygen uptake and reaction rates of enzyme systems handling glucose. In this role iodine indirectly exerts a tremendous influence on the body's total metabolism.

Plasma Thyroxine

The free thyroxine with its associated iodine is secreted into the blood stream and bound to plasma protein for transport to body cells as needed. After being used to stimulate oxidation in the cell, the hormone is degraded in the liver and the iodine is excreted in bile as inorganic iodine.

Clinical Needs
Abnormal Thyroid Function

Both hyperthyroidism and hypothyroidism affect the rate of iodine uptake and use, and subsequently influence the body's overall metabolic rate.

Goiter

Endemic colloid **goiter,** characterized by great enlargement of the thyroid gland, occurs in persons living where water and soil and thus locally grown foods contain little iodine. Some 800 million people live in iodine-deficient areas in underdeveloped countries of the world where endemic goiter is a large health problem. In such situations the iodine-starved thyroid gland cannot produce a normal quantity of thyroxine. As a result the blood level of the thyroid hormone is too low to shut off TSH secretion by the pituitary gland. The pituitary gland continues putting out TSH, and these large quantities of TSH continue to stimulate the thyroid gland, calling on it to produce the thyroxine that it cannot supply. In this iodine-deficient state, the only response that the thyroid makes is to increase the amount of thyroglobulin (colloid), which then accumulates in the thyroid follicles. Such a gland becomes increasingly engorged and may attain a tremendous size, weighing 500 to 700 g (1 to 1½ lb) or more (Fig. 8-4).

Iodine Overload

An excessive incidental dietary intake of iodine may occur occasionally through dairy products. These dairy sources include iodized salt licks for the animals and the use of iodophors, iodine-containing chemicals used to sanitize udders, milking machines, and milk tanks. Other iodine-containing compounds are the iodates used as dough conditioners in breads, erythrosine used as food colorings, and derivatives of iodine supplements added to animal feeds. Various case reports and population studies have indicated that levels of iodine through foods, dietary supplements, or topical medications may exceed by many times the RDA.[14]

Iodine Requirement

Tests for urinary iodide excretion are used to indicate iodine intake and status, as well as the risk for goiter and a wide spectrum of other iodine deficiency disorders. These disorders can range from severe **cretinism** with mental retardation to barely visible enlargement

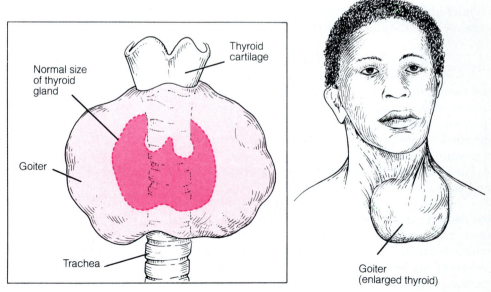

FIG. 8-4   Goiter. The extreme enlargement shown here is a result of extended duration of iodine deficiency.

Thyroid cartilage

Normal size of thyroid gland

Goiter

Trachea

Goiter (enlarged thyroid)

of the thyroid gland.[8] Balance studies indicate that an adult needs to ingest a minimum of 50 to 75 µg/day of iodine to maintain desirable tissue levels as measured by urinary excretion rates. Based on these findings, the current RDA standard sets an allowance for all adults of 150 µg/day to provide an extra margin of safety. An added 25 µg/day is recommended during pregnancy to cover fetal requirements. The extra need during lactation is 50 µg/day to meet infant growth needs. The demand is increased during periods of accelerated adolescent growth. Thus the allowance for older children ages 11 and above is set at 150 µg/day, the same as that for adult maintenance.

Food Sources of Iodine

Seafood provides a considerable amount of iodine. The quantity in natural sources varies widely depending on the iodine content of the soil and the iodine compounds used in food processing. The commercial iodizing of table salt (1 mg to every 10 g salt) provides a main dietary source.

Other Essential Trace Elements

Zinc

Zinc has come to nutritional prominence as an essential trace element with wide clinical significance. But much is still to be learned about the details of its metabolism. Its wide tissue distribution reflects its broad metabolic activity as a component of key cell enzymes. An adult's total zinc content ranges from 1.3 to 2.3 g and is distributed in many tissues including pancreas, liver, kidney, lungs, muscle, bone, eye (cornea, iris, retina, lens), and in endocrine glands and in prostate secretions and spermatozoa. The plasma zinc level is about 75 to 120 µg/dl (11.5 to 18.5 µmol/L).

Clinical Problems

Because of its widespread metabolic use, a number of clinical problems caused by zinc deficiency (see box, p 156) can occur.

Hypogonadism.   Diminished function of the gonads and dwarfism result from pronounced human zinc deficiency during critical growth periods.

Taste and smell defects.   Hypogeusia (diminished taste) and hyposmia (diminished smell) in a number of clinical situations are improved with zinc supplementation.

Wound healing.   The healing of wounds, or any other tissue injury from physiologic stress, inflammation, or hormonal changes, is retarded in zinc-deficient persons. This defect seems to be common in the average hospital, and patients benefit from zinc supplemen-

tation. Frequently, hospital diets, especially with poor consumption by ill persons, provide limited amounts of dietary zinc.

Chronic illness in aging.   Older persons with poor appetites who subsist on marginal diets in the face of unhealed wounds and debilitating illness are particularly vulnerable to zinc deficiency. As a result of such deficiency, they often suffer from reduced immune function.[15]

Malabsorption disease.   Zinc deficiency can occur with malabsorption diseases such as Crohn disease. The ulcerative lesions in the mucosal surface hinder the absorption of zinc, and zinc intake is low due to anorexia or selection of foods low in zinc.

Zinc Requirement and Food Sources

As with the trace element iron, an optimal intake of zinc in the U.S. population cannot be assumed. The current daily adult RDAs are set at 15 mg for men and 12 mg for women, because of their lower weight. The RDA table (see inside book covers) gives remaining allowances based on age and sex. The best sources of dietary zinc are seafood (especially oysters), meat, and eggs. Additional less rich sources are legumes and whole grains. Since animal food sources supply the major portion of dietary zinc, pure vegetarians, especially women, may be at risk for development of marginal zinc deficiency. Table 8-11 gives some comparative food sources of zinc.

Copper

This trace element has frequently been called the "iron twin." The two elements are metabolized in much the same way and share functions as cell enzyme components. Both are related to energy production and hemoglobin synthesis. Copper is widely distributed in natural foods, so a general dietary deficiency is rare. It has only been observed during total parenteral nutrition (TPN) feeding in a rare genetic disease. The RDAs estimate a safe and adequate range of dietary copper intake for adults at 1.5 to 3 mg/day, which regular U.S. diets supply. Copper is widely distributed in natural foods. Its richest sources are organ meats (especially

cretinism • A congenital disease resulting from absence or deficiency of normal thyroid secretion, characterized by physical deformity, dwarfism, mental retardatio, and often goiters.

goiter • Enlargement of the thyroid gland caused by lack of sufficient available iodine to produce the thyroid hormone, thyroxine.

CLINICAL APPLICATION   *Zinc Barriers*

Are people eating more zinc but absorbing it less? Current trends toward a "heart-healthy" diet may be the reason why. Some Americans may be at risk for developing a zinc deficiency, not because they are avoiding zinc-rich foods, but because they are choosing foods and supplements that reduce its availability for absorption. For example:

- Animal foods, rich in readily available zinc, are consumed less by an increasingly cholesterol-conscious public.
- Fiber, being promoted by some persons as a cardiovascular panacea, may create a negative zinc balance.
- Phytic acid, a component of fiber-rich foods, present another zinc antagonist, though its effect on zinc absorption is currently controversial.
- Vitamin-mineral supplements may contain iron/zinc ratios greater than 3:1 and provide enough iron to inhibit zinc absorption.

Other factors that reduce zinc availability include such unusual cravings as pica, the eating of nonfood material

such as clay, practiced primarily by children and pregnant women. Also, such clinical conditions as cystic fibrosis, alcohol cirrhosis, celiac disease, and diarrhea limit zinc absorption.

The risk for deficiency is greatest among pregnant and breast-feeding women. Low levels can reduce the amount of protein available to carry iron and vitamin A to the target tissues and reduce the mother's appetite and taste for foods. As a result, the fetus is at even greater risk for inadequate growth and development.

All these conditions, plus milling processes that remove excessive amounts of zinc from grains, have resulted in an average per capita intake of 12.5 mg/day. This is less than the 15 mg/day recommended for most persons, far less than the 20 to 25 mg/day recommended for pregnancy and lactation, respectively.

To put more zinc in individual diets:

- Include some form of animal food—meat, milk, and eggs—in the diet every day to ensure a minimal intake of zinc.

- Avoid extensive use of alcohol.
- Avoid "crash" diets.

Signs of zinc deficiency are still fairly rare in the United States, so there is no need for persons to overprotect themselves with massive doses. These large doses may compete with other elements such as iron and create still other deficiency problems. Excess zinc can lead to nausea, abdominal pain, and anemia. As with all other nutrients, too much of a good thing can sometimes be as bad as too little—or even worse.

REFERENCES

Moser-Veillon PB: Zinc: consumption patterns and dietary recommendations, *J Am Diet Assoc* 90(8):1089, 1990.

Rossander-Hulten L and others: Competitive inhibition of iron absorption by manganese and zinc in humans, *Am J Clin Nutr* 54:152, 1991.

Wisker E and others: Calcium, magnesium, zinc, and iron balances in young women: effects of a low-phytate barley-fiber concentrate, *Am J Clin Nutr* 54:553, 1991. ◆

---

liver), seafoods (especially oysters), nuts, and seeds, with smaller amounts in whole grains and legumes.

Manganese

The total adult body content of manganese is about 20 mg, occurring mainly in the liver, bones, pancreas, and pituitary. It functions like other trace elements as an essential part of cell enzymes that catalyze a number of important metabolic reactions. Manganese deficiency, evidenced by low serum levels, has been reported in diabetes and pancreatic insufficiency, as well as in protein-energy malnutrition states such as kwashiorkor. Toxicity occurs as an industrial disease syndrome, inhalation toxicity, in miners and other workers who have prolonged exposure to manganese dust. In such cases, excess manganese accumulates in the liver and central nervous system, producing severe neuromuscular symptoms that resemble those of Parkinson's disease. The RDA estimates a safe and adequate dietary intake of manganese at 2 to 5 mg/day, which regular U.S. diets supply. The best food sources of manganese are plant foods—cereal grains, legumes, seeds, nuts, leafy vegetables, tea, and coffee. Animal foods are relatively poor sources.

Chromium

The precise amount of chromium present in body tissues is not well defined because of difficulties in analysis. Although large geographic variations occur, the total body content is small, less than 6 mg. The highest concentrations have been found in skin, adrenal glands, brain, muscle, and fat. Serum levels are usually less than 10 mg/ml. Chromium functions as an essential component of the organic complex **glucose tolerance factor (GTF)**, which facilitates the action of insulin. The RDA standard estimates a safe and adequate intake of chromium for adults at a range of 50 to 200 µg/day. Brewer's yeast is a rich source. Good food sources include liver, cheddar cheese, and wheat germ. Most grain products provide additional sources.

Cobalt

Cobalt occurs in only minute traces in body tissues, and the main storage area is the liver. As an essential component of cobalamin (B_{12}), cobalt's only known function is associated with red blood cell formation. The normal cobalt blood level, representing the trace element in transit and in red blood cells, is exceedingly small, about 1 µg/dl. Cobalt is provided in the human

TABLE 8-11

Food Sources of Zinc (RDAs for Adults: Women, 12 mg; Men, 15 mg)

	Quantity	Zinc (mg)		Quantity	Zinc (mg)
Bread, cereal, rice, pasta			**Meat, poultry, fish, dry beans, eggs, nuts**		
Bran muffin, homemade	1 muffin	1.08	Almonds (roasted)	1 oz (22 nuts)	1.39
Bread, whole wheat	1 slice	0.42	Beef liver (fried)	3.5 oz	6.07
Cream of wheat (cooked)	¾ cup	0.24	Cashews (roasted)	1 oz	1.59
English muffin, plain	1 muffin	0.41	Chicken, dark (roasted, without skin)	3.5 oz	2.80
Oatmeal (cooked)	¾ cup	0.86	Chicken, light (roasted, without skin)	3.5 oz	1.23
Pasta, enriched (cooked)	1 cup	0.70	Chick-peas (boiled)	1 cup	2.51
Wheat flakes	1 cup	0.63	Clams, canned	3 oz	2.32
			Crab, Alaska king (steamed)	3 oz	6.48
Vegetables			Egg, whole	1 large	0.72
Artichoke (boiled)	1 med	0.43	Ham, canned (lean)	3.5 oz	1.93
Asparagus (boiled)	½ cup (6 spears)	0.43	Kidney beans (boiled)	1 cup	1.89
Avocado (raw)	1 med	0.73	Lentils (boiled)	1 cup	2.50
Broccoli (raw)	½ cup	0.18	Lima beans (boiled)	1 cup	1.79
Brussels sprouts (boiled)	½ cup (4 sprouts)	0.25	Lobster (steamed)	3 oz	2.48
Carrots (raw)	1 med	0.14	Oysters (steamed)	3 oz (12 med)	154.62
Collards (boiled)	½ cup	0.23	Peanuts (roasted)	1 oz	0.93
Kale (boiled chopped)	½ cup	0.15	Soybeans (boiled)	1 cup	1.98
Peas, green (boiled)	½ cup	0.95			
Potato (baked, with skin)	1 med	0.65	**Milk, dairy products**		
Tomato (raw)	1 med	0.13	Milk, skim	8 fl oz	0.98
			Milk, whole	8 fl oz	0.93
Fruits			Yogurt, whole	8 fl oz	1.34
Apricots (raw)	3 med	0.28			
Banana (raw)	1 med	0.19	**Fats, oils, sugar**		
Cantaloupe (raw)	½ cup	0.25	This food group is not an important source of zinc.		
Figs (dried)	10 figs	0.94			
Orange juice (fresh)	8 fl oz	0.13			
Orange, navel (raw)	1 med	0.08			

diet only by vitamin B_{12}. The human requirement is unknown but is evidently minute. For example, as little as 0.045 to 0.09 µg/day maintains bone marrow function in patients with pernicious anemia. Cobalt is widely distributed in nature. However, for our needs cobalt is obtained in preformed vitamin B_{12}, synthesized in animals by intestinal bacterial flora.

Selenium

Selenium is deposited in all body tissues except fat. Highest concentrations occur in liver, kidney, heart, and spleen. Serum levels are about 0.22 µg/dl. Selenium functions as an integral component of an antioxidant enzyme that protects cells and lipid membranes against oxidative damage. In this role, selenium balances with tocopherol (vitamin E), each sparing the other. This protective function is widespread, since the enzyme is found in most body tissues. Selenium also acts as a structural component, incorporated into the protein matrix of the teeth. The RDA standard estimates a safe and adequate adult intake of selenium at about 50 to 200 µg/day. Food sources vary with the selenium soil content. Usually good sources include sea-

food, legumes, whole grains, low-fat meats and dairy products, with smaller amounts in vegetables.

Molybdenum

The precise occurrence of molybdenum in human tissues and its clear coenzyme roles are under continuing investigation. The body tissue amount of molybdenum is exceedingly small, 0.1 to 1 µg/g of wet tissue. The largest amounts are deposited in liver, kidney, adrenal glands, and bone, with lesser but significant quantities in the lungs, spleen, and muscle. The RDA standard estimates a safe and adequate allowance for adults and older children of 75 to 250 µg/day.[8] The ranges for other age groups are derived on the basis of weight. The amount of molybdenum in foods varies considerably, depending on the environment in which the food

---

glucose tolerance factor (GTF) • A biologically active complex of chromium and nicotinic acid that facilitates the reaction of insulin with receptor sites on tissues.

is grown. In general, however, the richest sources include legumes, whole grains, milk, leafy vegetables, and organ meats. The poorer sources include fruits, stem and root vegetables, and muscle meats.

Fluoride

The trace element fluoride accumulates in all body tissues showing calcification, mostly in bones and teeth. In human nutrition fluoride functions mainly to inhibit dental caries. The principal cause of caries is acid dissolution of tooth enamel. This acid is produced by microorganisms feeding on fermentable carbohydrates adhering to the teeth after a meal or snack. Fluoride therapy enhances the ability of the tooth structure to withstand the erosive effect of the bacterial acid. Establishment of a fluoride requirement is difficult because it appears to be retained in the bones regardless of the intake level. The RDA adult standard estimates a need in the range of 1.5 to 4.0 mg/day. Fish, fish products, and tea contain the highest concentration of fluoride. Cooking in fluoridated water raises the level in many foods. The public health measure of fluoridation of public water supply to 1 ppm provides adequate amounts, and has largely been responsible for the remarkable decline in dental caries.

Probably Essential Trace Elements

The remaining trace elements that have been found in human tissue have less well-defined metabolic functions. But they have been found to be essential in animal nutrition and are probably essential in human nutrition in a similar manner as well, both as cofactors for cell enzymes in key metabolic reactions and as structural components in special tissues, for example, the role of boron with calcium in bone-building.[13] These 8 trace elements are silicon (Si), vanadium (V), nickel (Ni), tin (Sn), cadmium (Cd), arsenic (As), aluminum (Al), and boron (B). Apparently, most of these trace elements are needed in such minute amounts that primary dietary deficiency is highly unlikely. However, with increased use of long-term TPN therapy, induced deficiencies may be of increasing clinical concern.

WATER BALANCE

A number of the major minerals described in the first section of this chapter have basic functions as electrolytes in controlling the body's vital water balance. This collective function is fundamental to health and often a vital part of patient care. Thus, in brief summary here, we look at the three basic interdependent factors that control this balance: (1) the water itself, the solvent base for solutions, (2) the various particles (solutes) in solution in the water, and (3) the separating membranes that control the flow.

Water-Electrolyte Balance
Body Water Distribution

If you are a woman, your body is about 50% to 55% water. If you are a man, your body is about 55% to 60% water. The higher water content in most men is a result of their greater muscle mass. Striated muscle contains more water than any body tissue other than blood. The remaining 40% of a man's weight is about 18% protein and related substances, 15% fat, and 7% minerals. A woman's remaining body composition is about the same except for a somewhat smaller muscle mass and a larger fat deposit.

Water Functions

Body water performs three essential functions: (1) it helps give structure and form to the body through the turgor it provides for tissues; (2) it creates the water-based environment necessary for the vast array of chemical actions and reactions that comprise the body's metabolism and sustain life; and (3) it provides the means for maintaining a stable body temperature.

Water Compartments

Consider the water in your body in two compartments, as shown in Fig. 8-5: (1) the total water outside of cells—the extracellular fluid compartment (ECF) and (2) the total water inside of cells—the intracellular fluid compartment (ICF).

ECF. Water outside of cells makes up about 20% of the total body weight. It consists of four parts: (1) blood plasma, which accounts for about 25% of the ECF and 5% of body weight, (2) **interstitial fluid,** the water surrounding the cells, (3) secretory fluid, the water circulating in transit, and (4) dense tissue fluid, water in dense connective tissue, cartilage, and bone.

ICF. Water inside cells makes up about 40% to 45% of the total body weight. Since the body cells handle our vast metabolic activity, it is no surprise that the total water inside cells is about twice the amount outside.

Overall Water Balance: Intake and Output

The average adult metabolizes 2.5 to 3 L of water each day in a constant turnover balanced between intake and output. This water enters and leaves the body by various routes, controlled by basic mechanisms such as thirst and hormonal activity.

Water enters the body in three main forms: (1) preformed water as such and in other beverages that are consumed, (2) preformed water in foods that are eaten, and (3) metabolic water, a product of cell oxidation.

Water leaves the body through the kidneys, skin, lungs, and fecal elimination through the large intestine.

These routes of intake and output must be in con-

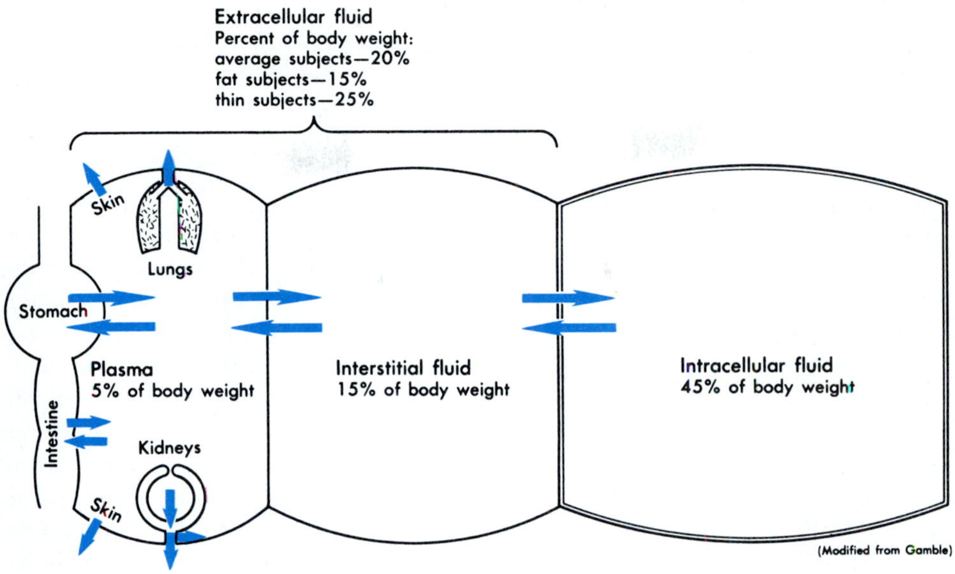

FIG. 8-5 Body fluid compartments. Note the relative total quantities of water in the intracellular compartment and in the extracellular compartment.

stant balance (Table 8-12). Abnormal conditions, such as diarrhea and dysentery, produce much greater losses, causing serious clinical problems if prolonged. Extensive loss of body fluids can be especially dangerous in infants and children. Their bodies contain a greater percentage of the total body water, and much more of the water is outside of cells and easily available for loss.

Forces Controlling Water Distribution

Forces that influence and control the distribution of body water revolve around two factors: (1) the **solutes,** particles in solution in body water, and (2) the separating membranes between water compartments.

A variety of particles with varying concentrations occur in the body. Two main types, electrolytes and plasma protein, control water balance.

Electrolytes

Several minerals provide major electrolytes for the body. In this role, these small inorganic elements are called **electrolytes** because they are free in solution and carry an electrical charge. These free, charged forms are ions, atoms or elements or groups of atoms that, in solution, carry either a positive or negative electrical charge. An ion carrying a positive charge is called a cation; examples are sodium (Na^+), a major cation of water outside cells, potassium (K^+), a major cation of water inside cells, calcium (Ca^{++}), and magnesium (Mg^{++}). Conversely, an ion carrying a negative charge is called an anion; examples are chloride (Cl^-), carbonate (HCO_3^-), phosphate ($HPO_4^=$), and sulfate ($SO_4^=$). Because of their small size, these ions or electrolytes can diffuse freely across body membranes. Thus they produce a major force controlling movement of water within the body.

TABLE 8-12
Approximate Daily Adult Intake and Output of Water

	Intake (replacement) mL/day		Output (loss) Obligatory (insensible) mL/day	Additional (according to need) mL/day
Preformed		Lungs	350	
Liquids	1200-1500	Skin		
In foods	700-1000	Diffusion	350	
Metabolism	200-300	Sweat	100	±250
(oxidation		Kidneys	900	±500
of food)				
		Feces	150	
TOTAL	2100-2800	TOTAL	1850	750
(approx. 2600 mL/day)		(approx. 2600 mL/day)		

electrolytes • A chemical element or compound, which in solution dissociates as ions carrying a positive or negative charge (for example, H^+, Na^+, K^+, Ca^{++}, Mg^{++}, and Cl^-, HCO_3^-, $HPO_4^=$, $SO_4^=$). Electrolytes constitute a major force controlling fluid balances within the body through their concentrations and shifts from one place to another to restore and maintain balance—*homeostasis.*

interstitial fluid • The fluid situated between parts or in the interspaces of a tissue.

solutes • Particles of a substance in solution; a solution consists and a dissloving medium (solvent), usually a liquid.

Plasma Proteins

Organic substances of large molecular size, mainly albumin and globulin of the plasma proteins, influence the shift of water in and out of capillaries in balance with their surrounding water. In this function, these plasma proteins are called colloids (Gr. *kolla*, glue) and form colloidal solutions. Because of their large size, these particles or molecules do not pass readily through separating capillary membranes. Therefore they normally remain in the blood vessels, where they exert **colloidal osmotic pressure (COP)** to maintain the vascular blood volume.

Organic Compounds of Small Molecular Size

Other organic compounds of small size, such as glucose, urea, and amino acids, diffuse freely but do not influence shifts of water unless they occur in abnormally large concentrations. For example, the large amount of glucose in the urine of a patient with uncontrolled diabetes mellitus causes an abnormal osmotic diuresis or excess water output.

Water and solutes move across the body's separating membranes by the basic physiologic mechanisms that operate fluid balances according to body need. These mechanisms include osmosis, diffusion, filtration, active transport, and pinocytosis.

Influence of Electrolytes on Water Balance
Measurement of Electrolytes

The concentration of electrolytes in a given solution determines the chemical activity of that solution. It is the number of particles in a solution that is the important factor in determining chemical combining power. Thus electrolytes are measured according to the total number of particles in solution, each one of which contributes chemical combining power according to its valence, rather than their total weight. The unit of measure commonly used is an equivalent. Since small amounts are usually in question, most physiologic measurements are expressed in terms of *milliequivalents*. The term refers to the number of ions—cations and anions—in solution, as determined by their concentration in a given volume. This measure is expressed as the number of milliequivalents per liter (*mEq/L*).

Losing By a Hair

Many Americans spend a great deal of money each year getting their hair analyzed. For a few strands of hair and a sizable fee they can find out if their potassium levels are low, their lead levels are high, or their sodium levels are just right. Or can they?

Hair is dead tissue. It starts out as living cells, full of minerals found in the rest of the body. When cells die, these minerals linger on. The dead cells are "glued" together with a sulfur-rich protein called *keratin* and continue to "grow" as a single strand of hair. On the other hand, claims notwithstanding, vitamins disappear when the cells die and are not found in hair. Yet even with the detection of minerals there are problems:

- Some minerals are lost when hair cells die. The keratin is so rich in sulfur that it masks the presence of some minerals and attracts others in levels that exceed those found in the body.
- Hair can be "contaminated" by shampoos, hard or soft water, dyes, or even air pollution, thereby throwing off laboratory calculations.
- Science just doesn't know what the relationship is between hair levels and blood levels for certain nutrients.
- Some persons don't even know how to wash hair samples before testing, so large amounts of contaminants get analyzed too.
- There are no standard lab values for minerals found in hair. Laboratories can simply state that levels are higher, lower, or the same as those seen previously.

TO PROBE FURTHER

But hair analysis is not totally worthless. Coroners use it all the time to find out if a person has died from arsenic, lead, or other poisons. Public health workers use it to compare mineral levels in populations in different parts of the country if they suspect that soil depletion, water contamination, or other environmental changes have affected nutrient levels in local food supplies. Also, it can help researchers and individual practitioners monitor changing nutrient levels over a period of time.

The usefulness of hair analysis in general practice, however, is overshadowed by strong condemnation from the American Medical Association and health professionals. This negative response comes not only because of its shortcomings, but also because mail-order hair analysis companies use it to diagnose conditions (that often don't exist) and "suggest" (being careful to avoid the term *prescribe*) treatments with a variety of supplements, which frequently just happen to be sold by the same companies doing the analysis, in amounts that are often potentially dangerous.

So, unless you're due for a haircut, have some money you don't need, and feel the need to purchase and use unnecessary supplements, hair analysis is probably not the most productive thing you could choose to do.

REFERENCES
Dormandy TL: Trace element analysis of hair, *Br Med J* 293:975, Oct 18, 1986.
Fosmire GJ: Report of the Public Information Committee, American Institute of Nutrition: Hair analysis to assess nutritional status, *Nutr Today* 21(5):31, 1986.

Electrolyte Balance

Electrolytes are distributed in the body water compartments in a definite pattern, which has physiologic significance. This distribution pattern maintains stable electrochemical neutrality in body fluid solutions. According to biochemical and electrochemical laws, a stable solution must have equal numbers of positive and negative particles. It must be electrically neutral. When shifts and losses occur, compensating shifts and gains follow to maintain this dynamic balance, essential electroneutrality.

Electrolyte Control of Body Hydration

As indicated, ionized sodium is the chief cation of ECF, and ionized potassium is the chief cation of ICF. These two electrolytes control the amount of water retained in any given compartment. The usual bases for these shifts in water from one compartment to the other are ECF changes in concentration of these electrolytes. The terms *hypertonic* and *hypotonic* dehydration refer to the electrolyte concentration of the water outside the cell, which in turn causes a shift of water into or out of the cell to maintain balance.

Influence of Plasma Protein on Water Balance
Capillary Fluid Shift Mechanism

Water is constantly circulated throughout the body by the blood vessels. However, it must get out of the vessels to service the tissues and then be drawn back into circulation to maintain the normal transporting flow. Two main opposing pressures—colloidal osmotic pressure *(COP)* from plasma protein (mainly albumin) and hydrostatic pressure (blood pressure) of the capillary blood flow—provide balanced control of water and solute movement across capillary membranes. The body maintains this constant flow of water and the materials it is carrying to and from the cell by means of a shifting balance of these two pressures. It is a filtration process operating according to the differences in osmotic pressure on either side of the capillary membrane.

When blood first enters the capillary system, the greater blood pressure forces water and small solutes (glucose, for example) out into the tissues to bathe and nourish the cells. The plasma protein particles, however, are too large to go through the pores of capillary membranes. Hence the protein remains in the vessel and exerts the now greater colloidal osmotic pressure that draws the returning fluid and its materials back into circulation from the cells. This process is called the **capillary fluid shift mechanism.** It provides one of the most important and widespread homeostatic mechanisms in the body to maintain water balance, without which cells would die.

Cell Fluid Control

Much as plasma protein provides colloidal osmotic pressure to maintain the volume of extracellular fluid,
cell protein helps to provide the osmotic pressure that maintains the volume of fluid inside the cell. Also, ionized potassium within the cell guards cell water in balance with ionized sodium guarding water outside the cell. This balance supports the flow of water, nutrients, and metabolites in and out of cells to sustain life.

Influence of Hormones on Water Balance
ADH Mechanism

The antidiuretic hormone (ADH), also called *vasopressin,* is secreted by the posterior lobe of the pituitary gland. It causes reabsorption of water by the kidney according to body need. Thus it is a water-conserving mechanism. In any stress situation with threatened or real loss of body water, this hormone is triggered to hold on to precious body water.

Aldosterone Mechanism

Aldosterone is primarily a sodium-conserving hormone, related in its operation to the renin-angiotensin system, but in doing this job it also exerts a secondary control over water loss. This mechanism's full name is the **renin-angiotensin-aldosterone mechanism,** because renin, an enzyme from the kidney, and angiotensin, the active product of its substrate (angiotensinogen) from the liver, are the intermediate substances used to trigger the adrenal glands to produce in turn the aldoste-

capillary fluid shift mechanism • Process that controls the movement of water and small molecules in solution (electrolytes, nutrients) between the blood in the capillary and the surrounding interstitial area. Filtration of water and solutes out of the capillary at the arteriole end and reabsorption at the venule end are accomplished by shifts in balance between the intracapillary hydrostatic blood pressure and the colloidal osmotic pressure exerted by the plasma proteins.

colloidal osmotic pressure (COP) • Pressure produced by the protein molecules in the plasma and in the cell. Because proteins are large molecules, they do not pass through the separating membranes of the capillary cells. Thus they remain in their respective compartments, exerting a constant osmotic pull that protects vital plasma and cell fluid volumes in these compartments.

renin-angiotensin-aldosterone mechanism • Three-stage system of sodium conservation, hence control of water loss, in response to diminished filtration pressure in the kidney nephrons: (1) pressure loss causes kidney to secrete the enzyme renin, which combines with and activates angiotensinogen from the liver; (2) active angiotensin stimulates of the adjacent adrenal gland to release the hormone aldosterone; (3) the hormone causes reabsorption of sodium from the kidney nephrons and water follows.

rone hormone. Both aldosterone and ADH are activated by stress situations such as injury or surgery.

To Sum Up

Minerals are inorganic substances that are widely distributed in nature. They build body tissues; activate, regulate, and control metabolic processes; and transmit neurologic messages.

Minerals are classified as: (1) major minerals, required in relatively large quantities, which make up 60% to 80% of all the inorganic material in the body, and (2) trace elements, required in quantities as small as a microgram, which make up less than 1% of the body's inorganic material. Seven major and 10 trace minerals are known to be essential in human nutrition, with another eight trace elements probably essential, and still others constantly being examined for possible essentiality.

Overall water balance in the body is controlled by fluid intake and output. The distribution of body fluids is mainly controlled by two types of solutes: (1) electrolytes, charged mineral elements and other particles derived from inorganic compounds and (2) plasma protein, mainly albumin, consisting of particles too large to pass through capillary membranes but capable of influencing the flow of fluid from one compartment to another. These solute particles influence the distribution of fluid passing across cell or capillary membranes, separating body fluid into its two compartments.

QUESTIONS FOR REVIEW

1. List the seven major minerals, describing physiologic function and problems created by dietary deficiency or excess.
2. List the 10 trace elements with proven essentiality for humans. Which have established RDA standards? Which have safe and adequate intake limits established? Why is it difficult to establish RDAs for everyone?
3. What accounts for the edema of starvation?
4. Why does potassium depletion occur in prolonged diarrhea?

REFERENCES

1. Eaton SB, Nelson DA: Calcium in evolutionary perspective, *Am J Clin Nutr* 54(suppl):281S, 1991.
2. Wisker E and others: Calcium, mangnesium, zinc, and iron balances in young women: effects of a low-phytate barley fiber concentrate, *Am J Clin Nutr* 54:553, 1991.
3. Fullmer CS: Intestinal calcium absorption: calcium entry, *J Nutr* 122:644, 1992.
4. Andon B and others: Spinal bone density and calcium intake in healthy postmenopausal women, *Am J Clin Nutr* 54:927, 1991.
5. Scrimshaw NS, Murray EA: The acceptability of milk and milk products in populations with a high prevalence of lactose intolerance, *Am J Clin Nutr* 48:342, 1988.
6. Bouillon R and others: Conference report: Consumer Development Conference—prophylaxis and treatment of osteoporosis, *Am J Med* 90:107, 1991.
7. Nelson ME and others: A 1-year walking program and increased dietary calcium in postmenopausal women: effects on bone, *Am J Clin Nutr* 53:1304, 1991.
8. Food and Nutrition Board, National Academy of Sciences–National Research Council: *Recommended dietary allowances,* ed 10, Washington, DC, 1989, National Academy Press.
9. Avioli LV: Calcium and phosphorus. In Shils ME, Young VR, eds: *Modern nutrition in health and disease,* ed 7, Philadelphia, 1988, Lea & Febiger.
10. Food and Nutrition Board, Committee on Diet and Health, National Research Council: *Diet and health: implications for reducing chronic disease risk,* Washington, DC, 1989, National Academy Press.
11. Mertz W: The essential trace elements, *Science* 213:1332, 1981.
12. Fairbanks VF, Beutler E: Iron. In Shils ME, Young VR, eds: *Modern nutrition in health and disease,* ed 7, Philadelphia, 1988, Lea & Febiger.
13. Lipschitz DA: The anemia of chronic disease, *J Am Geriatr Soc* 38:1258, 1990.
14. Pennington JAT: A review of iodine toxicity reports, *J Am Diet Assoc* 90(11):1571, 1990.
15. Sherman AR: Zinc, copper, and iron nutriture and immunity, *J Nutr* 122:604, 1992.

Guidelines for Trace Element Supplementation

Currently in the consumer marketplace, trace elements have become popular in both sales and discussions of supplementation. Are there any reasonable guidelines for supplementation based on reliable and current research?

Ten trace elements have generally been identified as essential for optimal health, although this designation for some of them still awaits a full scientific consensus. These elements are chromium, cobalt, copper, fluoride, iodine, iron, manganese, molybdenum, selenium, and zinc. Public health workers are concerned about toxic levels of several elements, especially arsenic, manganese, vanadium, and nickel. Nutritionists should also be concerned about toxicity, in terms of dietary and supplemental contributions leading to excess intake, as well as deficiency, in terms of deciding whether to eliminate factors interfering with bioavailability and to evaluate the possible need for supplements.

The following list may serve as a basic guide for examining the need for supplementation of the U.S. diet with trace minerals.

Iron is provided by organ meats, dried fruits, whole grains, fortified breakfast cereals, legumes, and dark green leafy vegetables. Men require 10 mg/day; women 15 mg. The RDA for pregnant women is doubled to 30 mg/day, but since this increased pregnancy requirement cannot be met by the iron content of usual U.S. diets or by the iron stores of many women, *daily iron supplements are recommended.* Other high-risk groups may need to supplement their diets: adolescent girls, low-income adolescent boys, athletes, and elderly blacks. Before recommending a supplement to these individuals, however, you will want to evaluate their intake of iron antagonists such as fiber and caffeine.

Iodine is provided by foods grown in iodine-rich soil, seafood, and iodized salt. Daily adult requirements are 150 μg/day, though the average intake is several times that amount because of the widespread use of iodine-containing compounds in the dairy and baking industries. Since greater levels can result in thyrotoxicosis, *supplementation is not recommended.*

Zinc is supplied by oysters, whole grains, legumes, nuts, and meats. The recommended intake is 15 mg/day for men; 12 mg/day for women. Pregnancy increases the need by only 3 mg/day, and lactation by 7 and 4 mg/day for early and later lactation, respectively, to avoid deficiency signs of slow growth, impaired taste and smell, poor wound healing, and skin problems. Others at risk include alcoholics and individuals on long-term low-calorie diets. It takes 3 to 24 weeks for symptoms to appear, but supplementation relieves deficiency symptoms in a matter of days. To avoid an overdose, characterized by gastrointestinal upset, nausea, and bleeding, eating habits should be checked for zinc antagonists, for example, an excessive intake of fiber or iron.

Copper is widely available in liver, oysters, shellfish, nuts, whole grains, and legumes. The average diet was previously believed to provide 2 to 5 mg/day, easily meeting the minimum RDA standard of 2 to 3 mg/day. Intake levels are now believed to range from less than 1 mg to no more than 2 mg/day, based on new analysis methods, thus placing a larger segment of the population at risk for developing a mild deficiency. Before recommending supplements, however, examine factors that reduce copper bioavailability, such as a low protein intake, or high levels of zinc, cadmium, fiber, or ascorbic acid.

Chromium is provided by brewer's yeast, animal products, and whole grains. Daily requirements have been estimated between 50 and 200 μg. Deficiency signs include resistance to insulin and other signs of diabetes. Supplementation not only reduces insulin resistance, but also increases HDL cholesterol, thereby offering some protection against coronary heart disease. Although reliable diagnostic tests have not been developed yet, it is estimated that current intakes fall below recommended levels. However, because it has shown effectiveness only in small, controlled studies, supplementation recommendations have not been made yet for any population groups.

Selenium is provided by fish, whole wheat, and plants grown in selenium-rich soil. RDAs of 70 and 55 μg/day are stated for men and women, respectively, but the average diet provides this much and more. Selenium is believed to offer protection against breast cancer. One group of researchers believes that optimal cancer protection is provided at levels of 150 to 300 μg/day, though the connection between blood levels in cancer patients and cancer-free individuals has not been established. In addition to cancer, selenium is believed to protect against heart disease, arthritis, heavy metal poisoning, sexual dysfunction, and aging. As there is no current evidence of selenium deficiency in the general population, *supplementation is not recommended.*

Manganese is provided by whole grains, green vegetables, and dried beans. Safe intake is estimated in the range of 2.5 to 5 mg/day. Deficiency signs in humans have not been reported, but signs of toxicity have. Toxicity is associated mainly with industrial exposure. However, the possibility of an excess suggests that *supplementation is not recommended.*

Silicon requirements for humans are not known, nor are reliable food sources. Deficiency has been associated with poor bone growth in chicks and statistically correlated with cardiovascular disease in humans. However, the need for supplementation has not been established.

Nickel is provided by legumes, cocoa, wheat, shellfish, milk, meats, and a variety of vegetables and fresh fruits. Requirements are estimated at about 75 μg/day, though U.S. intakes have been estimated between 300 and 600 μg/day. In light of this excessive intake, plus the existence of at least one sign of toxicity (a nickel-sensitivity dermatitis) *supplementation is not recommended.*

Vanadium requirements and reliable food sources are both unknown. However, it is estimated that the average American diet provides 1 to 2 mg/day. Some individuals are apparently sensitive to this amount, exhibiting severe depression. They improve when given megadoses of vitamin C, which blocks vanadium activity. The need for supplementation is not indicated because of its potential for toxicity in this sensitive population group.

REFERENCES

Gable CB: Hemochromatosis and dietary iron supplements: implications from U.S. mortality, morbidity, and health survey data, *J Am Diet Assoc* 92(2):208, 1992.

Hemminki E, Rimpela U: A randomized comparison of routine versus selective iron supplementation during pregnancy, *J Am Coll Nutr* 10(1):3, 1991.

Nielsen FH: New essential trace elements for the life sciences, *Biol Trace Elem Res* 26:599, 1990.

Nielsen FH: Nutritional requirements for boron, silicon, vanadium, nickel, and arsenic: current knowledge and speculation, *FASEB J* 5:2661, 1991.

Pennington JAT: A review of iodine toxicity reports, *J Am Diet Assoc* 90(11):1571, 1990.

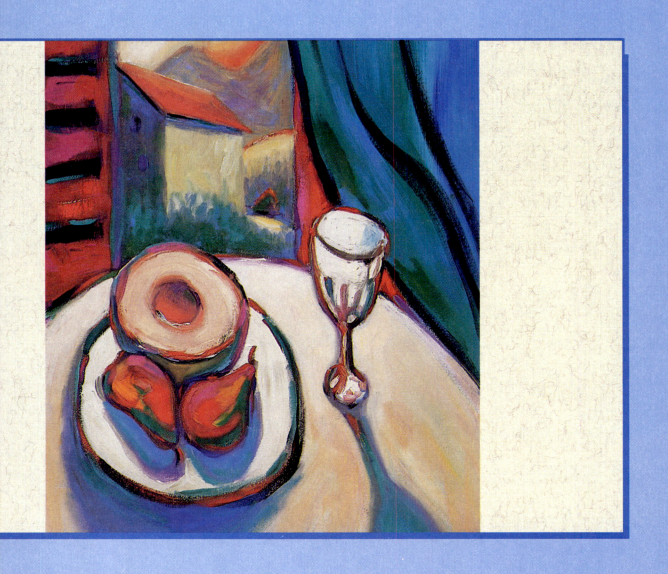

*C*ommunity Nutrition: The Life Cycle

PART

2

CHAPTER 9

The Food Environment and Food Habits

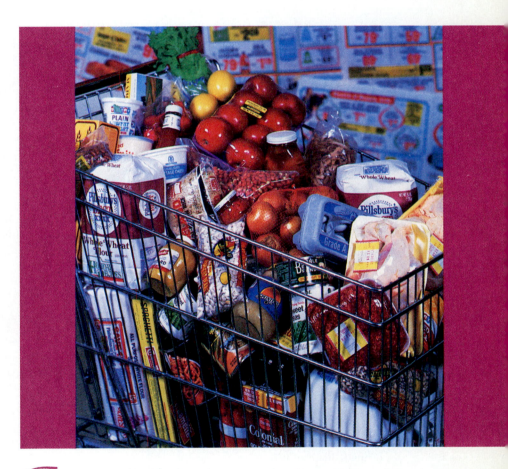

This chapter begins the second part of your study of nutrition with a two-chapter sequence on food habits and family nutrition counseling. Here we seek to apply the nutritional science principles you have learned to personal and family needs.

The science of human nutrition only comes alive in terms of personal need. Human compassion and concern are necessary, as well as practical guides and skills, to apply knowledge in a useful and helpful manner.

Here we begin with a look at our changing food environment and

169

the web of influences that determine personal food choices and habits.

The Ecology of Human Nutrition
The Food Environment and Malnutrition

Out of necessity our food habits are inevitably linked to our environment. As a result, our rapidly changing human environment with its problems of imbalance such as pollution and malnutrition often threaten health. The word **ecology** comes from a Greek word, *oikos,* meaning "house." Just as many factors and forces within a family interact to influence its members, so even greater forces in our physical environment and social system can interact to produce disease.

The public health significance of malnutrition, local to worldwide in scope, continues to grow.[1-3] Protein-energy malnutrition continues to rank first among the nutritional deficiency diseases in the world. Observation and experience have brought deepened awareness of two important interrelated facts: (1) having adequate food alone is not the complete answer, although it fulfills a fundamental need for all persons, and (2) a national high standard of living does not necessarily eliminate the problem of malnutrition. Even in the midst of plenty here in America, malnutrition exists.[4,5] It is found among vulnerable groups such as elderly and hospitalized persons. It is found among persons suffering from alcoholism and drug addiction. It is associated with poverty and homelessness. It is partner to a distorted obsession with thinness. Human misery and human waste of life from malnutrition, more stark in some regions of our country and the world than in others, occurs nonetheless in both world hemispheres. The extent of this human suffering is impossible to quantify.

At its fundamental biologic level, malnutrition results from an inadequate supply of nutrients to the cells. However, this lack of essential nutrients at the cell level is by no means a simple problem. It is caused by a complex web of factors: physical, psychologic, personal, social, cultural, economic, political, and educational. Each of these factors is more or less important at a given time and place for a given individual. If these factors are only temporarily adverse, the malnutrition may be short term, alleviated rapidly, and cause no long-standing results or harm to life. But if they continue unrelieved, malnutrition becomes chronic. Irreparable harm to life follows (see box below), and eventually death ensues. For the **epidemiologist** a triad of variables influences disease: (1) agent, (2) host, and (3) environment. These three factors describe malnutrition.

Agent

The fundamental agent in malnutrition is lack of food. Because of this lack, certain nutrients in food that are essential to maintaining cell activity are missing. As in-

---

CLINICAL APPLICATION   *Functional Consequences of Malnutrition*

In addition to specific disorders associated with deficiencies of particular nutrients, other human factors are related to malnutrition. These factors include immunocompetence, reproductive competence, work output, mental ability, and social or behavioral traits. The full impact of inadequate nutrition on these and more subtle aspects of human life and health is difficult to measure. And it is of particular concern in early childhood.

We have long assumed a linear relationship between intake and well-being, at least up to the point of adequacy. We have relied on body measurements, especially those measuring growth rates in children, to tell us how badly undernourished an individual or a population is. Measurements such as weight-for-height or height-for-age are compared with those of reference populations that are well nourished. Then degrees of malnutrition are defined in terms of that reference standard:(1) mild or first degree—75% to 90% of standard; (2) moderate, or second degree—60% to 75% of standard; and (3) severe, or third degree—less than 60% of standard.

We are now learning that a possible threshold of tolerance exists, and that a person may be able to adapt successfully to lowered intakes of kcalories up to a point, or threshold. If the kcalorie intake is chronically below this threshold, the individual is then likely to suffer functional disabilities, but if the kcalories consumed fall chronically below what is recommended and this threshold point, the individual lives a marginal life barely free of impairment.

Studies have validated that long-term severe malnutrition leads to stunting of mental and emotional as well as physical development. However, the effects of chronic malnutrition, even in the early years of life, may be reversible by improved diet and social-emotional care later in the child's development. Of course, serious deficits of food are often accompanied by poverty in other areas of life, and a family may not be capable of making up for the early years of hardship.

REFERENCES

Fuchs VR, Reklis DM: America's children: economic perspectives and policy options, *Science* 255(5040):41, Jan 3, 1992.

Grantham-McGregor S and others: Development of severely malnourished children who received psychosocial stimulation: six-year follow-up, *Pediatrics* 79:247, 1987.

Splett PL, Story M: Child nutrition: objectives for the decade, *J Am Diet Assoc* 91(6):665, 1991. ◆

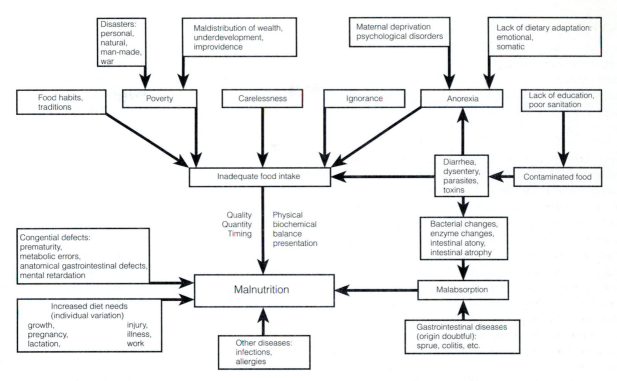

FIG. 9-1 The multiple etiology of malnutrition. (Modified from Williams CD: Malnutrition, *Lancet* 2:342, 1962.)

dicated, many factors may interact to cause or modify this lack of food: inadequate quantity and quality of food, insufficient amounts for children during critical growth periods, loss of supply through famine, poverty, maldistribution, war, or unwise choices made from foods available.

Host

The host is the person—infant, child, or adult—who suffers from malnutrition. Various personal characteristics may influence the disease: presence of other diseases, increased need for food during times of growth, pregnancy, or heavy labor, congenital defects or prematurity, and personal factors such as emotional problems and poverty.

Environment

Many environmental factors influence malnutrition. These include sanitation, social problems, culture, economic and political structure, and agriculture.

The classic interactive and tangled web of some of these factors leading to malnutrition, as experienced by pioneer British pediatrician Cecily Williams in her early work in Africa with kwashiorkor, is shown in Fig. 9-1. This debilitating web of malnutrition factors, in one combination or another, is still being experienced in numerous places around the world every day.[2,3]

Economic and Political Environment
Food Availability and Use

In any society, at both governmental and personal levels, food availability and use involve both money and politics. It is plainly evident that money is a basic necessity for getting an adequate food supply. Sometimes, however, the role of politics and government structure and policies is not always as evident. Nonetheless, both are always intertwined in securing human nutrition.[6]

Government Food and Agriculture Programs

In any country, food and agricultural programs at any level of government influence food availability and distribution. A number of factors may be involved, such as land management practices and erosion, water distribution and its consequent pollution from long-term use of questionable pesticides, food production and distribution policies, and food assistance programs for persons in need.

ecology • Relations between organisms and their environments.

epidemiology • The study of factors determining the frequency, distribution, and strength of diseases in population groups.

The Problem of Poverty

We are all made increasingly aware through the daily news that malnutrition, even famine and death, exists in many countries that are hard pressed by social conditions such as war, inequity, and desperate poverty. But even here, in the United States, one of the wealthiest nations, many studies document widespread hunger and malnutrition among the poor, especially among minority groups, with increasing numbers of infants and young children involved.[7] For example, black infants in the United States still have twice the chance of dying in their first year than white infants do, one of five U.S. children under age 18 lives in poverty, and black and Hispanic children are nearly three times more likely to live in poverty than white children.[7-9]

Tremendous problems exist among the poor and at times they seem almost insurmountable. Often a culture of poverty develops and is reinforced and perpetuated by society's values and attitudes, which wall off such persons more completely than do physical barriers. As a result of extreme pressures caused by living conditions, poverty-stricken persons become victims of negative attitudes and characteristics, feeling isolated and powerless and insecure, feelings that influence their use of community health services.

Isolation

Strong feelings of alienation from mainstream society are common among the poor. In many communities few if any channels of communications are open between the lowest income groups and the rest of society. In most instances a poor person responds to such feelings of alienation by further withdrawal. Each person feels isolated and alone and concludes that no one is really concerned. Hazards to health are inherent in poor housing and poor nutrition and are often compounded by distance from the sources of health care.

Powerlessness

It is ironic that often those persons most exposed to risks and emergencies have the fewest coping resources. Extreme frustration is inevitable and persons become overwhelmed. Why try, they conclude, if they have no control over the situation? Why plan, if there is no future different from today? In such a day-to-day struggle to exist, the poor person often sees little value in long-range preventive health measures.

Insecurity

Subjected to forces outside their control, poor individuals and families have little or no security. Insecurity and anxiety often incapacitate them. In such a setting, where hunger may be a constant companion, food—which has for poor people the same deep psychologic and emotional meaning that it has for all people—assumes even greater meaning than it has for persons who rarely know hunger.

Role of the Health Worker

How can concerned health workers help individuals and families conditioned by years of poverty or crushed by new poverty? In the face of such overpowering feelings of isolation, helplessness, and insecurity, what attitudes are necessary to be of real help? What methods and approaches are most likely to reach our clients and patients and supply their needs? Some basic principles can help.

Self-awareness

First, we must explore our own feelings about the poor. We must be aware of our own distorted vision, our own class values and attitudes. If we are to be agents of constructive change, true helping vehicles, we must first have some understanding of the person's situation and its broad social setting. We must also understand ourselves better and confront our own cultural conditioning and biases.

Rapport

Genuine warmth, interest, friendliness, and kindness grow from within. Rapport is that feeling of relationship between persons that is born of mutual respect, regard, and trust. This sense of relationship gives both helper and helped a deep feeling of working together. Its most basic ingredient is a concern for people and persons, a positive orientation toward human beings in general and concern for individuals in particular. It is born of a deep knowledge of what it means to be human.

Acceptance

This term is another way of stating the principle that one must begin where the client or patient is. Each person's own concerns should be the primary consideration. Often we work with other team specialists to cut through the maze of factors involved in a given situation before the client or patient is ready to accept or even to consider the health practice or diet counsel that is needed or desired. Much time may have to be spent, for example, in coming to understand the meaning of food to this person, before practical dietary matters can begin to be explored.

Listening

Here, more than elsewhere, the art of listening—positive, active, creative listening—is vital. Clients must tell their story in their own way, with no interruption by distracting statements or questions and no deflecting of the conversation to another's problems. This listening must also be observant. Sequence of statements, subjects introduced, areas of intense feeling, and areas ignored give clues to needs. Throughout we must proceed with sensitivity and create a relaxed, nonthreatening atmosphere, in which persons feel free to talk—*and we must listen*. The reason that some frustrated persons finally take their problems to the streets may well be that no one listens to them unless they do.

Development of Food Habits

In addition to these factors of poverty and politics, other aspects of our lives influence our food patterns. Food habits, like other forms of human behavior, do not develop in a vacuum. They result from many personal, cultural, social, and psychologic influences. For each of us these factors are interwoven to develop a whole, unique individual.

Cultural Influences
Strength of Personal Culture

Often the most significant thing about a society's **culture** is what it takes for granted in daily life. Culture involves not only the more obvious and historical aspects of a person's communal life, that is, language, religion, politics, technology, and so on, but also all the little habits of everyday living, such as preparing and serving food and caring for children, feeding them, and lulling them to sleep. These many facets of a person's culture are learned gradually as a child grows up in a given society. Through a slow process of conscious and unconscious learning, we take on our culture's values, attitudes, habits, and practices through the influence of our parents, teachers, and others. Whatever is invented, transmitted, and perpetuated, socially acquired knowledge and habits, we learn as part of our culture. These elements become internalized and entrenched.

Food in a Culture

Food habits are among the oldest and most deeply rooted aspects of many cultures and exert deep influence on the behavior of the people. The cultural and subcultural background determines what shall be eaten as well as when and how it shall be eaten. There is, of course, considerable variation. But rational or irrational, beneficial and injurious customs are found in every part of the world. Nevertheless, food habits are primarily based on food availability, economics, and personal food meanings and beliefs. Included among these influential factors are the geography of the land, the agriculture practiced by the people, their economic and marketing practices, their view about healthy or safe food, and their history and traditions. Within every culture certain foods are deeply infused with symbolic meaning. These symbolic foods are related to major life experiences from birth through death, to religion, to politics, and to general social organization. From early times ceremonies and religious rites have surrounded certain events and seasons. Food gathering, preparing, and serving have followed specific customs and commemorated special events of religious and national significance and heritage. Many of these customs remain today (see Issues and Answers, p. 189).

Social Influences
Social Organization

The study of human group behavior reveals numerous activities, processes, and structures by which social life goes on. Human behavior can be understood in terms of social phenomena and problems, such as social change, urbanism, rural life, the family, the community, race relations, delinquency, drugs, and crime. These social problems carry nutritional implications. Two aspects of social organization concern health professionals: class structure and value systems.

Class structure. The structure of a society is largely formed by groupings according to factors such as economic status, education, residence, occupation, or family. Within a given society many of these groups exist, and their values and habits vary widely. Subgroups develop on the basis of region, religion, age, sex, social class, health concerns, occupation, or political affiliation. Within these subgroups there may be still smaller groupings with distinct attitudes, values, habits. A person may be a member of several subcultural groups, each of which influences values, attitudes, and habits. Our democratic philosophy, as well as the humanitarian ideals on which the health professions have been nurtured, combine to make the reality of class differences difficult for us to accept.

Value systems. A society's value systems develop as a result of its history and heritage. Traditionally four basic premises have influenced American value systems and have affected attitudes toward health care and food habits:

- *Equality:* A high value on equality leads health workers to establish quality health care standards for all people, although in reality this does not always work out.
- *Sociality:* The high respect accorded to a social nature builds peer group pressures and status-seeking within social groups. Foods may be accepted because they are high status foods or rejected because they are low-prestige foods. Even the use of dietary supplements has been associated with the desire for prestige, along with health concerns.[6]
- *Success:* The esteem in which success is held often leads persons to measure life in terms of competitive superlatives. They want to set the best table, provide the most abundant supply of food for the family, or to have the biggest eater and the fattest baby of any in the neighborhood.
- *Change:* The value placed on change leads families and individuals to seek constant variety in their diets, to be geared for action, to be a mobile society, and to seek quick-cooking, conveniently prepared foods. In response to such marketing demands, food technologists continually produce an array of new food products.

Food and Social Factors

Food habits in any setting are highly socialized. These habits perform significant social functions, some of which may not always be evident. First, within social relationships, food is a symbol of social acceptance, warmth, and friendliness. People tend to accept food more readily from those persons they view as friends or allies. They accept advice about food from persons they consider to be authorities or with whom they can feel warm relationships.

Second, within family relationships, the primary social unit, strong food patterns develop. Food habits that are most closely associated with family sentiments are the most tenacious throughout life. Long into adulthood, certain foods trigger a flood of childhood memories and are valued for reasons totally apart from any nutritional value. Strong religious factors associated with food tend to have their origin and reinforcement within the family meal circle. Also, family income, community sources of food, and market conditions influence food habits and ultimately food choices. Persons eat foods that are readily available to them and that they have the money to buy.

Psychologic Influences
Social Psychology

Social psychology is concerned with (1) social interaction in terms of its effect on individual behavior and (2) the social influences of individual perception, motivation, and action. How does a particular individual perceive a given situation? What basic needs motivate action and response? What social factors surround a particular action? Issues of particular concern include the effect of culture on personality, the socialization of the child, differences in individuals in groups, group dynamics, group attitudes and opinions, and leadership. The methods of social psychology have made important contributions to nutrition, medicine, nursing, and allied health care, especially to problems of human behavior under stress.

Food and Psychologic Factors

Individual behavior patterns, specially those related to eating, result from many interrelated psychosocial influences. Factors that are particularly pertinent to the shaping of food habits are motivation and perception.

1. *Motivation.* People are not the same the world over. Those of differing cultures are not motivated by the same needs and goals. Even primary biologic drives such as hunger and sex are modified in their interpretation, expression, and fulfillment by many cultural, social, and personal influences. The kinds of food sought, prized, or accepted by one individual at one time and place are rejected by another living in different circumstances. For persons existing in a state of basic hunger or semistarvation, food is the whole perception and motivation. Such a person thinks, talks, and dreams about food. Under less severe circumstances, however, the concern for food may be on a relatively abstract level and may involve symbolism that is associated with other needs. For example, Maslow's classic hierarchy of human needs illustrates these human strivings.[10] He described five levels of need that operate in turn, building on the prior ones:

   - *Basic physiologic needs:* Hunger, thirst
   - *Safety needs:* Physical comfort, security, protection
   - *"Belongingness" needs:* Love, giving and receiving affection
   - *Recognition needs:* Self-esteem, status, sense of self-worth, strength, self-confidence, capability, adequacy
   - *Self-actualization needs:* Self-fulfillment, creative growth.

   Of course, these levels of need overlap and vary with time and circumstance. But we can use them to help us understand the needs of our clients and plan care accordingly.

2. *Perception.* To make sense out of an otherwise chaotic assortment of impressions, we perceive our environment in different ways. These perceptions enable us to live in an environment that feels relatively stable. However, perception also limits understanding. Every phenomenon that the outer world offers is filtered through our own social and personal lenses. In every experience of our lives, we perceive a blend of three facets: (1) the *external* reality, (2) the *message* of the stimulus that is conveyed by the nervous system to the integrative centers of the brain where thinking and evaluation go on, and (3) the *interpretation* we put on every part of our personal experience. A host of subjective elements—hunger, thirst, hate, fear, love, self-interest, values, temperament—influence our response to the outer world's phenomena.

On the basis, then, of personal motivation and perception, personal learning takes place. In the final analysis, each person must learn in his or her own way according to need. It is this very personal human dimension that makes a health professional's work profound. Persons learn because they have an urgent need to know. They learn because their curiosity is aroused. They learn because they want to make meaning out of their lives. They learn by exploring, making mistakes and correcting them, testing, verifying. All of these things individuals must do for themselves. This is true of everyone's learning. It is true of the learning we desire for our clients. It is true of our own learning.

Health Concerns: Misinformation and Food Safety

Food Misinformation

Unscientific statements about food and nutrition often mislead the public and contribute to poor food habits. Persons have often surrounded their cultural eating habits with myths of various sorts.[11] Some scientifically unsubstantiated beliefs about certain foods may be harmless, but others may have more serious implications for health and well-being. Claims about foods or supplements that are not based on scientific evidence, such as heavy use of vitamin supplements for general health maintenance, often mislead the public and contribute to poor food habits.[12] False information may come from folklore, or it may be built on half-truths, innuendos, and outright deception, as in cases of fraud.

In contrast, nutritional science is a growing body of knowledge built on vigorously examined scientific evidence. Concern for food safety and wholesomeness clearly existed long before the scientific method was known. Nonetheless, in this rapidly changing world, it is only on the sound basis of scientific knowledge that we may make wise food choices and recognize misinformation as such (see p. 179).

Types of Food Faddist Claims

Food faddists make exaggerated claims for certain types of food. These claims fall into four basic groups: (1) certain foods will cure specific conditions; (2) certain foods are harmful and should be avoided; (3) special food combinations are very effective as reducing diets or have special therapeutic effects; and (4) other "natural" foods can meet body needs and prevent disease. But there is a basic error. Examine these claims carefully. Notice that each one focuses on foods as such, not on the chemical components—the nutrients—that are the actual physiologic agents of life and health. It is true, of course, that certain individuals may be allergic to specific foods and obviously should avoid them. It is also true that certain foods have particularly high concentrations of certain nutrients and are therefore good sources of such nutrients. But it is the nutrients, not the specific foods, that have specific functions in the body. And furthermore, each of these nutrients may be found in a number of different foods. Persons require specific nutrients, never specific foods.

Why should the health worker be concerned about food faddism and its effects on food habits? What harm may food faddism do? Essentially, food fads involve three basic dangers that concern all members of the health care team.

- *Dangers to health:* Responsibility for one's health is fundamental. However, self-diagnosis and self-treatment can be dangerous, especially where health problems are concerned. When such action is based on questionable sources, the dangers are multiplied. By following such a course, a person with a real illness may fail to seek appropriate medical care. Many anxious patients who have cancer, diabetes, or arthritis have been misled by fraudulent claims of cures and postponed effective therapy. Superstitions that are perpetuated counteract scientific progress and sound health teaching.

- *Money spent needlessly:* Some of these foods and supplements used by faddists are harmless, but most are expensive. As much as $2.5 billion per year has been spent by consumers on nutrient supplements. Such money is wasted. When dollars are scarce, the family may neglect to buy foods that fill its basic needs, opting instead to purchase a "guaranteed cure" (see the Case Study, p. 187).

- *Distrust of the food market:* Our food environment is rapidly changing. We need intelligent concern and rational problem solving to meet nutritional requirements. A wise course is to select a variety of primary foods "closer to the source"—having minimal processing—adding a few carefully selected processed items for specific uses. Blanket erroneous teaching concerning food and health breeds public suspicion and distrust of the common food market and of food technology and agriculture in general. Each food product must be evaluated on its own merits in terms of individual needs. These needs include nutrient contribution, esthetic values, safety, and cost.

Groups Vulnerable to Food Fads

Food fads appeal especially to certain groups of people with particular needs and concerns. Among these are older adults, adolescents, obese persons, athletes, and those whose living depends on their physical appearance.

- *Older persons:* Fear of changes that come as youth and potency wane leads many middle-aged persons to grasp at exaggerated claims that some product will restore their youthful vigor. Elderly persons in pain and discomfort, perhaps living alone with chronic illness, may respond to the hope that the special supplement holds a sure cure.[13] Desperately ill and lonely individuals are easy prey for exaggerated health claims.

- *Young persons:* Figure-conscious adolescent girls and muscle-minded rapidly growing boys frequently respond to advertisements for crash programs to attain the perfect body. Young people, particularly those who are lonely or have exaggerated ideas of glamour, hope to achieve peer group acceptance by these means.

- *Obese persons:* One of the most disturbing and frustrating health problems in America is obesity. Obese persons, faced with a bewildering barrage of propaganda advocating diets, pills, and devices, are likely to respond to the fad of the moment to solve everything (see Chapter 6).
- *Athletes and coaches:* Athletes and their coaches are prime targets for those who push supplements. Always looking for the added something to give them the competitive edge, athletes tend to be lured by nutrition myths and hoaxs (see Chapter 14).
- *Entertainers:* Persons in the public eye, such as entertainers, are often gullible and easily believe false claims. They may look for certain foods, drugs, or dietary combinations that will help them retain the physical appearance and strength on which their careers depend.

These various groups are vulnerable for obvious reasons. No segment of the population, however, seems to be completely free from food faddism's appeal. Particularly in metropolitan areas, "health food" with its attendant supplements is a large industry, bigger in the United States than in any other country.[14]

The Answer

How do we respond to food habits associated with food faddism, misinformation, or even deception? What can health professionals do? What should they do? Several things merit consideration:

1. **Assess your own attitudes and habits.** We cannot counsel or teach others until we have first examined our own position. Instruction based on personal conviction, practice, and enthusiasm will achieve far more than teaching that says, in effect, "Do as I say, not as I do."
2. **Use reliable sources.** Two types of background knowledge are vital: (1) knowledge of the product and the persons behind it, and (2) knowledge of human nutritional physiology and the scientific method of problem-solving.
3. **Recognize human needs.** Observe these needs in yourselves and in others to understand how psychologic and cultural factors affect food habits. Consider the emotional needs that are symbolically fulfilled by foods, the eating of foods, and by the rituals surrounding the process. Respect personal needs. Welcome the positive power that food and eating rituals possess for filling these needs. Even when there is reason to believe that the client is using food as a crutch for emotional adjustment, the value of such an adjustment must be considered. A wise teacher of mine once put it well: "We must avoid 'breaking crutches' without providing alternative support."
4. **Be alert to community opportunities.** Grasp any opportunity that arises to present sound health information to groups or individuals, formally or informally. Learn of available community resources and use them. Develop communication skills. Avoid monotony. Use a well-disciplined imagination. Without these things, the message will not convince.
5. **Think scientifically.** We can teach young children to use the problem-solving approach to everyday situations. Children are naturally curious. With their eternal *"Why?"* they often seek evidence to support statements made to them. We need to teach them and ourselves the value of asking three significant questions: "What do you mean?" "How do you know?" and "What is your evidence?"
6. **Know responsible authorities.** The Food and Drug Administration (FDA) has the legal responsibility of controlling the quality and safety of food and drug products marketed in the United States. But it needs the vigilance of consumers to help fulfill so large a task. Other governmental, professional, and private organizations also provide resources for consumer education.

Influence of Food Safety Concerns on Food Habits

America's food supply has radically changed over the past years. These changes, which have swept the food-marketing system, are rooted in widespread social change and scientific advance. The agricultural and food processing industries have developed a wide variety of chemicals to increase and preserve our food supply and to create new products. In the process, however, critics have increasingly voiced concerns about how these changes have affected food safety, food habits, and the overall environment. Concerns center on pesticides and food additives.

Plant Pesticides and Animal Drugs

For the most part, over the past few decades, American agriculture has developed into a modern mechanized business structure. As a whole, it has brought large crop yields to feed a growing population. To accomplish this task, a growing chemical industry has supplied an increasing number of plant pesticides and herbicides to build large crops, as well as animal antibiotics and growth hormones to develop livestock for market. Large American agricultural corporations, as well as individual farmers, continue to use a number of chemicals to advance food production. They use them for a variety of reasons—to control a wide number of destructive insects, kill weeds, control plant diseases, stop fruit from dropping prematurely, cause leaves to fall and thus facilitate harvesting, make seeds sprout, keep seeds from rotting before they sprout, increase yield, and improve marketing quality.

Over time, however, problems from the frequent use

of pesticides have developed in four main areas: (1) pesticide residues on food, (2) leaching of the chemicals into ground water and surrounding wells, (3) increased exposure of farm workers to the strong chemicals, and (4) increased amount of chemicals required as insect tolerance for them develops. The task of assessing health risks for the thousands of pesticides in use or being developed is difficult. The current FDA routine screening assays detect only part of all U.S. pesticides.[15] Currently, an increasing number of concerned farmers, with help from soil scientists, are developing alternative systems of sustainable agriculture that do not rely on heavy pesticide use. Instead, they combine conservative practices and modern technology that protect resources, preserve the environment, reduce the need for toxic pesticides and herbicides, and are still profitable.[16,17]

Food Processing Additives

In addition, over the past few decades, chemicals intentionally added to foods during processing have become an integral part of our food supply. Our present variety of food market items would be impossible without them. For example, additives enrich food with added nutrients, produce uniform qualities of food products, standardize functional factors such as thickening and stabilization, preserve foods, improve flavor and texture. Table 9-1 lists some examples of these additives.

TABLE 9-1

Some Examples of Intentional Food Additives

Function	Chemical compounds	Common food uses
Acids, alkalis, buffers	Sodium bicarbonate	Baking powder
	Tartaric acid	Fruit sherbets
		Cheese spreads
Antibiotics	Chlortetracycline	Dip for dressed poultry
Anticaking agents	Aluminum calcium silicate	Table salt
Antimycotics	Calcium propionate	Bread
	Sodium propionate	Bread
	Sorbic acid	Cheese
Antioxidants	Butylated hydroxyanisole (BHA)	Fats
	Butylated hydroxytoluene (BHT)	Fats
Bleaching agents	Benzoyl peroxide	Wheat flour
	Chlorine dioxide	
	Oxides of nitrogen	
Color preservative	Sodium benzoate	Green peas
		Maraschino cherries
Coloring agents	Annotto	Butter, margarine
	Carotene	
Emulsifiers	Lecithin	Bakery goods
	Monoglycerides, diglycerides	Dairy products
	Propylene glycol alginate	Confections
Flavoring agents	Amyl acetate	Soft drinks
	Benzaldehyde	Bakery goods
	Methyl salicylate	Candy, ice cream
	Essential oils, natural extracts	Canned meats
	Monosodium glutamate	
Nonnutritive sweeteners	Saccharin	Diet packed canned fruit
	Aspartame	Low-kcalorie soft drinks
Nutrient supplements	Potassium iodide	Iodized salt
	Vitamin C	Fruit juices
	Vitamin D	Milk
	Vitamin A	Margarine
	B vitamins, iron	Bread and cereal
Sequestrants	Sodium citrate	Dairy products
	Calcium pyrophosphoric acid	
Stabilizers and thickeners	Pectin	Jellies
	Vegetable gums (carob bean, carrageenan, guar)	Dairy desserts and chocolate milk
	Gelatin	Confections
	Agar-agar	Low-kcalorie salad dressings
Yeast foods and dough conditioners	Ammonium chloride	Bread, rolls
	Calcium sulfate	
	Calcium phosphate	

A number of micronutrients and antioxidants are being added to processed foods, not for increasing the nutrient content but for their technical effects.[18]

Food additives have served many useful purposes, but problems also have developed. Initial control of food safety began in 1938 with the establishment of the Federal Food, Drug, and Cosmetic Act. Such control continued in 1960 with amendments regulating the use of food additives. These amendments created what has become known as the *GRAS list*—Generally Recognized As Safe additives. Rigid testing to determine their true safety, however, was lacking. Any additive developed after 1960 required this rigid testing before approval. The now famous Delany Clause, named for the congressman who proposed it, was attached in the final hours of congressional debate on the legislation. This clause banned food additives found to cause cancer "in man or animal." Today, however, advanced testing procedures and new knowledge of natural food constituents and metabolic processes make the zero-risk Delany clause seem outdated and inconsequential in terms of its intent over three decades ago.[19] The 1977 congressional directive to FDA to test the thousands of GRAS items is ongoing.[20]

Research has always been a large part of the FDA's work. Along with the United States Department of Agriculture (USDA) Agricultural Research Service, FDA scientists continually evaluate foods and food components through their own research (Fig. 9-2). In the past, FDA views and policies have varied with administrators and sometimes left much to be desired. Nevertheless, broader views more in tune with today's needs seem to prevail now.[21,22] Today people want to know more than just that a given food will not kill them. They want to know whether it has any positive nutritional value. Thus for a more health-conscious public and a changed marketplace, the FDA has currently developed expanded nutrition guidelines for food labels on a variety of food products.

FDA Food Labeling Regulations
Food Standards

For the past three decades the FDA has followed its truth in packaging regulations that dealt mainly with food standards. The basic standard of identity has required that labels on foods not having an established reference standard must list all the ingredients in the order of the amount found in the product. Other food standard information on labels has related to food quality, fill of the container, and enrichment.

Nutrition Information

In the mid-1970s, the FDA began describing general nutrition information on food labels, and some producers added limited information on their own in response to increasing market demand. Nutrients and food constituents that consumer groups wanted listed on labels included the macronutrients (carbohydrates, fat, and protein) and their total energy value (kcalories), key micronutrients (vitamins and minerals), sodium, cholesterol, and saturated fat.

New FDA Food Label Regulations

In November of 1990 a new law, the Nutrition Labeling and Education Act of 1990 (NLEA), was enacted by Congress and signed by the President. The NLEA requires mandatory labeling of most processed foods under the jurisdiction of the FDA and forms the core of the FDA's reform effort. It also includes voluntary labeling of fresh fruits, vegetables, and seafood. The USDA is responsible for standards and consumer information concerning other meat and poultry, as well as dairy products. Over a 3-year process, involving consumers and producers, as well as health professionals, the new food labels have emerged. Basic features of the new labeling regulations include guidelines to define the following items: kcalories and nutrients (see Clinical Application p. 179), descriptive terms, serving sizes and number of servings per container, health claims, and a standardized label format based on results of consumer research (see To Probe Further, p. 180).[23]

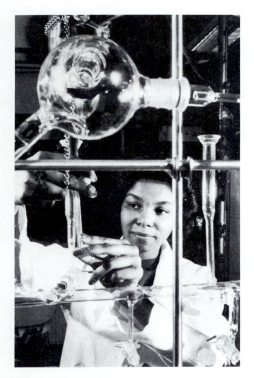

FIG. 9-2   Research in food chemistry. A chemist in the U.S. Department of Agriculture's Agricultural Research Service makes an adjustment on a molecular still used in a project to aid in manufacturing dry milk.

The Nutrition Labeling and Education Act was signed into law in November 1990 after being passed unanimously by Congress. Changes in this law mandate easy-to-understand labels for all foods, including fresh fruits and vegetables. In January 1993 the Food and Drug Administration (FDA) and the USDA's Food, Safety, and Inspection Service published the final regulations. The first major change in food labeling regulations since nutrition labeling was introduced about 20 years ago, went into effect in May 1993 (Fig. 9-3). Consumers should see the resulting new labels in the summer of 1994.

The most visible changes will be how food is advertised and marketed. Manufacturers will no longer be able to claim that a product does not contain an ingredient that has never been contained in that product. This means that products that never contained cholesterol will no longer be able to make the claim "no cholesterol." Descriptors—such as "light," and "low fat," or "reduced kcalories"—will have legal definitions that will be universal to all products.

The new label reference value, Daily Reference Value (DRV), replaces the USRDAs introduced in 1973 and based on 1968 Recommended Dietary Allowances (RDAs). DRVs will be listed for carbohydrates, proteins, total fat, saturated fat, fiber, cholesterol, sodium, and potassium. DRVs for energy sources (fats, carbohydrates, protein) will be based on percentages of 2000 kcal and DRVs for other food components will represent the uppermost limit that is considered desirable.

The following is a comparison of the information that has appeared on the old labels with the information that will appear on the new labels.

From the moment these new labels appear, consumers will begin asking dietitians and other health care professionals to interpret the new format and terms and the additional information provided. These new labels will be an important educational tool to assist in educating consumers. All health professionals, especially dietitians, must familiarize themselves with the new label content and meanings of the new terms and values.

REFERENCES

Boucher, N: Buyer beware. *Self* September: 148, 1992.

Cassel, JA: A nutrition label the public can understand—and count on. *Top Clin Nutr* 8(21):51, 1993.

Legislative Highlights: Final food labeling regulations. *JADA* 93(2):146, 1993. ◆

Nutrition Facts

Serving Size: 1/2 cup (114 g)
Servings Per Container: 4

Amount per Serving

kcalories 260
kcalories from Fat 120

	% Daily Value*
Total Fat 13 g	20%
Saturated Fat 5 g	25%
Cholesterol 30 mg	10%
Sodium 660 mg	28%
Total Carbohydrate 31 g	11%
Sugars 5 g	
Dietary Fiber 0 g	0%
Protein 5 g	

Vitamin A 4% • Vitamin C 1% • Calcium 15% • Iron 4%

*Percents (%) of a Daily Value are based on a 2,000 kcalorie diet. Your Daily Values may vary higher or lower depending on your kcalorie needs:

Nutrient	2,000 kcalories	2,500 kcalories
Total Fat	< 65 g	80 g
Saturated Fat	< 20 g	25 g
Cholesterol	< 300 mg	300 mg
Sodium	< 2,400 mg	2,400 mg
Total Carbohydrate	300 g	375 g
Fiber	25 g	30 g

1 g Fat = 9 kcalories
1 g Carbohydrate = 4 kcalories
1 g Protein = 4 kcalories

FIG. 9-3

What's old?	What's new?	What's old?	What's new?
Label information	**Label information**	**Terms with legal definitions**	**Terms with legal definitions**
Serving size (set by manufacturer)	Serving size (set by federal government)	Low kcalorie	Kcalorie free
		Reduced kcalorie	Sugar free
Servings per container	Servings per container	Diet	Sodium free (salt free)
Kcalories (total per serving)	Kcalories (total per serving)	Low sodium	Low sodium
	Kcalories from fat (total per serving)	Sodium free	Very low sodium
Protein, carbohydrate, fat (g per serving)	Protein, carbohydrate, fat (g per serving)	Very low sodium	Low kcalorie
	Saturated fat (g per serving)	Reduced sodium	Source of
	Cholesterol (mg per serving)		Reduced
	Complex carbohydrates (g per serving)		Light
	Sugars (g per serving)		Less
	Dietary fiber (g per serving)		More
			Fat free
			Low fat
Sodium (mg per serving)	Sodium (mg per serving)		Reduced fat
Percentage of USRDA for: protein, vitamin A, vitamin C, thiamin, riboflavin, niacin, calcium, and iron	Vitamin A (μg per serving)		Low in saturated fat
	Vitamin C (mg per serving)		Reduced saturated fat
	Calcium (mg per serving)		Cholesterol free
	Iron (mg per serving)		Low in cholesterol
	Percentage of daily recommended amount for:		Reduced cholesterol
	Total fat, saturated fat, unsaturated fat, cholesterol, total carbohydrates, complex carbohydrates, sugars, dietary fiber, sodium, potassium, vitamin A, vitamin C, calcium, and iron		Fresh
			Freshly

Government Food Safety Control Agencies

General Agency Controls

Several government agencies help control the safety and quality of our food supply. Concerned sections of the U.S. Department of Health and Human Services are the FDA and the Public Health Service (PHS). The USDA controls pesticide use in farming; related work is assigned to the Agricultural Research Service and the Consumer Marketing Service. The Federal Trade Commission and the National Bureau of Standards also protect the consumer. Of these various agencies, however, the one specifically controlling food safety is the FDA.

Food and Drug Administration (FDA)

The FDA is a law enforcement agency charged by Congress to ensure, among other things, that our food supply is safe, pure, and wholesome. The agency's current commissioner, who is both a physician and a lawyer, is speeding up the backlog of assessment work and strengthening the agency's credibility with tough enforcement.[21] The agency enforces federal food safety regulations through various activities including (1) food sanitation and quality control, (2) control of chemical contaminants and pesticides, (3) control of food additives, (4) regulation of movement of food

---

FDA Guidelines for Nutrition Labeling Regulations

TO PROBE FURTHER

The passage into law of the Nutrition Labeling and Education Act of 1990 gave evidence of the growing awareness and concern of the American people about food, nutrition, and health. The NLEA empowers the federal Food and Drug Administration to develop and enforce nutrition labeling regulations for the food industry and the public that help consumers make wise food choices.

The FDA label guidelines cover five main areas: nutrients and energy, serving sizes, definitions for terms used, label format, and health claims.

Nutrients and kcalories

The new label law requires a food product to provide nutrient and energy information for

- Protein (in terms of amino acid quality)
- Energy (as kcalories)
- Fat-soluble vitamins A, D, E, and K
- Water-soluble vitamins C, thiamin, riboflavin, niacin, pyridoxine (B_6), folate, and cobalamin (B_{12})
- Calcium, phosphorus, magnesium, iron, zinc, iodine, and selenium

On the label, the new standard reference term for nutrient-energy values is Reference Daily Intake (RDI). The RDIs are derived from the current 1989 RDAs and are population-based averages for all the age and sex groups of the current RDAs (excluding pregnant and lactating women, for whom the stated current RDAs apply). A second new reference term is Daily Reference Value (DRV), which designates the contribution a given product makes to meeting the nutrient RDIs. Thus the DRV of a given nutrient in a food product is the nutrient's content in that product expressed as a percentage of the RDI for that nutrient.

Serving sizes

A standardized reference serving size is set for 131 food categories in quantities customarily eaten. These portions are expressed in common household measures. The USDA has standardized serving sizes for 23 meat and 22 poultry product categories.

Descriptors

To improve communication between producers and consumers, everyone must work from the same FDA supplied dictionary. In this FDA dictionary, nine core terms that were previous points of confusion and concern are now precisely defined. These terms are free, low, light or lite, less, high, source of, more, fresh, and reduced. The development schedule calls for the appearance of these new labels in the marketplace by November 8, 1993.

Nutrition label format

The standardized nutrient labeling format provided by the FDA is mandatory for all food products and marketing agents. This format results from consumer research to develop sound nutrition information the consumer wants and readily understands. It serves as an important means of nutrition education. The FDA has also established voluntary labeling guidelines for fresh fruits, vegetables, and fish.

Health claims

The FDA guidelines indicate that any label health claim must be supported by substantial scientific evidence. Thus far, only four of the initial proposals meet this test and can be used: (1) sodium and hypertension, (2) calcium and osteoporosis, (3) lipids and cancer, and (4) lipids and cardiovascular disease. The FDA did not find, as yet, sufficient evidence to support claims concerning fiber and either cancer or cardiovascular disease.

REFERENCES

FDA staff: The new food label: your guide to better nutrition, *Nutr Today* 25(1):37, 1992.

Legislative News: Terms on food labels: ADA comments on proposals from FDA and USDA, *J Am Diet Assoc* 92(3):543, 1992.

Lewis CJ, Yetley EA: Focus group sessions on formats of nutrition labels, *J Am Diet Assoc* 92(1):62, 1992.

Liu J-Z, Guthrie HA: Nutrition labeling—a tool for nutrition education, *Nutr Today* 25(2):16, 1992.

across state lines, (5) nutrition and nutrition labeling of foods, (6) safety of public food service, and (7) safety of meat and milk. The most common means of enforcement is use of recalls and seizures of contaminated food.

The FDA's division of consumer education conducts an active program of protection through consumer education and general public information. Special attention is given to nutrition misinformation. Materials are prepared and distributed to individuals, students, and community groups. Consumer specialists work through all FDA district offices.

Foodborne Disease

Costs

Another large factor affecting food safety and food choice is foodborne disease. Many disease-bearing organisms inhabit our environment and can contaminate our food and water. Lapses in their control still occur, resulting in high incidences of illness, death, and economic costs. For example, U.S. estimates of foodborne disease are approximately 12.6 million cases each year costing $8.4 billion.[24,25] Microbiologic diseases, bacterial and viral, represent 84% of these U.S. costs, compared with 88% in Canada. The most economically significant U.S. diseases are salmonellosis and staphylococcal poisoning, costing annually $4 billion and $1.5 billion, respectively. Other costly types include listeriosis, trichinosis, *Clostridium perfringens* enteritis, and botulism. Botulism's high annual cost per case is $322,200, but the total impact is only $87 million because relatively few cases (270) occur.

Food Sanitation

Strict sanitation measures and rigid personal hygiene are essential. Throughout all preparation, the food and everything that touches it must be scrupulously clean. Cooking procedures and temperatures must be followed, all serving equipment must be kept clean, leftover food must be stored and reused appropriately or discarded, and garbage must be contained and disposed of in a sanitary manner. We know all these measures, but some persons do not always practice them. These rules are especially important for food handlers working in any phase of public food service operations, food processing and packaging plants, public markets, or delicatessen shops or counters. Also, persons with any infectious disease or hand injury, however small, should not work with food, but they sometimes do.

Bacterial Food Infections

Bacterial food infections result from eating food contaminated by large colonies of bacteria. Specific bacteria cause specific diseases. Three examples are salmonellosis, shigellosis, and listeriosis.

Salmonellosis. Salmonellosis is caused by the bacterium *Salmonella*, which is named for the American veterinarian-pathologist Daniel Salmon (1850-1914), who first isolated and identified species commonly causing human foodborne infections, *S. typhi* and *S. paratyphi*. These organisms grow readily in common foods such as milk, custards, egg dishes, salad dressings, and sandwich fillings. Seafood, especially shellfish such as oysters and clams, from polluted waters may also be a source of infection. A large number of recently reported U.S. cases have been traced to shell eggs.[26] Salmonellosis continues to be one of the main causes of foodborne disease worldwide.[27] Unsanitary handling of foods and utensils can spread the bacteria. Resulting cases of gastroenteritis may vary in intensity from mild diarrhea to severe attacks. Practices of immunization, pasteurization, and sanitary regulations involving community water and food supplies as well as food handlers help to control such outbreaks. Incubation and multiplication of the bacteria take time after the food is eaten, so symptoms of food infection develop slowly, usually 12 to 24 hours after ingestion.

Shigellosis. Shigellosis is caused by the bacterium *Shigella*, named for the Japanese physician Kiyoshi Shiga (1870-1957), who first discovered a main species of the organism—*S. dysenteriae*—during a **dysentery** epidemic in Japan in 1898. Shigellosis is usually confined to the large intestine and may vary from a mild transient disturbance in adults to fatal dysentery in young children. The bacteria grow easily in foods, especially in milk, a common carrier to infants and children. Reported outbreaks have been traced to uncooked tofu salad and to shredded lettuce and cabbage packaged for restaurants and the retail market.[28,29] The boiling of water or the pasteurization of milk kills the organisms, but the food or milk can easily be reinfected by unsanitary handling by a carrier. The disease is spread in much the same way as salmonellosis is transmitted, by unsanitary handling of food.

Listeriosis. Listeriosis is caused by the bacterium *Listeria*, named for the English surgeon Baron Joseph Lister (1827-1912) who first applied knowledge of bacterial infection to principles of antiseptic surgery in a benchmark 1867 publication, which led to "clean" op-

dysentery • A general term given to a number of disorders marked by inflammation of the intestines, especially of the colon, and attended by abdominal pain and frequent stools containing blood and mucus. The causative agent may be chemical irritants, bacteria, protozoa, or parasites.

erations and the development of modern surgery. Only within the past 10 years, however, has knowledge of the role of *Listeria* in directly causing foodborne disease in humans, both occasional illness and disease epidemics, increased and the major species causing human illness—*L. monocytogenes*—been identified.[30] Before 1981 *Listeria* was thought to be only an animal disease organism transmitted to humans only by direct contact with infected animals. Now we know that these organisms occur widely in the environment. In high-risk individuals such as elderly persons, pregnant women, infants, or persons with suppressed immune systems, the organisms can produce rare but often fatal illness, with severe symptoms such as diarrhea, flulike fever and headache, pneumonia, **sepsis, meningitis,** and **endocarditis.** Foodborne disease has been traced to a variety of foods including raw milk, raw eggs, seafood, chicken, turkey, meat, and meat products.[31,32]

Bacterial Food Poisonings

Food poisoning is caused by the ingestion of bacterial toxins that have been produced in foods by the growth of specific kinds of bacteria before the food is eaten. The powerful toxin is ingested directly and symptoms therefore develop rapidly, usually within 1 to 6 hours after the food is eaten. Two types of bacterial food poisoning are most commonly responsible, staphylococcal and clostridial.

Staphylococcal food poisoning. Named for the main causative organism, *Staphylococcus aureus,* staphylococcal food poisoning is by far the most common form of bacterial poisoning observed in the United States. Powerful preformed toxins contaminate the food, producing rapid illness within 1 to 6 hours after ingestion.[33] Symptoms come on suddenly—severe cramping and abdominal pain with vomiting and diarrhea, usually accompanied by sweating, headache, and fever. In some cases there may be shock and prostration. Recovery is fairly rapid, however, depending on the amount of toxin ingested. The source of contamination is usually an infection on the hand of a worker preparing the food, often minor or unnoticed. Foods that are particularly effective culture beds include custard- and cream-filled bakery goods, chicken and ham salads, processed meats, cheese, sauces, and combination dishes. The toxin makes no change in the normal odor, taste, or appearance of the food, so the person eating it is not warned.

Clostridial food poisoning. Named for the bacterium *Clostridium,* mainly *C. perfringens* and *C. botulinum,* clostridial food poisoning is caused by powerful toxins in contaminated foods. The *C. perfringens* spores are in soil, water, dust, refuse, virtually everywhere. The organism multiplies in cooked meat and meat dishes and develops its toxin in foods held for extended periods at warming or room temperatures. Thus, many reported outbreaks occur from food eaten in school cafeterias, college dining rooms, and restaurants. In each case, cooked meat was improperly handled in preparation and refrigeration. Control rests mainly on careful preparation and adequate cooking of meats, prompt service, and immediate refrigeration at sufficiently low temperatures. *C. botulinum* causes far more serious, often fatal food poisoning from eating food containing its powerful toxin. Depending on the dose of toxin taken and the individual response, the illness may vary from mild discomfort to death within 24 hours. Mortality rates are high. Vomiting, weakness, and dizziness are initial complaints. Progressively, the toxin irritates motor nerve cells and blocks transmission of neural impulses at the nerve terminals, causing gradual paralysis. Sudden respiratory paralysis with airway obstruction is the major cause of death, especially in infants and young children.[34]

C. botulinum spores are widespread in soil throughout the world and may be carried on harvested food to the canning process. Like all clostridia, this species is anaerobic (develops in the absence of air) or nearly so. The relatively air-free can and the canning temperatures (above 27° C [80° F]) provide good conditions for toxin production. The development of high standards in the commercial canning industry has eliminated this source of botulism, but cases still result each year, mainly from eating carelessly home-canned foods. Boiling for 10 minutes destroys the toxin (not the spore), so all home-canned food, no matter how well preserved, should be boiled at least 10 minutes before eating. In the United States, Alaska and Washington have the highest incidence. Alaska has the greater number of botulism cases due to native habits of eating uncooked or partially cooked meat that has been fermented, dried, or frozen.[35]

Table 9-2 summarizes these bacterial sources of food contamination.

Viruses

Illnesses caused by viral contamination are few compared to those caused by bacterial contamination. These include upper respiratory tract infections, such as colds and influenza, and infections from hepatitis A virus.[36] Explosive epidemics of infectious hepatitis have occurred in schools, towns, and other communities after fecal contamination of water, milk, or food. Contaminated shellfish from polluted waters have caused several outbreaks. Again, stringent control of community water and food supplies, as well as personal hygiene and sanitary practices of food handlers, are essential for prevention of disease.

TABLE 9-2

Selected Examples of Bacterial Foodborne Disease

Foodborne disease	Causative organisms (genus and species)	Food source	Symptoms and course
Bacterial food infections			
Salmonellosis	Salmonella S. typhi S. paratyphi	Milk, custards, egg dishes, salad dressings, sandwich fillings, polluted shellfish	Mild to severe diarrhea, cramps, vomiting; appears 12-24 hours or more after eating; lasts 1-7 days
Shigellosis	Shigella S. dysenteriae	Milk and milk products, seafood, salads	Mild diarrhea to fatal dysentery (especially in young children); appears 7-36 hours after eating; lasts 3-14 days
Listeriosis	Listeria L. monocytogenes	Soft cheese, poultry, seafood, raw milk, meat products (paté)	Severe diarrhea, fever, headache, pneumonia, meningitis, endocarditis; symptoms begin after 3-21 days
Bacterial food poisoning			
(Enterotoxins)			
Staphylococcal	Staphylococcus S. aureus	Custards, cream fillings, processed meats, ham, cheese, ice cream, potato salad, sauces, casseroles	Severe abdominal pain, cramps, vomiting, diarrhea, perspiration, headache, fever, prostration; appears suddenly 1-6 hours after eating; symptoms subside generally within 24 hours

Clostridial
  Perfringens enteritis
  Botulism
	Clostridium
	C. perfringens
	C. botulinum
		Cooked meats, meat dishes held at warm or room temperature
		Improperly home-canned foods; smoked and salted fish, ham, sausage, shellfish
			Mild diarrhea, vomiting; appears 8-24 hours after eating; lasts a day or less
			Symptoms range from mild discomfort to death within 24 hours; initial nausea, vomiting, weakness, dizziness, progressing to motor and sometimes fatal breathing paralysis

Changes in Personal Food Habits

Basic Determinants of Food Choice

We have discussed the broad areas of environment, culture and psychosocial development, as well as modern food safety concerns, in terms of their influence on food habits. Clearly, some of the basic determinants of food choice focus on a variety of interacting physical, social, and physiologic factors, as summarized in Table 9-3. It is difficult at best to change some of our own eating patterns for health needs or personal desires. It is even more difficult to help our health care clients modify some of their habits, although we understand their cultural patterns. Nonetheless, we need to maintain a sensitive, flexible appreciation of just how complex are the factors that influence choices persons make when they eat what they do.

Immigration and Ethnic Diversity

The story of immigration to the United States and our growing ethnic diversity is hardly a new one. It is indeed one of our fundamental themes. We have discussed the importance of these ethnic, cultural, and religious identities. In the United States we have many cultures and subcultures that have remained distinct or have become assimilated in varying degrees. Every group has contributed parts of its food habits to the general culture. In turn American food patterns have infused their own, so that lines of difference are less distinct.

Americans of a score of different ethnic backgrounds have enriched our overall cultural patterns. We find varied and intermingling foods and food patterns blending with those of our own particular background (see Issues and Answers, p. 189). However, sometimes

endocarditis • Inflammation of the endocardium, the serous membrane that lines the cavities of the heart.

meningitis • Inflammation of the *meninges,* the three membranes that envelop the brain and spinal cord, caused by a bacterial or viral infection and characterized by high fever, severe headache, and stiff neck or back muscles.

sepsis • Presence in the blood or other tissues of pathogenic microorganisms or their toxins; conditions associated with such pathogens.

TABLE 9-3		
Factors Determining Food Choices		
Physical factors	**Social factors**	**Physiologic factors**
Food supply available	Advertising	Allergy
Food technology	Culture	Disability
Geography, agriculture, distribution	Education, nutrition, and general	Health-disease status
Personal economics, income	Political and economic policies	Personal food acceptance
Sanitation, housing	Religion and social customs	Needs, energy or nutrients
Season, climate	Social class role	Therapeutic diets
Storage and cooking facilities	Social problems, poverty, or alcoholism	

this happy intermingling of different cuisines has a cost. It does not always occur without difficulty and cultural dislocation. Ethnic groups within the United States encounter a new world. Their life-styles often undergo dramatic alterations, and the cultural integrity of the group can be severely shaken. Every group adapts in a unique way specific to its original culture and to the historic circumstances in which it undergoes the change.

Changing American Food Patterns

Some traditional American food patterns are also changing. The stereotype of the all-American family with parents and two children eating three meals a day with a ban on snacking is no longer the common pattern. In the past two decades we have experienced far-reaching changes in our way of living and subsequently in our food patterns.

Households

The number of households is gradually increasing, and the alternate pattern of nontraditional households that are not families—that is, groups of unrelated persons or persons living alone—continues. By the year 2000 the average household size is expected to decline from 2.69 to 2.48, with husband-wife households decreasing from 58% to 53% of all households.[37,38] The number of children under age 5 will decline through this decade. The number of adults over age 65 will increase, and the greatest increase will be among those "oldest old" persons over age 85, who will have increased by 30%. The racial and ethnic population pattern will also have changed by the year 2000. Whites, not including Hispanics, will decline from 76% to 72% of the American population. Hispanics, the fastest growing population group, will increase from 8% to 11%. Blacks will increase from 12.4% to 13%. Other racial groups including Native Americans, Alaskan natives, Asians, and Pacific Islanders will increase from 3.5% to 4%.[38,39] These continuing trends indicate significant changes in the American social picture, part of a dynamic and rapidly changing society.

Working Women

The number of women in the work force continues to increase rapidly, a trend that is not likely to reverse. By the year 2000, women of all racial and ethnic groups will be the major source of new entrants into the labor market, comprising 47% of the total work force, compared to 45% in 1988.[38,40] Between 1988 and 2000 white men will comprise only 25% of the net growth of the labor force. There is a correlation between the education of women and their presence in the labor force; about 51% of college undergraduates are women. In general, women account for 30% of the enrollment in law schools, 25% in medical schools, 30% in business schools, and 12% in technical graduate schools. This phenomenon of working women is not restricted to one social, economic, or ethnic group. It is a widespread societal change, bringing with it changes in the functioning of the family. Working mothers rely on food items and cooking methods that save time, space, and labor.

Family Meals

Family meals are less common. Many persons rarely eat breakfast and lunch in the family setting, but family dinners occur about 75% of the time. Often both parents or the single parent works, and many late afternoon sports or other activities for children curtail the time available for meal preparation and having the whole family sit down to eat at the same time.

Health Consciousness

The interest of Americans in physical fitness continues. This has taken primarily two forms. First, there is more general nutrition awareness. Consumers have an increased interest in the nutrition content of their food, an expressed concern about a wholesome and safe food supply, and a strong support of the new nutrition labeling regulations. Interest in health claims on food products has increased, but there is some uncertainty about how to evaluate them. Second, there is more attention to weight watching, though not always through a healthy approach that includes regular meals with less fat combined with moderate regular physical exercise. More than half of the American population at any given time is on a weight-reducing diet. Consumers are interested in "light" foods perceived to be lower in kcalories.

Economy

More and more Americans are economizing on food. Many supermarket shoppers are changing their diets primarily to save money. Consumers are stocking up on bargains and cutting back on expensive convenience foods. They are buying items in larger packages and in bulk and doing much less store hopping for bargains, staying with the store they consider to have the lowest overall prices. Brand loyalty has declined, and the purchase of generic products has increased. Consumers look more carefully at labels to gain information about comparative products.

Gourmet Cooking

The use of gourmet foods and specialty ethnic dishes has risen, and food specialty shops have sprung up in every shopping center. Gourmet cooking has become a popular hobby, and entertaining guests at home over a gourmet meal often displays the chef's (male or female) skills in the elegance and quality of the food. This phenomenon parallels the general trend toward meals that are easy to fix, take little time, and fulfill the consumers' nutrition needs. Supermarkets are establishing special gourmet deli shops and specialty fast foods, take-out picnic baskets, and other creative items.

Fast Foods

Today approximately one third of all food that Americans eat is eaten away from home, much of it from fast food restaurants. About 46 million people eat at a fast-food restaurant each day, about one out of every 12 meals.[41] Several factors have contributed to this phenomenal increase in the use of fast food, including a greater number of working women, dual-career families, more diverse schedules of family members, an aging population, and an increasing number of one- and two-person households. Fast foods meet the needs of many people because they are quick, reasonably priced, and readily available. Also, currently these restaurants are responding to the health concerns of their customers by changing some of their practices, such as the continued trend toward the use of vegetable oils instead of animal fats for frying, an increase in the number of low-fat menu items, and more fruits and vegetables available at salad bars.[42] Food industry analysts even predict a future of increasing home delivery services, high-quality vending machine foods, and ready-to-eat packages for microwave-equipped homes and cars.[43]

To Sum Up

We all grow up and live our lives in a social context. We each inherit at least one cultural background and live in our particular society's social structure, complete with food habits and attitudes about eating. It is from a social perspective that we can best examine changes in food habits. We need to understand the effects on health that are associated with major social and economic shifts. We also need to understand current social forces to best help persons make new dietary changes that will benefit their health. We must meet concerns about food misinformation and food safety.

The United States has a long history of immigration. Every new group has adjusted to life in the new country in its own way. They have contributed a unique ethnic diversity to American life and food patterns.

Traditional American food patterns are changing in a number of ways. We increasingly rely on food technology in our fast, complex life. More women are working, households are getting smaller, more and more persons are living alone, and our meal patterns are different. We search for less fancy, lower cost food items, and also creative gourmet cooking. In general we are more nutrition and health conscious. Fast food outlets have increased and become a large factor in our changing food patterns.

QUESTIONS FOR REVIEW

1. Describe some ways in which environmental factors interact to produce malnutrition and give examples.
2. What is the meaning of culture? How does it affect our food patterns?
3. What are some social and psychologic factors that influence our food habits? Give examples of personal meanings related to food.
4. Why does the public tend to accept nutrition misinformation so easily? What groups are more susceptible? Select one such group and give some effective approaches you might use in reaching them with sound nutrition information.
5. How do food misinformation and concerns about food safety affect food habits?
6. What is the basis of concern about food additives and pesticide residues?
7. In what ways does ethnic diversity enrich American food patterns? Give several examples.
8. Name several trends in America's changing food patterns and discuss their implications for nutrition and health.

REFERENCES

1. Bloom BR: A new threat to world health, *Science* 239:9, Jan 1, 1988.
2. Jelliffe DB, Jelliffe EFP: Causation of kwashiorkor: toward a multi-factorial consensus, *Pediatrics* 90:110, 1992.

3. Umoh EJ: Malnutrition in Nigerian children, *J Am Diet Assoc* 91(6):655, 1991.

4. Wolgemuth JC and others: Wasting malnutrition and inadequate nutrient intakes identified in a multiethnic homeless population, *J Am Diet Assoc* 92(7):834, 1992.

5. Kerstetter JE and others: Malnutrition in the institutionalized older adult, *J Am Diet Assoc* 92(9):1109, 1992.

6. Cross AT: Politics, poverty, and nutrition, *J Am Diet Assoc* 87(8):1007, 1987.

7. Yankauer A: What infant mortality tells us, *Am J Pub Health* 80(6):653, 1990.

8. Splett PL, Story M: Child nutrition: objectives for the decade, *J Am Diet Assoc* 91(6):665, 1991.

9. Fuchs VR, Reklis DM: America's children: economic perspectives and policy options, *Science* 255(5040):41, Jan 3, 1992.

10. Maslow AH: *Motivation and personality*, New York, 1954, Harper & Row.

11. Harper AE: Nutrition: from myth to magic to science, *Nutr Today* 23(1):8, 1988.

12. Report: Use of vitamin and mineral supplements in the United States, *Nutr Rev* 48(3):161, 1990.

13. White-O'Connor B and others: Dietary habits, weight history, and vitamin supplement use in elderly osteoarthritis patients, *J Am Diet Assoc* 89(3):378, 1989.

14. Toufexis A: The new scoop on vitamins, *Time* 139(14):54, 1992.

15. Walker T: Better assay for pesticides tainting food, *Sci News* 139(19):293, 1991.

16. Regonold JP and others: Sustainable agriculture, *Sci Am* 262(6):293, 1991.

17. Council on Scientific Affairs, American Medical Association: Biotechnology and the American agriculture industry, *JAMA* 265(11):1429, 1991.

18. Waslien CI, Rehwoldt RE: Micronutrients and antioxidants in processed foods—analysis of data from the 1987 Food Additives Survey, *Nutr Today* 25(4):36, 1990.

19. Weisburger EK: Current carcinogen perspectives: de minimis, Delany, and decisions, *Sci Total Environ* 86:5, 1989.

20. Burdock GA and others: GRAS substances, *Food Tech* 44:78, 1990.

21. Gibbon A: Can David Kessler revieve the FDA? *Science* 252:200, 1991.

22. Iglehart JK: Health policy report: the Food and Drug Administration and its problems, *N Engl J Med* 325(3):217, 1991.

23. Report: Update—the Nutrition Labeling and Education Act of 1990, *J Am Diet Assoc* 91(9):1054, 1991.

24. Todd E: Preliminary estimates of costs of foodborne disease in the United States, *J Food Protect* 52:595, 1989.

25. Todd E: Epidemiology of the foodborne illness: North America, *Lancet* 336:788, 1990.

26. Centers for Disease Control: Salmonellosis outbreaks, *MMWR*, Dec 21, 1990.

27. Baird-Parker AC: Foodborne salmonellosis, *Lancet* 336:1231, 1990.

28. Lee LA and others: An outbreak of shigellosis at an outdoor music festival, *Am J Epidemiol* 133(6):608, 1991.

29. Satchell FB and others: The survival of *Shigella sonnei* in shredded cabbage, *J Food Protect* 53(7):228, 1990.

30. Donnelly CW: *Listeria*—an emerging foodborne pathogen, *Nutr Today* 25(5):7, 1990.

31. Genigeorgis CA and others: Prevalence of *Listeria* spp. in turkey meat at the supermarket and slaughterhouse level, *J Food Protect* 53(4):282, 1990.

32. Johnson JL and others: *Listeria monocytogenes* and other *Listeria* spp. in meat and meat products: a review, *J Food Protect* 53(1):81, 1990.

33. Tranter HS: Foodborne staphylococcal illness, *Lancet* 336:1044, 1990.

34. Schreiner MJ and others: Infant botulism: a review of 12 years' experience at the Children's Hospital of Philadelphia, *Pediatrics* 87(2):159, 1991.

35. Lancaster MJ: Botulism: north to Alaska, *Am J Nurs* 90(1):60, 1990.

36. Appleton H: Foodborne viruses, *Lancet* 336:1362, 1990.

37. Bureau of the Census: *Projections of households and families: 1886 to 2000*, Washington, DC, 1986, US Department of Commerce.

38. US Department of Health and Human Services, Public Health Service: *Healthy people 2000: national health promotion and disease prevention objectives*, Pub No 91-50212, Washington, DC, 1990, US Government Printing Office.

39. Spencer G: Projections of the population of the United States by age, sex, and race: 1985 to 2080, *Current Population Reports, Population Estimates and Projections*, Series P-25, No 1018, Washington, DC, 1989, US Department of Commerce, Bureau of the Census.

40. Kutscher RE: Projection 2000: overview and implications of the projections to 2000, *Monthly Labor Review*, Sept, 1987.

41. Price K and others: Fast foods: the current state of affairs, *Dietetic Curr* 18(4):1, 1991.

42. Shields JE, Young E: Fat in fast foods—evolving changes, *Nutr Today* 25(2):32, 1990.

43. Stanton JL: 2001: a food odyssey, *Food Nutr News* 65:29, 1990.

FURTHER READING

Aspenland S, Pelican S: Traditional food practices of contemporary Taos Pueblo, *Nutr Today* 27(2):6, 1992.
Grivetti LE: Clash of cuisines, *Nutr Today* 27(2):13, 1992.
Todhunter EN: Seven centuries of cookbooks—treasures and pleasures, *Nutr Today* 27(1):6, 1992.

Three interesting articles provide background for the early development of cultural food patterns in America: (1) preservation of a Native American food heritage, (2) the journal of Columbus and its record of native food patterns in the New World, and (3) a rich historical view of developing American food patterns in cookbooks of successive generations.

FDA staff: The new food label: your guide to better nutrition, *Nutr Today* 27(1):37, 1992.

This article provides details of the new food labeling regulations developed by the FDA.

Clydesdale FM: Meeting the needs of the elderly with foods of today and tomorrow, *Nutr Today* 26(5):13, 1991.
Hall RL: Food safety and biotechnology, *Nutr Today* 26(3):15, 1991.

Two food scientists provide helpful background concerning food safety and the trends in present and future foods.

CASE STUDY

Faddism and Economic Problems: A Young Family Trying to Cope

Helen Brown, age 20, and her husband Charles, age 21, live in a small flat in the low-rent district of the city with their three children—a boy of 3, a girl of 18 months, and their new baby of 6 weeks. Helen has gained more weight, so that she now weighs 93 kg (205 lb). Already she feels old and unattractive. She has always been rather dependent on her mother and lately on her husband. But now she seems less and less able to cope.

Charles works in a gas station during the day and sometimes gets extra mechanic work at night, but still he barely makes enough to meet expenses. Many bills are unpaid. The friction between Charles and Helen has increased, and Charles is frequently absenting himself from home.

Recently, about the time that Helen came home from the county hospital with the new baby, Helen's mother, Mrs. Miller, age 50, came to live with the Brown family. She had been living alone, but now because her arthritis was worse and had begun to cripple her more, she could no longer work or care for herself. There seemed no other place for her to go but to her daughter's home.

A district public health nurse in the county, Miss Jordan, was visiting Helen and her new baby for a 6-week checkup. When Miss Jordan arrived at the apartment, she found Helen distraught and in tears. Charles, she said, had gone off to work that morning, angrily saying that he might not return until she grew up and learned how to manage things better. Helen was wearing an old housecoat and her hair was uncombed. She had a formula bottle in her hand, seemingly not knowing quite what to do with it. The apartment was crowded and cluttered, dishes filled the small kitchen sink, and every available space seemed taken up with used utensils. The two older children were thin and fretful, hitting at each other over a toy both wanted and pulling at their mother's housecoat for her attention.

Although it was midmorning, the children had had no breakfast. The baby was crying in the crib in the corner of the room waiting for the bottle Helen was trying to fix. Helen's mother was lying on the sofa with her crutches nearby.

Miss Jordan offered to feed the baby, for which Helen seemed grateful. After the feeding Miss Jordan weighed the baby and found that she was not gaining weight as she should. Helen said that none of the formula seemed to agree with the baby and she was constantly spitting it up.

At this point someone knocked on the door. It was Mrs. Bryant who lived in the flat above. She was older than Helen, about 45, a loud and dominant-appearing woman. She was bringing a bottle of some food supplement to Helen. While Helen searched for $10, Mrs. Bryant enthusiastically told Miss Jordan about her special health food products.

"This is a special high-protein food supplement. It isn't sold through stores but only through special agents like me who know its real worth. You know, all this processed food you buy in markets is worthless. There's no food value left in it. It's no wonder everybody's half sick. It's all caused by bad diet. But this supplement will make the difference. It's a natural food substance, organically grown. It's the very thing Helen needs to get her strength back and help her lose weight. As for the children," she continued, "it's just what they need, too, to put some meat on their bones."

Then Mrs. Bryant turned to Helen's mother and patted her arm. "You poor dear. As soon as you start using this, too, a double dose daily for awhile, your arthritis will be cured."

As she was leaving, Mrs. Bryant said to Miss Jordan, "You look a little peaked yourself. You could use some, too. Here, let me leave this leaflet with you that tells all about it."

After Mrs. Bryant left, Helen explained that Charles' anger that morning resulted from her buying the expensive special food supplement when their family budget was so tight.

After talking briefly with Helen and her mother, Miss Jordan made definite arrangements to return the following week. As she drove away from the apartment building, she was thinking about her observations and the problems she had encountered in the Brown family. Already she had decided that when she returned to the district public health office, she would consult with the nutritionist and leave the supplement pamphlet with her to investigate. She also decided to speak with the psychiatric nursing consultant and a social worker in the social services department.

Questions to Guide Your Inquiry

1. Imagine you are the nutritionist or the nurse. What important questions come to your mind from your observations?

2. What problems do you identify? What are Helen's needs? What are her husband's needs?

3. What solutions do you propose? How would you involve other health department persons in your plan of action?

4. Consider each of the children. What growth and development needs—physical, psychosocial, as well as nutritional—does each child have? What food and feeding practices are related? (See age group needs in Chapter 12.)

5. What actions do you propose to meet each child's needs?

6. What are Mrs. Miller's needs? Do you think nutrition is related to arthritis? (See Chapter 26.)

7. Why is this family vulnerable to the "health food" sales pressures of the neighbor, Mrs. Bryant?

8. What food myths or misinformation did you find? What dangers are involved in such food fads or misinformation? Why does food faddism exist? What can health workers do about food fads?

9. What additional information would you need to work with this family toward some positive goals? What possible sources or means would you use to obtain this information?

The Spice of Ethnic Diversity in American Food Patterns

In the area of good food, the increasing ethnic diversity in the United States population is cause for celebration! Our taste buds celebrate the spice such ethnic diversity brings to American food patterns. Older American traditions from a variety of cultures mingle with more recent arrivals to provide a smorgasbord of ethnic experiences. Each reflects the culture in which it developed, based on both religious laws and regional influences.

Religious dietary laws

Jewish. Observance of Jewish food laws differs among the three basic groups within Judaism: (1) Orthodox, strict observance; (2) Conservative, less strict; and (3) Reform, less ceremonial emphasis and minimum general use. The basic body of dietary laws is called the *Rules of Kashruth.* Foods selected and prepared according to these rules are called *kosher,* from the Hebrew word meaning "fit, proper." Originally these laws had special ritual significance. Present Jewish dietary laws apply this significance to laws governing the slaughter, preparation, and serving of meat, to the combining of meat and milk, to fish, and to eggs. Various food restrictions exist.

1. *Meat.* No pork is used. Forequarters of other meats are allowed, as well as all commonly used forms of poultry. All forms of meat used are rigidly cleansed of all blood.
2. *Meat and milk.* No combining of meat and milk is allowed. Orthodox homes maintain two sets of dishes, one for serving meat and the other for meals using dairy products.
3. *Fish.* Only fish with fins and scales are allowed. These may be eaten with either meat or dairy meals. No shellfish or eels may be used.
4. *Eggs.* No egg with a blood spot may be eaten. Eggs may be used with either meat or dairy meals.

Many of the traditional Jewish foods relate to festivals of the Jewish calendar that commemorate significant events in Jewish history. Often special Sabbath foods are used. A few representative foods include:

- *Bagels:* Doughnut-shaped, hard yeast rolls
- *Blintzes:* Thin filled and rolled pancakes
- *Borscht (borsch):* Soup of meat stock, beaten egg or sour cream, beets, cabbage, or spinach. Served hot or cold.
- *Challah:* Sabbath loaf of white bread, shaped as a twist or coil, used at the beginning of the meal after the *kiddush,* the blessing over wine.
- *Gefullte (gefilte fish):* From a German word meaning "stuffed fish," usually the first course of Sabbath evening meal, made of fish fillet, chopped and seasoned and stuffed back into the skin or rolled into balls.
- *Kasha:* Buckwheat groats (hulled kernels), used as a cooked cereal or as a potato substitute with gravy.
- *Knishes:* Pastry filled with ground meat or cheese.
- *Lox:* Smoked, salted salmon.
- *Matzo:* Flat unleavened bread.
- *Strudel:* Thin pastry filled with fruit and nuts, rolled and baked.

Moslem. Moslem dietary laws are based on restrictions or prohibitions on some foods and promotion of others, derived from Islamic teachings in the Koran. The laws are binding and must be followed at all times, even during pregnancy, hospitalization, or travel. The general rule is that "all foods are permitted" unless specifically conditioned or prohibited.

1. *Milk products.* Permitted at all times.
2. *Fruits and vegetables.* Except if fermented or poisonous.
3. *Breads and cereals.* Unless contaminated or harmful.
4. *Meats.* Seafood including fish, shellfish, eels, and sea animals, and land animals except swine; pork is strictly prohibited.
5. *Alcohol.* Strictly prohibited.

Any food combinations are used as long as no prohibited items are included. Milk and meat may be eaten together, in contrast to Jewish kosher laws. The Koran mentions certain foods as being of special value: figs, olives, dates, honey, milk, and buttermilk. Prohibited foods in the Moslem dietary laws may be eaten when no other sources of food are available.

Among the Moslem people, a 30-day period of daylight fasting is required during Ramadan, the ninth month of the Islamic lunar calendar, thus rotating through all seasons. The fourth pillar of Islam commanded by the Koran is fasting. Ramadan was chosen for the sacred fast because it is the month in which Mohammed received the first of the revelations that were subsequently compiled to form the Koran and also the month in which his followers first drove their enemies from Mecca in AD 624. During the month of Ramadan, Moslems throughout the world observe daily fasting, taking no food or drink from dawn to sunset. Nights, however, are often spent in special feasts. First, an appetizer is taken, such as dates or a fruit drink, followed by the family's "evening breakfast," the *iftar.* At the end of Ramadan a traditional feast lasting up to 3 days climaxes the observance. Special dishes mark this occasion. There are delicacies such as thin pancakes dipped in powdered sugar, savory buns, and dried fruits.

Spanish (Hispanic) and Native American influences

Mexican. Food habits of early Spanish settlers and Indian nations form the basis of present food patterns of persons of Mexican (Hispanic) heritage who now live in the United States, chiefly in the Southwest. Three foods are basic to this pattern: dried beans, chili peppers, and corn. Variations and additions may be found in different places or among those of different income levels. Relatively small amounts of meat and occasional eggs are used. Fruit, such as oranges, apples, and bananas, or papayas and mangos are used, depending on availability. For centuries corn has been the basic grain used as bread in the form of torti-llas, flat cakes baked on a hot griddle. Some wheat is used in making tortillas; rice and oat are added cereals. Coffee is a main beverage. Major seasonings are chili peppers, on-ions, and garlic; the basic fat is lard.

Puerto Rican. The Puerto Rican people share a com-mon heritage with the Mexicans, so much of their food pattern is similar. They add tropical fruits and vegetables, many of which are available in their neighborhood mar-kets in the United States. A main type of food is *viandas*, starchy vegetables and fruits such as plantain and green bananas. Two other staples of the diet are rice and beans. Milk, meat, yellow and green vegetables, and other fruits are used in limited quantities, but dried codfish is a staple food. Coffee is a main beverage. Lard is the main cook-ing fat.

Native American. The Native American population, Indian and Alaskan Natives, is composed mainly of more than 500 federally recognized diverse groups living on res-ervations, in small rural communities, or in metropolitan areas. Despite their individual diversity, the various groups share a spiritual attachment to the land and a determina-tion to retain their culture. Food has great religious and social significance, and is an integral part not only of cel-ebrations and ceremonies but also of everyday hospitality, which includes a serious obligation for serving food. Foods may be prepared and used in different ways from region to region and vary according to what can be grown locally, harvested or hunted on the land or fished from its rivers, or is available in food markets. Among the Native Ameri-can groups of the southwest United States, the food pat-tern of the Navajo people, whose reservations extend over a 25,000 square mile area in the junction of three states—New Mexico, Arizona, and Utah—may serve as an ex-ample.

Historically, the Navajos learned farming from the early Pueblo people, establishing corn and other crops as staples. Later they learned herding from the Spaniards, making sheep and goats available for food and wool. Some families also raised chickens, pigs, and cattle. Currently, Navajo food habits combine traditional dietary staples with modern food products available from supermarkets and fast food restaurants. Meat is eaten daily—fresh mutton, beef, pork, chicken, or smoked or processed meat. Other staples include: bread—tortillas or fry bread, blue corn bread, and cornmeal mush; beverages—coffee, soft drinks and fruit-flavored sweet ades; eggs, vegetables—corn, po-tatoes, green beans, tomatoes; some fresh or canned fruit. Frying is a common method of food preparation; lard and shortening are main cooking fats. There is an increased use of modern snack foods high in fat, sugar, calories, and sodium, especially among children and teenagers.

Southern United States influences

African Americans. The black populations, especially in the southern states, have contributed a rich heritage of American food patterns, particularly to southern cooking as a whole. Like their moving original music of spirituals, blues, gospel and jazz, southern black food patterns were born of hard times, and developed through a creative abil-ity to turn any basic staples at hand into memorable food. Although regional differences occur, as with any basic food pattern, surveys indicate representative use of foods from basic food groups:

1. *Breads/cereals.* Traditional breads include hot breads such as biscuits, spoonbread (a soufflé-like dish of cornmeal mush with beaten eggs), cornmeal muf-fins, and skillet cornbread. Commonly used cereals are cooked cereals such as cornmeal mush, hominy grits (ground corn), and oatmeal. In general, more cooked cereal is used than ready-to-eat dry cereals.
2. *Eggs/dairy products.* Eggs are used and some cheese, but little milk, probably due to the greater preva-lence of lactose intolerance among blacks than among whites.
3. *Vegetables.* A frequent type of vegetable is leafy greens: turnip greens, collards, mustard greens, and spinach, usually cooked with bacon or salt pork. Cab-bage is used boiled or chopped raw with a salad dressing (cole slaw). Other vegetables used include okra (coated with cornmeal and fried), sweet pota-toes (baked whole or sliced and candied with added sugar), green beans, tomatoes, potatoes, corn, but-terbeans (lima), and dried beans such as black-eyed peas or red beans cooked with smoked ham hocks and served over rice. The black-eyed peas over rice is a dish called Hopping John, traditionally served on New Year's Day for good luck in the new year.
4. *Fruits.* Commonly used fruits include apples, peaches, berries, oranges, bananas, and juices.
5. *Meat.* Pork is a common meat, including fresh cuts and ribs, sausage, and smoked ham. Some beef is used, mainly ground for meat loaf or hamburgers. Poultry is used frequently, mainly fried chicken, and baked holiday turkey. Organ meats such as liver, heart, intestines (chitterlings), or poultry giblets (gizzard and heart) are used. When it is available, fish includes catfish, some flounder, and shellfish such as crab and shrimp. Frying is a common method of cooking; fats used are lard, shortening, or vegetable oils.
6. *Desserts.* Favorites include pecan, sweet potato, and pumpkin pie and deep-dish peach or berry cobblers; cakes such as coconut and chocolate; and bread pud-ding to use leftover bread.
7. *Beverages.* Coffee, apple cider, fruit juices, lemonade, iced tea, carbonated soft drinks, and buttermilk, a better-tolerated form of milk.

French Americans. The Cajun people of the southwestern costal waterways in southern Louisiana have contributed a unique cuisine and food pattern to America's rich and varied fare. It provides a model for learning about rapidly expanding forms of American ethnic food. The Cajuns are descendants of the early French colonists of Acadia, a peninsula on the eastern coast of Canada now known as Nova Scotia. In the prerevolutionary wars between France and Britain, both countries contended for the area of Acadia. However, after Britain finally gained control of all of Canada, fear of an Acadian revolt led to a forcible deportation of French colonists in 1755. After a long and difficult journey down the Atlantic coast, then westward along the Gulf of Mexico, a group of the impoverished Acadians finally settled along the bayou country of what is now Louisiana. To support themselves, they developed their unique food pattern from seafood at hand and what they could grow and harvest. Over time they blended their own French culinary background with the Creole cookery they found in their new homeland around New Orleans, which had descended from classical French cuisine combined with other European, American Indian, and African dishes. Thus the unique Cajun food pattern of the southern United States represents an ethnic blending of cultures using basic foods available in the area. Cajun foods are strong-flavored and spicy, with the abundant seafood as a base, usually cooked as stew and served over rice. The well-known hot chili sauce, made of crushed and fermented red chili peppers blended with spices and vinegar and sold worldwide under the trade name Tabasco sauce, is still made by generations of a Cajun family on Avery Island on the coastal waterway of southern Louisiana.

The most popular shellfish native to the region is the crawfish, now grown commercially in the fertile rice paddies of the bayou area. Other seafood used includes catfish, red snapper, shrimp, blue crab, and oysters. Cajun dishes usually start with a *roux* made from heated oil and flour mixed with liquid to form a sauce base, to which vegetables, then meat or seafood, and seasonings are added to form a stew. Vegetables used include onions, bell peppers, parsley, shallots, and tomatoes; seasonings are cayenne (red) pepper, hot pepper sauce (Tabasco), crushed black pepper, white pepper, bay leaves, thyme, and *filé* powder. *Filé* powder is made from ground sassafras leaves and serves both to season and to thicken the dish being made. Some typical Cajun dishes include seafood or chicken gumbo, jambalaya (dish of Creole origin, combining rice, chicken, ham, pork, sausage, broth, vegetables, and seasonings), red beans and rice, blackened catfish or red snapper (blackened with pepper and seasonings and seared in a hot pan), barbecued shrimp, breaded catfish with Creole sauce, and boiled crawfish. Breads and starches include French bread, hush puppies (fried cornbread-mixture balls), cornbread muffins, cush-cush (cornmeal mush cooked with milk), grits, rice, and yams. Vegetables include okra, squash, onions, bell peppers and tomatoes. Desserts include ambrosia (fresh fruits such as oranges and bananas with grated coconut), sweet potato pie, pecan pie, berry pie, bread pudding, or pecan pralines.

Eastern-Oriental food patterns

Chinese. Chinese cooks believe that refrigeration diminishes natural flavors. Therefore they select the freshest foods possible, hold them the shortest time possible, then cook them quickly at a high temperature in a *wok* with only small amounts of fat and liquid. This basic round-bottom pan allows control of heat in a quick stir-frying method that preserves natural flavor, color, and texture. Vegetables cooked just before serving are still crisp and flavorful when served. Meat is used in small amounts in combined dishes rather than as a single main entree. Little milk is used, but eggs and soybean products such as tofu add protein. Foods that have been dried, salted, pickled, spiced, candied, or canned may be added as garnishes or relishes to mask some flavors or textures or to enhance others. Fruits are usually eaten fresh. Rice is the staple grain used at most meals. The traditional beverage is unsweetened green tea. Seasonings include soy sauce, ginger, almonds, and sesame seed. Peanut oil is a main cooking fat.

Japanese. In some ways, Japanese food patters are similar to those of the Chinese. Rice is a basic grain at meals, soy sauce is used for seasoning, and tea is the main beverage. The Japanese diet contains more seafood, especially raw fish items called *sushi*. Many varieties of fish and shellfish are used. Vegetables are usually steamed; some are pickled. Fresh fruit is eaten in season, a tray of fruit being a regular course at main meals.

Southeast Asian. Since 1971, in the wake of the war in Vietnam, more than 340,000 Southeast Asians have come to the United States as refugees. The largest group are Vietnamese; others have come from the adjacent war-torn countries of Laos and Cambodia. They have settled mainly in California, with other groups in Florida, Texas, Illinois, and Pennsylvania. Their basic food patterns are similar. They are making an impact on American diet and agriculture, and Asian grocery stores stock many traditional Indo-Chinese food items. Rice, both long-grain and glutinous, forms the basis of the Indonesian food pattern, and is eaten at most meals. The Vietnamese usually eat rice plain in a separate rice bowl and not mixed with other foods, whereas other Southeast Asians may eat rice in mixed dishes. Soups are also commonly used at meals. Many fresh fruits and vegetables are used along with fresh herbs and other seasonings such as chives, spring onions, chili peppers, ginger root, coriander, turmeric, and fish sauce. Many kinds of fish and shellfish are used, as well as chicken, duck, pork, and beef. Stir-frying in a wok-type pan with a small amount of lard or peanut oil is a common method of cooking. A variety of vegetables and seasonings are used, with small amounts of seafood or meat added. Since coming to the United States, the Indonesians have made some diet changes that reflect American influence. These include use of more eggs, beef and pork, but less seafood, more candy and other sweet snacks, bread, fast foods, soft drinks, butter and margarine, and coffee.

Mediterranean influences

Italian food patterns. The sharing of food is an important part of Italian life. Meals are associated with warmth and fellowship, and special occasions are shared with families and friends. Bread and pasta are basic foods. Milk, seldom used alone, is typically mixed with coffee in equal portions. Cheese is a favorite food, with many popular varieties. Meats, poultry, and fish are used in many ways, and the varied Italian sausages and cold cuts are famous. Vegetables are used alone, in mixed main dishes or soups, in sauces, and in salads. Seasonings include herbs and spices, garlic, wine, olive oil, tomato puree, and salt pork. Main dishes are prepared by initially browning vegetables and seasonings in olive oil; adding meat or fish for browning as well; covering with such liquids as wine, broth, or tomato sauce; and simmering slowly on low heat for several hours. Fresh fruit is often the dessert or a snack.

Greek. Everyday meals are simple, but Greek holiday meals are occasions for serving many delicacies. Bread is always the center of every meal, with other foods considered accompaniments. Milk is seldom used as a beverage, but rather as the cultured form of yogurt. Cheese is a favorite food, especially *feta*, a white cheese made from the sheep's milk and preserved in brine. Lamb is a favorite meat, but others, as well as fish, are used also. Eggs are sometimes a main dish, never a breakfast food. Many vegetables are used, often as a main entree, cooked with broth, tomato sauce, onions, olive oil, and parsley. A typical salad of thinly sliced raw vegetables and feta cheese, dressed with olive oil and vinegar, is often served with meals. Rice is a main grain in many dishes. Fruit is an everyday dessert, but rich pastries, such as *baklava* are served on special occasions.

REFERENCES

Broussard-Marin L, Hynak-Hankinson MT: Ethnic food, the use of Cajun cuisine as a model, *J Am Diet Assoc* 89(8):1117, 1989.

Chau P and others: Dietary habits, health beliefs, and food practices of elderly Chinese women, *J Am Diet Assoc* 90(4):579, 1990.

For your information: A look at Japanese Dietary Guidelines, *J Am Diet Assoc* 90(11):1527.

Monsen ER: Respecting diversity helps America eat right, *J Am Diet Assoc* 92(3):282, 1992.

Nobmann ED and others: The diet of Alaska Native adults, *Am J Clin Nutr* 55:1024, 1992.

Nomani MZA and others: Effects of Ramadan fasting on plasma uric acid and body weight in healthy men, *J Am Diet Assoc* 90(10):1435, 1990.

Stowers SL: Development of a culturally appropriate food guide for pregnant Caribbean immigrants in the United States, *J Am Diet Assoc* 92(3):331, 1992.

CHAPTER 10

Family Nutrition Counseling: Food Needs and Costs

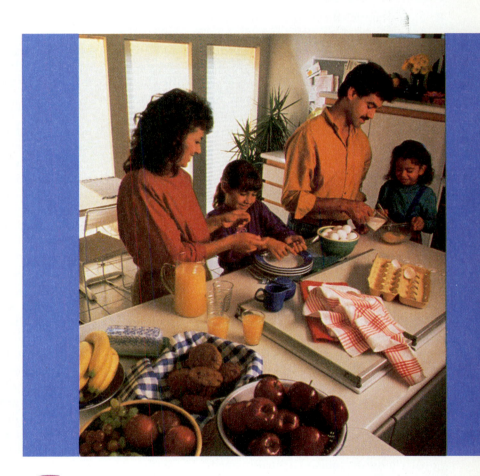

𝒯his chapter continues the two-chapter opening sequence on food habits and family nutrition counseling that introduces Part II of your study on Community Nutrition and the Life Cycle.

In the previous chapter we considered the food environment and influences that shape food habits. Here we continue with family counseling and education approaches to meeting health problems, frequently in the face of economic hardships.

Often in our clinics and communities we must interpret complex information in a variety of settings to meet numerous family health and nutrition needs. Here, then, we seek approaches and resources to help meet these needs.

Family Nutrition Counseling

Community health workers frequently need to apply the principles of health teaching in family nutrition counseling. Health and nutrition are inseparable, and the term *counseling* is appropriate. If we work with the family on the basis of counseling principles, various members are led to explore their own situation, to express their needs, and to find ways of meeting those needs that are best suited to their particular life situation. Our job is to help them explore their options and make decisions in the light of knowledge and personal support.

Person-Centered Goals

Realistic family diet counseling must be person-centered. It involves close attention to personal and family needs, nutrition and health problems, and food choices and costs. In our work we have three main goals: (1) to obtain basic information about the client and the living situation that relates to nutrition and health needs; (2) to provide basic health teaching to help meet these needs; and (3) to support the client and family in all personal efforts to meet needs through encouragement, reinforcement, general caring and concern, and practical resources. A basic skill that all health workers must learn, therefore, is the skill of talking with clients in a helpful manner.

Interviewing

Skills in interviewing are essential in health care. Interviewing does not necessarily mean only the more formal or structured history-taking activity. Frequently it means a purposeful planned conversation either in the hospital or clinic or home. It may be a simple telephone call to the home to determine ongoing needs or progress. General principles of interviewing should guide these activities, including the purpose or focus, means used to achieve the purpose, and measuring results.

Focus and Purpose

As indicated, the focus of all health care is the individual client and personal health needs. It may be a small intermediate goal relating to some aspect of the overall care, or it may be a long-term goal. Our ultimate purpose is to provide whatever help the individual or family may need to determine personal health needs and goals and to work with the person or family in finding ways of meeting these needs and goals.

Means Used to Achieve Purpose

Health workers use various means of accomplishing these purposes—building a helping relationship, creating a comfortable climate, and developing positive attitudes.

Relationship. Counseling is a dynamic person-centered process built upon a helping relationship. This is reflected in the common use of the word *services* for all health care–related activities.[1] The most important means of helping a person is establishing a relationship of mutual trust and respect. The most significant tool we ever have for helping others is ourselves. Our role is that of a helping vehicle. Within this kind of relationship, true healing can take place.

Climate. The kind of climate we create involves both the physical setting and the psychologic feelings involved. The physical setting should be as comfortable as possible in relation to space, ventilation, heating, lighting, and sitting or lying down. Other important factors include providing sufficient time for the interview, in a quiet setting free from interruptions and with sufficient privacy to ensure confidentiality. If it is in an office setting, the desk should be to the side, not between the therapist and client.

Attitudes. The word *attitude* refers to that aspect of personality that accounts for a consistent behavior toward persons, situations, or objects. Our attitudes are learned. Hence they develop from life experiences and influences. Because they are learned, they can be examined. We can become more aware of them. We can try to strengthen those attitudes that are desirable and constructive, and at the same time seek to change or modify those attitudes that are less desirable and more destructive. If a health worker is to be able to help meet clients' needs, certain attitudes are necessary components of behavior:

- *Warmth:* A genuine concern for the client or patient is displayed by interest, friendliness, and kindness. We convey warmth by being human and thoughtful.
- *Acceptance:* We must meet clients as they are and where they are. To accept the client does not necessarily mean approval of behavior. It does mean a realization that clients or patients usually regard their behavior as purposeful and meaningful. It may well be for them a means of handling stress. An attitude of acceptance conveys that a person's thoughts, ideas, and actions are important and worth attention simply because a person—a human being—has the right to be treated as having worth and dignity.
- *Objectivity:* To be objective is to be free from bias. It is having a nonjudgmental attitude. Of course, complete objectivity is impossible, but reasonable objectivity is certainly a goal that can be attained. We must be aware of our own feelings and biases and we should attempt to control them. The evaluation of a situation must be based on what is actually happening, the facts as we perceive them, not

on mere opinions, assumptions, or inferences.

- *Compassion:* This attitude enables us to feel with and for another person or oneself. It means accepting the impact of an emotion, holding it long enough to absorb its meaning, and entering into a kind of fellowship of feeling with the person who is moved by the emotion. There is nothing soft or easy in developing the attitude of compassion. It requires emotional maturity.

Measuring Results

Continuous and terminal evaluation of our interviews is an ongoing part of our activity. Evaluation is measuring how behavioral changes in the client and in ourselves are related to the needs and goals that have been identified. In summary, therefore, health workers will always be dealing with the following sequence of questions in interviewing:

1. *Need:* What is wrong? What is the health problem or need of the client or patient?
2. *Goal:* What does the client want to do about it? What is the client's immediate goal? What is the long-range goal?
3. *Information:* What information do I need to know to help the client? What does the client need to know to help take care of personal needs? What knowledge and skills are necessary to solve the health problem?
4. *Action:* What has to be done to help meet the need? What plan of action is best for solving the health problem and meeting the client's personal needs?
5. *Result:* What happened? What was the result of the action planned and carried out? Did it solve the problem or meet the need? If not, why not? What change in plan is indicated?

Important Actions of the Interview

Five important actions of an interview can be identified: observing, listening, responding, terminating, and recording. Each of these requires study, practice, and development of skills.

Observing

Ordinarily we do not deliberately and minutely look at all the persons we meet. However, in the care of persons with health needs the helping role requires such behavior. Our purpose is to gather information that will guide us in understanding clients or patients and their environment. Valid observation is a skill that is developed through concentration, study, and practice. Areas of such needed observation include the following:

Physiologic functioning and features. Refer to Table 1-1 (see p. 7) and review the clinical signs of nutritional status. Such features as these may be used as a basis for making detailed observations of physical features. Learning to take an organized look at the person may help develop greater accuracy and objectivity. We tend to see what we have the mindset, sensitivity, or awareness to see. Therefore, we need to develop certain sensitivities to detect pertinent details that can provide important clues to real needs.

Behavior patterns. Observe closely not only the physical features but also the immediate behavior of the client or patient in the health care situation. Attempt to look at the behavior in terms of its meaning to the person in relation to self-concept and the illness. From these observations, certain assumptions or educated guesses about immediate and long-term needs and goals can be made. But realize all the while that these are only assumptions and hence need to be validated and clarified with the client to determine whether they are indeed factual. This action helps us to understand our own feelings and rule out our own biases, prejudices, or distortions of the situation.

Environment. Observing the client's immediate environment in an organized manner is also helpful. This may be the home and community environment on a visit, or it may be the immediate environment in a clinic or hospital setting.

Listening

Hearing and listening are not the same thing. Hearing is purely a physiologic function, only the first phase of the listening process. The function of the listening is to hear, to identify the sound, to understand its meaning, and to learn by it.

Although the senses have amazing powers of perception, they are limited. The nervous system must constantly select and discriminate among the millions of bits of information it confronts. Listening is also limited. A large part of communication time is spent in listening, but the average person without special training has only about 25% listening efficiency. In other words, one hears only a small percentage of the total surrounding communication.

The task of the health worker is to learn the art of creative listening. First of all, we must learn to be comfortable as a listener. Usually our lives are so filled with activity and noise that to sit and listen quietly is often difficult. Actually, most of us have had little experience during our own development of being listened to, so that listening to others must be learned. We practice listening by staying close by, assuming a comfortable position, and giving our full attention to the person who is speaking. We show genuine interest by indicating agreement or understanding with a nod of the head or saying "Uh-huh," "I see," or "And then?" at the appropriate moments in the conversation. We must learn to remain silent when the other person's comment jogs some personal memory or parallel experience of our own. We learn to listen not only for words the client uses but also the repetition of key words, to the rise and fall of the tone of voice, to hesitant or aggressive expression of words and ideas, and to the softness or harshness of tone. We listen to the overall content of what is being said, to the main ideas being expressed, and to the topics chosen for discussion. We listen for the feelings, needs, and goals that are being stated. We learn to listen to the silences and to be comfortable with them, giving the person time to frame thoughts and express them.

Responding

The responses we give to the client or patient may be verbal or nonverbal. Nonverbal responses include signs and actions, such as gestures and movements, silences, facial expressions, nods of the head, and touch. Verbal responses make use of language—words and meanings (Table 10-1). But we must remember that we give our own meanings to the words we use. A word is only a symbol, not the thing itself. Thus we must give attention to our choice of words; we must "begin where the person is." And all the while we must provide a supportive environment for responses (see box below). Also, we must watch the level and pace of our speaking. Questions should be clear, concise, free from bias, and always nonthreatening. Sometimes a verbal response may be a simple restatement of what the client has said. This enables the person to hear the statement again, think about it and thus reinforce, expand, or correct it. At other times the response may be a reflection of what the expressed feelings seem to be. This enables the client to respond, to verify or to deny that this was indeed the feeling. We must never act on our assumptions about the client's feelings without verifying them first.

◆ **C**LINICAL **A**PPLICATION   *Creating a Supportive Nutrition Counseling Environment*

Over 50 years ago a sensitive physician expressed truths about the client/patient interview in a healing environment that are human verities today as much as then. Perhaps they are even more true in our far more complex world today. He reminds us anew that we must listen, really listen, to our clients and patients every day if we are to help them.

Listening

"Now hear this," he seems to be imploring us still. "We must listen," he is saying, "for what the client wants to tell us, for he does not want to tell us, and for what he cannot tell us. He does not want to tell things that are shameful or painful. And he cannot tell us his implicit assumptions that even he does not know." It sounds like creative listening, as a more modern philosopher and counselor, Carl Rogers, used to call it. This is no mere passive thing. It is an active counseling skill. Only by using it can we really hear and respond wisely.

Also, nutrition counselors may inadvertently close communication channels by failing to ask questions or otherwise verbally discouraging the client from expressing real concerns and expectations or by using body language that is distracting, inappropriate, or mis-

interpreted by the client because of cultural differences.

Questions and reflections

Questions or statements that reflect what the client says or feels and that encourage further expression are usually open-ended, making a simple yes-or-no response inadequate, or affective, reflecting feelings that the client may have implied but not expressed directly. Closed questions and self-directed statements do little to encourage the person to "open up" (see Table 10-1).

Body language

Body language can be distracting or intimidating, or it can make the client feel at home. The key is to understand the client's concept of the following communication factors:

*   *Personal space.* Americans like a lot of room. Try sitting next to the only passenger on a city bus and note the amount of anxiety created! In other cultures, such as the Middle East, closeness, even to the point of pushing and shoving, is considered acceptable behavior. Thus we must understand that our distance from our clients may affect their sense of comfort.

*   *Eye contact.* Americans show respect by looking at each other straight in the eye. Asians do the same by looking downward. Attempts to interchange these behaviors can be interpreted as being rude.
*   *Speech inflection.* The tone of voice and its loudness and inflection may be interpreted as threatening or comforting, depending on the region or country of origin of the listener.

You cannot always be aware of your clients' attitudes toward body language ahead of time. However, you can take note of any signs of uneasiness and at least invite them to discuss anything about the interview that may be causing concern.

Yes, Dr. Henderson, we still hear you. We can—and must—listen.

REFERENCES

Henderson L: Physician and patient as a social system, *N Engl J Med* 212:819, 1935.
Heppner PP and others: Carl Rogers: reflections on his life, *J Counsel Dev* 63:14, 1984.
Vickery CE, Hodges PAM: Counseling strategies for dietary management: expanded possibilities for effecting behavior change, *J Am Diet Assoc* 86(7):924, 1986. ◆

TABLE 10-1

Verbal Responses Used by the Helping Professions

Purpose of response	Type of response	Description
Clarification	Content	Counselor summarizes content of conversation up to that point
	Affective	Counselor paraphrases or defines concern that client has implied but not actually stated
Leading	Closed question	Question that can be answered with "yes" or "no" or with very few words
	Open question	Question that cannot be answered briefly; often triggers discussion or a flow of information
	Advice	Provision of an alternative type of behavior by counselor for client; may be an activity or thought
	Teaching	Information presented by counselor with intention of helping client acquire knowledge and skills to perform appropriate nutrition-related behaviors
Self-revealing	Self-involving	Response made to client's statements that reflects the personal feelings of counselor
	Self-disclosing	Response made to client's statements that reflects factual information about counselor
	Aside	Statement counselor makes to self

Terminating the Interview

The close of the interview should meet several needs. It may be used to summarize the main points covered or to reinforce learning. If contact with the client is to continue, it can include plans for the follow-up visits or activities. It should always leave the person with the sense that the health worker's concern has been sincere and that the door is always open for further communication, should the person so desire.

Recording

Some means of recording the important points of the interview should be arranged. This should be as unobtrusive as possible, with little note-taking, if any, during the interview itself and completion of the record immediately afterward. If some recording device is used, the client's permission must always be obtained. Give full assurance that identity will be erased and that the recording will only be used for a specific purpose, such as to help the health worker improve interviewing skills or to learn the health needs of a particular group of people, as in gathering research data.

Various members of the health team contribute information about the client or patient and the health problem in a system of written reports. This is the patient's chart, a legal document which in case of litigation could be used in court. There is an obligation to the client or patient to respect confidentiality and to determine what and how much information is shared and with whom. At the same time health workers have a responsibility for relaying to other health team members pertinent information to aid in the total planning of care.

What aspects, then, of the interview should be recorded? Data from two basic areas of communication are needed: (1) a description of the client or patient's general physical and emotional status and concerns, followed in some instances by judgment of the immediate and ongoing care needs; and (2) description of whatever care and teaching was given and results ob-

served. In addition, we may sometimes include follow-up plans made with the client or patient and the family, or notes concerning needs that were passed on to other health team members or to other agencies. Similar information is often communicated through oral team reports and various case conferences.

Nutrition History and Analysis
Personal Life Situation and Food Patterns

First, working closely with the nutritionist on the health care team, learn the family's situation and values and identify health and nutrition needs through a general nutrition history and its analysis. Several methods for such interviewing may be used, depending on the circumstances and the need, either separately or in combination.[2]

24-Hour recall. Ask the person to recall all food and drink consumed during the previous day, noting the nature and amount of each item. This method has disadvantages with some persons, such as elderly people or young children, whose memory may be limited, and it does not reveal long-term food habits. Simple food models in pictorial form can be used successfully to help quantify the reported food intake.[3]

Food records. Persons are asked to record their food intake for a brief period of time, usually about 3 days, or on certain days periodically.[4] Each person is taught how to describe the food items used singly or in combination, and how to measure amounts consumed. Often a 3-day record is used following an initial diet history as a periodic monitoring tool.

Food frequency. Use a structured questionnaire that lists common food items or food groups to obtain information about quantity and frequency of use.[5] This tool may be helpful in relation to a particular disease risk or incidence by helping to determine use of specific groups of foods over an extended period of time.

Name _____   Date _____

Height _____ Weight (lb) _____ (kg) _____ Age _____

Ideal weight _____

Referral
Diagnosis
Diet order
Members of household
Occupation
Recreation, physical activity

Present food intake	Place	Hour	Frequency, form, and amount checklist
Morning			Milk
			Cheese
			Meat
			Fish
			Poultry
Noon			Eggs
			Cream
			Butter, margarine
			Other fats
Evening			Vegetables, green
			Vegetables, other
			Fruits (citrus)
			Legumes
			Potato
			Bread—kind
			Sugar
			Desserts
			Beverages
Summary			Alcohol
			Vitamins
			Candy

FIG. 10-1   Nutrition history: activity-associated general day's food pattern. Also record general activity pattern throughout the day.

Diet history.   At the initial individual or family contact, a nutrition interview provides needed information for planning continuing care. Professional nutritionists and dietitians use a comprehensive form of this approach in a variety of clinical and community settings, usually evaluating their findings by detailed computer analysis.[6] Other health team members working with the dietitian may contribute helpful nutrition information through use of a simplified version, such as the activity-associated general day's food pattern given in Fig. 10-1. Most people eat in relation to activity or work throughout the day, where they are, what they are doing, and whom they are with at the time. So using such an activity-associated guide through the day gives both interviewer and client a structure, a beginning, middle, and end, and provides a series of memory jogs to flesh out the information in greater detail and permit constructive counseling. With respect to each item, questions are asked in terms of general habits—nature of food items, form, frequency, preparation, portion, seasoning—not in terms of a specific day's intake. All through such an interview important clues to food attitudes and values can be communicated. Note these for later thought and exploration. If your manner is in-

terested and accepting, the information should be valid and straightforward. Conversely, if you are judgmental and authoritarian, persons will probably tell you only what they think you want to hear.

Changing American Eating Behavior

A basic reason for using an activity-associated general day's food intake as the structure for a diet history is that America's eating behavior is changing from traditional patterns. Recent surveys indicate that current eating behavior has become much more fragmented into frequent light feedings—called "grazing" by many observers—than the traditional family meals. Actually, one study that compared American eating patterns over the past 15 years found that the smallest and fastest shrinking population segment is that group called "Happy Cookers" who still cook three square meals a day.[7] These investigators found that this traditional group now accounts for only 15% of the American population and that their numbers have declined 35% over the previous 15-year period. On the other hand, the largest and fastest growing segment, whom the researchers called the "Chase and Grabbits," is composed of those eating easily portable items that don't take much time to cook or consume. This group now accounts for 26% of the population and its numbers have swelled 136% over the past 15 years.

Plan of Care

On the basis of the diet history and review of any health problems requiring diet modification, a realistic personal food plan can be developed with the individual and family. Then any related follow-up care as needed can be developed. This may take the form of return visits to the clinic, home visits, consultation and referral with other members of the health care team, or use of community resources. Follow-up work requires patience and a steady focus on the goal, knowing that there are options, not just one way of reaching it. Imagination and good humor are invaluable. Take one step at a time. Guide the client and family in applied nutrition principles, give support as needed, help with adjustments of the plan, provide reinforcement of prior learning, and continue to add new learning opportunities as the family's needs develop.

The Teaching-Learning Process
Learning and Changed Behavior

There is far more to teaching and learning than merely dispensing information. But the myth still prevails in much of health education that if enough information is provided, harmful health practices will be changed. This is not the case. There is a vast difference between a person who has learned and a person who has only been informed. Learning must ultimately be measured in terms of changed behavior. As with counseling, valid education focuses not on the practitioner-teacher or the content, but on the personal learner. The health teacher's major task is to create situations in which clients and their families can learn, succeed, and develop self-direction, self-motivation, and self-care. These learning goals are especially important in dealing with adult patients and clients[8] (see To Probe Further, p. 200).

Aspects of Human Personality Involved in Learning

The teaching-learning experience involves three fundamental aspects of the human personality: thinking, feeling, and the will to act.

Thinking

We grasp information through our personal thinking process. We take in information selectively, then process and shape it according to our needs. The total thought process provides the background knowledge that is the basis for reasoning and analysis. The learner senses the contribution of this thinking to the learning process as "I know how to do it."

Feeling

In each of us specific feelings and responses are associated with given items of knowledge and situations. These emotions reflect desires and needs that are aroused. Emotions provide impetus, creating the tensions that spur us to act. The learner senses the contribution of emotion to the learning process as "I want to do it."

Will to Act

The will to act arises from the conviction that the knowledge discovered can fulfill the felt need and relieve the symptoms of tension. The will focuses the decision to act on the knowledge received so that attitude, value, thought, or pattern of behavior can be changed. The learner senses the contribution of the will to the learning process as "I will do it."

Principles of Learning

Learning follows three basic laws: (1) learning is *personal*, occurring in relation to perceived personal needs; (2) learning is *developmental*, building on prior knowledge and experience; and (3) learning means change, resulting in some form of *changed behavior*.

Individuality

Learning can only be individual. In the final analysis we must all learn for ourselves, according to our own needs, in our own way and time, and for our own purpose. The teacher must discover who the learner is by asking questions that clarify the learner's relationship to the problem. New approaches to realistic nutrition education can help teachers vary teaching-learning strategies to meet the differing needs of learners and learning situations.

Need Fulfillment

An important initial force in learning is personal **motivation.** Persons learn only what they believe will be useful to them, and they retain only what they think they need or shall need. The more immediately persons can put new learning to use, the more readily they grasp it. The more it satisfies their immediate goals, the more effective the learning will be.

Contact

Learning starts from a point of contact between prior experience and knowledge, an overlap of the new with the familiar. Find out what the individual already knows

motivation • Forces that affect individual goal-directed behavior toward satisfying needs or achieving personal goals.

Effect of Adult Learning Concepts on the Nutrition Interview

The adult client's openness to new knowledge, and even more so the ability to change behavior, is influenced by attitudes, educational background, physical characteristics, and economic situations. Teaching adults is quite different from teaching preadults.

We often say that a child is not a miniature adult, and we treat them accordingly. But we sometimes forget that an adult is not just a larger preadult person, and we may be condescending—even insulting—without being aware of it. This is equally true in the nutrition interview as in a more formal educational setting.

The successful counselor considers these seven most prevalent attitudes affecting the counseling session with an adult client or patient:

- *Clients want to be treated as adults.* Clients do not appreciate being reprimanded or talked down to.
- *Every client is an individual.* No matter how many clients you see with a particular health problem, each client wants to be treated as though his or her condition presents unique needs, which it surely does.
- *Most adult clients prefer objectivity and a businesslike approach.* Although warmth and empathy are appropriate, do not forget the fact that the counseling session is a role-playing situation. Some degree of formality, such as the use of titles and surnames, not first name familiarity, creates a structured environment to which most working adults are accustomed. If the client prefers a more relaxed atmosphere, he or she should be the one to steer the session in that direction.
- *Clients often resist change.* Change is threatening, especially when it involves something as personal as eating habits. An explanation of the need for change accomplishes more than insisting on change.
- *Some clients lack confidence.* Lack of education, fear of failure, distrust of the medical community, and other factors may reduce the client's confidence in his or her ability to follow diet plans. Patience, answering questions appropriately, and setting realistic goals may help promote a sense of confidence, as well as initiate therapy.
- *Some clients are overconfident.* Some clients expect too much from their diet plan or themselves. This is sometimes a mask for a fear of failure. Again, setting realistic goals may help the client become a bit more realistic and avoid disappointment.
- *Clients need positive reinforcement and feedback.* Some clients need help to overcome fear and anxiety and guidance to promote adherence to a food plan.

To accommodate educational factors, the counselor should consider the following:

TO PROBE FURTHER

- *Educational levels vary.* A lack of education may strip a client of the courage to ask questions or verbalize feelings and concerns. The counselor should make the client more comfortable by avoiding jargon and responding to every question on the level on which it is asked.
- *Isolated facts are difficult to remember.* The counselor must be familiar with the client's values and experiences to relate individual nutrition concepts, thus making them more meaningful.
- *Many adults have been exposed to years of incorrect or out-of-date information.* This may be difficult to overcome because of the effective teaching skills of persons dispensing misinformation. However, a professionally conducted session in which the correct information is presented in a nonintimidating way may be helpful in convincing the client that your message is more reliable than those provided by, for example, a television commercial.

Additional considerations include physical and economic factors such as the following:

- *Physical factors.* Physical factors affecting the counseling session, such as limited or no vision, limited hearing ability, illiteracy, or language barrier, may require more time, patience, or specially designed audiovisuals to facilitate learning. Involving a friend or family member in the session to interpret or learn may help reinforce the food behavior changes at home.
- *Economic factors.* Economic factors influence the outcome of counseling if the client believes that the new food choices are expensive. Explaining wise buying practices and the benefits of dietary changes versus the cost of continued health care, always in a supportive nonintimidating way may help the client overcome this anxiety. If cost is a barrier, the counselor may refer the client to a social worker or any social service organization that could provide assistance.

Above all, counselors and teachers of adult clients must treat them as the adults they are. Such wise practitioners develop approaches and methods that help their adult learners enhance their own creative thinking and problem-solving skills. At the beginning of every counseling or teaching, they strive to establish the empathy and good rapport that is essential for effective communication. Only in this way is sufficient information obtained about the client's concerns and expectations and learning needs to develop an effective plan for solving nutrition-related problems.

REFERENCES

Kicklighter JR: Characteristics of older adult learners: a guide for dietetics practitioners, *J Am Diet Assoc* 91(11):1418, 1991.

Meyer MK: Enhancing the client acceptance of nutrition counseling: understanding the service concept and developing a positive residual, *J Am Diet Assoc* 89(11):1655, 1989.

and to what past experiences the present situation can be related. Start the process of learning at this point. Search for the areas of association that are present, then relate your teaching to that point of contact.

Active Participation

Since learning is an active process through which behavior can change, learners must become personally involved. They must participate actively. Indeed, effective teaching strategies require active participation of learners to bring about desired changes in attitudes and behaviors.[9] One means of securing participation is through planned feedback. Feedback may take several forms:

1. Ask questions that require more than a "yes" or "no" answer and that reveal a degree of understanding and motivation, such as those in Table 10-1.
2. Use guided return demonstrations, which are brief periods in which procedures are practiced and skills discussed. Such guided practice develops ability, self-confidence, and security. It enables the learner to clarify the principles involved as a basis for decision making about particular situations and actions.
3. Have the learner try out the new learning in personal experiences outside the teacher-directed situation. Alternate such trials with return visits to review these experiences. Answer, or help the person to answer, any questions raised and provide continued support and reinforcement.

Appraisal

At appropriate intervals take stock of the changes that your clients have made in outlook, attitude, and actions toward their specific goals in health and nutrition care and education. Careful, sympathetic questioning may reveal any blocks to learning. In addition to speeding the learning process, such concern will show you whether you are communicating clearly, making contact, or choosing the best method. It may help you to recall principles that you may have glossed over. In the final analysis, the measure of success in teaching lies not in the number of facts transferred, but in the change for the better that has been initiated in your client.

In all, the nutrition educator who builds on clients' needs and goals, imparts a strong knowledge and interest in the subject, shows respect and concern for each individual in the program, and projects self-confidence, has the greatest chance for success. In the long run, clients following a personal goal-setting approach in their nutrition counseling and education will have more opportunity to develop self-care responsibility and personal choice than those following a purely diet-prescription approach[9] (see Issues and Answers, p

208). Initially the personal goal-setting approach may take longer, but it achieves far greater long-term results.

Family Economic Needs: Food Assistance Programs

In your counseling you will discover economic stress among many clients and their families. Some may need financial help. In such situations you will need to discuss available food assistance programs and make appropriate referrals, through your team nutritionist and social worker or directly to community agencies and programs involved.

Commodity Distribution Program

In the post-Depression years, legislation was initiated to stabilize agricultural prices. This legislation provided for the federal government to purchase market surpluses of perishable goods. Later the resulting accumulation of food stocks led to the creation of distribution programs as a means of disposing of the stored products (Fig. 10-2). Such surplus has been defined as either physical (exceeding requirements) or economic (prices below desired levels). Foods coming under these regulations include meat and poultry, fruits and vegetables, eggs, dried beans, and peas. Most of these items purchased under this program have been donated by the Food and Nutrition Service of the U.S. Department of Agriculture (USDA) to schools through the National School Lunch and School Breakfast Programs. Foods accumulated through other aspects of the legislation are price-supported basic and nonperishable items. These foods have been donated to child-feeding programs, summer camps, Indian reservations, trust

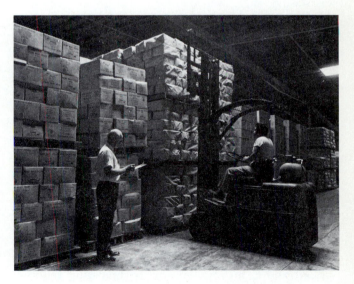

FIG. 10-2 Warehouse for food surplus goods used in Commodity Distribution Program.

territories, nutrition programs for the elderly, charities, disaster-feeding programs, and the Commodities Supplemental Food Program (Fig. 10-3).

Food Stamp Program

Also growing out of the post-Depression years, the Food Stamp Program was founded to help low-income families purchase needed food. The program became part of permanent legislation by the Food Stamp Act of 1964, which made the program available to all counties wishing to participate. The program has developed from a $13 million program in 1961 to one of nearly $12 billion in 1985.[10] Although it has suffered federal budget cuts through the 1980s, it remains the largest U.S. food assistance program. Under this program the participant is issued coupons or food stamps. The coupons are distributed to participating households, defined by the program as a group of people living in the same house who buy, store, and eat food together. These coupons are supposed to be sufficient to cover the household's food needs for 1 month. These households must have a net monthly income below the program's eligibility limit to qualify. This limit is quite low, and usually families who qualify simply aren't making enough money to buy food. Eligibility is based on gross, not actual net, income. For example, the Poverty Index Ratio (PIR) used, as that with the U.S. Department of Health and Human Services for its National Health and Nutrition Examination Survey (NHANES), is calculated on gross family income.[11,12] This PIR compares household income to three times the cost of the lowest USDA Thrifty Food plan. Households with a PIR of less than 1 are below the official poverty line.

Child Nutrition Programs

After the Commodities Supplemental Food Program was started, the government faced a glut of accumulated food items and needed a means of disposing of them. Then during World War II the military discovered a distressing rate of nutrition-related disorders that prevented a number of its draftees from serving in the army. Out of these two situations the National School Lunch Program of 1946 was born. From this initial program came all of today's child nutrition programs.

National School Lunch and Breakfast Program

These programs provide financial assistance to schools to enable them to provide nutritious lunches and breakfasts to all their students. The program allows poor children to eat free meals or meals at reduced prices, whereas other students pay somewhat less than the full cost of the meal. Commodity foods, as described above, are available to participating schools, and the programs usually entail minimal costs to the school district. All public and private nonprofit schools

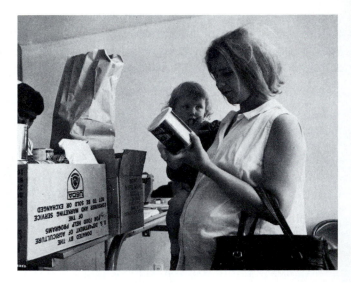

FIG. 10-3   Pregnant mother and her child participating in Commodities Supplemental Food Program.

are eligible to participate in the program if their average tuition per student does not exceed $1500. Children's residential institutions, preschools, and Head Start programs run as part of a school system are also eligible. Lunches served must fulfill approximately one third of the child's Recommended Dietary Allowance (RDA) for nutrients.

Child Care Food Program

This program provides USDA food commodities, cash equivalents, and meal reimbursements for most or all of the meal and administration costs of feeding children up to 12 years of age who are enrolled in organized child care programs. These settings include day care centers, recreation centers, settlement houses, and some Head Start programs. The children's eligibility for free and reduced-price meals is the same as for the school lunch and breakfast programs.

WIC

The Special Supplemental Food Program for Women, Infants, and Children, commonly called by its basic initials *WIC*, provides nutritious foods to low-income women who are pregnant or breast-feeding and to their infants and children under age 5. The food is either distributed free or purchased by free vouchers (Fig. 10-4). It is designed to supplement the diet with rich sources of iron, protein, and certain vitamins. The vouchers are good for such foods as milk, eggs, cheese, juice, fortified cereals, and infant formulas. The program includes funding to cover clinic visits for medical check-ups and for nutrition education and counseling by public health nutritionists. It is administered by the USDA through state health departments and Native

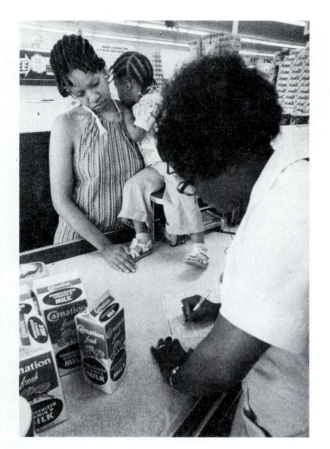

FIG. 10-4   Mother in WIC program using program vouchers at a supermarket to buy groceries.

American tribes, bands, or groups, run locally by public health facilities or organizations.

WIC participants must be pregnant or postpartum mothers (up to 6 months), lactating mothers (up to 12 months), or women having children under age 5. They must be at nutritional risk and must have an income under the reduced-price guidelines for the school lunch program. Factors indicating nutritional risk include evidence of an inadequate diet, poor growth patterns, a lack of nutrition understanding, or a medical history of nutrition-related problems, such as low birth weight or premature infants, pregnancy-induced hypertension (toxemia), spontaneous abortions (miscarriages), and anemia. Reports indicate that the prevalence of anemia among infants and children in low-income families has steadily declined over the past decade.[13] The decline is largely due to the positive impact of public health programs such as WIC, which includes both food support and continuing nutrition education. A recently developed "Simple-Easy" education plan provides the WIC client with the personalized action plans they need to achieve needed behavior change.[14] Also, WIC prenatal supplementation has helped reduce the incidence of low birth weight and raise the mean birth weight.

By the early 1980s, the WIC program served the needs of about 2 million persons who received benefits at just over 1000 clinics across the United States. Unlike the food stamp or school lunch programs, however, WIC is not an entitlement program. This means that eligibility does not automatically entitle one to benefits. There is an absolute ceiling each year on funding and therefore on participation.

Nutrition Program for Elderly Persons

Congress has provided two types of food programs to benefit the growing numbers of elderly citizens in the United States. Regardless of their income level, all persons over 60 years of age are eligible to receive meals from the Congregate Meals Program or the Home-Delivered Meals Program. Elderly persons often face many social, physical, and economic difficulties and do not eat adequately to fulfill their nutritional needs. Many of them suffer from isolation and social deprivation. The main difference in these two programs is their setting and social aspect. The Congregate Meals Program provides ambulatory elderly persons with a hot nourishing noon meal at a community center where they can share food once a day, 5 days a week, with a group of their peers at no charge. Free transportation is often provided. Social events and nutrition information accompany the meals. The nutrition education component often includes, for example, one of a special series of brief 10-statement self-check reviews of true-false questions, each designed to correct misconceptions about the relationship between diet and one of the common chronic diseases among the elderly.[15] In comparison, the Home-Delivered Meals Program, sometimes called Meals-on-Wheels, provides homebound elderly persons who have difficulty preparing their own meals with at least one nutritious meal delivered to them in their home Monday through Friday. A special concern in this program centers upon the very frail elderly persons being served who are most needy.[16] Both programs may accept voluntary contributions for meals from those who are able to do so.

All of these food assistance programs reviewed here provide a base of food security for many low-income families. However, studies indicate that family food shortages in general have increased during the past decade among low income families who are barely subsisting, as well as among participants in these government assistance programs who also experience food shortages, especially during the last week of each monthly cycle of stamps, coupons, or vouchers.[17] U.S. populations most at risk for these food shortages include the elderly, single-parent families, and children.

Food Buying Guides

General family nutrition counseling may also involve guidance in planning for control of family food costs.

USDA Food Plans

The USDA periodically issues low-cost food plans to serve as guides for food assistance programs. These plans are called liberal, moderate, low, and thrifty or very low-cost food plans, but in comparison to modern consumer food costs in general they are all low-cost plans. These very low-cost food plans are developed by nutritionists, economists, and computer experts at USDA on the basis of a predetermined level of spending appropriate to the prevailing policy identifying the poverty threshold. The lowest of all these low-cost plans is used to determine allotments of food stamp coupons to poor households.

Family Food Costs

A number of factors influence the way a family divides its food dollar. Some of these factors as listed here can help your client's family work out a household food plan.

1. Family income
2. Number, sex, ages, and general activities of family members
3. Any family food produced or preserved at home
4. Likes and dislikes of family members and special family dishes
5. Special dietary needs of any family member
6. Time, transportation, and energy for food shopping and preparation
7. Skill and experience in food management: planning, buying, cooking
8. Storing and cooking facilities in the home
9. Amount and kind of entertaining, if any
10. Meals eaten away from home
11. Value family places on food and eating

Good Shopping and Food Handling Practices

Today's American family spends more time shopping for food than cooking it. Food marketing is big business, and buying food for a family may seem to be a more complex affair than the preparation of food at home. A large American supermarket may stock some 8000 or more different food items, and more are being added daily. A single food item may be marketed in a dozen different ways at as many different prices. Frequently client families ask for more help with food buying than with any other aspect of fulfilling their diet needs, in terms of both cost and nutrition.[18,19] These four food handling practices will help to control costs.

Plan Ahead

Use market guides in newspapers, plan general menus, keep a kitchen supply checklist, and make out a market list ahead according to location of items in a regularly visited market. Such planning helps avoid impulse buying and extra trips.

Buy Wisely

Know the market, market items, packaging, grades, brands, portion yields, measures, and food value in a market unit. Watch for sale items and buy in quantity if it results in savings and the food can be adequately stored or used. Be cautious in selecting convenience foods. The added time saving may not be worth the added cost.

Store Food Safely

The kitchen waste that results from food spoilage and misuse can be controlled. Conserve food by storing items according to their nature and use, using dry storage, covered containers, and refrigeration as needed. Keep opened and partly used food packages at the front of the shelf for early use. Avoid plate waste by preparing only the amount needed by the family and use leftovers intelligently and creatively.

Cook Food Well

Retain maximum food value in cooking processes and prepare food with imagination and good sense. Give zest and appeal to dishes by using a variety of seasonings and combinations.

In all family nutrition counseling, however, we must remember that, as much as the family may have learned about nutrition, this is not always a primary factor. Family members usually eat because they are hungry or because the food looks and tastes good, not necessarily because it is nutritious.

The Best Food Buys
Vegetables and Fruits

In addition to minerals, these foods supply vitamins A and C, two nutrients found in surveys to be most often lacking in the average American diet. Give your clients the following guidelines:

1. Buy fresh items in season instead of out-of-season foods transported in from warmer, distant places.
2. Select fresh produce that is firm, crisp, and heavy for size. Medium size items are usually better buys than large, most of which may need to be discarded in preparation.
3. Distinguish between types of fresh produce defects. Small surface defects do not affect quality or food value and may cost less. Many or deep defects cause more waste, as does decay that is even slightly evident.
4. Compare cost of fresh produce sold by weight or count. The resulting price per item can be computed by each method of sale to make the best choice.
5. Avoid fancy grades in canned vegetables and fruits. Grading is based on shape, size, and perfection of pieces. Lower grades contain small, bro-

ken, or imperfect pieces but are equal in taste and food value, thus are good buys.

6. Buy vegetable and fruits in large cans, if family size warrants it.
7. Select low-cost dried foods. Dehydrated foods vary in price. Dried beans, peas, and lentils are excellent food buys. But specialty dried foods, such as potatoes or dried fruits, are usually more expensive than fresh ones.
8. Compare cost of frozen, canned, and fresh vegetable and fruit items. Frozen items are usually more expensive. However, specials and family-sized packages can be compared weight for weight with canned or fresh items in season.
9. Cook vegetables with care. Excess cooking water and time destroy or eliminate vitamins and minerals and rob the vegetable of color, texture, and taste. Such unappetizing food often goes uneaten and causes costly waste.

Breads and Cereals

Most bread and cereal products are well liked, inexpensive, and fit easily into meal plans. This group of foods, along with potatoes and other vegetables, provides complex carbohydrate, which nutritionists advise should be the staple food of most persons' diets. Whole-grain foods are good sources of dietary fiber and are high in important vitamins and minerals. They are also important sources of amino acids and, in combination with other grains and legumes, form complete or complementary proteins. Many foods in this group can be excellent bargains:

1. Whole-grain or enriched products are much more nutritious than refined grains and products and are usually no more expensive.
2. Enriched specialty breads, such as French or Italian, cost up to three times more than whole-grain bread with similar or better nutritive value.
3. Precooked rice is much more expensive than unprocessed and often lacks many of the nutrients lost in processing.
4. Many cereals have nutrients added. Cereals that advertise 100% of the RDA for vitamins and minerals are usually more expensive. If the diet is adequate, such levels of supplementation are unnecessary.
5. Ready-to-eat cereals and instant hot cereals and those packaged for individual servings are usually much more expensive. Buy grains in bulk if adequate storage can be provided.
6. Baked goods made at home, from scratch or even from some mixes, are usually much cheaper than bakery goods.
7. A large loaf of bread may not weigh more than a small loaf. Compare prices of equal weights of bread to find the better buy.

8. Try unusual forms of grains. For example, bulgur, buckwheat groats (hulled kernels), barley, and millet are excellent grains and can be used in many meals. Bulgur, which is cooked like rice, has a toastlike color, is rich in wheat flavor, and is equal in food value to whole wheat.

Protein Foods
Plant Proteins

Dried beans and peas, grains, nuts, and seeds are inexpensive sources of complementary proteins. Legumes and grains contribute different ratios of needed amino acids and in various mixes complement one another to provide food sources of complete protein (see Chapter 4). These foods store well, are versatile in preparation, low in fat, and free of cholesterol, which is purely an animal product. They are also good sources of vitamins and minerals, including iron, zinc, and the B vitamins. For example, tofu, a curd made from soybean milk, has been the low-cost protein backbone of the East Asian diet for more than 2000 years.

Eggs

Eggs provide high-quality complete protein and are sold according to grade and size, neither of which is related to food value. Egg grades are based on qualities such as firmness of egg white, appearance, and delicacy of flavor, not on food value or quality. Shell color varies with species and has no effect on quality.

Milk and Cheese

Dairy products are good sources of high-quality complete protein. However, whole milk products carry saturated fat, so distinguish among them those that are lower in fat as well as lower in price:

1. Fluid nonfat milk, buttermilk, and canned evaporated milk cost less than whole, fluid milk. Low-fat milks may be 1% or 2% butterfat; whole milk is 4%. To produce these lower fat milks, part of the butterfat is removed and dry milk solids are added. For example, 2% milk contains 135 kcal/cup (8 oz); whole milk contains 170 kcal/cup; nonfat milk contains 80 kcal/cup.
2. Nonfat dried milk is the best bargain of all forms. Reconstituted with water it provides a fluid nonfat milk at less than half the cost of fresh form. It can also be used in many ways in cooking to add valuable nutrition, as well as the base for making yogurt.
3. If family size warrants it, buy milk in large bulk containers.
4. If cheese is used often, buy it in bulk. It costs less per unit of weight and keeps better. Cheese standards set by the FDA are based on percentage of fat and moisture. The most commonly used, ched-

dar cheese (American, Daisy, Longhorn), is 50% fat and 30% moisture. Spread cheeses and imported cheeses are much more expensive.

4. Cottage cheese is an unripened, soft curd (80% moisture) and hence a rapidly perishable item. Buy it only as used to avoid waste from spoilage.

Poultry

Buy poultry by the whole bird. Usually the larger, more mature birds cost less than the young broilers and fryers, and they can be made equally tender with longer, moist cooking methods, such as braising, stewing, or pressure cooking.

Organ Meats

Liver, kidney, and heart carry many nutrients, especially iron, although liver is high in cholesterol. However, in some areas they may actually be more expensive than some other boneless cuts of meat. A good cookbook will have appetizing ways of cooking them for family acceptance.

Fish

This is sometimes a fairly expensive food in many areas, depending on the season and the kind. Shellfish is more costly. Less expensive packed styles of canned fish may be available. For example, tuna is packed according to sizes of pieces, with fancy or solid pack (large pieces) being most expensive.

Red Meats

Since meat is commonly one of the most costly food items, learn how it is graded, cut, processed, and marketed. Excellent learning material is available through the local county home advisor, USDA Extension Service. Avoid cuts with large amounts of gristle, bone, and fat. The lower grades provide good quality and less fat and cost less. A new, leaner form of beef, developed by genetic engineering and animal feeding changes, is beginning to enter our markets.[20]

Additional Resources

Farmers' Markets

In community farmers' markets local produce is made available directly to consumers. This outlet has the advantage of fresh produce at prices lower than those found in the supermarket. It also offers opportunities for socializing experiences between growers and consumers and gives a sense of community cohesion.

Consumer Cooperatives

Consumer cooperatives focus on the economics of food marketing as well as on the issues of nutrition and ecology. The newer food cooperatives usually deal in bulk sales of whole or minimally processed foods. Belonging to a food cooperative increases personal responsibility and individual choice, and brings food issues into the hands of the consumer. Many of these food cooperatives stress the purchase of locally grown foods, thus strengthening local farmers while providing very fresh foods for consumers.

Home Gardens

With a little effort any extra yard space may be turned into a home garden. Many persons are now turning to their backyards, interspacing vegetable plants among flowers and shrubbery in frontyards, using alloted community spaces, window boxes, planter boxes on porches, and even indoor potted plots to grow at least a portion of their own produce.

To Sum Up

A major role of health care professionals is to translate the large amount of nutrition information available so that it can meet the needs of clients and families. They must present it in such a way that it is easily understood, is retained and applied by the learner, and can be evaluated to improve its effectiveness and ability to meet continuing care needs. Valid health and nutrition education must focus on the needs of the learner. Goals for planning counseling and educational activities and the methods for meeting these goals must be based on identifiable client and family needs.

Families and individuals under economic stress need counseling concerning financial assistance. Various U.S. food assistance programs operate to help families in need. Referrals to appropriate agencies may be made. The nutrition counselor may also need to assist the family in planning the most economic and nutritious meals possible within their limited circumstances. The family may need help in learning good shopping and food handling practices—planning ahead, buying wisely, storing safely, and cooking appropriately to preserve nutritional values and make food appetizing.

QUESTIONS FOR REVIEW

1. Identify and describe the skills necessary for an effective nutrition counseling session.
2. Identify the basic principles of learning and describe how they may be used in planning nutrition education for one of your clients and family.
3. What government food assistance programs are available to help low-income families? What other local food resources are available in your community?
4. List and discuss the best food buys described in this chapter. How many of the recommended practices do you follow in selecting, storing, and preparing foods?

REFERENCES

1. Meyer MK: Enhancing the client acceptance of nutrition counseling: understanding the service concept and de-

veloping a positive residual, *J Am Diet Assoc* 89(11):1655, 1989.

2. Barrett-Connor E: Nutrition epidemiology: How do we know what they ate? *Am J Clin Nutr* 54(suppl):1825, 1991.

3. Posner BM and others: Validation of two-dimensional models for estimation of portion size in nutrition research, *J Am Diet Assoc* 92(6):738, 1992.

4. Larkin FA and others: Comparison of three consecutive-day and three random-day records of dietary intake, *J Am Diet Assoc* 91(12):1538, 1991.

5. Zulkifli SN: The food frequency method for dietary assessment, *J Am Diet Assoc* 82(6):681, 1992.

6. Hankin JH and others: Validation of a quantitative diet history method in Hawaii, *Am J Epidemiology* 133(6):616, 1991.

7. Morris B: Are squaremeals headed for extinction? *Wall Street Journal*, March 15, 1988.

8. Kicklighter JR: Characteristics of older adult learners: a guide for dietetics practitioners, *J Am Diet Assoc* 91(11):1418, 1991.

9. Johnson CC and others: Behavioral counseling and contracting as methods for promoting cardiovascular health in families, *J Am Diet Assoc* 92(4):479, 1992.

10. U.S. General Accounting Office: *Overview and perspectives on the Food Stamp Program*, Washington, DC, 1985, U.S. Government Printing Office.

11. National Center for Health Statistics: *Public use data tapes, NHANES, 1976-1980*, Hyattsville, MD, 1982, Office of Health Research Statistics and Technology, Department of Health and Human Services.

12. Wotecki CE and others: Selection of nutrition status indicators for field surveys: the NHANES III design, *J Nutr* 120:1440, 1990.

13. Yip R and others: Declining prevalence of anemia among low-income children in the United States, *JAMA* 258:1987, 1987.

14. Erickson K: Effective education: make it simple—make it easy, *J Nutr Ed* 23:40A, 1991.

15. Magnus MH: Self-check, group-check: congregate meal site nutrition education, *J Nutr Ed* 22:310D, 1990.

16. Development and current status of the home-delivered meals programs in the Unites States: Who is served? *Nutr Rev* 48(4):181, 1990.

17. Taren DL and others: Weekly food servings and participation in social programs among low income families, *Am J Public Health* 80(11):1376, 1990.

18. Borra ST, Wellman NS: 'Checking out' the supermarket shopper, *J Am Diet Assoc* 91(12):1511, 1991.

19. Carson CA and others: Putting nutrition on the grocery shelf, *J Am Diet Assoc* 92(2):159, 1992.

20. Sun M: Designing food by engineering animals, *Science* 240:136, April 8, 1988.

FURTHER READING

Kicklighter JR: Characteristics of older adult learners: a guide for dietetics practitioners, *J Am Diet Assoc* 91(11):1418, 1991.
Meyer MK: Enhancing the client acceptance of nutrition counseling: understanding the service concept and developing a positive residual, *J Am Diet Assoc* 89(11):1655, 1989.

These two articles provide helpful background for working with older adult clients and for understanding the full meaning of the word *service* as it refers to the real product of any true health care system.

Erickson K: Effective education: make it simple—make it easy, *J Nutr Ed* 23:40A, 1991.
Magnus MH: Self-check, group-check: congregate meal site nutrition education, *J Nutr Ed* 22:310D, 1990.

These two single-page gems illustrate excellent examples of nutrition education work in the WIC program for mothers and young children on the topic of iron/anemia, and in the Congregate Meal Program for older adults on the topic of nutrition and chronic disease.

ISSUES·AND·ANSWERS

A Person-Centered Model Applied to Diabetes Education

A recently developed **paradigm** for nutrition education called *holistic education* can well apply to teaching good self-care practices to clients with chronic disorders such as diabetes.

This approach draws from good management and good medicine: (1) it varies its style to meet the situation, and (2) it focuses on the whole person—mind-body-spirit, well-being, and wellness. Holistic education regards clients or patients as active partners in the mutual goal of good health care. And further, it teaches persons to use their "boxes and their bubbles"—an excellent thinking model. Our "box" is our rational left side of the brain. Our "bubbles" emerge from our intuitive right side of the brain. We need both. We need to combine rational processes and intuitive ones to build creative thinking skills. Activity that just provides information or shows techniques does not help clients build creative thinking skills for themselves.

Investigations of national patient education programs indicate that many of them provide information and skills training without incorporating learning theories in the design of the program. They also lack a systematic way of assessing and influencing learner attitudes.

Learning theories are usually based on the psychosocial needs of the persons involved as well as their educational needs. In this instance, the person with diabetes has the major responsibility for its day-to-day management to maintain health and avoid complications. Thus diabetes education serves as a model for all good nutrition education and counseling in health care. With approximately 75% of all treated persons with diabetes failing to follow their prescribed diets, we should examine what we are doing in designing instruction for the person with diabetes. Ask yourself these questions.

Is the teaching process effective? Does the teaching process take into account the following:
- How do people learn?
- What is worth learning?
- Who really is responsible for a person's health?
- What responsibilities for learning lie within the learner versus the instructor?

Is the learning process effective? Does the learning process consider the following:
- How significant is the condition to the person at that point in his or her life?
- Does the person have a sense of psychologic safety, that is, does the person feel accepted well enough to discuss diabetes control problems openly and honestly?
- How will the instructor know if the person's attitude has changed toward receiving or using new information?

These questions are important reminders to consider factors that influence learning behavior when planning any health care and education program. Although this may seem to be immediately beyond the realm of nutrition, it is extremely important in any aspect of the care plan and learning process precisely because self-care control of any chronic disease lies primarily in the hands of the person with the disease. This is especially true in diabetes care. No matter how much information is provided, it is ultimately up to the individual to decide what foods are selected, how much is eaten, and when it is consumed.

Diabetes educators, for example, often fail to consider major aspects of the person's own individual and unique personal life that may influence these decisions, such as family finances, work situation, or social activities. They may also fail to recognize the effect of these activities on the individual's sense of personal responsibility for his or her own health. This may also influence the type of instruction provided or even the decision to provide instruction at that time at all.

The educator must be able to assess the person's sense of responsibility and capacity for continuing self-care daily

TABLE 10-2

Levels of Personal Responsibility and Relevant Intervention Methods for Diabetes

Levels of personal responsibility	Client characteristics	Intervention method
1. Being diabetic is a disaster	Feels hopeless, helpless, defeated; self-care may be impossible	Educate family member or other caregivers
2. Being diabetic is a burden	Blames problem on others; expects others to feel sorry for him or her; feels angry, threatened	Provide emotional support; help client accept anger in order to move on
3. Being diabetic is a problem	Blames self as often as others; personal growth is possible	Reinforce attitudes that reflect sense of responsibility; examine irresponsibility; examine irresponsible attitudes in nonjudgmental way
4. Being diabetic is a challenge	Rarely blames others for problem; recognizes responsibility, but does not act on it; good self-care expected	Point out discrepancies between stated need and actual behavior
5. Being diabetic is an opportunity	Takes total responsibility for the problem; acts positively on decisions; optimal self-care is expected	Provide tools required for good self-care

A Person-Centered Model Applied to Diabetes Education—cont'd

and use this information to develop or revise instruction and counseling that leads to positive behaviors. Dietitians and other health care workers may benefit from the systematic methods of assessment that have already been developed in the field of clinical psychology. Therapists have identified five levels of responsibility and client characteristics, with possible intervention methods for each level, as shown in Table 10-2.

Such a system for assessing client attitudes has specific benefits. These benefits can guide client education in good self-care involving food habits not only in diabetes but also in other chronic conditions in families such as hypertension and cardiovascular disease. Benefits of such a system include:

1. It recognizes, and reinforces in the instructor, that the client is ultimately responsible for his or her health.
2. It gives the instructor an objective, measurable way of assessing client attitudes that can be compared and evaluated for progress.
3. It serves as a basis for selecting appropriate teaching methods or counseling techniques, which can then be changed to match the client's current level of responsibility.

REFERENCES

American Medical Association, Council on Scientific: Education for health, *JAMA* 263:1816, 1990.

Johnson CC and others: Behavioral counseling and contracting as methods for promoting cardiovascular health in families, *J Am Diet Assoc* 92(4):479, 1992.

Rinke WJ: Holistic education: a new paradigm for nutrition education, *J Nutr Educ* 18(4):151, 1986.

paradigm • A pattern or model serving as an example; a standard or ideal for practice or behavior based on a fundamental value or theme.

Nutrition During Pregnancy and Lactation

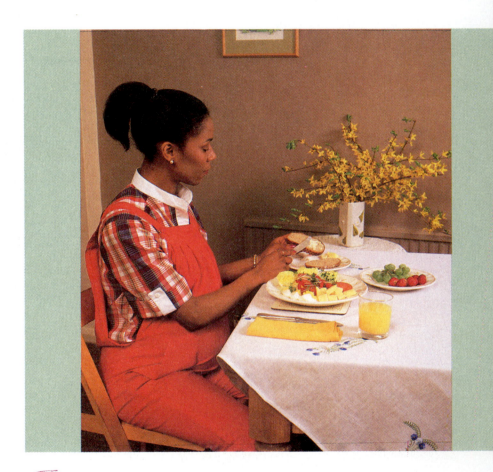

*I*n this chapter we begin a three-chapter sequence on nutrition in health care throughout the life cycle. In each chapter, we relate principles of nutrition to the remarkable process of human growth and development.

As we focus first on the beginning of new life, we examine the prenatal nutritional demands of the pregnant mother and her developing child within. Mother and child possess great powers of adaptation to meet these demands.

Here, then, we explore these tremendous physiologic changes during pregnancy and some possible complications. You will see how vital a role nutritional support plays in a successful course and outcome.

Maternal Nutrition and the Outcome of Pregnancy

Early Medical Practice

For centuries, in all cultures, a great body of folklore has surrounded pregnancy. Various traditional practices and diets have been followed, many of which have had little basis in fact, and much clinical advice has been based only on supposition. For example, early obstetricians even held the notion that semistarvation of the mother was really a blessing in disguise because it produced a small baby of light weight who would be easier to deliver. To this end they used diets restricted in kcalories, protein, water, and salt. Despite the lack of any scientific evidence to support such ideas, two erroneous assumptions, now known to be false, governed practice: (1) the parasite theory: whatever the fetus needs it draws from the stores of the mother despite the maternal diet; and (2) the maternal instinct theory: whatever the fetus needs, the mother instinctively craves and consumes.

Healthy Pregnancy

It is clear now that until recently much of the counsel given to pregnant women over the past few decades has been based more on tradition than on scientific fact. Increasing evidence indicates that positive nutritional support of pregnancy, rather than past negative restrictions born of limited knowledge and false assumptions, promotes a positive successful outcome with increased health and vigor of mothers and infants alike. This struggle over the past four decades, particularly to define the positive "healthy pregnancy," has not been easy. Jacobson describes such a healthy pregnancy in broader terms of mother and infant and family.[1] We are beginning to understand more now just what this really means, especially as we see around us the current fetal damages from malnutrition and drug abuse. We know that we must assess and support more fully the quality of life of each mother and her family if we are to approach the healthy pregnancy we desire for all mothers.

Directions for Current Practice

Clinical observations and developing science in both nutrition and medicine have provided directions for healthier pregnancies. They have refuted previous false ideas and laid a sound base for our current practice. A benchmark report of the National Research Council (NRC) first reflected this applied scientific base and led the way. This report, *Maternal Nutrition and the Course of Human Pregnancy*, was a clear turning point and provided undeniable direction for a new positive approach to the management of pregnancy.[2] Indeed, continuing research has reinforced this positive direction. On the basis of the significant NRC findings, guidelines for nutritional care of pregnant women were then issued by the American College of Obstetrics and Gynecology and the American Dietetic Association.[3,4] These reports have continued to provide guidelines for physicians, nutritionists, dietitians, and nurses in their prenatal care. We are reminded by these guides that a child is nutritionally 9 months old at birth, even older when we consider the significance of the mother's preconception status. Ancient Chinese wisdom has indeed embodied this truth in its counting of age at birth as 1 year.

Factors Determining Nutritional Needs

It is now evident from increased knowledge and the wide experience of many clinicians that maternal nutrition is critical to both the mother and the child. It lays the fundamental foundation for the successful outcome of pregnancy—a healthy and happy mother and child. Several vital considerations emerge as factors that determine the nutritional requirements of the mother during her pregnancy.

Age and Parity

The teenage mother adds her own immaturity and growth needs to those imposed on her by her pregnancy.[5] At the other end of the reproductive cycle, hazards increase with age. Also, the number of pregnancies, **parity,** and the time intervals between them greatly influence the mother's nutrient reserves, her increased nutritional needs, and the outcome of the pregnancy.

Preconception Nutrition

The mother brings to each pregnancy all of her previous life experiences, including her diet and food habits. Her general health and fitness and her state of nutrition at the time of conception are products of her lifelong dietary habits and her genetic heritage.

Complex Physiologic Interactions of Gestation

Three distinct biologic entities are involved during **gestation:** the mother, the **fetus,** and the **placenta.** To-

---

fetus • The unborn offspring in the postembryonic period, after major structures have been outlined; in humans the growing offspring from 7 to 8 weeks after fertilization until birth.

gestation • The period of embryonic and fetal development from fertilization to birth; pregnancy.

parity • The condition of a woman with respect to having borne viable offspring.

placenta • Special organ developed in early pregnancy that provides nutrients to the fetus and removes metabolic waste.

gether they form a unique biologic whole. Constant metabolic interactions go on among them. Their functions, while unique, are at the same time interdependent. It is this unique biologic **synergism** that nourishes and sustains the pregnancy.

Basic Concepts Involved

As a result of our increased knowledge of pregnancy and nutrition, we can provide better nutritional guidance. Three basic concepts form a fundamental framework for assessing maternal nutrition needs and for planning supportive prenatal care for both parents.

Perinatal Concept

The prefix *peri-* comes from the Greek root meaning "around, about, or surrounding." Thus the word *perinatal* refers more broadly to the scope of factors that surround a birth than merely the 9 months of the physical gestation. Certainly, as nutrition knowledge and understanding have increased, health professionals realize that all of a woman's life experiences surrounding her pregnancy need to be considered. Her nutritional status and food patterns, which have developed over a number of years, and the degree to which she has established and maintained nutritional reserves are all important factors. Cultural and social influences have shaped beliefs and values of both parents about pregnancy. All of these influences come to bear upon any pregnancy.

Synergism Concept

The word *synergism* is a term used to describe biologic systems in which the cooperative action of two or more factors produces a total effect greater than and different from the mere sum of the parts. In short, a new whole is created by the unified, joint effort of blending the parts in which each part makes more powerful the action of the others. Of the many biologic and physiologic examples of synergism, pregnancy is a prime case in point. Maternal organism, fetus, and placenta combine to produce a new whole, a system not existing before and producing a total effect greater than and different from the sum of the parts, all for the sole purpose of sustaining and nurturing the pregnancy and its offspring. Physiologic measures change. Blood volume increases, cardiac output increases, ventilation rate and tidal volume of breathing increase, and basal metabolic rate increases. The physiologic norms of the nonpregnant women do not apply.

Thus the normal physiologic adjustments of pregnancy cannot be viewed as pathologic with application of treatment procedures for that same type of response in the nonpregnant state. For example, a normal physiologic generalized edema of pregnancy is a protective response. It reflects the normal increase in total body water necessary to support the increased metabolic

work of pregnancy and is associated with enhanced reproductive performance.

Life Continuum Concept

In a real sense, throughout her life a woman is providing for the ongoing continuum of life through that food that she eats. Each child obviously becomes a part of this continuing process during the pregnancy, when the mother's diet directly sustains growth. But in the broader sense both parents carry over their nutritional heritage, practices, and beliefs in the teaching of their growing children, who in the next generation pass on this heritage both genetically and culturally.

Positive Nutritional Demands of Pregnancy

Basic Nutrient Allowances and Individual Variation

The period of gestation is an exceedingly rapid growth period. During this brief 9-month period, the human life grows from a single fertilized egg cell (ovum) to a fully developed infant weighing about 3 kg (7 lb). On the basis of this intense physiologic growth and development of the fetus, what nutrients must the mother supply? What must her diet provide to meet the nutritional demands of the fetus and of her own changing body during this critical period of human growth?

Throughout the pregnancy there is an increased need for all the basic nutrients, as indicated by the current Recommended Dietary Allowances (RDAs) outlined by the NRC (Table 11-1).[5] But it is important to remember that these are guidelines, and individual variances in need must be examined for each pregnancy, including body size, activity, and multiple pregnancy. Also, quantitative need for nourishment of pregnant adolescents must be noted.[6] The need for individual counseling and for correct use of the RDAs as guidelines is clearly stated by the NRC: "They are not called 'requirements,' because they are not intended to represent merely literal (minimal) requirements of average individuals, but to cover substantially the individual variations in the requirements of healthy people."[5] In considering the needs of the healthy pregnant woman, we will review here the nutrient elements in terms of general amounts of increased intake indicated, why this increase is recommended, and how it may be obtained in basic foods.

Energy Needs

Kcalories must be sufficient to (1) supply the increased energy and nutrient demands by the increased metabolic workload, including some maternal fat storage and fetal fat storage to ensure an optimal newborn size for survival, and (2) spare protein for tissue building. A minimum of about 36 kcal/kg is required for efficient use of protein during pregnancy. The current

TABLE 11-1

RDAs of Some Selected Nutrients for Pregnancy and Lactation (National Research Council, 1989 Revision)

Nutrients	Nonpregnant girl 11-14 yr 46 kg 101 lb	Nonpregnant girl 15-18 yr 55 kg 120 lb	Nonpregnant woman 25 yr 63 kg 138 lb	During pregnancy All ages	Lactation (600 ml/day) First 6 months	Lactation (750 ml/day) Second 6 months
Kcalories	2200	2200	2200	No change in the first trimester; add 300 kcal/day for second and third trimesters	2840	2710
Protein (g)	46	44	50	Add 10 g/day	Add 15 g/day	Add 12 g/day
Calcium (mg)	1200	1200	800	1200 mg throughout		
Iron (mg)	15	15	15	30 mg throughout	15	15
Vitamin A (μg RE)	800	800	800	800 μg RE throughout	1300	1200
Thiamin (mg)	1.1	1.1	1.1	1.5 mg throughout	1.6 mg throughout	
Riboflavin (mg)	1.3	1.3	1.3	1.6 mg throughout	1.8	1.7
Niacin (mg NE)	15	15	15	17 mg NE throughout	20 mg NE throughout	
Ascorbic acid (mg)	50	60	60	70 mg throughout	95	90
Vitamin D (μg)	10	10	5	10 μg throughout	10 μg throughout	

RDA standard recommends an additional amount of energy, 300 kcal during the second and third trimesters of rapid growth, making a total of about 2200 to 2500 kcal, about a 10% to 15% increase over the mother's general prepregnant need. This amount may be insufficient for active, large, or nutritionally deficient women, who may need as much as 2500 to 3000 kcal. Remember that a minimum of 1800 kcal is required just to avoid negative nitrogen balance, to say nothing of the added pregnancy and activity needs. This primary positive emphasis on sufficient kcalories is critical to ensure nutrient and energy support of the pregnancy. Appropriate weight gain during the pregnancy indicates whether sufficient kcalories are being provided.

Protein Needs

The total amount of protein recommended for the pregnant woman is about 60 g/day, an increase of about 10 to 15 g/day. Protein, with its essential nitrogen, is the nutrient basic to tissue growth. Nitrogen balance studies give some indication of the large amounts of nitrogen used by the mother and child during pregnancy and emphasize the importance of maternal reserves to meet initial needs even before the pregnancy is confirmed. More protein is necessary to meet tissue demands posed by (1) rapid growth of the fetus, (2) enlargement of the uterus, mammary glands, and placenta, (3) increase in maternal circulating blood volume and subsequent demand for increased plasma proteins to maintain colloidal osmotic pressure and circulation of tissue fluids to nourish cells, and (4) formation of **amniotic fluid** and storage reserves for labor, delivery, and lactation.

Milk, egg, cheese, and meat are complete protein foods of high biologic value. Protein-rich foods also contribute other nutrients such as calcium, iron, and B vitamins. Additional protein may be obtained from legumes and whole grains, with lesser amounts in other plant sources.

Mineral Needs

All of the major and trace minerals play roles in maternal health. Two that have special functions in relation to pregnancy—calcium and iron—deserve particular attention.

Calcium

The pregnant woman needs 1200 mg of calcium daily, an increase of 400 mg/day for women age 25 or older, to match the general recommendation for all adolescents and young women ages 19 to 25. Calcium is the essential element for the construction and maintenance of bones and teeth. It is also an important factor in the blood-clotting mechanism and is used in normal muscle action and other essential metabolic activities. The rapid fetal mineralization of skeletal tissue during the final period of rapid growth demands more calcium.

amnionic fluid • The watery fluid within the membrane enveloping the fetus, in which the fetus is suspended.

synergism • The joint action of separate agents in which the total effect of their combined action is greater than the sum of their separate actions.

Dairy products are a primary source of calcium. Some increase in milk or equivalent in milk foods (cheese, or nonfat milk powder used in cooking) is recommended. Additional calcium is obtained in whole or enriched cereal grains and in green leafy vegetables.

Iron

The pregnant woman needs 30 mg/day of iron, a 50% increase over her general needs. Some pregnant women may need supplementary iron in addition to increased dietary sources to meet the additional requirement of pregnancy. The iron cost of pregnancy is high. With increased demands for iron, often insufficient maternal stores, and inadequate provision through the usual diet, a daily supplement of 30 to 60 mg of iron may be prescribed. If the woman is anemic at conception, a larger therapeutic amount of 120 to 200 mg of iron is recommended.

To obtain the needed amount of iron, check the percentage of elemental iron in the iron preparation being used. For example, the commonly used compound ferrous sulfate is a hydrated salt ($FeSO_4$ $7H_2O$), which contains 20% iron. It is usually dispensed in tablets containing 195, 300, or 325 mg of the ferrous sulfate compound. Each tablet, then, would contain 39, 60, or 65 mg of iron, respectively. Thus to supply a regular daily supplement of 60 mg of iron, one 300-mg tablet of ferrous sulfate is required, and for a therapeutic dose of 120 mg iron, two 300-mg tablets are required.

However, there are problems with routine iron supplementation for all pregnant women, such as unpleasant gastrointestinal side effects and less motivation to maintain a good diet. Also, there may be imbalances with other trace elements, such as zinc, which competes with iron for absorption. Actually, excess iron intake when not needed may mask inadequate pregnancy-induced hemodilution, a normal pregnancy adaptation that puts less strain on the maternal heart, minimizes hemoglobin loss with blood loss at delivery, and increases nutrient flow to the fetus. Thus, some prenatal clinics are currently following revised protocols that prescribe regular prenatal vitamins with iron at the first clinic visit. Then individual additional iron supplementation is used only if hemoglobin falls to 10.5 g/dl or less at any time during the pregnancy. This practice seems to be supported by current trials.[6,7]

During pregnancy, the maternal circulating blood volume normally increases from 40% to 50%, and may increase more with multiple births. An individual mother's iron supplement need must be assessed accordingly. Maternal iron is also needed to supply iron stores for the developing fetal liver. Adequate maternal iron stores also help fortify the mother against serum iron losses at delivery.

It is no surprise, then, that our major food source of iron by far is liver. Its use can be encouraged by suggesting appetizing ways of preparing it. Other food sources include meat, legumes, dried fruit, green vegetables, eggs, and enriched bread and cereals (see list of iron-containing foods in Chapter 8).

Vitamin Needs

Increased amounts of vitamins A, B-complex, C, and D are needed during pregnancy. If these needs are met, sufficient amounts of vitamins E and K are also available.

Vitamin A

The daily amount of vitamin A recommended for pregnancy is 800 μg of retinol equivalents (RE), a continuance of the woman's regular need. For most women in the United States, no extra amount is needed. However, malnourished, underweight women, as well as those with multiple pregnancies, need more. Vitamin A is an essential factor in cell development, maintenance of strong epithelial tissue, tooth formation, and normal bone growth. Liver, egg yolk, butter and fortified margarine, and dark green and yellow vegetables and fruits are good food sources.

B Vitamins

There is a special need for the various B vitamins during pregnancy. These are usually supplied by a well-balanced diet that is increased in quantity and quality to supply needed energy and nutrients. The B vitamins are important as coenzyme factors in a number of metabolic activities related to energy production, tissue protein synthesis, and function of muscle and nerve tissue. Therefore they play key roles in the increased metabolic work of pregnancy.

There is a special increased metabolic need for folate during pregnancy. Folate deficiency usually occurs in conjunction with general malnutrition, making the pregnant woman in high-risk, low-socioeconomic conditions especially vulnerable. A specific megaloblastic anemia caused by maternal folate deficiency sometimes occurs and warrants supplementation of the diet with folic acid. This added amount is particularly needed where such demands are greater, as in a multiple pregnancy. The RDA standard recommends a supplement of 400 μg/day of folate, more than twice the regular adult need of 180 μg/day, to prevent such deficiencies.

Vitamin C

Special emphasis must be given to the pregnant woman's need for ascorbic acid. Vitamin C is essential to the formation of intercellular cement substance in developing connective tissues and vascular systems. It also increases the absorption of iron that is needed for the increasing quantities of hemoglobin. The RDA standard recommends 70 mg/day for the pregnant woman, an increase of 10 mg/day over the regular adult need of 60 mg/day. Additional food sources such as citrus fruit and other vegetables and fruits should be included in the mother's diet.

Vitamin D

Adults who lead active lives involving adequate exposure to sunlight probably need little additional vitamin D. However, during pregnancy the increased need for calcium and phosphorus presented by the developing fetal skeletal tissue requires additional vitamin D to promote the absorption and utilization of these minerals. The recommended amount for pregnancy is 10 µg cholecalciferol (400 IU)/day. Food sources include fortified milk, liver, egg yolk, and fortified margarine.

Dietary Patterns: General and Alternative
General Daily Food Pattern

A variety of familiar foods usually supplies the mother's need for added nutrients and makes eating a pleasure. The increased quantities of essential nutrients needed during pregnancy may be met in many ways by planning around a daily food pattern and using key types of suggested core foods. A general daily food pattern that meets basic nutrient needs is suggested in Table 11-2. Compare the increases in each food group suggested for the pregnant or lactating adolescent or woman during the reproductive cycle with the basic amounts for the nonpregnant woman. It indicates increased amounts of basic foods during pregnancy to meet increased key nutrient needs. It may be used as a guide, with additional foods added according to individual energy needs and personal desires. This pattern represents the "orthodox middle-class American diet." It has been labeled the "biomedically recommended prenatal diet," which is generally used worldwide by most health professionals in industrialized, affluent countries.

Alternative Food Patterns

With the increasing ethnic diversity in our American culture, it is especially important to use the mother's personal cultural food patterns in dietary counseling. We are indeed ethnocentric if we rigidly adhere to the orthodox pattern previously discussed as the pattern for all pregnant women. It is itself but one alternative diet pattern among many others from different cultures, belief systems, and life-styles. We need to remind ourselves sometimes that an extreme unquestioning

---

TABLE 11-2

Daily Food Guide for Women

Food group	One serving equals		Nonpregnant 11-24 yr	Nonpregnant 25+ yr	Pregnant/ lactating
Protein foods	**Animal protein:**	**Vegetable protein:**	5	5	7
Provide protein, iron, zinc, and B vitamins for growth of muscles, bone, blood, and nerves; vegetable protein provides fiber to prevent constipation	1 oz cooked chicken or turkey 1 oz cooked lean beef, lamb, or pork 1 oz or ¼ cup fish or other seafood 1 egg 2 fish sticks or hot dogs 2 slices luncheon meat	½ cup cooked dry beans, lentils, or split peas 3 oz tofu 1 oz or ¼ cup peanuts, pumpkin, or sunflower seeds 1½ oz or ⅓ cup other nuts 2 tbsp peanut butter	A half serving of vegetable protein daily		One serving of vegetable protein daily
Milk products			3	2	3
Provide protein and calcium to build strong bones, teeth, and healthy nerves and muscles and to promote normal blood clotting	8 oz milk 8 oz yogurt 1 cup milk shake 1½ cups cream soup (made with milk) 1½ oz or ⅓ cup grated cheese (like cheddar, Monterey, mozzarella, or Swiss)	1½-2 slices presliced American cheese 4 tbsp Parmesan cheese 2 cups cottage cheese 1 cup pudding 1 cup custard or flan 1½ cups ice milk ice cream, or frozen yogurt			

Recommended minimum servings

NOTE: The Daily Food Guide for Women may not provide all the kcalories you require. The best way to increase your intake is to include more than the minimum servings recommended.

Adapted from California Department of Health Services, Maternal and Child Health: *Nutrition during pregnancy and postpartum period: a manual for health care professionals,* Sacramento, 1990, CDHS.

Continued.

TABLE 11-2

Daily Food Guide for Women—cont'd

			Recommended minimum servings		
			Nonpregnant		Pregnant/ lactating
Food group	One serving equals		11-24 yr	25+ yr	
Breads, cereals, grains					
Provide carbohydrates and B vitamins for energy and health nerves; also provide iron for healthy blood; whole grains provide fiber to prevent constipation	1 slice bread 1 dinner roll ½ bun or bagel ½ English muffin or pita 1 small tortilla ¾ cup dry cereal ½ cup granola ½ cup cooked cereal	½ cup rice ½ cup noodles or spaghetti ¼ cup wheat germ 1 4-inch pancake or waffle 1 small muffin 8 medium crackers 4 graham cracker squares 3 cups popcorn	7 Four servings	6 of whole grain products daily	7
Vitamin C-rich fruits and vegetables					
Provide vitamin C to prevent infection and to promote healing and iron absorption; also provide fiber to prevent constipation	6 oz orange, grapefruit, or fruit juice enriched with vitamin C 6 oz tomato juice or vegetable juice cocktail 1 orange, kiwi, or mango ½ grapefruit or cantaloupe ½ cup papaya 2 tangerines	½ cup strawberries ½ cup cooked or 1 cup raw cabbage ½ cup broccoli, brussels sprouts, or cauliflower ½ cup snow peas, sweet peppers, or tomato puree 2 tomatoes	1	1	1
Vitamin A-rich fruits and vegetables					
Provide beta-carotene and vitamin A to prevent infection and to promote wound healing and night vision; also provide fiber to prevent constipation	6 oz apricot nectar or vegetable juice cocktail 3 raw or ¼ cup dried apricots ¼ cantaloupe or mango 1 small or ½ cup sliced carrots 2 tomatoes	½ cup cooked or 1 cup raw spinach ½ cup cooked greens (beet, chard, collards, dandelion, kale, mustard) ½ cup pumpkin, sweet potato, winter squash, or yams	1	1	1
Other fruits and vegetables					
Provide carbohydrates for energy and fiber to prevent constipation	6 oz fruit juice (if not listed above) 1 medium or ½ cup sliced fruit (apple, banana, peach, pear) ½ cup berries (other than strawberries) ½ cup cherries or grapes ½ cup pineapple ½ cup watermelon	¼ cup dried fruit ½ cup sliced vegetable (asparagus, beets, green beans, celery, corn, eggplant, mushrooms, onion, peas, potato, summer squash, zucchini) ½ artichoke 1 cup lettuce	3	3	3
Unsaturated fats					
Provide vitamin E to protect tissue	⅛ medium avocado 1 tsp margarine 1 tsp mayonnaise 1 tsp vegetable oil	2 tsp salad dressing (mayonnaise-based) 1 tbsp salad dressing (oil-based)	3	3	3

pursuit of "science as magic" may well lead us to label any alternative practice as unscientific and unreasonable, thus closing our minds to some possibly fruitful avenues of scientific exploration. We must always remember that specific nutrients, not specific foods, are required for a successful pregnancy and that these nutrients are found in a wide variety of food choices. If we are wise we will encourage our clients to use foods that serve their nutritional needs, whatever those foods might be. A number of resources have been developed to serve as guides for a variety of alternative food patterns, ethnic and vegetarian.

In essence, then, two important principles govern the diet: (1) that the pregnant woman eat a sufficient quantity of food and (2) that she eat regularly, avoiding any habit of fasting or skipping meals, especially breakfast following the night's fast during sleep.

General Dietary Problems
Functional Gastrointestinal Problems
Nausea and Vomiting

These symptoms are usually mild and short-term. The condition is known as morning sickness of early pregnancy because it occurs more often on arising than later in the day. At least 50% of all pregnant women, most of them in their first pregnancy, experience this condition, beginning during the fifth or sixth week of the pregnancy and usually ending about the fourteenth to sixteenth week. A number of factors may contribute to the situation. Some are physiologic, based on hormonal changes that occur early in pregnancy. Others may be psychologic, based on situational tensions or anxieties about the pregnancy itself. Still others may be dietary problems, based on poor food habits. Simple treatment generally improves food toleration. Small frequent meals and snacks, fairly dry and consisting chiefly of easily digested energy-yielding foods, such as carbohydrates (mainly starches), are usually more readily tolerated. Also, it sometimes helps to avoid cooking odors as much as possible. Liquids are best taken between meals instead of with meals.

Hyperemesis

In a small number of pregnant women, about 3.5 per 1000 pregnancies, a severe form of persistent nausea and vomiting occurs that does not respond to usual treatment. This condition, hyperemesis, begins early in the pregnancy and may last throughout. It may develop into the more serious pernicious form of **hyperemesis gravidarum.** This persistent condition causes severe alterations in fluids and electrolytes, weight loss, and nutritional deficits, sometimes requiring alternative feeding by enteral or parenteral methods to sustain the pregnancy (see Chapter 18).[8] If the condition is unchecked, the mother is usually hospitalized and re-

ceives peripheral parenteral nutrition, followed by careful oral refeeding or tube feeding. In any case, continued personal support and reassurance are important.

Constipation

The complaint of constipation is seldom more than minor but contributes to discomfort and concern. Placental hormones relax the gastrointestinal muscles, and the pressure of the enlarging uterus on the lower portion of the intestine may make elimination somewhat difficult. Increased fluid intake and the use of naturally laxative foods containing dietary fiber, such as whole grains, fruits and vegetables, dried fruits (especially prunes and figs), and other fruits and juices generally induce regularity. Laxatives should be avoided.

Hemorrhoids

A fairly common complaint during the latter part of pregnancy is that of hemorrhoids. These are enlarged veins in the anus, often protruding through the anal sphincter. This vein enlargement is usually caused by the increased weight of the fetus and the downward pressure it produces. The hemorrhoids may cause considerable discomfort, burning, and itching. Occasionally, they may rupture and bleed under pressure of a bowel movement, causing the mother still more anxiety. The problem is usually controlled by the dietary suggestions given for constipation. Also, sufficient rest during the latter part of the day may help relieve some of the downward pressure of the uterus on the lower intestine.

Heartburn or Gastric Pressure

The related complaints of heartburn or a full feeling are sometimes voiced by pregnant women. These discomforts occur especially after meals and are usually caused by the pressure of the enlarging uterus crowding the stomach. Gastric reflux of some of the food mass, now a liquid chyme mixed with stomach acid, may occur in the lower esophagus, causing an irritation and burning sensation. Obviously, this common complaint has nothing to do with heart action, but is so called because of the proximity of the lower esophagus to the heart. The full feeling comes from general gastric pressure, lack of normal space in the area, a large meal, or gas formation. These complaints are usually remedied by dividing the day's food into a series of small meals and avoiding eating large meals at any time. Comfort is also improved by wearing loose-fitting clothing.

> **hyperemesis gravidarum** • Severe vomiting during pregnancy that is potentially fatal.

Effects of Iron Supplements

During pregnancy an iron supplement in the form of ferrous sulfate may be given to counteract the physiologic dilution anemia of pregnancy because of the increased circulating blood volume. The effects of added iron medication include gray or black stools and sometimes nausea, constipation, or diarrhea. To help avoid food-related effects, the iron supplement should be taken an hour before a meal or two hours after with liquid such as water or orange juice but not with milk or tea. The iron effect in the body is increased with vitamin C and decreased with milk, other dairy foods, eggs, whole grain bread and cereal, and tea.

Weight Gain During Pregnancy
General Amount of Weight Gain

Healthy women produce healthy babies over a wide range of total weight gain. It is the individual assessment of need and the quality of the weight gain that is paramount. Optimal weight gain from a quality diet throughout pregnancy makes an important contribution to a successful course and outcome. It should not be a problem or a source of contention. An average weight gain during pregnancy is about 11 to 14 kg (25 to 30 lb). Around this average many individual variations occur. There is no specific rigid norm or restriction to which all women should be held regardless of individual needs. Such a course is obviously unwise and unscientific. Current recommendations are therefore usually stated in terms of ranges to accommodate variances in needs. An initial base for evaluation, however, may be the average weight of the products of pregnancy as shown in Table 11-3. In addition to the components of growth and development usually attributed to a pregnancy, an important part is maternal stores. This laying down of extra adipose fat tissue is necessary for maternal energy reserves to sustain rapid fetal growth during the latter half of pregnancy and for labor and delivery and maintaining lactation after birth. About 2 to 3.5 kg (4 to 8 lb) of adipose tissue are commonly deposited for these needs. A current report of the National Academy of Sciences, *Nutrition During Pregnancy,*

recommends setting weight gain goals together with the pregnant woman according to her prepregnant nutritional status and weight-for-height[6]:

1. Normal weight women: 11.5 to 16.0 kg (25 to 35 lb)
2. Underweight women: 13.0 to 18.0 kg (28 to 40 lb)
3. Overweight women: 7.0 to 11.5 kg (15 to 25 lb)

The recommendation for adolescent mothers is that they should strive for the upper end of the range, 16 kg (35 lb). A woman carrying twins should have a target weight gain of 16 to 20.5 kg (35 to 45 lb).

Quality of Weight Gain

The important consideration, as indicated, lies in the nutritional quality of the gain.[9] Specifically, the foods consumed should be nutritious and meet the nutrient requirements, not contribute only empty kilocalories. Also, there has been failure in some cases to distinguish between weight gained as a result of edema and that due to deposition of fat—maternal stores for energy to sustain rapid fetal growth during the latter part of pregnancy and energy for lactation to follow. Analysis of the total tissue gained in an average pregnancy shows that the largest component, 62%, is water. Fat accounts for 31% and protein for 7%. Water is also the most variable component of the tissue gained, accounting for a range of 8 kg (18 lb) to as much as 11 kg (24 lb). Of the 8 kg of water usually gained, about 5.5 kg (12 lb) is associated with fetal tissue and other tissues gained in pregnancy. The remaining 2.5 kg (6 lb) accumulates in the maternal interstitial tissues.[10] Gravity causes the maternal tissue fluids to pool more in the lower extremities, leading to general swelling of the ankles, which is seen routinely in pregnant women. This fluid retention is a normal adaptive phenomenon designed to support the pregnancy and exert a positive effect on fetal growth. The connective tissue becomes more **hygroscopic** due to the estrogen-induced changes in the ground substance. The connective tissue thus becomes softer and more easily distended to facilitate delivery through the cervix and the vaginal canal. Also, the increased tissue fluid during pregnancy provides a means for handling the increased metabolic work and circulation of numerous metabolites necessary for fetal growth.

Clearly, severe kcaloric restriction is potentially harmful to the developing fetus and the mother. It is inevitably accompanied by restriction of the vitally needed nutrients essential to the growth process. Thus *weight reduction should never be undertaken during pregnancy.* To the contrary, sufficient weight gain should be encouraged with the use of a nourishing diet as outlined.

Rate of Weight Gain

On the whole, about 1.0 to 2.3 kg (2 to 5 lb) is an average weight gain during the first trimester. Thereaf-

---

TABLE 11-3

Approximate Weight of Products of Normal Pregnancy

Products	Weight
Fetus	3400 g (7.5 lb)
Placenta	450 g (1 lb)
Amniotic fluid	900 g (2 lb)
Uterus (weight increase)	1100 g (2.5 lb)
Breast tissue (weight increase)	1400 g (3 lb)
Blood volume (weight increase)	1800 g (4 lb) (1500 ml)
Maternal stores	1800-3600 g (4-8 lb)
TOTAL	10,850-12,650 g (10.8-12.7 kg; 24-28 lb)

ter, a weight gain of about 0.5 kg (1 lb) per week, more or less, during the remainder of the pregnancy is usual, although some women may need to gain more. There is no scientific justification for routinely limiting weight gain to lesser amounts. Moreover, an individual woman who needs to gain more should not have unrealistic grid patterns imposed upon her. It is only unusual patterns of gain, such as a sudden sharp increase in weight after the twentieth week of pregnancy, which may signal abnormal water retention, that should be monitored closely, especially if it occurs in conjunction with blood pressure elevation and proteinuria.

Weight Gain Related to Sodium Intake

Sometimes in relation to weight gain, questions are raised about the use of salt during pregnancy. A regular moderate amount of dietary sodium is needed for two essential reasons: (1) it is the major mineral required for controlling the extracellular fluid compartment; and (2) this vital body water is increased during pregnancy to support its successful outcome. Current practice usually follows a regular diet with moderate sodium intake, 2 to 3 g/day, with light use of salt to taste. Limiting sodium beyond this general use is contrary to physiologic need in pregnancy and is unfounded. The NRC and professional obstetric guidelines have labeled routine salt-free diets and diuretics as potentially dangerous.[2-4] Maintaining the needed increase in circulating blood volume during pregnancy requires adequate amounts of sodium and protein.

High-Risk Mothers and Infants
Identify Risk Factors Involved

To avoid the consequences of poor nutrition during pregnancy, a first procedure is to identify mothers at risk (see Clinical Application, p. 220). In a joint report, the American College of Obstetrics and the American Dietetic Association have issued a set of risk factors as shown in Table 11-4 that identify women with special nutritional needs during pregnancy.[4] These nutrition-related factors are based on clinical evidence of inadequate nutrition. However, rather than waiting for clinical symptoms of poor nutrition to appear, a better approach would be to identify poor food patterns that will bring on nutritional problems and prevent these problems from developing.[10] On this basis, three types of dietary patterns predict failure to support optimal maternal and fetal nutrition: (1) insufficient food intake, (2) poor food selection, and (3) poor food distribution throughout the day. These patterns, added to the list of risk factors in Table 11-4, are much more sensitive for nutritional risk.

Plan Personal Care

Once early assessment identifies risk factors, practitioners can then give more careful attention to these

TABLE 11-4
Nutritional Risk Factors in Pregnancy

Risk factors present at the onset of pregnancy	Risk factors occurring during pregnancy
Age	Low hemoglobin or hematocrit
15 years or younger	Hemoglobin less than 12 g
35 years or older	Hematocrit less than 35 mg/dl
Frequent pregnancies; three or	Indadequate weight gain
more during a 2-year period	Any weight loss
Poor obstetric history or poor fe-	Weight gain of less than 1 kg
tal performance	(2 lb) per month after the
Poverty	first trimester
Bizarre or faddist food habits	Excessive weight gain: greater
Abuse of nicotine, alcohol, or	than 1 kg (2 lb) per week after
drugs	the first trimester
Therapeutic diet required for a	
chronic disorder	
Inadequate weight	
Less than 85% of standard	
weight	
More than 120% of standard	
weight	

women. By working closely with each mother and her personal food pattern and living situation, the nutritionist can develop a food plan with her to ensure an optimal intake of energy and nutrients to support her pregnancy and its successful outcome.

Recognize Special Counseling Needs

Several special needs require sensitive counseling. These areas of need include the age and parity of the mother, any use of harmful agents such as alcohol, cigarettes, or drugs, and socioeconomic problems.

Age and Parity

Pregnancies at either age extreme of the reproductive cycle pose special problems. The adolescent pregnancy carries many social and nutrition-related risks. Imposed on a still immature teenage body are the additional demands of the pregnancy. The obstetric history of a woman is expressed in terms of number and order of pregnancies, or her **gravida** status. **Nulligravidas** (no prior pregnancy) 15 years old and younger are especially at risk, since their own growth is incomplete, so sufficient weight gain and the quality of their diet are particularly important.[11,12] Sensitive counseling provides both information and emotional support. It

---

gravida • A pregnant woman.

hygroscopic • Taking up and retaining moisture readily.

nulligravida • A woman who has never been pregnant.

CLINICAL APPLICATION

Who Will Have the Low-Birth-Weight Baby?

The number of babies weighing less than 2500 g (5 lb) at birth is on the rise. It is a leading cause of infant mortality in the United States. It also contributes to poor cognitive abilities and learning problems in the school-age children who survive.

Perinatal nutritionists are well aware of the dietary factors that may influence this increase, especially poor weight gain during pregnancy. The prevalence of that turn-of-the-century adage to "grow the baby to fit the pelvis" continues to influence some physicians, nurses, and expectant mothers alike to limit prenatal weight gain to 9 kg (20 lb) or less to avoid obstetric problems, especially at delivery. This practice is harmful and is refuted by recent evidence that a gain of 11 to 15 kg (25 to 35 lb) is correlated with birth weights of greater than 2500 g (5 lb).

The obsession with weight control during pregnancy can lead to harmful restrictions of vital energy and nutrients. Weight reduction should *never* be attempted during pregnancy. Such regimens are extremely dangerous to the fetus. Even the common practice of skipping breakfast, especially late in pregnancy, may potentially impair intellectual development by inducing a ketotic, pseudostarvation state very quickly. Increased ketoacidosis from fat breakdown can cause neurologic damage to the fetus.

Nondietary factors influencing the incidence of low-birth weight (LBW) or premature babies have been identified in numerous studies:

- Rise in number of older primigravidas (that is, over 35 years of age)
- Rise in number of teenage pregnancies
- Low socioeconomic status, low educational level
- History of obstetric problems, such as prior LBW birth or reproductive loss
- Poor nutritional status, including low prepregnant weight for height, low energy intake during pregnancy, low hemoglobin level and hematocrit, inadequate early weight gain
- Clinical problems such as pregnancy-induced hypertension (PIH)
- Behavioral/environmental risk factors, smoking, alcohol and drug abuse
- Single marital status (often an indicator of low economic status)
- Technologic advances in neonatal care, which keep premature infants alive longer
- Race: nonwhites have higher rates of LBW infants than whites do, which is more a function of poverty, limited education, or young age rather than race as such

To reduce the risk of LBW infants in populations being served by your facility, you may want to do the following:

- Explain the rationale for gaining around 11 to 15 kg (25 to 30 lb).
- Discourage the use of cigarettes, alcohol, and drugs.
- Monitor excessive weight gain and sodium intake in older primigravidas, who are often at risk for prenatal essential hypertension and obesity.
- Explore eating habits of adolescents in the local community, working with the girl and her significant others to incorporate nutrient-dense foods into her meal and snack selections.
- Keep abreast of federal, state, and local supplemental food programs (for example, WIC) available to low-income women to ensure an adequate intake of nutrients and kilocalories.
- Encourage regular eating patterns throughout pregnancy.

REFERENCES

Hack M and others: Effect of very low birth weight and subnormal head size on cognitive abilities at school, *N Engl J Med* 325(4):231, July 25, 1991.

Haughton B and others: Public health nutrition practices to prevent low birth weight in eight southeastern states, *J Am Diet Assoc* 92(2):187, 1992.

Joyce T: The dramatic increase in the rate of low birthweight in New York City: an aggregate time-series analysis, *Am J Pub Health* 80(6):682, 1990.

Saigal S and others: Cognitive abilities and school performance of extremely low birth weight children and matched control children at age 8 years: a regional study, *J Pediatr* 118:118, May, 1991. ◆

should involve family or other persons significant to the young mother. On the other hand, the older **primigravida** (first pregnancy), over 35 years of age, also requires special attention. She may be more at risk for hypertension, either preexisting or pregnancy induced, and may need more attention to rate of weight gain and amount of sodium used, as well as any drug therapy prescribed.[13,14] In addition, several pregnancies within a limited number of years leave a mother drained of nutritional resources and entering each successive pregnancy at a higher risk. Counseling may well include discussions of acceptable means of contraception and nutrition information and support.

Social Habits: Alcohol, Cigarettes, and Drugs

These three personal habits cause fetal damage and are contraindicated during pregnancy. Extensive or habitual alcohol use leads to the well-described and documented fetal alcohol syndrome (FAS), which is currently a leading cause of mental retardation. Cigarette smoking during pregnancy is also contraindicated. Harmful substances in tobacco cause fetal damage and special problems of placental abnormalities, including prematurity and low birth weight (see Clinical Application above), due largely to impaired oxygen transport. Counseling with mothers who smoke should certainly stress the importance of quitting.

Drug use, both recreational and medicinal, also poses numerous problems. Self-medication with over-the-counter drugs carries potential adverse effects. The use of street drugs is especially hazardous, exposing the developing fetus to the risks of addiction and AIDS from the mother's use of contaminated needles. Dangers come not only from the drug itself or contaminated needles but also from the impurities such street drugs contain. In addition, drug abuse from megadosing with basic nutrients such as vitamin A during pregnancy may also bring fetal damage.[15] Especially dangerous are drugs made from vitamin A compounds that are prescribed for severe acne, such as the retinoids isotretinoin (Accutane) and etretinate, which have caused spontaneous abortion of malformed infants in women who conceived during such acne treatment.[16] Thus the use of these drugs without contraception is definitely contraindicated.

Caffeine

Although milder in its effect, depending on extent of use, than agents discussed above, caffeine is still a widely used drug that can cross the placenta and enter fetal circulation. Its use at pharmacologic levels has been associated with with low birth weight. A pharmacologic dose of caffeine—250 mg—is contained in 2 cups of coffee, 3.5 cups of tea, or five 12-oz colas, so such use is not recommended.[17] Most responsible health agencies have recommended that pregnant women avoid caffeine-containing beverages and that products containing caffeine be plainly labeled to inform consumers.

Socioeconomic Problems

Special counseling is required for women and young girls living in low-income situations or extreme poverty. Numerous studies and clinical observations indicate that lack of prenatal care, often associated with racial prejudices and fears as well as poverty, places the expectant mother in grave difficulty.[18,19] Special counseling, sensitive to personal needs, is required to help plan resources for care and financial assistance. Resources include programs such as WIC and the Commodity Distribution Program, both of which are described in Chapter 10.

Complications of Pregnancy

Anemia

Anemia is common during pregnancy. It is often associated with a normal maternal blood volume increase of about 50% and a disproportionate increase in red cell mass of about 20%.[20] About 10% of all women in large prenatal clinics in the United States have hemoglobin concentrations of less than 10 g/dl and a hematocrit reading below 32%. Anemia is far more prevalent among the poor, many of whom live on diets barely adequate for subsistence. However, anemia is by no means restricted to lower economic groups.

Iron-Deficiency Anemia

A deficiency of iron is by far the most common cause of anemia in pregnancy. The total cost of a single normal pregnancy in iron stores is large—about 500 to 800 mg. Of this amount nearly 300 mg is used by the fetus. The remainder is used in the expanded maternal blood volume and its increased red blood cells and hemoglobin mass. This iron requirement exceeds the available reserves in the average woman. Thus, in addition to including iron-rich foods in the diet, a daily supplement of 30 to 60 mg is recommended. Treatment of highly deficient states requires more, daily therapeutic doses of 120 to 200 mg, which is usually continued for 3 to 6 months after the anemia has been corrected to replenish the depleted stores.

Folate-Deficiency Anemia

A less common megaloblastic anemia of pregnancy results from folate deficiency. During pregnancy, the fetus is sensitive to folate inhibitors and therefore has increased metabolic requirements for folate. To prevent this anemia, the RDA standard recommends 400 µg of folate daily. Women with poor diets will need supplementation to reach this intake goal.

Hemorrhagic Anemia

Anemia caused by blood loss is more likely to occur during labor and delivery rather than during pregnancy. Blood loss may occur earlier, as a result of abortion or ruptured tubular pregnancy. Most patients undergoing these physiologic problems receive blood by transfusion, and iron therapy may be indicated for adequate replacement hemoglobin formation.

Pregnancy-Induced Hypertension (PIH)
Relation to Nutrition

A number of clinicians have presented clinical and laboratory evidence that pregnancy-induced hypertension (formerly labeled toxemia) is a disease principally affecting young mothers with their first pregnancy. It is especially related to diets poor in protein, kcalories, calcium, and salt. Such malnutrition affects the liver and its metabolic activities. Whatever its underlying causes and multiorgan effects, nutritional support of the pregnancy is, as always, a primary concern. Certainly, as many practitioners have observed, PIH is classically associated with poverty, inadequate diet, and

---

primigravida • A woman pregnant for the first time.

little or no prenatal care. Much of the PIH problem, which seems to develop early from the time of implantation of the fertilized ovum into the uterine lining, may be reduced by good prenatal care from the beginning of the pregnancy, which inherently includes attention to sound nutrition.[21,22] It is this sound nutritional status, which a woman brings to her pregnancy and maintains throughout, that provides her with optimal resources for adapting to the physiologic stress of gestation. Her fitness during pregnancy is a direct function of her past good state of nutrition and her optimal nutrition throughout pregnancy.

Clinical Symptoms

PIH is defined according to its manifestations, which generally occur in the third trimester. These symptoms are hypertension, abnormal and excessive edema, albuminuria, and in severe cases convulsions or coma, a state called **eclampsia.**

Treatment

Specific treatment varies according to the individual patient's symptoms and needs. Optimal nutrition is a fundamental aspect of therapy in any case. Emphasis is given to a regular diet with adequate dietary protein and calcium. Correction of plasma protein deficits stimulates the capillary fluid shift mechanism and increases circulation of tissue fluids, with subsequent correction of the **hypovolemia** (see Chapter 8). In addition, adequate salt and sources of vitamins and minerals are needed for correction and maintenance of metabolic balance.

Maternal Disease Conditions

Preexisting clinical conditions in the mother further complicate pregnancy. In each case, management of these conditions is based on general principles of care related both to pregnancy and to the particular disease involved. Examples of three such maternal conditions are reviewed here. They are hypertension, diabetes mellitus, and phenylketonuria.

Hypertension

Preexisting hypertension in the pregnant woman can cause considerable maternal and fetal consequences. Many of these problems can be prevented by initial screening and continued monitoring by the prenatal nurse, with referral to the clinical nutritionist for plan of care. The hypertensive disease process begins long before signs and symptoms appear and later symptoms are inconsistent. Risk factors for hypertension before and during pregnancy are given in Table 11-5. Nutritional therapy centers on (1) prevention of weight extremes, underweight or obesity, (2) correction of any dietary deficiencies and maintenance of optimal nutritional status during pregnancy, and (3) management

TABLE 11-5		
Risk Factors in Pregnancy-Induced Hypertension		
Before pregnancy		**During pregnancy**
Nulligravida		Primigravida
Diabetes mellitus		Large fetus
Preexisting condition (hypertension, renal or vascular disease)		Glomerulonephritis
Family history of hypertension or vascular disease		Fetal hydrops
Diagnosis of pregnancy-induced hypertension in a previous pregnancy		Hydramnios
Dietary deficiencies		Multiple gestation
Age extremes		Hydatidiform mole
20 years or younger		
35 years or older		

of any related preexisting disease such as diabetes mellitus or hyperlipidemia.[23] Sodium intake may be moderate but should not be unduly restricted because of its relation to fluid and electrolyte balances during pregnancy and its controversial therapy in hypertension in general. Initial and continuing client education and a close relationship with the nurse-nutritionist care team contribute to successful management of the hypertension and prevent problems that may occur.

Diabetes Mellitus

The management of diabetes in pregnancy presents special problems. Today, however, improved expectations for the diabetic mother's pregnancy constitute one of the success stories of modern medicine.[24] Contributing factors to this improved outlook include advances in technology for monitoring fetal development, increased knowledge of nutrition and diabetes, and especially management refinements in tight blood glucose control through self-monitoring. Routine screening is necessary to detect gestational diabetes, and team management is required for preexisting insulin-dependent diabetes mellitus (IDDM). During pregnancy, glycosuria is not uncommon because of the increased circulating blood volume and its load of metabolites. Gestational diabetes occurs in 2% to 13% of the pregnant population.[25] But only 20% to 30% of these women showing this pregnancy-induced abnormal glucose tolerance subsequently develop diabetes. Nonetheless, follow-up is important because of the higher risk these women carry for fetal damage during this gestational period. Refer to Chapter 21 for a detailed discussion of diabetes care.

Maternal Phenylketonuria

Successful detection and management of phenylketonuria (PKU) babies through U.S. newborn screening programs in all states has ensured their normal growth and development to adulthood. PKU is a genetic meta-

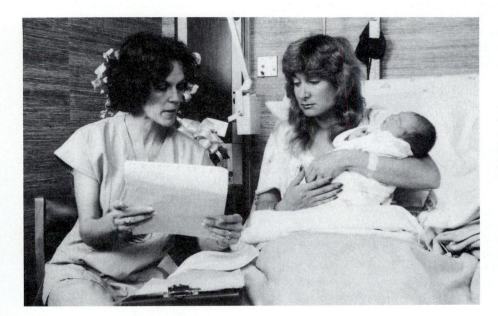

FIG. 11-1   Nurse discussing post-partum and infant care with new mother.

bolic disease due to a missing enzyme for the metabolism of the essential amino acid phenylalanine. It is controlled by a special low-phenylalanine diet initiated at birth. Now a new generation of young women with PKU since birth are beginning to have children of their own. However, maternal PKU presents potential fetal hazards. Experience has shown how crucial it is for the mother to follow a strict low-phenylalanine diet prior to conception, whenever possible, to minimize risks of fetal damage in the early cell differentiation weeks of pregnancy.[26]

Nutrition During Lactation

Current Breast-Feeding Trends

An increasing number of mothers in America and other developed countries are choosing breast-feeding for their infants (see To Probe Further, p. 224). Several factors have contributed to this choice: (1) more mothers are informed about the benefits of breast-feeding (Fig. 11-1); (2) practitioners recognize the ability of human milk to meet infant needs (Table 11-6); (3) maternity wards and alternative birth centers are being modified to facilitate successful lactation; and (4) community support is more available, even in work places. Exclusive breast-feeding by well-nourished mothers can be adequate for periods ranging from 2 to 15 months. Solid foods are usually added to the baby's diet at about 6 months of age.

Nutritional Needs

The physiologic needs of lactation are greater than those of pregnancy, and they demand adequate nutritional support (see Tables 11-1 and 11-2). The basic nu-

tritional needs for lactation include the following additions to the mother's prepregnant needs.

Protein

The RDA standard for protein needs during lactation is 65 g/day during the first 6 months and 62 g/day during the second 6 months. This is an increase of about 15 to 20 g/day from the regular needs of the adolescent girl (44 to 46 g/day) and the adult woman (46 to 50 g/day).

Energy

The recommended kcaloric increase is 500 kcal more than the usual adult allowance. This makes a daily total of about 2500 to 2700 kcal. This additional energy need for the overall total lactation process is based on three factors:

Milk content.   An average daily milk production for lactating women is 850 ml (30 oz). Human milk has a kcal range of 20 to 70 kcal/oz or an average of 24 kcal/oz. Thus 30 oz of milk has a value of about 700 kcal.

Milk production.   The metabolic work involved in producing this amount of milk requires from 400 to 450 kcal. During pregnancy the breast is developed for

---

eclampsia • Advanced pregnancy-induced hypertension (PIH), manifested by convulsions.

hypovolemia • Abnormally decreased volume of circulating blood in the body.

Breast-Feeding: The Dynamic Nature of Human Milk

There is no question that human milk is the ideal first food for human infants. Its dynamic nature changes to match the infant's growth needs. The mother's choice to breast-feed her infant depends on a number of factors, however, especially for new mothers who often need information and counseling from early in the pregnancy.

TO PROBE FURTHER

Even premature infants can thrive on human milk. Mothers and physicians have sometimes been reluctant to consider breast-feeding for babies born prematurely or delivered by cesarean section, fearing that there may be some negative effect on the quantity or quality of human milk. This uncertainty about the nutritional quality of mother's milk has also led them to encourage adding formula or solid foods to the diet to make sure the baby is well fed. These practices are usually unnecessary. They often contribute to allergies, obesity, and digestive problems because of the extra stress placed on an immature gut.

Breast milk for the preterm infant

Levels of nutrients in mother's milk shift according to the gestational age of the infant at birth. The preterm infant is often spared its mother's milk by some hospital workers because they think of it as mature milk, having too little protein and too much lactose to meet the child's needs. An analysis of the nutritional quality of preterm milk, however, reveals energy and fat concentrations that are 20% to 30% higher, protein levels 15% to 20% higher, and lactose levels 10% lower than those found in mature milk. Premature milk can meet the preterm infant's needs.

Breast milk during weaning

Nutrient levels continue to change with time to match changing growth patterns and developing digestive abilities. Mother's milk does provide sufficient kilocalories and nutrients to keep babies well-fed without supplemental formula or food. Even when the infant is being weaned, the nature of human milk ensures adequate nutrients, just in case the new, solid-food diet can't meet the child's needs. Human milk collected during gradual weaning has been found to have higher concentrations of protein, sodium, and iron. Lactose levels are lower, possibly so that higher amounts of kilocalories can be supplied by fats, a more concentrated source.

Breast milk and the cesarean section infant

The quality of human milk is not influenced by the way the baby comes into the world. Many women fear that a baby born by cesarean section cannot be nursed, because they think that this method of delivery delays or prevents the production of mature milk. Milk production is stimulated by the release of the placenta, which occurs whether the delivery is vaginal or not. Studies confirm that there is no significant difference in the length of time it takes for mature milk to come in after vaginal and cesarean deliveries.

Thus premature or cesarean deliveries should not discourage women from breast-feeding. Mothers should not underestimate the nutritive quality of their milk simply because it does not appear as rich and thick as cow's milk. After all, cow's milk is made for young calves who are up and running around after birth and have a much shorter, faster growth period. But for the human infant, in both nutritional and immunologic terms, breast milk remains the best milk.

Mothers' fact and fancy about breast-feeding

In early counseling, mothers do express a variety of concerns about breast-feeding, some of which are-valid and some not. These are a few such statements:

"My breasts aren't big enough." When it comes to breast-feeding, all women are created equal. The only parts of the breast that participate in milk production are the glandular and nervous tissue, as well as the nipple; these are basically the same in healthy women. The only difference between a 32A and a 42DD is the amount of fat the breast contains.

"Breast-feeding causes cancer." Actually, in recent years, investigators have been looking to breast-feeding as a possible means of preventing breast cancer. At this point, no studies exist that convincingly show that breast-feeding either helps or hinders a woman from developing this disease.

"Breast-feeding will ruin my figure." Breast-feeding might actually help a woman regain her figure more quickly. Because the caloric demand of breast-feeding exceeds that of the nonpregnant woman by about 500 kcal, a slightly faster rate of weight loss might be expected. Furthermore, oxytocin, the hormone manufactured to stimulate milk production, also stimulates uterine contractions, helping reduce the uterus to its prepregnant size more rapidly.

"Breast-feeding is painful." It can be if the baby is nursed infrequently or the mother's hygienic practices leave much to be desired. However, if milk is not allowed to collect in the breast to the point of engorgement, if the nipples are kept clean and dry, and if proper latch-on techniques are used while nursing, the chances for having a painful experience will be relatively small.

"Breast milk isn't nutritious." The thin, bluish appearance of breast milk has some women convinced that it is no more nourishing than water. Let them look at Table 11-6; they'll be pleasantly surprised at how well breast milk meets the nutritional needs of the infant.

"I can't go to work/school if I breast-feed." Breast milk can be stored for 24 hours in the refrigerator or several months in the freezer. Many working mothers take advantage of this by expressing their milk and storing it for use by a baby-sitter. In fact, women often express milk on their breaks at school or work. (Some employers even provide breast pumps at the work place.) Not only does this relieve the pressure of buildup, but it also allows the milk to be stored for later use at home.

Other women would like to breast-feed but are worried about special "what if" situations, such as:

"What if I need a cesarean section?" The method of delivery does not affect the quality or quantity of milk pro-

duced. And the baby can be held in such a way (the football hold) that he or she does not rest on the mother's abdominal stitches.

"What if the baby is premature?" Mother's milk changes to meet the infant's needs at all stages of development.

"What if the baby has a birth defect such as Down syndrome?" This baby can be nursed; however, it does require time, patience, and the use of slightly different nursing techniques. The mother should be told about the special nursing needs of this infant to avoid disappointment or a feeling of failure in case breast-feeding becomes impractical for her particular living situation.

"What if I have twins?" Believe it or not, it has been done. It takes time, patience, and good coordination, but it can be done. Triplets, however, are another matter altogether. Women have successfully nursed triplets, but often they did very little else until the babies were weaned. This mother will need emotional support whether she attempts to nurse or, finding the amount of time and patience required overwhelming, is forced to bottle-feed.

Some women may purposefully choose to breast-feed to avoid pregnancy. But this is by no means a dependable contraception method. The more well-nourished women of the world tend to be more fertile and have been less than pleasantly surprised to find themselves pregnant and breast-feeding at the same time. Women who breast-feed must understand that the lack of a menstrual period during lactation does not mean they cannot become pregnant. Contraceptives, preferably barrier types, may be required if another pregnancy is not desired at that time.

Advantages and barriers to breast-feeding

These factors need to be reviewed with each individual mother in her particular situation. Only on this basis can she make the informed decision best for the baby and for her.

There are many nutritional, physiologic, psychologic, and practical advantages to breast-feeding:
1. *Human milk changes* to meet changing nutrient and energy needs of both the newborn and the maturing infant during the first months of life. It is always there in the correct form to meet the growing infant's needs.
2. *Fewer infections,* since the mother transfers certain antibodies or immune properties in human milk to her nursing infant. Also, there is no exposure of the infant to infectious organisms in the environment that can contaminate preparation and equipment for bottle-feeding, especially in poorer living situations.
3. *Fewer allergies and intolerances,* especially in allergy-prone infants, since cow's milk contains a number of potentially allergy-causing proteins that human milk does not have.
4. *Ease of digestion,* since human milk forms a softer curd in the gastrointestinal tract that is easier for the infant to digest.
5. *Convenience and economy,* since the mother is free from the time and expense involved in buying and preparing formula, and her breast milk is always ready and sterile.
6. *Psychologic bonding,* since the mother and infant relate

TO PROBE FURTHER

to one another during feeding, regular times of rest and enjoyment, cuddling, and fulfillment.

Despite the advantages of breast feeding, some women do have to deal with perceived barriers associated with misinformation, personal feelings of modesty, family pressures, or outside employment.

1. *Misinformation,* a major barrier, creates negative impressions and ideas. Women in today's world often lack positive role models in extended families or experienced friends with whom they can discuss their feelings and obtain much practical guidance. Experienced breast-feeding mothers can fill this need, especially for young first-time mothers.
2. *Personal modesty and anxiety,* or a fear of appearing immodest in breast exposure, may hinder some young mothers from breast-feeding. Sensitive counseling, especially with a positive role model as described, can help to allay some of these personal fears. Most of women's breast-feeding is in the privacy of the home, rather than around others, so early support during initial experiences would be helpful.
3. *Family pressures,* especially from the husband, not to breast-feed have strong influence on the young first-time mother, even though she may want to do so. Initial counseling and education about breast-feeding should include both parents whenever possible. Reasons for negative attitudes can be explored and misinformation clarified with sound education.
4. *Outside employment,* with a limited maternity leave and job loss if the mother does not return to work at that time, can complicate the mother's decision, even though she may want to breast-feed her baby. However, if the mother does have the will, there are ways to do both. After breast-feeding is well established during her maternity leave, she can regularly express milk by hand or with a breast pump into sterile disposal nursing bags to use with disposal holder, cap, and nipple ensemble. Rapid chilling and strict sanitation are required, but can be planned, given the commitment. Some companies provide child care facilities for their employees, recognizing this modern need as good business. And the mother can plan occasional formula feeds to fill in with the sustained breast-feeding.

All of these approaches to breast-feeding have real rewards for the infant. In addition, they can strengthen the mother's confidence in her own maternal capabilities. The importance even of these intangible benefits should not be underestimated.

REFERENCES

Armotrading DC and others: Impact of WIC utilization rate on breast-feeding among international students at a large university, *J Am Diet Assoc* 92(3):352, 1992.

Ghaemi-Ahmadi, S: Attitudes toward breast-feeding among Iranian, Afghan, and Southeast Asian immigrant women in the United States: implications for health and nutrition education, *J Am Diet Assoc* 92(3):354, 1992.

Jason J: Breast-feeding in 1991, *N Engl J Med* 325(14):1036, Oct 3, 1991.

Kistin N and others: Breast-feeding rates among Black urban low-income women: effect of prenatal education, *Pediatrics* 86(5):741, 1990.

TABLE 11-6
Nutritional Components of Human Milk (per 100 ml)

Milk component	Colostrum	Transitional	Mature	Cow's milk
Kilocalories	57.0	63.0	65.0	65.0
Vitamins, fat-soluble:				
A (μg)	151.0	88.0	75.0	41.0
D (IU)	—	—	5.0	2.5
E (mg)	1.5	0.9	0.25	0.07
K (μg)	—	—	1.5	6.0
Vitamins, water-soluble:				
Thiamin (μg)	1.9	5.9	14.0	43.0
Riboflavin (μg)	30.0	37.0	40.0	145.0
Niacin (μg)	75.0	175.0	160.0	82.0
Pantothenic acid (μg)	183.0	288.0	246.0	340.0
Biotin (μg)	0.06	0.35	0.6	2.8
Vitamin B_{12} (μg)	0.05	0.04	0.1	0.6
Vitamin C (mg)	5.9	7.1	5.0	1.1

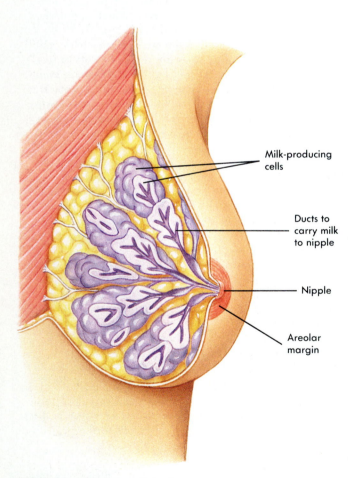

FIG. 11-2   Anatomy of the breast.

Milk-producing cells

Ducts to carry milk to nipple

Nipple

Areolar margin

this purpose, stimulated by hormones from the placenta, forming special milk-producing cells called lobules (Fig. 11-2). After birth the mother's production of the hormone prolactin continues this milk-production process, which the suckling infant stimulates. Thus milk production depends on the demand of the infant. The suckling infant stimulates the brain's release of the hormone oxytocin from the pituitary gland to initiate the let-down reflex for the release of the milk from storage cells to travel down to the nipple. This reflex is easily inhibited by the mother's fatigue, tension, or lack of confidence, a particular source of anxiety in the new mother. She may be reassured that a comfortable and satisfying feeding routine is usually established in 2 to 3 weeks (Fig. 11-3).

Maternal adipose tissue storage.   The additional energy need for lactation is drawn from maternal adipose tissue stores deposited during pregnancy in normal preparation for lactation to follow in the maternal cycle. Depending on the adequacy of these stores, additional energy input may be needed in the lactating woman's daily diet.

Minerals

The RDA standard for calcium during lactation is 1200 mg/day, the same as for the nonpregnant adolescent girl and the young adult woman, but a 400-g increase from the regular adult need of 800 mg. The calcium needs of the breast-feeding mother are not greater than those needed during pregnancy. The increased amount of calcium that was required during gestation for the mineralization of the fetal skeleton is now diverted into the mother's milk production. Iron, because it is not a principal mineral component of milk, need not be increased for the production of milk.

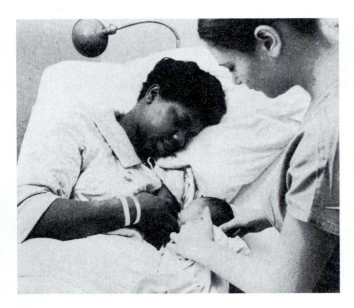

FIG. 11-3 Breast-feeding the newborn infant. Note that the nurse, in assisting the mother, avoids touching the infant's outer check so as not to counteract his natural rooting reflex at the touch of the breast.

In addition, for the breast-feeding infant, the American Academy of Pediatrics recommends a fluoride supplement of 0.25 mg/day, because lactating mothers produce milk that is low in fluoride (about 16 μg/L).[27]

Vitamins

The RDA standard for vitamin C during lactation is 95 mg/day during the first 6 months and 90 mg/day for the second 6 months. This is a considerable increase from the regular 50 to 60 mg/day for adolescent girls and 60 mg/day for adult women. Increases over the mother's prenatal intake are also recommended for vitamin A, since it is a constituent of milk, and for the B-complex vitamins, because they are involved as coenzyme factors in energy metabolism. The quantities of vitamins needed therefore invariably increase as the kcalorie intake increases.

Fluids

Adequate fluid intake is needed, but contrary to common beliefs additional fluid beyond this need does not increase the mother's milk supply. Additionally, it is difficult to drink when one is not thirsty; natural thirst guides sufficient intake. The more critical factor necessary for successful milk production is the increased energy intake. The basis for this increased caloric need is described in the previous discussion. Additional beverages such as juices and milk contribute both fluid and kcalories.

Rest and Relaxation

In addition to the increased diet, the nursing mother requires rest, moderate exercise, and relaxation. Both parents may benefit from counseling focused on reducing the stresses of their new family situation, as well as meeting their own personal needs.

To Sum Up

Pregnancy involves synergistic interactions among three distinct biologic entities: the fetus, the placenta, and the mother. Maternal needs reflect the increasing nutritional needs of the fetus and the placenta, as well as the need to meet maternal needs and to prepare for lactation. An optimal weight gain of about 11 kg (25 lb), or more as needed, is recommended during pregnancy to accommodate the rapid growth taking place. Even more significant than the actual weight gain, though it must be sufficient, is the quality of the diet.

Common problems occurring during pregnancy include nausea and vomiting, heartburn, and constipation. In most cases they are easily relieved without medication by simple, often temporary changes in the diet. Serious problems with pregnancy may be associated with preexisting chronic maternal conditions, for example, diabetes mellitus, or conditions arising as a result of physical or metabolic demands of pregnancy, for example, iron-deficiency anemia and PIH. Unusual or erratic eating habits, age, parity, prepartum weight status, and low income are among the many related factors that also place the mother at risk for complications.

The ultimate goal of prenatal care is a healthy infant and a mother physically capable of breast-feeding her child, should she choose to do so. Human milk provides essential nutrients in quantities required for optimal infant growth and development. It also supplies immunologic factors that offer protection against infection. Lactation requires an increase in kcalories beyond the needs of pregnancy. Adequate fluid intake is guided by the mother's natural thirst.

QUESTIONS FOR REVIEW

1. List and discuss five factors that influence the nutritional needs of the woman during pregnancy. Which factors would place a woman in a high-risk category? Why?
2. List six nutrients that are required in larger amounts during pregnancy. Describe their special role during this period. Identify four food sources of each.
3. Identify two common problems associated with pregnancy and describe the dietary management of each.
4. List and describe the screening indicators and risk factors for hypertension and diabetes mellitus during pregnancy.
5. List and discuss five major nutritional factors of lactation.

REFERENCES

1. Jacobson HN: A healthy pregnancy: the struggle to define it, *Nutr Today* 23(1):30, Feb 1988.

2. Food and Nutrition Board, Committee on Maternal Nutrition, National Research Council–National Academy of Sciences: *Maternal nutrition and the course of human pregnancy,* Washington, DC, 1970, National Academy Press.

3. American College of Obstetricians and Gynecologists, Committee on Nutrition: *Nutrition in maternal health care,* Chicago, 1974, The College.

4. American College of Obstetricians and Gynecologists and American Dietetic Association, Task Force on Nutrition: *Assessment of maternal nutrition,* Chicago, 1978, The College and Association.

5. Food and Nutrition Board, National Academy of Sciences–National Research Council: *Recommended dietary allowances,* ed 10, Washington, DC, 1989, National Academy Press.

6. Hemminki E, Rimpala U: A randomized comparison of routine versus selective iron supplementation during pregnancy, *J Am Coll Nutr* 10(1):3, 1991.

7. Barclay BA: Experience with enteral nutrition in the treatment of hyperemesis gravidarum, *Nutr Clin Pract* 5:153, 1990.

8. Susser M: Maternal weight gain, infant birth weight, and diet: causal sequences, *Am J Clin Nutr* 53:1384, 1991.

9. King JC: Dietary risk patterns during pregnancy, *Nutr Update* 1:206, 1983.

10. Johnson CS and others: Pregnancy weight gain in adolescents and young adults, *J Am Coll Nutr* 10(3):185, 1991.

11. Skinner JD, Carruth BP: Dietary quality of pregnant and nonpregnant adolescents, *J Am Diet Assoc* 91(6):718, 1991.

12. Sibai BM: Chronic hypertension in pregnancy, *Clin Perinatol* 18(4):833, 1991.

13. Walker JJ: Hypertensive drugs in pregnancy, *Clin Perinatol* 18(4):845, 1991.

14. New York State Department of Health: Use of supplements containing high-dose vitamin A, *JAMA* 257:1292, 1987.

15. Watson RR: Vitamin A and teratogenesis: recommendations for pregnancy, *J Am Diet Assoc* 88(3):364, 1988.

16. Fenster L and others: Caffeine consumption during pregnancy and fetal growth, *Am J Public Health* 81(8):1023, 1991.

17. Hansell MJ: Sociodemographic factors and quality of prenatal care, *Am J Public Health* 81(8):1023, 1991.

18. Schneck ME and others: Low-income pregnant adolescents and their infants: dietary findings and health outcomes, *J Am Diet Assoc* 90(4):555, 1990.

19. Mitchell MC, Lerner E: Maternal hematologic measures and pregnancy outcomes, *J Am Diet Assoc* 92(4):484, 1992.

20. Repke JT: Prevention of preeclampsia, *Clin Perinatol* 18(4):779, 1991.

21. Zuspan FP: New concepts in the understanding of hypertensive diseases during pregnancy, *Clin Perinatol* 18(4):653, 1991.

22. Sanderson SL and others: Successful hyperlipemic pregnancy, *JAMA* 265(14):1858, 1991.

23. Jovanovic-Peterson L, Peterson CM: Diabetes manipulation as a primary treatment strategy for pregnancies complicated by diabetes, *J Am Coll Nutr* 9(4):320, 1990.

24. Hadden DR: Geographic, ethnic, and racial variations on the incidence of gestational diabetes mellitus, *Diabetes* 34 (suppl):8, 1985.

25. Waisbren SE and others: Psychosocial factors in maternal phenylketonuria: prevention of unplanned pregnancies, *Am J Public Health* 81(3):299, 1991.

26. American Academy of Pediatrics, Committee on Nutrition: Fluoride supplementation, *Pediatrics* 177:758, 1986.

27. Dusdieker LB and others: Prolonged maternal fluid supplementation in breast-feeding, *Pediatrics* 86(5):737. 1990.

FURTHER READING

Jack BW and Culpepper L: Preconception care, risk reduction and health promotion in preparation for pregnancy, *JAMA* 264(9):1147, 1990.

These caring physicians discuss the priority of the 1990s, as identified in the Institute of Medicine's *Preventing Low Birthweight,* through preconception nutrition assessment, improving risk status, and preparing families for childbearing.

Carruth BR, Skinner JD: Practitioners beware: regional differences in beliefs about nutrition during pregnancy, *J Am Diet Assoc* 91(4):435, 1991.

Horner RD and others: Pica practices of pregnant women, *J Am Diet Assoc* 91(1):34, 1991.

These articles provide information about various food beliefs and practices that need to be investigated during the prenatal period.

Haughton B and others: Public health nutrition practices to prevent low birth weight in eight southeastern states, *J Am Diet Assoc* 92(2):187, 1992.

This article reviews the problem of low birth weight, a leading cause of infant mortality in the United States, and the efforts of a group of public health nutritionists in the southern Region IV of the US Department of Health and Human Services to assess and reduce the problem.

CASE STUDY

A Baby for the Delgados

Felicia Delgado is a 19-year-old married primigravida who tested positive for urinary human chorionic gonadotropin (HCG) 2 weeks ago. Mrs. Delgado is 151 cm (5 ft, 5 in) tall with an average pregravid weight of 57 kg (125 lb). Current gestational age: 6 weeks. Her history for chronic disorders and other serious health programs is negative.

During her initial diet interview, Mrs. Delgado indicated that the pregnancy was unplanned. She seemed especially worried about the effects of her diet on the baby. As college students, she and her 21-year-old husband had erratic meals, dominated by junk food. Mrs. Delgado's 24-hour diet history revealed an inadequate intake of dark green or yellow vegetables and milk products, as well as meat or eggs and citrus fruits. The couple realized that these types of foods were an important part of a nutritious diet but are inexperienced as cooks and feel they lack the time and money to prepare healthful meals every day.

At the end of the initial counseling session, the nutritionist told the couple about a series of prenatal group discussions conducted by members of the clinic's perinatal health team, including sessions on pregnancy, labor and delivery, and the care and feeding of the infant. These are attended primarily by a mixture of experienced parents and young, first-time parents-to-be and are offered as a means of introducing practical aspects of pregnancy and parenting.

The Delgados attended every prenatal group meeting and kept all consequent diet-counseling sessions. Their food choices improved in time, and Mrs. Delgado's weight gain progressed normally, to a total of 12 kg (28 lb) by the time of delivery. The Delgados had a healthy 4 kg (8 lb, 2 oz) baby girl.

Questions for Analysis

1. What health professional ideally should be included on the health care team caring for Mrs. Delgado? Describe the significance of each role to the outcome of her pregnancy. What roles do Mr. and Mrs. Delgado have?
2. What nutritional deficiencies would you expect in Mrs. Delgado's diet? What practical problems would you expect her to encounter in attempting to improve her diet?
3. Write a 1-day meal plan for Mrs. Delgado, taking into account her life-style and schedule, as well as the amounts of nutrients considered adequate for pregnancy.
4. Write a lesson plan for a group session on nutrition during pregnancy. Include a general description, behavioral objectives, content outline. Include a general description, behavioral objectives, content outline, teaching methods and materials, and evaluation tool(s) you would use.
5. Would you encourage Mrs. Delgado to breast-feed? If so, why? What factors would you expect might discourage her for trying? How would you discuss these factors?
6. Write a lesson plan for an infant feeding session, addressing breast- and bottle-feeding methods. Include the components listed in questions 3 and 4.

Drug Use and the Outcome of Pregnancy

Since the tragic discovery a number of years ago of the teratogenic effects of thalidomide, the interest in the effects of drugs used during pregnancy has risen dramatically among health workers and the general public. The tragic consequences of inappropriate drug use make it of essential that the nutritionist or nurse, while obtaining a dietary history, also gather a complete history of drug use, both licit and illicit, to warn the mother of the potential dangers involved and have her discuss in detail any prescribed drugs with her physician. Listed here are descriptions of the effects of a variety of common drugs on the pregnant woman, the fetus, and the outcome of pregnancy.

Alcohol

No safe level of alcohol consumption has yet been found for pregnant women, despite a recent claim that pregnant women can safely have up to two drinks a day. Even moderate social drinking has been associated with subclinical signs of fetal alcohol syndrome (FAS). This disorder is characterized by growth retardation, malformed facial features, joint and limb abnormalities, cardiac defects, mental retardation, and, in serious cases, death. FAS signs have been seen in tests with rats as early as the human equivalent of the third week of gestation, when most women are unaware of their pregnancies. Thus moderate to heavy drinking among sexually active women of childbearing age may carry potential danger.

The nutritional problems of FAS are similar to those seen in chronic alcoholism. A zinc deficiency has specifically been associated with congenital defects and impairs immune function among children born to alcohol abusers. Alcohol has also induced signs of secondary hyperparathyroidism in pregnant animals, thus potentially affecting serum calcium levels.

Psychotropic drugs

A number of drugs have routinely been prescribed for female patients to treat a variety of neuroses and psychoses. If taken during pregnancy, they exhibit teratogenic effects.

Lithium has recently been associated with an increased risk for Epstein's anomaly (a rare cardiovascular abnormality), goiter, diabetes insipidus, as well as neonatal toxic disturbances such as cyanosis, hypothermia, and bradycardia. A diminished suck reflex will impede attempts to nourish the infant exposed to lithium in utero.

Diazepam (Valium) is associated with an abnormal fetal heart rate. The neonate risks delivery by cesarean section, with oral-facial malformations, a depressed Apgar score, and a reluctance to feed. Rats exposed to diazepam in utero have exhibited abnormal motor skills and arousal processes.

Tricyclic antidepressants (for example, imipramine) have led to morphologic and behavioral abnormalities in rats.

Anticonvulsants

Phenytoin (Dilantin, Hydantoin) is prescribed to control seizures caused by epilepsy and other conditions. Even though this drug has caused malformations in the offspring of rats, physicians are reluctant to discontinue it for their patients with epilepsy during pregnancy. Because only 7% of children born to mothers using the drug develop malformations, and significantly more develop malformations and developmental disabilities when the mother's epilepsy goes untreated, this may be one case in which prenatal drug use is more beneficial than not using it.

Caffeine

Apparently it is wise to avoid this very commonly used stimulant, at least during pregnancy. Pregnant women who are heavy coffee drinkers are considered at risk for miscarriages, premature deliveries, and small-for-gestational-age infants. Therefore intake of caffeinated foods, beverages (coffee, tea, cocoa, cola), and medications should be curtailed.

Marijuana

Evaluation of the effects of street drugs (marijuana, LSD, heroin, methadone) on nutritional status is difficult because of multiple drug use, uncertain purity, unknown dosage and timing, and inadequate nutritional status of many drug users. A 1982 report on a study of marijuana use in 35 pregnancies revealed a higher incidence of meconium staining (which could relate to fetal damage), poor prenatal weight gain, very short (less than 3 hours) or prolonged labor, operative delivery (cesarean, forceps, or vacuum), and other perinatal problems among marijuana users. Although the researchers admitted flaws in their study (for example, the use of subjects who chose to participate or not), the outcome indicates a need to investigate these potentially fatal effects further.

Nicotine

Cigarette smoking has been well documented for its association with low-birth-weight infants, impairment of mental and physical growth, and increased potential mortality. The dietary implications of prenatal smoking are presented in at least one study showing that, although the smokers may eat more than nonsmokers, they still deliver smaller babies. In addition, nicotine's ability to increase heart rate, blood pressure, and fat breakdown compromises the health and nutritional status of mother and infant alike.

Thus, with the exception of those used to treat individuals with seizure disorders or natural replacement therapy (for example, insulin for persons with type I diabetes), drugs should be avoided at all costs during pregnancy to ensure the health of the mother and a safe and healthy outcome of the pregnancy. The nutrition counselor would

Drug Use and the Outcome of Pregnancy—cont'd

be well advised to keep up with the most recent findings regarding medications (prescribed, over-the-counter, and street drugs) to evaluate the nutritional status of the mother using them and warn her of the potential harm they may pose for her and her baby.

REFERENCES

Fenster L and others: Caffeine consumption during pregnancy and fetal growth, *Am J Pub Health* 81(4):458, Apr 1991.

Frank DA and others: Cocaine and marijuana use during pregnancy by women intending and not intending to breast-feed, *J Am Diet Assoc* 92(2):215, 1992.

Petitti DB, Coleman C: Cocaine and the risk of low birth weight, *Am J Pub Health* 80(1):25, Jan, 1990.

Serdula M and others: Trends in alcohol consumption by pregnant women, *JAMA* 265(7):876, Feb 20, 1991.

Nutrition for Growth and Development

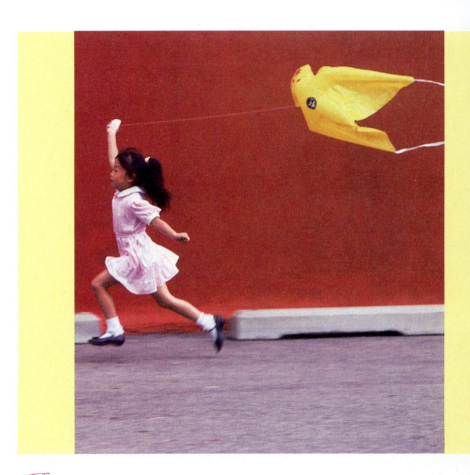

*I*n this second chapter in our life cycle series, we look at growing infants, children, and adolescents. We consider their physical growth and their inseparable psychosocial development at each progressive stage.

This unified growth and development nurtures the integrated nature of the child into that of the adult. The *whole* process produces the *whole* person.

Here, within this dual framework, we consider food and feeding as as a vital part of the whole development of the child. In each age group, we relate nutritional needs and the food that supplies them to the normal physical maturation and psychosocial development achieved at each stage.

Human Growth and Development
Individual Needs of Children

Growth may be defined as an increase in size. Biologic growth of an organism occurs through cell multiplication. Development is the associated process in which growing tissues and organs take on increased complexity of function. Both of these processes are part of one whole, forming a unified inseparable concept of growth and development. Through these changes a small dependent newborn is transformed into a fully functioning independent adult. However, each child is a unique individual with individual needs. This is a paramount principle in working with children. Thus we must always seek to discover these individual human needs if we are to help each child reach his or her greatest growth and development potential.

Normal Life Cycle Growth Pattern

The normal human life cycle follows four general stages of overall growth and development:

Infancy

Growth velocity is rapid during the first year of life, with the rate tapering off in the latter half of the year. At age 6 months an infant has probably doubled the birth weight and at 1 year may have tripled it.

Childhood

In the latent period of childhood between infancy and adolescence, the growth rate slows and becomes erratic. At some periods there are plateaus. At other times small spurts of growth occur. The overall **growth deceleration** affects appetite accordingly. At times children will have little or no appetite, and at other times they will eat voraciously. Parents who know that this is a normal pattern relax and do not make eating a battleground with their children.

Adolescence

With the beginning of puberty the second **growth acceleration** period occurs. Because of the hormonal influences involved, enormous physical changes develop. These changes include the development of long bones, sex characteristics, and fat and muscle mass.

Adulthood

In the final stage of a normal life cycle, growth levels off on the adult plateau. Then it gradually declines during old age—the period of senescence.

Measuring Childhood Physical Growth
Growth Charts

Children grow at widely varying individual rates. In clinical practice a child's pattern of growth is compared with **percentile** growth curves derived from measurement of numbers of children throughout the growth years. Contemporary **growth chart grids** have been developed by the National Center for Health Statistics (NCHS) and reflect a broad base for growth patterns in children today. These charts are based on data from large numbers of a nationally representative sample of children. Two age intervals are used: birth to 36 months and 2 to 18 years, with separate curves for boys and for girls (see Appendix H).

Anthropometry

Practitioners use **anthropometry** to monitor a child's growth, with the growth charts and other clinical standards as reference. A number of methods and measures may be employed.

Weight and height. These are common general measures of physical growth. They provide a basic measure but give only a crude index of growth without showing finer details of individual variations. They are used mainly to look for patterns of growth over time, as the individual child's pattern is plotted on the related age group chart. The recumbent length of infants and small children is measured initially, then standing height as they grow older.

Body circumferences and skin folds. The head circumference is a valuable measure in infants but is seldom taken routinely after 3 years of age. Measures of abdomen, chest, and leg at its maximal girth of the calf are usually included at periodic intervals. Other measures for monitoring muscle mass growth and **body**

---

anthropometry • The science of measuring the size, weight, and proportions of the human body.

body composition • The relative sizes of the four basic body compartments that make up the total body: lean body mass (muscle mass), fat, water, and bone.

growth acceleration • Period of increased speed of growth at different points of childhood development.

growth chart grids • Grids comparing stature (length), weight, and age of children by percentile; used for nutritional assessment to determine how their growth is progressing. The most commonly used grids are those of the National Center for Health Statistics (NCHS), published by the Fels Research Institute.

growth deceleration • Period of decreased speed of growth at different points of childhood development.

growth velocity • Rapidity of motion or movement; rate of childhood growth over normal periods of development, as compared with a population standard.

percentile • One of 100 equal parts of a measured series of values; rate or proportion per hundred.

composition include the midarm circumference and the triceps skinfold at the same point. Using these two measures, the midarm muscle circumference can be calculated easily (see Chapter 16). Skin fold measures, including a number of body sites, are done with special calipers and require skill and practice for accuracy. Longitudinal growth studies in research centers employ many measures of development in addition to these basic monitoring ones used in general practice.

Clinical Signs

Various clinical signs of optimal growth may be observed as measures of a child's nutritional status. These include such factors as general vitality; a sense of well-being; good posture; healthy gums, teeth, skin, hair, and eyes; muscle development; and nervous control. Refer to Table 1-1 (Chapter 1) for a review of these general signs and observations.

Laboratory Tests

In addition, other measures of growth can be obtained by various laboratory tests. These may include studies of blood and urine to determine levels of hemoglobin, vitamins, and similar substances (see Appendix J). X-ray films of the hand and wrist may be used to measure degree of bone development.

Nutritional Analysis

A nutritional analysis of general eating habits (see Chapter 10) provides helpful information for assessing growth needs. A diet history form (see Fig. 10-1) and food value tables (see Appendix A) may be used. In clinical practice, however, diet evaluations are usually done by computer. The nutritionist uses information from a variety of methods for a basic food intake analysis to use in diet counseling with the parents.[1,2]

Mental and Psychosocial Development
Mental Growth

Measures of mental growth usually involve abilities in speech and other forms of communication, as well as the ability to handle abstract and symbolic material in thinking. Young children think in very literal terms. Then, as they develop in mental capacity, they can handle more than single ideas and form constructive concepts.

Emotional Growth

Emotional growth is measured in the capacity for love and affection, as well as the ability to handle frustration and its anxieties. It also involves the child's ability to control aggressive impulses and to channel hostility from destructive to constructive activities.

Social and Cultural Growth

Social development of a child is measured in terms of the ability to relate to others and to participate in group living and cultural activities. These social and cultural behaviors are first learned through relationships with parents and family, all of which have much influence on food habits and feeding patterns. As the child's horizon broadens, relationships are developed with those outside the family, with friends, and with others in the community, at school or at church or at other social gatherings. For this reason a child's play during the early years is a highly purposeful activity.

Nutritional Requirements for Growth
Energy Needs

During childhood the demand for kcalories is relatively great. However, there is much variation in need with age and condition. For example, the total daily kcaloric intake of a 5-year-old child is spent in the following ways: (1) about 50% supplies basal metabolic requirements (BMR); (2) 5% is involved in the thermic effect of food (TEF) that is eaten, that is, in the work of digestion, absorption, and general stimulation of metabolism; (3) various physical activities require about 25%; (4) 12% is needed for tissue growth; and (5) about 8% is represented in fecal loss. Of these kcalories, carbohydrate is the primary energy source, and is also important to spare protein for its essential growth needs rather than having it spent for energy. Fat kcalories are important as backup energy sources, but particularly as sources of essential fatty acids such as linoleic acid needed for growth. However, an excess of fat, especially from animal sources, should be avoided.

Protein Needs

Protein provides the essential building materials for tissue growth—amino acids. As a child grows, the requirements per unit of body weight gradually decrease. For example, during the first 6 months of life an infant requires 2.2 g/kg of body weight. This amount gradually decreases until adulthood, when protein needs are only about 0.8 g/kg. Usually the healthy, active, growing child will consume the necessary amount of kcalories and protein in the variety of foods provided.

Water Requirements

The infant's relative need for water is greater than that of the adult. The infant's body content of water is 70% to 75% of the total body weight, whereas in the adult water constitutes only about 60% to 65% of the total body weight. Also, a large amount of the infant's total body water is *outside* the cell and more easily lost. The child's water need is related to the kcaloric intake and the urine concentration. Generally an infant drinks daily an amount of water equivalent to 10% to 15% of body weight, whereas the adult's daily amount equals 2% to 4% of the body weight. A summary of approximate daily fluid needs during the growth years is given in Table 12-1.

TABLE 12-1

Approximate Daily Fluid Needs During Growth Years

Age	ml/kg
0-3 months	120
3-6 months	115
6-12 months	100
1-4 years	100
4-7 years	95
7-11 years	90
11-19 years	50
>19 years	30

Mineral and Vitamin Needs

In your previous study of minerals and vitamins, you learned of their essential roles in tissue growth and maintenance and in overall energy metabolism. Positive childhood growth and development depend on an adequate amount of these essential substances. For example, rapidly growing young bones require calcium and phosphorus. An x-ray film of a newborn's body would reveal a skeleton appearing as a collection of disconnected, separate bones requiring mineralization. Calcium is also needed for the developing teeth, muscle contraction, nerve irritability, blood coagulation, and heart muscle action. Another mineral of concern is iron, essential for hemoglobin formation. The infant's fetal store is diminished in 4 to 6 months. Thus solid food additions at that time help supply needed iron. Such initial foods as enriched cereal and egg and later meat accomplish this. The use of iron-fortified formulas and foods, especially by high-risk children enrolled in the WIC program, has greatly reduced the incidence of iron-deficiency anemia among children.

Excess amounts of two vitamins, A and D, are of concern in feeding children. Excess intake of these vitamins may occur over prolonged periods because of misunderstanding, ignorance, or carelessness. Parents must be carefully instructed to use only the amount directed and no more. These excesses bring clear toxic symptoms:

1. *Vitamin A.* Symptoms of toxicity from excess vitamin A include lack of appetite, slow growth, drying and cracking of the skin, enlargement of the liver and spleen, swelling and pain of long bones, and bone fragility.
2. *Vitamin D.* Symptoms of toxicity from excess vitamin D include nausea, diarrhea, weight loss, excess urination especially at night, and eventual calcification of soft tissues, including those of renal tubules, blood vessels, bronchi, stomach, and heart.

A summary of the overall nutritional needs for growth, as recommended by the National Research Council (NRC), is given in Table 12-2.

Stages of Growth and Development: Age Group Needs

The Stages of Human Life

Throughout the human life cycle food and feeding not only serve to meet nutritional requirements for physical growth, but they also relate intimately to personal psychosocial development. The nutritional age-group needs of children cannot be understood apart from the child's overall maturation as a unique person. Over the past 30 years, Erikson's theory of human development has come to play a significant role in our view of the human life cycle.[3] A leading American psychoanalyst, Erikson has contributed much insight to our understanding of human personality and growth throughout critical periods of our development.

Psychosocial Development

Erikson has identified eight stages in human growth and a basic psychosocial developmental problem for the crisis the person struggles with at each stage. The developmental problem at each stage has a positive ego value and a conflicting negative counterpart:

1. *Infant*—Trust versus distrust
2. *Toddler*—Autonomy versus shame and doubt
3. *Preschooler*—Initiative versus guilt
4. *School-age child*—Industry versus inferiority
5. *Adolescent*—Identity versus role confusion
6. *Young adult*—Intimacy versus isolation
7. *Adult*—Generativity versus stagnation
8. *Older adult*—Ego integrity versus despair

Given favorable circumstances, a growing child develops positive ego strength at each life stage and therefore builds increasing inner resources and strengths to meet the next life crisis. The struggle at any age, however, is not forever won at that point. A residue of the negative remains, and in periods of stress, such as an illness, regression in some degree usually occurs. But as the child gains mastery at each stage of development, assisted by significant positive relationships of support, integration of self-controls takes place. Various related developmental tasks surround each of these stages. This is learning that, when accomplished, contributes to successful resolution of the core problem.

Physical Growth

The developmental tasks of childhood food choices and feeding practices are intimately related. Food habits do not develop in a vacuum. They flow as an integral part of physical and psychosocial development. In this section we relate these two influences to the general age group's developmental characteristics.

At each of the age group stages of childhood we discuss, food and feeding practices are integrated and associated with the normal physical and psychosocial maturation. Various neuromuscular motor skills enable the child to accomplish related physical activities. Psy-

TABLE 12-2

RDA for Growth (National Research Council, 1989 version)

		Weight		Height		Energy	Protein	Fat-soluble vitamins			
	Age(yr)	(kg)	(lb)	(cm)	(in)	(kcal)	(g)	Vit. A (μg RE)	Vit. D (μg)	Vit. E (mg α-TE)	Vit. K (μg)
Infants	0-0.5	6	13	60	24	650	13	375	7.5	3	5
	0.5-1	9	20	71	28	850	14	375	10	4	10
Children	1-3	13	29	90	35	1300	16	400	10	6	15
	4-6	20	44	112	44	1800	24	500	10	7	20
	7-10	28	62	132	52	2000	28	700	10	7	30
Males	11-14	45	99	157	62	2500	45	1000	10	10	45
	15-18	66	145	176	69	3000	59	1000	10	10	65
Females	11-14	46	101	157	62	2200	46	800	10	8	45
	15-18	55	120	163	64	2200	44	800	10	8	55

chosocial development influences food attitudes, behavior, patterns, and habits.

Infant (Birth to 1 Year)

Physical Characteristics of a Full-Term Infant

The full-term infant is born after successful growth and development during a normal gestation period of about 40 weeks (280 days), weighing approximately 3.2 kg (7 lb). During the first year of life, the infant grows rapidly, from this average birth weight to a 1-year-old child ready to walk and weighing about 9 kg (20 lb). Thus energy requirements during this first year of tremendous growth are high.

Full-term infants have the ability to digest and absorb protein, a moderate amount of fat, and simple carbohydrate. They have some difficulty with starch, since amylase, the starch-splitting enzyme, is not being produced at first. However, as starch is introduced, this enzyme begins to function. The renal system functions well, but more water relative to size is needed than in an adult to manage urinary excretion. Their first baby teeth do not erupt until about the fourth month, so initial food must be liquid or semiliquid. They have limited nutritional stores from gestation, especially in iron. Thus they need supplements of vitamins and minerals, first in concentrated drops and later in semisolid food additions to their first food—breast milk or a substitute infant formula. The newborn's **rooting reflex** and somewhat recessed lower jaw are natural adaptations for feeding at the breast.

Psychosocial Development

The core psychosocial developmental task during infancy is the establishment of trust versus distrust. Much of the infant's early psychosocial development is **tactile** in nature, from touching and holding, especially in feeding. Feeding is the infant's main means of establishing human relationships. The close mother-infant bonding in the feeding process fills the basic need to build trust. The need for sucking and the development of the oral organs—lips and mouth—as sensory organs represent adaptations to ensure an adequate early food intake for survival. As a result, food becomes the infant's general means of exploring the environment and is one of the early means of communication. As muscular coordination involving the tongue and the swallowing reflex develops, infants gradually learn to eat a variety of semisolid foods, beginning at about 6 months of age. As physical and motor maturation develop, they begin to show a desire for self-feeding. When these stages of development occur, the exploration of new powers should be encouraged. If their needs for food and love are fulfilled in this early relationship with the mother, father, or other feeding adult, as well as in broadening relationships with other family members, trust is developed. They evidence this trust by an increasing capacity to wait a bit for feedings until they are prepared.

Breast-feeding

The ideal food for the human infant is human milk. It has specific characteristics that match the infant's nutritional requirements during the first year of life. The process of breast-feeding today, as in the past, is successfully initiated and maintained by most women who try. However, sometimes there are problems, as well as a high degree of variability among nursing mothers as to frequency of feedings and intake and growth indexes. Thus, in providing support for mothers who want to breast-feed their babies, experienced nutritionists and nurses, many of whom are certified professional lactation counselors, advise flexibility rather than a rigid approach.

The mother's breasts, or mammary glands, are highly specialized secretory organs, as indicated in the previous chapter and illustrated in Fig. 11-1. They are com-

Water-soluble vitamins						Minerals							
Vit. C (mg)	Thiamin (mg)	Riboflavin (mg)	Niacin (mg NE)	Vit. B_6 (mg)	Folate (μg)	Vit. B_{12} (μg)	Calcium (mg)	Phosphorus (mg)	Magnesium (mg)	Iron (mg)	Zinc (mg)	Iodine (μg)	Selenium (μg)
30	0.3	0.4	5	0.3	25	0.3	400	300	40	6	5	40	10
35	0.4	0.5	6	0.6	35	0.5	600	500	60	10	5	50	15
40	0.7	0.8	9	1.0	50	0.7	800	800	80	10	10	70	20
45	0.9	1.1	12	1.1	75	1.0	800	800	120	10	10	90	20
45	1.0	1.2	13	1.4	100	1.4	800	800	170	10	10	120	30
50	1.3	1.5	17	1.7	150	2.0	1200	1200	270	12	15	150	40
60	1.5	1.8	20	2.0	200	2.0	1200	1200	400	12	15	150	50
50	1.1	1.3	15	1.4	150	2.0	1200	1200	280	15	12	150	45
60	1.1	1.3	15	1.5	180	2.0	1200	1200	300	15	12	150	50

posed of glandular tissue, fat, and connective tissue. The secreting glandular tissue has 15 to 20 lobes, each containing many smaller units called lobules. In the lobules secretory cells called alveoli or acini form milk from the nutrient material supplied to them by a rich capillary system in the connective tissue. During pregnancy the breasts are prepared for lactation. The alveoli enlarge and multiply and toward the end of the prenatal period secrete a thin, yellowish fluid called **colostrum.** As the infant grows, the breast milk develops, adapting in composition to meet growth needs.

Breast milk is produced under the stimulating influence of the hormone prolactin from the anterior pituitary gland. After the milk is formed in the mammary lobules by the clusters of secretory cells (alveoli or acini), it is carried through converging branches of the **lactiferous ducts** to reservoir spaces called **ampullae** under the **areola,** the pigmented area of skin surrounding the nipple. Two other pituitary hormones, principally oxytocin and to a lesser extent vasopressin, stimulate the ejection of the milk from the alveoli to the ducts, releasing it to the baby. This is commonly called the let-down reflex. It causes a tingling sensation in the breast and the flow of milk. The initial sucking of the baby stimulates this reflex. The newborn rooting reflex, oral needs for sucking, and the basic hunger drive usually induce and maintain normal relaxed breast-feeding for the healthy mother.

The mother should follow the baby's lead with an on-demand schedule. The baby's continuing rhythm of need establishes feedings, usually about every 3 to 4 hours. The mother can feed the baby for about 5 to 10 minutes on each breast, burping the baby gently between each period of sucking to expel swallowed air and noting when the baby is satisfied and then removing him from the breast. The nipple should air dry to prevent irritation and soreness. Interval use of a pacifier provides more sucking if needed.

The mother's diet and rest are important factors in establishing lactation and breast-feeding. Table 11-2 indicates a balanced diet to support ample milk production, including food choices from various food groups for meals and snacks. Natural thirst guides adequate fluid intake. Adequate rest and relaxation for the mother are essential. She should be guided not to allow an undue concern about the usually slow rate of weight loss after childbirth to lead her to curtail her diet and thus compromise her milk supply. This energy supply is especially important in the early weeks of establishing the regular milk production. Afterward, a

ampullae • A general term for a flasklike wider portions of a tubular structure; spaces under the nipple of the breast for storing milk.

areola • A defined space; circular area of different color surrounding a central point, such as the darkened pigmented ring surrounding the nipple of the breast.

colostrum • Thin yellow fluid first secreted by the mammary gland a few days before and after childbirth, preceding the mature breast milk. It contains up to 20% protein including a large amount of lactalbumin, more minerals and less lactose and fat than does milk, and immunoglobulins representing the antibodies found in maternal blood.

lactiferous ducts • Branching channels in the mammary gland that carry breast milk to holding spaces near the nipple ready for the infant's feeding.

rooting reflex • A reflex in a newborn in which stimulation of the side of the cheek or the upper or lower lip causes the infant to turn its mouth and face to the stimulus.

tactile • Pertaining to the touch.

gradual weight loss occurs naturally, but the mother should not unrealistically expect a rapid return to her prepregnant weight.[4] Breast-feeding is simple and enjoyable for the healthy, relaxed mother and infant. A nutritionally adequate diet ensures ample milk production. Infant supplements of vitamins K and D are usually given, but supplements of iron and fluoride are controversial.

However, for the premature and low-birth-weight baby, feeding through the first year of life poses more problems. These special needs are discussed in Issues and Answers (p. 249).

Bottle-feeding

Formula feeding by bottle may be preferred by some mothers. If the mother does not choose breast-feeding or stops early, bottle-feeding of an appropriate formula is an acceptable alternative. A variety of commercial formulas that approximate human milk composition are available. Several types of constituent protein are used, as shown in Table 12-3, including cow's milk base, soy protein, **casein hydrolysate, elemental** amino acids, or meat base. Some of the milk-based formulas are whey-adjusted to more nearly approximate the protein ratio in human milk. Standards for levels of nutrients required in infant formulas are based on recommendations from the American Academy of Pediatrics. Currently, minimum levels are established for 29 nutrients, and maximum levels for nine nutrients.[5]

When formula is given, the baby should be cradled in the arm, as in breast-feeding. The close human touch and warmth are important. When the infant is obviously satisfied, extra milk should not be forced, regardless of the amount remaining in the bottle. Any remaining formula should be thrown away and not refrigerated for reuse. Infants usually take the amount of formula they need. Today most infants are fed on a so-called demand schedule, which works out to be about every 3 to 4 hours. A healthy infant will soon establish an individual pattern according to growth requirements.

Cow's Milk

Regular unmodified cow's milk is not suitable for infants for three reasons: (1) it causes gastrointestinal bleeding; (2) its **renal solute load** is too heavy for the infant's renal system to handle, leaving too small a margin of safety for maintaining water balance during illness, diarrhea, or hot weather; and (3) it affects iron status, not only because of the gastrointestinal bleeding and blood loss but also because it is low in iron and its high calcium and phosphorus levels inhibit iron absorption.[6] In addition, infants should not use reduced fat milks, such as nonfat or 2% fat, for two reasons: (1) insufficient energy is provided to support requirements, causing body fat to be used to make up the deficit; and (2) linoleic acid in the fat portion of milk is the essential fatty acid needed for growth and development of body tissues. A specific form of eczema has been observed in infants deficient in linoleic acid, and a low-fat diet in infancy may harm physical and intellectual development.[7] To meet the special needs of in-

---

TABLE 12-3

A Comparison of Types of Formulas Manufactured for Full-Term Infants

Type of formula used		Protein content	Fat content	Carbohydrate content
Milk-based routine	Source:	Nonfat cow's milk	Vegetable oils	Lactose
	g/100 kcal:	2.2-2.3	5.4-5.5	10.4-10.8
	% Kcal:	9	48-50	41-43
Whey-adjusted routine	Source:	Nonfat cow's milk plus demineralized whey	Vegetable and oleo oils	Lactose
	g/100 kcal:	2.2	5.4	10.8
	% Kcal:	9	48	43
Soy isolate/cow's milk sensitivity	Source:	Soy isolate	Vegetable oils	Corn syrup solids and/or sucrose
	g/100 kcal:	2.7-3.2	5.1-5.6	9.9-10.2
	% Kcal:	12-13	45-51	39-40
Casein hydrolysate/protein sensitivity, galactosemia	Source:	Casein hydrolysate	Corn oil or corn oil and MCT*	Tapioca starch and glucose, sucrose, or corn syrup solids
	g/100 kcal:	2.8-3.3	3.9-4.0	13.1-13.6
	% Kcal:	11-13	35	52-54
Meat-based cow's milk sensitivity, galactosemia	Source:	Beef hearts	Sesame oil and beef heart fat	Tapioca starch and sucrose
	g/100 kcal:	4.0	4.8	9
	% Kcal:	16	47	37

*Medium-chain triglycerides.

TABLE 12-4

TABLE 12-4

Guideline for Adding Solid Foods to Infant's Diet During the First Year*

When to start	Foods added	Feeding
Fifth to sixth month	Cereal and strained cooked fruit	10 AM and 6 PM
	Egg yolk (at first, hard boiled and sieved; soft boiled or poached later)	
	Strained, cooked vegetable and strained meat	2 PM
	Zwieback or hard toast	At any feeding
Seventh to ninth month	Meat: beef, lamb, or liver (broiled or baked and finely chopped)	10 AM and 6 PM
	Potato: baked or boiled and mashed or sieved	

Suggested meal plan for age 8 months to 1 year or older

7 AM	Milk	240 ml (8 oz)
	Cereal	2-3 tbsp
	Strained fruit	2-3 tbsp
	Zwieback or dry toast	
12 NOON	Milk	240 ml (8 oz)
	Vegetables	2-3 tbsp
	Chopped meat or one whole egg	
	Puddings or cooked fruit	2-3 tbsp
3 PM	Milk	120 ml (4 oz)
	Toast, zwieback, or crackers	
6 PM	Milk	240 ml (8 oz)
	Whole egg or chopped meat	
	Potato: baked or mashed	2 tbsp
	Pudding or cooked fruit	2-3 tbsp
	Zwieback or toast	

*Semisolid foods should be given immediately before milk feeding. One or two teaspoons should be given at first. If food is accepted and tolerated well, the amount should be increased to 1 to 2 tablespoons per feeding.

NOTE: Banana or cottage cheese may be used as substitution for any meal.

fants, the American Academy of Pediatrics recommends breast milk or formulas up to 1 year of age, with a gradual addition of appropriate foods beginning at 6 months. There is no need for currently marketed special formulas for older infants and they are an added expense.[8]

Beikost: Solid Food Additions

No nutritional need exists for introducing solid foods to infants earlier than 4 to 6 months of age.[9,10] Earlier use may contribute to allergies. Nutritional and medical authorities agree that for the first 6 months of life the optimal single food for the infant is human milk, or alternative feeding of appropriate formula. Until that time the infant does not need any additional food and is not able to fully handle them. On the contrary, there are advantages to delaying the introduction of solid foods until this time. Six-month-old infants have reached the stage of development in which they can communicate desire and interest in food and thus participate in the feeding process. Self-feeding efforts begin first with a whole hand **palmar grasp**, and then a more refined **pincer grasp** is developed by the end of the first year. There is also less tendency at this time to overfeed the infant. As solid food is gradually added, the amount of milk consumed is reduced accordingly.

No one sequence of food additions must be followed.

casein hydrolysate formula • Infant formula with base of hydrolyzed casein, major milk protein, produced by partially breaking down the casein into smaller peptide fragments, making a product that is more easily digested.

elemental formula • A nutrition support formula composed of simple elemental nutrient components that require no further digestive breakdown and are thus readily absorbed. Infant formula produced with elemental, ready to be absorbed components of free amino acids and carbohydrate as simple sugars.

palmar grasp • Early grasp of the young infant, clasping an object in the palm and wrapping the whole hand around it.

pincer grasp • Later digital grasp of the older infant, usually picking up smaller objects with a precise grip between thumb and forefinger.

renal solute load • Collective number and concentration of solute particles in a solution carried by the blood to the kidney nephrons for excretion in the urine. These particles are usually nitrogenous products from protein metabolism and the electrolytes Na^+, K^+, Cl^-, and HPO_4^{--}.

A general guide is given in Table 12-4. Individual responses and needs may be a basis for choices, as food becomes a source of enjoyment and a new means of bonding warm family relationships. Single foods are given first, one at a time in small amounts, so that adverse reactions can be identified. The traditional initial transition food is fortified infant cereal mixed with a little milk or formula, then fruits, vegetables, egg, potato, and finally meat. Small amounts are given at first, usually offered before the milk feeding. Over time the child will learn to eat and enjoy a wide variety of foods, which is the basic goal. Many commercial baby foods are available, prepared today without the formerly used ingredients of sugar, salt, or monosodium glutamate. Some mothers prefer preparing their own baby food. This can easily be done by cooking and straining vegetables and fruits in a clean environment, freezing a batch at a time in ice cube trays, then storing the cubes in plastic bags in the freezer. Then a single cube can be reheated conveniently for use at a feeding.

Two basic principles should guide the feeding process: (1) necessary nutrients are needed, not any specific food; and (2) food is a main basis of early learning. Food not only serves for physical sustenance but also supplies other personal development and cultural needs. Good food habits begin early in life and continue as a child grows older. By the time infants are approximately 8 or 9 months old, they should be able eat family foods—chopped, cooked foods, simply seasoned—without needing special infant foods. Throughout the first year of life the infant's needs for physical growth and psychosocial development will be met by breast milk or formula, a variety of solid food additions, and a loving, trusting relationship between parents and child (Fig. 12-1).

Toddler (1 to 3 Years)
Physical Characteristics and Growth

After the rapid growth of the first year the growth rate of children slows. But although the rate of gain is less, the pattern of growth produces significant changes in body form. The legs become longer, and the child begins losing baby fat. There is less body water and more water inside the cells. The young child begins to look and feel less like a baby and more like a child. Energy demands are fewer because of the slackened growth rate. However, important muscle development is taking place. In fact, muscle mass development accounts for about one half the total gain during this period. As the child begins to walk and stand erect, more muscle is needed to strengthen the body. There is special need, for example, for big muscles in the back, the buttocks, and the thighs. The overall rate of skeletal growth slows, but there is more deposit of mineral rather than lengthening of the bones. The increased mineralization strengthens the bones to support the increasing weight. The child has 6 to 8 teeth at the beginning of the toddler period. By 3 years of age the remainder of the deciduous teeth have erupted.

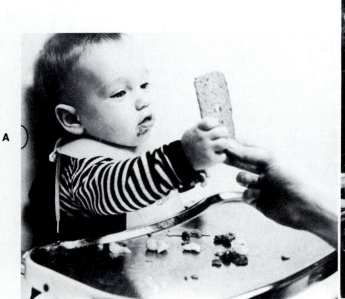
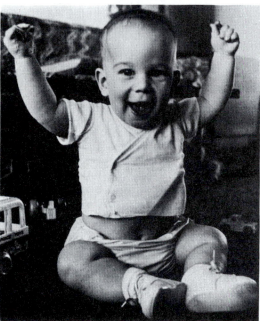

FIG. 12-1   A, This 6-month-old boy is taking a variety of solid food additions and is developing wide tastes. Here feeding has become a bond of relationship between parent and child and is serving as a source not only of physical growth but also of psychosocial development. **B,** Optimum physical development and security are evident, the result of sound nutrition and loving care.

◆ | CLINICAL APPLICATION | *Toddler Eating Made Simple*

Parents waste a lot of time coaxing, arguing, begging, and even threatening their 2- to 5-year-olds to eat more than 1½ green peas at dinner. You can help them save time by developing child-feeding strategies based on the developmental needs of their toddlers.

The first step is to remind them that their children are not growing as fast as they did during the first year of life. Consequently, they need less food. Also, a child's energy needs are sporadic. Parents should watch toddlers' activity levels. Food should be provided to help their bodies keep up with the myriad of activities they have planned each day.

Next, offer a few suggestions that make child-feeding easier:
- Serve small portions, not much more than a baby-food jar could hold. Let them ask for seconds if they're still hungry.
- Guide them in serving themselves small amounts. This takes a while because, like adults, children's eyes tend to be bigger than their stomachs. Constant, gentle reminders will eventually help them learn when to stop.
- Keep quick-fix, nutritious foods around for off-hour meals. The term *snack* isn't appropriate for the amount of food some youngsters put away between meals. To keep from turning into a permanent short-order chef,

the parent should consider keeping food such as fruit, cheese, and peanut butter to serve between meals and to provide essential nutrients.
- Don't put away the main meal before serving dessert. Amazing but true: some children will ask for main meal foods after finishing dessert, if they're still hungry.
- Avoid overseasoning. If it's too spicy, no amount of screaming and cajoling will make them eat it.
- Don't force foods that the child dislikes. Individual food dislikes usually don't last very long. If the child shuns one food, offer a similar one—if it's available at that meal; for example, a fruit if the child shuns vegetables. If not, ignore it and don't worry about malnutrition. At this rate, there's little chance of deficiency signs cropping up soon.
- Enroll the child in nursery school. Because food is not always available in the classroom, toddler students learn to eat at regular times. They also tend to try foods that are abhorred at home, probably because of peer pressure of a desire to impress a new authority figure—the teacher.
- Be patient. While adults are discussing world events over broccoli, toddlers are learning how to pick it up with their forks.

Remember that beginning at about age 4 young children are able to perceive relationships of food to positive concepts of health and nutrition. They are ready to learn more about food in these positive relations, so cash in on these rapidly developing capacities and explorations.

Also, remember that the child's social and emotional environment surrounds food and positive attitudes and behaviors relate to improved dietary quality.

Yes, toddlers might take longer; they might not eat. But with flexibility, time, patience, and a sense of humor, however, most parents find they can get enough nutrients into their children to keep them healthy and happy throughout the preschool years.

REFERENCES

Satter EM: *Child of mine: feeding with love and good sense,* Palo Alto, California, 1986, Bull Publishing Co.

Satter EM: *How to get your kid to eat . . . but not too much,* Palo Alto, California, 1987, Bull Publishing Co.

Singleton JC and others: Role of food and nutrition in the health perceptions of young children, *J Am Diet Assoc* 92(1):67, 1992.

Stanek K and others: Diet quality and the eating environment of preschool children, *J Am Diet Assoc* 90(11):1582, 1990. ◆

Psychosocial Development

The psychosocial development of toddlers is pronounced. The core developmental problem they struggle with is the conflict of autonomy versus shame. Each child has a profound increasing sense of self, of being a distinct and individual person apart from the parents, not just an extension of them. As physical mobility increases, the sense of **autonomy** and independence increases. A growing curiosity leads to much exploration of the environment, and increasingly the mouth is used as a means of exploring. Touch is important, providing the means of learning what objects are like. Often the constant use of "no" is not a perverse negativism as much as it reflects a significant struggle with newly emerging ego needs in conflict with the parents' control efforts. The child wants to do more and more, but the attention span is fairly short and interest shifts to other things.

Food and Feeding

Physical growth and psychosocial development during the toddler period influence nutrient needs (Table 12-2) and food patterns (see the Clinical Application above).

Energy. The need for kcalories is not high due to the relatively decreased growth rate after the first year of life. The energy need now increases very slowly in small spurts. At about 1 year of age children need approximately 850 to 1000 kcal, and only 1300 to 1500

autonomy • The state of functioning independently, without extraneous influence.

kcal by age 3. From age 1 to 2 some children do not eat as much as they did in the second half of infancy. Parents will avoid conflict with their toddler about eating if they remember this normal decreased need for kcalories, due to the slowed growth rate, and the child's necessary struggle for autonomy and selfhood, which often involves refusal of food. But they will eat when they are hungry.

Protein.   In relation to energy (kcalories) needs, protein needs are relatively increased. The toddler requires a total of about 16 g/day. Muscle and other body tissues grow rapidly. At least half of this protein should be of animal origin, because animal protein has high biologic value. This does not mean that meat itself is necessary. Studies of children in Southern California families following a balanced lactoovovegetarian diet have shown that they grow just as well and attain similar heights as do their nonvegetarian counterparts.[11]

Minerals.   Calcium and phosphorus are needed for bone mineralization. The bones are strengthening to keep pace with the muscle development and increasing activity. Iron is needed to maintain adequate hemoglobin levels in an increasing blood volume as the body size increases.

Food choices.   About 2 to 3 cups of milk daily are sufficient for the young child's needs. Sometimes excess milk intake, a habit carried over from infancy, may exclude many solid foods from the diet. As a result, the child may lack iron and develop a so-called milk anemia. On the other hand, a child may dislike milk as a beverage and replacement can be made in soups, puddings, or custards, or dry milk can be used in cooked cereals, mashed potatoes, meatloaf, and the like. Offering the child an increasing variety of foods will help to develop good food habits, for such food habits are learned and there is little opportunity for learning if a child is not exposed to a wide variety of foods. An emphasis on refined sweets is best avoided, reserving them for special occasions, not for habitual use nor bribes to get a child to eat.

Summary Principles

Two important principles, which parents should know and understand, can guide wise feeding practices during this period:

1. The child needs fewer kcalories but relatively more protein and minerals for physical growth. Therefore a variety of foods should be offered in smaller amounts to provide key nutrients. Young children of mothers working outside the home meet these nutritional needs for growth just as well. A study of a large sample of U.S. children has shown that maternal employment status has no detrimental effects on young children's diets.[12]

2. The child is struggling for selfhood in normal psychosocial development. This struggle often takes the form of refusal of food and a desire to do things for self before being fully able to do them completely. If parents are patient, offer a variety of foods in small amounts, and encourage some degree of food choice and self-feeding in the child's own ceremonial manner, eating can be a happy positive means of development. It can help satisfy the child's growing need for independence and ritual. Parents need to maintain a calm, relaxed attitude of sympathetic interest, to understand the child's struggle and give help where needed. But they must be careful to avoid both overprotection and excessive rigidity.

Preschooler (3 to 6 Years)

Physical Characteristics and Growth

As shown in normal childhood growth charts (see Appendix H), each child tends to settle into a regular genetic **growth channel** as physical growth continues in spurts. On occasion the child bounds with energy. Play is hard play—running, jumping, and testing new physical resources. At other times the child will sit for increasing periods of time engrossed in passive types of activities. Mental capacities are developing and there is more thinking and exploring of the environment. Energy needs, about 1800 kcal/day, as well as specific nutrients, as shown in Table 12-2, need emphasis. Protein requirements continue to increase as the child grows older. Preschool children need about 24 g/day of good, quality protein such as found in milk, egg, meat, and cheese. They continue to need calcium and iron for storage. Since vitamins A and C may be lacking in the diets of growing preschool children, a variety of fruits and vegetables should be provided.

Psychosocial Development

Each age group builds on the previous one. The core psychosocial developmental problem preschool children struggle with is essentially that of initiative versus guilt. They are beginning to develop the superego— the conscience. As powers of active movement increase, they have increasing imagination and curiosity. This very capacity often leads them into troubled feelings about their changing attitudes, especially toward parents. This a period of increasing imitation and of sex identification. The little boy imitates his father or other male role models. The little girl imitates the mother or other female role models. In their play much of this becomes evident in the use of grown-up clothes and role-playing in domestic or job situations. Wise parents will avoid sex stereotyping responses, especially during this formative period. Self-feeding skills increase and eating assumes greater social aspects. The family mealtime is an important means of socialization and sex identification, as the children imitate their parents and others at the table.

Food and Feeding

The preschool child is beginning to form definite responses to various types of foods:

1. *Vegetables and fruits.* Fruits are usually well liked. However, of all the food groups, vegetables usually are less well liked by children, yet these foods contain many vitamins and minerals needed for growth. Where there is space or opportunity, involving the young child in planting and growing vegetables in a small garden is an excellent early learning experience. Trips to the market can also help the child see a variety of shapes and colors in vegetables and discover new ones, as each in turn can be prepared at home in a variety of tasteful ways. Children usually dislike strong vegetables such as cabbage and onions. They have a keen sense of taste, so flavor and texture are important. They like pieces of crisp raw vegetables or fruits to eat as finger foods. Tough strings cause problems, and tough parts are hard to manage and therefore should be removed. For example, it is easy to break a crisp piece of celery and remove the strings before giving it to the child. Children also react to consistency of vegetables, disliking them overcooked.

2. *Milk, cheese, egg, and meat.* It is helpful if children can set their own goals in quantities of food. Portions need to be relatively small. Often children can pour their own milk from a small pitcher into a small glass and subsequently drink more. The quantity of milk needed usually declines during these years. The child will drink 2 or 3, rarely 4, cups of milk during the day. Smaller children like their milk more room temperature, not icy cold. Also, they prefer it in small glasses that hold about 4 to 6 oz rather than in large, adult-sized glasses. Cheese is liked as a good finger food or snack. Egg is usually well liked if cooked with sufficient body to pick up with the fingers, such as scrambled or boiled. Meat should be tender, easy to chew or cut; hence ground meat is popular, but it must be well cooked to make it safe.

3. *Grains.* The wide variety in which grains can be eaten adds to their appeal to children, who enjoy various breads, cereals, and crackers.

4. *Temperature.* Since children prefer their foods lukewarm, not hot, some foods may remain on their plates and become dry and gummy and so be refused. Thus very small portions should be served at first.

5. *Single foods.* Children usually prefer single foods

to combination dishes such as casseroles or stews. This a period of language learning for children. They like to learn names of foods, and be able recognize and name them from their shape, color, texture, taste. So these identifiable characteristics need to be retained as much as possible.

6. *Finger foods.* Children like to eat food they can pick up with their fingers. Frequently when appetites lag, fruits can be substituted for vegetables. Often a variety of raw fruits and vegetables cut in finger sized pieces and offered to children for their own selection provides a resource of needed nutrition.

7. *Food jags.* Because of developing social and emotional needs, preschool children frequently follow "food jags," eating only a particular food. This may last for several days. But it is usually short-lived and is of no major consequence.

The preschool period is one of increasing growth for the young child. Lifetime food habits are forming. Food continues to play an important part in the developing personality, and group eating becomes significant as a means of socialization. The social and emotional environment and companionship at mealtimes greatly influence the young child's food intake and quality of the diet.[13] The child learns food patterns at the family table or in group situations away from home. For example, if the family is vegetarian, they will need to give special attention to the child's energy and protein needs for growth. The child may be involved in a child care or preschool situation in which group eating occurs. Food habits of preschoolers are greatly affected by peer modeling, and food preferences grow according to what the group is eating. In such situations the child learns a widening variety of family food habits and forms new social relationships and food patterns. Current study shows that young children also include a relationship to health in their perceptions of food and are more ready to understand and learn more about food, nutrition, and health than we had previously thought.[14]

The School-Age Child (6 to 12 Years)
Physical Characteristics and Growth

The school-age period has been called the latent time of growth. The rate of growth slows, and body changes occur gradually. However, resources are being laid down for the rapid adolescent growth ahead. Sometimes this has been called the lull before the storm. By now the body type has been established, and growth

growth channel • The progressive regular growth pattern of children, guided along individual genetically controlled channels, influenced by nutritional and health status.

rates vary widely. Girls usually outdistance boys in the latter part of this period.

Psychosocial Development

The core psychosocial developmental problem children struggle with during these early school years is the tension between industry versus inferiority. They have widening horizons, new school experiences, and challenging learning opportunities. They develop increased mental powers, ability to work out problems, and face competitive activities. They develop abilities to cooperate in group activities and begin to experience a sense of adequacy and accomplishment, and sometimes the frustration of not winning. The child begins moving from a dependence on parental standards to those of peers, first steps in preparing for coming maturity and self-growth. Pressures are generated for self-control of a growing body. These pressures produce changes in previously learned habits, and negative attitudes sometimes expressed are evidence of these struggles for growing independence. There is a temporary disorganization of previous learning and personality, a sort of loosening up of the pattern for the inevitable changes ahead in adolescence. It is a diffuse period of gangs, cliques, hero worship, pensive daydreaming, emotional stresses, and learning to get along with other children.

Food and Feeding

The slowed rate of growth during this period results in a gradual decline in the food requirement per unit of body weight. This decline continues up to the latter part of the period just before approaching adolescence. Likes and dislikes are a product of earlier years. Family food attitudes are imitated, but increasing outside activities often compete with family mealtimes and family conflicts arise. Research has firmly established the close relation of sound nutrition and childhood learning. Breakfast is particularly important for a school child. It breaks the fast of the sleep hours and prepares the child for problem-solving and memory spans in the learning hours at school. The School Breakfast and Lunch Programs provide nourishing school meals that many children would not otherwise have (see Chapter 10). In school a child can observe many food attitudes and taste new foods that he or she may not normally know or accept. Some traditional favorite foods of American children are listed in Table 12-5.

The school-age child has increasing exposure to influences on food habits. Television becomes a strong source of food selection. There are positive learning opportunities in the classroom, particularly when parents provide support and reinforcement at home and nutrition education is integrated into other activities.

Adolescent

Physical Characteristics and Growth

During the adolescent period, with the onset of puberty, the final growth spurt of childhood occurs. Maturation during this time varies so widely that chronologic age as a reference point for discussing growth ceases to be useful, if indeed it ever was. **Physiologic age** becomes more important in dealing with individual boys and girls. It accounts for wide fluctuations in metabolic rates, food needs, scholastic capacity, and even illness. These capacities can be more realistically viewed only in physiologic growth terms.

The profound body changes in the adolescent period result from hormonal effects regulating the development of the sex characteristics. The rate at which these changes occur varies widely and is particularly distinct in growth patterns that emerge between the sexes. In girls the amount of subcutaneous fat deposit increases, particularly in the abdominal area. The hip breadth increases, and the bony pelvis widens in preparation for reproduction. A pelvic girdle of subcutaneous fat results.[15] This is often a source of anxiety to many figure-conscious young girls. In boys physical growth is mani-

TABLE 12-5

Favorite Food Choices of American Children (Listed in Order of Preference)

Breakfast	Lunch or dinner	Vegetables	Fruits	Beverages	Desserts	Sandwiches
Cereal	Steak or roast beef	Corn	Apple	Cola or soda	Ice cream	Peanut butter and jelly
Pancakes and waffles	Pizza	Carrots	Orange	Milk	Cake	Meat or cold cuts
Eggs	Spaghetti	Beans	Peach	Fruit punch	Pie	Ham
French toast	Chicken	Tomatoes	Grapes	Root beer	Pudding	Tuna fish
Toast	Hamburger	Peas	Banana	Juices (other than orange)	Gelatin dessert	Cheese
Sweet rolls	Fish	Greens, collards or spinach	Watermelon	Orange juice	Banana split	Bacon, lettuce, and tomato
Doughnuts	Macaroni and cheese	Potatoes	Pear	Lemonade	Brownie	Roast beef

Adapted from survey data of Lamme AJ, Lamme LL: Children's food preferences, *J Sch Health* 50(7):397, 1980.

fested more by an increased muscle mass and long-bone growth. His growth spurt is slower than that of the girl, but he soon passes her in weight and height.

Psychosocial Development

Adolescence is an ambivalent period full of stresses and strains. On the one hand teenagers look back to the securities of earlier childhood; on the other they reach for the maturity of adulthood. The core psychosocial developmental problem adolescents struggle with is that of identity versus role diffusion. The search for self begun in early childhood reaches its climax in the identity crisis of the teen years. The profound body changes associated with sexual development cause changes in body image and resulting tensions in maturing girls and boys. Individual variance is great in response to these tensions, depending on the resources that have been provided for them in earlier developmental years.

The identity crisis of the adolescent years, largely revolving around sexual development and preparation for an adult role in a complex industrialized and technologic society, produces many psychologic, emotional, and social tensions. The actual period of rapid physical growth is relatively short, only 2 or 3 years. However, the attendant psychosocial development continues over a much longer period. The pressure for peer group acceptance is strong, and fads in dress and food habits are common. Also, in a technically developed society such as in the United States, where high values are placed on education and achievement, prolonged preparation for careers often delays marriage and family far beyond the initiation of the reproductive years. Social tensions and family conflicts are created. These conflicts may have nutritional consequences as teenagers eat away from home more often and develop a snacking pattern of personal and peer group food choices.

Food and Feeding

With the rapid growth of adolescence come increased demands for energy, protein, vitamins, and minerals.

Energy. Kcaloric needs increase with the metabolic demands of growth and energy expenditure. Although individual needs vary, girls require fewer kcalories than boys, or about 2200 kcal/day; boys need 2500 to 3000 kcal/day. Sometimes the large appetite characteristic of this rapid growth period leads adolescents to satisfy their hunger with snack foods that are high in sugar and fat and low in essential protein.

Protein. Adolescent growth needs for protein are increased, especially during the pubertal changes in both sexes and for the developing muscle mass in boys. Girls require 44 to 46 g/day; boys need 45 to 59 g/day to sustain daily need and maintain nitrogen reserves.

Minerals. The calcium requirement for all adolescents is increased to 1200 mg/day to meet the demands of bone growth. In fact, adolescence is a crucial time for the development of bone mass, under the influence of increasing sexual hormones, especially of estrogen in girls. Current studies provide new insight into possible genetic mechanisms that determine peak bone density.[16] Menstrual iron losses in the adolescent girl predispose her to simple iron-deficiency anemia. Young female athletes, such as gymnasts and runners, who begin their training before menarche, develop secondary amenorrhea and, in turn, reduced bone mineral density.[17]

Vitamins. The B vitamins are needed in increased amounts, especially by boys, to meet the extra demands of energy metabolism and muscle tissue development. Intakes of needed vitamins C and A may be low because of erratic food intake, especially in vegetables and fruits. A high incidence of folate deficiency has been found among adolescent girls, with a positive relationship to megaloblastic anemia—low red blood cell folate and hemoglobin levels—all of which responded to supplement therapy of 400 μg of folate daily for 2 months.[18]

Eating Habits

Physical and psychosocial pressures influence adolescent eating habits (see To Probe Further, p. 246). By and large, boys fare better than girls. Their large appetites and the sheer volume of food they consume usually ensure intake of adequate nutrients. But the adolescent girl may be less fortunate. Two factors combine to place her under pressures concerning body weight.

Physiologic sex differences. Because of the girl's physiologic sex differences associated with fat deposits during this growth period and her comparative lack of physical activity, she may gain excess weight easily.

Social and personal tensions. Social pressures and tensions concerning figure control sometimes cause adolescent girls to follow unwise, self-imposed crash diets for weight loss. In some cases actual self-starvation regimens may result in complex and far-reaching eating disorders such as anorexia nervosa and bulimia (see Chapter 6). Usually these problems, which may assume

---

physiologic age • Rate of biologic maturation in individual adolescents that varies widely and accounts more for wide and changing differences in their metabolic rates, nutritional needs, and food requirements than does chronologic age.

Food Habits of Adolescents

TO PROBE FURTHER

Teenagers have gained the reputation of having the worst eating habits in the world. Is this justified? Here's a closer look at the actual eating habits of American adolescents during the last 15 years.

- *Skipping meals.* A study of California teenagers revealed that lunch—not breakfast, as most people assume—was the meal most frequently skipped. Breakfast was skipped most frequently by obese children, however. In all cases the frequency of regular meals increased with income and social status.
- *Snacking.* Another study indicated that 12- to 16-year-olds met or exceeded their RDA per 100 kcal for protein, riboflavin, and vitamin C through between-meal foods. Vitamin A, calcium, and iron levels fell considerably below the standard.
- *Fast foods.* Having a limited range of items, fast food restaurant menus are more likely to be lacking one or more essential nutrients. They are generally considered to be inadequate in calcium and vitamin A and too high in kilocalories, saturated fats, and sodium. Current marketing practices will continue to attract the young, who often consider fast food restaurants as popular hangouts to escape the demands of an ever-encroaching adult world. Thus it is likely that these places will influence the nutritional quality of adolescent meals for some time.
- *Unusual food choices.* Teenagers are likely to eat any type of food at any time of the day. Studies have shown that they are as likely to have barbecued chicken for breakfast as pancakes for dinner. These food choices are only unusual in terms of the time of day at which they are consumed, however, and usually present no threat to health or nutritional status.
- *Alcohol consumption.* As adolescents approach the drinking age in their locale, alcohol begins to provide a more significant portion of their total caloric intake. As they begin to drink at younger and younger ages, even a mild form of abuse coupled with the elevated nutritional requirements of adolescence may compromise their nutritional status, especially in terms of folic acid, which is destroyed by excessive amounts of alcohol. Subclinical damage to the intestinal mucosa caused by chronic alcohol use could also influence the absorption of other nutrients.

In general the adolescent diet may be no worse than the average adult diet, although intakes of calcium, vitamin A, iron, and ascorbic acid are usually seriously inadequate during these years, especially among girls. In addition, eating habits and social pressures have made this age group susceptible to at least two important nutritional problems: obesity and anorexia nervosa.

- *Obesity.* Obesity affects approximately 10% to 20% of the adolescent population. As in adults, an excessive intake of kilocalories is less often the cause than lack of exercise. Concern about personal appearance could make the adolescent more reluctant than an adult to participate in activities (team sports, dance classes) that are popular ways of controlling weight.
- *Anorexia nervosa.* This serious eating disorder is considered the flip side of the weight management coin. It usually affects achievement-oriented, affluent girls, although the problem now crosses socioeconomic and sexual barriers. The self-induced starvation is often attributed to an obsession with attaining a slim figure—a desire that goes as far as to result in self-starvation, emaciation, and serious health problems, including amenorrhea.

The food habits of adolescents reflect a reduced influence of parents on eating habits, increased peer pressure or desire to conform, extrasensitivity to appearance, and elevated needs for energy. The nutrition counselor must remember these influences when helping adolescents and their families plan food patterns that will enhance health and meet growth requirements during the teenage years.

REFERENCES

Bigler-Daughten S, Jenkins RM: Adolescent snacks: nutrient density and nutritional contribution to total intake, *J Am Diet Assoc* 87(12):1678, Dec 1987.

Frank GC and others: A food frequency questionnaire for adolescents: defining eating patterns, *J Am Diet Assoc* 92(3):313, 1992.

Witschi JC and others: Sources of fat, fatty acids, and cholesterol in the diets of adolescents, *J Am Diet Assoc* 90(10):1429, 1990.

---

severe proportions, involve a distorted self-image and a morbid, irrational pursuit of thinness, even when the actual body weight is normal or below age norms.[19] Even in less clinical situations, constant dieting among teenage girls can bring varying degrees of poor nutrition at the very time in life when their bodies need to be building reserves for potential reproduction. The harmful effects that bad eating habits can have on the future course of a pregnancy are clearly indicated in many studies relating preconception nutritional status to the outcome of gestation (see Chapter 11).

To Sum Up

Growth and development depend on nutrition to support heightened physiologic and metabolic processes. Nutrition, in turn, depends on a multitude of social, psychosocial, cultural, and environmental influences that affect individual growth potential throughout the life cycle.

Four types of growth are usually measured during each phase of development: physical, mental, emotional, and sociocultural. Each type of growth is evaluated in assessing the child's nutritional status and planning an effective counseling approach. Nutritional needs change with each growth period.

Infants experience rapid growth. They have relatively immature digestive systems and limited ability to absorb and excrete metabolites efficiently. Breast-feeding is preferred during the first 6 months of life. Solid foods are not needed, nor can they be handled, until about 4 to 6 months of age.

Toddlers (ages 1 to 3 years), preschoolers (ages 3 to 6 years), and school-age children (ages 6 to 12 years) experience a slowed and erratic latent growth of childhood. Their energy requirements per unit of body weight are not as great as the infant's. Their nutritional needs center on protein for growth with attendant minerals and vitamins. Social and cultural factors influence the development of food habits.

Adolescents (ages 12 to 18 years) experience a second large growth spurt before reaching adulthood. This rapid growth is accompanied by sexual maturation as well as physical growth. Increased kcaloric and nutrient needs on the average are easier for boys to achieve than for girls, who frequently feel social and peer pressures to restrict food intake for weight control. This pressure may inhibit their ability to acquire the nutritional reserves necessary for later reproduction.

QUESTIONS FOR REVIEW

1. How is physical growth measured? What signs are used to measure mental, emotional, and sociocultural growth?
2. What factors are responsible for the major differences in nutritional and feeding needs of the preterm and full-term infant?
3. Why is breast-feeding the preferred method for feeding infants? Outline some dietary needs for the new breast-feeding mother and techniques for feeding the baby. Describe techniques for teaching a new bottle-feeding mother. Describe some types of commercial formulas that would provide appropriate alternative feeding.
4. Outline a general schedule for a new mother to use as a guide for adding solid foods to her infant's diet during the first year of life.
5. What changes in physical growth and psychosocial development influence eating habits in the the toddler, preschool child, and school-age child? How do these factors influence the nutritional needs of each age group?
6. What factors influence the changing nutritional needs of adolescents? Who is usually at greater nutritional risk during this phase—boys or girls? Why? What nutritional deficiencies may be associated with this vulnerable age?

REFERENCES

1. Treiber FA and others: Dietary assessment instruments for preschool children: reliability of parental responses to the 24-hour recall and a food frequency questionnaire, *J Am Diet Assoc* 90(6):814, 1990.
2. Gurrahie EJ and others: The value of debriefing mothers of 3- to 7-year-old children when analyzing children's food desires, *J Am Diet Assoc* 91(6):710, 1991.
3. Erikson E: *Childhood and society*, New York, 1963, WW Norton.
4. Potter S and others: Does infant feeding method influence maternal postpartum weight loss? *J Am Diet Assoc* 91(4):1991.
5. Foman SJ, Zeigler EE: Nutrients in infant formulas, *J Nutr* 119:1763, 1989.
6. Zeigler EE and others: Cow milk feeding in infancy: further observations on blood loss from the gastrointestinal tract, *J Pediatr* 116:11, 1990.
7. Eck LH and others: Characteristics of families feeding infants low-fat milk, *Top Clin Nutr* 5(2):1990.
8. Foman SJ and others: Formulas for older infants, *J Pediatr* 116:690, 1990.
9. Shulman RJ and others: Impact of dietary cereal on nutrient absorption and fecal nitrogen loss in formula-fed infants, *J Pediatr* 118:39, 1991.
10. Report: introduction of solid foods and total energy intake in exclusively breast-fed infants, *Nutr Rev* 48(7):280, 1990.
11. Sabaté J and others: Attained height of lacto-ovo vegetarian children and adolescents, *Eur J Clin Nutr* 45:51, 1991.
12. Johnson RK and others: Effect of maternal employment on the quality of young children's diets: the CSF II experience, *J Am Diet Assoc* 92(2):213, 1992.
13. Stanek K and others: Diet quality and the eating environment of preschool children, *J Am Diet Assoc* 90(11):1582, 1990.
14. Singleton JC and others: Role of food and nutrition in the health perceptions of young children, *J Am Diet Assoc* 92(1):67, 1992.
15. Hammer LD and others: Impact of pubertal development on body fat distribution among white, Hispanic, and Asian female adolescents, *J Pediatr* 118:975, 1991.
16. Ott SM: Bone density in adolescents, *N Engl J Med* 325(23):1646, 1991.
17. Baer JT, Taper LJ: Amenorrheic and eumenorrheic adolescent runners: dietary intake and exercise training status, *J Am Diet Assoc* 92(1):89, 1992.
18. Tsui JC, Nordstrom JW: Folate status of adolescents: effects of folic acid supplementation, *J Am Diet Assoc* 90(11):1551, 1990.
19. Casper RC, Offer D: Weight and dieting concerns in adolescents: fashion or symptom? *Pediatrics* 86(3):384, 1990.

FURTHER READING

McConnell PE, Shaw JB: Position of The American Dietetic Association: Child nutrition services, *J Am Diet Assoc* 93(3):334, 1993.

Newman V: Position of The American Dietetic Association: Promotion and support of breast-feeding, *J Am Diet Assoc* 93(4):466, 1993.

These two reports provide background for the supportive positions of ADA concerning the important contribution of breast-feeding to the nutritional well-being of infants, and the nutritional support of various child nutrition services to the growth and development of young children. In each case, the basis of the position is made clear and recommendations are made for actions to implement it.

Splett PL, Story M: Child nutrition: objectives for the decade, *J Am Diet Assoc* 91(6):665, 1991.

Basing their observations on the national nutrition goals and objectives, these public health nutritionists describe the societal changes that have placed increasing numbers of our children at risk for nutrition-related health problems and outline specific related national health objectives.

CASE STUDY

Nutrition Program for Adolescents

Amanda Spencer is a graduate student of clinical nutrition assigned to the "Save Our Senior High" Project in Oakdale, a metropolitan community of 300,000 located in the northwestern United States. A representative of the city's educational advisory board approached her institution for assistance in developing a program that addresses three major problems faced by the majority of high school students: (1) popularity of fad diets among athletes, (2) obesity, and (3) iron-deficiency anemia.

Amanda and other members of her class met with students learning other health professions (medicine, dentistry, nutrition, nursing, social work), as well as several student representatives from the high school, to plan the program. After they developed goals and objectives, they decided that the nutrition topics would be addressed in a series of workshops entitled "Nutrition and Physical Fitness," "Food for the Teen Years," and "Snack Facts."

The program was introduced to the students through an advanced bulletin distributed at the largest high school in the city, where the project was to begin. The bulletin included an article written by Amanda, "Teenage Nutrition: A Seeming Paradox." This article responded to a common concern expressed by adolescents: the apparent preoccupation of school officials with the students' food habits when they, as a group, looked and usually felt very healthy.

Her article stirred a tremendous interest in the student population. Attendance at each session was high, and the discussions were lively. The evaluation results were positive. In reviewing the evaluative data and low cost of the project, the city council asked Amanda and her classmates to repeat the program at two other high schools where these problems were also prevalent. The council approached the school board about the possibility of including the project in the citywide high school curriculum for the coming year.

Questions for Analysis

1. Outline the content of Amanda's article to reflect major points that you would have included.
2. Write a class outline for each workshop, including objectives, major topics, and questions you would expect from the students. What teaching methods and materials would you expect to be most effective in each workshop?
3. What outside influences on eating habits would you expect in this student population? How effective would you expect this educational program to be in influencing a change of behavior in eating habits?
4. Aside from in-school nutrition education programs, describe possible tactics for influencing the eating habits of teenagers.

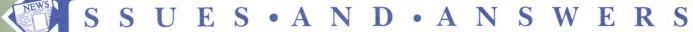
Feeding the Premature Infant

Babies born too soon or too small are surviving longer and with fewer serious physical and psychologic problems than before. Despite improvements in health, however, premature infants still present a number of problems that affect the feeding process: a poor sucking reflex; difficulty in swallowing, sucking and breathing; small gastric capacity; reduced intestinal motility; tiring easily from eating and being handled; and increased nutrient requirements for catch-up growth. Thus the health team involved in the care of premature and small-for-dates infants is faced with a myriad of decisions to be made to overcome these feeding difficulties.

Should the infant be tube-fed?

Infants born before the thirty-fourth week of gestation are routinely given human milk or formula by tube (gavage, nasogastric, transpyloric) for up to several weeks after birth. Even older babies, born between 34 and 37 weeks of gestation, may receive some tube-feedings. This is believed to overcome sucking and swallowing difficulties, to slow gastric motility, and to prevent fatigue. Even in the hands of the most skilled nursing personnel, however, this method creates grave potential hazards. These dangers include irritation of the stomach and esophagus, gastric perforation, and excessive vagal stimulation, reflux, and aspiration, which may outweigh any problems caused by bottle-feeding.

In an attempt to minimize the potential complications in very-low-birth-weight (VLBW) infants weighing less than 1500 g (3⅓ lb) at birth, some medical centers have established nutritional care protocols based on tube-feedings. Once infants are medically stable, usually 3 to 4 days after admission, they are given half-strength formula, which is gradually increased as tolerated for 7 to 10 days or until weight gain begins. Criteria for beginning oral feedings are based on the absence of complications associated with enteral feedings—abdominal distention, reflux, diarrhea, and gastric residue. Infants treated in this manner in various studies have done well, although they tend to lose more weight at first and take a bit longer to regain their birth weights than anticipated.

Other workers have tried to avoid the complications of enteral feeding completely by initiating bottle-feedings as soon after birth as possible. Researchers have found that small-for-gestational-age (SGA) infants could sustain appropriate weight gain through bottle-feeding, even when bottles were given on demand. This response, however, has been observed in infants who were larger and healthier, weighing 1800 to 2500 g (4 to 5½ lb) at birth, than those treated by the previous tube-feeding protocol.

The advantages of one method over the other cannot be calculated in terms of weight gain because of the lack of standard growth rates established for different states of prematurity. However, since both methods have been suc-

cessful, clinical practitioners should consider the patient's degree of illness, gestational age, and potential for imitating intrauterine growth from that age, without imposing stress on the metabolism and excretory system, when weighing the decision to recommend tube-feedings or oral feedings for premature or SGA infants.

Should the infant's feeding be by schedule or on demand?

The trend toward on-demand feeding of full-term infants has grown with evidence of their ability to control caloric intake and avoid the effects of overfeeding or underfeeding. Premature infants, as indicated, have similar skills. Workers have even found that feeding on demand results in an adequate fluid and nutrient intake in less time than scheduled feedings among infants over 7 days old with birth weights of 1500 to 1800 g (3⅓ to 4 lb).

A modified-demand feeding method has been effective in infants with eating-related central nervous system disorders, lethargy, hyperbilirubinemia, and heart problems.

The resistance to on-demand feedings in premature or full-term infants during the hospital stay has often come from staff and administrators who think it would disrupt hospital routine. Cost-saving studies may make some administrators seriously reconsider the practicality of rigidly scheduled routines, despite the effectiveness of such feedings for babies with special needs.

Should the infant be breast-fed or bottle-fed?

A variety of formulas reflect the estimated nutrient needs of low-birth-weight babies (see Table 12-6). These have been used safely, promoting weight gain similar to that expected in utero. Human milk was previously not considered for preterm infants because nutrient levels in mature milk were thought to be too low to meet the infant's needs. More recently studies have found that preterm milk is higher in protein, sodium chloride, magnesium, and iron than mature milk and may be uniquely developed for preterm infants. Breast milk also offers immunologic protection as well as easy digestibility. However, the preterm infant relying solely on breast milk will require supplements of calcium and phosphorus to ensure adequate bone growth. Although requirements are not known, vitamins D and C and folic acid supplements are also recommended. Sodium supplements may also become necessary for infants weighing less than 1200 g (2.8 lb) because they are susceptible to hyponatremia.

What feeding practices should be followed during the infant's first year?

The most common feeding mistakes practiced by parents of full-term infants include introducing solid food before 4 months of age, introducing cow's milk before 6 to 12 months of age, serving solids in the nursing bottle, and serving low-fat milk before 2 years of age. Parents of premature infants may be more anxious to follow these practices to encourage growth. Unfortunately their negative ef-

Feeding the Premature Infant—cont'd

fects on the health of full-term infants are exaggerated in the preterm child.

Parents must be reminded that their 4-month-old who was born 2 months prematurely is physiologically a 2 month-old and will present the same tongue-thrust reflex that is a sign of lack of preparedness for spoon-feedings in a full-term 2- month-old. Parents should be encouraged to follow recommended infant feeding practices (see pp. 236-240) on the basis of the child's physiologic, or corrected, age rather than on the chronologic age.

In summary, current trends in feeding premature infants include:

- More bottle-feeding and breast-feeding to avoid the potential hazards of tube-feeding
- More on-demand feeding to prevent overfeeding or underfeeding and reduce health care costs
- At-home feeding practices based on corrected chronologic age rather than birth age, using the preferred practice of delaying the start of solid foods until corrected age of 4 months, cow's milk until corrected age of 12 months, and low-fat milk until at least corrected age of 2 years

In other words, premature babies are given more credit for their abilities to handle foods in ways similar to those of full-term infants.

REFERENCES

Bhatia J, Rassin DK: Feeding the premature infant after hospital discharge: growth and biochemical responses, *J Pediatr* 118:515, 1991.

Cooke R and others: Vitamin D and mineral metabolism in the very low birth weight infant receiving 400 IU of vitamin D, *J Pediatric* 116:423, 1990.

Fenton TR and others: Nutrition and growth analysis of very low birth weight infants, *Pediatrics* 86(3):378, 1990.

Kien CL and others: Effects of lactose intake on nutritional status in premature infants, *J Pediatr* 116:446, 1990.

TABLE 12-6

Nutritional Value of Special Formulas and Human Milk for the Preterm Infant

Nutritional component	Advisable intake Birth weight 1.0 kg (2.2 lb)	1.5 kg (3.3 lb)	Human milk content Preterm	Mature	Standard formulas Enfamil* Similac† SMA‡	Special premature formulas Enfamil Premature with whey*	Similac Special Care†	"Preemie" SMA‡
Kilocalories/dl			73	73.0	67.0	81.0	81.0	81.0
Protein (g/100 kcal)	3.1	2.7	2.6§	1.5	2.2	3.0	2.7	2.5
Vitamins, fat-soluble								
D (IU/120 kcal/kg/day)	600.0	600.0	—	4.0	70-75	75.0	180.0	76.0
E (IU/120 kcal/kg/day)	30.0	30.0	—	0.3	2-3	2.0	4.0	2.0
Vitamins, water-soluble								
Folic acid (μg/120 kcal/kg/day)	60.0	60.0	—	8.0	9-19	36.0	45.0	14.0
Vitamin C (mg/120 kcal/kg/day)	60.0	60.0	—	7.0	10.0	10.0	45.0	10.0
Minerals								
Calcium (mg/100 kcal)	160.0	140.0	40.0	43.0	66-68	117.0	178.0	92.0
Phosphorus (mg/100 kcal)	108.0	95.0	18.0	20.0	49-66	58.0	89.0	49.0
Sodium (mEq/100 kcal)	2.7	2.3	1.5‖	0.8	1.0-1.8	1.7	1.9	1.7

*Mead Johnson Nutritional Division, Evansville, Ind.
†Ross Laboratories, Columbus, Ohio.
‡Wyeth Laboratories, Philadelphia.
§Range: 1.9-2.8 g/100 kcal.
‖Range: 0.9-2.3 mEq/100 kcal.

CHAPTER 13

Nutrition for Adults: Early, Middle, and Later Years

CHAPTER OUTLINE

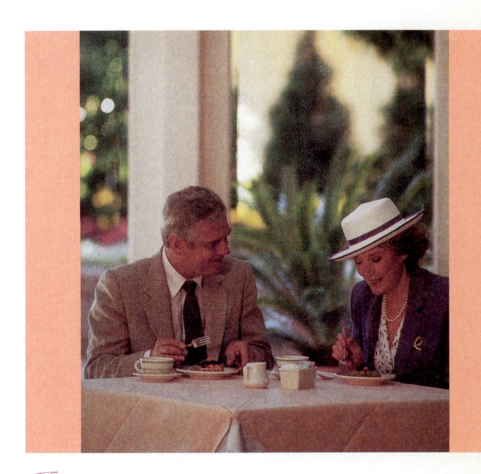

In this chapter, we complete our three-chapter sequence on nutrition through the life cycle. After the tumultuous adolescent years come the challenges, problems, and opportunities of maturity during adulthood.

Today when adolescents come of age, they have lived only about a quarter of their potential life span. They face a changing world of accelerated pace and complexity. America reflects these changes in its aging and increasingly diverse population.

Here we review adulthood—its early, middle, and later years. We look at each stage in terms of maturing needs and the role of nutrition in health concerns.

TABLE 13-1

RDA for Adults (National Research Council, 1989 Version)

	Age(yr)	Weight (kg)	Weight (lb)	Height (cm)	Height (in)	Energy (kcal)	Protein (g)	Vit. A (μg RE)	Vit. D (μg)	Vit. E (mg α-TE)	Vit. K (μg)
Males	19-24	72	160	177	70	2900	58	1000	10	10	70
	25-50	79	174	176	70	2900	63	1000	5	10	80
	51+	77	170	173	68	2300	63	1000	5	10	80
Females	19-24	58	128	164	65	2200	46	800	10	8	60
	25-50	63	138	163	64	2200	50	800	5	8	65
	51+	65	143	160	63	1900	50	800	5	8	65

Adulthood: Continuing Human Growth and Development

Aging Throughout the Life Cycle

Aging is a positive concept. It starts at conception and ends at death. It encompasses the whole of life, not merely its latter stages. Indeed, every stage has its unique potential and fulfillment, and the periods of adulthood—young, middle, and older—are no exception. Basic human needs continue, although in changing patterns, as persons mature and grow older.

Throughout your study, it is important to view continuing adult growth as a positive changing period of maturing human life. Two important concepts are significant parts of the whole process:

- **The individual.** Although gradual aging throughout the adult years has group influences in a society, it is at the core an *individual* process.
- **The total life.** Although it changes at each stage of the life span, aging is a *total life* process.

These two basic concepts govern the needs of these years—physiologic, psychosocial, socioeconomic, and nutritional.

Coming of Age in America

Young adults coming of age in America are experiencing extensive population and technology changes during this decade that affect their personal and working lives. And with our increasing life span and the growing number of older adults in our population, the personal, social, and health care needs are being felt in all our lives. The recent report of the U.S. Department of Health and Human Services, *Healthy People 2000: National Health Promotion and Disease Prevention Objectives*, projects **demographic** changes we can expect in our society over the 1990s that will affect all adults and families.[1] The report summarizes these changes in terms of our total population and households, age distribution, racial and ethnic composition, economic expansion, and immigration by the year 2000:

- **Population and households.** The U.S. population will have grown by about 7% to nearly 270 million. Average size of households will decline from 2.68 to 2.49, and two-parent households, from 58% to 53%.
- **Age distribution.** The U.S. population will be older, with an average age of more than 36; 35 million people (13%) will be over age 65. The fastest growing group, the "oldest-old"—those over age 85—will increase 30% to a total of 4.6 million. The number of children under age 5 will decline from more than 18 million to fewer than 17 million.
- **Racial and ethnic composition.** Proportion of whites—not including Hispanic Americans—will decline from 76% to 72%, and the fastest growing group—the Hispanics—will rise from 8% to 11.3%, representing more than 31 million. The proportion of blacks will increase from 12.4% to 13.1%, and other racial groups—Native Americans, Alaska Natives, Asians, and Pacific Islanders—will increase from 3.5% to 4.3%.
- **Economic expansion.** A shift in birth rates will decrease the number of young job seekers, and more jobs will require technical skills. Work force entry rates will be highest among women of all racial and ethnic backgrounds, making them almost half (48%) of the total work force. Occupations most likely to grow include service, technical, sales, professional, and management.
- **Immigration.** Up to 6 million people will probably be added to the American population by immigration, with the East and West coasts receiving most of them.

Shaping Influences on Adult Growth and Development

Within this broader, rapidly changing world, today's adults are growing and developing in many divergent ways. In terms of our interest in nutrition and health at each life stage, however, four basic areas of adult life shape its general path: physical, psychosocial, socioeconomic, and nutritional.

Water-soluble vitamins							Minerals						
Vit. C (mg)	Thiamin (mg)	Riboflavin (mg)	Niacin (mg NE)	Vit. B_6 (mg)	Folate (μg)	Vit. B_{12} (μg)	Calcium (mg)	Phosphorus (mg)	Magnesium (mg)	Iron (mg)	Zinc (mg)	Iodine (μg)	Selenium (μg)
60	1.5	1.7	19	2.0	200	2.0	1200	1200	350	10	15	150	70
60	1.5	1.7	19	2.0	200	2.0	800	800	350	10	15	150	70
60	1.2	1.4	15	2.0	200	2.0	800	800	350	10	15	150	70
60	1.1	1.3	15	1.6	180	2.0	1200	1200	280	15	12	150	55
60	1.1	1.3	15	1.6	180	2.0	800	800	280	15	12	150	55
60	1.0	1.2	13	1.6	180	2.0	800	800	280	10	12	150	55

Physical

Overall physical growth of the human body, governed by its genetic potential, levels off with physical maturity in the late teens and early adult years. Now physical growth is no longer marked by increasing numbers of cells and body size. Rather, it is the vital process of **replication**, growing new cells constantly to replace old ones to maintain body structure and function, increasing learning and strengthening mental capacities. Then at older ages, physical growth gradually declines. Individual vigor reflects the health status of preceding years.

Psychosocial

Here we pick up the threads of Erikson's eight stages of human personality development introduced in Chapter 12 at the beginning of the life cycle (see p. 235). Three remaining developmental tasks of personal psychosocial growth characterize the adult years: (1) young adults—intimacy vs isolation, (2) middle adults—generativity vs self-absorption, and (3) older adults—integrity vs despair. Individual adults at each age experience these struggles in some way, including their influence on life-style and health.

Socioeconomic Status

We all grow up and live our lives in a social and cultural context. Now, as indicated, our world is rapidly changing. We are experiencing major social and economic shifts, and most adults and their families are feeling the strain in some way. These pressures directly influence food security and health.

Nutritional Needs

Basic energy and nutrient needs of individual adults in each age-group, of course, vary according to living and working situations. However, current RDA standards for healthy adults, as shown in Table 13-1, reflect general needs and serve as a point of ready reference for comparing these needs in our discussion.

Adult Age-Group Needs: Health Promotion and Disease Prevention

Early Adult: 18 to 40 Years

Physical Characteristics

After the turbulent physical growth and sexual development of the preceding adolescent years, the young adult's body growth pattern levels off into a state of adult *homeostasis*. Finely regulated gene control of neural and hormonal activity and feedback maintain a stable internal environment of "body wisdom." The body functions are fully developed, including sexual maturation and reproductive capacity.

Psychosocial Development

In the early adult years, every person is launched, for better or worse, as a socially mature individual. The core psychosocial growth task each young adult must resolve is the problem of *intimacy vs isolation* (Fig. 13-1). It is a time of physical maturity, of becoming comfortable with the physical self generally, and of increasing adult role demands. If positive development is achieved, the person can build intimate relationships leading to self-fulfillment, either in marriage or in other personal relationships. If these psychosocial

---

demographic • The statistical data of a population, especially those showing average age, income, education, births, deaths, and so on.

replicate • To make an exact copy; to repeat, duplicate, or reproduce. In genetics, replication is the process by which double-stranded DNA makes copies of itself, each separating strand synthesizing a complementary strand. Cell replication is the process by which living cells, under gene control, make exact copies of themselves a programmed number of times during the life span of the organism. The process can be reproduced in the laboratory with cultured cell lines for special studies in cell biology.

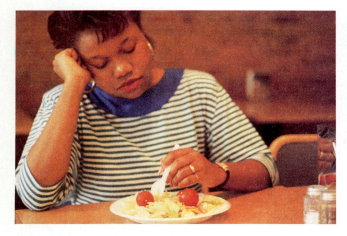

FIG. 13-1   The early adult years center on the core problem of intimacy versus isolation.

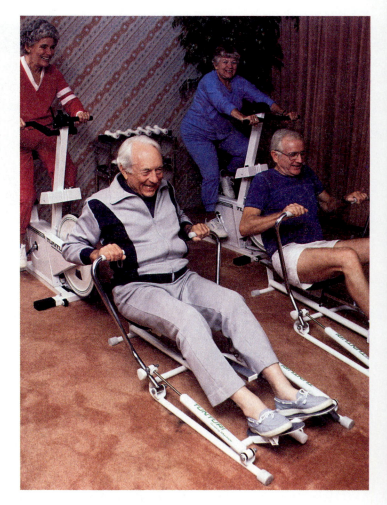

FIG. 13-2   Energy needs vary according to degree of activity.

strengths have not been developed in the previous years of growing up, the person may become increasingly isolated from others.

Socioeconomic Status

The early adult years reflect the social and economic pressures of continued education to prepare for adult responsibilities and career beginnings, of establishing one's own home, of parenthood and starting young children on their way through the same life stages, and of early struggles to make one's way in the world. Given the changing economic environment in today's world, many young adults face difficulties in meeting these basic goals of education, work, and family.

Nutritional Needs

All of these physical, psychosocial, and socioeconomic factors influence nutritional needs. Distinct differences in growth patterns that emerged between males and females during adolescence are strengthened in adult bodies. The young man's larger muscle mass and long bone growth are established. The young woman's wider hip breadth and pelvic girdle of subcutaneous fat, genetically designed to support reproduction, continue to prompt concerns and sometimes unwise actions in relation to social pressures for thinness that contribute to insufficient nutritional support. Nutritional needs of this period center on energy, protein, and the micronutrients.

1. **Energy.** The RDA energy standard for young men is 2900 kcal/day, and for young women, 2200 kcal/day (see Table 13-1). The larger male body size and muscle mass require more energy to maintain, especially because the lean muscle mass is the most metabolically active tissue in the body composition. The adult resting energy expenditure (REE) per unit of body weight, a measure of metabolic rate, differs by about 10% between the genders.[2] The re-

mainder of the energy need is for physical activities (Fig. 13-2), which is much smaller than that for metabolic needs. The height and weight reference figures in Table 13-1 are not meant to imply ideal ratios. They are actual **medians** for the designated age-group reported by a large national nutrition and health survey. Women require additional energy to support pregnancy and lactation (see Chapter 11).

2. **Protein.** The RDA standard for protein during the early adult years is 58 g/day for men and 46 g/day for women. These allowances are based on a daily protein intake of approximately 0.8 g/kg body weight for both genders, which many American adults exceed. By age 25 protein needs are 63 g/day for men and 50 g/day for women. An additional 10 g/day of protein is needed for pregnancy; an added 15 g/day is needed for lactation.

3. **Minerals.** The RDA standard for minerals during adulthood is sufficient if provided on a regular basis by a well-balanced diet. Two minerals, calcium and iron, need emphasis. In the current RDA val-

ues, the calcium allowance has been increased from 800 to 1200 mg/day for young adults to ensure peak skeletal bone mass, which is attained by approximately age 35.[3] Iron is another mineral often lacking in poor diets, resulting in iron-deficiency anemia. Women require more iron intake to offset iron loss from menstrual blood loss, so their RDA for iron is 15 mg/day; for men, it is 10 mg/day. Iron requirements for pregnancy are doubled, 30 mg/day, which is difficult to attain by diet, so a supplement is usually needed. No increase is needed during lactation.

4. **Vitamins.** The vitamin needs of young adults are usually met by regular, well-balanced diets. Problems in some individuals may relate more to inadequate regular intake rather than to increased need. A well-selected, mixed diet usually supplies all the vitamins in normally needed quantities.

Middle Adult: 40 to 65 Years

Physical Characteristics

Physical maintenance established during the early adult years continues into the middle adult years. However, the cell replication rate begins to decline slowly and a gradual cell loss starts. Depending on the degree of physical activity, which may be less during these years, the body fat proportion may begin to increase. This is especially seen in postmenopausal women, in turn increasing weight concerns. In addition, periodic physical examinations and laboratory tests showing increased blood lipid levels may indicate early risks of chronic heart disease.

Psychosocial Development

Persons in the middle adult years face the psychosocial problem of *generativity*—active involvement in some way, usually with family and grandchildren or in community groups—*vs self-absorption*. The children are now adults themselves, grown and gone to make their own lives. For some, these years have been called the "empty nest." For many, however, it is an opportunity to expand personal growth—"it's my turn now" (Fig. 13-3). There is a realistic coming to terms with what life is all about, together with a sharing of stored learnings by passing on life's teachings to younger persons. It is a regeneration of one's life in the lives of young people following in the same way. To the degree that these inner struggles are not won, there is an increasing self-absorption, a turning in on oneself, and a withering rather than a regenerating spirit of life.

Socioeconomic Status

With a changing economy in the marketplace and increasing technology in business and manufacturing, shifts in the nature of employment bring increased job loss for workers or "outplacement" for executives and managers. No longer can employees expect job secu-

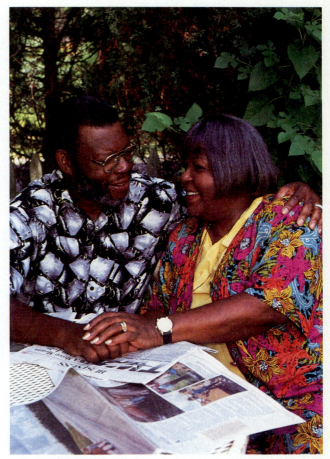

FIG. 13-3   Middle adult years can often be a time to expand personal growth.

rity with the same company all their working lives to retirement with a hefty pension at age 65. For adults in the middle of their working lives, supporting families and planning for the future, such financial problems can be devasting. In addition, the numbers of "new poor" families only increase the poverty problem.

Nutritional Needs

The energy and protein needs of the earlier adult years continue, but calcium allowances return to 800 mg/day (see Table 13-1). There is increasing evidence, however, that postmenopausal women need an increased intake of calcium to prevent bone mass calcium loss that follows the loss of protective estrogens in menopause, when osteoporosis risk is increased. Physical activity tends to decrease, adding to weight problems and increased vulnerability to fads that promise youth and vigor.

median • In statistics, the middle number in a sequence of numbers.

Later Adult: 65 to 85 Years

Physical Characteristics

The later adult years generally bring a gradual waning of physical vigor, work capacity, and strength. Usually physical activity decreases, along with overall energy balance needs and metabolic requirements. With increasing age, the body composition changes. Total body water, bone mass, and lean body mass decrease, and body fat mass increases. Weight gain commonly occurs in postmenopausal women, a pattern that continues into later years and frustrates many.[6] Older persons are "fatter" in body composition for any given relative weight, when compared with younger persons of the same weight, and the fat distribution—especially in men—centers mainly in the central abdominal area.[7]

Psychosocial Development

The final core psychosocial development problem between *integrity vs despair* is resolved in the later adult years. Depending on a person's resources at this point, a sense of wholeness and completeness predominates or a sense of bitterness and revulsion and of wondering what life was all about deepens. If the outcome of life's basic experiences has been positive, the individual arrives at older age a rich person—rich in the wisdom of the years. Building on each previous level, psychosocial growth now reaches its personal positive resolution.

But some of our older patients will not have resolved each of the core developmental problems along the way. They still struggle with those same problems with which they wrestled in previous stages of life. Thus they arrive at the middle and older years poorly equipped to deal with the adjustments of aging and health problems. On the other hand, many will have been enriched by life's human experiences in their maturing process. In turn they bring enrichment to our lives, and the resulting relationship is rewarding.

Socioeconomic Status

Older adults often face retirement with a limited fixed income in a changing economy. Others may have no stable income source and lack economic security. As a result, studies consistently show significant differences in nutritional intake between older persons with low and high socioeconomic statuses, with those in low economic circumstances having poorer diets.[8] Living alone may also influence food intake, because social isolation may cause depression and lack of incentive or ability to procure and prepare food. This is true of inner-city elderly persons and homebound rural older adults.[9,10] Many of them experience economic and social deprivation.

Nutritional Needs

The current RDAs for older adults generally remain the same as those for all adults above age 50, with some distinctions:

1. **Energy.** The basic energy allowance for all adults beyond age 50 is calculated at 1.5 times the REE. This makes the average need of men (77 kg) 2300 kcal/day and of women (65 kg) 1900 kcal/day, with a normal variation of ±20%.[2] Energy needs of older adults beyond age 75 are likely to be somewhat less because of reduced body size, REE, and activity. Light to moderate activity is encouraged to maintain muscle mass and well-being. The sharp decline in activity frequently seen in elderly persons is not inevitable and certainly not desirable.

2. **Protein.** The daily protein allowance remains the same beyond age 50, based on approximately 0.75 to 0.8 g/kg body weight for both genders. This makes the average allowance for men 63 g/day and for women 50 g/day.[2] The older adult body has a gradually decreasing lean body mass. Thus this continuing basic protein allowance is higher per unit of lean body mass for older adults and should allow for some decrease in utilization efficiency.

3. **Minerals.** Daily mineral allowances remain the same as for middle adults.[2] However, some evidence indicates that older adults—especially postmenopausal women—may need increased amounts of calcium to continue to protect against bone calcium loss and the development of osteoporosis.[3]

4. **Vitamins.** Daily vitamin allowances also remain essentially the same as those for middle adults. Basic needs are met with regular, well-balanced diets. Individual problems may occur with inadequate intake or during illness.

Oldest-Old: 85+ Years

U.S. Census Bureau Projections

All projections and our personal experiences indicate that as a population we are growing older. The oldest adult group among us is the fastest growing, but because this is so recent and rapid a phenomenon historically, this "oldest-old" group is the least understood. To distinguish the changing nature of the older adult population, the U.S. Census Bureau is now using three classifications instead of one: (1) the *young-old*—ages 65 through 74, (2) the *old-old*—ages 75 through 84, and (3) the *oldest-old*—ages 85 and beyond. In projecting life expectancies for men and women in the United States, the Census Bureau issues estimates based on three levels of predicted mortality: low, middle, and high.[11] The estimates for the low and middle levels of predicted mortality by the years 2020 and 2040 are given in Table 13-2. The Census Bureau also projects that over 1 million Americans will be 100 years or older in the year 2040. Given the rapid pace of biomedical research, many scientists working in this field think it is more likely that the actual numbers will surpass all of the Census Bureau projections.[12]

TABLE 13-2

U.S. Census Bureau Population Projections for Adults Over Age 85, for the Years 2020 and 2040 (based on low and middle estimates of predicted mortality)

Level of predicted mortality	Number of Americans age 85 and over (millions)	
	2020	2040
Middle mortality	6.7	12.2
Low mortality	8.6	17.8

From Spencer G: *Projection of the population of the United States by age, sex, and race: 1988 to 2080,* Bureau of the Census, Current Population Reports, Series P-25, No 1018, Washington, DC, 1989, US Government Printing Office.

Nutritional Needs

A growing consensus among clinicians and nutritionists caring for these older persons is that the current RDA values for adults at age 50, which actually vary little from those for younger adults, do not necessarily meet the highly individual and differing needs of persons aged 85 and beyond.[13] Elderly persons differ from younger adults in the way they absorb some nutrients, gastric acidity, overall nutrient use, exercise response, body composition changes with age, and how these changes influence nutritional needs.[14] For example, in comparison with needs of younger adults, they probably need more or less of several nutrients:

- Less *vitamin A,* because they store more and use it less efficiently
- More *vitamin D,* because they make it less efficiently and have less sun exposure
- More *pyridoxine (B6),* because their increased sensitivity to depletion affects function of the nervous system and immune system
- More *cobalamin (B12),* because their decreased ability to make stomach acid limits its absorption

In addition, some elderly persons—often women, with small bodies and low daily energy intakes of about 1000 to 1200 kilocalories—may require prudent supplementation to the diet to help meet their overall nutritional needs.[14]

Positive Health Promotion: Dietary Pattern for Adult Health

Two basic food guides, issued by the USDA and the U.S. Department of Health and Human Services, can serve as patterns for planning healthful diets for adults of any age-group. These are the Food Guide Pyramid, which provides a visual pattern for food choices from five basic food groups, and the U.S. Dietary Guidelines, which provides a general set of seven simple statements that summarize a sound approach to reducing risks for America's leading health problems. Both of these guides are described in Chapter 1. They emphasize the two basic keys to healthful diet planning and food behavior at any age—moderation and variety.

The Aging Process

Basic Gerontology Research

Basic research in **gerontology** is moving rapidly to enable us to understand better the physical aging process, in terms of length and quality.

Length of Life

Over the past century, the general life expectancy of Americans has almost doubled from 40 to nearly 80 years.[15] Scientists agree that most of the advance thus far has resulted from the "easier" gains in reducing deaths of infants and young children and mothers in childbirth, and that the "harder" work of increasing life expectancy lies ahead in learning more about the normal aging process, apart from the diseases of aging.[15,16] Currently, the new tools of molecular biology of cells allow basic biomedical research to focus on the difficult task of separating out the many factors that cause cells to grow old. Studies thus far clearly support the theories that oxidative cell damage by free cell radicals has an influence in the aging process and that this damage may also be responsible for behavior deficits in aging.[17] Ongoing research suggests a critical connection between the general functional decline of **senescence** and the "growing old" of human cells, which involves gene control and a biologic limit to cell replication rather than a chronologic age.[18] Studies such as these are beginning to separate the diseases of age from the normal process of aging and lay the groundwork for a lengthened and improved ending of the human life span.[16]

Quality of Life

The U.S. demographic reports of a lengthened life span and a rapidly growing older population have forced a primary attention to the quality of that extended life. Many researchers in the field are calling this longer life phenomenon "a new stage in the epidemiologic history of developed nations."[16] We are truly looking at a phenomenal future of increased numbers of elderly persons and elevated health care costs. For example, the first of the World War II "baby

gerontology • Study of the aging process and its remarkable progressive events.

senescence • The process of growing old; a consequence of advancing age or of a premature aging process from disease.

boomers"—that population hump moving through our midst—turn 85 in the year 2031. Then by 2040, when the average baby boomer will be 85, Medicare spending for the population 65 years and older could reach from $147 to $212 billion (in 1987 dollars).[12] Overall, the number of persons in the United States aged 85 and older is now growing six times faster than the rest of the population, and the cost of caring for disabled persons in that group is expected to double in the next decade.[19]

As a result of these projected needs, medical research has shifted its agenda for the 1990s to a revitalized study of aging, so that gerontology is reported to be a "growth industry."[19] Top-priority research at the National Institutes of Health centers on the study of abnormal cell proliferation and the neurosciences related to brain aging. A related top priority in clinical **geriatrics** research targets the prevention and treatment of disabilities in older persons. This means a focus on nonfatal, but highly disabling, age-dependent conditions of frailty—arthritis, osteoporosis, such sensory impairments as blindness, and Alzheimer's disease.[12,16]

General Biologic Changes in Aging

The general biologic process of growth and gradual decline extends over the entire life span. It is conditioned by all previous life experiences and the imprint of these experiences on individual genetic heritage.

Nature of Biologic Change

During middle and older adulthood, there is a gradual cell loss and reduced cell metabolism, with a related gradual reduction in the performance capacity of most organ systems. These changes—both physical and mental—may occur rapidly in one organ system and slowly in others, and individuals vary widely in the rate and order in which these changes occur.[20] But in general, lean body mass continues an age-related decline that accelerates in later life. For example, by age 70 the kidneys and the lungs lose about 10% of their weight, the liver loses 18%, and skeletal muscle diminishes by 40%, in comparison with values in young adults. Also, an important, overall reduction in the body's reserve capacities takes place. An important cause is the gradual reduction in cellular units. For example, functioning units of the kidney—the nephrons—are lost as the "aging Western kidney," which evolved in prior ages of vastly different food intake needs, now responds to our modern high-protein diet (see Chapter 22).

Effect of Biologic Change on Food Patterns

Some resulting physiologic factors may affect food patterns. For example, secretion of digestive juices is diminished, and motility of the gastrointestinal tract is decreased. This contributes to decreased absorption and use of nutrients. Sensory perceptions of taste, smell,

and vision also diminish, although these responses are highly individual.[21] These senses influence appetite and the amount of food consumed, so food for older adults generally needs more—not less—enhancement in seasoning. In addition, along with these biologic changes often comes an increased concern about body functions, increasing social stress, personal losses, and diminished social opportunities to maintain self-esteem. All of these responses can affect food intake.

Individuality of the Aging Process

The biologic changes in aging are general. But in reality, persons in the advancing years of life display a wide variety of individual reactions. We all simply get old at different rates. Every person bears the imprint of individual trauma and accumulation of disease experience, and we grow older at our own individual and unique gene-controlled nature and rate of aging. All of these factors directly affect individual aging. We can discuss aging and its nutritional needs in general terms, but individual situations and needs vary widely and must always be individually assessed. Actually, as we increasingly realize, the greatest influence of nutrition on the aging process takes place in earlier growth years when resources for later times are being built. Thus nutrition's most effective role is in growth and middle years, which prepare each one of us to meet the gradually declining metabolic processes of older age.

Individuality in Nutritional Needs of Elderly Persons

Energy

The reduced basal metabolic requirements caused by losses in functioning cells and reduced physical activity combine to create less energy demand as age advances. Some studies have indicated that the concept of a limited, less rich diet—"undernutrition without malnutrition"—may actually lengthen life.[22] Individual needs vary with body size and physical activities, but an average estimate of energy need is about 1800 kcal/day, more or less.

There are major gaps in our knowledge of energy and nutrient needs of elderly persons. For example, nutrient uptake by cells may decline with aging, so that older persons may need higher plasma levels to maintain optimal tissue concentrations. Also, because living situations vary widely among older adults, much more information is needed on their daily life activities and the degree of energy they may be capable of expending. Kilocalorie requirements are highly individual, according to activity. Primary consideration must be given to the living situation of the person and the degree of activity in various phases of life. Perhaps the simplest criterion for judging adequacy of kilocaloric intake is the maintenance of *normal* weight. However, there is current rethinking of traditional standards for appropriate weight based in life insurance weight-for-height tables (see Chapter 6). Recent assessment of these and other data has raised the possibility that the greatest longevity is not associated with the conventional "desirable" weight but with levels 10% to 25% greater. This view has obvious nutritional implications in terms of optimal energy intake for adults of all ages. To meet these energy needs, adults need ample carbohydrates but limited fats.

1. **Carbohydrates.** The optimal need for energy from carbohydrate is unknown, but it is usually recommended that at least 50% to 55% of daily kilocalories in the diet come from carbohydrate foods, mostly complex carbohydrates, such as starches. Easily absorbable sugars are used, and generally carbohydrate metabolism is not disturbed. The fasting blood sugar level is essentially normal in elderly persons. They can choose freely among carbohydrate foods, according to individual needs, desires, and physical responses. Current findings indicate that much of the observed carbohydrate intolerance of older persons may be caused by factors other than biologic aging per se and that diet and exercise modifications can substantially curtail age-related glucose intolerance and insulin resistance.

2. **Fats.** Generally, Americans eat too much fat, sometimes amounting to as much as 40% of their diet's kilocalories. Fat intake is best limited to about 20% of the total kilocalories. Some fat is needed as a source of energy, important fat-soluble vitamins, and essential fatty acids. A resonable goal is to avoid large quantities of fat, with more emphasis on the quality of the smaller amount of fat consumed, using mostly plant sources rather than animal fats. Digestion and absorption of fats may be somewhat delayed in elderly persons, but these functions are not greatly disturbed with age. There is no need to be unduly restrictive. Sufficient fat for food palatability aids appetite. Excessive fat, however, should be avoided because of the delayed absorption capacity of elderly persons.

Protein

There is a basic need for quality protein, though not in excessive amounts, to meet the needs of adults in our society:

1. **Basic needs.** The usual daily adult protein intake continues to meet the aging individual's need—about 0.8 g/kg of body weight. Even this amount provides an allowance for wide variation in individual needs. Also, although protein may be increased during illness or convalescence or during a wasting disease, the overall mass of actively metabolizing tissue decreases with age. There is inadequate research information on what levels of dietary pro-

tein can best perserve the lean body mass and tissue function of the aging adult. We need to know whether populations receiving 0.8 g/kg body weight of protein or less show any accelerated losses of lean body mass. It is possible that to maintain nitrogen balance, elderly persons need relatively more protein as their total energy intake is reduced.

2. **Protein quality.** Protein needs are influenced by two basic factors: (1) the biologic value of the protein, based on the quantity and ratio of its essential amino acids, and (2) adequate kcaloric value of the diet. It is estimated that about 25% to 50% of protein intake should come from animal sources, the only foods that are "complete" proteins with all the essential amino acids, with the remainder coming from plant protein sources. In a vegetarian diet, careful supplementary mixtures of plant proteins—with additions of acceptable milk and egg protein—must be selected to ensure adequate quality protein intake. Protein should supply from 15% to 20% of the day's total kilocalories. Healthy older adults do not need supplemental amino acid preparations. They are an expensive and inefficient source of nitrogen.

Vitamins

Traditionally, nutrient standards have indicated that additional vitamin intake in the healthy adult is unnecessary, and that although tissue stores may gradually decrease with normal aging, there is no difference in requirement from that for normal adults. However, a growing concern among geriatric family physicians and researchers studying nutritional needs in elderly persons is that these older adults have different nutrient needs from those of their younger counterparts.[14] Some individual problems may stem from inadequate normal intake, rather than from an increased need. In most cases, a mixed diet of moderation and variety usually supplies needs. Increased therapeutic needs in illness should be evaluated on an individual basis.

Minerals

Usually increased minerals are not needed in normal aging. The same adult allowances are sufficient if provided on a continuing basis by a well-balanced diet. However, several essential minerals must be emphasized in diets for elderly persons, including calcium and iron, because of their relation to osteoporosis and anemia. Some individuals may need increased attention and encouragement to ensure adequate dietary

geriatrics • Branch of medicine specializing in medical problems associated with old age.

sources of these minerals among their daily food choices.

Water

Too often the vital need for water in older adults is overlooked. The normal thirst mechanism sometimes diminishes with age, and dehydration can easily occur.[23] About 1 in 5 elderly persons suffer from *xerostomia,* dry mouth caused by a severe reduction in the flow of saliva, which in turn affects their food intake.[24] This condition may be associated with the use of certain medications, autoimmune diseases, or radiation therapy to the head and neck. Conscious attention to adequate fluid intake, not dependent on normal thirst, is an important aspect of health maintenance and care.

Nutrient Supplementation

Healthy adults of any age who regularly consume healthful diets rarely need added nutrient supplementation. However, elderly persons are at greater nutritional risk and often benefit from prudent, individually assessed supplementation—especially women, the oldest-old, persons in poor health, and those having in-

adequate energy intake, living alone, lacking social support or mobility, and having insufficient money for food.[14,25,26] There is some indication, however, that certain specific nutrient supplementation might be a rational approach to improve cognitive function in disoriented older adults (see box below).[27,28] And in illness or debilitated states, supplementation may well be needed to replenish losses.

Health Care and Clinical Needs

Successful Aging

Many older Americans are not only living longer, but also aging well. Thay have vigor and vitality and are often involved in positive health maintenance programs with such names as "Successful Aging."[29] Even 80% of individuals over age 85 with disabilities and infirmities and with an average age of nearly 90 are not in nursing homes but are able to live in the community, alone or with friends or family, in residential settings, or in adult foster care in private homes.[30] A recent 9-year study of 1598 urban elderly persons in Ohio shows that two to eight times as many impaired or disabled per-

---

Food for Thought Among Elderly Persons

TO PROBE FURTHER

Among elderly persons, as well as others, it is a common observation that poor mental function and malnutrition go hand in hand. Although scientists have not yet figured out the precise connections, they find a strong correlation between nutritional deficiencies and poor **cognitive** performance and memory among elderly persons. A study of 260 noninstitutionalized adults over the age of 60 reveals that those with poor nutritional food intakes scored poorly on special tests that measure nonverbal abstract thinking ability and memory. Protein, vitamin C, and various B vitamins—folate, niacin, pyridoxine, riboflavin, thiamin, and B_{12}—emerged as the nutrients of particular significance to the subjects' ability to think and remember.

Researchers are reluctant at this point to say, on the basis of such studies, that poor nutritional status causes poor thinking abilities and memory loss. A number of factors may intervene:

- Persons with poor memories may forget to take a vitamin pill. Those who don't recognize objects or shapes may have such difficulties preparing meals that they often fail to eat, leading to a poor nutritional status.
- Educated persons may be more inclined to take nutritional supplements and, because of their experience in taking tests, score better than average.
- In a population of basically healthy elderly persons, a subgroup may have undetected clinical problems that contribute to poor mental performances.

There is no doubt that mental problems in elderly per-

sons, including mental retardation, affect diet practices in residents of intermediate- or long-term care facilities and group homes and require regular developmental disability consultation with trained professionals. Less clear is just how poor nutritional status may precipitate, aggravate, or prolong mental problems in elderly persons. Some more obvious nutrient candidates involved are precursors for neurotransmitters: the four amino acids tyrosine, tryptophan, threonine, and histidine, as well as choline. Other candidates are nutrients affecting the metabolism of neurotransmitters: pyridoxine, vitamin C, thiamin, copper, and iron. Then still other candidates are nutrients with general effects on brain metabolism: glucose, folate, cobalamin, nicotinic acid, riboflavin, zinc, potassium, and magnesium.

Thus we can make a strong presumptive case for the potential importance of nutritional status in the mental abilities of older adults. But what we lack is precise knowledge of the possible mechanisms involved, which probably act in concert with many other contributory factors.

REFERENCES

Hodkinson HM: Diet and maintenance of mental health in the elderly, *Nutr Rev* 46:79, 1988.

Mercer KC, Ekvall SW: Comparing the diets of adults with mental retardation who live in intermediate care facilities and in group homes, *J Am Diet Assoc* 92(3):356, 1992.

Raskind M: Nutrition and cognitive function in the elderly, *J Am Med Assoc* 249(21):2938, 1983.

sons are cared for in the community as in institutions.[31] However, for many older individuals in nursing homes or hospitals and in the community, malnutrition is too often present and requires personal care and prevention.

Malnutrition
Incidence

Protein-energy malnutrition among elderly persons has been shown to occur in up to 59% of nursing home residents and as many as 65% of hospitalized medical and surgical patients, and it varies some 5% to 22% in outpatients over 70 years old.[32-34] One 10-year chart survey of almost 3000 outpatients aged 60 and above attending a large medical clinic in New York identified nearly 100 malnourished persons weighing less than 45.5 kg (100 lb). Half of these older clients had no physician-recorded diagnosis of malnutrition or weight loss, and three fourths had no physician-prescribed nutrition supplement or nutrition assessment referral. Thus malnutrition, with or without a contributory disease, is all too common among elderly persons living in the community, and often a specific nutritional diagnosis is not made.

Warning Signs and Preventive Care

Warning signs can alert us to early malnutrition in elderly persons. If heeded, they are crucial to preventing unnecessary and sometimes irreversible weight loss.[32,35,36]

1. **Physical signs.** Recent unintended weight loss, perhaps associated with eating problems, such as tooth loss or poorly fitting dentures; dry mouth from decreased salivary secretions; diminished sensory perceptions, such as taste, smell, or sight; difficulty swallowing; mental confusion
2. **Multiple medications.** Long-term use of multiple medications, often termed "polypharmacy," with actions and side effects that are often unexplained to patient and family and that interact with food or nutrients or reduce appetite
3. **Psychosocial signs.** Grief from loss of spouse or family and friends; depression; loneliness or living alone; homebound with lack of sunlight; increased use or abuse of alcohol, which often displaces food intake
4. **Economic problems.** Low socioeconomic status, lack of sufficient money for food, inadequate housing, homelessness
5. **Food-related difficulties.** Disability affecting food shopping or preparation and eating, missed meals and snacks or fluids, food wasted or rejected, insufficient food stores at home, lack of fruits and vegetables or fortified whole-grain products, poor nutrition knowledge, lack of ethnic "comfort foods" that increase interest in eating

Nutrition Screening Initiative

The Nutrition Screening Initiative (NSI) is a 5-year program to promote routine nutrition screening in all U.S. community health and medical care settings, working through a network of registered dietitians, public health and clinical nutritionists, physicians, other health care professionals, the public, and policymakers.[37] This initial multidisciplinary project of the American Dietetic Association, the American Academy of Family Physicians, and the National Council on the Aging has first targeted the warning signs of malnutrition in older Americans, because of the large burden that their poor nutritional status has in the U.S. population. Based on an initial comprehensive survey of research in gerontology and geriatrics and a consensus of leaders to establish goals, warning signs of malnutrition within a framework of the following seven basic risk factors were identified[38-40]:

· Inappropriate food intake
· Poverty
· Social isolation
· Dependency or disability
· Acute or chronic diseases or conditions
· Chronic medication use
· Advanced age

NSI has developed a public awareness checklist for warning signs of poor nutritional health, "Determine Your Nutritional Health," including a nutrition information sheet based on the word *DETERMINE*, as a mnemonic device to convey the basic nutrition information in a way that can be easily remembered.[41] In addition, screening tools and a directional manual for health professionals in their assessment and care-planning work with older clients have also been developed.*

Clinical Problems
Chronic Diseases

Physicians specializing in geriatrics and clinical nutritionists working with older adults increasingly relax their strict "medically indicated" diets, especially for elderly patients in long-term care facilities. At these older

---

cognitive · Pertaining to the mental processes of perceptions, memory, judgment, and reasoning, as contrasted with emotional and volitional processes.

---

*Copies of all of these documents and materials—background research survey; report of the multidisciplinary consensus conference in Washington, DC; the public awareness checklist "Determine Your Nutritional Health" in English and Spanish; the screening tools and manual for professionals; and a summary brochure that describes the NSI project—are available through the NSI office: Nutrition Screening Initiative, 2626 Pennsylvania Ave, NW, Washington, DC 20037; (202)625-1662.

ages the finer points of diets for lowering cholesterol or managing non–insulin-dependent diabetes mellitus are not the caring physician's and dietitian's major concern. In many older individuals, such highly restrictive diets lead to decreased food intake and serious weight loss and are thus inappropriate. Instead, the general practice is to follow a regular diet—well-balanced nutritionally with a variety of food choices and some moderation in fats and sweets, as indicated for us all (see Chapter 1).

Disability

Currently, major attention in research and clinical practice has turned to improving the functional disabilities and infirmities that some elderly persons experience. The goal is to add quality of life to these extended years. For example, increased work in the field of musculoskeletal problems, such as arthritis and osteoporosis, relates malnutrition to increased falls and fractures by measures of many nutritional markers. Research has shown that programs for patients with osteoporosis and arthritis to teach them about the disease and its management can make a difference in these patients' lives.[42,43] Both individual and group sessions—including nutrition assessment and counseling, physical therapy, medical evaluation, and treatment—have a positive impact on patients' general physical and psychologic well-being, helping them to cope with the pain and chronic nature of the condition.

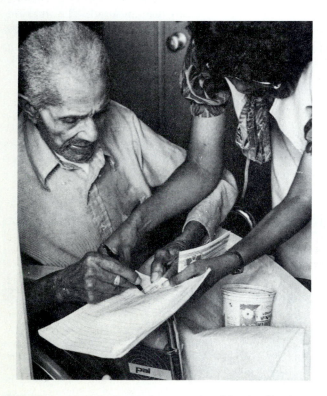

FIG. 13-4 Elderly disabled man assisted by the Food Stamp Program to obtain needed food.

Community Resources
Government Programs for Older Americans

The regular government food assistance programs for individuals and families also provide support for older Americans. These include the Food Stamp Program (Fig. 13-4) and the surplus agricultural commodities distribution program (see Chapter 10). These programs provide needed foods and food-buying extension for many older adults. However, the single greatest impact on the growing field of nutritional gerontology has been the Older Americans Act, which created the National Nutrition Program for Older Americans.[44,45]

Older Americans Act—Title VII and Title III

In 1972 the Nutrition Program for Older Americans, Title VII of the Older Americans Act, was authorized by Public Law 92-258. The program was developed to meet the nutritional and social needs of persons 60 years of age and older who (1) could not afford adequate diets, (2) were unable to prepare adequate meals at home, (3) had limited mobility, or (4) were isolated and lacked incentive to prepare and eat food alone. The original program provided such services as outreach, escort and transportation, health care, information and referral, health and welfare counseling, and nutrition and consumer education. In 1978 amendments were authorized by Public Law 95-478, which coordinated nutrition services with other services for older people. Under this amended Act, Title III-C, the services funded after 1980 included the provision of meals, both congregate and home-delivered, and related nutrition services and education.

1. **Congregate meals.** The program provides older Americans, particularly those with low incomes, nutritionally sound meals at low cost in senior centers and other public or private community facilities. Older adults can gather for a hot noon meal and receive not only food, but also social support. They also receive sound food and nutrition information to help dispel nutrition myths and misinformation, to which elderly persons are often vulnerable.[46]

2. **Home-delivered meals.** For those persons who are homebound through illness or disability, meals are delivered by couriers to the home. This service provides nutritional needs and human contact and support. Often the courier is the only person with whom the homebound individual has contact during the day. For elderly homebound participants in both urban and rural areas, many of whom have poor diets, this single hot meal 5 days a week provides their main source of food intake.[47]

USDA Research Centers

The USDA, in collaboration with universities, is establishing human nutrition research centers on aging, which are authorized by Congress to study nutrition's role in aging. Current investigations include such areas as protein needs in aged persons, the nutritional status of elderly men and women, and the prevention and slowing of osteoporosis.

USDA Extension Services

The USDA operates agricultural extension services in state universities and county agencies. Through these agencies, county home advisors provide communities with much practical nutrition material and counseling for older adults and community workers.

Public Health Departments

Skilled health professionals work in the community through local and state public health departments. Health guidance for elderly persons is available through their resources. The public health nutritionist is a significant member of the health care team and provides counseling and nutrition education services, community program planning, and oversight of food service facilities in nursing homes licensed by the state (see box below). Counseling is also provided concerning the various food assistance programs available (see Chapter 10).

Professional Organizations and Resources
National Council on the Aging

The National Council on the Aging, established in 1950, is located in Washington, D.C. It is an organization for professionals and volunteers that works on many fronts to improve the quality of life for older

---

CLINICAL APPLICATION
Improving the Nutritional Status of Elderly Persons in Long-Term Care Facilities

Over the past three decades the number of nursing home beds has increased from about 880,000 to 1.5 million, and the need by the year 2000 is expected to exceed 3.5 million. Take a look at the following statistics on those who reside in long-term care facilities:

- 80% are 75 years of age or older.
- 50% cannot feed themselves.
- 85% have moderate to severe protein-energy malnutrition, which decreases their response to rehabilitative efforts.

Residents of long-term care facilities have a wide spectrum of needs, and food is a critical issue. Daily meals become particularly significant to residents, a fact that some facilities with otherwise excellent care in nursing and imaginative cultural programs sometimes fail to realize in their food service. The use of full-time dietitians can often change this situation.

Improvements in the nutritional status of residents as a result of professional nutrition services by qualified nutrition specialists has been documented many times. These skilled and sensitive persons address the following factors in quality care that must be present to ensure the optimal nutritional status of their clients:

Administrative activities

- Developing cyclic menus based on nutritional requirements and reflecting the needs and desires of that population

- Training staff to ensure proper food preparation, including appetizing seasonings and creative uses for foods that require changes in consistency from thin liquids to ground foods
- Working with nursing staff, speech therapists, and food service staff regarding the nutritional needs of patients suffering from dysphagia

Clinical activities

- Conducting nutritional assessments of residents on admission and at regularly scheduled intervals thereafter
- Encouraging use of appropriate consistency and texture of foods (e.g., not using pureed foods when ground foods can be used and not using ground foods when chopped foods can be used)
- Making accurate calculations of diets for persons with insulin-dependent diabetes mellitus (IDDM) and renal failure
- Discouraging abuse of alcohol, nicotine, and drugs
- Developing resident education programs, such as appropriate physical activity to increase a sense of well-being
- Encouraging eating by recognizing cultural diversity in ethnic food patterns; considering individual food preferences; satisfying the desire for "something sweet" with products made from appropriate sweeteners; occasional planning of special events,

such as picnics, which may include family members; creating a homelike atmosphere in the dining hall with appealing menus and regular food in the more current move away from "special diets"; preparing meals in the residential area to "entice" residents with the aroma; using color schemes and china patterns with soothing tones; using special menus for festive events and special parties, such as Octoberfest and luaus; holding monthly birthday parties with live music and a party menu or a family dinner party with special orders from a "Touch of Class" menu

The overall goal of such quality food management is simple—"to get people to eat." The most nutritious meal in the world is not good unless it is eaten.

REFERENCES

Endres J and others: Acceptance and consumption of crystalline fructose menu items by institutionalized elderly persons, *J Am Diet Assoc* 90(3):431, 1990.

Gallagher FA: Elegance adds appeal to nursing home foodservice, *J Am Diet Assoc* 90(12):1632, 1990.

Herbelin K: Techniques for supporting food choices of residents in long-term–care facilities, *J Am Diet Assoc* 92(6):718, 1992.

Samolsky S and others: Feeding the Hispanic hospital patient: cultural considerations, *J Am Diet Assoc* 90(12):1707, 1990.

Americans. It maintains a nonprofit central national resource for research, planning, training, information, technical assistance, advocacy, program and standards development, and publications that relate to all aspects of aging, including nutrition. Currently, this organization is working with the American Dietetic Association and the American Academy of Family Physicians to develop and implement the national project for identifying older Americans at risk for malnutrition, the Nutrition Screening Initiative.

American Geriatric Society

This professional organization of physicians engaged in medical care of elderly patients promotes research in geriatrics to advance scientific knowledge of the aging process and the treatment of its diseases. A number of nurses and other health professionals are associate members. The society publishes the *Journal of the American Geriatrics Society*.

The Gerontological Society

This society's membership includes a wide number of interested health professionals. Its committee on aging has stimulated increased interest among other related organizations and community and government agencies in gerontology and the problems of aging persons in our society. This organization publishes the *Journal of Gerontology*.

Community Groups

Local community groups representing health professions—such as the medical society, nursing organizations, and dietetic associations—sponsor a variety of programs to help meet the needs of elderly persons in their communities. In addition, qualified nutritionists and registered dietitians in private practice are available in most communities for individual counseling and community program support. Senior citizens' centers in local communities also provide a broad range of services and available nutrition education and counseling.

Volunteer Health Organizations

Many activities of volunteer health organizations, such as the American Heart Association and the American Diabetes Association, relate to the health and nutrition needs of older persons. These organizations include professional and public members. They operate at national and community levels to fund and conduct research and education.

To Sum Up

The challenge of meeting the nutritional needs of the older population is compounded by the lack of needed research in this area; the interaction of current and past

social, economic, and psychologic factors; and the wide range of individual differences in the biologic process of aging.

Nutritional requirements should, at least in part, be based on biologic changes caused by aging—reduced speed of conduction for nerve impulses, reduced blood flow and pulmonary function, reduced tissue mass in several organs, and so on. Current nutrient and energy standards, however, lack specific research on older adult needs and thus are based mainly on extrapolations of data available for younger adult populations, as well as requirements to counteract chronic disease processes prevalent in aging, such as cardiovascular disease.

Major illnesses found in elderly persons are often associated with malnutrition and weight loss. Malnutrition may be associated with a number of factors, such as underlying illness, fad diets, and poverty. It may also stem from various conditions affecting food intake, such as oral problems (dry mouth, infections, lack of teeth, poorly fitting dentures, and swallowing difficulty), psychosocial problems resulting from isolation, and other personal factors contributing to boredom or apathy. The Nutrition Screening Initiative (NSI)—a national project conducted by The American Dietetic Association, the American Academy of Family Physicians, and the American Council on the Aging—is currently working in many communities to identify those elderly persons at risk for malnutrition and to help educate individuals and communities in preventive care.

QUESTIONS FOR REVIEW

1. Briefly describe five main ways the U.S. population is changing. Illustrate how these changes may have touched your own life or the life of someone you know. How do you think these changes may influence persons' diets or their nutrition and health status?

2. Describe the influence of physical, psychosocial, socioeconomic, and nutritional factors on adult growth and development. Give examples from the experience of any adult you may know.

3. Select any one of the adult age-groups and describe the basic needs of this group in the adult life span in terms of physical growth, psychosocial development, socioeconomic status, and related nutritional needs.

4. Describe two basic U.S. food guides developed as patterns for planning healthful diets. How might you use them in helping a middle-aged couple on a limited income to improve their poor food intake pattern?

5. Distinguish between the two terms *gerontology* and *geriatrics*. Describe current research goals and activities in these fields in relation to length and quality of life.

6. Describe some of the general biologic changes in aging. How may these changes affect eating, food choices, and nutritional status?

7. Identify five basic warning signs of malnutrition in older

adults. Give examples describing how each of these situations lead to poor nutrition. Give some ways that each situation might be improved to prevent malnutrition.

8. What is the current national Nutrition Screening Initiative (NSI)? Describe what you may know thus far about its purpose, goals, methods, or materials. Why do you think such a project is important in the lives of elderly Americans during the 1990s?

9. Describe the government programs for older Americans and other community resources for nutrition and health needs.

REFERENCES

1. US Department of Health and Human Services, Public Health Services: *Healthy people 2000: National health promotion and disease prevention objectives*, Pub No 91-50212, Washington, DC, 1990, US Government Printing Office.

2. Food and Nutrition Board, National Academy of Science—National Research Council: *Recommended dietary allowances*, ed 10, Washington, DC, 1989, National Academy Press.

3. Anderson JJB: Dietary calcium and bone mass through the life cycle, *Nutr Today* 25(2):9, 1990.

4. Svendsen OL and others: Measurement of body fat in elder subjects by dual energy x-ray absorptiometry, *Am J Clin Nutr* 53:1117, 1991.

5. Blanchard J and others: Comparison of methods for estimating body composition in young and elderly women, *J Gerontol* 45(4):B119, 1990.

6. Wing RR and others: Weight gain at the time of menopause, *Arch Intern Med* 151:97, 1991.

7. Schwartz RS and others: Body fat distribution in healthy young and older men, *J Gerontol* 45(6):M181, 1990.

8. Ryan VC, Bower ME: Relationship of socioeconomic status and living arrangements to nutritional intake of the older person, *J Am Diet Assoc* 89(12):1805, 1989.

9. Roe DA: In-home nutrtional assessment of inner-city elderly, *J Nutr* 120:1538, 1990.

10. Smiciklas-Wright H and others: Nutritional assessment of homebound rural elderly, *J Nutr* 120:1535, 1990.

11. Spencer G: *Projections of the population of the United States by age, sex and race: 1988 to 2080*, Bureau of the Census, Current Population Reports, Series P-25, No 1018, Washington, DC, 1989, US Government Printing Office.

12. Schneider EL, Guraluik JM: The aging of America: impact on health care costs, *JAMA* 263(17):2335, 1990.

13. Andres R, Hallfrisch J: Nutrient intake recommendations needed for the older American, *J Am Diet Assoc* 89(12):1739, 1989.

14. Lehr D and others: Practical nutritional advice for the elderly. I. Evaluation, supplements, RDAs, *Geriatrics* 45(10):26, 1990.

15. Gibbons A: Gerontology research comes of age, *Science* 250:622, 1990.

16. Olshansky SJ and others: In search of Methuselah: estimating the upper limits of human longevity, *Science* 250:634, 1990.

17. Floyd RA: Oxidative damage to behavior during aging, *Science* 254:1597, 1991.

18. Goldstein S: Replicative senescence: the human fibroblast comes of age, *Science* 249:1129, 1990.

19. Gibbons A: Aging research: a growth industry, *Science* 252:1483, 1991.

20. Chernoff R, Lipschitz D: *Health promotion and disease prevention in the elderly*, vol 35, Aging, New York, 1988, Raven Press.

21. Weiffenbach JM and others: Oral sensory changings in aging, *J Gerontol* 45(4):M121, 1990.

22. Weindruch R , Walford R: *The retardation of aging and disease by dietary restrictions*, Springfield, Ill, 1989, Charles C Thomas.

23. Hoffman NB: Dehydration in the elderly: insidious and manageable, *Geriatrics* 46(6):35, 1991.

24. Rhodus NL, Brown J: The association of xerostomia and inadequate intake in older adults, *J Am Diet Assoc* 90(12):1688, 1990.

25. Murphy S and others: Factors influencing the dietary adequacy and energy intake of older Americans, *J Nutr Educ* 22(6):284, 1990.

26. McIntosh WA and others: The relationship between beliefs about nutrition and dietary practices of the elderly, *J Am Diet Assoc* 90(5):671, 1990.

27. Raskind M: Nutrition and cognitive function in the elderly, *JAMA* 249(21):2939, 1983.

28. Hodkinson HM: Diet and the maintenance of mental health in the elderly, *Nutr Rev* 46:79, 1988.

29. Fries JF: The sunny side of aging, *JAMA* 263(17):2354, 1990.

30. Kane RA and others: Adult foster care for the elderly in Oregon: a mainstream alternative to nursing homes? *Am J Pub Health* 81(9):1113, 1990.

31. Ford AB and others: Impaired and disabled elderly in the community, *Am J Pub Health* 81(9):1207, 1991.

32. Morley JE: Anorexia in older patients: its meaning and management, *Geriatrics* 45(12):59, 1990.

33. Miller DK and others: Abnormal eating attitudes and body image in older undernourished individuals, *J Geriatr Soc* 39(5):462, 1991.

34. Manson A and Shea S: Malnutrition in elderly ambulatory medical patients, *Am J Pub Health* 81(9):1195, 1991.

35. Davies L, Knutson KC: Warning signals for malnutrition in the elderly, *J Am Diet Assoc* 91(11):1413, 1991.

36. Fischer JF , Johnson MA: Low body weight and weight loss in the aged, *J Am Diet Assoc* 90(12):1697, 1990.

37. Hess MA: ADA as an advocate for older Americans, *J Am Diet Assoc* 91(7):847, 1991.

38. Dwyer JT: *Screening older Americans' nutritional health: current practices and future possibilities*, Washington, DC, 1991, Nutrition Screening Initiative.

39. White JV and others: *Nutritional Screening Initiative: toward*

a common view, Washington, DC, 1991, Nutrition Screening Initiative.

40. White JV and others: Consensus of the Nutrition Screening Initiative: risk factors and indicators of poor nutritional status in older Americans, *J Am Diet Assoc* 91(7):783, 1991.

41. White JV and others: Nutrition Screening Initiative: development and implementation of the public awareness checklist and screening tools, *J Am Diet Assoc* 92(2):163, 1992.

42. Gold DT and others: Treatment of osteoporosis: the psychologic impact of a medical education program on older patients, *J Am Geriatr Soc* 37(5):1989.

43. Gold DT and others: Osteoporosis in late life: does health locus of control affect psychosocial adaption? *J Am Geriatr Soc* 39(7):670, 1991.

44. O'Shaughnessy C: *Older Americans Act Nutrition Program,* Washington, DC, 1990, Congressional Research Service, Library of Congress.

45. Carlin JM: Nutritional gerontology: a new and growing field, *J Am Diet Assoc* 90(12):1665, 1990.

46. Hutchings LL, Tinsley AM: Nutrition education for older adults: how Title III-C Program participants perceive their needs, *J Nutr Educ* 23(2):53, 1991.

47. Stevens DA and others: Nutrient intake of urban and rural elderly receiving home delivered meals, *J Am Diet Assoc* 92(6):714, 1992.

FURTHER READING

Haines PS and others: Eating patterns and energy and nutrient intakes of US women, *J Am Diet Assoc* 92(6):698, 1992.

Hertzler AA, Frary R: Dietary status and eating out practices of college students, *J Am Diet Assoc* 92(7):867, 1992.

These two articles survey food patterns of young adults in college and young middle adults to age 50, comparing practices of eating out on the fast-food track, in restuarants, and in the home mix pattern and relating nutritional needs to each group.

Davies L, Knutson KC: Warning signals for malnutrition in the elderly, *J Am Diet Assoc* 91(11):1413, 1991.

Fischer J, Johnson MA: Low body weight and weight loss in the aged, *J Am Diet Assoc* 90(12):1697, 1990.

These two articles provide important information about the serious problems of malnutrition in older adults. The first describes the work of two dietitians with gerontology nutrition at a large university medical center in London under the National Health Service system; the second provides a comprehensive review of elderly malnutrition in America under a besieged health care system in need of reform.

White JV and others: Nutrition Screening Initiative: development and implementation of the public awareness checklist and screening tools, *J Am Diet Assoc* 92(2):163, 1992.

In this article the working committee guiding the 5-year NSI project on malnutrition in elderly Americans reviews the results of the 1991 NSI Consensus Conference and follow-up development of the public awareness checklist and screening tools.

Can We Eat to Live Forever?

The world is getting older. Our life span has extended from age 45 at the turn of the century to nearly 80 years today. It is expected to climb even higher.

We owe this lengthening of life to the conquest of infectious disease, the provision of safer work settings, and the development of more effective medical technology. In short, we have largely conquered our external environment. It's time we conquered our *inner* environment—through proper nutrition.

Scientists are beginning to consider the importance of nutrition in combatting the physical deterioration that accompanies old age: a 10% loss of kidney and lung tissue, 18% loss of liver tissue, 40% loss of skeletal tissue, and as much as 25% (12% in men) loss of bone by the seventh decade of life. You would think that they could simply make biochemical calculations to find optimal blood levels for nutrients that could retard these losses and make recommendations for dietary intake. However, achieving an optimal diet among elderly persons is much more complex than that.

Sensory deprivation

Elderly persons tend to live alone. Such physical and emotional isolation tends to diminish the desire to eat. When this is combined with the progressive deterioration in sight, smell, touch, and hearing that occurs in some older adults, attempts to prepare meals are not only frustrating, they are dangerous.

Taste and smell

Oral infections, poor hygiene, and a reduced salivary flow rate contribute to the increased difficulty in tasting and smelling. To what extent does this affect the desire to eat? No one knows. Some scientists say the effect is little, suspecting poor research techniques in studies of this problem. Others believe it is serious enough to warrant further research to arrest ongoing losses.

Bone and tooth loss

Approximately one half of all adults have lost their teeth by age 65. The main culprit is periodontal disease. Researchers are beginning to look at this problem as a possible manifestation of osteoporosis, or weakened bone. They are focusing the study of calcium on the following:

- *Calcium RDAs.* Some suggest that 1200 to 1500 mg/day of calcium may be necessary to prevent calcium loss, rather than the current RDA of 800 mg.
- *Phosphate.* Calcium and phosphorous maintain an inverse ratio in the blood. Processed foods contribute heavily to phosphate levels in the American diet and are suspected of promoting calcium resorption from bone.
- *Megavitamins.* Excessive vitamin A levels have been associated with a greater loss of bone in elderly persons.

Studies of elderly subjects usually reveal that many use vitamin supplements, with some adding additional amounts of vitamin A. This warrants further study.

- *Protein.* America's obsession with meat may harm aging bones, because a high protein intake results in increased loss of calcium in the urine.

Kilocaloric needs

It has repeatedly been reported that elderly persons fail to consume recommended amounts of kilocalories. However, based on animal studies, some researchers claim that a restricted diet also makes people live longer, but this has not been proved and is still controversial. An even more recent reassessment of the effect of body weight suggests that we should all weigh 10% to 25% more than we do to live longer. Because the reassessment does not associate body size with detrimental habits, such as smoking, it is also controversial.

Gastrointestinal problems

Reduced production of digestive juices, less peristaltic activity, and reduced mucosal surface area all work to inhibit nutrient absorption and promote such digestive disorders as constipation.

Drugs

The prevalence of chronic disease means a prevalence of prescription and over-the-counter drug use. Drugs, either individually or in combination with each other, can alter taste, appetite, and other factors and affect nutritional status.

Poverty

Many elderly persons either cannot work or are coerced into retirement. For these reasons they tend to be among the poorest citizens in the United States. As a result, even those individuals in good health often lack the money to shop, the transportation to reach a shopping area, or adequate food preparation and storage equipment to maintain a reasonably healthful diet.

Based on the information available thus far, the most nutritionally supportive environment for elderly persons is one in which they do the following:

- Have company for meals, such as at congregate meal sites, as well as family support and friends
- Have foods with pleasant but distinctive aromas and flavors
- Consume meals that are lower in protein-rich and processed foods; are higher in fiber-rich foods (complex carbohydrates and a variety of fresh fruits and vegetables) and calcium (from nonbovine as well as bovine sources, to avoid excessive protein levels); and provide a moderate amount of kilocalories
- Avoid supplements, especially of vitamin A, unless medically indicated
- Avoid unnecessary drugs and be informed of the action and side effects of every drug they take

Can We Eat to Live Forever?—cont'd

- Are subsidized financially or placed in living situations (senior centers or private homes with roommates) that provide some financial, emotional, and nutritional support

Although these may seem like reasonable recommendations for any age-group, elderly persons present such a myriad of long-standing compounding factors that a wide variety of service and professional assistance may be needed to avoid nutritional deficits. Thus counselors who hope to promote a nutritionally supportive environment for elderly clients must themselves maintain a network of professional sources available for referrals and must work together as a team to meet the unique needs of older persons.

REFERENCES

Fischer J, Johnson MA: Low body weight and weight loss in the aged, *J Am Diet Assoc* 90(12):1697, 1990.

Hoffman NB: Dehydration in the elderly: insidious and manageable, *Geriatrics* 46(6):35, 1991.

Rhodus NL, Brown J: The association of xerostomia and inadequate intake in older adults, *J Am Diet Assoc* 90(12):1688, 1990.

Rolls BJ, McDermott TM: Effects of age on sensory-specific satiety, *Am J Clin Nutr* 54:988, 1991.

CHAPTER 14

Nutrition and Physical Fitness

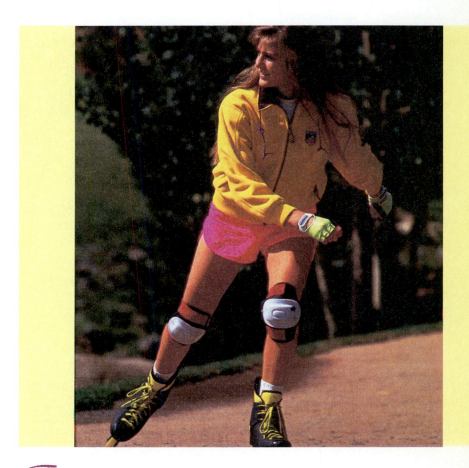

This chapter is the first of a two-chapter sequence on health maintenance through the life cycle. Here we begin with nutrition and physical fitness. In an increasingly technologic society, building physical activity into our busy lives requires commitment and effort. However, it is a vital cornerstone in the preventive approach to controlling our modern "chronic diseases of civilization."

First, we examine how nutrition works in energy fuels and muscle action. Then we apply these principles to athletic performance and building a reasonable and appropriate personal exercise program.

Modern Civilization, Chronic Disease, and Physical Activity

Modern Developed Nations and Diseases of Civilization

Over thousands of years our marvelous human bodies have developed from earlier ages of human history when survival depended on constant exercise and energy expenditure. Now, over only the few past generations, the developed nations of the world have come to live in very different circumstances. Our high-technology societies demand little, if any, physical activity in our work and in our life-style. As a result, our health has been paying a price. Our inactivity contributes to a host of modern ills, so-called diseases of civilization, including coronary heart disease, diabetes, hypertension, osteoporosis, and obesity.[1]

Health Toll of Inactivity

American workers and leaders, students and teachers, and parents and children seem to be increasingly aware of the health toll of our inactivity. According to some estimates, 100 million Americans now practice some form of regular exercise, a twofold increase over the past two decades. Walking and swimming are our most popular outdoor activities, with bicycling and jogging

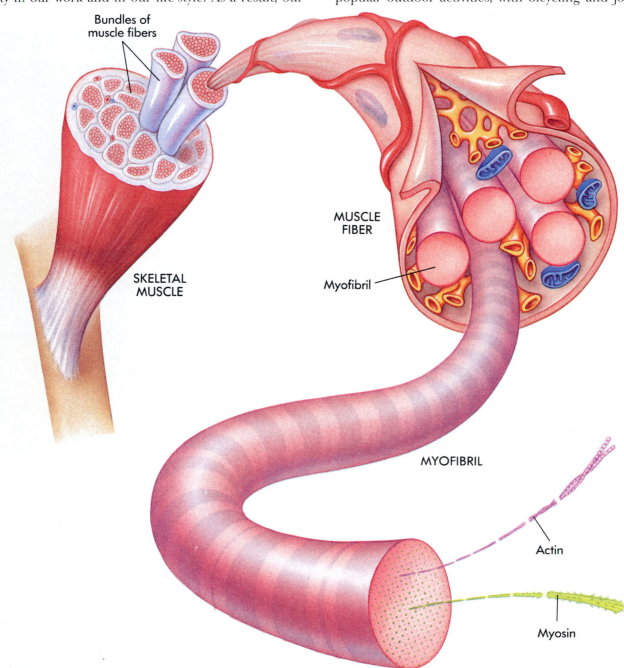

FIG. 14-1   Skeletal muscle, showing the progressively smaller bundles within bundles.

close behind. And in relation to the big business of athletics, we have seen the new speciality of sports medicine develop.

Nonetheless, in everyday life, the need for exercise is serious. The modern health care approach of prevention, as well as the necessity of dealing with chronic disease, demands positive attention to the related roles of nutrition and physical fitness in health care. Exercise has currently emerged as an effective therapy, along with nutritional care and weight management, in the control of hypertension, diabetes, and elevated blood lipid levels.[2-4] Whatever level of exercise or active pursuits a person is able to do, even a limited beginning builds into consistent habits. For many, it is a matter of life and health.

Energy Sources for Physical Activity
The Nature of Energy

You will recall from Chapter 6 that the term *energy* refers to the body's ability, or power, to do work. The energy required to do body work takes several different forms: mechanical, chemical, electric, light, radiant, and heat. Energy, like matter, can be neither created nor destroyed. It can only be changed into another form and constantly cycled in the body and environment. We also speak of energy as **potential** (stored) or **kinetic** (active). Potential energy is stored energy, ready to be used. Kinetic energy is active energy, being used to do work. Energy balance in physical activity requires a base of sound nutrition to supply the **substrate** fuels, which—along with oxygen and water—meet widely varying levels of energy demand for body action.

Muscle Action: Fuels, Fluids, and Nutrients
Muscle Structures

The synchronized action of millions of specialized cells and structures that make up our skeletal muscle mass make possible all forms of physical activity. A finely coordinated series of small bundles within the muscle fibers (Fig. 14-1), triggered by nerve endings, produce a smooth symphony of action through simultaneous and alternating contraction and relaxation. These successively smaller muscle structures include the following:

1. **Skeletal muscle.** The largest bundle in the series is the complete muscle. Each particular muscle is composed of muscle fibers called **fasciculi.**
2. **Muscle fiber.** In turn each muscle fiber is composed of bundles of still smaller strands called **myofibrils.**
3. **Myofibril.** Each single myofibril strand of the muscle fiber is made up of the smallest of all the fiber bundles, called **myofilaments.** Contraction occurs here.
4. **Myosin** and **actin.** Finally, within each myofilament are the contractile proteins, **myosin** and **actin,** which are the smallest moving parts of every muscle.

Muscle Action

Inside the cell membrane these contractile proteins, myosin and actin, are arranged in long parallel rows. These parallel rows slide together and mesh tightly when the muscle contracts and then pull apart when the muscle relaxes, allowing the muscle to shorten or lengthen as needed. When a specific motor nerve impulse excites these molecules of myosin and actin in a myofilament, they mesh together and thereby shorten the muscle. This contraction of the muscle bundles occurs instantly and simultaneously. Then periods of relaxation occur between contractions. This alternating process continues until muscle fatigue builds up and the muscle can no longer respond. Muscle fatigue occurs for two reasons: (1) the supply of *glycogen*, the immediate muscle fuel, is exhausted and thus insufficient to sustain the required chemical reaction, and (2) *lactic acid*, the metabolic product of this chemical muscle reaction, accumulates during sustained high levels of exercise and cannot be removed fast enough.

Fuel Sources

Phosphate bonds form high-energy compounds in body metabolism (see Chapter 2). The main high-energy compound of the body cells is *adenosine triphosphate (ATP)*. It has rightly been called the "energy currency" of the cell. Various forms of energy are called on for successive energy needs:

1. **Immediate energy.** High-power or immediate energy demands over a short time depend on ATP's ready availability within the muscle tissue. This

---

actin • Myofibril protein whose synchronized meshing action in conjunction with **myosin** causes muscles to contract and relax.

fasciculi • A general term for a small bundle or cluster of muscle, tendon, or nerve fibers.

kinetic • Energy released from body fuels by cell metabolism and now active in moving muscles and energizing all body activities.

myofibril • Slender thread of muscle; runs parallel to the muscle fiber's long axis.

myofilaments • Threadlike filaments of actin or myosin, which are components of myofibrils.

myosin • Myofibril protein whose synchronized meshing action in conjunction with **actin** causes muscles to contract and relax.

potential • Energy existing in stored fuels and ready for action, but not yet released and active.

substrate • The specific organic substance on which a particular enzyme acts to produce new metabolic products.

amount is used up rapidly and a backup compound, *creatine phosphate (CP),* is made available. These high-energy phosphate compounds, however, will sustain all-out exercise for only about 5 to 8 seconds.

2. **Short-term energy.** If an activity lasts longer than between 30 seconds and 2 minutes, *muscle glycogen* supplies the continuing need. Although the amount of available glycogen is small, it is an important rapid source of energy for brief muscular effort.

3. **Long-term energy.** Exercise continuing for more than 2 minutes requires an oxygen-dependent or *aerobic* energy system. A constant supply of oxygen in the blood is necessary for continued exercise. Special cell organelles, the *mitochrondria,* located within each cell, produce large amounts of ATP. The ATP is produced mainly from glucose and fatty acids and supplies continued energy needs of the body.

Fluids

An increased intake of water is essential in the course of exercise. A deficiency can be dangerous, because it limits capacity greatly. As exercise continues, the body temperature increases as part of the energy produced is released as heat. To control this temperature increase, the body shunts as much heat as possible to the skin, where it is released in sweat. Over time, and especially in hot weather, this excessive sweating can lead to *dehydration.* This is a serious complication.

Nutrients

The fuel nutrients also become depleted during continued exercise. As energy demands increase, the body burns blood glucose and muscle glycogen to provide energy. With prolonged exercise, levels of these nutrients fall too low to sustain the body's continued demands. Fatigue follows, and exhaustion threatens.

Oxygen Use and Physical Capacity

Oxygen Consumption

The most profound limitation to exercise is a person's ability to deliver oxygen to the tissues for use in the production of energy. This vital ability depends on the fitness of the pulmonary and cardiovascular systems. Because the heart is a muscle, exercise strengthens and enlarges it, enabling it to pump more blood per beat, a capacity called **stroke volume.** The **cardiac output,** how much the heart pumps out in a given period, depends on the amount of blood per contraction and on the *cardiac rate,* the number of contractions in a given time. In general, then, a person's **aerobic capacity** depends on the degree of fitness and body composition.

1. **Body fitness.** Physical fitness is defined in terms of aerobic capacity, which depends on the body's abil-ity to deliver and use oxygen in sufficient quantities to meet the demands of increasing levels of exercise. Oxygen uptake increases with exercise intensity until either the demand is met or the ability to supply it is exceeded. This maximal oxygen (O_2) uptake, or aerobic capacity, is called the **VO_2 max**—maximal uptake volume of oxygen.[5] This capacity determines the intensity and duration of exercise that a person can perform. From the resting level, there is a steep rise in oxygen consumption during the first 3 minutes of exercise. In about 6 minutes the rate levels off into a steady state, indicating an equilibrium between the energy required by the exercising muscles and the aerobic energy-producing system. This aerobic capacity of an individual is measured in terms of milliliters of oxygen consumed per kilogram of body weight per minute. Thus persons of differing sizes can be compared equally.

2. **Recovery period.** During exercise, to accommodate the body's increased energy demands, the heart rate increases and breathing becomes deeper and more rapid. After exercise stops, these functions do not immediately return to their preexercise levels, especially if the exercise has been strenuous. This recovery takes time, because the body must replenish its "oxygen debt."

3. **Body composition.** Gender differences in aerobic capacity reflect the gender differences in body composition. In general, men have a higher aerobic capacity because of their larger lean body mass, the active metabolic body tissue. These highly metabolic tissues of the body thus use more oxygen than do other tissues, such as fat. When oxygen consumption is expressed only in terms of lean body mass instead of body weight, however, men and women have the same aerobic capacity. But women carry more body fat, a gender difference in body composition that serves critical biologic functions. Apart from stored adipose fat fuel, essential structural and functional body fat in women is about 12% of their body weight; in men it is only 3%. And because women must, of course, carry their entire body weight as part of their total work load, their performance will be affected accordingly.

4. **Genetic influence.** A person's aerobic capacity is determined mainly by genetics. But the genetic heritage is influenced, as indicated, by body composition, which is associated with gender, and by aerobic training and age. Before puberty, lean body mass is about equal in boys and girls of comparable body size, but it increases rapidly in boys at puberty due to the anabolic effect of testosterone. Maximal aerobic capacity then peaks at 18 to 20 years of age and declines gradually thereafter, largely due to age-related losses in lean body mass.[5]

Diet and Exercise: Fluids and Nutrients
Role of Water and Nutrients in Exercise

Along with oxygen, an increased intake of water and nutrients is necessary in the course of exercise. Water is essential in any exercise, but especially in prolonged exercise.[6] A deficiency of water is dangerous and limits exercise capacity greatly. As exercise continues the body temperature increases dramatically, because part of the energy produced by the processes of glycolysis is released as heat. To control this increased heat, the body shunts as much water as possible to the skin, where it escapes in perspiration. Over time, and especially in hot weather, this excessive water loss from perspiration leads to dehydration. This is a serious complication limiting the intensity and duration of exercise.

Nutrients also become depleted during continued exercise as the body draws on its stored energy. As demands for cell ATP increase, the body metabolizes blood glucose and muscle glycogen to provide energy via anaerobic glycolysis. With prolonged exercise of greater intensity, however, the levels of these nutrients fall too low to sustain the body's demands. Fatigue follows, muscle failure occurs because of lactic acid build-up, and exercise cannot continue.

Energy-Yielding Macronutrients

Our diet supplies the necessary fuel substrate from the three energy-yielding macronutrients for meeting our energy needs. We need carbohydrate and fat as basic fuels but depend little on protein. General needs apply to all individuals, but the young person—especially the growing child—has some special needs.

Protein
Protein as a Fuel Substrate

Protein is usually discounted as a fuel substrate in energy production during exercise. Although some amino acids can feed into the cell's basic energy cycle, the extent of this input during exercise is minimal. There is evidence that some amino acid breakdown occurs during exercise, and there is some nitrogen loss in sweat. But authorities agree that under normal circumstances, protein makes a relatively insignificant contribution to energy during exercise. In endurance events, however, somewhat more protein may be used, especially when carbohydrate resources are exhausted.[7]

Protein in the Diet

Most experts recommend 0.8 to 1.0 g protein/kg body weight to meet general needs of the active person. This amounts to the general RDA standard for adults, which contributes about 10% to 12% of the kilocalories in the diet. Most Americans eat about twice this amount of protein, putting a taxing load on the kidneys and the liver. Nitrogen consumed in excess of need must be excreted. This requires an increased production of urea, which contributes to dehydration, a serious factor during strenuous exercise. High-protein diets can also lead to increased excretion of calcium in the urine.

Fat
Fat as Fuel Substrate

In the presence of oxygen, fatty acids are oxidized to provide energy. The rate at which this can occur is determined in part by the rate of mobilization of fatty acids from storage. But all stored fat is not alike. Actually, the body stores fat in two ways: (1) as *depot* fat in adipose tissue, which is destined for transport back and forth to other tissues as needed for energy, and (2) as *essential* fat in metabolically active tissue, such as bone marrow, heart, lungs, liver, spleen, kidneys, intestines, muscles, and nervous system, which is reserved in these places for necessary structural and functional use only. Although storage depot fat in men and women is roughly comparable, essential fat reserves make the big difference—they are about four times greater in women.

Free fatty acids, the fat fuel, are stored with glycerol as triglycerides in the body's adipose tissue. The enzyme *lipoprotein lipase* mobilizes these stores of fatty acids. This lipase is stimulated by exercise. Its activity is affected by levels of hormones also involved in exercise, especially growth hormone and epinephrine.

Fat in the Diet

It is important to recognize that fat as a fuel substrate is not drawn from the diet directly, but from the body's stored adipose fat. Dietary fat is not necessary to maintain these body fat stores, because excess kilocalories in the diet will be stored as fat, regardless of their di-

aerobic capacity • Milliliters of oxygen consumed per kilogram of body weight per minute; influenced by body composition.

cardiac output • Total volume of blood propelled from the heart with each contraction; equal to the stroke putput multiplied by the number of beats per the time unit used in the calculation.

stroke volume • The amount of blood pumped from a ventricle (chamber of the heart releasing blood to body circulations) with each beat of the heart.

VO₂max • Maximal uptake volume of oxygen during exercise; used to measure the intensity and duration of exercise a person can perform.

etary source. We do not need to eat in excess of our dietary needs to burn fat, and there is no danger of depleting our fat stores before exercise has proceeded to exhaustion. Thus there is little basis for increased levels of fat in the diet. On the other hand, however, some fat in the diet is needed, especially as a source of the essential fatty acid linoleic acid. In an apparent attempt to imitate the low-fat diet of the now-famous runners, the Tarahumara Indians of the mountains of Mexico, some compulsive runners in other countries have virtually eliminated fat from their diets, inducing a dangerous linoleic acid deficiency. Because the heart muscle prefers fatty acids—especially linoleic acid—as an energy source, there have been reports of deaths from cardiac arrest in some of these cases (see box, p. 275). Although some dietary fat is necessary, it should not exceed 25% to 30% of the total daily kcaloric intake.

Carbohydrate

Carbohydrate as Fuel Substrate

Although fat and protein have their special roles to play in maintaining general health, the major nutrient for energy support in exercise is carbohydrate. Carbohydrate fuels come from two sources: the circulating blood glucose and glycogen stored in muscle and liver.

Carbohydrate in the Diet

Because carbohydrates are the major energy nutrient, they should contribute about 60% of the daily kcaloric intake. Complex carbohydrates (starches) are preferable to simple carbohydrates (sugars). Starches provide a sustained source of blood glucose, as well as glycogen storage. Simple sugars supply important daily energy, especially for athletes who may require as much as 5000 kcal/day, and also contribute to glycogen storage. However, in some persons, simple carbohydrates may contribute to the danger of subsequent hypoglycemia.

In repeated bouts of intense exercise, diets low in carbohydrate have proved to be incapable of restoring tissue glycogen levels.[5] A low-carbohydrate diet decreases the capacity for work, which intensifies over time. Conversely, a high-carbohydrate diet restores glycogen concentrations to their regular levels. Numerous studies have shown poor exercise performance in persons who eat low-carbohydrate diets. Athletes especially experience fatigue, ketoacidosis, dehydration, and hypoglycemia. However, cyclists given carbohydrate feedings before and during exercise maintained glucose concentrations and rates of glucose oxidation necessary to exercise strenuously and thus were able to delay fatigue.[8,9]

Sometimes athletes use a glycogen-loading food plan, as shown in Table 14-1, to build up glycogen reserves for endurance events. This modern depletion-tapering plan extends fuel reserves and avoids the potential side

TABLE 14-1

Modified Depletion-Taper Precompetition Program for Glycogen Loading

Day	Exercise	Diet
1	90-minute period at 70%-75% V_{0_2} max	Mixed diet, 50% carbohydrate (350 g)
2-3	Gradual tapering of time and intensity	Diet above continued
4-5	Tapering of exercise time and intensity continues	Mixed diet, 70% carbohydrate (550 g)
6	Complete rest	Diet above continued
7	Day of competition	High-carbohydrate preevent diet

From Wright ED: Carbohydrate nutrition and exercise, *Clin Nutr* 7(1):18, 1988.

effects, such as extra water storage in muscles, caused by the formerly-used classic glycogen-loading program. In general, during the 3 days before a competition, athletes need to consume about 65% of their energy intake as complex carbohydrates or 550 g/day of carbohydrates, whichever is greater.[10]

Regulating Micronutrients

Vitamins and Minerals as Fuel Substrate

Vitamins and minerals cannot be used as fuel substrates. They are not oxidized or used up in the process of energy production. They are essential in the energy production process but only as catalytic cofactors in enzyme reactions.

Vitamins and Minerals in the Diet

Increased exercise levels are not correlated with increased dietary needs for vitamins or minerals beyond the RDAs. A well-balanced diet will supply adequate amounts of vitamins and minerals, and exercise may well improve the body's efficient use of them. For example, because athletes have a dietary need for energy, their larger kcaloric intake from good food sources automatically increases their general intake of vitamins and minerals. Multivitamin and mineral supplementation does not improve physical performance in healthy athletes who eat a well-balanced diet. And certainly the potential side effects from megavitamin supplements are well known (see Chapters 7 and 8). However, *therapeutic* iron supplements may be necessary for some athletes who experience anemia (see box, p. 275).

Exercise and Energy

Physically active persons, especially athletes, need more fuel. Exercise raises the body's kcaloric need. Also, exercise has the benefit of helping to regulate appetite to meet these needs. At mild-to-moderate levels of exercise, persons have actually been shown to eat less than inactive persons do. This may relate to an internal "set

Some women athletes—especially runners and gymnasts, who enter their highly competitive and demanding sport during preadolescence and early adolescence—experience anemia and amenorrhea during heavy training and endurance events. A reduced hemoglobin (Hb) level in an athlete's blood means reduced oxygen-carrying capacity, with obvious implications for aerobic capacity and ability to sustain an exercise work load. Absence of menses or delayed puberty in young girls means less protective estrogen and a higher risk of low bone density and stress fractures.

The definition of anemia has been set at a Hb value of less than 12 g/dL for women (normal is 14). (For men, anemia results when the Hb value is less than 14 g/dL; normal is 16). We know little, however, about the relative influence of Hb levels *within* the normal range on athletic performance. Some suggest that athletes' Hb levels should be higher for optimal performance, although excessive concentrations of Hb lead to increased blood viscosity and a decreased rate of flow. Maintenance of normal Hb levels at least of women has been proposed.

Although frank anemia is rare among competitive athletes, low normal values are typical. Heavy exercise may include transient anemia during the initial weeks of training, with the Hb level eventually stabilizing at the low end of normal. Strenuous continued exercise is also associated with low iron stores in athletes, which pose long-term problems.

Possible causes of so-called sport anemia include (1) a diet inadequate in iron, (2) decreased iron absorption, and (3) increased iron losses. Current studies of athletes have revealed that some diets are low in iron. Decreased iron absorption and increased loss are additional causes that add to the problem. Women athletes have cyclic menstrual loss of iron unless they experience amenorrhea. Recent studies have also shown significant amounts of iron lost in profuse sweating. Another possibility is occasional *intravascular hemolysis,* the rupture of red blood cells (RBCs) caused by the stresses of heavy exercise. This effect may be transient or chronic. It is manifested as free Hb in the urine but has not been reported often.

Another factor in athletes' low-normal Hb levels may be *hemodilution.* Strenuous training leads to an increase in plasma volume and absolute quantity of Hb, but the increases may not be proportional—plasma volume increases more than does the Hb level. Hemodilution with increased iron loss and increased RBC turnover may account for the prevalence of low-normal values among athletes. Obviously this situation is complicated if the diet is inadequate in bioavailable iron, as is sometimes found.

Amenorrhea is defined in studies as absence of menses entirely, or less than two periods in a year. The normal hormonal functioning of estrogen initiates and controls the female reproductive cycle at puberty around age 12. When athletic training begins at an early age before normal menarche, this normal growth and development pattern is delayed, along with the secondary gender characteristics shaping the female figure, as evidenced in the small, flat bodies of young gymnasts. Older amenorrheic adolescent runners have usually entered training after menarche, then stopped menstruating after beginning their running program. Menstrual abnormalities in athletic women are usually associated with (1) reduced body fat, (2) age of menarche, (3) intensity of the training and competing program, and (4) nutritional inadequacies from weight loss efforts. Most dietary studies indicate an inadequate intake of two key nutrients—iron and calcium.

In cases of both delayed and interrupted menses, normal estrogen levels are depressed. Estrogens cause increased osteoblastic activity (bone growth) to help ensure rapid adolescent bone development and mature bone maintenance. Thus the young amenorrheic athlete is faced with a constant juggling act. On one hand, she may lack sufficient estrogen activity to stimulate the usual bone growth pattern. On the other hand, she often lacks adequate dietary calcium and iron as she restricts her diet in a constant struggle with growth, strength, weight, optimal body fat, and intense exercise. As a result, she may be doubly at risk for low bone density and stress fractures, as well as for "sports anemia."

Perhaps the journalist's poignant question after covering young women athletes in Olympic competition may well echo our own: "Old too soon, wise too late?"

REFERENCES

Baer JT, Tapir LJ: Amenorrheic and eumenorrheic adolescent runners: dietary intake and exercise training status, *J Am Diet Assoc* 92(1):89, 1992.

Benardot D and others: Nutrient intake in young, highly competitive gymnasts, *J Am Diet Assoc* 89(3):401, 1989.

Highet R: Athletic amenorrhea, *Sports Med* 7:82, 1989.

Myburgh KH: Low bone density is an etiologic factor for stress fractures in athletes, *Ann Intern Med* 113:754, 1990.

Press A: Old too soon, wise too late? *Newsweek* CXX(6):22, 1992.

Weaver CM, Rajram S: Exercise and iron status, *J Nutr* 122:782, 1992. ◆

point" regulating the amount of body fat the person will carry. According to this theory (see Chapter 6), the set point is raised—that is, more body fat is stored—when the individual becomes inactive. In any case, when exercise levels rise above mild or moderate amounts to strenuous levels, kcaloric needs also rise to supply needed fuel.

Even for the athlete, however, there is no significantly greater need for protein or fat than for a nonactive person. Carbohydrate is the preferred fuel and critical foodstuff for the active person. These carbohydrates should mainly be complex in form at an intake that will not only meet increased energy needs, but also supply added vitamins and minerals. The following ratio is the approximate dietary composition recommended for support of physical activity:

> Protein: 10% to 15% of total kilocalories (1.0 to 1.5 g/kg)
> Fat: 30% of total kilocalories
> Carbohydrate: 55% to 60% of total kilocalories (or remainder of kilocalories to meet energy needs)

Nutrition and Athletic Performance

Athletes, Coaches, and Nutritional Practices

Misinformation

Athletes and their coaches are particularly susceptible to myths and magic claims about foods and dietary supplements. They search relentlessly for the competitive edge (see box, p. 275). Knowing this, marketers unremittingly exploit this search, making this group particularly vulnerable. Manufacturers sometimes make distorted and false claims for products. For example, pangamic acid—marketed a few years ago as "vitamin B_{15}" but not a vitamin at all—carried claims about its ability to enhance oxygen transport during exercise. Naturally, if there were such a compound, it would be of interest to athletes and their trainers. However, scientific research has exposed these claims as unfounded.

Myths

In addition to specific fraud, the world of athletics is beset with superstitions and misconceptions. Some of these myths include the following:
- Athletes need protein for energy.
- Extra protein is needed to build bigger and stronger muscles.
- Muscle tissue is broken down during exercise, and protein supplements are needed to replace this breakdown.
- Vitamin supplements are needed to enable athletes to use more energy.
- Vitamins and minerals are burned up in workouts and training sessions.
- Electrolyte solutions are needed during exercise to replace sweat losses.

- A pregame meal of steak and eggs ensures maximal performance.
- Sugar is needed before and during performance to enhance energy levels.
- Drinking water during exercise will cause cramps.

Pregame Meal

Traditionally, steak and eggs have been the ritual foods for the precompetition meal. However, if such a meal is eaten less than 6 hours before the athletic event, it will still be in the stomach during the event. Protein and fat delay the emptying of the stomach, and neither contributes to the glycogen stores needed during exercise. On the contrary, the ideal pregame meal is now known to be a light, low-fat, low-protein meal high in complex carbohydrate (starches) and eaten 2 to 4 hours before competition. This allows the body time to digest, absorb, and transform it into stored glycogen. Such a high-carbohydrate pregame meal is illustrated in Table 14-1. A high-carbohydrate diet with a minimum of 500 g/day is recommended throughout training. For competition days, a diet containing about 600 g/day is needed. Tables 14-2 and 14-3 may be used to calculate these diets. Small amounts of carbohydrate-containing foods or drinks may be consumed up to a brief time before the event without affecting the performance. A total carbohydrate intake of 1 to 5 g/kg body weight taken from 5 minutes to 4 hours before the exercise has been found to enhance performance.[10]

Hydration: Water and Electrolytes

Water

Dehydration can be a serious problem for athletes. Its extent depends on the intensity and duration of the exercise, the surrounding temperature, the level of fitness, and the preexercise or pregame state of hydration. It is most severe in endurance events. For example, marathon runners sometimes collapse from dehydration. They may also have other problems, such as cramps, delirium, vomiting, hypothermia, or hyperthermia—all caused by dehydration. By planning carefully before the event and replacing fluids along the way, the athlete can prevent many of these problems. Mandatory weighing before and after the event is done, and each pound (2.2 kg) of weight lost is replaced by 16 oz (480 to 500 ml) of fluid.[10]

1. **Cause.** About 60% of the energy from the breakdown of glucose is released as heat. In minimal physical exercise this heat production maintains desirable body temperature. But during heavier exercise it exceeds the body's needs and sometimes its heat tolerance. Sweating is our main mechanism for dissipating body heat. The major source of fluid lost in sweat is plasma fluid. Endurance events can cause the loss of several liters of water as sweat, which is

TABLE 14-2

Grams of Carbohydrates in Typical Foods

Food group	Carbohydrates per serving (g)	Food item
Starchy vegetables, breads, cereals	15	*One serving:* ½ cup dry breakfast cereal; ½ cup cooked breakfast cereal; ½ cup cooked grits; ½ cup cooked rice; ½ cup cooked pasta; ½ cup baked beans; ½ cup corn; ½ cup beans; 1 small baked potato; ½ bagel; ½ English muffin; 1 slice bread; ¾ oz pretzels; 6 saltine crackers; 2 four-inch diameter pancakes; 2 taco shells
Vegetables (carrots, green beans, broccoli, cauliflower, onions, spinach, tomatoes, vegetable juice)	5	*One serving:* ½ cup cooked vegetables; 1 cup raw vegetables; ½ cup vegetable juice
Fruits	15	*One serving:* ½ cup fresh fruit; ½ cup fruit juice; ¼ cup dried fruit; 1 small apple; 4 apricots; ½ banana; 12 cherries or grapes; ½ grapefruit; 1 nectarine; 1 orange; 1 peach; 1¼ cups watermelon
Milk	12	*One serving:* 1 cup milk; 8 oz plain low-fat yogurt
Sweets*	15	*One serving:* ½ slice plain cake; 2 small cookies; 3 gingersnaps; ½ cup ice cream; ¼ cup sherbet

From American Diabetes Association, American Dietetic Association: Exchange lists for meal planning, Chicago, 1986, The Association.

*NOTE: Also high in fat.

TABLE 14-3

A 600-g Carbohydrate Diet*

Menu	Carbohydrates (g)
Breakfast	
1 orange	14
2 cups oatmeal	50
1 cup skim milk	12
2 bran muffins	48
Snacks	
¾ cup chopped dates	98
Lunch	
Lettuce salad:	
1 cup romaine lettuce	2
1 cup garbanzo beans	45
½ cup alfalfa sprouts	5.5
2 tbsp French dressing	2
3 cups macaroni and cheese	80
1 cup apple juice	28
Snack	
2 slices whole wheat toast	26
1 tsp margarine	—
2 tbsp jam	14
Dinner	
2 oz turkey breast (no skin)	—
2 cups mashed potatoes	74
1 cup peas and onions	23
1 banana	27
1 cup skim milk	12
Snack	
1 cup pasta	33
2 tsp margarine	—
2 tbsp Parmesan cheese	—
1 cup cranberry juice	36
TOTAL	628

*This diet provides 4000 kcals, of which 61% are from carbohydrates (628 g), 14% are from protein (139 g), and 26% are from fat (118 g). A carbohydrate/protein/fat ratio of 60:15:25 is a good goal when planning a diet to aid athletic performance.

pulled from the plasma fluid to control body heat. Unless this amount is replaced, serious consequences can follow.

1. **Prevention.** The thirst mechanism fails to keep pace with the body's increased need for fluid during exercise. The dehydrated person, therefore, must push fluids. To prevent dehydration, athletes are advised to drink more water than they think is needed, without dependence on the normal thirst mechanism. Cold water, about the temperature inside a refrigerator, is absorbed more quickly from the stomach. It is important to speed rehydration and to minimize the discomfort that a full stomach gives the athlete. Small cups of cold water—or mild solutions of saline and glucose during longer ultra-events, such as 50-mile runs, 100-mile cycling, or triathlons—should be consumed frequently.[11] Until quite recently, it was thought that drinking water immediately before or during an athletic event would cause cramps. There is no basis for this claim.

Electrolytes

A number of special "sports drinks" (see box, p. 279) are now being marketed, with the indication that the electrolytes lost in sweat must be replaced. This is true, but how? Sweat is more dilute than our internal fluids, and thus we lose proportionately—not just absolutely—much more water than anything else. Adding electrolytes and sugar to water simply delays its emptying from the stomach. In most instances, water is the rehydration fluid of choice. Electrolytes are replaced with the athlete's next meal. However, during longer and more demanding endurance events—especially in a warm environment—one of the newer mild saline and glucose (6% solution) sports drinks that has a rapid gastric emptying and intestinal absorption time may be used.[12]

Training and Precompetition Abuses Among Athletes

Weight Control Measures

The sport of wrestling has a long history of widely fluctuating weight patterns among its athletes. Wrestlers often restrict food and fluid intake to certify for a weight classification that is below their off-season weight, seeking to gain advantages in strength, speed, and leverage over a smaller opponent.[13] This practice of "making weight" still seems to be an ingrained tradition that produces large, frequent, and rapid weight loss and regain cycles, with methods such as dehydration, severe food restriction, and loss of food and fluid through induced vomiting and use of laxatives and diuretic drugs. Such disordered eating affects normal growth, and progressive dehydration impairs regulation of body temperature and cardiovascular function. Other sports, such as bodybuilding and gymnastics, often follow similar routines, especially before competition.[14,15] Young preadolescent girls in gymnastics, for example, are forced to maintain a small body size in the face of advancing age. Therefore they increasingly reduce food intake and body fat, sometimes developing eating disorders. As a result, a cascade of events may follow—impaired growth, delayed puberty, and induced amenorrhea from low estrogen levels, a complicating factor in bone development and later osteoporosis.[15] A similar pattern has been observed among young runners.[16]

Drug Abuse

From ancient Greek runners and discus throwers in the first Olympian contests to top competitors from world nations in today's Olympic events, athletes have experimented with various **ergogenic** aids in their eternal search for the competitive edge or the perfect body. Modern athletes—from national league football players to their aspiring high school counterparts—are doing the same thing, trying to find the magic potion in everything from bee pollen and seaweed to freeze-dried liver flakes, gelatin, amino acid supplements, and ginseng.[17] Such efforts have been worthless in most cases, but fortunately not particularly harmful. However, in the case of the group of drugs called anabolic-androgenic steroids, which are now epidemic in the sporting world, great danger and even death lies ahead for the user.[18] These illegal drugs must be obtained through a black market network, which adds legal jeopardy and street preparation impurities to the drug's inherent dangers to personal health. These dangers have included reported death from fatal cardiac arrest, acute heart attack, and cancer of the liver and prostate.[18] Abuse of steroids in the United States has now moved from early use among bodybuilders and has invaded almost all areas of athletics, becoming epidemic among football players and increasingly common among young junior and senior high school boys. In addition, other abuses amplify the dangers of steroids. For example, a large dosage of a diuretic—such as furosemide (Lasix, 80 to 120 mg)—is taken on the day of drug testing to dilute the urine and decrease the risk of detection. Also, large megadoses of vitamins and minerals become abused drugs and as such are used as ergogenic aids in all areas and levels of sports. Such megadoses of nutrients alter normal metabolic processes and cause severe disturbances. Little or no government regulation of the industry and poor production quality control result in variable strength products and contamination during processing.[18]

Building a Personal Exercise Program

Health Benefits

In various other chapters we discuss physical activity in relation to different health problems. These chapters can be referred to for questions about particular conditions. Here we summarize health benefits of aerobic exercise for some of these conditions.

Coronary Heart Disease

Aerobic exercise increases heart size and strength, improving its stroke volume and resulting blood circulation. An increased stroke volume means that the heart puts out more blood with each beat, so it needs to pump fewer times per minute to circulate the same amount of blood. This represents a long-term reduction in the heart's work load. This improved pulmonary and body circulation enhances the oxygen-carrying capacity of the blood and sustains the overall blood volume. Exercise also raises blood levels of high-density lipoproteins (HDLs), creating a more favorable ratio of HDLs to low-density lipoproteins (LDLs), which carry cholesterol loads to cells (see Chapter 20).

Diabetes Management

Exercise helps control diabetes by enhancing the action of insulin through an increased number of insulin re-

Sort Out the Sports Drinks Saga

TO PROBE FURTHER

The first of the so-called sports drinks hit the market running about 25 years ago, and now these beverages have spawned a multimillion-dollar industry. Their claims abound, and sorting them out is not always easy for athletes and their coaches, who forever seek that prize of the competitive edge.

The current saga of the sports drinks began with a solution called Gatorade, a beverage its developers named for their university's football team. They reasoned that if they analyzed the perspiration of their players, they could replace the lost minerals and water in a drink containing some flavoring, coloring, and sugars to make it acceptable, and it would taste better and do a better job than plain water. Although it has been highly profitable for the university and for the manufacturer, most athletes simply do not need it. Physically fit athletes engaged in regular nonendurance exercise do as well if they consume plain water and get their minerals from their regular diets.

However, what long-term endurance athletes do need, especially in hot weather, is water and fuel—carbohydrates. For example, a runner in a long-distance marathon perspires 2% to 6% of his or her weight, thereby losing so much water that his or her body cannot keep cool enough and the overall system overheats, leading to heatstroke and collapse. Also, without adequate carbohydrate replacement, the muscles soon run out of glycogen stores and slow down. But simply adding sugar to water holds the fuel sugar in the stomach longer, where it does the body tissues no good for immediate needs.

To meet the body's dual need during such marathon events, a second category of sports drinks has now developed, using glucose polymers instead of so much sugar and less sodium. These short chains of about five glucose molecules, known as maltodextrins, are produced in the breakdown of starch. These drinks are less concentrated, are only slightly sweetened and flavored, and leave the stomach rapidly, thus making them ideal as a continuing fuel source for the endurance athlete. Two such products in this category, marketed in powdered mix form, are Ross Lab's Exceed and Coca-Cola's Max. But these products cannot be found in supermarkets. They are provided mainly through pharmacies to professionals working with serious athletes.

Other sports drinks to enter the market have been Gatorade clones—such as the product Recharge—which claims to add no sugar, yet supplies an ample amount of it as fructose and glucose in its fruit juice base. And still another category has emerged in such products as Gear Up, which adds to its base of 10 fruit juices 10 vitamins in amounts yielding 137% of the RDAs in a single 10-oz bottle and contains no minerals. All of these extra vitamins do not help your performance at all, and on a hot day a perspiring athlete could easily consume a megadose in four or five bottles.

So sort out the claims of sports drinks. They are not for everyone. For the long run, special ones meet needs of the athlete in endurance events. But for nonendurance activities, most persons don't need them. After all, water is the best solution for regular needs—and it costs far less.

REFERENCES

Coleman E: Sports drink research, *Food Technol* 45:104, 1991.

Coyle EF: Carbohydrate supplementation during exercise, *J Nutr* 122:788, 1992.

Millard-Stafford M and others: Carbohydrate-electrolyte replacement during a simulated triathlon in the heat, *Med Sci Sports Exerc* 22(5):621, 1990.

Murray R and others: Carbohydrate feeding and exercise: effect of beverage carbohydrate content, *Eur J Appl Physiol* 59:152, 1989.

---

ceptor sites and by stimulating insulin-balancing hormones, such as glucogon. This effect is particularly useful in the management of non–insulin-dependent diabetes mellitus (NIDDM) in obese adults. However, in the management of insulin-dependent diabetes mellitus (IDDM), the nature and scheduling of physical activity must be balanced with food and insulin to prevent hypoglycemic reactions. But such management can be done and is a healthful tool of self-care (see Chapter 21).

Weight Management

Exercise is extremely beneficial in weight management, because it helps to regulate appetite, increases the basal metabolic rate, and reduces the fat deposit "set point" level. Together with a well-planned diet, physical exercise corrects the energy balance in favor of increased energy output and decreased energy intake (see Chapter 6). A simple, well-defined walking program can reduce the amount of body fat, even without any noticeable changes in dietary intake.[19] Thus exercise by itself has a significant effect on reducing fat and increasing lean body content.

Stress Management

Exercise is a positive alternative activity to reduce excess stress-related eating. It also provides a physical out-

ergogenic • Tendency to increase work output; various substances that increase work or exercise capacity and output.

let for working off the hormonal physiologic events produced in the body by stress, thus helping to reduce a major risk factor in the development of chronic disease (see Chapter 15).

Bone Disease

Exercise helps increase bone mineralization, thus reducing the risk of bone weakness and of potential osteoporosis (see Chapters 8 and 26).

Mental Health

Exercise stimulates the production of brain opiates, which are associated with a decreased susceptibility to pain. These substances contribute to an improved mood, including a sense of exhiliration or kind of "high."

Assessment of Personal Health and Exercise Needs

There are many kinds of exercise. Choosing those kinds which are best depends on individual health and personal needs, the aerobic benefits involved, and personal enjoyment.

Health and Personal Needs

In planning an exercise program, it is important to assess individual health status, personal needs, present level of fitness, and resources required. What do you want to gain from your exercise? How much time can you commit to it? How much, if anything, does it cost? Perhaps it is even more important to ask yourself what you like to do. If the exercise you choose isn't fun, you will soon stop doing it, and it will benefit no one. Also, it is wise to start slowly and build gradually rather than risk injury and discouragement. Moderation and regularity are key guides in planning.

Beneficial Level of Exercise

To build aerobic capacity, the level of exercise must raise the pulse rate to within 70% of maximal heart rate. Unless you have had an exercise tolerance or stress test and know precisely what your maximal exercising heart rate is, a rule of thumb is to determine your cardiac rate by subtracting your age from 220 (Table 14-4). This calculation estimates your maximal heart rate, and 70% of this figure tells you the rate to which you want to raise your pulse in the course of exercise. This rate should then be maintained for an uninterrupted period of at least 20 minutes and be practiced at least three times per week to have aerobic benefits. Check your resting pulse before starting the exercise period, then again during and immediately afterward, to monitor your progress in developing your maximal exercising heart rate and aerobic capacity.

Types of Physical Activity

General Exercise

There are many exercises from which you may choose. Many of them are enjoyable and healthful but do not reach aerobic levels. For example, golf is a passion for many, but it is far too slow and sporadic to be aerobic. Also, most sports in the hands of amateurs—rather than those with fast-paced extraordinary skill to provide sustained exercise—are too slow-paced to be aerobic. These include tennis, football, baseball, and basketball. Weight lifting develops and strengthens muscles but is not an aerobic exercise.

Aerobic Exercise

Forms of exercise that can be sustained at a necessary level of intensity to provide aerobic benefits include such activities as swimming, running, jogging, bicycling, and the recently popular aerobic dancing routines and

---

TABLE 14-4

Target Zone Heart Rate According to Age to Achieve Aerobic Physical Effect of Exercise

Age	Maximal attainable heart rate (pulse: 220 minus age)	Target zone	
		70% Maximal rate	85% Maximal rate
20	200	140	170
25	195	136	166
30	190	133	161
35	185	129	157
40	180	126	153
45	175	122	149
50	170	119	144
55	165	115	140
60	160	112	136
65	155	108	132
70	150	105	127
75	145	101	124

TABLE 14-5

Aerobic Exercises for Physical Fitness (Maintained at Aerobic Level for at Least 20 Minutes)

Type of exercise	Aerobic forms
Ball playing	Handball
	Raquetball
	Squash
Bicycling	Stationary
	Touring
Dancing	Aerobic routines
	Ballet
	Disco
Jumping rope	Brisk pace
Running or jogging	Brisk pace
Skating	Ice-skating
	Roller-skating
Skiing	Cross-country
Swimming	Steady pace
Walking	Brisk pace

workouts (Table 14-5). Perhaps the simplest and most popular form of stimulating exercise is *walking*. If the pace is fast enough to elevate your pulse and it is maintained for at least the required 20 minutes, walking can be an excellent form of aerobic exercise. It is convenient and requires no equipment other than good walking shoes. It is also emotionally satisfying to many persons for whom running, swimming, cycling, and dancing may not be most appropriate.

Preparation for Exercise

Once a sport or exercise has been chosen, adequate preparation is essential. Safety precautions must be observed. Runners and joggers need appropriate shoes; cyclists need good helmets. Before exercising, stretch the muscles to prevent stress and injury. Similarly, take time after completing the exercise to cool down. Many exercise-related injuries, such as pulled muscles and stress fractures, are related to inadequate preparation. It is also possible to exercise beyond the limits of tolerance. Incidences of injuries in running, for example, start rising dramatically at the 25-miles-per-week marker. Some studies have compared the personality profiles of compulsive runners with those of anorexic persons (see Issues and Answers, p. 283). Certainly a level of compulsion that comes to dominate one's life is *unhealthful*. In short, listen to your own body. When you are tired, rest. When you hurt, stop. When the level of exercise is no longer a challenge and you want to increase it somewhat, do so—but only then.

To Sum Up

The energy molecule of the body is adenosine triphosphate (ATP), and the powerhouse of the cell is the mitochondrion. The cell's storehouse of energy is creatine phosphate (CP). These two high-energy phosphate compounds are in limited supply. They can provide energy for only a brief initial period and need to be replenished for exercise to continue. This added supply is made available by anaerobic glycolysis, with added energy made available for continued exercise by the body's aerobic system of energy production. The process of glycolysis metabolizes only carbohydrate substrate, furnished either by blood glucose or stored glycogen. Dietary carbohydrate is necessary to replenish these fuel sources. Protein contributes little to total energy production for exercise, whereas the body's ability to burn fat as fuel depends on the level of fitness. The higher the body's efficiency in using oxygen, the more fatty acids will contribute to the energy supply. Even in the best-trained athletes, fatty acid oxidation must be accompanied by glucose metabolism.

Contrary to popular belief, the protein needs of the diet are not increased by exercise and neither is the body's need for vitamins and minerals. Exercise does increase the body's need for kilocalories and water. Cold water taken in small, frequent amounts is the best way to prevent dehydration in endurance events. Electrolytes lost in sweat are replaced by a continuing diet of adequate quality and quantity. Adding electrolytes or sugar to water delays its emptying from the stomach and thus delays rehydration.

The optimal diet for the active person is 10% to 15% of the kilocalories from protein, 25% to 30% from fat, and 55% to 60% from carbohydrate. The pregame meal for athletes should be small, requiring little or no protein or fat and relying mainly on complex carbohydrate (starches).

The health benefits of general and aerobic exercise are many and increase with practice. The minimal level of aerobic exercise for cardiovascular health elevates the heart rate to 70% of maximum for a sustained period of at least 20 minutes at least three times per week. Excellent aerobic exercises include sustained fast walking, swimming, jogging, running, and aerobic dancing or workouts. Approach any exercise sensibly, and choose those activities which are enjoyable.

QUESTIONS FOR REVIEW

1. What are the component muscle structures, and how do they produce muscle action?
2. What type of substrate fuel does the body use for immediate energy needs? Short-term needs? Long-term needs?
3. How does oxygen relate to physical activity capacity and aerobic effect?
4. Outline the nutrition and physical fitness principles you would discuss with a client who is an athlete. Plan a diet for this client that would meet nutrient and energy needs.
5. Why is fluid balance vital during exercise periods? How is water and electrolyte balance achieved?
6. Describe the dangers of anabolic steroids used by some athletes for bulking muscles and gaining an edge in strength over an opponent.
7. How would you conduct a counseling session for a patient with coronary heart disease about the role of exercise in cardiovascular health? For an overweight client with non–insulin-dependent diabetes mellitus (NIDDM)?

REFERENCES

1. Sigh VN: A current perspective on nutrition and exercise, *J Nutr* 122:760, 1992.
2. Gordon NF, Scott CB: Exercise and mild essential hypertension, *Prim Care* 18(3):683, 1991.
3. Tjoa HI, Kaplan NM: Nonpharmacologic treatment of hypertension in diabetes mellitus, *Diabetes Care* 14(6):449, 1991.
4. Merrill GF, Friedricks GS: Plasma lipid concentrations

in college students performing self-selected exercise, *J Am Coll Nutr* 9(3):226, 1990.

5. Guyton AC: *Textbook of medical physiology,* ed 8, Philadelphia, 1991, WB Saunders.

6. Barr SI, Gestill DL: Water: can the endurance athlete get too much of a good thing? *J Am Diet Assoc* 89(11):1629, 1989.

7. Paul G: Dietary protein requirements of physically active individuals, *Sports Med* 8:154, 1989.

8. Sherman WM and others: Carbohydrate feedings 1 h before exercise improves cycling performance, *Am J Clin Nutr* 54:866, 1991.

9. Coyle EF: Carbohydrate supplementation during exercise, *J Nutr* 122:788, 1992.

10. Hoffman CJ, Coleman E: An eating plan and update on recommended dietary practices for the endurance athlete, *J Am Diet Assoc* 91(3):325, 1991.

11. Lindeman AK: Eating and training habits of triathletes: a balancing act, *J Am Diet Assoc* 90(7):993, 1990.

12. Millard-Stafford and others: Carbohydrate-electrolyte replacement during a simulated triathalon in the heat, *Med Sci Sports Exerc* 22(5):621, 1990.

13. Steen SN, Brownell KD: Patterns of weight loss and regain in wrestlers: has the tradition changed? *Med Sci Sports Exerc* 22(4):470, 1990.

14. Kleiner SM and others: Metabolic profiles, diet, and health practices of championship male and female bodybuilders, *J Am Diet Assoc* 90(7):962, 1990.

15. Benardo D, Czerwinski C: Selected body composition and growth measures of junior elite gymnasts, *J Am Diet Assoc* 91(1):29, 1991.

16. Baer JT, Taper LJ: Amenorrheic and eumenorrheic adolescent runners: dietary intake and exercise training status, *J Am Diet Assoc* 92(1):89, 1992.

17. Lamb DR, Wardlaw GM: *Sports nutrition, Nutri-News,* St Louis, 1991, Mosby–Year Book.

18. Kleiner SM: Performance-enhancing aids in sport: health consequences and nutritional alternatives, *J Am Coll Nutr* 10(2):163, 1991.

19. Bergman EA, Boyungs JC: Indoor walking program increases lean body composition in older women, *J Am Diet Assoc* 91(11):1433, 1991.

FURTHER READING

Barr SI, Costill DL: Water: can the endurance athlete get too much of a good thing? *J Am Diet Assoc* 89(11):1629, 1989.
Hoffman CJ, Coleman E: An eating plan and update on recommended dietary practices for the endurance athlete, *J Am Diet Assoc* 91(3):325, 1991.
Moses K, Manore MM: Development and testing of a carbohydrate monitoring tool for athletes, *J Am Diet Assoc* 91(8):962, 1991.

These three articles provide important information concerning water intake for the athlete, as well as excellent eating plans and monitoring tools.

Hickson JF and others: Nutrition and the precontest preparations of a male bodybuilder, *J Am Diet Assoc* 90(2):264, 1990.
Kleiner SM and others: Metabolic profiles, diet, and health practices of championship male and female bodybuilders, *J Am Diet Assoc* 90(7):962, 1990.

These authors take us backstage in the world of bodybuilders to learn of their myths and practices in relation to diet, weight control, and drug use.

The Winning Edge—or Over the Edge?

Athletes, their coaches, and our entire culture have become increasingly aware that the percentage of body fat vs the percentage of lean body mass is a major influence on athletic performance. Each extra pound of body fat an athlete carries into competition is nonproductive weight. It is the muscles—the lean body mass—that provide the strength, agility, and endurance required to win.

Because of this, athlete strive to achieve as low a percentage of body fat as possible while still maintaining good health. In reaching for such a goal, however, many young athletes develop an abhorrence of body fat, resulting in food aversion and the undertaking of excessive weight-loss regimens. These self-generated excesses are commonly reinforced by those surrounding the young athletes: coaches, teammates, and perhaps the most demanding of all, parents.

Such an all-consuming focus results in compulsive behaviors, leading the young person to set unrealistic goals and resulting in abusive weight losses. The fear of failure—failure to make the team, failure in competition, and failure to live up to others' expectations—pushes athletes in their campaign to beat the opponent, have a low level of body fat, and win a particular contest by a large, decisive amount.

Fortunately, such excessive voluntary weight losses in young athletes are not usually caused by chronic emotional problems. The reasons typically are more superficial, resulting from an accumulation of immediate, short-term goals and concerns. These athletes usually respond well to counseling and can reverse the excessive behavior with the support of concerned friends and teammates.

Yet for some individuals, excessive, compulsive fixation on lean body mass and the loss of body fat becomes obsessive and enduring. For example, a compulsive runner's ideal of 5% body fat is regularly found only in ballet dancers, gymnasts, fashion models, and victims of anorexia nervosa. Our culture reinforces this "positive" attribute of beauty: slimness in women, physical prowess in men. When a susceptible individual enters a time of stress in search for a firm identity, however, he or she may turn toward our cultural stereotypes to provide this self-concept. For women this stress is usually encountered in adolescence, when being physically attractive becomes important in dating. For men the sense of self is more closely tied to their vocational and sexual effectiveness, both of which are related to their physical abilities. Thus the test of a man's abilities tends to occur more often in adulthood, which may result in his preoccupation with physical fitness as a way to deny any decline in strength or ability. This may be why the majority of compulsive runners—those who feel they must run despite everything, including injury or ill health—are men.

Although our culture views compulsive dieting—as occurs in anorexia nervosa—as a serious, emotional disorder, compulsive training is seen as a positive personality trait showing dedication. In reality, both may be symptomatic of unstable self-concepts and attempts to establish a firm sense of identity. They are perceptual disorders: whereas the anorexia victim always sees herself as fat, the compulsive runner always sees himself as out of shape. Such compulsive training becomes the whole life, although it is unnatural, not really living, to be pushed by whatever means possible, legal or sometimes illegal. No goal, once attained, is sufficiently satisfying. If 5% body fat is achieved, the person strives for 4%. Such striving, often despite physical indications against it, has even resulted in permanent disabilities and death, sometimes from cardiac arrest caused by a linoleic acid deficiency. These driven individuals have a strict sense of self-denial and are unable to enjoy any of life's more passive, receptive pleasures.

Although physical fitness and athletic accomplishments may be admirable goals, the thrill of victory for a small percentage of participants may be a hollow one, if the victory is at the expense of their health and peace of mind. The ability to slow down, stop, and smell the roses may mean more in the long run to the quality and quantity of a person's life than the color of a coveted ribbon or medal that may be won.

REFERENCES

Clark N: How to approach eating disorders among athletes, *Top Clin Nutr* 5(3):41, 1990.

Kantrowitz B and others: Living with training, *Newsweek* CXX(6):24, 1992.

Williams M: *Beyond training: how athletes enhance performance legally and illegally*, Champaign, Ill, 1989, Leisure Press.

CHAPTER 15

Nutrition and Stress Management

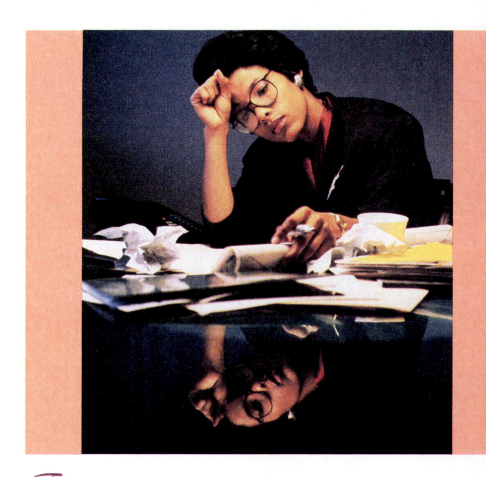

This chapter concludes Part II on the relation of nutrition to the life cycle and health maintenance. In the previous chapter we looked at the role of physical activity in maintaining health. Here we consider the fact of stress in our modern competitive society and its effect on health and nutrition.

Here we seek to understand what stress does to our bodies and how the body adapts, so we can apply these principles to nutrition support needs. Then we examine ways in which inevitable life stress may be managed to help us develop more successful coping skills, and thus reduce this health-disease risk factor in our lives.

Role of Stress as a Health-Disease Risk Factor

Stress of Modern Society and Disease

Modern society is fast-paced and competitive. Its pressures and problems within the rapidly changing environment of a complex technologic age affect air, water, and food. Just as the pebble dropped into the still surface of a body of water sends out ever-widening ripples in all directions, so modern life's stresses—either physical or psychosocial—send out waves that wash over the human body, often contributing further to disease and malnutrition.

These automatic physiologic waves that sweep through the body are built-in adaptive responses to stress triggered through our neuroendocrine system. Through some 40,000 or more years of human development, this physiologic reaction has readied the body to confront or escape danger—the familiar "fight or flight" response. But this response is not well adapted to today's high-pressured and sedentary modern society and life-style. Often we can neither fight nor flee. Yet the same set of physiologic responses continue to be triggered, as if our lives were actually threatened. And indeed they often are, because these repeated physiologic reactions are linked to reduced immune function and the emergence of our so-called diseases of civilization—coronary heart disease, cancer, diabetes, and hypertension.

Stress and Nutrition Care Planning

The classic work of Canadian physician Hans Selye[1,2] clearly shows the close relationship of stress to the risk and incidence of disease. He called stress "the wear and tear in the human machinery which accompanies any vital activity."[2] Over the years of his monumental work, he established the basic pattern of individual physiologic response to a given stress agent. Different reactions in different persons depend on *conditioning factors,* which can inhibit or enhance one or more stress effects. These factors may be internal or built-in, such as genetic predisposition, age, or gender. Or they may be external or manageable, such as poor diet or alcohol and other drug abuse. Numerous other investigators have reinforced the validity of Selye's early foundation work with applications in many areas of health and disease. Thus stress management has become a necessary consideration in nutrition assessment and care planning based on identified human needs. It is an essential component in current health-promotion programs.

Human Needs: The Process of Life Changes and Events

Constant change and balance are both basic to the ongoing process of life. The changing human body gives evidence of the dynamic interior metabolism interacting with the changing exterior environment. Normal physiologic stress is a vital part of this interaction. For example, during pregnancy, normal physiologic stress adapts the maternal body to support fetal growth and prepare for birth. Also, normal stress of inserted muscles on bones helps maintain calcium balance, and the general stress of pain warns of injury or illness.

However, it is severe, prolonged, relentless, uncontrolled stress—be it physical or psychosocial hunger or pain—that contributes to exhaustion of resources and illness or death, because the adaptability of individuals given no relief is finite. Such debilitating stress may relate to four basic areas of human need, to which health team workers must always be sensitive in order to identify individual stresses requiring assessment and care: (1) life cycle growth and development, (2) health-disease status, (3) stress-coping balance, and (4) general human needs for self-fulfillment. All of these areas involve nutritional concerns.

Life Cycle Growth and Development Continuum

From the beginning of life at conception to its ending at death, a steady one-way integrated continuum of physical growth and psychosocial development proceeds. As we have seen in previous chapters, each stage of human life brings unique physical characteristics and psychosocial maturation. Both of these are integral aspects of every person's total life and health. Over the past 30 years, we have gained much understanding of the development of the human personality and its coping resources through the work of the American psychoanalyst Erik Erikson.[3] Through his studies, Erikson identified eight stages of human growth and development from infancy to old age and the psychosocial struggles at each stage (see Chapters 12 and 13). Given favorable life circumstances, people develop positive internal resources to meet life's inevitable crises. Although in periods of increased stress some regression may occur, generally the child and then the adult integrates self-controls and strengths in relation to physical maturation and develops neuromuscular and mental skills. But to the degree that individual life circumstances have not been favorable, stresses multiply and contribute to health problems.

Health-Disease Spectrum

Throughout the life cycle, persons move back and forth across a spectrum of degrees of health and disease. Many fortunate ones remain on the positive side of good health because of their "luck of the draw" in genetic heritage, and they live relatively healthy lives free from major disease. Others less fortunate experience varying degrees of disease or injury. Individual responses depend on personal resources—physical and mental, as well as psychosocial and economic. Thus the determination of any person's health and nutrition status will always involve data from two sources:

1. **Subjective data.** Such information as perceived pain, tolerances, feelings about health status or care, and personal perceptions of problems, goals, and priorities is vital for planning valid personal care. This important primary information is gained from talking with and listening to the person and the family.

2. **Objective data.** Also important is quantified information indicating body functions and capacities. This information comes from various technologic sources, such as laboratory, x-ray, or other tests; performance measures; nutrition analyses; physical findings; and clinical and behavioral observations and tests.

Too often health professionals may dwell mainly in the area of modern medical technology and its multitude of procedures and tests, perhaps because they feel more skilled and comfortable and less vulnerable here. But all the while, especially in high-risk populations, significant roots of disease lie in the subjective area of personal stresses and needs—economic, psychosocial, and mental pressures, as well as physical ones.

Stress-Coping Balance

Stress is a fact of life. Thus there must also be a coping balance to maintain positive health. In *physiologic stress*, either normal or abnormal, a number of automatic physiologic responses maintain the body in a state of dynamic balance or *homeostasis*. For example, to meet the physiologic stress of disease, injury, shock, or physical exertion, various homeostatic mechanisms automatically respond to restore the body's normal metabolism. Similarly, in *psychosocial stress*, a person uses learned mental defense mechanisms, which may or may not be constructive in the circumstances. For example, such defenses as rationalization, compensation, suppression, depression, withdrawal, or substitution are developed during growing years to cope with stress, relieve tension, and preserve the inner self-concept. Often such learned reactions are the only means of making a painful situation psychologically tolerable, but some are less constructive than others.

Basic Human Needs

Human needs and motives, including nutrition-related ones, are highly personal. People are not the same the world over. Those of differing cultures and life circumstances are not motivated by the same needs and goals. Even primary biologic drives, such as hunger and sex, are modified in their expression by many cultural, social, and personal influences. A hierarchy of human needs, such as that developed by American psychologist Abraham Maslow (see Chapter 9), helps us understand human strivings.[4] Through his classic work with persons showing characteristics of positive mental

health behavior, he described five levels of common human needs, each having priority at different times depending on personal circumstances:

- Basic physiologic needs: hunger, thirst
- Safety needs: physical comfort, security, protection
- "Belongingness" needs: giving and receiving love and affection
- Self-esteem needs: self-worth, status, capability
- Self-actualization needs: self-fulfillment, creative growth

Of course these levels of need overlap and vary with the particular situation and time. Nonetheless, they help us understand basic human needs and plan nutrition and health care accordingly, especially in times of stress.

The Nature of Stress
Perception of stress

Individual responses to stress vary according to its reality and how it is perceived. The word "perception" comes from the Latin verb *perceptio*, which means literally "to take in" or to comprehend. We constantly take in through our senses a chaotic assortment of impressions. We make sense out of this chaos through our brain's interpretation of it all, which enables us to live in an environment that feels relatively stable. But perception also limits understanding, because everything the outer world offers is understood through a social and personal lens. We perceive every life experience through a blend of three factors: (1) the actual external *reality*, (2) the *message* of the stimulus that is conveyed by the nervous system to the brain's integrative centers where thinking and evaluation go on, and (3) the *interpretation* that we put on every bit of information. A host of subjective elements—such as hunger, thirst, hatred, fear, self-interest, values, and temperament—influence responses to everything the outer world presents.

Common Life Stressors

As indicated, common life stressors are twofold in nature: (1) physical or physiologic stress, and (2) psychologic or socioeconomic stress. The first form of stress may come from injury, disability, disease, or physical abuse. The second form may come from emotional pressures, verbal abuse, or lack of financial resources. Undoubtedly, emotional tension from multiple causes is the most common agent of human stress. It can contribute to serious conditions, such as cardiovascular and gastrointestinal diseases, diabetes, and cancer, especially if the body is conditioned by malnutrition, faulty diet, or poor housing and homelessness. This is often the case with high-risk families in the grip of poverty. Ultimately, the effect of any life stressor will depend upon three influencing characteristics of the stress: (1) its strength, whether it is relatively mild with minor consequences or severe with major results, (2) its duration, whether it is fairly transient or is long term and relentless, and (3) the strength of resisting forces, the personal coping resources—whether they are strong, relatively positive and constructive, or whether they are more negative, pessimistic, and destructive.

Physiologic-Metabolic Response to Stress

When any form of stress occurs, the body automatically responds to defend itself from harm. Selye called this common physiologic response to stress the *general adaptive syndrome.*[2] An understanding of this automatic "cascade of physiologic events" provides an essential base for (1) identifying needs and resources, (2) planning nutritional support, both immediate and long-term, and (3) rebuilding metabolic reserves. This immediate reaction of the body to stress involves actions of the combined neuroendocrine systems through three progressive stages of physiologic response (Fig. 15-1).

Combined Actions of the Neuroendocrine System

Both parts of the nervous system, the central nervous system and the autonomic or sympathetic nervous system, constantly control and modulate reactions of the body to sensory stimuli and stress. Together with a large array of hormones and other chemical messengers, the overall neuroendocrine system provides a vast network of conscious and unconscious reactions to protect the body.[5]

Conscious Response: Central Nervous System

Certain processes in the body are under conscious direction. The person decides to behave or act in a certain way to a given situation. In response to conscious decisions and directions, the brain and central nervous system send messages to the muscles, which in turn carry out the specific actions involved. For example, the person may choose to eat some available food, take a walk, read a book, call a friend on the phone, watch television, or do some other conscious act.

Unconscious Response: Autonomic Nervous System

Other processes, such as breathing and the pumping of the heart muscle, are essential to life and must always go on. Thus such actions are automatically programmed and regulated. This essential control is managed by the autonomic, or sympathetic, nervous system.

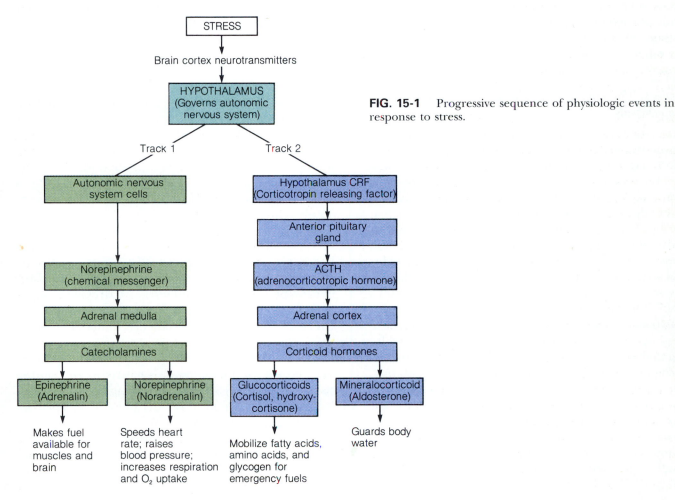

FIG. 15-1   Progressive sequence of physiologic events in response to stress.

For many years, Western science considered the autonomic functions to be beyond the reach of conscious control. However, Eastern traditions have evidenced such phenomena in "holy men" who are able to slow their heart rate, control blood pressure and respiration, or show no evidence of pain in response to apparently painful stimuli. It has only been in recent years that Western medicine has shown interest in conscious control over unconscious processes and has been able to put forth theories about it with scientific credibility.

Combined Neuroendocrine Response

In response to stress, the autonomic nervous system and its integrated hormones and other chemical messengers mobilize the body's reserves for protection. It is this immediate and continuing automatic physiologic response that Selye called the general adaptive syndrome.[1,2] From his research, Selye identified three stages of this generalized response process: (1) *initial alarm reaction,* in which the body's force's are mobilized for action, (2) *adaptation-resistance stage,* in which energy reserves are adjusted or rebuilt, and (3) *exhaustion stage,* in which resources give out if severe stress continues unrelieved. These stages overlap in the body's response to daily life stressors reflecting the intensity of the person's life situation. The rate of stress and its automatic physiologic response is increased during nervous tension, physical injury, infections, muscular work, or any other strenuous activity as a major defense mechanism that increases resistance to stressful agents.

Stage I: The Initial Alarm Reaction to Stress
Brain Signals

In this first stage, the body's forces are mobilized for action. In response to a perceived threat, the brain instantly triggers the release of chemical messengers, *neurotransmitters,* in the brain cortex. These messengers then relay impulses along neuron tracks in the brain's outer edge to the *hypothalamus,* the "primitive" brain at the head of the brain stem that governs autonomic body functions, such as breathing, heart rate, blood pressure, digestion, hormonal balance, and many other vital activities. This part of the brain, the hypothalamus, has been called the "automatic pilot" or the "brain's brain." On instant receipt of the stress message, the hypothalamus immediately triggers still other chemical messengers and hormones along two separate, yet integrated, tracks to adapt the body's normal physiology to changes needed to combat the danger.[5] In Fig. 15-1, you can trace these brain signals and message relays along their two tracks and note the body's important protective physiologic effects. Some liken this chain of events to a train switching freight at different stations. Others compare it to a symphony. No human creation is sufficiently well-orchestrated, complex, and efficient

to compare with this remarkable system of control as the body is readied for crisis.

Stage II: Resistance and Adaptation to Stress

After the initial alarm reaction, if the particular stress has not been so strong that continued exposure overwhelms the person's coping resources, a second stage of resistance and adaptation follows. Here energy reserves are adjusted and rebuilt, allowing a certain tolerance to build up.

Hormonal Feedback Mechanism

The body's normal hormonal feedback mechanism now comes into play to shut off continued output of the initiating hormonal agent and thus return blood levels of hormones from various target glands back to their normal levels. For example, during the initial alarm reaction, thyroid hormone and adrenal cortex corticoids—which manage massive immediate metabolic needs—flood the circulation and raise blood levels of these substances. Then, in this second stage of response, these high levels in turn feed back to the controlling master gland—the pituitary—to now shut off or lower its triggering hormones—thyroid stimulating hormone (TSH) to the thyroid gland and adrenocorticotropic hormone (ACTH) to the adrenal glands—for a period of automatic adjustment back to normal balance.

Rebuilding Reserves

As a result of the massive alarm reaction, normal body reserves are rapidly depleted. The blood becomes concentrated with metabolic materials, and there is marked loss of body weight. A period of restoration must eventually follow. This period allows the glands and other body tissue reserves to rebuild, the blood dilution to resume normal levels, and the body weight to return toward normal. This vital rebuilding process obviously requires positive nutritional support.[6]

Adaptive Homeostasis

The level of this adaptation to the initial or chronic stress depends, of course, on the extent of the stress and the person's coping powers. The stress reaction is generalized throughout the body, always resulting in this general adaptive syndrome identified by Selye.[2] This is true no matter what type of stress is applied. Under the influence of stress, some higher-risk persons may develop such conditions as gastric ulcers, cardiovascular disease, hypertension, headache, or neurosis, depending on the nature of their physical and psychosocial makeup and situation. When stress is superimposed on persons made vulnerable by nutritional deficiency, disorder, or disease, the effect is to make a bad situation worse. Often this is the case—for example, in

---

◆ | **C**LINICAL **A**PPLICATION | *Identifying Patients at Nutritional Risk*

In 1974 the health care industry was introduced to a new phrase—iatrogenic, or physician-induced, malnutrition. The term was not coined to imply malicious intent or disregard for patients' welfare, but to point out that malnutrition may result from emphasis on complex modern treatments while fundamental principles of nutrition are forgotten. Since then, various studies have shown that protein-kilocalorie malnutrition affects roughly one half of the patients in general medical and surgical wards in U.S. teaching hospitals. Patients with evidence of malnutrition have been shown to have significantly longer hospital stays, higher mortality rates, and greater frequency of surgical complications. Early identification of patients at risk and the provision of adequate kilocalories, protein, and micronutrients prevent a potential prolonged, complicated, or even catastrophic hospital course. The patient at risk nutritionally has one or more of the following characteristics:

- Severely underweight—less than 80% of standard for height
- Severely overweight—greater than 120% of standard for height (The risk involves the erroneous assumption that kilocalorie restriction benefits the acutely ill obese patient.)
- Recent loss of 10% or more of usual body weight (this includes those who are dieting)
- Substance abuse, especially alcohol abuse
- Nothing by mouth (NPO) for more than about 5 days while being given simple intravenous solutions (dextrose or saline)
- Protracted nutrient losses, such as occurs in malabsorption or short bowel syndrome, fistulas, draining abscesses or wounds, or renal dialysis

- Increased metabolic demands, such as occurs with trauma, burns, or sepsis
- Taking drugs—such as steroids, immunosuppressants, and antitumor agents—that have antinutrient or catabolic properties

Presence of any of these characteristics is a warning that the patient is at increased risk of malnutrition. Absence of these conditions, however, does not mean that malnutrition does not exist or cannot occur.

REFERENCES

Butterworth CE: The skeleton in the hospital closet, *Nutr Today* 9:4, 1974.

Halevy J, Bulvik S: Severe hypophosphatemia in hospitalized patients, *Arch Intern Med* 148:153, 1988.

Weinsier RL and others: Handbook of clinical nutrition, ed 2, St Louis, 1989, Mosby–Year Book. ◆

---

high-risk populations suffering chronic stress of poverty and malnutrition or the malnutrition seen in some hospitalized patients (see box above).

Stage III: Exhaustion of Stress-Coping Resources

After still more prolonged exposure to stress, the adaptation powers of the body weaken and a final stage of exhaustion follows. If the stress is severe enough and applied long enough, particularly if disease compounds it, the person's adaptation energy becomes exhausted and must be restored if life is to continue.

Immunity

Persons under stress of life events experience depressed immune function and increased vulnerability to disease. This is true of both physiologic disease and psychosocial pressure, which can bring crises both large and small. Renewed research activity in nutritional immunology has resulted, and current studies indicate that the stress of protein-energy malnutrition brings atrophy to lymphoid tissue, especially the thymus gland.[7,8] This process of lymphoid tissue loss is also associated with a deficiency of vitamin A.[9] Investigators are finding that the stress of malnutrition particularly depresses one of the immune functions, that of the activity of the "natural killer cells." These important cells

are members of the T cell population of lymphoid cells, the **lymphocytes,** a type of white blood cell making up a major component of the body's remarkable defense system.[5] Together with a companion B cell population of lymphoid cells, which produce **antibodies** for defense against disease agents, these lymphocytes come from precursor cells in the bone marrow (Fig. 15-2).

The T cells make up the majority of the circulating pool of small lymphocytes in blood and lymph and in certain areas of the lymph nodes and spleen. A T cell recognizes invading substances by means of specific

---

antibody • Any of numerous protein molecules produced by B cells as a primary immune defense for attaching to specific related **antigens;** animal protein made up of a specific sequence of amino acids that is designed to interact with its specific antigen during an allergic response or to prevent infection.

lymphocytes • Special white cells from lymphoid tissue that participate in humeral and cell-mediated immunity.

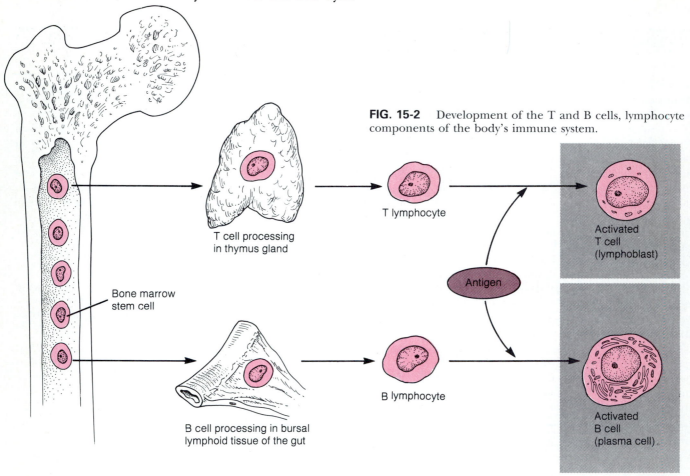

FIG. 15-2   Development of the T and B cells, lymphocyte components of the body's immune system.

special receptors on its surface. On contact with an **antigen**—any foreign intruder or "nonself"; an alien substance such as a virus—the T cells immediately multiply and initiate specific cellular immune responses: (1) they activate the **phagocytes,** special cells that have intracellular killing and degrading mechanisms for destroying invaders, and (2) they release chemical mediators that start the inflammatory process. Some T cells can even do more by becoming "killer cells" themselves and attacking antigens directly. These special double-duty cells have been called "helper cell independent cytotoxic T lymphocytes," abbreviated more graphically to the name HIT cells.

Disease

Researchers studying crisis-related immunity have concluded that heightened and sustained stress can suppress immune function. But whether or not this condition leads to disease depends on individual conditioning factors, such as poor health and nutrition (see box, p. 291), exposure to infectious disease, and general physiologic and psychologic resources.[6,7] These studies suggest that stress-related immunosuppression has its most significant consequences in elderly persons and others who have preexisting deficiencies in the immune system.

Death

The exhaustion stage of response to stress cannot be maintained for long periods, because body systems begin to wear out in their ability to cope. If resources are not restored and the stress is relentless and prolonged, finally the body's energy sources are depleted and death follows. Intervention must occur earlier to reduce stress, prevent disease, and promote health. A vital part of such intervention is nutritional support.

Life Cycle Stress: High-Risk Population Groups

Life Cycle Stress Periods

At each stage of the human life cycle, specific physiologic and psychosocial developments create nutrition-related stress for both the physical body and the person. In previous chapters we have discussed some of the general stress factors that might intervene along the way, such as poor eating habits, bizarre diets, extreme vegetarianism, substance abuse as with alcohol and drugs, megadoses of food supplements, nutrient imbalances, eating disorders, lack of exercise or extreme exercise, and poor mental attitude. Nutritional needs must be met within the total life context at any particular point. Added stress may be imposed by physical

Interactive Cycle: Stress, Nutritional Status, and Immunity

Stress wears many faces and shows itself in different forms. It imposes an interactive cycle of physiologic events involving nutritional status and the body's line of defense, its all-important immune system. The full effects of stress on nutrient needs and immunity is yet to be fully understood, because the stressor and our responses to it are difficult to measure. But we do know that continued stress is like a run on the metabolic bank, soon exhausting its resources and defenses.

A number of important questions need answers. Precisely how does the neuroendocrine-metabolic cascade triggered by stress affect our need for specific nutrients? How does stress affect our long-term health and well-being? To answer these questions, we need to know just what the role of stress is in our utilization of nutrients and just what effect our nutrient status has on our response to stress.

Although we do not have all the answers yet to questions about the interactive nature of stress, nutritional status, and immunity, we do have now enough information to emphasize the importance of optimal nutrition in guarding against disease and promoting a rapid recovery when it does occur. Some nutritional factors play lead roles in this overall process:

- **Energy.** Stress may increase the body's basal caloric need as much as 200%. The stress hormones act to increase body heat production and when this heat is released it is not available to the body as chemical energy for cell metabolism. Then weight loss beyond what could be explained by decreased appetite and food intake occurs. This caloric inefficiency induced by stress accounts for the dramatic increase in energy intake need, which may rise as much as 10-fold in severely traumatized persons. And if fat fuel stores are inadequate, the individual may not survive. In this case, thin is not beautiful; thin is deadly.
- **Protein.** Stress may increase the body's basal protein need from 60% to as much as 500%. The integrity of body tissues involved in the body's immune system, such as the skin and the mucosal tissue, depends on adequate protein. Mucosal immunity especially depends on the protection of its mucosal secretions, which constantly bathe the body cavities and orifices. These secretions contain a variety of biochemical and immunologic factors. The antibodies formed require protein.
- **Fat.** Dietary fatty acids, notably linoleic and arachidonic acids, influence prostaglandin synthesis by macrophages. In turn, these prostaglandins can stimulate and suppress other cellular and humoral immune functions as needed.
- **Vitamins.** We have long known that vitamin A functions in the maintenance of healthy epithelial tissue, such as the outer skin and the inner mucosal tissue. Vitamin A-deficient persons have fewer goblet cells and less protective mucus production with fewer component immunoglobulin factors. Work with vitamin C has shown that it enhances phagocytosis activity by macrophages, and in vitamin C deficiency protective macrophage mobilization and aggregation are impaired. Deficiencies of vitamins A and B_{12} and folate all impair T cell production response. Antibody production in the spleen after an antigen challenge has been found to be impaired in animals deficient in vitamins A, E, and pyridoxine. Megadoses of vitamin E have been associated with suppression of B cell functions. In addition, because of their key functions as coenzymes in energy and protein metabolism, thiamin, riboflavin, and niacin requirements are increased in response to stress.
- **Minerals.** Deficiencies of zinc impair T cell proliferation and responsiveness. Iron deficiencies affect humoral immunity.

These examples make it clear that nutritional status influences immunity and response to stress. On this foundation we can build our practice now. The challenge ahead for nutrition scientists is to further define and quantify nutrition's interactive role in both stress and immunity, and further clarify the exquisite mechanisms involved.

REFERENCES

Berdanier CD: The many faces of stress, *Nutr Today* 22(2):12, 1987.

Ross AC: Vitamin A and protective immunity, *Nutr Today* 27(4):18, 1992.

---

trauma, injury, disease, or disability. Other stress may relate to the workplace, the rapidly changing environment, or increasing social isolation in a profoundly changing society (see box above). And for many the overriding pain of poverty leads to physical, psychosocial, and mental health problems.

Here we review briefly some of the stress factors through the life cycle and consider approaches to nutritional care. Then in the remaining parts of the chapter, we explore ways of managing high-risk stress as a

antigen • Any foreign or "non-self" substances—such as toxins, viruses, bacteria, and foreign proteins—that stimulate the production of **antibodies** specifically designed to interact with them.

phagocytes • Cells that ingest microorganisms, other cells, or foreign particles; macrophages.

means of more positive nutritional support and health promotion in general.

Pregnancy
Physiologic and Psychosocial Stress

As indicated in Chapter 11, enormous physiologic changes occur in the pregnant woman's body to sustain and support a healthy pregnancy and its outcome, a healthy baby. But pregnancy also presents added psychologic and socioeconomic stress to both parents as they face changing social and personal roles and financial responsibilities. Many parents have matured physically and emotionally through their own growth and development to meet these changing life needs. But others lack these resources and face greater stress. This is especially true, for example, in teenage pregnancies. Also, cultural and social influences have shaped values and beliefs of both parents about pregnancy. Genetic heritage and previous life experiences and food habits have determined the mother's current health and nutritional reserves to meet the physiologic stress of her pregnancy. All of these conditioning factors are important.

High-Risk Pregnancy: Added Stress Factors

A number of added stress factors can contribute to a high-risk pregnancy and a potential poor outcome. Some of these stressors are present when the pregnancy begins. These include (1) age extremes for reproduction—teenagers aged 15 or younger and women aged 35 or older, (2) frequent pregnancies—three or more during a 2-year period, and (3) poor obstetric history and fetal performance. These risks are further compounded by the stress of poverty, lack of prenatal care, and harmful personal habits. These harmful habits include abuse of alcohol, resulting in the well-known fetal alcohol syndrome; abuse of drugs, resulting in addicted infants; the smoking of cigarettes, an increasing habit among teenage girls, resulting in low–birth-weight infants; and bizarre or faddist food habits that deny essential nutrients to the fetus. Such behaviors contribute to fetal damage, inadequate maternal weight gain, and low–birth-weight infants. These preexisting maternal risk factors require special personal counseling and nutritional guidance (see Chapter 11).

High-Risk Pregnancy: Clinical Complications

Further physiologic and personal stress may be added by clinical complications of the mother's pregnancy. These complications include anemia, pregnancy-induced hypertension, and preexisting maternal disease, such as insulin-dependent diabetes mellitus (IDDM) or maternal phenylketonuria (MPKU). Special team care (see Chapter 11) is needed in these complicated pregnancies to provide specific individual nutritional support.

Infant Growth and Development
Physiologic and Psychosocial Stress

Normal growth demands place both physiologic and psychosocial stress on the infant. Birth itself is a stressor. After the period of rapid fetal growth, the full-term neonate moves quickly at birth from a warm, protective, and supportive uterine environment to the stress of the external world, literally cut off from its former umbilical nourishment. Survival depends on immediate adaptation. Not only is physiologic nourishment by either breast-feeding or appropriate formula required, but also psychosocial nurturing by loving care for both physical comfort and emotional support. Indeed, feeding becomes the twofold link to survival by supplying essential nutritional support and the main means of establishing human relationships.

High-Risk Infants

Not all infants, however, are so fortunate in their development and growth experience during the stress of these early critical fetal-neonatal-infant periods of life. They carry the additional stress of developmental problems or disease. Tiny babies born prematurely or small for gestational age have low birth weights (LBWs) and may have some form of intrauterine growth retardation (IUGR). The subgroup IUGR refers to term babies born at 37 or more weeks of gestation, having both weight and length problems. The premature subgroup refers to preterm LBW babies born before week 37 of gestation. In general, the morbidity and mortality rates are significant in these LBW babies. High rates of LBW coexist in adverse socioeconomic circumstances, another stress and human toll of poverty.[10]

Other high-risk infants may have birth defects. And still others experience a general failure to thrive. This growth failure can be attributed to both organic defect possibilities and nonorganic factors contributing to the stress of defective mother-infant interaction.[11] Decreased energy intake causes the lack of appropriate weight gain. But defective mother-infant interaction can cause not only decreased energy intake, but also developmental delay and abnormal behaviors. All of these high-risk infants are subjected to greatly increased physiologic and psychosocial stress and bring added emotional stress to their parents and families. All of them require much special care and nutritional support. Careful nutrition and social assessment are needed to identify underlying causes of the associated feeding problems, so that appropriate care can be planned.

Childhood Growth and Development
Physiologic and Psychosocial Development

During the period of latent childhood growth between infancy and adolescence, the child's growth rate slows and becomes more erratic—steady but in spurts. Nonetheless, continued growth places metabolic stress demands on the young body that gradually increase the energy and nutrient needs. In the early school years especially, growth rates vary widely because resources are being laid down for the rapid adolescent growth ahead. During these years, children need not only physiologic nutrition support, but also psychosocial nurturing as they progressively gain personal strengths of autonomy, initiative, and industry through supportive family relationships and other broadening social experiences. Food and mealtimes become an increasingly important means of socialization.

High-Risk Children

Added physiologic and psychosocial stressors increase health risks for children. For example, such stressors may be associated with growth failure, developmental disability, or inheritance of chronic disease.

1. **Growth failure.** The growth potential of an individual is genetically determined. If conditions are favorable, each child will grow according to his or her own predetermined growth curve, or channel. Unfavorable stressful conditions deflect a child away from this individual predetermined growth curve. The extent of the stress and growth failure depends on the severity of the unfavorable conditions and how long the child is exposed to them without adequate relief, leaving the child stunted and wasted. Depending on the extent of damage and the quality of rehabilitation, a high-energy diet with appropriate amounts of protein and trace elements may restore a child to his or her growth channel.

2. **Developmental disability.** Developmentally disabled children are at high risk of nutritional deficiency and multiple health problems.[12] They have sustained chronic physical or mental impairments during the growth years from numerous causes, including such conditions as cerebral palsy, spina bifida, and Down's syndrome. Now, in addition, we have new problems with infants born to mothers who used alcohol—that is, fetal alcohol syndrome (FAS)—or used cocaine and crack extensively during pregnancy or who have AIDS and have transmitted the virus to their infants.[13] Myriad psychosocial, economic, and physical stressors face these children and their families. A team of specialists is needed to provide care, with the team nutritionist determining nutritional needs and using available resource persons and agencies as indicated. The development of these children to their highest physical, mental, and emotional potential is based on optimal nutrition.[14,15]

3. **Inheritance of chronic disease.** Children born with various metabolic disorders of genetic origin, such as phenylketonuria (PKU), are now able to develop normally through the use from birth of a special formula and diet that controls the intake of specific nutrients for which the corresponding specific enzyme is missing or inadequate. Also, a number of the lipid disorders and essential hypertension, which underlie potential development of coronary heart disease, are familial. Children in such genetically high-risk families carry a strong risk for developing these chronic diseases. Thus pediatricians and nutritionists advise the adoption of prudent family eating patterns that control fat, cholesterol, and sodium intake. The stress of childhood obesity, a growing risk problem, is also receiving more attention.

Adolescent Growth and Development
Physiologic and Psychosocial Stress

The flooding hormones of puberty rapidly increase the stress of adolescent growth and sexual maturation. This is an ambivalent period full of stressors and strains as these older children struggle to find their own identities and self-images and reach adult maturity. Individual adolescents vary greatly in response to these stressful tensions, depending on the supportive resources provided for them in their earlier developmental years. The identity crisis of "growing up" both physically and emotionally is necessary preparation for an adult role in a complex society. There is little wonder that this period is fraught with stress and its problems, many of which are carried into adulthood unresolved. This whole maturation process has never been easy. But in today's rapidly changing world it seems even more profound and produces many psychologic, emotional, and social tensions.

High-Risk Adolescents

Many young girls, pressured by family and society to maintain the thin "ideal" figure, add the stress of constant dieting to their already increased physiologic demands of accelerated adolescent growth. Some develop a distorted perception of their body image with resulting serious semistarvation eating disorders of *anorexia nervosa* or *bulimia nervosa*, as discussed in Chapter 6. Also, an increasing number of adolescent girls are experiencing the multiple health risks and stresses of teenage pregnancies. Lacking education or skills, they face uncertain futures of rearing their young children as a single parent, unprepared to provide financial or emotional support. The added stress of poverty often results.

Two other sources of physiologic and psychosocial stress bring health risks during the teen years and compromise nutritional status. These are excessive athletic training and abuse of alcohol and other drugs.

1. **Athletics.** The challenge and excitement of team sports sometimes push young preadolescents and adolescents to place added health risks on their bodies. Pressure to be admired by peers, to achieve ap-

proval of coaches or parents, or to follow in the footsteps of a favored older brother or sister may lead some boys and girls to exceed their physical capacity and sustain serious injury. The constant search for the "competitive edge" may lead to dietary misinformation and exploitation, with consequent nutritional problems.

2. **Alcohol and other drug abuse.** As adolescents approach the drinking age in their community, alcohol becomes a means of appearing more adult and may assume an increasing share of the total energy intake. Pressured by peer groups, some begin to drink at younger and younger ages and reach the stage of addiction by adolescence. Even mild alcohol abuse in the face of the increased nutritional requirements of adolescence can compromise nutritional status. For example, the important B vitamin folate is destroyed by excessive alcohol.[16] The extent of excessive social drinking, as well as teenage alcoholism in susceptible persons, presents a serious risk to life and health, especially when combined with highway driving, as often occurs after parties. Other drug abuse and addictions have also brought devastating results to many young lives. Many have become addicted as early as elementary school, bringing physical and mental illness, malnutrition, disease, and death. A large part of any alcohol or other drug abuse rehabilitation program must be optimal nutrition support.

Adulthood and Aging
Physiologic Stress of Aging

The biologic changes of aging are general, but persons in the advancing years of life experience the physiologic stress of aging in different ways, depending in large measure on their health status. They display a wide variety of individual reactions to normal body stress. They simply get old at different rates and in different ways. On top of individual genetic heritage, each person bears the unique imprint of health and disease experience. This combination has a direct effect on individual aging. But in any case the body's physical resources gradually decline, and the risk of disease and dependency increases.

Psychosocial Problems

In young and middle adulthood, personal stress relates mainly to striving to find one's way in the world with family and career. Greater stress and risks develop if disease, disability, or poverty is present. The population of older adults aged 85 and older is growing, so the stress related to health concerns and needs of this expanding age-group is also increasing. As biologic changes occur, there often comes concern about the loss of body functions, decreased capacities, increasing social stress and isolation (see Issues and Answers, p. 302), personal losses, and diminished social opportuni-

ties. Financial pressures and a decreasing sense of acceptance and accomplishment cause many elderly persons mental stress and loss of personal values. Many feel inadequate. Often they are lonely, restless, unhappy, and uncertain. The greater part of the aging process in any area is culturally determined. Unfortunately, in many instances Western culture imposes a set of negative roles on persons as they reach older age. All of these sources of stress, both physical and psychosocial, increase health risks and vulnerability to disease and malnutrition in the aging population. Persons in the fast-growing "oldest-old" group over age 85 are particularly vulnerable.

The Stress of Physical Trauma and Disease

At any age the presence of injury, disease, and disability adds more stress—with increased health and nutrition risks—to the general strains of human growth and development. These high-risk persons are found in hospitals and clinics, medical and rehabilitation centers, community agencies, and homes. In each case, special nutritional care and support are needed to help reduce risks and manage stress. Comprehensive nutrition assessment is needed to identify these high-risk patients and plan their care. Extended disabling conditions bring with them still more stress and require continued nutritional support (see Chapter 26).

Childhood Disease

Growing children are vulnerable to various forms of *protein-energy malnutrition,* especially children from poor homes and stressed families. The problem of child abuse in such stressed families is serious and adds more risk to their physical and emotional health, even to their lives. An underlying malnutrition is easily compounded by the stress of hospitalization and disease. Children with gastrointestinal problems that hinder food intake and use are at special risk of growth retardation. For example—malabsorption disease, which often becomes chronic over time—prevents absorption of needed nutrients and stunts growth (see Chapter 19). Metabolic diseases such as insulin-dependent diabetes mellitus (IDDM) and other genetic disorders carry risks of complications involving various organ systems and require special individual management (see Chapter 21). Hypermetabolic diseases, such as cancer, may threaten life and require vigorous nutritional support (see Chapter 25).

Traumatic Injury and Disability

Persons of any age sustaining critical trauma, such as extensive burns (see Chapter 23), spinal cord injury, or other serious injuries and disabilities (see Chapter 26) experience extreme physiologic and psychosocial stress and are at special risk. They require both immediate care and long-term rehabilitation by a nutrition support team of specialists. Three important factors guide this individual nutrition support: (1) the need to replenish the large catabolic losses, (2) the demand for essential anabolic tissue healing, and (3) the need for extensive personal support. The plan of care for these stressed high-risk patients and its outcome depend on (1) age—elderly persons and children are more vulnerable, (2) health condition—any preexisting condition, malnutrition, or disease, such as diabetes or cardiovascular or renal problems, complicates care, and (3) wound severity—location, extent, and time elapse before treatment influence risk and prognosis.

Chronic Diseases of Aging

Added stress and health risks among adults include chronic diseases of aging or any of the multiple risk factors for such diseases. For example, coronary heart disease—the major cause of death in the United States and most other Western societies—is a multifaceted disease with numerous risk factors, as summarized in Table 15-1. Some of these risks involve personal characteristics that we cannot control, such as our genetic heritage. Others are background conditions that can be screened and treated. But in the middle, and most important, are those personal behaviors that we learn and, with motivation, can change. One of these learned behaviors is our degree of ability to cope with life's stresses. This relation of stress to chronic conditions—such as hypertension and coronary heart disease—has been determined by numerous studies, and more attention is being given to stress reduction in health-promotion programs.[17,18] Other learned behaviors are harmful habits we can seek to change. Most of these interventions to reduce risk involve in some way food patterns and nutrition. All of these high-risk persons require special nutritional care and support.

Stress Related to Work, Increased Exercise, and Environment

Many persons experience increased stress and health risk from the nature of their jobs, intensive exercise, and environmental factors. Increasing awareness of these problems, preventive measures to reduce risks, and health care for exposed persons have begun to develop through work-site programs, sports medicine practice, and community health programs.

Stress of the Workplace
Work-Site Hazards

Increased physical risks and stresses occur in labor-intensive jobs and those with safety and health hazards, such as use of heavy machinery or hazardous tools and working at heights. Poor lighting and ventilation, as well as smoking, present health risks in offices and industrial plants and offices. Because computers have

TABLE 15-1

Multiple Risk Factors in Cardiovascular Disease

Personal characteristics (no control)	Learned behaviors (intervene and change)	Background conditions (screen and treat)
Gender	Stress and coping	Hypertension
Age	Cigarette smoking	Diabetes mellitus
Family history	Sedentary life-style	Hyperlipidemia (especially
	Obesity	hypercholesterolemia)
	Food habits	
	Excess fat	
	Excess sugar	
	Excess salt	

largely replaced typewriters in business offices, data entry operators using video display terminals are experiencing eyestrain, headache, and musculoskeletal pains from repetitive strain injury, as well as emotional and mental stress.[19] Two special high-risk groups are (1) migrant farm workers, whose lives involve multiple physical, psychologic, and socioeconomic stress factors, and (2) workers in electronic and chemical industries and those handling radioactive materials. Such groups of workers may be exposed to hazardous chemicals or other carcinogenic substances.

Management-Employee Relations

Often in positions of management are persons with the so-called "Type A" behavior pattern, characterized by intense striving for achievement, competitiveness, impatience, time urgency, overcommitment to professional activities, and excessive drive and hostility.[20] The well-known "executive syndrome" of stress-related ills—peptic ulcer, heart disease, hypertension, diabetes, and alcohol and other drug abuse—can result from the competitive pressures of managing a business. Sometimes in today's business world, these pressures are reflected in deteriorating management-employee relations and mounting stress from our jobs. A study by the National Center for Health Statistics indicates that more than half of the 40,000 workers surveyed reported increasing job stress.[21] Much of this stress, often involving dislocation and uncertainty, is spilling over to affect workers' personal lives and health. In this age of a technologic service economy and the business office, many workers are saying "my job is killing me" and naming a tyrannical boss as the main culprit. These job-related ills also affect workers suffering economic hardships, unemployment, or underemployment.

The Stress of Heavy Exercise

Aside from heavy labor on the job, many persons in athletics and intensive physical fitness programs also experience physical stress and therefore risk injury (see Chapter 14). Heavy athletic exercise places great stress on the body. Heavy body-contact team sports, especially in the big business of professional teams where high stakes in money and competition are involved, carry tremendous pressure and risk of disabling injury. For every "star" there are hundreds of battered bodies who never make top billing or income. And every team member's playing life is short. Also, compulsive persons in individual athletic activities, such as running, or those in strenuous physical fitness programs can experience severe injury. Compulsive striving, often despite physical indications against it, has resulted in permanent disabilities.

Stress of Environmental Factors

Persons exposed to a variety of environmental stressors have additional health risks. Air and water pollution are two of the prices we have paid for our advanced technologic society. Health problems accumulate over time, for example, when buried radioactive or chemical wastes leach out into ground water and contaminate public water sources, or when automobile and factory emissions contaminate air and increase respiratory problems. As target organisms develop tolerance levels, the ever-increasing use of pesticides in agriculture has accumulated, further exposing farm workers and consumers to a variety of potentially dangerous chemicals (see Chapter 9).

Poverty, Psychosocial Stress, and Mental Health

The High-Risk Problem of Poverty

Poverty and Hunger

We are all made increasingly aware through the daily news, or personal contact and experience in our own communities, of the growing world and U.S. economic cycle of poverty. A recent report of the U.S. Census Bureau in September 1992 revealed that the number of persons below the official poverty level increased from 31.5 million in 1989 to 35.7 million in 1991, the highest total since 1964.[22] We also know through personal contact and experience in our own communities that poverty and its physiologic and psychosocial toll on human lives are hard realities for many persons. As we discussed in previous chapters, extreme poverty and its ever-present companion hunger—even to famine and death—exist in a number of the world's nations, fanned by war and ethnic or class barriers. But the social roots of poverty and its harvest of hunger do not stop at our borders. In the United States, one of the wealthiest countries on earth, many studies document a "growing epidemic" of hunger and malnutrition among the poor. A 1986 Physician Task Force on Hunger in America found that in the United States alone at least 20 million persons—12 million of whom are children—suffered from hunger, but the current rate for children has increased—one child in every four un-

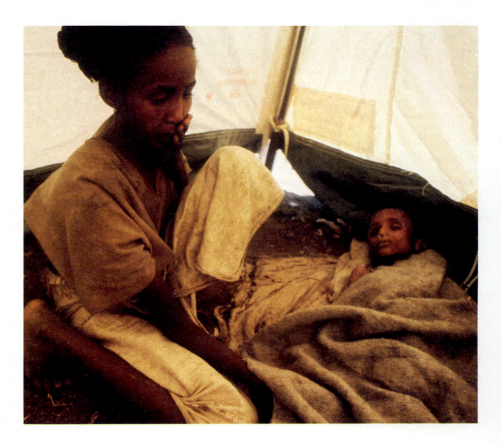

der 6 years of age is poor.[23] In the past, hunger has been viewed mainly as a problem of overpopulation. World population has just passed the 5 billion mark and grows daily. Now, however, hunger is recognized as more than just a problem of numbers of people. It is also seen as a major problem, with economic and social and political roots, resulting in an increasing gap between the rich and the poor, within and between countries.

Poverty and Politics

A number of socioeconomic and political factors have contributed to the plight of the millions of Americans living at or below the poverty line. These include economic displacement and underemployment and unemployment, homelessness, marital breakup, poor health, alcoholism and other drug abuse, functional illiteracy, mental illness, and wage discrimination based on gender and race.[23] As is true in any system, those holding political power at any given time and place determine the economic, agricultural, and food distribution policies that reflect their ideology and may or may not meet the needs of the people involved. Many of the persons living at or below the poverty line, some of them homeless, must rely regularly on soup kitchens and food banks to supplement their meager diets. For many concerned Americans, hunger in the United States is a troubling problem. As records show for most Americans, this problem was virtually eliminated during the 1970s but has reemerged and spread rapidly with new government administrations in the 1980s and early 1990s, indicating that the roots of hunger are mainly political and socioeconomic—rather than technical—because we have available resources for feeding all Americans.[24] This relentless stress of poverty imposes large health risks on individuals and families, especially the growing numbers of young children caught in its grip.

The Psychosocial Stress of Poverty

Tremendous human problems exist among the poor, problems that at times seem almost insurmountable. Often a "culture of poverty" develops and is reinforced and perpetuated by society's values and attitudes. Such attitudes serve to wall off poor persons more completely than do physical barriers. As a result of the extreme pressures and stress caused by their living conditions, poverty-stricken persons become victims of negative attitudes and behaviors that influence their use of community health services.

These psychosocial stressors of poverty further increase health risks of persons involved. It is small wonder that they often become frustrated with despair, caught in a vicious cycle of feelings of isolation, insecurity, and powerlessness. As health workers, we must begin with self-awareness of personal social values and attitudes, if we are to be true "helping vehicles" and agents of constructive change. Only then can we establish a genuine rapport within which we can work together. And we must *listen*—positively, actively, and creatively. Refer back to Chapter 9 and reread the discussion about the ecology of human nutrition and the twin problems of poverty and malnutrition. We need to constantly resensitize ourselves to these human problems and never view them in the abstract, but in terms of the human lives they represent.

Mental Health Needs and Problems

For many persons, life stresses produce increased risk of mental health problems. Clinicians see many of these problems daily in primary health care. An increasing number of these disorders are found in the substance abuse–dependency category, centering on alcohol and drugs. Other problems include phobias and affective disorders, such as depression. All of these mental health problems involve a large high-risk population and have implications for public health, food behaviors, and nutritional status.

At special risk are persons in long-term institutional care facilities for both physical and mental disorders. Often, increased numbers of patients and inadequate staff personnel result in limited individual attention with increased stress of nutrition and health problems.

Also, the stress of increasing prison populations is taking its toll on inmates' lives and the lives of their families. Increased prison sentencing, much of it drug-related, has increased prison populations to highly crowded conditions, making a bad situation worse. According to a Bureau of Justice Statistics report, at the end of 1989 state prisons nationwide held a record 610,000 inmates, 63,000 more than at the same time the year before, and the trend is expected to continue.[25] Officials estimate that just keeping up with this level of growth would require building the equivalent of a 1000-bed prison every 6 days. Such high-stress settings multiply physical and mental health risks, and individual nutrition needs often suffer.

High-Risk Stress Management

As we have seen, a key factor in the development of disease and risk of poor nutrition is stress, both physiologic and psychosocial. This basic risk factor permeates human life with positive and negative effects. The goal of health promotion, therefore, centers on managing stress in positive ways by, (1) identifying high-risk persons, (2) recognizing key elements in daily stress management, and (3) planning appropriate methods of reducing stress and its health risks. This positive approach applies not only to the lives of our clients and patients, but also to our own. The familiar "burnout" syndrome is not uncommon.

Key Elements in Daily Stress Management
Personal Approaches

Building positive resources on a personal level for managing daily stress includes attention to key coping factors, such as having a sense of being in control of one's life, developing positive personality characteristics, and engaging in self-assessment.

1. **Control of personal life.** Many studies with population groups, as well as laboratory research with animals, indicate that stress is better tolerated and provokes fewer negative physiologic effects if the person has a measure of control over it. Some stressors in life can be changed; many cannot. But the ultimate control lies within: *we choose how we respond.*

2. **Role of personality.** Positive personality characteristics—such as hopefulness, a positive outlook or general life orientation, and ability to "go with the flow"—have been found to correlate with a better ability to deal with life's stressors and with a lowered risk of illness. On the other hand, a rigid, "uptight" approach to life places persons at much higher risk. This high-risk type of person is generally characterized by two basic behaviors: (1) a compulsion to work too hard—characterized by trying to do too much in one space of time and expecting a great deal from self and others beyond reasonable levels, and (2) free-floating hostility—characterizing by losing one's temper easily, being impatient, and struggling against time and other people.[26] This behavior may not be easy to change. After all, it is basically the single-minded competitive productivity that American business and society rewards. But for happier and more healthful living, some change on a personal level is worth the effort. Perhaps society needs to make some profound changes in its approach to work and management style, human fulfillment, dignity, and reward.

3. **Self-assessment.** Ask yourself some important questions: Do you know how you typically react? Do you know what level of stress you are operating under? Do you know what direction you seem to be taking? Then, after such introspection, you can seek alternative ways of changing your stress pattern: (1) determine your own priorities and values in life, (2) avoid those stressors which can be avoided, and (3) displace stressors that cannot be eliminated with other positive activities to strengthen your coping ability and develop more constructive, relaxed behavior. These positive activities include a focus on key elements that help displace and reduce stress: diet, exercise, relaxation, and personal interest areas, as described in the following social approaches.

Social Approaches

Human beings are by nature social beings and need other people in their lives to sustain positive health. Although persons at times may cherish quiet times alone, there are no true hermits. Everyone needs some kind of social support system, a network of friends and family to count on when help is needed. Everyone needs some kind of meaningful group support, such as church, school or special course, community group, sports team, personal interest or hobby groups, music groups or choruses, computer clubs, political groups, volunteer work, or social clubs. There are many ways to develop a sense of belonging. This feeling of having something to contribute and having someone to turn to is critical as a buffer from unavoidable life stresses.

Methods of Reducing Stress and Health Risks
Positive Health Promotion

The preventive approach to developing positive health means making changes wherever necessary to build positive attitudes and habits. This life-style approach includes actions in three main areas—exercise, relaxation, and diet—to reduce stress-related risk factors and promote health.

Physical Activities

A number of activities to build physical fitness are described in Chapter 14, including aerobic exercise for strengthening heart and lung action. But there are many more beneficial effects of physical exercise. Exercise can improve both mental and physical health through the following:

- Draining off accumulated excess chemical messengers, catecholamines and hormones, triggered by the primitive "fight or flight" response to stress
- Increasing the rate and efficiency of body metabolism
- Decreasing body fat deposits and thereby helping to maintain a healthful weight
- Increasing blood levels of high-density lipoproteins (HDLs), which help control serum cholesterol levels and decrease risk of coronary heart disease
- Helping to dissipate anger and hostility
- Improving overall health and well-being, thereby decreasing risk of illness and its physiologic and psychologic stress
- Inducing a meditation-like state, bringing a sense of detachment and mental relaxation
- Brightening the mood and helping maintain a positive outlook

Aerobic exercise best achieves these benefits (see Chapter 14). Effective types of exercise include swimming, running, jogging, bicycle riding, team or individual sports, "aerobics" class or other group workouts, and walking. Walking must be brisk and sustained for about 30 to 40 minutes to become aerobic in effect. Walking is the best constant exercise—simple, regular, sustained. It benefits the heart, lungs, weight, and state of mind. Take time along the way to notice where you are as you walk, be it wonders of nature along country trails or interest in human activity on city streets.

Relaxation Exercises

Relaxation is the needed counterbalance with physical activity as a means of reducing stress and its high-risk effects. It helps to dissipate and diminish the harmful internal physiologic effects of stress. The ways people "unwind" are as varied as the people themselves. But a personally satisfying means of relaxing is important to everyone. Even persons with turbulent and demanding lives have learned to find little daily "time out" opportunities that create islands of peace to help break the cycle of chronic stress. For many persons, though, this attitude and ability do not come easily or naturally. Our Puritan work ethic heritage, a fast-paced and demanding life-style, and the too often overriding cultural values on money and material goods as a measure of success lock one into mind sets, habits, and ways of thinking and behaving that are self-destructive. Further, a rigid and rapid life-style cultivates some negative ways people physically reinforce stress in their lives and ways in which they "take it out" on others around them and on their own bodies. Muscle tension is a common example, as are headaches, backaches, and leg cramps—all classic symptoms of stress overload.

A number of useful techniques are available that focus on ways one can *learn* to relax. With *practice*, a necessity for any learning, persons can not only feel relaxed, but also help control such autonomic functions as breathing, pulse rate, blood pressure, electric brain impulses, and peripheral blood circulation, as well as relax muscle tensions. These relaxation techniques include biofeedback, progressive muscle relaxation exercises, clinical hypnosis, and meditation with visual imagery. Today a number of medical centers are studying the induced relaxation response, used with meditation and guided imagery together with other techniques, to help treat health problems. They have found strong evidence that the calming effects of these relaxation techniques relieve stress and, in doing so, support the body's immune system. Although individual methods of relaxation vary, a significant personal pattern can meet individual needs. In essence, persons must change their lives and rethink their values to some degree if they want to avoid such risks as an early and possibly fatal heart attack—or, better still, if they simply want to have a happier life.

Diet

First, a word of warning. Despite the great amount of food misinformation available today from many sources, there is no "wonder cure" for stress. Beware the wonder-food or supplement claim, the so-called magic properties of any specific nutrient or food. Instead seek a basic balanced dietary pattern that is both nutritionally sound and personally satisfying.

1. **Nutritional balance.** In general, human beings need to eat a balanced diet that provides sufficient energy to maintain a healthful weight and supplies all the necessary macro- and micronutrients. Although no clear scientific evidence as yet relates specific nutrients to stress, interest and concern are increasing among scientists and clinicians working in the area that stress—difficult to quantify because of its many faces—may well affect nutrient needs in ways we do not yet fully understand.[8] It is true, of course, that in cases of debilitation and malnutrition, more nutrient-dense foods are needed to replenish stores. But in most instances of usual daily-living stress patterns, a reasonable and regular diet of sound nutrition in satisfying food choices is the need. As we discussed in Chapter 9, a complex web of many different factors influences food choices, as indicated in Table 15-2. Being aware of these influences may help in making more positive choices. Whatever the choices may be, the well-nourished person has a much better means of displacing stress—be it high-risk illness, disappointment, or job demands—and maintaining a strong immunity against disease.

   So the simple admonition to "eat right," which involves many variations in food choices and follows wise health promotion guidelines, is in fact a simple prescription that society would do well to incorporate into a new life-style, along with some daily form of exercise and relaxation.

2. **Food and mood.** We all know from personal experience that mood influences the food that we eat. Sometimes either overeating or loss of appetite is associated with periods of depression or disappointment. There is a place for "comfort foods" in dealing with stress. Plan for their wise use in times of need.

3. **Food pattern and pace.** Food habits are hard to change. They are always tied to life-style. Many per-

---

TABLE 15-2

Factors Determining Food Choices

Physical factors	Social factors	Physiologic factors
Food supply available	Advertising	Allergy
Food technology	Culture	Disability
Geography, agriculture, distribution	Education (nutrition and general)	Health-disease status
Personal economics, income	Political and economic policies	Heredity
Sanitation, housing	Religion and social custom	Personal food acceptance
Season, climate	Social class, role	Needs, energy, or nutrients
Storage and cooking facilities	Social problems, poverty, or alcoholism	Therapeutic diets

sons eat rapidly and irregularly and suffer both physical and emotional consequences. Persons are better able to deal with stress if they simply slow their eating to savor the food, eat smaller "mini-meals" more frequently, and avoid the rich, heavy meals that often make up the typical food pattern. Moderation and variety are the key. Begin with breakfast, needed by the body after the overnight fast, and continue through the day with small amounts of food to refuel the body at regular intervals. Avoid the excesses Americans tend to eat of fat, salt, and sugar, and in some cases caffeine, mostly in the form of coffee. Individual sensitivity to caffeine is highly variable, but it is a stimulant drug that many consider to be abused.

Socioeconomic Needs

In cases of economic stress, various food assistance programs may help supply needed food (see Chapter 10). Other community programs such as food banks and public meals help fill emergency needs.

Hypermetabolic Needs

Additional energy and nutritive demands are created by the physiologic stress of hypermetabolic conditions, such as traumatic injury, surgery, infection, or cancer. The magnitude of the metabolic response varies (see Chapter 23). But in any case it underscores the importance of good pre-stress nutritional status on a regular basis.

To Sum Up

The modern world is demanding and complex. It exposes human beings to many stressors and risk factors that affect nutritional status and health, both physical and emotional. Among these risk factors, stress plays a major role. It triggers a cascade of primitive automatic physiologic events, designed as a "fight or flight" mechanism to protect the body through the general alarm and adaptive responses. But in a modern stress-filled world, this reaction only compounds the problem and contributes to illness. Throughout life, physiologic and psychosocial stress attends growth and development, with special high-risk persons being pregnant women, infants, young children, adolescents, and elderly persons.

At any age, additional stressors may increase health risks for vulnerable persons. These include physical trauma and disease, disability, environmental problems, the multiple problems of poverty and the general economic stress of minority populations, and mental problems. High-stress management involves both personal and social approaches, based on identified individual and family needs, goals, and expectations. Methods of reducing stress and health risks focus on positive promotion of health and nutrition and helping to build greater effective coping capacity through sound diet, relaxation, and physical activity, with a strengthened personal support system.

QUESTIONS FOR REVIEW

1. Describe the general adaptive syndrome identified by Selye, which the body activates in response to stress, in terms of the physiologic events in each of its three stages. Why does this response create problems in today's modern society?
2. Identify sources of physiologic and psychosocial stress in each of the growth and development stages of the life cycle. Select several of these problems, describe their nature, and outline general care.
3. Describe additional high-risk stress conditions that may occur throughout the life cycle, giving approaches to planning nutrition and health care. Give special attention to the problem of poverty.
4. Identify and describe key elements in daily stress management and methods of reducing stress and health risks.

REFERENCES

1. Selye H: *The stress of life,* New York, 1956, McGraw-Hill.
2. Selye H: Hunger and stress, *Nutr Today* 5(1):2, 1970.
3. Erikson E: *Childhood and society,* New York, 1963, WW Norton.
4. Maslow AH: *Motivation and personality,* New York, 1954, Harper & Row.
5. Guyton AC: *Textbook of medical physiology,* ed 8, Philadelphia, 1991, WB Saunders.
6. Berdanier CD: The many faces of stress, *Nutr Today* 22(2):12, 1987.
7. Beisel WR: History of nutritional immunology: introduction and overview, *J Nutr* 122:591, 1992.
8. Chandra RK: Protein-energy malnutrition and immunological responses, *J Nutr* 122:597, 1992.
9. Ross AS: Vitamin A and protective immunity, *Nutr Today* 27(4):18, 1992.
10. Fenton TR and others: Nutrition and growth analysis of very low birth weight infants, *Pediatrics* 86(3):378, 1990.
11. Tsang RC, Nichols BL: *Nutrition during infancy,* Philadelphia, 1988, Hanley & Belfus.
12. Thommessen M and others: Energy and nutrient intakes of disabled children: do feeding problems make a difference? *J Am Diet Assoc* 91(12):1522, 1991.
13. Lucas BL: Serving infants and children with special health care needs in the 1990s—are we ready? *J Am Diet Assoc* 89(11):1599, 1989.
14. Hine RJ and others: Early nutrition intervention services for children with special health care needs, *J Am Diet Assoc* 89(11):1636, 1989.
15. Kozlowski BW, Powell JA: Position of The American Dietetic Association: Nutrition services for children with special health care needs, *J Am Diet Assoc* 89(8):1133, 1989.

16. Tsui JC, Nordstrom JW: Folate status of adolescents: effects of folic acid supplementation, *J Am Diet Assoc* 90(11):1551, 1990.

17. Boone JL: Stress and hypertension, *Prim Care* 18(3):623, 1991.

18. Monsen ER: Reversing heart disease through diet, exercise, and stress management: an interview with Dean Ornish, *J Am Diet Assoc* 91(2):162, 1991.

19. Pickett CWL, Lees REM: A cross-sectional study of health complaints among 79 data entry operators using video display terminals, *J Soc Occup Med* 41(3):113, 1991.

20. Bennett P, Carroll D: Stress management approaches to the prevention of coronary heart disease, *Br J Clin Psychol* 29:1, 1990.

21. Miller A and others: Stress on the job, *Newsweek* CXI(17):40, Apr 25, 1988.

22. Rennert L: Poverty in the US hits worst level since 1964, *The Sacramento Bee* 272:1, Sept 4, 1992.

23. Hinton AW and others: Position of The American Dietetic Association: domestic hunger and inadequate access to food, *J Am Diet Assoc* 90(10):1437, 1990.

24. Wardlaw G: Hunger and undernutrition in the world, *Nutri-News*, Aug 1990.

25. Langan PA: America's soaring prison population, *Science* 251:1568, 1991.

26. Rime B and others: Type A behavior pattern: specific coronary risk factor or general disease-prone condition? *Br J Med Psychol* 62:229, 1989.

FURTHER READING

Cohen BE: Food security and hunger policy for the 1990s, *Nutr Today* 25(4):23, 1990.

Cotugna N, Vickery CE: Nurturing social responsibility: nutrition students volunteer in hunger projects, *J Am Diet Assoc* 92(3):297, 1992.

Wolgemuth JC and others: Wasting malnutrition and inadequate nutrient intakes identified in a multiethnic homeless population, *J Am Diet Assoc* 92(7):834, 1992.

These three articles focus on the problem of homelessness and the malnutrition this lack of food security brings, as well as efforts being made to find solutions.

Monnsen ER: Reversing heart disease through diet, exercise, and stress management: an interview with Dean Ornish, *J Am Diet Assoc* 91(2):162, 1991.

The editor of this journal provides some interesting highlights of the San Francisco study of heart disease, which involved a strong focus on stress management.

Ross AC: Vitamin A and protective immunity, *Nutr Today* 27(4):18, 1992.

This author provides helpful guidance for understanding the workings of the human immune system and the vital role of nutritional status and key nutrients to maintaining this vital defense against the stress of disease.

Social Isolation, Stress, and Health

Part of being human is the social activity of eating. Even on the occasions when we eat alone, we are experiencing the social web of our culture in the nature of the food and the meanings it has for us. It is small wonder, then, that food intake and social relationships are inevitably interwoven with nutritional status and health. When deprived of these significant relations, we experience the stress of social isolation and our health suffers.

But, you may well ask, what is new about these associations? We've seen before that isolated persons, especially older ones, seem to have more health problems. This is true. Scientists interested in this issue have long noted such associations between social relationships and health. But the reasons behind their observations have been far less clear, raising still more unanswered cause and effect questions. For example, does the lack of satisfying social relationships itself cause people to become ill or die? Or are people with ill health just less likely to establish and maintain significant social relationships? Or is there some other causal factor, such as a *misanthropic* personality—which predisposes persons to "hate human beings" in general and leads to lowered capacity to form quality social relationships in particular—that makes persons become ill or die? A growing body of evidence, however, is beginning to bring some answers. It is revealing the significant impact of social isolation stress on health and its role as an important risk factor of growing concern in our rapidly changing society.

Background studies

The concept of "social support" first appeared in the mental health literature of the mid-1970s and was linked to the rapidly developing field of research on stress and its psychosocial and physiologic associations with the causes of health and illness. There was growing recognition that chronic disease in an aging population and changing society was caused not by a single factor, such as a microbe—as had often been the case in the past—but rather by multiple behavioral, environmental, biologic, and genetic factors, which combined over time to produce illness or death. Both population studies and clinical research began to bring some answers.

Population studies. Compelling evidence from an early 1965 baseline study of 4775 urban adults in Alameda County, California, aged 30 to 69, which surveyed four types of social ties—marriage, extended family and friends, church, and other formal or informal group affiliations—indicated that lack of social relationships constitutes a major risk factor for mortality. Similar population studies followed in other places such as Tecumseh, Michigan; Evans County, Georgia; Gothenberg, Sweden; and rural eastern Finland. Though methods and results varied and raised further questions for study, the finding that social rela-

tionships predict mortality for men and women in a wide range of populations, even after adjustment for medical risk factors involved, was remarkably consistent.

Clinical studies. There was also growing evidence from clinical research with both animals and humans that variations in social contacts produce both psychologic and physiologic effects that could, if prolonged, produce in turn serious illness or death. Based on a wide range of studies through the 1970s and early 1980s, a psychophysiologic theory was proposed—reinforcing Selye's earlier work on stress—to explain how social relationships and contacts can promote health and protect against disease. This broad base of studies suggests that social relationships and contacts mediate their effect through the *amygdala*, a small oval-shaped complex of nuclei within the tip of the brain's temporal lobe connected through the limbic cortex to the hypothalamus. This mediation acts to: (1) activate the anterior hypothalamic zone, stimulating release of human growth hormone, and (2) inhibit the posterior hypothalamic zone, depressing secretion of ACTH, cortisol, catecholamines, and associated sympathetic autonomic nervous system activity. These mechanisms are consistent with the impact of social relations on illness or death from a wide range of causes, as well as adverse effects on the growth and development of infants and young children who are deprived of these early satisfying social contacts and fail to thrive. Overall, evidence from physiologic and psychosocial studies and clinical experience are steadily reinforcing the theory for the impact of social relationships on health.

Risk factor for health

The growing evidence of social relationships as a cause or risk factor in illness and death from a wide range of diseases is probably stronger than the evidence that led to the designation of Type A behavior pattern as a risk factor for coronary heart disease. The evidence on social relationships and health increasingly equals that of cigarette smoking established in the Surgeon General's 1964 report. Although the current evidence firmly establishes a lack of social relationships as a risk factor in illness or death, three basic questions require further investigation: What precise mechanisms and processes link social relationships to health? What "levels of exposure" to social relationships determine these effects? How can we lower the prevalence of relative social isolation in our modern society or lessen its harmful effects on health?

Linking mechanisms

Over the past decade, social support research has established the supportive quality of social relationships, especially their capacity to buffer or moderate the harmful effects of stress and other health hazards. But recent experimental studies with animals and humans seem to indicate that social relationships have generally beneficial effects

Social Isolation, Stress, and Health—cont'd

on health, not solely or primarily attributable to their buffering effects, and that there may be aspects of social relationships other than their supportive quality that accounts for these positive effects. Current investigators point to our need to understand better the social, psychologic, and biologic processes that link quality and quantity of social relationships to health. Social support is only one of these processes, whether it is in the form of emotional nurturing, practical help, or information. But social relationships may also affect health, because they regulate or integrate human thought, feelings, motivation, and behavior in ways that promote health. Current views suggest that social relationships affect health by (1) fostering a sense of meaning or wholeness to life or (2) facilitating health-promoting behaviors, such as eating a sound diet; getting proper sleep; exercising regularly; using alcohol appropriately, if at all; avoiding cigarette smoking and use of other harmful drugs; adhering to medical regimens; and seeking appropriate medical care.

Determinants of social relationships

Clearly, both biology and personality affect persons' health and the quality and quantity of their social relationships. Current research shows that social relationships have a predictive, and arguably causal, association with health in their own right. But the quality and extent of a person's social relationships is also a function of broader social forces. Whether we are employed, married, attend church, belong to organizations, frequently see friends or relatives, and the nature of these contacts, are all determined in part by our positions in the larger social structure. This social structure is further stratified by age, race, gender, and socioeconomic status and is organized in terms of residential communities, work organizations, and larger political and economic structures. Surveys indicate that those persons generally less socially integrated in our society are the poor, the elderly, and blacks. Also, our changing social patterns of having fewer children, living longer, and moving frequently affect opportunities for work, marriage, living and working in different settings, making friends, and seeing relatives. And all of these social patterns are themselves subject to larger economic and political change, which can directly affect persons' social relationships.

To verify this research base concerning the significant association of social relationships to health, we have only to look around us at our rapidly changing society and the effects of these changes in persons' lives over the past few decades. In contrast with the 1950s, for example, adults today are less likely to be married, belong to voluntary organizations, or visit informally with others and more likely to be living alone and to live longer. These far-reaching social changes mean that in the 21st century, soon to be upon us, we will see a steady increase in the number of older people who lack spouses or children, the very persons to whom they would turn for social support.

It is indeed ironic that we are just now learning the full impact of social relationships on our health and well-being, at a time of great social change when we have an increasing likelihood of losing some of our more traditional social supports. The implications of the stress of increasing social isolation are obvious for community health care programs and resources, which will help meet these changing needs.

REFERENCES

Cohen S, Syme SL: *Social support and health*, New York, 1985, Academic Press.

House JS, Landis KR, Umberson D: Social relationships and health, *Science* 241:540, 1988.

Walker D, Beauchene RE: The relationship of loneliness, social isolation, and physical health to dietary adequacy of independently living elderly, *J Am Diet Assoc* 91(3):300, 1991.

PART

3

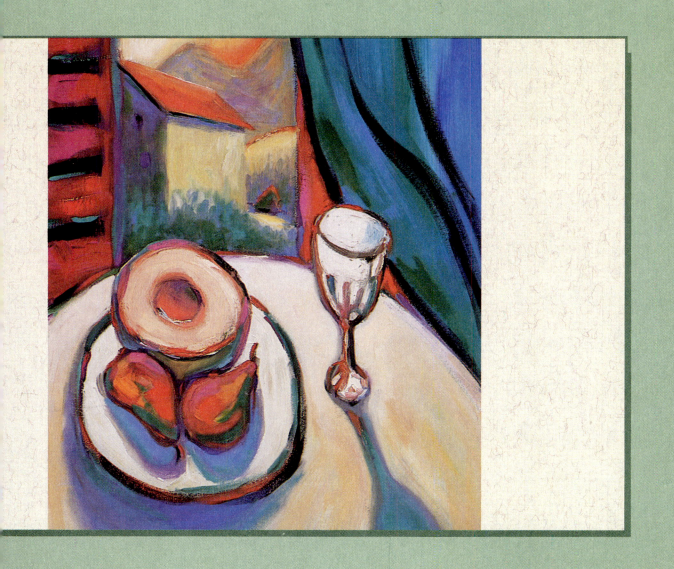

*I*ntroduction to Clinical
Nutrition

CHAPTER 16

Nutritional Assessment and Therapy in Patient Care

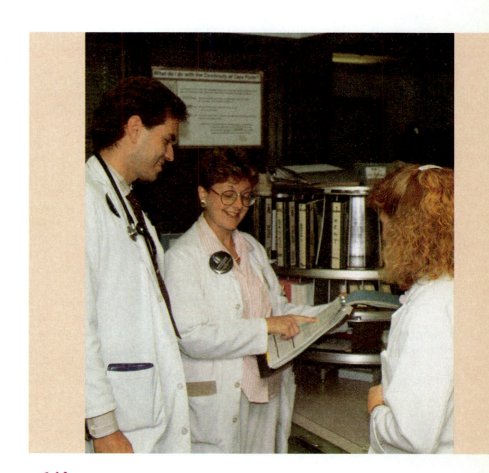

$\mathcal{W}$ith this chapter we begin our final study sequence on clinical nutrition. In this concluding section we apply the principles of nutritional science and community nutrition discussed in the previous sections to nutritional needs in disease.

Here we focus on the essential first step in comprehensive nutritional care—assessing nutritional needs and goals as the first step in planning sensitive and valid patient care. Wherever the place of care and whatever the need, the health care team of practitioners, patient, and family work together to support the healing process and promote health.

The Therapeutic Process

Role of Nutrition in Clinical Care

Persons face acute illness or chronic disease and its treatment in a variety of settings: the acute care hospital, the long-term rehabilitation center, the extended care facility, the clinic, the private office, and the home. In all instances nutritional care is fundamental. It is vital support for any medical treatment. Frequently it is the primary therapy in itself. About 2500 years have passed since Hippocrates admonished us to pay closer attention to this significant connection between nutrition and disease, but we are only now, in more modern scientific times, beginning to catch a glimmer of the real depth of his valuable instruction.

Comprehensive nutritional assessment provides the necessary data for appropriate nutritional therapy based on identified needs. Clinical nutritionists, all registered dietitians (RDs), many with advanced degrees in nutritional science, use their expertise and skills to make sound clinical judgments and work effectively with the clinical care team. Together these professionals provide an essential component for successful medical treatment. They assist the patient in recovery from illness or injury, help the person maintain follow-up care to promote health, and also help to control health care costs.

Stress of the Therapeutic Encounter

In the modern hospital setting, the therapeutic encounter between health care providers and their patients occurs under stressful conditions at best. Several factors can contribute to the nutritional toll.

Bed Rest

Even though the reason for the hospitalization may indicate the need for bed rest, at the same time the bed rest itself can bring detrimental effects on the body's physiology.[1] For example, after just 3 days of lying supine in bed, the body begins to lose its resistance to the pull of gravity and continuing inactivity diminishes muscle tone, bone calcium, plasma volume, and gastric secretions, bringing some impairment of glucose tolerance and shifts in body fluids and electrolytes.

Hospital Malnutrition

Hospital, or **iatrogenic,** malnutrition has been widely documented. First, hospitalized patients with hypermetabolic and physiologic stress of illness or injury are at particular risk for malnutrition from their increased needs for nutritional support. In addition, a fundamental problem is lack of adequate admission nutrition screening or follow-up monitoring to identify patients at malnutrition risk and to provide essential nutrition support immediately.[2] Other problems of hospital routine also contributing to lack of adequate nourishment include (1) highly restricted diets remaining on order and unsupplemented too long, (2) unserved meals because of interference of medical procedures and clinical tests, and (3) unmonitored lack of patient appetite.

Hospital Setting and System

Each injured or ill patient is a unique person and requires special treatment and care. At the same time a sometimes formidable array of staff persons seek to determine needs and implement what each perceives to be appropriate care. It is no surprise that the course does not always run smoothly or that patients often feel intimidated and powerless. Sometimes our complex system and highly specialized technology get in the way and we lose sight of our reason for being—to meet individual human needs and personal care.

Constant open and validating communication is essential, both among the health team members and between the health care provider and the patient and family. At such times we need to remind ourselves of the fundamental ethical principles guiding all our patient care.[3] These principles should ensure that all we do must:

- *Benefit* the patient
- Do no *harm*
- Preserve the patient's *autonomy*
- *Disclose* full and truthful information for patient decisions concerning personal care
- Provide *social justice*

Such ethical behavior is based on the overriding fundamental principles of right action found within the Anglo-American law, which emphasizes the basic rights of privacy and free choice.[4] Continuing open communication provides the basis for such ethical practices among the health team members and between the health care providers and the patient and family. It is especially important for many stressed elderly patients.[5] In this team effort for quality nutritional care, the clinical dietitian (a clinical nutrition specialist), with the physician, carries the primary responsibility. The nurse and other primary care practitioners provide essential support.

Focus of Care: The Patient

Patient-centered Care

The primary principle of nutritional practice, then, too often overlooked in the many routine procedures of the hospital setting, is evident: to be valid, nutritional care must be person centered. In this renewed partnership **paradigm** for patient-centered health care, the patient must always be the senior partner.[6,7] It must be based on initial identified needs, updated constantly with the patient, with continuing results monitored in relation to therapy goals. This is necessary, of course, to provide essential physical care. But it is also necessary to support the patient's personal needs for maintaining self-esteem and control as much as possible. In addition, a second fundamental fact needs emphasis: despite all methods, tools, and technologies described here or elsewhere, the most therapeutic tool you will ever use is yourself. It is to this seemingly simple yet profoundly personal healing encounter that you bring yourself and your skills.

Health Care Team

In the setting of the individual medical center, with its strengths and despite its shortcomings and within the essential team care provided, the clinical nutritionist must care for the patient's fundamental nutritional needs in a close relationship with medical and nursing care. Sensitive communication skills are essential for all ages and degrees of health problems. Determining the patient's nutritional care needs is the initial and ongoing responsibility.

Phases of the Care Process

Five distinct yet constantly interacting phases are essential in the therapeutic care process.

1. *Assessment: database.* A broad base of relative information about the patient's nutritional status, food habits, and life situation is necessary for making accurate initial assessments. Useful background information may come from a variety of sources, such as the patient, the patient's chart, family or other relatives and friends, oral and written communication with other hospital personnel or staff, and related research. A number of valuable assessment tools have been developed, some of which are described here.
2. *Analysis: problem list.* A careful analysis of all data collected determines specific patient needs. Some needs will be immediately evident. Others will develop as the situation unfolds. On the basis of this analysis, a list of problems may be formed to guide continuing care activities.
3. *Planning care: needs and goals.* Valid care is based on identified problems. The plan must always be based on personal needs and goals of the individual patient, as well as the identified medical care requirements or options discussed with the patient and family.
4. *Implementing care: actions.* The patient care plan is put into action according to realistic and appropriate activities within each situation. For example, nutritional care and education will involve decisions and actions concerning an appropriate food plan and mode of feeding, as well as the training and education needs of the patient, staff, and family who will carry it out.
5. *Evaluating and recording care: results.* As every care activity is carried out, results are carefully checked to see if the identified needs have been met. Ap-

propriate revisions of the care plan can be made as needed for continuing care. These results are carefully recorded in the patient's medical record. Clear documentation of all activities is essential.

In our discussion here, we look at each of these phases in terms of quality nutritional care. We focus on methods and tools of nutrition assessment, practical management of nutritional therapy and care, maintenance of effective medical records, and ways of ensuring quality standards of nutritional care.

Nutritional Assessment and Analysis

The Purpose and Process of Collecting Nutritional Data

The fundamental purpose of nutritional assessment in general clinical practice is to determine (1) the overall nutritional status of the patient, (2) current health care needs, both physical and psychosocial as well as personal, and (3) related factors influencing these needs in the person's current life situation. The first step in nutritional assessment, as with assessing any situation to determine needs and actions, is to collect pertinent information—a data base—for use in identifying needs. The clinical nutritionist, assisted by other health team members as needed, uses several basic types of activities for nutritional assessment of patients' needs, often called the *ABCD* approach:

- **A**nthropometrics
- **B**iochemical tests
- **C**linical observations
- **D**iet evaluation and personal histories

Each part of this approach is important because no single parameter alone directly measures individual nutritional status or determines problems or needs. Further, the overall resulting picture must be interpreted within the context of personal social and health factors that may alter nutritional requirements. Only with this type of comprehensive evaluation can nutrition assessment become the real index to the quality of life that it should be. Since such a comprehensive history is a fundamental tool for planning health care, history taking is a primary skill for all health professionals. A broad number of tests may be used for research purposes in a large facility with access to highly sophisti-

---

iatrogenic • Describes a medical disorder caused by physician diagnosis, manner, or treatment.

paradigm • A pattern or model serving as an example; a standard or ideal for practice or behavior based on a fundamental value or theme.

cated equipment. However, the precedures outlined here provide a good base in general practice.

Anthropometrics

Skill gained through careful practice is necessary to minimize the margin of error in making body measurements. Selection and maintenance of proper procedures and equipment, as well as attention to careful technique, are essential in securing accurate data.

Weight

Hospitalized patients should be weighed at consistent times, for example, before breakfast after the bladder has been emptied. Clinic patients should be weighed without shoes in light, indoor clothing or an examining gown. For accuracy, use regular clinic beam scales with nondetachable weights. An additional weight attachment is available for use with very obese persons. Metric scales with readings to the nearest 20 g provide specific data. However, the standard clinic scale is satisfactory. Check all scales frequently and have them calibrated every 3 or 4 months for continued accuracy.

After careful reading and recording of the patient's weight, ask about the usual body weight and compare it with standard height and weight tables (see Chapter 6). Interpret present weight in terms of percentage of usual and standard body weight for height. Check for any recent weight loss: 1% to 2% in the past week, 5% over the past month, 7.5% during the previous 3 months, or 10% in the past 6 months is significant. More than this rate can be severe. A check of unexplained weight loss in elderly persons is particularly important, since it may be a clue to depression or a wasting disease such as cancer and needs to be on record and followed up.[8,9] Values charted in the patient's record should indicate percentage of weight change.

Height

If possible use a fixed measuring stick or tape on a true vertical flat surface. If one is not available, the movable measuring rod on the platform clinic scales may be used with reasonable accuracy. Have the patient stand as straight as possible, without shoes or cap, heels together, and looking straight ahead. The heels, buttocks, shoulders, and head should be touching the wall or vertical surface of the measuring rod. Read the measure carefully and compare it with previous recordings. Note the growth of children or the diminishing height of adults. Metric measures of height in centimeters provide accurate data.

Body Mass Index (BMI)

The weight and height measures are used to calculate the patient's body mass index: weight (kilograms) divided by height (meters)^2. This ratio is commonly used in evaluating obesity states in relation to risk factors.

Details of this calculation, conversion factors, and reference values are described in Chapter 6.

Body Frame

Two added measures have recently been developed to answer questions about the arbitrary categories of body frame size for height and weight used in the current tables of the Metropolitan Life Insurance Company.[10]

Elbow breadth. New standards of weight and body composition by frame size and height have been developed with frame size based on measurement of elbow breadth.[11] With patient's arm extended and forearm bent upward to form a 90° angle, elbow breadth is measured with a specially developed instrument such as the Frameter, which measures the distance in centimeters between the two outer bony landmarks (medial and lateral epicondyles of the humerus). An anthropometric kit with all materials and references is available from the research and development group (Health Products, 2126 Ridge, Ann Arbor, MI 48104).

Wrist circumference. This is a measure of height divided by wrist circumference (in centimeters).[12] With the patient's right hand extended and using a nonstretchable metric tape, measure the wrist circumference at the joint just distal (toward the fingers) to the bony wristbone protrusion (the styloid process). Interpret results by the following standard:

Frame size	Male ratio values	Female ratio values
Small	10.4	11.0
Medium	9.6-10.4	10.1-11.0
Large	9.6	10.1

Body Measures

In general clinical practice, the clinical nutritionist uses two basic body measurements—the mid–upper arm circumference and the triceps skin fold thickness—and from these calculates a third measure, the mid arm muscle circumference. First, using a nonstretchable centimeter tape, locate the midpoint of the upper arm on the nondominant arm, unless it is affected by edema. The midarm circumference (MAC) is measured at this midpoint and read accurately to the nearest tenth of a centimeter and recorded. The resulting measure is compared with previous measurements to note possible changes. Second, using a standard millimeter skin fold caliper, take a measure of the triceps skin fold thickness (TSF) at this same midpoint of the upper arm. This measure provides an estimate of the subcutaneous fat reserves. Then, together with the midpoint circumference value at this same point, the midarm muscle circumference (MAMC) is calculated by the following formula:

$$\text{MAMC (cm)} = \text{MAC (cm)} - [3.14 \times \text{TSF (cm)}]$$

If desired, the TSF may be left in millimeters, as measured with the calipers, and the value of the factor (pi; π) in the formula changed to 0.314.

This final derived value gives an indirect measure of the body's skeletal muscle mass, a good indicator of body composition. Finally, to interpret the patient's measurements for monitoring nutritional status, these values are compared as percentages of standards in reference tables (Appendix I).

Alternative Measures for Nonambulatory Patients

Several alternative measures can provide values for estimating height and weight of persons confined to bed.

Total arm length. With the patient holding the arm straight down by the side of the body, and using a nonstretchable metric tape, measure the arm length from attachment at the shoulder to the end of the arm at the wrist. Reference standards indicate relation of this measure to height equivalents.[13] This is also a useful alternative to standing body height when body conditions distort usual standing height of ambulatory patients. For example, this measure is helpful with older persons, in whom a general thinning of weight-bearing cartilages, the bent-knee gait, and a possible **kyphosis** of the spine may make standing height measurement inaccurate.

Armspan. The full armspan measure is an alternate to height in adults, especially practical for elderly persons. Tests indicate that it may give a more accurate result than height in calculating BMI in elderly patients.[14] Using a flexible metric tape, measure full armspan from fingertip to fingertip in centimeters, passing the tape in front of the clavicles. A recumbent half-span measure from fingertip to body midline at the sternal notch may be used with patients having limited movement in one arm, then doubled to achieve the same result.

Knee height. With the patient lying in the supine position and left knee and ankle each bent at a 90-degree angle, the knee height is measured with a special caliper.[15] A simple comparative measure of knee to floor height in the sitting position, from the outside bony point just under the kneecap, indicating head of the tibia, down to the floor surface, may also be used.[16] The knee height (KH) measurement is then used to calculate the value for deriving body height equivalent:

Height (women) = [(1.83 × KH) − (0.24 × age)] + 84.88
Height (men) = [(2.02 × KH) − (0.04 × age)] + 64.19

Calf circumference. With the patient in the same supine position and left knee bent at a 90-degree angle, and using nonstretchable metric tape, measure the calf circumference (CC) at the largest point. This measurement is then used with three other values—knee height (KH), midarm circumference (MAC), and subscapular skin fold (SSF)—to derive body weight value[15,17]:

Weight (women) = (1.27 × CC) + (0.87 × KH)
                  + (0.98 × MAC) + (0.4 × SSF) − 62.35
Weight (men) = (0.98 × CC) + (1.16 × KH)
                + (1.73 × MAC) + (0.37 × SSF) − 81.69

Biochemical Tests

A number of laboratory tests are available for studying nutritional status. The most commonly used ones for assessing and monitoring nutritional status and planning nutritional care in clinical practice are listed here. General ranges for normal values are given in standard texts.

Measures of Plasma Protein

Basic measures include serum albumin, hemoglobin, and hemocrit. Additional ones may include prealbumin (PAB), a thyroxine-binding protein, serum transferrin, or total iron-binding capacity (TIBC) and ferritin.

Measures of Protein Metabolism

Basic 24-hour urine tests are used to measure urinary creatinine and urea nitrogen levels. These materials are products of protein metabolism. The patient's 24-hour excretion of creatinine is interpreted in terms of ideal *creatinine* excretion for height, the creatinine-height index (CHI) (Table 16-1). Comparison is made with standard values for this index. The patient's 24-hour urea nitrogen excretion is used with the calculated dietary nitrogen intake over the same 24-hour period to calculate nitrogen balance:

N balance = (protein intake ÷ 6.25) − (urinary urea N + 4)

The formula factor of 4 represents additional nitrogen loss through the feces and skin. Urinary urea nitrogen excretion reflects metabolism of dietary nitrogen, as the nitrogen balance formula indicates, and is a measure of the adequacy of protein nutrition.

Measures of Immune System Integrity: Anergy

Basic measures are made of lymphocyte count. Additional measures may be made by skin testing, observing delayed sensitivity to common recall antigens such as mumps or purified protein derivative of tuberculin (PPD). Skin tests are read at 24 and 48 hours, with

---

kyphosis · Increased, abnormal convexity of the upper part of the spine; hunchback.

TABLE 16-1

Ideal Weight and Urinary Creatinine Values for Height (Adults)*

Height (cm)	Females Weight (kg)	Females Creatinine (mg)	Males Weight (kg)	Males Creatinine (mg)
140	44.9			
141	45.4			
142	45.9			
143	46.4			
144	47.0			
145	47.5		51.9	
146	48.0		52.4	
147	48.6	828	52.9	
148	49.2		53.5	
149	49.8		54.0	
150	50.4	852	54.5	
151	51.0		55.0	
152	51.5		55.6	
153	52.0	878	56.1	
154	52.5		56.6	
155	53.1	901	57.2	
156	53.7		57.9	
157	54.3	922	58.6	1284
158	54.9		59.3	
159	55.5		59.9	
160	56.2	949	60.5	1325
161	56.9		61.1	
162	57.6		61.7	
163	58.3	979	62.3	1362
164	58.9		62.9	
165	59.5	1005	63.5	1387
166	60.1		64.0	
167	60.7	1040	64.6	1421
168	61.4		65.2	
169	62.1		65.9	
170		1075	66.6	1465
171			67.3	
172			68.0	
173		1111	68.7	1516
174			69.4	
175		1139	70.1	1552
176			70.8	
177		1169	71.6	1589
178			72.4	
179			73.3	
180		1204	74.2	1639
181			75.0	
182			75.8	
183		1241	76.5	1692
184			77.3	
185			78.1	1735
186			78.9	
187				1776
188				
189				
190				1826

*1959 Metropolitan Life Insurance Company Standards corrected for nude weight without shoe heels.

Data from Jeffe DB: *The assessment of the nutritional status of the community*, Geneva, 1966, World Health Organization.

greater than 5 mm considered positive and the presence of one positive test indicating intact immunity.

Clinical Observations

Keen observation is made of possible malnutrition signs as well as those evident through vital signs and physical examination.

Clinical Signs of Malnutrition

Careful attention to physical signs of possible malnutrition provides an added dimension to the overall assessment of general nutritional status (see To Probe Further, p. 314). A guide for a general examination of such signs is given in Table 16-2. A careful description of any such observations is documented in the patient's medical record.

Vital Signs and Physical Examination

Other physical data may include pulse rate, respiration, temperature, and blood pressure. A study of the common procedures of a normal physical examination will provide useful background orientation.

Diet Evaluation and Personal Histories

A careful nutrition history, including nutritional information related to living situation and other personal, psychosocial, and economic problems, is a fundamental part of nutrition assessment. But obtaining accurate information about basic food patterns and actual dietary intake is not a simple matter. However, a sensitive practitioner may obtain useful information by using one or more of the basic tools described here.

Specific 24-Hour Food Record

For hospitalized patients, a record of food intake over a specific 24-hour period may be needed for tests such as a nitrogen balance study or for monitoring energy and nutrient intake. A careful explanation of purpose and procedure for the patient and staff is needed. However, such a brief recall or record in general practice has limited value in determining overall basic food habits.

Diet History

General knowledge of the patient's basic eating habits is needed to determine any possible nutritional deficiencies. In conjunction with the patient's usual living situation and related food attitudes and behaviors, social and family history, and medical history with current status and treatment, the nutrition interview provides an essential base for further personal nutrition counseling and planning of care (Fig. 16-1). For example, an activity-associated day's food intake pattern, using guides discussed in Chapter 10 (Fig. 10-1), can provide a useful tool for obtaining a fairly valid picture of food habits and eating behaviors. In addition to food

TABLE 16-2

Clinical Signs of Nutritional Status

Body area	Signs of good nutrition	Signs of poor nutrition
General appearance	Alert, responsive	Listless, apathetic, cachectic
Weight	Normal for height, age, body build	Overweight or underweight (special concern for underweight)
Posture	Erect, arms and legs straight	Sagging shoulders, sunken chest, humped back
Muscles	Well-developed, firm, good tone, some fat under skin	Flaccid, poor tone, undeveloped, tender, "wasted" appearance, cannot walk properly
Nervous control	Good attention span, not irritable or restless, normal reflexes, psychologic stability	Inattentive, irritable, confused, burning and tingling of hands and feet (paresthesia), loss of position and vibratory sense, weakness and tenderness of muscles (may result in inability to walk), decrease or loss of ankle and knee reflexes
Gastrointestinal function	Good appetite and digestion, normal regular elimination, no palpable (perceptible to touch) organs or masses	Anorexia, indigestion, constipation or diarrhea, liver or spleen enlargement
Cardiovascular function	Normal heart rate and rhythm, no murmurs, normal blood pressure for age	Rapid heart rate (above 100 beats/min tachycardia), enlarged heart, abnormal rhythm, elevated blood pressure
General vitality	Endurance, energetic, sleeps well, vigorous	Easily fatigued, no energy, falls asleep easily, looks tired, apathetic
Hair	Shiny, lustrous, firm, not easily plucked, healthy scalp	Stringy, dull, brittle, dry, thin and sparse, depigmented, easily plucked
Skin (general)	Smooth, slightly moist, good color	Rough, dry, scaly, pale, pigmented, irritated, bruises, petechiae
Face and neck	Skin color uniform, smooth, healthy appearance, not swollen	Greasy, discolored, scaly, swollen, skin dark over cheeks and under eyes, lumpiness or flakiness of skin around nose and mouth
Lips	Smooth, good color, moist, not chapped or swollen	Dry, scaly, swollen, redness and swelling (cheilosis), or angular lesions at corners of the mouth or fissures or scars (stomatitis)
Mouth, oral membranes	Reddish pink mucous membranes in oral cavity	Swollen, boggy oral mucous membranes
Gums	Good pink color, healthy, red, no swelling or bleeding	Spongy, bleed easily, marginal redness, inflamed, gums receding
Tongue	Good pink color or deep reddish in appearance, not swollen or smooth, surface papillae present, no lesions	Swelling, scarlet and raw, magenta color, beefy (glossitis), hyperemic and hypertrophic papillae, atrophic papillae
Teeth	No cavities, no pain, bright, straight, no crowding, well-shaped jaw, clean, no discoloration	Unfilled caries, absent teeth, worn surfaces mottled (fluorosis), malpositioned
Eyes	Bright, clear, shiny, no sores at corner of eyelids, membranes moist and healthy pink color, no prominent blood vessels or mount of tissue on sclera, no fatigue circles beneath	Eye membranes pale (pale conjunctivae), redness of membrane (conjuncitival infection), dryness of infection, Bitot's spots, redness and fissuring of eyelid corners (angular palpebritis), dryness of eye membrane (conjunctival xerosis), dull appearance of cornea (corneal xerosis), soft cornea (keratomalacia)
Neck (glands)	No enlargement	Thyroid enlarged
Nails	Firm, pink	Spoon-shaped (koilonychia), brittle, ridged
Legs, feet	No tenderness, weakness, or swelling; good color	Edema, tender calf, tingling, weakness
Skeleton	No malformations	Bowlegs, knock-knees, chest deformity at diaphragm, beaded ribs, prominent scapulas

Modified from Williams SR: Nutritional guidance in prenatal care. In Worthington-Roberts BS, Vermeersch J, Williams SR: *Nutrition in pregnancy and lactation,* St Louis, 1993, Mosby.

and nutrition information, drug therapy data from the medical record or the patient and family is important to determine any possible drug-nutrient interaction involved or any teaching needed by the patient (see Chapter 17).[19] Research carefully all prescriptions and over-the-counter drugs the patient is using.

Periodic Food Records

At various times, a 3- to 7-day food record is a helpful tool for assessing food patterns, especially when used to follow up a comprehensive initial diet history or counseling instructions for a special therapeutic diet required. A 3-day record is generally sufficient for determining overall food, energy, and nutrient intake. A number of appropriate software programs are available that make final computer analysis a simple matter (see Issues and Answers, p. 320). But, of course, the accuracy of the computer analysis depends entirely on the accuracy of the food record. Sometimes a food frequency questionnaire is helpful to determine food use

Nutritional Assessment: When Being Objective Does Not Always Mean Being Objective

TO PROBE FURTHER

Nutritionists, and other health professionals, like numbers. To identify malnutrition, they monitor serum levels of liver-secreted plasma proteins, such as albumin and transferrin, take anthropometric measurements, and determine creatinine-height indexes and cell-mediated immunity response. One study now suggests that these numbers do not add up to the accuracy of the clinical examination in determining a patient's nutritional status.

Researchers from the University of Toronto and Toronto General Hospital suggest that objective measurements may sometimes be inaccurate because they are influenced by several factors: (1) the effects of the disease process itself (rather than the distinct issue of malnutrition) on changes in nutrient levels, (2) delayed response to nutritional depletion (or repletion) because of the relatively long half-lives of such indexes as serum albumin and transferrin, and (3) the wide range of confidence limits in nutritional measurements.

These workers found that two physician clinical evaluators were able to agree on the nutritional status of 81% of 59 surgical patients examined independently. The history, emphasizing weight loss, edema, anorexia, unusual food intakes, and so on, and the physical examination, stressing jaundice, muscle wasting, edema, conditions of oral structures, and similar findings, provided enough information for them to come to conclusions that agreed with objective evaluations.

Does this mean that laboratory tests should be placed in semiretirement, limited to use in epidemiologic surveys instead of evaluating individuals? These researchers think they should, but they do acknowledge that accurate assessment tests do exist, such as total body nitrogen and total body potassium, although these are not generally available. They also suggest the possibility of combining several known indexes to make a more sensitive one, even though this lends itself to the possibility of leaving out one measurement that could have an important effect on the calculations.

However, they do emphasize an important point: nutritional status is as dependent on what you *see* as what you read on a laboratory sheet.

REFERENCES

Baker JP and others: Nutritional assessment: a comparison of clinical judgment and objective measurements, *N Engl J Med* 306(16):969, 1982.

Detsky AS and others: What is subjective global assessment of nutritional status? *J Parenteral Enteral Nutr* 11:8, 1987.

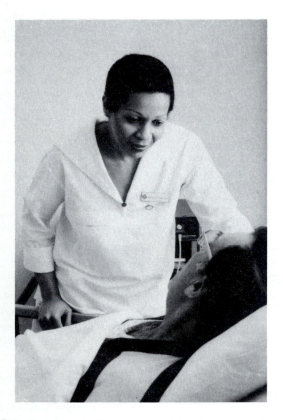

FIG. 16-1   Interviewing of patient to plan personal care.

over an extended period of time, which provides useful data, especially in combination with specific food records.[20]

Analyzing Nutritional Data

Valid patient care planning requires analysis of all nutritional data collected. On this basis problems requiring solutions can be identified. A detailed analysis of the nutrition information helps determine nutritional diagnosis, any primary or secondary nutritional disease, and any underlying nutrition-related conditions.

Nutritional Diagnosis

All the various nutritional data for each patient, collected by the clinical nutritionist and other team members through the broad assessment activities described, must be carefully analyzed to reach a valid nutritional diagnosis and plan of care. Every health team member participates in this analysis through various communications, discussions, case conferences, records, and reports (Fig. 16-2). The nutritional diagnosis requires information about all aspects related to the patient's needs: nutrient deficiencies, underlying disease requiring a modified nutrient or food plan, any personal cultural, ethnic, or economic needs, as well as mode of feeding and dietary mangement.

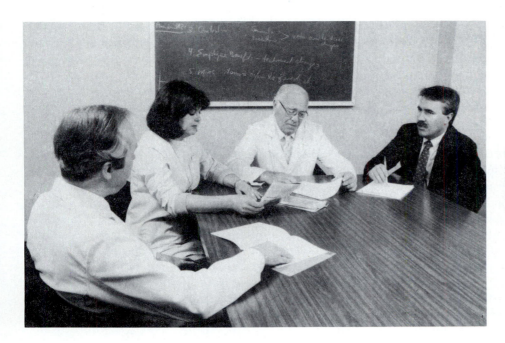

FIG. 16-2   The health team conference for planning patient care. Physician, nurse, clinical nutritionist, and social worker review patient's progress and needs.

Primary and Secondary Nutritional Disease

The clinical nutritionist coordinates these nutrition activities and carries a major responsibility on the health care team for interpreting nutrition-related data and making decisions and recommendations concerning any primary or secondary nutritional states. Primary deficiency disease results from a lack of essential nutrients in the diet, for whatever reason. Secondary deficiency disease results from one or more barriers to the use of the nutrients after they are consumed in food. This inability to use a given nutrient may stem from digestive or malabsorption problems or from lack of specific cell enzymes. Such problems may be caused by conditions such as lactose intolerance, celiac disease, inflammatory bowel disease, cell metabolism defects in genetic disease, chemotherapy, or radiation treatments.

Nutrition-related Conditions

Related chronic disease problems with nutrition involvement will also be considered. These include such conditions as heart disease, hypertension, cancer, diabetes, and liver and renal disease. Surgery also imposes nutrition demands and modifications. Any quantifiable data collected can be analzed by computer. Two major nutritional tasks in which the computer excels are (1) baseline screening to identify persons at risk of malnutrition because of their disease, injury, or life-style, and (2) analysis of intake to monitor effectiveness of ongoing treatment. Laboratory data may be handled in a similar manner, with general patterns of change monitored over time. Careful appraisal of medical and personal data from histories, records, reports, and interviews will help focus on various needs and problems

and provide a realistic picture of nutritional and eating difficulties.

Problem List

On the basis of this careful analysis, a problem list is usually developed. Around such a list, realistic and relevant personal care may be planned. Every aspect of the patient's needs is considered. In a conference with the health care team, the patient, family, and any other significant persons, personal goals are determined for care. These goals help establish priorities for immediate as well as long-term care.

Nutritional Intervention: Food Plan and Management

Basic Concepts of Diet Therapy

Normal Nutrition Base

A therapeutic diet is always based on the normal nutritional requirements for a particular patient. It is modified only as the specific disease in the specific individual necessitates. In planning and counseling for nutritional care this is an important initial fact to grasp and impart to patients and clients. For example, it is a great source of encouragement to the parents of a newly diagnosed diabetic child to know that the food plan will be based on individual growth and development needs and will make use of regular foods.

Disease Application

The principles of a special therapeutic diet will be based on modifications of the nutritional components of the normal diet as a particular disease condition may require. These changes may include the following types of modifications: (1) modification of one or more of the basic nutrients—protein, carbohydrate, fat, minerals, and vitamins; (2) modification in energy value as expressed in kilocalories; (3) modification in texture or seasoning, such as liquid or low residue.

Individual Adaptation

A therapeutic diet may be theoretically correct and have well-balanced food plans, but if these plans are unacceptable to the patient, they will not be followed. A workable plan for a specific person must be based on individual food habits within the specific personal life situation. This can be achieved only through careful planning with the patient, or with the parents of a child requiring a special diet, based on an initial interview to obtain a diet history, knowledge of personal food habits, living conditions, and related factors. In this way, diet principles can be understood and motivation secured to follow through. Whatever the problems, nutritional care is valid only to the extent that it involves this kind of knowledge, skills, and insights. Individual adaptations of the diet to meet individual needs are imperative for successful therapy.

Routine House Diets

A schedule of routine "house" diets, based on some type of cycle menu plan, is usually followed in hospitals for those patients not requiring a special diet modification. According to general patient need and tolerance, the diet order may be liquid (clear liquid or full liquid, with milk used on the full liquid diet), soft (no raw foods, generally somewhat bland in seasoning), and regular (a full, normal-for-age diet). Occasionally an interval step between soft and regular may be used (a light diet). Sample menus from hospital staff dietitians may be compared to note differences.

Managing the Mode of Feeding

Depending on the patient's condition, the clinical nutritionist may manage the diet by using any one of four feeding modes.

1. **Enteral:** *oral diet.* As long as possible, of course, regular oral feeding is preferred. Supplements are added if needed. According to the patient's condition, there may also be need for assistance in eating.
2. **Enteral:** *tube feeding.* If a patient is unable to eat but the gastrointestinal tract can be used, tube feeding may provide needed nutritional support. A number of commercial formulas are available or a blended formula may be calculated and prepared.
3. **Parenteral:** *peripheral vein feeding.* If the patient cannot take in food or formula via the gastrointestinal tract, intravenous feeding will be needed.

Solutions of dextrose, amino acids, vitamins, and minerals, with intermittent lipid formula, can be fed through peripheral veins when the need is not extensive or long term.

4. **Parenteral:** *total parenteral nutrition (TPN).* If the patient's nutritional need is great and support therapy may be required for a longer time, feeding through a large central vein is needed. Placement of this tube is a special surgical procedure. More concentrated special solutions can be used and monitored by a nutrition support team. The formulas are determined by the nutritionist and the physician, prepared by trained pharmacists, and administered by specially trained nurses. This skilled nutritional support team is essential for successful therapy.

Details of these various modes of feeding are given in Chapter 18, as they apply to different conditions.

Evaluation: Quality Patient Care
General Considerations

When the nutritional care plan is carried out, patient care activities need to be considered in terms of the nutritional diagnosis and treatment objectives, and the extent to which each of the care activities helps to meet the particular goals of the patient and the family. This evaluation is both continuous and terminal and requires careful, objective documentation (see Clinical Application, p. 317). It seeks to validate care while it is being given as well as to determine the effectiveness of a particular course of care. Various areas need to be investigated:

- *Estimate the achievement of nutritional therapy goals:* What is the effect of the diet or mode of feeding on the illness or the patient's situation? Is there need for any change in the nutrient ratios of the diet or formula as originally calculated, in the meal distribution pattern, or in the feeding mode?
- *Judge the accuracy of intervention actions:* Is there need to change any of the nutritional care plan components? For example, is there need for a change in the type of food or feeding equipment, environment for meals, procedures for counseling, or types of learning activities for nutrition education and self-care procedures?
- *Determine patient's ability to follow prescribed nutritional therapy:* Are there any hindrances or disabilities that prevent the patient from following the treatment plan? What is the impact of the nutritional therapy on the patient, the family, or the staff? Were the necessary nutrition assessment procedures for collecting nutrition data carried out correctly? Do the patient and family understand the information given for self-care? Have the community resources required by the patient and family been available

Nutritional Assessment and Therapy for a Patient with Cancer

Esther Landau is a 160 cm (5 ft, 4 in) tall, medium frame, 43-year-old patient recovering from a *gastrectomy* performed 8 days ago to treat gastric cancer. Her weight has dropped gradually for the past 4 months from an average of 59 kg (130 lb) before her illness began. She continues to follow a full liquid diet, consuming 60 to 120 ml (2 to 4 oz) of milk every few hours, plus 1 or 2 soft-boiled eggs each day. Today she informed the nutritionist that she consumed a total of 721 ml (24 oz) of milk and 2 eggs.

In reviewing Mrs. Landau's records, the nutritionist found the following nutritional assessment data: weight 47.3 kg (103 lb); triceps skin fold, 10 mm; and midarm circumference, 17 cm. Laboratory values include serum albumin, 3.0 g/dl; total iron-binding capacity (TIBC), 230 μg/dl; lymphocytes, 1200 cells/m^3 (23%); hematocrit, 35%, and hemoglobin, 10.5 g/dl. Urinalysis (24 hours) included urea nitrogen, 16 g; and creatinine, 1.75 g. Skin tests were pending.

After reviewing the data, the nutritionist calculated nitrogen balance, transferrin, and creatinine-height index, which were recorded on the pa-

tient chart. Basal energy expenditure needs and kilocalories and protein needed to overcome catabolism were also calculated, along with estimates for additional vitamin and mineral requirements.

The clinical nutritionist noted that the physician had ordered chemotherapy for the patient, continuing after discharge, and recommended the use of TPN, also to be continued after discharge, as a means of meeting Mrs. Landau's nutritional needs. In addition, the nutritionist planned ways of meeting any feeding problems that often accompany chemotherapy, such as sore mouth, nausea, and food intolerances. Following a carefully prepared protocol developed by the hospital nutritional support team, both Mrs. Landau and her husband were instructed in procuring and using the home TPN treatment. The nutritionist also provided follow-up counseling for Mrs. Landau and her husband at the office and in the group sessions for cancer patients and their families.

Questions for analysis

1. Use a nutritional assessment data summary sheet from your hospital (or

design your own) to record pertinent data given in this case study. What additional data would you collect? How would it be obtained?

2. For each test listed on your data sheet, explain what it measures and how that information contributes to an understanding of Mrs. Landau's status.

3. What specific nutritional needs can you identify in this case? List them in order of priority.

4. Calculate Mrs. Landau's nitrogen balance and transferrin for day 8. Why are these indices important to assessing her nutritional status?

5. What is Mrs. Landau's creatinine-height index? How does it reflect her nutritional status?

6. Interpret Mrs. Landau's anthropometric data, including your calculations of her midarm muscle circumference.

7. What skin tests were probably ordered? How would the results contribute to the assessment of her nutritional status?

8. What nutritional problems do you expect Mrs. Landau to encounter after discharge? How could they be resolved? What community agencies might contribute to her sense of well-being after discharge? ◆

---

and convenient for use? Has any needed food assistance program been sufficient to meet needs for the patient's ongoing care?

Quality Patient Care
PSROs

Over the past two decades, since the establishment of Professional Standards Review Organizations (PSROs) in 1972, there has been an increased emphasis on setting practice standards and forming hospital patient care review committees to monitor the delivery of quality patient care.[21,22] In addition, at present an increased focus on cost control in managed health care reforms is leading to mechanisms for effectively evaluating patient care programs on the basis of (1) cost effectiveness and (2) provision of nutritional services by the most qualified personnel.[23]

Quality Care Models

Within clinical nutrition, standards for both professional and support level staff have been developed in a

number of medical care settings. These models of quality care have established specific standards for (1) identifying patients who require increased nutritional support or nutrition education, (2) determining patient care priorities and spelling out the degree of care required, and (3) defining role responsibilities for carrying out each part of the care plan. These models have been applied to specific patient care needs, such as a standard of practice for quality assurance in nutritional care for patients with cancer.

---

enteral • A mode of feeding that uses the gastrointestinal tract, oral or tube feeding.

parenteral • A mode of feeding that does not use the gastrointestinal tract, but instead provides nutrition by intravenous delivery of nutrient solutions.

DRGs

With increasing concerns about health care costs, a system of preset payment for hospitalized Medicare patients according to specific diagnosis-related groups (DRGs) was developed at Yale University and was based on designated major categories (MCDs). This prospective payment control plan was first applied to government funded Medicare patients, but in today's world of economic realities some form of this management scheme is fast becoming a part of practice for the majority of hospitalized patients, as well as those in home care and extended care facilities.[24] Such increasing inevitable emphasis on cost containment brings a new demand for accountability by all health care professionals and managers.

Collaborative Roles of the Nutritionist and Nurse

The clinical nutritionist or dietitian works closely with the nurse in managing the nutritional care of patients. At varying times, depending on need, the nurse may provide valuable nutrition assistance as coordinator, interpreter, or teacher. Skills in consultation and referral are therefore essential.

Coordinator

Nurses can coordinate special services or treatment required because of their close relationship to patients and their constant attendance. The nurse may help schedule activities to prevent conflicts or secure needed consultation for the patient with the dietitian, social worker, or other health team member. Sometimes hospital malnutrition exists simply because meals are constantly being interrupted by various procedures, staff interviews, or medical rounds.

Interpreter

Because of a close relationship with the patient, the nurse can help reduce tension by careful, brief, easily understood explanations concerning various treatments and plans of care. This will include basic interpretation of the therapeutic diet from the clinical nutritionist or the physician and of the resulting food selections on the tray. The nurse may sometimes assist the patient in making appropriate selections from the menus provided.

Teacher or Counselor

One of the nurse's most significant roles is that of health care educator and counselor. There will be innumerable informal opportunities during daily nursing care for planned conversation about sound nutrition principles, reinforcing the counseling of the clinical nutritionist. In addition, according to patient situations, the nurse may work with the clinical nutritionist during periods of instruction about principles of the patient's diet therapy in relation to the disease process. The nurse will work in close cooperation with the clinical nutritionist and the physician to coordinate nutritional and medical management of the patient's illness into overall nursing care. At all times the nurse will work closely with the hospital's clinical nutrition staff to support and reinforce primary nutrition education, as well as discharge planning for follow-up care.[25] These clinical staff nutrition experts will always be excellent resources for needed nutrition consultation and referral.

Clearly, learning about the hospitalized patient's nutritional needs is a continuing activity beginning with admission. It should follow through and include plans for continuing application in the home environment. Follow-up care may be provided by the hospital's clinic dietitian, by consultation with clinical nutritionists in community private practice, by public health nutritionists and nurses, or by referrals to community agencies and resources.

To Sum Up

The basis for an accurate assessment of the patient's nutritional needs begins with the individual patient and family. Physical as well as psychologic, social, economic, and cultural factors in and out of the clinical setting all play a role in evaluating the patient's health status and any possible problems with adherence to a nutritional care plan.

Nutritional assessment is based on a broad foundation of pertinent data, including food and drug uses and values. The effectiveness of an assessment based on analysis of these data depends in turn on effective communication with the patient, family members, and significant others in the development of an appropriate care plan, as well as with other members of the health care team. The patient's medical record is a basic means of communication among health care team members.

Nutritional therapy, based on a combination of the personal and physiologic needs of the patient, requires a close working relationship among nutrition, medical, and nursing staff in the health care facility. The nurse's schedule offers many opportunities to reinforce nutritional principles of the diet. Nutritional therapy doesn't end with the patient's discharge. Outpatient nutrition services, appropriate social services, and food resources in the community help meet continuing needs of patients and their families.

QUESTIONS FOR REVIEW

1. Identify and discuss the possible effects of various psychologic factors on the outcome of nutritional therapy.
2. Outline a general procedure for assessing the nutritional needs and building a care plan for a 65-year-old wid-

ower hospitalized with coronary heart disease (see Chapter 20 if necessary). Include community agencies the patient could be referred to for follow-up care, services, and information.
3. Describe six commonly used anthropometric procedures, five blood tests, and two urine tests commonly used for nutritional status information in terms of significance of the measure or test—what is being measured and what the results tell you.
4. Select six clinical signs used to assess nutritional status and describe what each sign shows in a malnourished person and why.
5. Describe the nature and purpose of quality assurance plans for standards of nutritional care.

REFERENCES

1. Rubin M: The physiology of bed rest, *Am J Nurs* 88(1):50, Jan 1988.
2. Kamath SK and others: Hospital malnutrition: a 33-hospital screening study, *J Am Diet Assoc* 86(2):203, Feb 1986.
3. Bone RC: Ethical principles in critical care, *JAMA* 263(5):696, 1990.
4. Monsen ER and others: Ethics: responsible scientific conduct, *Am J Clin Nutr* 54:1, 1991.
5. Anderson EG: Getting through to elderly patients, *Geriatrics* 46(5):74, 1991.
6. Gilbert J: Partnership: a new paradigm for health care, *Hospitals* 64:72, 1990.
7. Koska MT: Patient-centered care: can your hospital afford not to have it? *Hospitals* 64:48, 1990.
8. Thompson MP, Morris LK: Unexplained weight loss in the ambulatory elderly, *Am J Geriatr Soc* 39:497, 1991.
9. Kubena KS and others: Anthropometry and health in the elderly, *J Am Diet Assoc* 91(11):1402, 1991.
10. Himes JH, Bouchard C: Do the new Metropolitan Life Insurance weight-height tables correctly assess body frame and body fat relationships? *Am J Pub Health* 75(9):1076, 1985.
11. Frisancho AR: Nutritional anthropometry, *J Am Diet Assoc* 88(5):553, May 1988.
12. Nowak RK, Schultz LO: A comparison of two methods for the determination of body frame size, *J Am Diet Assoc* 87(3):339, March 1987.
13. Mitchell CO, Lipschitz DA: Arm length measurement as an alternative to height in nutritional assessment of the elderly, *J Parenteral Enteral Nutr* 6(3):226, March 1982.
14. Kwok T, Whitelaw MN: The use of armspan in nutritional assessment of the elderly, *J Am Geriatr Soc* 39:492, 1991.
15. Chumlea WC, Roche AF, Mukherjee D: *Nutritional assessment of the elderly through anthropometry*, Columbus, Ohio, 1987, Ross Laboratories.
16. Haboubi NY and others: Measurement of height in the elderly, *J Am Geriatr Soc* 38:1008, 1990.
17. Chumlea WC and others: Prediction of body weight for the nonambulatory elderly from anthropometry, *J Am Diet Assoc* 88(5):564, May 1988.
18. Graham AW: Screening for alcoholism by life-style risk assessment in a community hospital, *Arch Intern Med* 151:958, 1991.
19. Travato A and others: Drug-nutrient interactions, *Am Fam Physician* 44(5):1651, 1991.
20. Zulkifli SN, Yu SM: The food frequency method for dietary assessment, *J Am Diet Assoc* 92(6):686, 1992.
21. Herbelin K: Quality assessment and assurance in a long-term care facility: meeting current federal requirements, *J Am Diet Assoc* 89(10):1499, 1989.
22. Edelstein SF: Using thresholds to monitor dietetic services: the JCAHO 10-step process for quality assurance, *J Am Diet Assoc* 91(10):1261, 1991.
23. Splett P: Assessing effectiveness of nutrition care: prerequisite for cost-effectiveness analysis, *Top Clin Nutr* 5(2):26, 1990.
24. Sandall MJ, Massey LK: The impact of the diagnosis-related groups/prospective payment system on nutrition needs in home health and extended care facilities, *J Am Diet Assoc* 89(10):1444, 1989.
25. Weddle DO and others: Inpatient and post-discharge course of the malnourished patient, *J Am Diet Assoc* 91(3):307, 1991.

FURTHER READING

Clay G, Bouchard C, Hemphill K: A comprehensive nutrition case management system, *J Am Diet Assoc* 88(2):196, Feb 1988.

This article describes an excellent nutrition assessment and management system model featuring (1) decreased charting time, (2) precise documentation, (3) nutritional diagnosis tool for intervention therapy, (4) quality care standard, (5) computer adaptation, and (6) quality assurance audits.

Posner BM and others: Validation of two-dimensional models for estimation of portion size in nutrition research, *J Am Diet Assoc* 92(6):738, 1992.

This article describes nutrition assessment methods and tools with practical models for estimating food intake amounts.

Chumlea WC and others: *Nutrition assessment of the elderly through anthropometry*, Columbus, Ohio, 1987, Ross Laboratories.

Gussler JD, ed: Nutrition screening and assessment as components of hospital admission. In *Eighth Ross Roundtable on Medical Issues*, Columbus, Ohio, 1987, Ross Laboratories.

These two manuals continue to provide background for using alternate techniques and calculations for nutrition assessment and monitoring of nonambulatory hospitalized elderly patients.

Selecting Nutrient Calculation Computer Software

In our modern age of electronics, the computer has become a standard tool for rapid calculation procedures. In clinical and community nutrition practices as well as population studies, it saves valuable time and provides a precise nutrient analysis of an individual's reported food intake.

Certainly computerized nutrient analyses are time savers from the previous tedious manual calculations using published food value tables. But just how precise are the results? This depends on the heart of any nutrient analysis software program—its nutrient database.

Over the past few years of computer use by clinicians, researchers, and educators, it has become increasingly evident that the quality of the nutrient database on which all calculations are based determines the quality of the resulting output. Experts in this field at the University of Minnesota's Nutrition Coordinating Center have provided important questions that may be used in evaluating the nutrient database in any software package being considered for purchase.

Does the database contain all foods and nutrients of interest?

Most databases contain the most common foods, but you may require particular foods such as ethnic, vegetarian, or fast-food items, brand name products, and infant or nontraditional foods. The number of food items in a database does not necessarily indicate how comprehensive the system is. And adding your own foods to the database requires considerable effort.

Is the database complete for nutrients of interest?

Missing values are common in available software packages and often are not flagged, so you may be unaware of this source of error. Inappropriate patient counseling may result. Such missing value errors in small items such as spices or other condiments may not matter, but a missing value for total saturated fatty acids in a fast-food hamburger because the food manufacturers have not supplied it is not acceptable.

Do foods included in the database provide sufficient specific data to accurately assess nutrients of interest?

For example, if total fat and fatty acids are of concern, separate database entries must be included for such items as regular, low-fat, and nonfat dairy products and brand name high-fat items such as margarines and salad dressings. In other cases inclusion of food items according to preparation method, or of any dietary supplements for vitamin-mineral calculations, may be required.Is the nutrient database current with the changing marketplace and availability of new nutrient data?

The USDA routinely releases updates of the *Agricultural Handbook No. 8,* the common source of data for nutrient calculation systems, as new information is available. Information from food manufacturers is also available. A well-maintained software product's database should include all such data updates, and the vendor should supply information about frequency of updating and sources of data.

Are manufacturers contacted routinely for new information or reformulations of existing products?

This question extends the previous question to emphasize the still too frequent neglect of brand-name product updating practices of software developers. Routine contact with food manufacturers is essential to maintaining an acceptable quality standard.

What quality control procedures are used to ensure database accuracy?

Because there are thousands of values for nutrients and seemingly endless amounts of nonnutrient information, for example, food-specific serving sizes, the margin for error is great and built-in maintenance procedures for checking such errors should be present.

Vendors of nutrient calculation software packages should be able to give answers to these important questions. Ask before you buy!

REFERENCES

Buzzard IM and others: Considerations for selecting nutrient-calculation software: evaluation of the nutrient database, *Am J Clin Nutr* 54:7, 1991.

Schakel SF and others: Sources of data for developing and maintaining a nutrient database, *J Am Diet Assoc* 88:1268, 1988.

CHAPTER 17

Drug-Nutrient Interactions

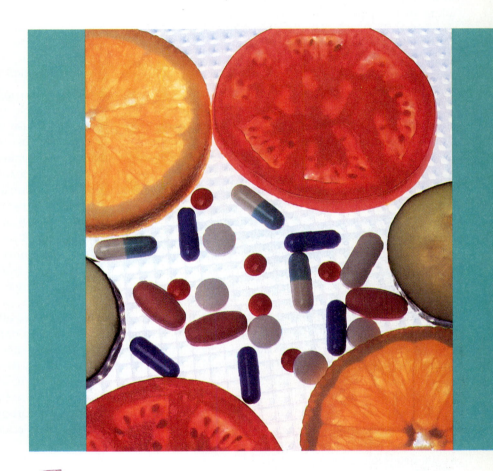

In this chapter, continuing our clinical nutrition sequence, we look briefly at some main effects of combining food and nutrients with drugs. We will see how these interactions affect nutritional therapy.

Today consumers are generally better informed about drug misuse. However, many are dangerously uninformed or misinformed about the specific drugs they may be taking, especially in relation to the food they eat.

All members of the health care team must have a basic knowledge of drug actions and nutrition to make the wisest and most effective use of drugs and nutritional therapy. Here we examine some of these drug-nutrient effects and how these interactions affect our nutritional therapy and education.

Drug-Nutrient Problems in Modern Medicine

Problem Significance: Causes, Extent, Effects

Increasing complexity and specialization mark our modern medical world. Every specialty field easily becomes isolated from many other interacting factors in the care of clients and patients that fall outside its primary area of expertise. These medical specialists who prescribe medications, pharmacists who fill these prescriptions, or nurses who administer them may not be fully aware of the impact of a particular drug in an individual patient's nutritional state. They are often unaware of the patient's diet and how it may influence the drug's effects. Similarly, a clinical dietitian may provide a diet description and food plan and not be fully aware of the client's medication program and its implications for sound nutritional care (see Clinical Application, p. 323).

Today consumers are generally better informed about misuse of drugs, both prescription and over-the-counter nonprescription ones. However, in our overmedicated society, many persons are often dangerously uninformed or misinformed about the specific drugs they may be taking, especially in relation to the food they eat.

The field of nutrient-drug interaction is indeed complex and confusing. We face a drug-oriented medical environment and a bewildering array of drug items. Every year American physicians prescribe and pharmacists dispense a total amount of drugs sufficient to provide seven individual medications for each woman, man, and child in the United States. To this amount we can then add the large volume of nonprescription drugs that Americans purchase over the counter. Some concerned persons have come to view our overmedicated society with alarm. Knowledgeable and concerned pharmacologists indicate that outside of extremely serious illness, most general medical problems can be treated with less than 25 drugs. The World Health Organization (WHO) has estimated that only some 150 to 200 drugs are actually needed to take care of almost all ordinary illnesses around the world. Yet on our American market there are about 54,000 drugs, many of them only slight variations of other drugs, the so-called me too drugs.

Drug Use and Nutritional Status

Elderly Persons at Risk

All of us, at any age, risk harmful drug or drug-nutrient interactions. However, elderly persons are particularly vulnerable.[1-3] Several things contribute to this increased risk among the elderly:

- They are likely to be taking more drugs for longer periods of time to control chronic diseases.
- Their drugs are likely to be more toxic.
- They respond to drugs with greater variability.
- They have less capability to handle drugs efficiently.
- Their nutritional status is more likely to be deficient.
- They are more likely to make increased errors in self-care because of illness, mental confusion, or lack of drug information.

As a result of these problems, concerned physicians, nutritionists, pharmacists, and nurses are increasingly working together as a team to provide drug and nutritional education and therapy on a sounder basis. A number of drug-nutrient interactions demand this type of teamwork in patient care. To meet this need, team process guides have been developed for various conditions.[4,5]

General Hospital Malnutrition

Studies of hospital malnutrition have revealed a number of possible mechanisms of nutrient-drug interaction that cause nutrition problems. Results of these studies give us information on contributing causes to this general malnutrition. Such causes are especially prevalent in hospitalized patients and require informed therapy.[6,7] Nutrient-drug mechanisms that influence nutrition status include those affecting the following:

- Decreased intestinal absorption
- Increased renal excretion
- Competition or displacement of nutrients for carrier protein sites
- Interference with synthesis of necessary enzyme, coenzyme, or carrier
- Hormonal effects on genetic systems
- The drug delivery system
- Components in drug formulation

In general, drugs are usually grouped according to primary action. Here we review briefly various effects of drugs on food and nutrients and effects of food and nutrients on drugs. In each case we give some examples for your reference in patient care.

Drug Effects on Food and Nutrients

Drug Effects on Food Intake

Increased Appetite

The following drugs have an effect of increasing the appetite.[1,8,9]

Antihistamines.   These drugs can lead to marked increase in appetite and subsequent weight gain. One of these agents, both an antihistamine and a serotonin antagonist, is cyproheptadine hydrochloride (Periactin).

Psychotropic drugs.   Some of the tranquilizers may lead to hyperphagia, or excessive eating (see Issues and Answers, p. 332). Those which lead to weight gain when

◆ **C**LINICAL **A**PPLICATION   *The Proof of the Pudding. . .*

The senses of taste and smell greatly affect our responses to various foods. The loss of these senses may drive persons to constantly seek elusive satisfaction by overeating, or it may stop them from eating entirely. In either case the pleasure of eating has gone and nutritional status suffers. Patients taking drugs that affect taste and smell need counseling concerning food choices, combinations, and seasonings that can help overcome this difficulty.

Some drugs affecting taste and smell include the following:

Anesthetics, local—benzocaine, cocaine, procaine

Antibiotics—amphotericin B, ampicillin, griseofulvin, lincomycin, streptomycin, tetracyclines

Anticoagulant—phenindione

Antihistamine—chlorpheniramine maleate

Antihypertensive agents—captopril, diazoxide, ethacrynic acid

Antiinfectious agent—metronidazole

Cholesterol-lowering agent—clofibrate

Hypoglycemic agent—glipizide

Psychoactive agents—carbamazepine, lithium carbonate, phenytoin, amphetamines

Toothpaste ingredient—sodium lauryl sulfate

Indeed, the proof of the pudding—our food—is in the taste, which is easily affected by a variety of drugs, resulting in diminished appetite and necessary food intake. Patients taking these drugs benefit from counseling about these taste effects, along with other effects, and ways of counteracting them in food selection, seasoning, and serving.

REFERENCES

Roe DA: *Diet and drug interactions,* ed 2, New York, 1989, AVI Books.

Powers D, Moore A: *Food-medication interactions,* ed 6, Phoenix, Ariz, 1988, Food-Medication Interactions.

Trovato A and others: Drug-nutrient interactions, *Am Fam Physician* 44(5):1651, 1991. ◆

---

given to psychotic patients may have the opposite effect on geriatric patients. Some of these drugs include chlordiazepoxide hydrochloride (Librium), diazepam (Valium), chlorpromazine hydrochloride (Thorazine), and meprobamate (Equanil). As with the tranquilizers, tricyclic antipressants such as amitriptyline hydrochloride (Elavil) may promote appetite and lead to significant weight gain.

Steroids. Anabolic steroids, including testosterone, promote nitrogen retention, increased lean body mass, and subsequent weight gain. Some athletes and body builders form habits of drug abuse with steroids to obtain these characteristic effects, but harm their bodies in the process.

Decreased Appetite

The following drugs have the effect of depressing the appetite.[1,8,9]

Amphetamines. These drugs act as stimulants to the central nervous system and have the effect of depressing the desire for food, thus leading to marked loss of weight. For this reason they have been used in the past as appetite-depressant drugs in the treatment of obesity. However, long-term use of these drugs in such treatment has caused problems, including addiction, since in most cases appetite itself is not the primary cause of the excess weight. For this reason, amphetamines are rarely used now for this purpose. Children taking amphetamines show dose-dependent growth retardation.

Insulin. A rapid drop in blood sugar, hypoglycemia, can be induced by insulin. This effect is not marked by hunger but often causes nausea, weakness, and aversion to foods. The hypoglycemic reaction is distinct from the effect of general insulin use in the management of diabetes, which may bring a feeling of hunger as nutrient metabolism is improved.

Alcohol. Abuse of alcohol can lead to loss of appetite, reduced food intake, and malnutrition. Alcoholism requires health risk screening and significant nutritional support in rehabilitation efforts.[10,11] The anorexia, or loss of appetite, can stem from various effects of alcoholism, such as gastritis, lactose intolerance, hepatitis, cirrhosis, ketosis, pancreatitis, alcoholic brain syndrome, drunkenness, and withdrawal symptoms. The resulting reduced food intake can then lead to malnutrition, which further complicates the anorexia by causing deficiencies of thiamin, zinc, or protein.

Taste Changes

A loss of taste, or dysgeusia, may be caused by a number of drugs. For example, the chelating agent D-penicillamine is used in the treatment of conditions such as heavy metal poisoning, rheumatoid arthritis, and cystinuria. The side effect of taste loss occurs as the agent also binds zinc and causes a drug-induced zinc deficiency. Other drugs affecting taste acuity include diuretics and anticancer agents such as methotrexate and doxorubicin hydrochloride (Adriamycin), as well as agents used to treat Parkinson's disease. Even a 1-g dose of aspirin increases perception of a bitter taste. Sodium lauryl sulfate, a substance often used in toothpaste to make it clean teeth better, can make orange juice taste bitter. A number of other drugs can also affect taste and smell. Thus, when any of these drugs are used, discussion of these sensory effects with the patient and use of food seasonings to enhance taste and smell is useful.

Nausea

Many drugs have the effect of decreasing appetite because they contribute to nausea and vomiting. For example, cardiac glycosides, digitalis, and related drugs can produce nausea if used in relatively large amounts. A number of drugs used in cancer chemotherapy (see Chapter 25) have similar effects and can contribute to malnutrition and weight loss.

Bulking Effects

Various agents, such as methyl cellulose and other dietary fiber products, can interfere with absorption of nutrients and contribute to their loss.[12] These bulking agents can also contribute to decreased intake of food by creating a sense of fullness and lack of desire for food intake. For this reason they have sometimes been used as adjunct therapy in weight management.

Drug Effects on Nutrient Absorption and Metabolism

Increased Absorption

A number of drugs can increase nutrient absorption and thus benefit nutritional status. For example, cimetidine (Tagamet), a gastric antisecretory agent, helps patients with bowel resection. The drug reduces gastric acid and volume output; lowers duodenal acid load and volume; reduces jejunal flow; maintains pH of secretions; decreases fecal fat, nitrogen, and volume; and thus improves absorption of protein and carbohydrates. This drug is therefore helpful in the treatment of various gastrointestinal disorders including peptic ulcer disease (see Chapter 19).

Decreased Absorption

A number of drugs contribute to primary malabsorption. Colchicine, for example, a drug used in the treatment of gout, leads to vitamin B_{12} deficiency, causing megaloblastic anemia. Alcohol abuse provokes malabsorption of thiamin and folic acid, causing peripheral neuritis and anemia. Laxatives produce severe malabsorption, leading to conditions such as osteomalacia. Secondary malabsorption may also be drug induced. Some drugs inhibit vitamin D absorption, leading to malabsorption and consequent deficiency of calcium. For example, the antibiotic neomycin causes tissue changes in the intestinal villi, precipitates bile salts, prevents fat breakdown by inhibiting pancreatic lipase, and decreases bile acid absorption. These effects lead to ste-

atorrhea and failure to absorb the fat-soluble vitamins A, D, E, and K. Malabsorption of vitamin D in turn leads to a calcium deficiency. Other drugs cause malabsorption of folic acid or impair its utilization causing malabsorption of still other nutrients. Methotrexate, for example, used in cancer chemotherapy, is a folic acid antagonist that impairs the intestinal absorption of calcium.

Summaries of the drugs causing primary and secondary nutrient malabsorption are given in Tables 17-1 and 17-2.

Mineral Depletion

Certain drugs can lead to mineral depletion through induced gastrointestinal losses or renal excretion.[13]

Diuretics. Diuretic drugs are intentionally used to reduce levels of excess tissue water and sodium. But they may also result in loss of other minerals, such as potassium, magnesium, and zinc. Potassium deficiency brings weakness, anorexia, nausea, vomiting, listlessness, apprehension, and sometimes diffuse pain, drowsiness, stupor, and irrational behavior. On the contrary, potassium-retaining diuretics, such as spironolactone, as well as overuse of potassium supplementation cause the opposite effect of hyperkalemia.

Chelating agents. Penicillamine attaches to metals and leads to deficiency of such key trace elements as zinc and copper.

Alcohol. The abuse of alcohol can lead to diminished levels of potassium, magnesium, and zinc.

Antacids. These commonly used over-the-counter medications are of concern because they can produce phosphate deficiency, with symptoms of anorexia, malaise, **paresthesia,** profound muscle weakness, and convulsions as well as calcification of soft tissues from the prolonged hypercalcemia.

Aspirin. Salicylates such as aspirin (acetylsalicylic acid—ASA) can induce iron deficiency by causing low-level blood loss from erosions in the stomach or intestinal tissue when taken incorrectly (see To Probe Further, p. 326).

Vitamin Depletion

Certain drugs act as metabolic antagonists and cause deficiencies of the vitamins involved.

Vitamin antagonists. Various drugs have been used successfully to treat disease because they are antagonists of certain vitamins and thus can control key metabolic reactions in which that vitamin is involved. For example, coumarin anticoagulants inhibit regeneration

TABLE 17-1

Drugs Causing Primary Nutrient Malabsorption

Drug	Use	Nutrients lost	Action
Cholestyramine	Holds bile acid; hypocholesterolemic agent	Fat; fat-soluble vitamins A, D, and K; vitamin B_{12}; iron	Binding agent for bile salts and nutrients
Colchicine	Antigout agent	Fat; vitamin B_{12}; provitamin A (carotene); lactose; sodium, potassium	Enzyme damage; inhibits cell division; structural defect
Methyldopa	Antihypertensive agent	Vitamin B_{12}, folic acid; iron	Unclear; possible autoimmune action
Mineral oil	Laxative	Fat-soluble vitamins A, D, and K; provitamin A (carotene)	Nutrients dissolve in oil and are lost in feces
Neomycin	Antibiotic	Fat; vitamin B_{12}; nitrogen; lactose, sucrose; sodium, potassium, iron, calcium	Binds bile salts; lowers pancreatic lipase; structural defect
Para-aminosalicylic acid	Antituberculosis agent	Fat; folic acid, vitamin B_{12}	Blocks mucosal uptake of vitamin B_{12}
Phenolphthalein	Laxative	Calcium, potassium; vitamin D	Rapid intestinal transit; loss of structural tissue integrity
Potassium chloride	Potassium replacement	Vitamin B_{12}	Lowered ileal pH
Salicylazosulfapyridine (Azulfidine)	Antiinflammatory agent (ulcerative colitis)	Folic acid	Blocks mucosal uptake of folic acid

Adapted from Roe DA: Interactions between drugs and nutrients, *Med Clin North Am* 63:985, 1979; and Roe DA: *Diet and drug interactions*, ed 2, New York, 1989, AVI Books.

TABLE 17-2

Drugs Causing Secondary Malabsorption of Calcium

Drug	Use	Action
Phenytoin, phenobarbital, primidone	Anticonvulsant agents	Accelerated vitamin D metabolism
Diphosphonates	Paget's disease (increased bone resorption and deformity)	Vitamin D hormone ($[1,25[OH]_2D_2]$) formation decreased
Glucocorticoids, such as prednisone	Collagen disease; allergies	Calcium transport decreased
Glutehimide	Sedative	Impaired calcium transport
Methotrexate	Leukemia	Folic acid antagonist—acute deficiency of the vitamin

Adapted from Roe DA: Interactions between drugs and nutrients, *Med Clin North Am* 63:985, 1979; and Roe DA: *Diet and drug interactions*, ed 2, New York, 1989, AVI Books.

of vitamin K, which is necessary for blood clotting. Also, some cancer chemotherapy drugs such as methotrexate have multiple antagonist effects on folate metabolism, thus inhibiting the synthesis of cell reproduction substances—deoxyribonucleic acid and ribonucleic acid (DNA and RNA)—and protein. In a similar manner, the antimalaria drug pyrimethamine inhibits the action of folate in protein synthesis. A list of vitamin antagonist drugs is given in Table 17-3.

Hypovitaminosis from use of oral contraceptives. Some women using oral contraceptive agents (OCA) have developed subclinical deficiencies of the vitamins folate, riboflavin, pyridoxine (B_6), cobalamin (B_{12}), and ascorbic acid (C). OCAs induce a greater demand for these vitamins. Table 17-4 includes a list of some of these effects on nutritional status.

Special Adverse Reactions

Several reactions are related to specific drug interactions with particular nutrients.

Monoamine oxidase inhibitors (MAOIs). These antidepressant drugs increase the vascular effect of simple **vasoactive** amines, such as tyramine and dopamine, from food.[15,16] The resulting tyramine syndrome is marked by headache, pallor, nausea, and restlessness. With increased absorption, symptoms may escalate to apprehension, sweating, palpitations, chest pain, fever, and increased blood pressure, at times, though rarely, to the extent of hypertensive crisis and stroke. A low tyramine food list (see Chapter 25) is provided for use by any patient taking one of these antidepressant drugs.

---

paresthesia • Abnormal sensations such as prickling, burning, and crawling of skin.

vasoactive • Having an effect on the diameter of blood vessels.

The Pain Reliever Doctors Recommend Most

TO PROBE FURTHER

Aspirin has a venerable history. Being a buffered form of salicylic acid, it is a modified version of an ancient folk remedy, willow bark, used for many hundreds of years for fever, aches, and pain. The acetyl group in acetylsalicylic acid makes aspirin easier on the stomach than willow bark.

Aspirin is an analgesic agent, an effect enhanced in combination with caffeine, that is used for relief of minor aches and pains. Its mechanism of action is through inhibition of certain *prostaglandins* (see Chapter 3), which have a profound influence on a spectrum of physiologic functions, including blood clotting, blood pressure, the inflammatory process, contraction of voluntary muscles, and transmission of nerve impulses.

Studies implicate aspirin in alleviating many disorders, dangers, and discomforts, including the following:

- The risk of repeated *transient ischemic attacks (TIAs),* little strokes, is reduced by 50% in men (but not women) who have already had one.
- Many studies indicate that aspirin is effective in reducing risk for *myocardial infarction,* a heart attack.
- Aspirin is one of the most effective antiinflammatory drugs and is effective in the long-term treatment of *arthritis.*
- Aspirin may play a role in inhibiting the spread of some *cancers* through its action of inhibiting production of prostaglandin E_2.
- Aspirin's effect as an anticoagulant is important in the treatment of *phlebitis* and other clot-related disorders.
- Aspirin may be effective in promoting *sleep.* Many scientists now believe aspirin is as effective as most prescription sedatives, and it has far fewer and less serious side effects.
- Diabetic patients who take aspirin may have a lower risk of developing *retinopathy.*

It is important to remember that aspirin is a drug. Many of the benefits of aspirin stem from its systemic, wide-reaching effects on metabolism, which may have unforeseen short- and long-term detrimental results. We do know that aspirin is to be strictly avoided by persons with hemophilia. Also, allergic reactions to aspirin can be severe. Aspirin seems to be implicated in asthma. Children are especially vulnerable to side effects and should not be given aspirin without a physician's instructions.

Aspirin is an irritant to the stomach and intestine. Its continuous use is associated with low-level chronic loss of iron caused by mucosal erosion. This can lead to iron-deficiency anemia.

Aspirin has been linked to birth defects, especially when it is taken later in the course of pregnancy. It increases risk of infant and neonatal mortality, low birth weight, and intracranial hemorrhage.

The best way to take aspirin is on an empty stomach with a full glass of water. This is important: the absorption of aspirin is facilitated by a large volume of liquid and inhibited by the presence of food. In addition, taking aspirin—especially on an empty stomach—without a large fluid intake invites erosion of the stomach lining. But aspirin should never be taken when using alcohol because it increases the bioavailability of alcohol, raises the blood concentration, and thus the effect of alcohol on brain centers.

REFERENCES

Griffith HW: *Complete guide to prescription and non-prescription drugs,* ed 5, Los Angeles, 1988, The Body Press, Price Stern Sloan.

Koch PA and others: Influence of food and fluid ingestion on aspirin bioavailability, *J Pharm Sci* 67(11):1533, 1978.

Roine R and others: Aspirin increases blood alcohol concentrations in humans after ingestion of ethanol, *JAMA* 264(18):2406, 1990.

Schachtel BP and others: Caffeine as an aspirin adjuvant, *Arch Intern Med* 151:733, 1991.

Flushing reaction. A number of drugs react with alcohol to produce a **flushing reaction** along with **dyspnea** and headache (Table 17-5). Central nervous system depressants, including hypnotic sedatives, antihistamines, phenothiazines, and narcotic analgesics, may cause a loss of consciousness if taken in combination with alcohol. Extreme caution must be exercised with these medications, and patients should be alerted to the dangers of mixing them with alcohol.

Hypoglycemia. Drugs such as chlorpropamide (Diabinese) and similar oral medications used to control non–insulin–dependent diabetes mellitus (NIDDM) (see Chapter 21) are hypoglycemic agents. They precipitate a rapid release of insulin, which may provoke a hypoglycemic reaction. This response of a rapidly reduced blood glucose level is especially strong when the drugs are used with alcohol. The symptoms of hypoglycemia include weakness, mental confusion, and irrational behavior. If not treated, loss of consciousness can follow.

Disulfiram reaction. The drug **disulfiram,** commonly called Antabuse, is used in the treatment of alcoholism. It combats alcohol consumption by producing extremely unpleasant side effects when taken with alcohol. Within 15 minutes flushing ensues, followed by headache, nausea, vomiting, and chest or abdominal pain. Other drugs, including aldehyde dehydrogenase inhibitors, may have this similar disulfiram effect.

TABLE 17-3

Examples of Drugs That Act as Vitamin Antagonists

Target vitamin	Drugs
Vitamin K	Coumarin anticoagulants
Folic acid	Methotrexate
	Pyrimethamine
	Triamterene
	Trimethoprim
Vitamin B$_6$	Cycloserine
	Hydralazine
	Isoniazid
	Levodopa

Adapted from Roe DA: Interactions between drugs and nutrients, *Med Clin North Am* 63:985, 1979; and Roe DA: *Diet and drug interactions,* ed 2, New York, 1989, AVI Books.

disulfiram • White to off-white crystalline antioxidant; inhibits oxidation of the acetaldehyde metabolized from alcohol. It is used in the treatment of alcoholism, producing extremely uncomfortable symptoms when alcohol is ingested following oral administration of the drug.

dyspnea • Labored, difficult breathing.

flushing reaction • Short-term reaction resulting in redness of neck and face.

TABLE 17-4

Interactions Between Oral Contraceptive Agents (OCA) and Vitamins and Minerals Affecting Nutritional Status

Nutrient affected by OCA	Effect	Clinical result
Vitamins		
Retinol (vitamin A)	Impairs liver storage; increases plasma binding	Unclear
Pyridoxine (vitamin B$_6$)	Alters metabolism of tryptophan and vitamin B$_6$	Abnormal protein metabolism; mood changes
Cobalamin (vitamin B$_{12}$)	Reduces vitamin B$_{12}$ serum levels	Unclear
Folic acid	Reduces red cell concentration; increases folate-binding protein	Megaloblastic anemia
Minerals		
Copper	Increases plasma levels of ceruloplasmin	Unclear
Iron	Increases serum levels of transferrin	Unclear
Zinc	Reduces serum levels of zinc	Unclear

Data adapted from Butterworth CE Jr, Weinsier RL: *Malnutrition in hospital patients: assessment and treatment.* In Goodhart RS, Shilis ME, eds: *Modern nutrition in health and disease,* ed 6, Philadelphia, 1980, Lea & Febiger.

TABLE 17-5

Adverse Drug Reactions Caused by Alcohol and Specific Foods

Type of reaction	Drugs	Alcohol/foods	Effects
Flushing	Chlorpropamide (diabetes) Griseofulvin Tetrachlorethylene	Alcohol	Dyspnea, headache, flushing
Disulfiram reaction	Aldehyde dehydrogenase inhibitors: Disulfiram (Antabuse) Calcium carbimide Metronidazole Nitrofurantoin Sulfonylureas	Alcohol Foods containing alcohol	Abdominal and chest pain, flushing, headache, nausea and vomiting
Hypoglycemia	Insulin-releasing agents: Oral hypoglycemic drugs	Alcohol Sugar, sweets	Mental confusion, weakness, irrational behavior, unconsciousness
Tyramine reaction	Monoamine oxidase inhibitors (MAOIs): Antidepressants such as phenelzine Procarbazine Isoniazid (isonicotinic acid hydrazide)	Foods containing large amounts of tyramine: Cheese Red wines Chicken liver Broad beans Yeast	Cerebrovascular accident (CVA), flushing, hypertension

Adapted from Roe DA: Interactions between drugs and nutrients, *Med Clin North Am* 63:985, 1979; and Roe DA: *Diet and drug interactions,* ed 2, New York, 1989, AVI Books.

Food and Nutrient Effects on Drugs

Food Factors Affecting Drug Absorption

The absorption of drugs is a complex matter. Food can affect eventual drug absorption in a number of ways.

Solution

Before an orally administered tablet or capsule can dissolve, it must first disintegrate. The drug's absorption, either from solution in acid gastric secretions or in the more alkaline medium of the intestine, may be more or less complete depending on its degree of solubility. The drug then passes through the intestinal mucosa and liver circulation before entering systemic circulation. Here it may be subject to metabolism, deactivation, and elimination through the so-called first-pass mechanism. Food may affect eventual drug absorption at any of these points.

Stomach Emptying Rate

The composition of the diet affects the rate at which the food enters the small intestine from the stomach. Delayed emptying of food from the stomach has the effect of doling out small portions of a drug, creating more optimal saturation rates on the absorptive sites in the small intestine. Fats, high temperatures, and solid meals prolong the time the food stays in the stomach. Food usually increases secretion of bile, acid, and gut enzymes. It also enhances intestinal motility and splanchnic blood flow. Drugs may adsorb to certain food particles.

Clinical Significance

Whether these effects have clinical significance depends on the extent of the effect and the nature of the drug. A small change in absorption is critical for a drug with a steep dose-response curve but perhaps unnoticeable for a drug with a wide range of effective concentrations. In general, the amount of absorption is clinically more important than the rate, since it has more impact on the steady-state plasma concentration of the drug after multiple doses. Table 17-6 gives some examples of drugs that are better utilized when taken without food and those which should be taken with food.

Food Effects on Drug Absorption

Increased Drug Absorption

Various circumstances contribute to the increased absorption of a drug.

Dissolving characteristics. When a drug does not dissolve rapidly after it has been taken, the time it remains in the stomach with food is prolonged. This increased time in the stomach may increase its effective dissolution and consequent absorption.

TABLE 17-6	
Food Effect on Drug Absorption	
Absorption reduced by food	**Absorption delayed by food**
Amoxicillin	Acetaminophen
Ampicillin	Amoxicillin
Aspirin	Aspirin
Demethylchlortetracycline	Cephalexin
Doxycycline	Cephradine
Isoniazid	Digoxin
Levodopa	Furosemide
Methacycline	Sulfadiazine
Oxytetracycline	Sulfamethoxazole
Penicillin G, V(K)	Sulfamethoxypyridazine
Phenethicillin	Sulfanilamide
Phenobarbital	Sulfisoxazole
Propantheline	
Rifampin	
Tetracycline	

Adapted from Roe DA: Interactions between drugs and nutrients, *Med Clin North Am* 63:985, 1979; and Roe DA: *Diet and drug interactions,* ed 2, New York, 1989, AVI Books.

Gastric emptying time. Delayed emptying of food from the stomach can have the effect of doling out small portions of a drug, creating more optimal saturation rates on the absorption sites in the small intestine.

Nutrients. Some nutrients promote absorption of certain drugs. For example, high-fat diets increase absorption of the antifungal drug griseofulvin. This drug is fat soluble, and high-fat diets stimulate the secretion of bile acids, which aid in absorption of the drug. Vitamin C, as well as gastric acid, enhances iron absorption. Also, citrus juices increase absorption of the antihypertensive drug nifedipine, as do meals with hydralazine.[17,18]

Blood flow. Food intake increases splanchnic blood flow, the circulation to the abdominal visceral organs. This increased circulation stimulates absorption.

Nutritional status. In addition to the presence of specific nutrients, nutritional status may also affect bioavailability of certain drugs in different ways. For example, the antibiotic chloramphenicol is absorbed more slowly in children with protein-energy malnutrition, but elimination of the drug is slower in well-nourished children. In both cases the effect is a net increased bioavailability of the drug.

Decreased Drug Absorption

The absorption of some drugs is delayed or reduced by the presence of food.

Aspirin. The absorption of aspirin is reduced or delayed by food, so it should be taken on an empty stomach with ample water, preferably cold (see To Probe Further, p. 326). Because aspirin increases the effect of alcohol, however, it should not be taken with alcohol.[19] In addition, caffeine enhances the analgesic effect of aspirin.[20]

Tetracycline. Nutritional status may also have an impact on drug absorption. For example, tetracycline absorption is impaired in malnourished individuals. Absorption of this commonly used antibiotic is also hindered when it is taken with milk, as well as with antacids or iron supplements. The drug combines with these materials to form new insoluble compounds that the body cannot absorb, causing loss of the minerals involved, calcium or iron.[15,16]

Phenytoin. The presence of protein inhibits the absorption of phenytoin. Carbohydrate increases its absorption, but fat has no impact.

Food Effects on Drug Distribution and Metabolism
Carbohydrate and Fat

Dietary carbohydrate and fat, especially their relative quantities, influence liver enzymes that metabolize drugs. For example, the presence of fat increases the activity of diazepam (Valium). Fat increases the concentration of the unbound active drug by displacing it from binding sites in plasma and tissue protein.

Licorice

Licorice, a sweet-tasting plant extract used in making chewing tobacco, candy, and certain drugs, causes sodium retention and increased hypertension.[21,22] A person being treated for hypertension needs to avoid any licorice-containing product. The active ingredient in licorice is glycyrrhizic acid from the name of its natural plant source, *Glycyrrhiza glabra*, meaning "sweet root," a member of the legume family. An analog of this active part of licorice is marketed under the trade names Biogastrone and Duogastrone, which are widely used, especially in Europe, for healing gastric ulcers, but hypertension is a side effect.

Indoles

The **indoles** in **cruciferous** vegetables (cabbage, Brussels sprouts, broccoli, cauliflower) can speed up the rate of drug metabolism. They apparently induce mixed-function oxidase enzyme systems in the liver.

Cooking Methods

The method of cooking foods may alter the rate of drug metabolism. Charcoal broiling, for example, increases hepatic drug metabolism through enzyme induction.

Changes in Intestinal Microflora

Changes in intestinal microflora related to the amount of dietary protein or fiber, for example, may influence intestinal drug metabolism.

Vitamin Effects on Drug Action
Drug Effectiveness

Pharmacologic doses, large megadoses beyond nutritional need, of vitamins decrease blood levels of drugs when vitamins interact with the drugs. For example, large doses of folate or pyridoxine can reduce the blood level and effectiveness of such anticonvulsive drugs as phenytoin (Dilantin) or phenobarbital, which are used for seizure control. Unwise self-medication with large doses of vitamins can cause severe toxic complications. On the other hand, vitamins themselves may become important medications when used as part of the medical treatment for a secondary deficiency induced by a childhood genetic or metabolic disease. Such is the case with biotin in treating certain organic acidemias, or riboflavin in treating certain defects in fatty acid metabolism.

Control of Drug Intoxication

Riboflavin is useful in treating boric acid poisoning. Boric acid combines with the ribityl side chain of riboflavin and is excreted in the urine. Also, vitamin E combats pulmonary oxygen toxicity. Premature human infants at risk for development of bronchopulmonary dysplasia by oxygen treatment have been protected by vitamin E administration during the acute phase of respiratory distress requiring oxygen treatment.

Nutrition-Pharmacy Team
Decades of Change

A decade or so ago hospitalized patients as a whole were less severely ill than they are today. Now, however, reflecting our more complex medical system and economic reform efforts, patients that are hospitalized are more acutely ill. They are more at risk for nutritional deficits and more likely to develop malnutrition, which leads to increased lengths of stay and higher costs. In

---

cruciferous • Bearing a cross; botanical term for plants belonging to the botanical family *Cruciferae* or *Brassicaceae*, the mustard family, so-called because of crosslike, four-petaled flowers; name given to certain vegetables of this family, such as broccoli, cabbage, Brussels sprouts, and cauliflower.

indole • A compound produced in the intestines by the decomposition of tryptophan; also found in the oil of jasmine and clove.

the 1960s and 1970s hospitals were beginning to develop multidisciplinary nutrition support committees to administer special enteral and parenteral feeding plans for more seriously ill persons. This was a form of nutritional care that required key roles of the clinical pharmacist and the clinical dietitian.[23] At the same time, the body of scientific knowledge advanced and more drugs were developed to match the advance. Thus the task of monitoring food and drug interactions also became more complex and required team responsibilities. It was soon recognized that coordinating pharmacy, food service, and clinical nutrition minimized adverse drug-nutrient interactions.

Current Trends

The movement in hospitals and other key health care facilities today is a shift in focus toward key processes and functions, such as drug-nutrient interactions in this case, rather than the traditional strictly compartmentalized tasks of departments. Current standards focus still on departmental or service roles. But this is changing because of economic necessity as well as philosophy of care. This changing focus is being shaped, for example, in the work of the Joint Commission on the Accreditation of Healthcare Organizations (JCAHO).[23]

By 1994 JCAHO's accreditation manual will reflect this philosophy that key functions often involve different disciplines coming together, partners with clearly defined responsibilities. The team of clinical nutritionist and clinical pharmacologist is clearly one of these partnerships.[24] The current JCAHO guideline, Standard 6.18, mandates the monitoring of drug therapy by clinical dietitians responsible for diet therapy and counseling with patients about adverse drug-nutrient interactions.[25]

In fact, programs are already being developed in medical centers such as the comprehensive program initiated by the clinical nutrition staff at the University of Maryland Medical System in Baltimore.[26] In this program the departments of clinical nutrition, pharmacy, and nursing have coordinated responsibilities in the process of monitoring and counseling on potential drug-food-nutrient interactions. As computer capabilities are expanded into the twenty-first century, computer-generated flagging, monitoring systems, and printouts provide more commonly used tools for rapid communication. Then, as the Baltimore group has shown, partnerships of clinical nutrition-pharmacy-nursing professions and their patients in relation to drug-nutrient interactions will become routine. Further JCAHO directives will require such specific responsibilities.

To Sum Up

The field of nutrient-drug interaction is in its infancy. More research is needed to sort out complicated relationships and possible effects. Drugs can have multiple effects on the body's absorption, metabolism, retention, and nutrient status. They can provoke adverse reactions in combination with certain foods and can influence appetite, either repressing it or artificially stimulating it. Drugs can either increase an individual's absorption of nutrients or, more commonly, decrease absorption, sometimes leading to clinical deficiences. Drugs can also induce mineral and vitamin deficiencies by their mode of action.

Just as drugs affect our use of food, food affects our use of drugs. Food can affect the absorption of drugs in a variety of ways. Foods also have an effect on subsequent distribution and metabolism of drugs. Vitamins may interfere with drug effectiveness, especially if they are taken in large doses. On the other hand, large doses of specific vitamins can be effective in countering certain toxicity conditions or a specific secondary deficiency induced by a genetic disease.

QUESTIONS FOR REVIEW

1. Name four ways food may affect drug use and give examples of each.
2. If your patient were using a prescribed MAOI such as tranylcypromine sulfate (Parnate), what foods would you instruct him to avoid?
3. What is the most effective way to take aspirin? With what type of liquid? With or without food? Why?
4. What foods would you suggest to a hypertensive patient on the diuretic drug hydrochlorothiazide (HCTZ) as good sources of potassium replacement?
5. Outline suggestions you would discuss with a patient experiencing a drug-induced taste loss. How would you explain the cause of the taste loss?
6. How does cimetidine (Tagamet) help improve the nutritional status of persons with gastrointestinal disease?

REFERENCES

1. Roe DA: Diet, nutrition and drug reaction. In Shils ME, Olson JA, Shike M, eds: *Modern nutrition in health and disease,* ed 8, Philadelphia, 1993, Lea & Febiger.
2. Roe DA: *Diet and drug interactions,* ed 2, New York, 1989, AVI Books.
3. Magnus MH, Roe DA: Computer-assisted instruction on drug-nutrient interactions for long-term caregivers, *J Nutr Educ* 23(1):10, 1991.
4. Roe DA: Process guides on drug and nutrient interactions for health care providers and patients. I. An overview, *Drug-Nutrient Interactions* 5(3):131, 1987.
5. Roe DA: Process guides on drug and nutrient interactions in arthritics, *Drug-Nutrient Interactions* 5(3):135, 1987.
6. Kamath SK and others: Hospital malnutrition: a 33-hospital screening study, *J Am Diet Assoc* 86(2):203, 1986.
7. Torum B: Protein-energy malnutrition. In Shils ME, Olson JA, Shike M, eds: *Modern nutrition in health and disease,* ed 8, Philadelphia, 1993, Lea & Febiger.

8. Clayman CB, ed: *The American Medical Association guide to prescription and over-the-counter drugs*, New York, 1988, Random House.

9. Griffith HW: *Complete guide to prescription and nonprescription drugs*, Los Angeles, 1988, The Body Press, Price Stern Sloan.

10. Graham AW: Screening for alcoholism by life-style risk assessment in a community hospital, *Arch Intern Med* 151:958, 1991.

11. Biery JR and others: Alcohol craving in rehabilitation: assessment of nutrition therapy, *J Am Diet Assoc* 91(4):463, 1991.

12. Roe DA, Kalkwarf H, Stevens J: Effect of fiber supplements on the apparent absorption of pharmacological doses of riboflavin, *J Am Diet Assoc* 88(2):212, Feb 1988.

13. Murray JJ, Healy MD: Drug-mineral interactions: a new responsibility for the hospital dietitian, *J Am Diet Assoc* 91(1):66, 1991.

14. Masse PG: Nutrient intakes of women who use oral contraceptives, *J Am Diet Assoc* 91(9):1118, 1991.

15. Trovato A and others: Drug-nutrient interactions, *Am Fam Physician* 44(5):1651, 1991.

16. Farrington E, Litteral J: Pediatric drug monitoring: clinically important drug-nutrient reactions, *Pediatr Nurs* 16(6):594, 1990.

17. Bailey DG and others: Interaction of citrus juices with felodipine and nifedipine, *Lancet* 337:268, 1991.

18. Semple HA and others: Interactions between hydralazine and oral nutrients in humans, *Ther Drug Monit* 13:304, 1991.

19. Roine R and others: Aspirin increases blood alcohol concentration in humans after ingestion of ethanol, *JAMA* 264(18):2406, 1990.

20. Schachtel BP and others: Caffeine as an analgesic adjuvant, *Arch Intern Med* 151:733, 1991.

21. Morris DJ and others: Licorice, chewing tobacco, and hypertension, *N Engl J Med* 151:733, 1991.

22. Baker ME, Fanestil DD: Liquorice as a regulator of steroid and prostaglandin metabolism, *Lancet* 337:428, 1991.

23. Hard R: Food service, pharmacy team up for nutrition, *Hospitals* 65:46, 1991.

24. Kessler DA: Communicating with patients about their medications, *N Engl J Med* 325(23):1650, 1991.

25. Joint Commission on the Accreditation of Healthcare Organizations: *Accreditation manual for hospitals*, Oakbrook, Ill, 1990, JCAHO.

26. Lasswell AB, Loreck ES: Development of a program in accord with JCAHO standards for counseling on potential drug-food interactions, *J Am Diet Assoc* 92(9):1124, 1992.

FURTHER READING

Ahmed FE: Effects of nutrition on the health of the elderly, *J Am Diet Assoc* 92(9):1102, 1992.

Kerstetter JE and others: Malnutrition in the institutionalized adult, *J Am Diet Assoc* 92(9):1109, 1992.

These excellent companion articles speak to the twin problems of malnutrition and polypharmacy—multiple drug use among elderly persons.

Clayman CB, ed: *The American Medical Association guide to prescription and over-the-counter drugs*, New York, 1988, Random House.

Clayman CB, ed: *Know your drugs and medications,* The American Medical Association Home Medical Library Series, Pleasantville, NY, 1991, Dorling Kindersley and Reader's Digest.

These two resources, prepared for public education and patient-professional reference, provide useful information about effects and interactions of drugs in common use.

ISSUES·AND·ANSWERS

The Calming of America?

American medicine has many names for the psychoactive drugs that act on the mind to dull its reactions. These drugs interact dangerously with alcohol and in some cases common foods. Perhaps the name that best fits the effect of these drugs is *tranquilizer,* from a Latin root meaning "calm, quiet." This meaning signifies the escape many persons seek from a turbulent, confusing world.

We live in an age of stress, often called the "Era of Anxiety." We also live in a culture committed to instant cures and the avoidance of discomfort. Often instead of probing the causes of our problems and striving to alter the conditions that develop them, we believe that somehow we must never feel uncomfortable. If we do, we take something for it. We seek the magic potion to ease the pain and often the symptoms.

To what extent do we actually use such antianxiety drugs in our search for relief? According to the National Academy of Sciences, some 8.5 million Americans take prescription sleeping pills at least once a year. Two million Americans take them every night for at least 2 months at a time. A study conducted by the National Institute on Drug Abuse indicated that 17 million Americans have used stimulants, 28 million have taken sedatives, and 51 million, nearly one out of every four, have taken tranquilizers.

America's single most widely prescribed tranquilizer drug is diazepam (Valium). For example, in one recent year, 3.2 billion pills were sold legally, up 50% from the year before and enough to provide every man, woman, and child in the United States with 145 pills a year. It is still widely prescribed for depression, along with others such as chlorpromazine and lithium. It is difficult to explain just why Valium has been such a frequently prescribed psychoactive drug in the United States. Certainly from a scientific or a pharmacologic viewpoint, no superior effectiveness has been proved. Its popularity can probably be explained by an aggressive marketing program. The large amount of drug available has led to increased black market exposure and easy street usage.

Valium belongs to a group of psychoactive drugs, first introduced in 1960, called *benzodiazepines.* These antianxiety drugs bind to specific receptor sites in the brain. Their clinical effects are mediated through the central nervous system. For some time scientists have sought the identity of the body's natural compound that occupies these receptor sites in the brain. Now pharmacologists report purification of this natural substance. Paradoxically they have discovered that this new 104–amino acid brain peptide not only blocks the receptor binding action of the antianxiety drugs but also appears to induce anxiety, indicating that it is not a natural tranquilizer but has just the opposite effect. This newly identified compound has been named *diazepam-binding inhibitor (DBI)* peptide. These scientists suggest that the naturally occurring DBI acts to trigger anxiety-associated behavior. Drugs such as Valium seem to achieve their antianxiety effect by getting in the way of this naturally occurring, anxiety-producing brain peptide.

Antianxiety drugs such as Valium, can cause several interactions and side effects relate to nutrition counseling needs.

Alcohol. Tranquilizers and alcohol do not mix. These drugs enhance the effects of alcohol and other central nervous systems (CNS) depressant drugs that slow down the nervous system. Other CNS depressant drugs include over-the-counter antihistamines or medicine for hay fever, other allergies, or colds, prescribed anticonvulsants such as Dilantin, pain medications, and narcotics. Long-term use of alcohol also induces liver enzyme changes, leading to more rapid metabolism and reducing the effect of drugs detoxified by the liver. Thus in the alcoholic person benzodiazepines may be metabolized more rapidly so increasingly larger doses may be needed to achieve the desired effect.

Weight gain. Persons taking these antianxiety drugs often experience a great increase in appetite, with subsequent weight gain. This may bring added concern and require general weight management counseling.

Gastrointestinal problems. Some general side effects, ranging from heartburn, nausea, and vomiting to constipation and diarrhea, interfere with food intake and utilization. Individual counseling relating to food choice, combinations, and forms may be needed.

Pregnancy/lactation. Some cases of birth defects from benzodiazepine use in the first 3 months of pregnancy have been reported. Continued use during pregnancy may cause fetal dependency with withdrawal side effects after birth. During lactation these drugs may cause unwanted side effects in the infant.

A more recently introduced antidepressant drug, Prozac, has widespread positive use, primarily because it is relatively free from side effects. Tranquilizer use is frequently encountered in clinical practice so nutrition counseling must cover their interactions with food and other drugs, including alcohol.

Current research at the National Institute of Mental Health is encouraging. The studies of psychiatrist Robert Post seem to indicate that repeated severe depressive episodes affect gene-modulated brain changes more permanently so that preventive drug therapy should be used more in recurrent illness. Early maintenance therapy may prevent the painful recurrences and the more lasting brain cell changes. Post indicates that the key thing now is to match the patient with the right type of medication, and in the long run there will be better medications to match with patients.

REFERENCES

Griffith HW: *Complete guide to prescription and non-prescription drugs,* ed 5, Los Angeles, 1988, The Body Press, Price Stern Sloan.

Holden C: Depression, *Science* 254:1450, 1991.

$\mathscr{C}$HAPTER 18

Feeding Methods: Enteral and Parenteral Nutrition

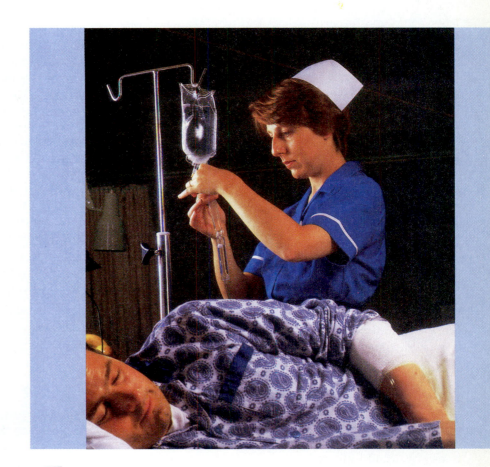

$\mathscr{I}$n this chapter we look at alternate modes of feeding to provide nutrition support for patients with special needs. We examine ways of feeding when the gastrointrestinal tract can still be used—enteral nutrition. Then we review the alternative of nutrient feeding directly into the vein when the gastrointestinal tract cannot be used—parenteral nutrition.

Protein-energy malnutrition is a serious concern in hospitalized patients, especially those with hypermetabolic illness or injury. Often a highly personalized aggressive nutritional program provided by the skilled hospital nutrition support team is lifesaving.

Here we compare these two special feeding methods. We see their various formulas, solutions, and delivery systems for use in hospital and home.

Enteral Feeding in Clinical Nutrition
Nutritional Support Needs

The lack of adequate nutrition to meet metabolic demands is increasingly recognized as a serious concern in medical and surgical patients. A number of surveys have shown that as many as 50% of surgical patients and 44% of medical patients suffer significant protein-energy malnutrition.[1] Persons with underlying chronic disease or traumatic injury are particularly at risk. Elderly persons are especially vulnerable. These patients range widely from those with sudden severe burns or other critical injury to those developing alcoholic hepatitis or with a malignant cancer. In all such cases with the gastrointestinal tract functioning, **enteral** nutrition support provides a front line to restore or, in the case of sudden injury, to maintain an optimal state of nutrition.

Questions do not center on the effectiveness of enteral nutrition support, even feeding by tube if needed, for this has been proved. Rather, current questions center on the most appropriate formula for each patient's specific disease state, the preferred method of formula delivery, and in the case of tube feeding, the causes and extent of possible tube-related complications.[1]

Modes of Enteral Nutrition Support

Even though they have a functioning gastrointestinal tract, some patients cannot restore or maintain a good nutritional status because they cannot eat enough regular food to sustain themselves. They need to take in more nutrient-dense nourishment. Two routes of enteral nutrition support are possible—oral or tube.

Oral Supplements

Depending on the patient's condition the initial option may be to add an oral general energy-nutrient food supplement such as Ensure (Ross) with or between meals. In addition, the energy value of foods in the regular diet may be increased as tolerated with added sauces, seasonings, and dressings. More frequent, less bulky, concentrated small meals may be helpful, making every bite count.

Tube Feeding

If sufficient oral intake of food and supplemental formula is not possible, then the second option is enteral nutrition by tube feeding, either as a supplement or as the complete meal.

Assessment and Patient Selection

Clinical experience has shown that underlying malnutrition carries its own substantial risk of illness and death above and beyond that associated with the patient's primary disease.[2] Thus a general assessment program at hospital admission should be routine procedure to identify those already in states of malnutrition as well as those at risk of potential malnutrition because of their underlying disease or injury. Metabolic activity factors (MAFs) (see Chapter 23) have been recognized and coded according to their added stress on the clinical state—disease, trauma, surgery, or sepsis. Also, the clinical dietitian, as well as other professionals in the hospital caring for the patient, who may discover eating problems or disorders and refer them to clinical nutrition, evaluates malnutrition risks in the current hospitalization and in conference with the attending physician may refer the patient to the nutrition support team for assessment and follow-up care. Basic factors indicating need of nutritional support for medical-surgical patients are the inability to eat for more than 7 to 10 days or maintenance on low kcalorie intravenous fluids for 10 days or more. Table 18-1 provides guidelines the nutrition support team uses for making decisions concerning the choice of feeding mode required.

After patients in need of nutritional support have been identified and the indicated mode of feeding is enteral nutrition, the choices of formula and delivery system follow.

Enteral Formulas
Complete Enteral Formulas
Blender Mixed or Commercial

Our current age of advanced nutritional science and technology has brought a variety of commercial formu-

TABLE 18-1
Questions Guiding Choice of Enteral Nutrition Tube-Feeding Route

Can the gastrointestinal tract be used safely?
  No   Use parenteral nutrition.
  Yes Proceed with enteral nutrition.
Is there adequate intestinal absorption?
  No   Use defined formula diet.
  Yes Use protein isolate diet.
Will nutritional support last longer than 4 to 6 weeks?
  No   Use nasoenteric tube feeding.
  Yes Use enterostomy tube feeding.
Is the patient at risk for aspiration?
  No   Use shorter nasogastric or gastrostomy tube.
  Yes Use longer duodenal or jejunal tube.
Is nutritional support providing adequate nutrient delivery?
  No   Add small vein peripheral parenteral nutrition.
  Yes Continue present formula tube feeding and route.

las and smaller, safer feeding tubes. The question of a blender-mixed formula seldom arises. However, in some instances of home enteral feeding, the patient or family may want to explore the possible use of a home blender-mixed diet. Although there may be emotional comfort in the use of home-prepared food, they need to know the problems involved. These problems involve its physical form, safety, and digestion and absorption:

1. *Physical form:* Foods broken down and mixed in a blender generally yield a **viscous** solution that is difficult to feed through a tube. Thus because of particle size and tendency to stick to the tube, a large-bore feeding tube that is more uncomfortable is required.
2. *Safety:* Such blender-mixed formulas carry problems of bacterial growth and inconsistent nutrient composition from settling out of solid components.
3. *Digestion and absorption:* The blended food formula requires a fully functioning digestion and absorption system to digest the food and absorb its released nutrients. Some patients have gastrointestinal deficits that require nutrients with varying degrees of predigestion (hydrolysis) or smaller molecular structure.

In overall comparison, then, commercial formulas provide a sterile, homogenized solution suitable for more comfortable small-bore feeding tubes and ensure a fixed profile of nutrients in intact or predigested form.

TABLE 18-2

Common Carbohydrate Forms in Commercial Enteral Nutrition Formulas

Starch—polysaccharides

Modified food starch
Hydrolyzed cereal solids
Tapioca starch
Pureed vegetables: green beans, peas, carrots

Glucose polymers*

Glucose polysaccharides
Glucose polymers
Glucose oligosaccharides
Maltodextrins
Corn syrup, corn syrup solids

Disaccharides

Sucrose—from starch hydrolysis
Lactose—from milk
Maltose—from starch and oligosaccharide hydrolysis

Monosaccharides

Glucose (dextrose)
Fructose

---

*From partial hydrolysis of cornstarch.

Nutrient Components

Carbohydrates

About half of the kcalories in the American diet come from carbohydrates, starches and sugars, the body's primary energy source. Although the large starch molecules are well tolerated and easily digested by most patients, their relative insolubility creates problems in most formulas. Thus the smaller saccharides formed by partial or complete hydrolysis of cornstarch are common formula components. In addition to the simple sugars glucose and sucrose, the carbohydrate components include intermediate glucose polymers of varying chain lengths of glucose units. These intermediate products of hydrolysis may be glucose polysaccharides of more than 10 glucose units or glucose oligosaccharides of only a few, about 2 to 10 glucose units, as shown in Table 18-2.

The disaccharide lactose is often deleted in the manufacture of nutrition support formulas because of primary (inherited lactase deficiency) and secondary (mucosal damage, enzyme deficiency) lactose intolerance in many malnourished individuals, as well as a relative deficiency following gastrointestinal surgeries. Some of these various causes of lactase deficiency indicating use of a lactose-free formula are shown in Table 18-3.

Protein

The protein content of standard enteral formulas is most critical because it maintains the body cell mass and its major functions (see Chapter 4). The biologic quality of dietary protein depends on its amino acid profile, especially its relative proportions of essential amino acids (see Table 4-5). Traumatized, catabolic, or seriously undernourished patients require at least 40% of the total amino acid intake as essential amino acids to restore and maintain desired nutritional status.[3] To supply these needs, three major forms of protein are used in nutrition support enteral formulas: intact proteins, hydrolyzed proteins, and crystalline amino acids. Table 18-4 shows some common sources of protein in standard commercial formulas and examples of conditions for which they are used.

Intact proteins. Intact proteins are the complete and original forms as found in foods, although protein

---

enteral • A mode of feeding that uses the gastrointestinal tract, oral or tube feeding.

viscous (viscid) • Physical property of a substance dependent on the friction of its component molecules as they slide by one another; viscosity.

TABLE 18-3
Classes of Lactose Deficiency

Primary: inherited

Racial, ethnic
Genetic

Secondary: enzyme deficiency, mucosal damage

Fasting
Malnutrition
Inflammatory bowel disease
Infections (gastroenteritis, cholera)
Medications (colchicine, neomycin)
Radiation

Relative deficiency

Gastric surgery
Short bowel syndrome

TABLE 18-4	
Common Protein Forms in Commercial Enteral Nutrition Formulas and Examples of Use	
Protein forms	**Examples of use**
Intact protein	*Use intact protein with:*
Milk protein: casein isolates, lact-albumin, whey Sodium and calcium caseinates Soy protein isolates Pureed beef Egg white solids	Normal small intestine absorption capacity Normal pancreatic enzymes
Hydrolyzed protein	*Use hydrolyzed protein with:*
Casein, lactalbumin, whey Soy protein Meat protein, collagen	Reduced absorbing surface Disorders of amino acid transport Pancreatic insufficiency
Crystalline amino acids	*Use crystalline amino acids with:*
L-Amino acids	Liver failure Kidney failure

isolates such as lactalbumin and casein from milk are intact proteins that have been separated from their original food source.

Hydrolyzed proteins. Hydrolyzed proteins are those protein sources that have been broken down by enzymes into smaller protein fragments and amino acids. These smaller products—tripeptides, dipeptides, and free amino acids—are absorbed more easily into the blood circulation, but the larger peptides must be broken down further before they can be absorbed.

Crystalline amino acids. Pure crystalline amino acids are easily absorbed, but because of their small size they increase the osmotic effect of the formula. Also, they adversely affect the formula taste and, if used as an oral supplement, require flavoring aids or different forms to improve palatability, for example, liquid beverage, pudding, frozen slush, or popsicle.

Fat

The major role of fat in a nutrition support enteral formula is to supply a concentrated energy source. The major forms of fat used in standard formulas are butterfat in milk-based mixtures; vegetable oils from corn, soy, safflower, or sunflower; the specially produced medium-chain triglycerides (MCT), monoglycerides, and diglycerides; and lecithin. The vegetable oils supply a rich source of essential fatty acids, especially linoleic acid. Current research is leading to the development of alternate structured lipids from various combinations of short-chain fatty acids, medium-chain fatty acids, and omega-3 fatty acids (see Chapter 3).[4,5]

Vitamins and Minerals

To provide complete nutrition, standard whole diet commercial formulas include sufficient vitamins and

minerals for nutrient requirements when energy needs are fully met.

Physical Properties

After the initial choice of a formula according to nutritional requirements and individual gastrointestinal function, attention is given to certain physical properties of formulas that may affect tolerance. These physical properties are osmolality (based on the concentration of the formula), kcalorie-nutrient density, and residue. Individual intolerance is reflected in gastric retention with abdominal distention and pain, diarrhea, or constipation. These problems, of which diarrhea is the most common, are often unrelated to the formula itself but may result from inappropriate tube-feeding techniques or drug interactions (see Issues and Answers, p. 351).

Medical Foods for Special Needs

Certain formulas designed for special nutritional therapy are called medical foods. The U.S. Food and Drug Administration (FDA) first recognized the concept of medical foods as distinct from drugs in 1972, when the first such special formula was developed for treatment of the genetic disease phenylketonuria (PKU) in newborns (see Chapter 19). During these early years as medical research developed an increasing number of special formulas, the definition of **"medical foods"** remained rather murky between labels of food or drug. In 1988 Congress amended the Orphan Drug Act to include medical foods, defining them as food specifically formulated for use under medical supervision for primary treatment of metabolic-genetic disease having distinctive nutritional requirements based on recognized scientific principles.[6] The Orphan

Drug Act Amendment to include and define medical foods has now been incorporated into the reformed Nutrition Labeling and Education Act of 1990. In addition to metabolic-genetic medical foods, four other categories of special medical food formulas have been developed: (1) end-stage renal disease, (2) hepatic disease, (3) pulmonary disease, and (4) hypermetabolic stress states.[6]

Modular Enteral Formulas

The commercial complete enteral formula products for tube feeding are designed with a fixed ratio of nutrients to meet general standards for nutritional needs. However, some patients' particular needs are not met by these standard fixed-ratio formulas, and they require an individualized modular formula. Such an individual formula is planned, calculated, prepared, and administered with the combined expertise of the nutrition support team, with the clinical dietitian on the team having the major responsibility. The modules vary from a single nutrient to a combination of several nutrients. For example, they may be single modules of carbohydrate, fat, and protein or either combined or single vitamins and minerals.

The advances in modular formula products for planning and calculating nutrition support have made possible more specific nutrient-energy combinations. Using these modules, the clinical dietitian can tailor an individual formula to meet underlying disease needs in conditions such as diabetes, congestive heart failure, renal failure, or liver disease.

Enteral Nutrition Delivery Systems

Feeding Equipment
Feeding Tubes

Recent advances in science and technology have made possible the enteral nutrition delivery systems used today. Modern small-bore nasoenteric feeding tubes made of softer, more flexible polyurethane and silicone materials have replaced former large-bore stiff tubing. These modern feeding tubes are more comfortable for patients and easily carry the variety of nutrient materials now available in enteral nutrition support formulas. Also, these nasoenteric tubes can be inserted not only into the stomach but also beyond the pyloric valve into the small intestine, duodenum or jejunum (Fig. 18-1). These lower placements are used to avoid dangers of vomiting and aspiration by patients on ventilators or for those who are restrained, have a depressed gag reflex, or are comatose. These longer tubes have weighted tips to hold them in place. Insertion and correct placement are guided by radiographic visualization.[7,8]

Containers and Pumps

Additional parts of the enteric tube-feeding system are the formula container and often an infusion pump. A number of containers and feeding sets are available. Clinical dietitians and nurses working with patients on tube feedings need to know details of their comparative advantages and limitations. For example, containers that hold a large volume of formula, as much as 1 L, may be convenient for the nursing staff, but if they are not used within a limited time they are subject to bacterial contamination. Sets that attach to the manufacturer's container reduce contamination. Also, an accurate flow rate must be controlled. A pump may be needed for more accurate control, which is essential for feedings that go directly into the small intestine or for more viscous formulas.

In the final analysis, whatever the type of formula and equipment used, microbiologic quality control programs maintained by enteral nutrition support services at all institutions are essential.[9,10] Such quality standards of practice reduce bacterial counts significantly, thus improving patient tolerance to enteral feeding and reducing complications of infection, diarrhea, and sepsis.

Alternate Routes of Formula Delivery

The nasoenteric route described is usually indicated for short-term therapy in many clinical situations. However, for long-term feedings, enterostomies—surgical placement of the tube at progressive points along the gastrointestinal tract—are the preferred route.[7]

Esophagostomy

A cervical esophagostomy is often placed at the level of the cervical spine to the side of the neck after head and neck surgeries for cancer or traumatic injury. This removes the discomfort of the nasal route and the entry point can be concealed easily under clothing.

Gastrostomy

A gastrostomy tube may be surgically placed in the stomach if the patient is not at risk for aspiration.

Jejunostomy

A jejunostomy tube is surgically placed in the duodenum, the middle section of the small intestine, if the patient is at risk for aspiration. This procedure is indicated for patients who lack a competent gag reflex or who have gastric cancer or gastric ulcerative disease.

Monitoring the Tube-Fed Patient

The nutrition support team carefully monitors all patients who are being nourished by tube feeding. The

---

medical foods • Specially formulated nutrient mixtures for use under medical supervision to treat various metabolic diseases.

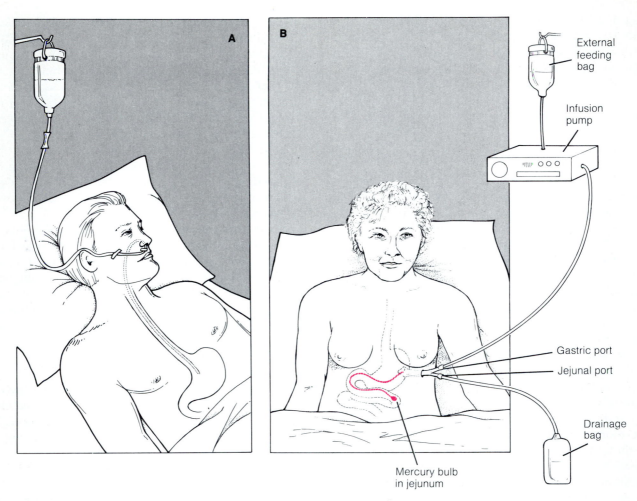

FIG. 18-1   Types of tube feeding. **A,** Common nasogastric feeding tube. **B,** Gastrostomy-jejunal enteral feeding tube.

nursing staff administering the formula to the patient checks for gastric residuals or gastric emptying rate, noting any signs of abdominal distention or bloating, and monitors usual vital signs—temperature, pulse, and respiration. Attending nurses also monitor the flow rate and record the intake and output of formula and fluid, as well as observe and report any individual patient responses to the formula.

The nutrition support team clinical dietitian monitors tolerance for the formula, state of hydration, and nutritional status response following laboratory test panels commonly included in nutrition support assessment protocols (see p. 343). Also monitored are any other special test results related to the patient's disease status or metabolic complications, such as insulin-dependent diabetes mellitus (IDDM), traumatic injury, or sepsis.

Formula Tolerance

Gastrointestinal signs of vomiting, abdominal distention or bloating, and frequency and consistency of bowel movements are noted. If these occur, the feeding may need to be adjusted to a less concentrated formula that is fed more slowly with continuous rather than intermittent bolus feeding until tolerance improves and symptoms subside. Daily blood and urine tests for glucose and acetone during the first week or so, according to protocol, reflect carbohydrate tolerance. Patients who are diabetic or those who are severely stressed with sepsis may have difficulty metabolizing carbohydrate and are monitored closely.[11] Rather than reducing the formula carbohydrate needed for energy, sometimes insulin is given as indicated.

Hydration Status

Daily weights, compared with a baseline weight before starting the formula, along with daily *separate* input-output measures and records of formula and water are essential. Sudden weight changes indicate hydration imbalance and need to be investigated. Signs of dehydration include weight loss, poor skin turgor, dry mu-

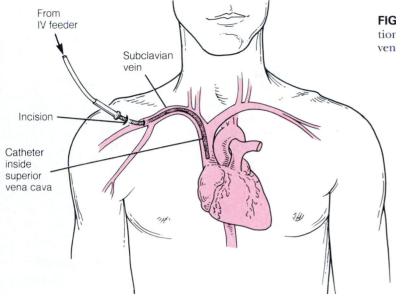

FIG. 18-2 Catheter placement for total parenteral nutrition (TPN) made for feeding via subclavian vein to superior vena cava.

From IV feeder

Subclavian vein

Incision

Catheter inside superior vena cava

cous membranes, low blood pressure from decreased blood volume, and increased levels of serum protein, blood cells, and hematocrit. Signs of overhydration include weight gain, edema, jugular vein distention, and elevated blood pressure.

Regular protocol monitoring includes serum tests for glucose, potassium, sodium, chloride, albumin, complete blood cell counts, and blood urea nitrogen along with periodic tests for urine specific gravity. Dehydration indicators include elevated blood levels of sodium, chloride, glucose, and urea and elevated levels of hematocrit and urine specific gravity. Severe dehydration is critical and life threatening. It can be prevented by careful monitoring and supplying the patient's daily fluid requirements with needed water given through the tube. If it does occur, the feeding is stopped and intravenous rehydration with a 5% glucose solution usually follows. In addition, the nutrition support clinical dietitian monitors the patient's nutritional response with regular assessments.

Documentation of the Enteral Nutrition Tube Feeding

The patient's medical record is always one of the most essential means of careful communication among the members of any health care team (see Chapter 16). It is especially necessary for nutrition support teams in monitoring each tube-fed patient and responding rapidly to individual reactions and needs. Divisions of team responsibilities vary, but the team clinical dietitian, usually a certified nutrition support specialist with advanced academic and clinical preparation, is involved in actions and documentation related to (1) all ongoing nutritional analyses of the actual formula intake, (2) tolerance of the formula and any complications, (3)

recommendations for corrective actions in formula changes, tubing, method and rate of delivery, and (4) education for patient and family.

Parenteral Feeding in Clinical Nutrition

Basic Technique

Applied to nutritional therapy, **parenteral** nutrition refers to any feeding methods other than by the normal gastrointestinal route. Specifically, in current medical and nutritional usage, it refers to the special feeding method of infusing basic predigested nutrient elements directly into the blood circulation through certain veins when the gastrointestinal tract cannot be used. Depending on the nutrition support need, two routes are available:

- *Central parenteral nutrition (CPN):* The use of a large central vein, usually the subclavian vein leading directly into the rapid blood flow of the superior vena cava to the heart, to deliver concentrated solutions that supply full nutritional support for longer periods (Fig. 18-2)
- *Peripheral parenteral nutrition (PPN):* The alternate use of a smaller peripheral vein, usually in the arm, to deliver less concentrated solutions for brief periods (Fig. 18-3)

parenteral • A mode of feeding that does not use the gastrointestinal tract, but instead provides nutrition by intravenous delivery of nutrient solutions.

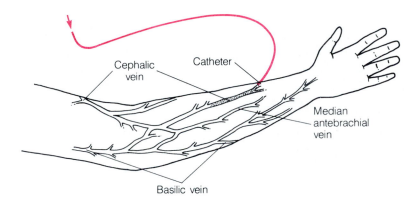

Cephalic vein

Catheter

Median antebrachial vein

Basilic vein

FIG. 18-3   Peripheral parenteral nutrition feeding into small veins in the arm.

Since the development over the past two decades of this basic surgical technique of inserting venous catheters into specific veins for feeding basic nutrients, parenteral nutrition has provided a major advance in critical patient care. It serves the needs of patients with major illness from traumatic injury or extensive debilitating disease. It combats actual or potential malnutrition and meets hypermetabolic nutritional demands. When the patient's condition is further complicated by inability to eat or take enteral tube feeding, nutritional status can be improved and maintained over extended periods solely through intravenous feeding. Hypertonic solutions of essential nutrients can be fed into the greater, rapid blood flow of a large central vein, avoiding the vascular inflammation and thrombosis potential of such concentrated solutions in smaller vessels. Thus, individually required amounts of life-sustaining nourishment, which is otherwise not available, are delivered. This complete sustaining of individual nutritional requirements through intravenous feeding has been termed *total parenteral nutrition (TPN)*.

TPN Development

Largely through the pioneering work of American surgeon Stanley Dudrick and his associates, the current era of parenteral nutrition found its direction in the early 1970s.[12,13] In the later 1970s and 1980s, development of the surgical technique, equipment, and solutions to meet the increased nutritional requirements of catabolic illness and injury has led to its current widespread use.[14,15]

Over the past two decades since its early development, TPN has provided not only brief periods of concentrated nutrition rehabilitation but also an ongoing life support system, a veritable artificial gut, for some individuals on a continuing basis for at least 10 years. Many studies in the past few years have demonstrated the effectiveness of carefully administered TPN by a highly skilled nutrition support team to wisely selected patients. Also, clinical experience has shown that PPN

can be used in many cases as a viable alternative for brief periods, or it may be used in conjunction with oral intake or tube feeding. This is frequently the case in transition feeding. The nutritional support team's clinical dietitian assesses the patient's nutritional status, calculates the nutritional needs, and then designs an appropriate parenteral solution to be recommended to the physician. Currently, a wide spectrum of nutrient solutions and delivery systems exist from which individual nutritional therapy can be planned to meet the clinical problems presented. Nutrition support team pharmacists mix each individual patient solution, and after surgical placement of the indwelling venous catheter, nutrition support nurses administer the individualized solution to the patient.

Indications for Parenteral Nutrition Support

Three basic factors govern decisions about the use of parenteral nutrition: availability of the gastrointestinal tract, degree of malnutrition, and degree of hypermetabolism or catabolism.[16] Risks are involved as well as considerable increase in costs. Thus careful assessment of each of these considerations is imperative.

Availability of the Gastrointestinal Tract

Certainly the long-standing medical adage—"If the gut works, use it!"—applies here. However, if major abdominal injury, for example, has made this natural pathway totally unusable, an alternate means of sustaining nutrition and life is an obvious necessity. In other cases the gut may be unavailable because of obstruction, **fistulas,** or malignant disease. In still other cases the patient may be unable to eat because of coma, severe anorexia and self-starvation, or mental disturbance.

Degree of Malnutrition

Any medical treatment has less chance of success if the patient is malnourished. Many studies have indicated that far more general malnutrition exists among hos-

TABLE 18-5

Patient Situations Imposing Need for TPN

Patient with limited or impossible use of gut	Metabolic rate, degree of catabolism (nitrogen loss per 24 hr)	Degree of malnutrition*
Situation 1	Normal (0-8g)	Normal
Situation 2	Moderate (8-15g)	Moderate
Situation 3	Severe (15g)	Severe

*In terms of percent of normal standards by nutritional assessment.

pitalized patients than was previously assumed. Also, it is now clear that disease imposes an even greater threat to positive nutritional status. Thus the assessment of nutritional status becomes an important part of overall care, especially for hospitalized patients (see Chapter 16). For the severely malnourished patient, especially those facing problems such as major organ failure or extensive surgery, serious consideration of TPN is indicated (Table 18-5).

Degree of Hypermetabolism or Catabolism

When a patient is suffering from major trauma or severe sepsis from radiation or chemotherapy enteritis in treatment for malignant disease (see Chapter 25), the rate of catabolism, or inability to absorb nutrients, may take a devastating toll on the body's resources. This toll as measured by nitrogen balance studies may range up to 15 g of nitrogen over 24 hours. The loss may be even more severe in some patients such as athletes with large lean body masses and extensive injuries. Catabolic periods seem inevitable following extensive surgery and large losses of body resources. The extent of these increased demands is seen in the increased nutritional requirements, especially in energy demand.

Basic Rules for TPN Use

With these three basic considerations in mind, most clinicians have formed general rules to guide TPN decisions as the preferred means of therapy. Some combinations of these factors are illustrated in Table 18-5. Two basic rules have evolved that form the basis for choice of TPN.

The "Rule of Five"

If a patient has had no food for 5 days and is likely not to be able to eat for another 5 days, TPN must be considered then rather than waiting until malnutrition has developed. It is an easier task to maintain positive nutrition than to replenish body stores from malnutrition losses. Starvation effects on the body, even during relatively brief periods, are well documented.[14] The small amount of glycogen stored in the liver, 50 to 75 g, is a crucial immediate energy source but can maintain normal glucose levels for only about 12 hours. Amino ac-

ids from body tissue proteins are then deaminated to provide blood glucose and substrate for needed metabolic functions with a urinary nitrogen loss of 10 to 15 g/day. Also, fatty acids are mobilized from the body's adipose tissues to provide keto acids as the principal fuel for the heart, brain, and other vital organs.

Weight Loss Rule

Any patient who has lost 7% of usual body weight over 2 months and who is deprived of oral nutrition for 5 to 7 days or longer is a candidate for TPN.

Patient Candidates for Parenteral Nutrition

TPN

On the basis of these general considerations, a number of patient situation examples suggest a need for vigorous TPN support:

- *Preoperative preparation of severely malnourished patients:* Congenital anomalies causing gastrointestinal disorders, stricture or cancer of the esophagus and swallowing difficulty, cancer of the stomach, severe peptic ulcer disease, or gastric obstruction
- *Postoperative surgical complications.* Prolonged ileus and obstruction, stomal dysfunction, short bowel syndrome, enterocutaneous, biliary, or pancreatic fistulas, and peritoneal sepsis
- *Inflammatory bowel disease:* Intractable gastroenteritis, regional enteritis (for example, acute Crohn's disease, see Chapter 19), ulcerative colitis, extensive diverticulitis, and radiation enteritis
- *Inadequate oral intake or malabsorption:* Malignant neoplasms and chemotherapy or radiation therapy, acute and relapsing pancreatitis, hypermetabolic states, major trauma, and massive burns, coma, hepatic insufficiency, or encephalopathy, and chronic malnutrition or anorexia nervosa

PPN

Generally, decisions to use PPN instead of TPN are based on comparative energy demands and anticipated time of use. PPN is usually the choice in the following situations:

- *Energy needs:* No more than 2000 kcal/day required
- *Time of use:* No more than 10 days of therapy needed

Nutrition Assessment

The nutrition support team clinical dietitian provides initial nutritional assessment and ongoing monitoring

fistula • Abnormal passageway, usually between two internal organs, or leading from an internal organ to the surface of the body.

of nutritional status. Initial assessment data supply the necessary basis for (1) identifying patients requiring special therapy, (2) calculating their nutritional requirements, and (3) determining the specific nutrient formulas to meet these requirements. Once therapy begins, careful monitoring helps maintain optimal therapy and avoid metabolic complications.

Guidelines for Nutrition Assessment

Necessary nutrition assessment is done by the standard ABCD approach—**a**nthropometrics, **b**iochemical laboratory data, **c**linical observations, **d**ietary evaluations—together with comprehensive detailed histories. These methods are described in detail in Chapter 16. Specific guidelines for parenteral nutrition support, depending on individual needs and clinical situations, include the following six procedures.

1. *Classify degree of weight loss.* Use measures of current body weight and height. Interpret actual body weight (ABW) in terms of desirable body weight for height (DBW), usual body weight (UBW), and amount of recent weight change:

   Percent desirable weight = ABW ÷ DBW × 100
   Percent usual body weight = ABW ÷ UBW × 100
   Percent weight change = UBW − [ABW ÷ UBW] × 100

   Compare the patient's amount of recent weight change with the values indicating malnutrition given in Table 18-6.

2. *Estimate body fat stores and skeletal muscle mass.* Use measure of triceps skin fold (TSF) and standard reference tables (Appendix I) for TSF data. Estimate body fat stores using measures of mid–upper arm circumference (MAC) to derive value for mid–upper arm muscle circumference (MAMC) and compare with standard reference tables. This gives an estimate of the patient's muscle mass interpreted as a percentage of the standard:

   MAMC (cm) = MAC (cm) − [0.314 × TSF (mm)]

3. *Estimate lean body mass.* Use the creatinine-height index (CHI) as an estimate of overall lean body mass. Compute the patient's CHI by using the daily urinary creatinine excretion value determined by laboratory analysis of a 24-hour urine collection. Compare this value with the ideal creatinine value for the patient's height in centimeters from standard tables (see Chapter 16). This gives an effective index of the patient's overall muscle mass and total lean body mass.

4. *Calculate degree of catabolism.* Measure the degree of catabolism by calculating the daily nitrogen balance, using the patient's protein intake for the day (food or formula) and the laboratory analysis of the urinary urea nitrogen output in a 24-hour urine collection for the same day:

   N balance = N intake (protein intake ÷ 6.25)
   − N loss (urinary urea N + 4)

5. *Estimate immune function.* Use the total lymphocyte count or the percentage of lymphocytes in the total white blood cell (WBC) count to determine general function of the patient's immune system. Compare this with the values in Table 18-7.

   Total lymphocyte count = Percent lymphocytes × WBC ÷ 100

   Delayed sensitivity skin testing is occasionally used with hospitalized patients at risk for **anergy** as a means of detecting cellular immune status (see Chapter 16).

6. *Measure plasma protein compartment.* Measure serum transferrin directly or, using laboratory analysis of total iron-binding capacity (TIBC), calculate the value for transferrin, the body's iron transport protein compound:

   Transferrin (mg/dl) = [TIBC (µg/dl) × 0.8] − 43

The serum albumin measure (half-life of 21 days) provides additional long-term data concerning the body's visceral protein mass. However, a decreased transferrin value (half-life 10 days) is a more sensitive marker of recent malnutrition. Prealbumin (half-life 2 days) is the most sensitive marker of current status. Compare these serum values obtained for the patient with values in Table 18-7.

TABLE 18-6

Indication of Severe Protein-Kcalorie Malnutrition According to Percentage of Recent Weight Loss

Body weight loss (%)	Time period
2	1 week
5	1 month
7.5	3 months
10	6 months

TABLE 18-7

Determination of Protein-Kcalorie Malnutrition by Plasma Values

Laboratory data	Normal values	Degree of malnutrition Moderate	Severe
Serum albumin (g/dl)	3.5	2.1-3	<2.1
Serum transferrin (mg/dl)	180-260	100-150	<100
Total lymphocyte count			
per mm³	1500-4000	800-1200	<800
% WBC	20-53		

TABLE 18-8

Monitoring Protocol for TPN

Baseline tests

CBC:	Hb	Nitrogen balance	SGOT
	Hct	Fe and TIBC	Alkaline phosphatase
	RBC indexes	FBS	Serum osmolality
	WBC differential count	BUN	Cholesterol
	Platelets	Creatinine	Triglycerides
Na^+	Ca^{++}	Uric acid	Urinalysis
K^+	PO_4	PT	Chest x-ray film
Cl^-	Mg^{++}	PTT	ECG
CO_2		Prealbumin	Body weight (kg)
		Albumin	Height (cm)
Skin tests (PPD, mumps, cocci)		Total protein	
		Bilirubin	

Stabilization tests (daily for first 5-7 days)

Fractional urine (sugar and acetone) every 6 hours; simultaneous blood
  sugar first and second days
Body weight
Intake and output record
Nitrogen balance
Serum electrolytes
Blood glucose
Prealbumin

Follow-up routine

Daily	Fractional urine (sugar and acetone)
	Body weight
	Intake and output
Three times a week	Electrolytes (Na^+, K^+, Cl^-, CO_2)
	Prealbumin
Once a week	CBC: Platelets PT Mg^{++}
	RBC indexes Ca^{++}
	Creatinine PO_4
	BUN
Once a month	Repeat baseline tests
	Add serum vitamin B_{12}, folate, Zn^{++}

CBC, Complete blood cell count; *Hb,* hemoglobin; *Hct,* hematocrit; *RBC,* red blood cell; *WBC,* white blood cell; *PPD,* purified protein derivative of tuberculin; *TIBC,* total iron-binding capacity; *FBS,* fasting blood sugar; *BUN,* blood urea nitrogen; *PT,* prothrombin time; *PTT,* partial thromboplastin time; *SGOT,* serum glutamic oxaloacetic transaminase; *ECG,* electrocardiogram.

Baseline and Monitoring Assessment for TPN

Baseline nutritional data before starting TPN provide a means of measuring effectiveness of treatment. At designated periods during therapy, certain tests are repeated to monitor the patient's course and avoid metabolic complications. Specific protocols vary in different medical centers. However, a general guide for such standard monitoring data is summarized in Table 18-8. All baseline and monitoring data are recorded in the patient's chart, along with all TPN solution orders.

Clinical Recommendations

Generally, clinicians give primary importance to two major monitoring procedures: (1) constant evaluation of kcalorie intake to ensure adequacy of the energy

TABLE 18-9

Example of Basic TPN Formula Components

Components	Amounts
Basic solution	
Crystalline amino acids	2.75%
Dextrose	25%
Additives	
Electrolytes	
Na	50 mEq/L
Cl	50 mEq/L
K	40 mEq/L
HPO_4	25 mEq/L
Ca	5 mEq/L
Mg	8 mEq/L
Vitamins	
Multiple (MV)	1.7 ml conc./L
Vitamin C (per day)	500 mg
Trace elements solution (per day)	
Zn	3 mg
Cu	1.6 mg
Cr	2 μg
Se	120 μg
Mn	2 μg
I	120 μg
Fe	1.5 μg
Other additives (as needed)	
Regular insulin	0-25 U/L
Heparin	1000 U/L

base to meet metabolic demands and (2) regular measure of protein-nitrogen adequacy to meet tissue rebuilding needs. Nutrition support teams are increasingly using the laboratory test for **prealbumin (PAB)**—normal value 15.7 to 29.6 mg/dl—as the most sensitive rapid plasma protein marker of current malnutrition status and response to nutritional support because of its rapid turnover and half-life of only 2 days.[11,17]

Parenteral Solutions

The TPN Prescription

The TPN prescription and plan of care are based on the calculation of basic nutritional requirements plus additional needs resulting from the patient's degree of catabolism, malnutrition, and any activity. An example of a basic TPN formula plan is shown in Table 18-9.

---

anergy • Diminished immunologic reactivity to specific antigens.

prealbumin (PAB) • Plasma protein with short life used as a biochemical measure for assessing current nutritional status.

This same principle guides nutritional therapy in any feeding mode. Nutritional needs are fundamental—energy (kcalories), protein, electrolytes, minerals, and vitamins.

Energy Requirements

The energy needs of critically ill patients are great, even as high as twice the normal basal rates in the case of major trauma such as massive burns.[18] Energy requirements from three sources must be met: basal energy expenditures (BEE); added energy cost of catabolism, fever, and malnutrition, the metabolic activity factor (MAF) (see Chapter 23); and any physical activity.

Basal Energy Expenditure

An estimate of the adult patient's energy needs for basal tissue metabolism is commonly calculated by the classic Harris-Benedict equations, which involve measures of weight in kilograms, height in centimeters, and age in years[19]:

Women: BEE = 655 + [9.6 × weight (kg)]
           + [1.7 × height (cm)] − [4.7 × age (yr)]
Men: BEE = 66 + [13.7 × weight (kg)]
           + [5.0 × height (cm)] − [6.8 × age (yr)]

The term *resting energy expenditure (REE)* is often used interchangeably with BEE in discussing basal energy needs. For practical purposes they are synonymous and are calculated by the same equations. Recent studies of the effect of age on response to TPN reinforce the fact that depleted body composition in malnourished patients over age 65 is restored more slowly than in younger adults and requires a greater kcaloric intake.[20]

Additional Energy Requirements

In addition to basal energy needs, total kcalorie requirements reflect the large energy drain of the illness or injury. Physiologic stress demands sufficient kcalories to combat the hypermetabolism and its resulting catabolic state and weight loss. If any large degree of malnutrition exists, even more kcalories are needed. Total energy requirements must also include any muscular or physical activity. This need varies considerably depending on the patient's condition, respiratory status, fever or sepsis, and extent of mobility.

In comparison with normal needs, the general range of energy requirements for hospitalized patients on parenteral nutrition support varies with the degree of added metabolic stress:

- Normal needs—25 to 30 kcal/kg/day
- Elective surgery—28 to 30 kcal/kg/day
- Severe injury—30 to 40 kcal/kg/day
- Extensive trauma or burns—45 to 55 kcal/kg/day

Protein Requirements

Nitrogen Balance

The function of protein in health is to sustain tissue growth and maintenance. In healthy adults this ideal

---

A 50% Solution to Protein Loss in Trauma Victims?

TO PROBE FURTHER

The need for protein in patients suffering from various forms of trauma such as severe injuries, sepsis, severe burns, or major surgery is accentuated by the high stress metabolic response to injury and the acute catabolism that this stress triggers. These patients often require TPN to supply needed nutritional support. The metabolic stress effect is indicated by elevated amino acid levels in the blood from the increased gluconeogenesis and catabolism. High levels of the branched-chain amino acids (BCAAs), valine, leucine, and isoleucine have been seen. These are known to help slow down protein catabolism in the body. They also take part in gluconeogenesis and are easily used as energy substrates in muscle. With all these health-promoting activities, do BCAAs have a therapeutic effect when added to the diet?

Some researchers seem to think so. They have tried different concentrations of BCAAs in infused solutions used with patients recovering from major abdominal surgery to see which was most helpful in achieving or preserving nitrogen balance. Of the three concentrations—15.6%, 50%, and 100%—the 50% solution, when given as part of the formula feeding, seemed most effective in preserving nitrogen balance without elevating any amino acids to abnormally high levels. However, before this solution becomes standard therapy, any adverse effects need to be avoided by careful analysis of plasma amino acid levels and evaluation of clinical outcome.

Recent studies, using 19% and 44% solutions of BCAAs with admixtures of dextrose and lipid emulsion as nonnitrogen kcalories for a fuel base, found little difference in nitrogen retention, and no significant clinical advantage over use of a standard amino acid formulation. As yet, continuing study has not been promising enough to justify the much greater cost of the BCAA-enriched formula, which is about five times that of a standard amino acid solution. For the present, BCAA supplementation is being used as a tool for research study, but not yet for nutrition support in stressed, critically ill patients.

So the question remains.

REFERENCES

Heyman MB: General and specialized parenteral amino acid formulations for nutrition support, *J Am Diet Assoc* 90(3):401, 1990.

Scholten DJ and others: Failure of BCAA supplementation to promote nitrogen retention in injured patients, *J Am Coll Nutr* 9(2):101, 1990.

state is reflected in nitrogen equilibrium. In illness, however, catabolism is reflected by negative nitrogen balance, that is, more nitrogen loss than intake, indicating wasting of tissue protein. Thus the goal of nutritional therapy in illness is to maintain positive nitrogen balance, constantly monitored by accurate nitrogen balance studies, to counteract the catabolic deterioration.[21]

Essential Amino Acids

The quality of the protein intake in terms of equivalent essential amino acids is fundamental to tissue synthesis (see To Probe Further, p. 344). The essential amino acids must be present in the optimal ratio for best use of the individual amino acids.

Ratio of Nitrogen to Nonprotein Kcalories

To protect the nitrogen sources (the amino acids) and make them available for tissue synthesis, sufficient nonprotein energy sources must be present to meet the increased kcaloric need. Carbohydrates are necessary to promote incorporation of plasma amino acids into muscle tissue protein. For optimal use, the normal adult diet sustains a ratio of 150 nonprotein kcal/1 g of nitrogen. To meet the metabolic stress of critical illness with minimal activity, this ratio should be 150 to 200 kcal/1 g of nitrogen. In terms of protein, the requirements in illness reflect these increased needs:

Catabolic state: Weight (kg) × 1.2 to 1.5 g protein
Healthy state: Weight (kg) × 0.8 to 1.0 g protein

Electrolyte Requirements

Special electrolyte profiles are required in intracellular and extracellular fluid for all tissues to maintain normal water balances throughout the body (see Chapter 8). These balances must be maintained during illness in the face of metabolic imbalances. For example, active tissue synthesis requires phosphate and potassium and is also influenced by available sodium and chloride ions. Monitoring of individual electrolyte status supplies the data needed to determine daily electrolyte requirements.

In general, the basic electrolyte needs for a 3000 kcal intake (3-L solution) are approximately the following:
- Chloride (Cl): 150 mEq
- Potassium (K): 120 mEq
- Sodium (Na): 120 to 150 mEq
- Phosphate (HPO$_4$): 60 to 75 mEq
- Magnesium (Mg): 24 to 36 mEq
- Calcium (Ca): 6 to 15 mEq

Vitamin and Mineral Requirements

Vitamin and mineral needs are based on normal standards (see current RDAs listed inside front covers), with increases according to metabolic states. Individual nu-

trients may be added as needed to cover increased metabolism and depletion states. Attention to necessary trace elements is especially important. Patients on long-term TPN have shown deficiencies of iron, zinc, and copper, and more recently significant deficiences of selenium, chromium, and molybdenum have occurred.[22] Trace element supplements of zinc and copper are needed especially by patients with severe burns because of their essential roles in wound healing during the acute recovery period.[23] The prescribed TPN solution reflects these needs and additions.

Preparation of the TPN Solution

A number of differing strength solutions of the basic nutrients are available for use by the TPN team in formulating individual nutritional needs, including protein, nonprotein energy, electrolytes, vitamins, and minerals.

Protein-Nitrogen Source

In the TPN solution, protein-nitrogen need is supplied by essential and nonessential crystalline amino acids. Standard commercial amino acid solutions produced by various manufacturers range in concentration from 3% to 11.4%, but the general standard product is the 8.5% solution.

In addition, two recent types of specialized amino acid solutions have been formulated, although they are more expensive than standard solutions and their superiority remains unclear. One type is enriched with the three BCAAs—isoleucine, leucine, and valine and designed for patients with extensive trauma and severe catabolic stress or with liver failure who have shown low plasma levels of these three amino acids. The other type is enriched with essential amino acids and is designed to prevent development of hyperuremia in patients with acute renal failure.

However, for most TPN patients a usual amino acid need is supplied by a 4.25% dilution achieved by the use of 1 L of standard 8.5% amino acid solution mixed with 1 L of dextrose solution.

Nonprotein Energy Source (Kcalories)

Nonprotein kcalories in TPN solutions protect protein (amino acids) for tissue synthesis demands. The major energy needs are supplied by glucose and lipid solutions.
1. *Glucose (dextrose):* Glucose is the most common and least expensive source of kcalories used for parenteral nutrition support. Hypertonic 50% to 70% solutions are available for use in TPN formulations. The most commonly used standard is the 50% solution. Glucose used in parenteral nutrition support is commercially available as dextrose monohydrate ($C_6H_{12}O_6H_2O$), which has an energy value of 3.4 kcal/g, not the energy value of

4 kcal/g of the regular dietary glucose form ($C_6H_{12}O_6$).

2. *Lipids.* Lipid emulsions provide a concentrated energy source, 9 kcal/g, as well as the essential fatty acid, linoleic acid. Lipids also have practical values associated with their effects on respiratory gas (carbon dioxide and oxygen) exchange, autoimmune disease, and vascular disease.[24] About 4% to 10% of the daily kcaloric intake should consist of fat emulsion to prevent fatty acid deficiency. A 500-ml bottle of 10% or 20% fat emulsion provides 555 kcal (1.1 kcal/ml) or 1000 kcal (2.0 kcal/ml), respectively.[25] Available commercial products use lipid emulsions of soybean and safflower oil combined or soybean oil alone.

Traditionally, lipid emulsions were fed separately. More recently, however, with improved solutions and equipment, in some cases lipids have been combined with the dextrose and amino acid base and called a 3-in-1 **admixture**.[26] With the additional modules of electrolytes and vitamins and adequate fluid, the whole feeding is identified as a *total nutrient admixture (TNA)*. Stable TNAs have also been prepared successfully for pediatric use.[27] Current refinements in products and technique have allowed various admixtures of lipids, carbohydrates, and protein in a common bag, complete with adequate fluid and electrolytes and either single or multiple forms of vitamins and trace elements. Newer alternative lipid sources include forms such as short-chain fatty acids, medium-chain fatty acids, omega-3 fatty acids, and blended or structured lipids.[5]

Electrolytes

Electrolytes in TPN formulas are based on the usual requirements for normal electrolyte balance with adjustments according to individual patient monitoring. Commercial amino acid formulations are available with or without added electrolytes. If electrolytes are present in the amino acid solution, they must be taken into account when calculating additions for a specific patient requirement. Three actions are basic in managing individual needs: (1) correct any preexisting deficits immediately; (2) recognize and replace excessive fluid and electrolyte losses to prevent chronic deficits; and (3) monitor and determine electrolyte needs daily.[28]

Vitamins

The Nutrition Advisory Group of the American Medical Association has established guidelines for parenteral administration of 12 vitamins: A, D, E, thiamin, riboflavin, niacin, pantothenic acid, pyridoxine, folate, biotin, cobalamin, and ascorbic acid. Multivitamin preparations based on these guidelines are available. Vitamin K is not a component of any formulation for adults. If it is needed for individual maintenance, it is added to the solution. Any larger deficit is treated by periodic intramuscular injection as needed.

Trace Elements

The American Medical Association has also set guidelines for the addition of four trace elements in TPN solutions: zinc, copper, manganese, and chromium. To these four elements, some manufacturers add selenium in a separate product. Single mineral products are also available for each of these trace elements. Iron is not routinely added. If it is needed by an individual patient, it is administered apart from the TPN admixture.[28] Caution is needed in adding minerals to the TPN solution. Incompatabilities of certain electrolytes and other components may form insoluble substances that separate out, depending on ion concentration and solution pH.

Parenteral Nutrition Delivery System

Equipment

Strict aseptic technique throughout the entire TPN administration by all the special nutrition support team members involved is absolutely essential. This includes (1) the solution preparation by the pharmacist, (2) the surgical placement of the venous catheter by the physician, and (3) the care of the catheter site and all external equipment and administration of the solution by the nurse. At every step of the TPN process, strict infection control is one of the primary team responsibilities.[29,30]

Venous Catheter

Surgical placement of the venous catheter is done by the physician, a surgeon, at the bedside, using local anesthesia. Commercially prepared sterile kits contain all the necessary equipment items for gaining access to a large central vein for feeding the nutrition support solution directly into the central blood circulation. Flexible silicone catheters are available in different lengths and calibers.[31] Smaller, shorter catheters (15 to 25 cm) are designed for use in the hospital. Larger, longer catheters such as the 1.6-mm caliber Hickman catheter are designed for long-term intermediate or home use. The catheter is passed through the outer vein, usually the subclavian vein, into the central superior vena cava, which leads directly into the heart (Fig. 18-2). In the vena cava the catheter tip lies so that concentrated solutions, five times the concentration of blood plasma, can be infused at a rate of 2 to 3 ml/min and can be immediately diluted by a large blood flow of 2 to 5 L/min, a dilution factor of at least a thousand.[31] The continuing development of TPN has led to new catheters and insertion techniques that have greatly reduced catheter-related complications. Commercial ster-

◆ CLINICAL APPLICATION | TPN Administration

Of all the various ways of nourishing the human body—normal eating, liquid diets, enteral nutrition, parenteral nutrition—TPN requires the highest degree of skilled and precise administration. The risk of potentially life-threatening complication and infection is ever present. The role of the trained nutrition support nurse is central in successful TPN. The nutrition support nurse administers the TPN solution according to the nutrition support team protocol, monitoring the entire TPN system frequently to see that it is operating accurately.

Specific clinical protocols will vary somewhat, but they usually include the following points:

- *Start slowly.* Give the patient time to adapt to the increased glucose concentration and osmolality of the solution.
- *Schedule carefully.* During the first 24 hours give 1 to 2 L by continuous drip. The slow rate is usually regulated by an infusion pump.
- *Monitor closely.* Note metabolic effects of glucose (blood glucose levels not to exceed 200 mg/dl) and electrolytes.

- *Increase volume gradually.* After the first day, increase by 1 L/day to reach desired daily volume.
- *Make changes cautiously.* Watch the effect of all changes and proceed slowly.
- *Maintain a constant rate.* Keep to the correct hourly infusion rate, with no catch-up or slow-down effort to meet the original volume order.
- *Discontinue slowly.* Discontinue TPN feeding gradually, reducing rate and daily volume about 1 L/day. ◆

---

ile dressing kits for continuing nursing care have also aided aseptic technique and infection control.

Infusion Devices

Various infusion devices control the solution flow rate and maintain an accurate flow range. Infusion pumps may be used to deliver the solution at a constant rate to prevent metabolic complication. Strict asepsis throughout the delivery system is essential. Protocols for external delivery system tubing changes guided by infection control monitoring include maintenance of sterility of the catheter hub and and tubing junction.[32]

Solution Administration

During the administration of the TPN solution, each patient has individual responses and needs for adjustments, according to fluctuations and changes in the illness or injury and the concentrated feeding. The skilled nutrition support nurse checks frequently to see that the entire TPN delivery system is operating accurately according to the support team protocol (see Clinical Application above).

Monitoring

In the hands of a well-trained TPN team, risks have been minimized and complications controlled by constant team effort. Specific protocols, updated periodically as needed, guide continuing assessment and monitoring. Related solution adjustments by the nutrition support team are made according to metabolic and nutritional needs.

Home Nutrition Support

Home Enteral Nutrition

Patient Selection

Home enteral nutrition tube feeding is not useful to all patients. But for those who require continued tube feeding to meet their clinical and nutritional needs, it provides a physiologic, safe, and relatively simple and less costly method of replenishing and maintaining nutrition support. Recent rapid developments in enteral formulas and tube-feeding equipment have now simplified home feeding and made it easier to manage. As a result, the number of patients using tube feeding for home enteral nutrition continues to grow as a means of cutting hospital costs and allowing earlier family support at home. Home care requires training of both patient and family.

Teaching Plan

Educating the patient and family for home care is usually a team responsibility of the nutrition support clinical dietitian and nurse. First, the clinical dietitian determines the patient's current nutrient and fluid requirements, selects the formula, complete or modular,

admixture • A mixture resulting from adding or mingling another ingredient; a combination of two or more substances that are not chemically united or that exist in no fixed proportion to each other.

computes formula amounts to be used, and outlines the feeding schedule. Then the dietitian and the nurse develop and carry out a teaching plan together, which includes the following topics and related tasks in preparing patients and families for discharge on home enteral feeding[33]:

- The nature of the formula, its rationale and preparation
- The feeding process, equipment, and pump function
- How to flush the tube and care for the tube site
- How to recognize formula intolerance
- How to avoid complications
- How to give medications with the feeding

The nutrition support clinical dietitian is responsible for the tasks that assess needs and determine the formula components and their preparation. The nurse is usually responsible for tasks related to feeding process and equipment. Then the dietitian and the nurse share the teaching tasks related to formula intolerance, complications, and medications. In reality, it is basically team teaching throughout. The nutrition support team clinical pharmacist may share the final topic on medications.

A teaching manual with illustrations is produced by the nutrition support team to guide the teaching-learning process and for continuing reference at home. The teaching plan should should start as soon as the decision for home feeding is made. A social worker should join the team to (1) schedule a separate counseling visit to determine any personal, psychosocial, or economic problems with the care and (2) confer with the nutrition support team to help work them out.

Finally, the teaching plan should allow 2 full days before discharge for the patient and family to practice with the support nurse and for the clinical dietitian to observe the patient (1) administering the formula and (2) recording all necessary information about formula and fluid intake, formula tolerance, and complications. Directions for this record are included in the home care manual. Records are reviewed regularly by home support team specialists providing follow-up care at home and in the clinic.

Follow-up Monitoring

The plan for follow-up monitoring should follow the specific protocol schedule developed by the nutrition support team for laboratory, clinical, and nutritional assessments. In early home visits the clinical dietitian and nurse team check progress and troubleshoot any problems that need to be worked out or that require adjustments in the formula or feeding plan.

Home Parenteral Nutrition

Experience from home use of other long-term medical care equipment, such as that for renal dialysis, has led to the concept of self-infusion of parenteral nutrients at home. Following the pattern given for home enteral nutrition, a full patient and family TPN education plan with supervised practice is essential. In the hands of selected, well-trained patients and their families, home TPN allows mobility and travel. It has offered special promise in long-term management of conditions such as severe abdominal injury or chronic severe inflammatory bowel disease. Special equipment, solutions, and guidelines for training selected patients and families have been developed and are successfully being used in a number of cases.

To Sum Up

For patients with functioning gastrointestinal tracts, enteral nutrition support has proved to be a potent tool against present or potential malnutrition. This nutritional support is achieved by a regular oral diet with nutrient-energy supplementation or alternately by tube feeding when the patient cannot, will not, or should not eat. Modern commercial products provide complete formulas or separate nutrient modules for individualizing a formula mixture to meet special needs. Companion advances in tube-feeding technology have provided extended tube-feeding systems of two types: (1) longer nasoenteric tubes reaching the duodenum and jejunum of the small intestine and (2) surgical enterostomies in which tubes are placed at progressively extended positions along the gastrointestinal tract. New systems of formulas, tubing and container systems, and electric pumps, together with a comprehensive teaching plan for patient and family and follow-up monitoring by the clinical team, have allowed home enteral feeding to increase rapidly.

For patients with critical hypermetabolic injury or illness or obstruction that makes the gastrointestinal tract unavailable, parenteral nutrition support acts as an artificial gut, an alternate lifeline. This feeding method depends heavily on biomedical technology for the development of tubes, bags, pumps, and other equipment for feeding nutrients directly into veins for blood circulation to the cells. The route of entry may be a large central vein for full feeding over a long period of time or a smaller peripheral vein for feeding less concentrated solutions for a shorter period of time. Home parenteral nutrition support is being successfully used by selected well-trained patients, with the support of equally well-trained families and constant clinical back-up.

QUESTIONS FOR REVIEW

1. Describe several types of patient situations in which enteral nutrition support may be indicated. What nutrition assessment procedures may help to identify these individuals?

2. Describe the nutrient components of a typical complete enteral formula. How does it differ from a modular formula?

3. What are medical foods? In what types of cases are they used?

4. Define parenteral nutrition and identify examples of conditions in which it would be used.

5. The following questions apply to the case of a man referred to nutrition support services. Imagine you are caring for this patient:

   a. A previously healthy 45-year-old man, while on a long transport haul as a truck driver, suffered an accident in which he sustained a severe abdominal injury requiring extensive surgical repair and leaving the gastrointestinal tract unavailable for use for an undetermined period of time. He is referred to the nutritional support team for follow-up TPN. Early in this care he asks you how this feeding works. How would you describe and explain the TPN feeding process?

   b. What nutritional status assessment procedures would be done and how would you explain to him the nature and purpose of each measure?

   c. From your study of this chapter, outline your estimate of his basic nutritional needs to serve as a basis for determining his TPN therapy.

   d. List the typical components of a basic TPN formula that he may require, and describe the purpose of each to help reassure him of its adequacy and importance.

   e. Sufficient energy (kcalories) intake is essential to immediately meet his metabolic needs after surgery. Assume a normal preinjury weight and height and an added metabolic activity factor (MAF) for stress of 1.5 times his basal energy expenditure (BEE). Calculate his total kcalorie need, using the Harris-Benedict equation for BEE and adding the MAF stress need.

   f. Define *prealbumin* and describe why it is a primary test for monitoring the effectiveness of the TPN formula in meeting his nutritional support needs for recovery.

REFERENCES

1. Benya R, Morbarham S: Enteral alimentation: administration and complications, *J Am Coll Nutr* 10(3):209, 1991.

2. Rombeau JL, Caldwell MD: *Enteral and tube feeding*, Philadelphia, 1990, WB Saunders.

3. Bell SJ and others: A chemical score to evaluate the protein quality of commercial parenteral and enteral formulas: emphasis on formulas for patients with liver failure, *J Am Diet Assoc* 91(5):586, 1991.

4. Bell SJ and others: Alternate lipid sources for enteral and parenteral nutrition: emphasis on formulas for patients with liver failure, *J Am Diet Assoc* 91(1):74, 1991.

5. Gottschlich MM: Selection of optimal lipid sources in enteral and parenteral nutrition, *Nutr Clin Prac* 7(4):152, 1992.

6. Talbot JM: Guidelines for the scientic review of enteral food products for special medical purposes, *J Parenter Enteral Nutr* 15(suppl3):100S, 1991.

7. Monturo CA: Enteral access device selection, *Nutr Clin Prac* 5(5):207, 1990.

8. Caufield KA and others: Technique for intraduodenal placement of transnasal enteral feeding catheters, *Nutr Clin Prac* 6(1):23, 1991.

9. Fagerman KE: Limiting bacterial contamination of enteral nutrient solutions: six-year history with reduction of contamination at two institutions, *Nutr Clin Prac* 7(1):35, 1991.

10. Fagerman KE: Microbiologic standards for enteral nutrient solutions overdue in the United States, *J Am Diet Assoc* 92(3):336, 1992.

11. Bernstein LH: Monitoring quality of nutrition support, *Diet Curr* 19(2):1, 1992.

12. Dudrick SJ and others: Can intravenous feeding as the sole means of nutrition support growth in the child and restore weight loss in an adult? *Ann Surg* 169:974, 1969.

13. Dudrick SJ: A clinical review of nutritional support of the patient, *Am J Clin Nutr* 33(suppl):1191, June 1982.

14. Rhoads JE, Dudrick SJ: History of intravenous nutrition. In Rombeau JL, Caldwell MD, eds: *Parenteral nutrition: clinical nutrition*, vol 2, Philadelphia, 1986, WB Saunders.

15. Fischer JE, ed: *Total parenteral nutrition*, Boston, 1991, Little, Brown.

16. De Chicco RS, Matarese LE: Selection of nutrition support regimens, *Nutr Clin Prac* 7(5):239, 1992.

17. Sawicky CP and others: Adequate energy intake and improved prealbumin concentration as indicators of the response to total parenteral nutrition, *J Am Diet Assoc* 92(10):1266, 1992.

18. Ireton-Jones CS, Baxter CR: Nutrition for adult burn patients: a review, *Nutr Clin Prac* 6(1):3, 1991.

19. Harris JA, Benedict FG: *A biometric study of basal metabolism*, Washington, DC, 1919, Carnegie Institution of Washington.

20. Shizzal HM and others: The effect of age on the caloric requirements of malnourished individuals, *Am J Clin Nutr* 55:783, 1992.

21. Konstantinides FN: Nitrogen balance studies in clinical nutrition, *Nutr Clin Prac* 7(5):231, 1992.

22. Fleming CR: Trace element metabolism in adult patients requiring total parenteral nutrition, *Am J Clin Nutr* 49:573, 1989.

23. Cunningham JJ and others: Zinc and copper status of severely burned children, *J Am Coll Nutr* 10(1):57, 1991.

24. Sax HC: Practicalities of lipids: ICU patient, autoimmune disease, and vascular disease, *J Parenter Enteral Nutr* 14(suppl 5):223, 1990.

25. Torosian MH, Daly JM: Solutions available. In Fischer JE, ed: *Total parenteral nutrition*, ed 2, Boston, 1991, Little, Brown.

26. Warshawsky KY: Intravenous fat emulsions in clinical practice, *Nutr Clin Prac* 7(4):187, 1992.

27. Bullock L and others: Emulsion stability in total nutrient admixtures containing a pediatric amino acid formulation, *J Parenter Enteral Nutr* 16(1):64, 1992.

28. La France RJ, Miyagawa CI: Pharmaceutical considerations in total parenteral nutrition. In Fischer JE, ed: *Total parenteral nutrition*, ed 2, Boston, 1991, Little, Brown.

29. Cahill SL, Benotti PN: Catheter infection control in parenteral nutrition, *Nutr Clin Prac* 6(2):65, 1991.

30. Thompson B, Robinson LA: Infection control of parenteral enteral nutrition solutions, *Nutr Clin Prac* 6(2):49, 1991.

31. Flowers JF and others: Catheter-related complications of total parenteral nutrition. In Fischer JE, ed: *Total parenteral nutrition*, ed 2, Boston, 1991, Little, Brown.

32. Davis CL: Nursing care of total parenteral and enteral nutrition. In Fischer JE, ed: *Total parenteral nutrition*, ed 2, Boston, 1991, Little, Brown.

33. Skipper A, Rotman N: A survey of the role of the dietitian in preparing patients for home enteral feeding, *J Am Diet Assoc* 90(7):939, 1990.

FURTHER READING

Bower RH: Nutritional and metabolic support of critically ill patients, *J Parenter Enteral Nutr* 14(5 suppl):257S, 1990.
Morales E and others: Dietary management of malnourished children with a new enteral feeding, *J Am Diet Assoc* 91(10):1233, 1991.

These two articles provide interesting background about the research and development that prepares a commercial nutrition support formula for market.

Frankenfield DC, Beyer PL: Dietary fiber and bowel function in tube-fed patients, *J Am Diet Assoc* 91(5):590, 1991.

These authors provide an excellent review of the metabolism and function of fiber in conjunction with tube feedings, and the use of fiber in enteral formulas to treat constipation and diarrhea in tube-fed patients.

DeChicco RS, Matarese LE: Selection of nutrition support regimens, *Nutr Clin Prac* 7(5):239, 1992.

These experienced nutrition support clinical dietitians provide an excellent review of the process used to determine whether a patient needs nutrition support, what type of feeding access and techniques should be, and how and when to make the transition back to oral feedings.

Heyman MB: General and specialized parenteral amino acid formulations for nutrition support, *J Am Diet Assoc* 90(3):401, 1990.

This gastroenterologist's comprehensive review of the state of the art in amino acid formulations, especially for pediatric nutrition support, provides a clearer understanding of evolving special amino acids and why their use should be approached with caution. Standard solutions, he concludes, will provide adequate protein for most adults and children.

Sawicky CP and others: Adequate energy intake and improved prealbumin concentration as indicators of the response to total parenteral nutrition, *J Am Diet Assoc* 92(10):1266, 1992.

This article illustrates the monitoring focus on total intake of kcalories and the rapid-feedback rise of serum prealbumin as primary focus for determining effectiveness of TPN therapy.

Troubleshooting Diarrhea in Tube-Fed Patients: A Costly Chase

Clinicians seem to agree generally that diarrhea is one of the most common complications associated with tube feeding, yet the reported incidence ranges widely from as little as 2% to as much as 63% in general patient populations and as high as 68% in intensive care patients. Questions that relate to this wide variance and that plague investigators apparently center on definition and cause. But the ultimate bottom line for patient and family and their health insurers if they have any is the price of the clinical search for the culprit. As we shall see, it is in fact a costly chase.

Problem of definition

It would appear on the surface that the question of what diarrhea is, is easy to answer. We've all had some experience, more or less. However, a valid clinical research study demands more—a precise operational definition on which to establish a research design and evaluate results. Judging from reports, investigators have not been able to agree on a definition, methods of reporting the extent of the diarrhea, the length of time tube-fed patients were monitored, and the sample of patients that were studied.

In fact, a current report of a 3-month study clearly indicates that the messy state of defining and reporting diarrhea in tube-fed patients resembles that of the disorder itself. These investigators—using the usual diarrhea criteria of frequency, consistency, and quantity—found as many as 14 different definitions in their review of studies in the scientific literature, no doubt accounting for the varying incidence reported. Of course the tube-fed patients, if asked, could have easily defined their diarrhea in terms of the psychologic and physical discomfort involved, as could their nurses in terms of increased cleanup work and concern for the patient.

Problem of cause

Reported causes of diarrhea in tube-fed patients also vary. These concerns usually center first on the formula itself, often followed by numerous adjustments in components and concentrations that only cloud the picture further and make the search for the actual culprit more difficult. A variety of conflicting causes associated with the complication of diarrhea have been reported, including not only the formula itself but also medications or some aspect of the patient's condition.

Formula. Possible formula factors relate to osmolality or concentration and to rate of delivery. However, conflicting reports have shown no increase in the incidence of diarrhea when the formula concentration varied widely from 145 to 430 mOsm, and no significant association has been made between malabsorp-

tion and formula *osmolality* or rate of delivery. Formulas providing 30% or more of total kcalories as fat have been associated with a higher incidence of diarrhea, whereas those providing 20% fat rarely were involved. Further study of fat composition is needed, specifically comparing medium- versus long-chain triglycerides and omega-3 versus omega-6 fatty acids. Studies of the role of fiber in tube feedings have also been conflicting. Reviewers have found that the studies thus far have been few, the models used variable, the limitations substantial, and the conclusions of the investigators mixed.

Bacterial contamination. Studies have demonstrated that the problem of diarrhea does not lie in the quick assumption that the formula as such was at fault but in the reality that bacterial contamination, frequently *Clostridium difficile* toxin, of the formula or feeding equipment was the cause. This problem may result from lack of careful aseptic technique in handling the formula and equipment or from failing to follow manufacturers' guidelines for appropriate hang times for formulas—usually no longer than 8 hours for systems set up by the nursing staff and 24 hours for systems prefilled with formula by the manufacturer and attached by connections. The less any system is handled and opened, the less chance there is for contamination. Bacteria are easily introduced where the delivery tubing connects with the patient's feeding tube and whenever the system is open.

Patient's condition. Malnourished or critically ill patients are more susceptible to mucosal tissue breakdown, depressed serum albumin levels, and malabsorption leading to diarrhea. The hypoalbuminemia contributes to reduced colloidal osmotic pressure within blood vessels (see Chapter 8). This loss of osmotic pressure in turn leads to edema of the intestinal mucosa, malabsorption, and diarrhea. Use of an easily absorbed elemental enteral formula is probably helpful, at least until the nutritional status improves sufficiently to progress to a standard intact-protein formula. Albumin may be given intravenously, but unless there is adequate nutritional support the body uses the infused albumin for energy rather than tissue rebuilding. In addition, periods of stress, including sepsis and central nervous system insults, can result in decreased motility of the gastrointestinal tract, including ileus. Such decreased motility contributes to bacterial overgrowth.

Medications. Multiple medications routinely given to hospitalized patients have been related to diarrhea. Antibotics are most often associated, but this practice coexists with poor patient condition, multiple organ failure, and therefore with diarrhea. In general, drug reactions may relate to the metabolically active agent or to another ingredient added for its physical properties in the form of the drug, for example, tablet or liquid as the following case illustrates.

Troubleshooting Diarrhea in Tube-Fed Patients: A Costly Chase—cont'd

The case of the costly chase

A recently reported case of unexplained diarrhea in a tube-fed patient illustrates the difficult, and often costly, search for the cause. A 55-year-old man, whom we call "Max," suffered an aortic aneurysm and had emergency surgery to repair it. In the intensive care unit, the postoperative course was complicated by respiratory problems requiring ventilator assistance. He was given a bronchodilator drug, theophylline, in tablet form, crushed and given by nasogastric tube with water. When Max was able to take nourishment, an isotonic formula given by enteral tube feeding was started and the crushed theophylline tablets were changed to a sugar-free theophylline solution. Within a day, Max began to have progressive abdominal distention and continuous liquid diarrhea. To rule out an abdominal catastrophe related to the aneurysm or surgery, a computed abdominal tomography scan (see Chapter 6), an aortogram, and a colonoscopy were done, but all of these studies were normal.

Despite discontinuation of the enteral feeding, the distention and diarrhea continued. Stool specimens were tested for fecal leukocytes, parasites, and *Clostridium difficile* toxin, and an enteric pathogen culture was prepared. All were nondiagnostic. Extensive additional serum and urine tests, as well as a sigmoidoscopy with rectal biopsy, gave no clue. Then stool electrolytes and osmolality measures suggested an osmotic diarrhea. Because Max was not receiving enteral feedings, his physicians thought a secretory bacterial toxin was probably causing the continuing diarrhea, so the previous studies were repeated to confirm the osmotic nature of the diarrhea. In addition, all the medications were reviewed, but none appeared to be the cause.

At this point, because the continued diarrhea prohibited enteral feeding and Max needed nourishment, total parenteral nutrition (TPN) was ordered. This move immediately brought an automatic Nutrition Support Service consultation, which included further assessment of medications. This evaluation revealed that the sugar-free theophylline solution was 65% sorbitol. Sorbitol is a polyhydric alcohol used as a sweetener in many sugar-free products such as dietetic foods and chewing gum. There was no information about sorbitol on the label or package insert of the drug for the physicians to know these facts, and because sorbitol was not thought to be an active agent, this information could be obtained only by contacting the manufacturer.

Fortunately for Max, however, the nutrition support team did know and found the hidden culprit in his medication. The nutritionist knew that sorbitol in larger doses is a laxative! After calculations of the regular daily amount of the theophylline Max was taking, he was receiving nearly 300 g of sorbitol daily when the usual laxative dose was only 20 to 50 g. The nutritional support team immediately recommended that this sorbitol-sweetened solution of theophylline be discontinued and that a sorbitol-free form of the medication be used instead. Almost immediately the diarrhea began to decrease and in 3 days was gone.

The extent of this costly chase was revealed in Max's hospital bill. He had continued to receive the faulty drug for almost half of his 3-month hospital stay, during which time the diarrhea prevented enteral feeding and he had to have the more expensive TPN. The TPN cost $4860 more than the enteral feedings would have cost for the same period. In addition, all the extensive investigations to find the cause of the diarrhea cost $4250, which together with all the indirect costs for extra days of care and supplies made a total hospital bill of about $170,000.

The causes of diarrhea in tube-fed patients are many, but in the hands of a skilled nutritional support team, the formula is seldom one of them. It is often found in the medications. Just remember what this medication's hidden ingredient—sorbitol—cost Max.

REFERENCES

Benya R, Mobarhan S: Enteral alimentation administration and complications, *J Am Coll Nutr* 10(3):209, 1991.

Bliss DZ and others: Defining and reporting diarrhea in tube-fed patients—what a mess! *Am J Clin Nutr* 55:753, 1992.

Bokus S: Troubleshooting your tube feedings, *Am J Nurs* 91:24, May, 1991.

Frankenfield DC, Beyer PL: Dietary fiber and bowel function in tube-fed patients, *J Am Diet Assoc* 91(5):590, 1991.

Guenter PA and others: Tube feeding–related diarrhea in acutely ill patients, *J Parenter Enteral Nutr* 15(3):277, 1991.

Hill DB and others: Osmotic diarrhea induced by sugar-free theophylline solution in critically ill patients, *J Parenter Enteral Nutr* 15(3):332, 1991.

CHAPTER 19

Gastrointestinal Diseases

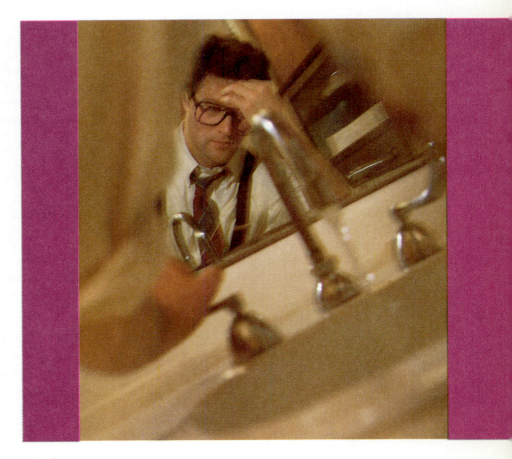

In this chapter, we consider diseases of the gastrointestinal tract and its surrounding accessory organs, the liver, gallbladder, and pancreas. In health, the digestion and absorption of our food is accomplished by a series of intimately interrelated actions of these organ systems. To the extent that disease or malfunction at any point interferes with this finely meshed process, nutritional therapy must modify food intake accordingly.

However, surrounding every stomach is a person. The gastrointestinal tract is a sensitive mirror of the individual human condition. Its physiologic function reflects physical and psychologic conditioning.

Thus, here we relate these basic functions and the healing process not only to the nutritional therapy indicated but also to the individual's personal needs.

Nutritional Management

When food is taken into the mouth, the act of eating stimulates the gastrointestinal tract into accelerated action. Throughout the digestive process, highly coordinated systems and interactive functions respond (see Chapter 5, Fig. 5-1). Secretory functions provide the necessary environment and agents for chemical digestion and move the food mass along. Absorptive functions carry the released nutrients through the body's circulation and nourish the cells. Psychologic factors influence the overall individual response pattern. This highly individual and interrelated functional network forms the basis for nutritional therapy in disease or malfunction.

After food is taken into the mouth, masticated, and swallowed, the esophagus conducts the food mass to the stomach by peristalsis and gravity. The gastroesophageal sphincter muscle at the entry to the stomach forms a controlling valve. It relaxes to receive the food, then closes to hold each bolus for digestive action of enzymes in the gastric acid mix. Then a number of small intestine and accessory organ conditions may interfere with normal food passage and create malabsorption problems. These overall conditions vary widely from brief periods of functional discomfort to serious disease and complete obstruction. Nutritional therapy in any case is adapted to the degree of dysfunction in choice and feeding mode.

Problems of the Mouth and Esophagus
Mouth Problems
Tissue Inflammation

The tissues of the mouth often reflect a person's basic nutritional status. In malnutrition they deteriorate and become inflamed, more vulnerable to local infection or injury, causing pain and difficulty with eating. These conditions in the oral cavity include (1) gingivitis, inflammation of the gums, involving the mucous membrane with its supporting fibrous tissue circling the base of the teeth; (2) stomatitis, inflammation of the oral mucosa lining the mouth; (3) glossitis, inflammation of the tongue; and (4) cheilosis, a cracking and dry scaling process at the corners of the mouth affecting the lips and corner angles, making opening the mouth to receive food difficult.

These oral tissue problems may also be nonspecific and unrelated to nutritional factors. In some cases, gingivitis and stomatitis occur in mild form in relation to another disease or to stress. Occasionally a severe form of acute necrotizing ulcerative gingivitis occurs. It is caused by a specific infectious bacterium *Fusobacterium nucleatum,* often in conjunction with a spirochete *Treponema vincentii,* and is also known as Vincent's disease, from the Paris physician Henri Vincent (1862-1950), who first identified the disease process. The gums around the bases of the teeth become puffy, shiny, and tender, overlapping the teeth margins. Affected gums often bleed, especially during tooth brushing. This is a serious condition that destroys gum tissue and the supporting tissues of the teeth, and requires a course of antibiotic treatment.

Food intake in these mouth conditions often decreases because of the pain. Maintaining adequate nutrition then becomes a major problem. Generally, patients are given high-protein, high-kcalorie liquids and then soft foods, usually nonacidic and without strong spices to avoid irritation. Temperature extremes may also be avoided if they cause pain. The diet is gradually advanced to unrestricted foods according to individual toleration and is often supplemented with vitamins. In severe disease, the use before meals of a mouthwash containing a mild topical local anesthetic helps relieve the pain of eating.

Dental Problems

The incidence of dental caries has recently been reduced in children and young adults. However, it is still present in many older adults, especially those unable to afford regular dental care, and causes tooth loss and chewing problems. In older adults, some 65 million in the United States alone, periodontal disease is a major cause of tooth loss.[1] Especially if dental caries is untreated, or if dental hygiene is poor, gum tissue at the base of the teeth becomes damaged and pockets form between the gums and the teeth. Dental plaque forms from a sticky deposit of mucus, food particles, and bacteria. The plaque hardens into calculus, a mineralized coating developed from the plaque and saliva. These hardened particles then collect in the pocket openings at the base of the teeth, where the bacteria attack the periodontal tissue. The result is bacterial erosion of bone tissue surrounding affected teeth and subsequent tooth loss. Preventive care, of course, through daily dental care with fluoridated toothpaste, careful flossing, and periodic plaque removal by the dentist and dental hygienist is the best approach. Extensive tooth loss leads to the need for replacement by dentures. In many elderly people these dentures become ill fitting and hinder adequate chewing. All of these dental problems need to be reviewed in any patient's nutritional history so that food textures and forms can be adjusted to individual needs.

Salivary Glands and Salivation

Disorders of the salivary glands affect eating, because saliva carries an amylase that begins starch breakdown and is vital in moistening the food to facilitate chew-

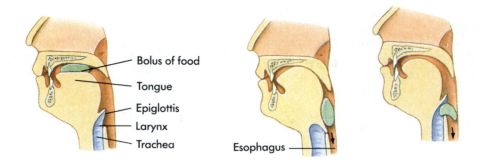

FIG. 19-1   Parts of mouth, pharynx, and esophagus involved in the swallowing process.

ing. Problems may arise from infection, such as the mumps virus that attacks the parotid gland. Other problems come from excessive salivation, which occurs in numerous disorders affecting the nervous system such as Parkinson's disease and from local disorders such as mouth infections or injury. It may arise from any disease or drug that causes overactivity of the parasympathetic division of the autonomic nervous system, which controls the salivary glands.

Conversely, lack of salivation, which causes dry mouth, may be a temporary condition caused by fear, salivary gland infection, or action of anticholinergic drugs that hinder the normal action of neurotransmitters. Permanent dry mouth is rare but does occur in Sjögren syndrome, a symptom complex of unknown cause that is thought to be an abnormal immune response. It occurs in middle-age older women and is marked by xerostomia (dry mouth), enlargement of the parotid glands, and is often associated with rheumatoid arthritis. It may also result from radiation therapy. There is difficulty in swallowing and speaking, interference with taste, and tooth decay. The extreme mouth dryness may be partially relieved by spraying the inside of the mouth with an artificial saliva solution.

Swallowing Disorders

The process of swallowing involves highly integrated actions of the mouth, pharynx, and esophagus (Fig. 19-1). Swallowing difficulty, known medically as dysphagia, is a fairly common problem with a wide variety of causes. It may be only temporary, as a piece of food lodged in the back of the throat, for which the **Heimlich maneuver** is appropriate first aid, or it may be involved with insufficient production of saliva and xerostomia. Such dysfunctional swallowing often causes children and adults alike to aspirate food particles, in turn causing coughing and choking episodes. The problem is usually referred to a special interdisciplinary team providing care.[1-3] The team includes physician, nurse, clinical dietitian, physical therapist, and especially the occupational therapist, who has had special training in swallowing problems.[1] Thin liquids are the most diffi-

cult food form to swallow, so various foods, such as baby rice cereal, and commercial agents are used for thickening liquids for individuals with dysphagia.[4,5]

Esophageal Problems
Central Problems

The esophagus is a long, muscular tube lined with mucous membranes that extends from the pharynx, or throat, to the stomach (Fig. 19-1). It is bounded on both ends by circular muscles, or sphincters, that act as valves to control food passage. The upper sphincter remains closed except during swallowing, thus preventing airflow into the esophagus and stomach. Disorders along the tube that may disrupt normal swallowing and food passage include esophageal spasm, uncoordinated contractions of the esophagus; esophageal stricture, a narrowing caused by a scar from previous inflammation or ingestion of caustic chemicals or a tumor; and esophagitis, an inflammation. These problems hinder eating and require medical attention through dilation, stretching procedures or surgery to widen the tube, and drug therapy.

Lower Esophageal Sphincter Problems

Defects in the operation of the lower esophageal sphincter (LES) muscles may come from changes in the smooth muscle itself or from the nerve-muscle hormonal control. In general, these LES problems arise from spasm, stricture, or incompetence.

Heimlich maneuver • A first-aid maneuver to relieve a person who is choking from blockage of the breathing passageway by a swallowed foreign object or food particle. Standing behind the person, clasp the victim around the waist, placing one fist just under the sternum (breastbone) and grasping the fist with the other hand. Then make a quick, hard, thrusting movement inward and upward.

TABLE 19-1

Dietary Principles for Care of Achalasia

Principles	Foods included
Energy nutrients	Moderate protein and carbohydrates and increased fat to help reduce LES pressure and gastric section
Texture	Liquid or semisolid food as tolerated
	Moderate to low fiber if it aids swallowing
Temperature	No very hot or very cold foods
Irritants	No citrus juices to injure mucosa if retained
	No highly spiced foods to irritate if retained
Meal pattern	Frequent, small meals as tolerated
Eating pace	Eat slowly in small bites and swallows

Adapted from Zeman FJ, Ney DM: *Applications of clinical nutrition,* Englewood Cliffs, NJ, 1988, Prentice Hall.

Spasms occur when the LES muscles maintain an excessively high muscle tone, even while resting, and thus fail to open normally when the person swallows. This condition is called **achalasia,** from its unrelaxed muscle state. It is also known as cardiospasm, from the proximity of the heart, although it has no relation at all to heart action. Patient symptoms include swallowing problems, frequent vomiting, a feeling of fullness in the chest, weight loss from eating difficulty, serious malnutrition, and pulmonary complications and infection caused by aspiration of food particles, especially during sleep hours.

Surgical treatment involves dilating the LES or slitting the muscle, an esophagomyotomy, which improves the stricture but not the peristalsis. Postoperative course starts with oral liquids and progresses to a regular diet within a few days according to toleration. General guidelines for nutritional management are given in Table 19-1.

Gastroesophageal Reflux Disease

Ongoing lower LES problems lead to chronic gastroesophageal reflux disease (GERD). Clinicians view this situation of "acid setting up shop in the esophagus" as serious and difficult as peptic ulcer disease in the stomach and duodenum for both the patient and the physician.[6] The true incidence of GERD is uncertain because many cases go undetected, and it is estimated that only the tip of the iceberg of chronic sufferers are seen clinically.[7] Regurgitation of the acid gastric contents into the lower part of the esophagus creates constant tissue irritation. The acid and pepsin cause tissue erosion with symptoms of substernal burning, cramping, pressure sensation, or severe pain. Symptoms are aggravated by lying down or by any increase of abdominal pressure, such as that caused by tight clothing. The condition is related to (1) an incompetent (lacking strength and ability, nonfunctioning) gastroesophageal sphincter, (2) frequency and duration of the acid reflux, and (3) inability of the esophagus to produce normal secondary peristaltic waves to prevent prolonged contact of the mucosa with the acid pepsin. A hiatal hernia may or may not be present.

Clinical symptoms. The most common symptom is **pyrosis,** a frequently severe heartburn, occurring 30 to 60 minutes after eating. U.S. surveys report that this common symptom occurs in 33% of persons with GERD at least once a month and in 7% daily.[7] Sometimes substernal pain radiates into the neck and jaw or down the arms. In addition to hiatal hernia, the acid reflux may be caused by pregnancy, obesity, pernicious vomiting, or nasogastric tubes. Other symptoms include iron deficiency anemia with chronic bleeding and aspiration, which may cause cough, dyspnea, or pneumonitis.

Complications. The most common complications are *stenosis* and esophageal ulcer. Also, significant **gastritis** in the herniated portion of the stomach may cause **occult bleeding.**

TABLE 19-2

Dietary Care of Gastroesophageal Reflux

Outcome	Action
Decrease esophageal irritation	Avoid common irritants such as coffee, carbonated beverages, tomato and citrus juices, and spicy foods
	Avoid any foods such as rich desserts that may cause heartburn
Increase lower esophageal sphincter pressure	Increase protein foods
	Decrease fat to about 45 g/day or less; use nonfat milk
	Avoid strong tea, coffee, and chocolate if poorly tolerated
	Avoid peppermint and spearmint
Decrease reflux frequency and volume	Eat small, frequent meals
	Sip only a small amount of liquid with meal; drink mostly between meals
	Avoid constipation; straining increases abdominal pressure reflux
Clear food materials from the esophagus	Sit upright at the table or elevate the head of bed
	Do not recline for 2 hours or more after eating

Adapted from Zeman FJ, Ney DM: *Applications of clinical nutrition,* Englewood Cliffs, NJ, 1988, Prentice Hall.

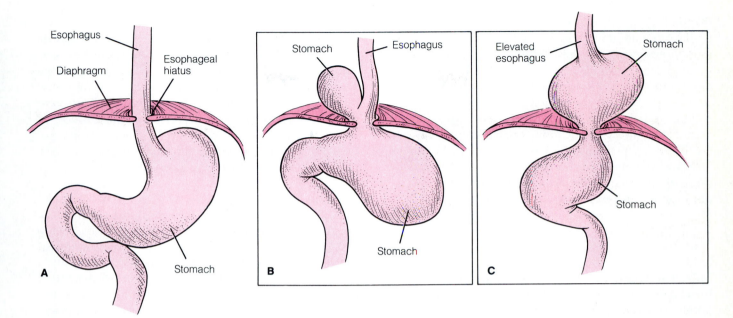

FIG. 19-2   Hiatal hernia compared with normal stomach placement. **A,** Normal stomach. **B,** Paraesophageal hernia (esophagus in normal position). **C,** Esophageal hiatal hernia (elevated esophagus).

Treatment.   Obesity is often a precipitating factor. Thus weight reduction is essential. The patient must avoid lying down immediately after eating and must sleep with the head of the bed elevated. Frequent use of antacids helps control the symptoms. From 85% to 90% of the patients respond to weight reduction and conservative measures. Table 19-2 summarizes these management principles.

Hiatal Hernia

The esophagus normally enters the chest cavity at the hiatus, an opening in the diaphragmatic membrane, and immediately joins the upper portion of the stomach. A hiatal hernia occurs when a portion of the upper part of the stomach at this entry point of the esophagus protrudes through the hiatus alongside the lower portion of the esophagus (Fig. 19-2). Food is easily held in this herniated area of the stomach and mixed with acid and pepsin, then it is regurgitated back up into the lower part of the esophagus. Gastritis can occur in this herniated portion of the stomach, as indicated, and cause bleeding and anemia. The reflux of gastric acid contents causes symptoms similar to those described above. Since obesity is frequently associated with hiatal hernia, weight reduction is a primary need. Avoiding tight clothing helps relieve discomfort. Patients will need to avoid leaning over or lying down immediately after meals and should sleep with the head of the bed elevated. Antacids help relieve the burning sensation. Large hiatal hernias or smaller sliding hernias may require surgical repair.

Problems of the Stomach and Duodenum: Peptic Ulcer Disease

Incidence

Peptic ulcer disease was uncommon in the previous century, but began to increase greatly during the early part of the 1990s. In the 1940s at least 10% to 15% of men were reported to have duodenal ulcers, with unreported cases in women and children adding to those figures.[8] The increase seems to have peaked about the mid-1950s, due to increased knowledge of the disease process and rapid progress in its medical management over the past 15 to 20 years. Possible genetic implications appear from the fact that about 40% of the adults and 50% of the children affected have strong family histories of peptic ulcer disease.[9] Yet in spite of the re-

achalasia • Failure to relax the smooth muscle fibers of the gastrointestinal tract at any point of juncture of its parts; especially failure of the esophagogastric sphincter to relax when swallowing, due to degeneration of ganglion cells in the wall of the organ. The lower esophagus also loses its normal peristaltic activity. Also called cardiospasm.

gastritis • Inflammation of the stomach.

occult bleeding • Obscure, difficult to detect, concealed from observation; such a small blood loss that it can be detected only by a microscope or chemical test.

pyrosis • Heartburn.

markable progress in knowledge and care, peptic ulcer remains a common, chronic, and recurring disease, most prevalent of the gastrointestinal diseases.[8] Now, with an aging population, an increasing number of older adult patients have the disease. The physiologic stress of illness and the added psychologic stress contribute to stress erosive gastritis and stress ulceration.[10-12] Major complications of peptic ulcer disease are bleeding, perforation, and obstruction, but these are rare with modern management. Less than 2% of the patients under treatment experience such a complication in any given year.[8]

Etiology

Peptic ulcer is the general term for an eroded mucosal lesion in the central portion of the gastrointestinal tract. The areas affected include the lower portion of the esophagus, the stomach, and the first portion of the duodenum, the duodenal bulb. Esophageal and gastric ulcers are less common. Most ulcers occur in the duodenal bulb, where gastric contents emptying into the duodenum through the pyloric valve are most concentrated. Gastric ulcers occur usually along the lesser curvature of the stomach. Peptic ulcer itself is a **benign** disease. Gastric ulcers, however, are more prone to develop into **malignant** disease.

In the past few years clinicians have seen a revolution in an understanding of the pathophysiology of peptic ulcer disease.[13,14] Three basic causative factors prevail.[15]

Gastric Acid and Pepsin

There is hypersecretion of gastric hydrochloric acid and pepsinogen, which the acid quickly converts to the strong active protein enzyme pepsin. The amount of acid varies, but the classic medical dictum—"no acid, no ulcer"—still holds.

Nonsteroidal Antiinflammatory Drugs (NSAIDs)

Widely used NSAIDs, the most commonly known of which is ibuprofen (Advil, Motrin), as well as the common analgesic aspirin (acetylsalicylic acid, ASA), irritate the gastric mucosa and cause bleeding, erosion, and ulceration, especially with prolonged or excessive use. The NSAID group of drugs are so named to distinguish them from the corticosteroids, synthetic variants of the natural adrenal hormones. The NSAIDs include a dozen antiinflammatory drugs.

Helicobacter pylori *Infection*

H. pylori are common spiraling, rod-shaped bacteria inhabiting the gastrointestinal area around the pyloric valve, the lower gastric antrum, and the upper duodenal bulb. Infection by this organism is a major determinant of chronic active gastritis. Mounting evidence indicates that it is a necessary ingredient, along with acid and pepsin, in the ulcerative process.

Clinical Symptoms

Basic symptoms of peptic ulcer are increased gastric tone and painful hunger contractions when the stomach is empty. In duodenal ulcer, the amount and concentration of hydrochloric acid is increased. In gastric ulcer it may be normal. Nutritional deficiencies are evident in low plasma protein levels, anemia, and loss of weight. Hemorrhage may be the first sign in some patients. Diagnosis is based on clinical findings, x-ray tests, or visualization by fiberoptic gastroscopy.

Medical Management

In treating patients with peptic ulcer disease, the physician has four basic goals: (1) to alleviate the symptoms, (2) to promote healing, (3) to prevent recurrences, and (4) to prevent complications. In addition to general traditional measures, the recently expanded knowledge base and development of a number of new drugs have increased the physician's available management tools.

General Therapeutic Measures

Adequate rest, relaxation, and sleep have long been a foundation for general care of peptic ulcer disease to enhance the body's natural healing process. Positive stress coping and relaxation skills, which help patients deal with personal psychosocial stressors, can be learned and practiced. Simple encouragement to talk about anxieties, anger, and frustrations helps to make patients feel better, and as soon as they are able, appropriate physical activity helps work out tensions. Habits that contribute to ulcer development, such as smoking and alcohol use, should be eliminated. Common drugs such as aspirin and NSAIDs should be avoided.

Drug Therapy

Current medical management of peptic ulcer disease has a wider choice of drugs to control underlying physiologic causes and clinical symptoms and to support healing. In various ways, five types of drugs now suppress gastric acid and pepsin secretion, protect mucosal tissue, buffer acid, and eliminate infection.

- *Histamine H_2-receptor antagonists:* These agents, commonly called H_2-blockers, are popular drugs for controlling gastric acid secretion. They competitively block the cell entry and function of histamine. Normally histamine attaches to its specific cellular **receptors** (type H_2) on the acid-producing parietal cells of the gastric mucosa and mediate their secretion of hydrochloric acid. Thus their blocking action effectively controls acid and pepsin because the inactive pepsinogen requires the acid for activation. Two examples of these drugs are cimetidine (Tagamet) and ranitidine (Zantac).
- *Proton pump inhibitors:* This new class of drugs, more potent than the H_2-blockers, also suppresses gastric acid, but by a different action. Without competi-

tion, they irreversibly prevent action of a key enzyme that actively secretes hydrogen ions needed for hydrochloric acid (HCl) production. Without available H+ ions, the HCl cannot be made. Then, without the acid, ulcers heal rapidly. Thus far the first drug of this type to be approved for use with ulcers resistent to convential therapy is omeprazole.

- *Mucosal protectors:* Drugs of this type act as cytoprotective agents by helping the stomach heal itself. They produce a gellike suspension that binds to the ulcer base and covers it and the surrounding normal mucosal tissue to protect the involved tissue from from harm while it heals.[16] This drug also forms complexes with pepsin that inactivate the pepsin.[13,14] An example of this type of drug is sucralfate.
- *Antacids:* These well-known substances counteract or neutralize acidity. Usually, magnesium-aluminum compounds, such as Mylanta II or Maalox TC (therapeutic choice) are the antacids of choice in treating peptic ulcer disease. This type of drugs is effective and relatively safe when used properly.[17]
- *Antibiotics:* Drugs of this type are used to control the *H. pylori* infection associated with peptic ulcer disease. Although the organism is easily suppressed, it seems to be more difficult to eradicate.[13,14] However, combinations of these agents being used include drugs such as amoxicillin or tetracycline, metronidazole (a bacterial and protozoan killer), and bismuth.

Other drugs for general needs include acetaminophen (Tylenol) to replace aspirin or NSAIDs. Also, if needed briefly for mild sedation to aid the initial need for relaxation and sleep, a tricyclic antidepressant such as amitriptyline (Elavil) may be prescribed.

The main challenge now is to develop a maintenance therapy that prevents recurrence of the disease.[18] Currently the best approach seems to include continuous low-dose drug therapy, intermittent full-dose treatment, or symptomatic self-care with the same agents used to heal the ulcer. Success rates hinge on the relative strengths of risk factors that influence recurrence (Table 19-3).

Nutritional Management

The revolutionary advance in knowledge of peptic ulcer disease and development of drugs for its medical management have also brought welcome reevaluation of the role of nutrition in its basic care. There is now both medical and nutritional agreement that the old restrictive bland milk-based diet routines of the past, long since known to be ineffective and potentially harmful, have no role in the modern management of peptic ulcer disease.[13,14,19] Instead, a positive nutrition approach and basic dietary principles guide our current practice.

Current Positive Nutrition Approach

The current nutritional practice is that of basic health maintenance or preventive approach in overall health care today.[20] As with any disease process involving tissue injury, the prime nutritional requirement is clear: sufficient energy-nutrient intake supplied by a regular well-balanced diet to support the primary medical management of (1) tissue healing and (2) tissue maintenance of structural and functional integrity. Initial and periodic nutritional assessment is needed to determine energy-nutrient status and any area of individual need.

Dietary Principles

The basic nutrition principles of a well-balanced diet are found in the regular guidelines of the RDA energy-nutrient standards and the U.S. Dietary Guidelines for health promotion (see Chapter 1). In addition to the major goal of optimal nutritional support, a second dietary goal is to avoid stimulating excess acid secretion and directly irritating the gastric mucosa. Only a few related food factors or habits have been shown to cause excess acid secretion and irritation:

- *Meal pattern:* Eat three regular meals a day without

TABLE 19-3

Recurrent Peptic Ulcer Risk Factors

Chance of recurrence	Risk factors
Possible	Positive family history
	Emotional stress
	Continued use of concentrated alcohol
Good	History of recurrences and complications
	Continued use of aspirin and other NSAIDs
	Increased *Helicobacter pylori* infection
Strong	Poor compliance with maintenance diet-drug plan
	Continued smoking (10 or more cigarettes/day)
	Gastric acid hypersecretion

Adapted from Earnest DL: Maintenance therapy in peptic ulcer disease, *Med Clin North Am* 75(4):1013, 1991.

---

benign • Not malignant or recurrent; favorable for recovery.

malignant • An abnormal condition such as a tumor, that tends to become progressively worse and results in death.

receptor • Any one of various specific protein molecules in surface membranes of cells and cell organelles, to which complementary molecules, such as hormones, neurotransmitters, drugs, viruses, or other antigens or antibodies, may become bound.

frequent snacks, especially at bedtime. Any food intake stimulates more acid output.

- *Food quantity:* Avoid stomach distention with large quantities of food at a meal.
- *Milk intake:* Avoid drinking milk frequently. It stimulates significant gastric acid secretion, has only a transient buffering effect, and its animal fat content is undesirable. Also, the milk sugar lactose creates problems of abdominal cramping, gas, and diarrhea for many persons with lactose intolerance caused by a deficiency of the enzyme lactase (see Chapter 2).
- *Seasonings:* Individual tolerance is the rule. However, several agents have caused variable results and may need to be watched: hot chili peppers, black pepper, and chili powder.
- *Dietary fiber:* There is no evidence for restricting dietary fiber. Some fibers, especially soluble forms, are beneficial.
- *Coffee:* Avoid regular and decaffeinated coffee. Coffee stimulates acid secretion and may cause dyspepsia. The comparative effect of regular tea and colas may be milder with some persons, but these beverages also stimulate acid secretion.
- *Citric acid juices:* These juices may induce gastric reflux and discomfort in some persons.
- *Alcohol:* Avoid alcohol in concentrated forms, such as 40% (80 proof) alcohol. Other less concentrated forms of wine, taken with food in moderate amounts, are tolerated well by some patients. Avoid beer; it has been shown to be a potent stimulant of gastric acid. For patients who find it particularly difficult to avoid alcohol and coffee completely, some physicians have suggested they may try a small serving of wine with dinner occasionally, or a small cup (*demitasse*) of coffee at the close of the meal to minimize the acid secretion.
- *Smoking:* The habit of smoking is often associated with food intake. It is best eliminated completely at any time. It not only affects gastric acid secretion but also influences the effectiveness of drug therapy.
- *Food environment:* Finally, consider the food environment. Eat slowly and savor the food in a calm environment. Respect individual responses or tolerances to specific foods experienced at any time. Remember that the same food may evoke different responses at different times depending on the stress factor.

Personal Focus

Sound nutritional management plays an important supportive role in the total medical care of persons with peptic ulcer disease. The individual must be the focus of treatment. The patient is not "an ulcer," but a person with an ulcer. The course of the disease is conditioned by the patient's unique makeup and life situation. And the presence of the ulcer in turn affects the patient's life. In the long run, a wide range of foods, attractive to the eye and the taste, and regular, unhurried eating habits provide the best course of action.

Small Intestine Diseases

Conditions of Malabsorption and Diarrhea
General Diarrhea

General diarrhea may result from basic dietary excesses. There may be fermentation of sugars involved or excess fiber stimulation of intestinal muscle function.[21] In other cases it may result from a specific food-borne infectious organism or from acute food poisoning with bacterial toxin (see Chapter 9). In the case of lactose intolerance, the accumulated concentration of undigested lactose in the intestine, due to lack of the enzyme lactase, creates increased osmotic pressure. This pressure effectively draws water into the gut and stimulates hypermotility, abdominal cramping, and diarrhea (see Chapters 2 and 8). Milk treated with lactase enzyme is tolerated by these persons without the difficulty encountered with regular milk. Secretory, osmotic, and inflammatory processes in the intestine result in increased losses of fluid and electrolytes from diarrhea (see Issues and Answers, p. 383).[22]

Malabsorption

There are multiple causes of a malabsorption condition.[23] Some of these causes include the following:
- *Maldigestion problems:* Pancreatic disorders, biliary disease, bacterial overgrowth, ileal disease (inflammatory bowel disease)
- *Intestinal mucosal changes:* Mucosal surface alterations, intestinal surgery such as resections that shorten the bowel, lymphatic obstruction, intestinal stasis
- *Genetic disease:* Cystic fibrosis with its complications of pancreatic insufficiency and lack of the pancreatic enzymes lipase, trypsin, and amylase
- *Intestinal enzyme deficiency:* Lactose intolerance caused by lactase deficiency (see Chapter 2)
- *Cancer and its treatment:* Absorbing surface effect of radiation and chemotherapy (see Chapter 25)
- *Metabolic biochemical defects:* Absorbing surface effects of pernicious anemia or gluten-induced enteropathy (celiac sprue)

Here we briefly review four of these malabsorptive conditions—celiac sprue, cystic fibrosis, inflammatory bowel disease, and short bowel syndrome.

Celiac Sprue
Metabolic Defect

In 1889 a London physician named Gee observed a number of malnourished children having extensive fatty diarrhea, steatorrhea, and distended abdomens. He gave the name "celiac" to the general clinical condition from the Greek word *kolia,* meaning "belly" or "abdomen." It was not until the mid-1950s that the Dutch pediatrician Dicke and his associates discovered the causative agent. Their tissue studies confirmed that the gliadin fraction of the protein gluten in wheat produced the fat malabsorption, and further that what had been called celiac disease in children and nontropical sprue in adults was a single disease, thus called now celiac sprue.[24] As currently used, the alternate terms *celiac disease* and *gluten-sensitive enteropathy* are synonymous with celiac sprue. In all cases, such diseased tissues consistently show an eroded mucosal surface lacking the number and form of normal villi and having few microvilli. This erosion effectively reduces the absorbing surface by as much as 95%.

Studies thus far clearly show that gluten somehow interacts with and damages the intestinal mucosa, but the primary mechanism remains obscure.[24] Current investigations indicate a biochemical metabolic defect probably involving an enzyme deficiency and a genetic

base. It is now apparent that the steatorrhea (about 80% of the ingested fat appears in the stools) and the progressive malnutrition are secondary effects caused by the primary biochemical reaction to gliadin in sensitive persons.

Nutritional Management

The goal of nutritional management is to control the dietary gluten and prevent malnutrition. The diet is better defined as low gluten rather than gluten free, since it is impossible to remove all the gluten completely and usually a small amount is tolerated by most patients. Wheat and rye are the main sources of gluten; it is also present in oats and barley. Thus these four grains are eliminated from the diet. Corn and rice are the substitute grains used. Parents of children with this condition need special instructions about food products to avoid, what constitutes a basic meal pattern, and recipes for food preparation. Careful label-reading habits must be discussed, since many commercial products use the offending grains as thickeners or fillers, and parents' knowledge of gluten-containing food products

---

TABLE 19-4

Low-Gluten Diet for Children with Celiac Disease

Dietary principles

- K-calories—high, usually about 20% above normal requirement, to compensate for fecal loss
- Protein—high, usually 6 to 8 g/kg body weight
- Fat—low, but not fat-free, because of impaired absorption
- Carbohydrates—simple, easily digested sugars (fruits, vegetables) should provide about one half of the kcalories
- Feedings—small, frequent feedings during ill periods; afternoon snack for older children
- Texture—smooth, soft, avoiding irritating roughage initially, using strained foods longer than usual for age, adding whole foods as tolerated and according to age of child
- Vitamins—supplements of B vitamins, vitamins A and B in water-miscible forms, and vitamin C
- Minerals—iron supplements if anemia is present

Food groups	Foods included	Foods excluded
Milk	Milk (plain or flavored with chocolate or cocoa) Buttermilk	Malted milk; preparations such as Cocomalt, Hemo, Postum, Nestle's chocolate
Meat or substitute	Lean meat, trimmed well of fat Eggs, cheese Poultry, fish Creamy peanut butter (if tolerated)	Fat meats (sausage, pork) Luncheon meats, corned beef, frankfurters, all common prepared meat products with any possible wheat filler Duck, goose Smoked salmon Meat prepared with bread, crackers, or flour
Fruits and juices	All cooked and canned fruits and juices Frozen or fresh fruits as tolerated, avoiding skins and seeds	Prunes, plums (unless tolerated)
Vegetables	All cooked, frozen, canned as tolerated (prepared *without* wheat, rye, oat, or barley products); raw as tolerated	Any causing individual discomfort All prepared with wheat, rye, oat, or barley products
Cereals	Corn or rice	Wheat, rye, oat, barley; any product containing these cereals
Breads, flours, cereal products	Breads, pancakes, or waffles made with suggested flours (cornmeal, cornstarch; rice, soybean, lima bean, potato, buckwheat)	All bread or cracker products made with gluten; wheat, rye, oat, barley, macaroni, noodles, spaghetti; any sauces, soups, or gravies prepared with gluten flour, wheat, rye, oat, or barley
Soups	Broth, bouillon (no fat or cream; no thickening with wheat, rye, oat, or barley products); soups and sauces may be thickened with cornstarch	All soups containing wheat, rye, oat, or barley products

is highly variable and influences the child's attitudes toward dietary compliance.[25] With an increasing number of processed foods being marketed, as well as increasing use of ethnic foods in Western society, it is difficult to detect all foods containing gluten, so a home test kit for gluten has been developed.[26] Good dietary management varies according to the child's age, pathologic conditions, and clinical status. Generally, a dietary program based on the low-gluten diet given in Table 19-4 may be followed. In a small subgroup of patients, the symptoms persist despite strict adherence to the diet. In rare instances, persons with such a refractory form of the disease respond only to parenteral nutrition support.[24]

Cystic Fibrosis
Genetic-Metabolic Defect

Cystic fibrosis is inherited as an autosomal recessive trait mainly in white populations in which 1 in 20 is a carrier and now 1 in 2500 newborns is affected.[27] It occurs rarely in other populations, for example, 1 in 17,000 black live births and 1 in 90,000 Asian live births. It is the most common fatal genetic disease in North America. In past years, children carrying the disease have generally lived to about age 10, dying from complications such as chronic obstructive pulmonary disease with progressive damage to airway epithelial cells and pancreatic insufficiency from fibrosis and resulting lack of pancreatic enzymes. Improved management of the disease based on increasing scientific knowledge has helped push the life expectancy up into the 30s. Currently, a screening test for newborns helps detect the disease early. Then early intervention and support by a skilled cystic fibrosis team of health care specialists can accurately assess individual needs, help families cope, and develop an appropriate therapeutic plan.[27,28]

In the summer of 1989 the cystic fibrosis gene was discovered, and shortly thereafter continuing studies disclosed the underlying biochemical defect.[29,30] The normal gene's large protein product, composed of 1480 amino acids in five domains (see Chapter 4), controls the opening and closing of ion channels that actively transport chloride ions across epithelial cell membranes. Scientists have named this large protein for its function, cystic fibrosis transmembrane conductance regulator (CFTR).[30] The mutant cystic fibrosis gene cannot produce this controlling protein product CFTR. Thus because of the resulting defective epithelial ion transport, chloride is trapped in the cells and excess sodium is also absorbed. This imbalance leads to the thickened mucus formation and clinical effects in the various organ systems involved.

Clinical Symptoms

The classic clinical symptoms of cystic fibrosis include the following effects in body organ systems[31,32]:

1. *Thick mucus in the lungs* that accumulates and clogs air passages, damages the epithelial tissue of these airways, and leads to chronic obstructive pulmonary disease (COPD) and frequent respiratory infections, both contributing to increased metabolism and increased energy-nutrient needs
2. *Pancreatic insufficiency* caused by progressive clogging of pancreatic ducts and functional tissue degeneration, resulting in lack of normal pancreatic enzymes protein-splitting trypsin, chymotrypsin, and carboxypeptidase, the fat-splitting lipase, and the starch-splitting amylase; progressive loss of functional insulin-producing beta cells in the islets of Langerhans, resulting in insulin-dependent diabetes mellitus (IDDM)
3. *Malabsorption* of undigested food nutrients and extensive malnutrition and stunted growth
4. *Biliary cirrhosis* caused by progressive clogging of bile ducts producing biliary obstruction and functional liver tissue degeneration
5. *Salt (NaCl) concentration* increased in the body perspiration, resulting in salt depletion

Nutritional Management

Current nutritional management of cystic fibrosis follows new guidelines developed by a consensus committee of the U.S. Cystic Fibrosis Foundation (CFF).[31] This more aggressive nutritional management program, used in all the CFF centers throughout the United States, results from three factors: (1) increased knowledge of the disease process, (2) early diagnosis and intervention, and (3) improved therapeutic products such as replacement pancreatic enzymes in the form of capsule-encased enteric-coated microspheres—(beads) that correct the maldigestion and help support energy-nutrient growth needs.[33] The overall goal is to support normal nutrition and growth for all ages. This management program is based on an initial and ongoing schedule for assessment, including anthropometrics, laboratory studies, and nutrition evaluation (Table 19-5). Related therapy is then outlined in five levels according to individual assessment results and nutritional care needs and actions (Table 19-6).[34] Directions for calculating energy needs for cystic fibrosis patients, basal metabolic rate (BMR) and daily energy requirements (DER), physical activity and disease status are included in Appendix M.

Inflammatory Bowel Disease
Nature and Incidence

The general term *inflammatory bowel disease (IBD)* is now used to apply to two intestinal conditions having similar symptoms but different underlying clinical problems—Crohn's disease and ulcerative colitis. Both of these conditions produce extended mucosal tissue lesions, although these lesions differ in extent and na-

TABLE 19-5

Basic Nutritional Assessment for Nutritional Management of Cystic Fibrosis

Key assessments	Monitoring schedule and indications		
Anthropometry		**Biochemical data**	
Weight	Every 3 months or as needed for growth evaluation and routine care	CBC†	Yearly routine care, interim as needed to detect deficiencies, iron status
Height (length)		TIBC,† serum iron, ferritin	
Head circumference (until age 2)		Plasma/serum retinol, alpha-tocopherol	
Midarm circumference		Albumin, prealbumin	As indicated, weight loss, growth failure, clinical deterioration
Triceps skin fold		Electrolytes, acid-base balance	Summer heat, prolonged fever
Midarm muscle circumference (derived)*			
		Dietary evaluation	
		Dietary intake	As indicated, history and food records, full energy-nutrient analysis
		3-day fat balance study‡	As indicated, weight loss, growth failure, clinical deterioration
		Anticipatory guidance	Yearly, interim as needed according to growth or situational needs

*See Chapter 16 for equations.
†*CBC*, Complete blood count; *TIBC*, total iron-binding capacity.
‡Three-day food records for analysis of fat intake; stool collections for analysis of fat content and degree of malabsorption.
Adapted from CFF consensus report; Ramsey B et al: Nutrition assessment and management in cystic fibrosis; a consensus report, *Am J Clin Nutr* 55:108, 1992.

TABLE 19-6

Levels of Nutritional Care for Management of Cystic Fibrosis

Levels of care	Patient groups	Nutrition actions
Level I—Routine care	All	Diet counseling, food plans, enzyme replacement, vitamin supplements, nutrition education, exploration of problems
Level II—Anticipatory guidance	Above 90% ideal weight-height index, but at risk of energy imbalance; severe pancreatic insufficiency, frequent pulmonary infections, normal periods of rapid growth	Increased monitoring of dietary intake, complete energy-nutrient analysis, increased kcaloric density as needed; assess behavioral needs; provide counseling, nutrition education
Level III—Supportive intervention	85%-90% ideal weight-height index, decreased weight-growth velocity	Reinforce all the above actions, add energy-nutrient–dense oral supplements
Level IV—Rehabilitative care	Consistently below 85% ideal weight-height index, nutritional and growth failure	All of the above plus enteral nutrition support by nasoenteric or enterostomy tube feeding (see Chapter 18)
Level V—Resuscitative or palliative care	Below 75% ideal weight-height index, progressive nutritional failure	All of the above plus continuous enteral tube feedings or TPN (see Chapter 18)

Adapted from CFF consensus report: Ramsey B et al: Nutrition assessment and management in cystic fibrosis: a consensus report, *Am J Clin Nutr* 55:108, 1992.

ture. However, they have been classed medically in a single group because they are similar in their clinical symptoms and management.[35,36] The incidence of these diseases, especially Crohn's disease, has increased worldwide. For example, a recent epidemiologic study in Denmark over a 25-year period indicated a sixfold increase in Crohn's disease, present in all ages and both sexes.[35] Crohn's disease is particularly prevalent in in-

dustrialized areas of the world. It also appears among otherwise low-risk persons who move from rural to urban centers. These factors suggest a role for pathogenic agents in the environment. Its incidence is highest among teenagers, with a secondary peak at ages 55 to 60. Although epidemiologic and clinical studies continue to advance knowledge of the disease processes involved, the precise causes of these two inflammatory bowel diseases remain unknown. Some evidence indicates that genetic factors may predispose persons to the development of IBD: (1) its increased incidence among children whose parents have IBD; (2) its incidence in certain close knit population groups; and (3) the high rate of IBD among identical twins as compared to fraternal twins.[37,38]

Ulcerative colitis and Crohn's disease have severe, often devastating tissue effects and nutritional consequences. But they can be distinguished by two main differences: (1) anatomic distribution of the inflammatory process and (2) the nature of tissue changes involved. First, Crohn's disease occurs in any part of the intestinal tract. In contrast, ulcerative colitis is confined to the colon and rectum. Second, in Crohn's disease, the inflammatory tissue changes become chronic and can involve any part of the intestinal wall and may penetrate the entire wall. Often this extensive tissue involvement leads to partial or complete obstruction and to **fistula** formation.[36] On the other hand, the tissue changes in ulcerative colitis are usually acute, lasting brief periods, and are limited to the mucosal and submucosal tissue layers of the intestinal wall.

Clinical Symptoms

A chronic bloody diarrhea is the most common clinical symptom, occurring at night as well as during the day. Ulceration of the mucous membrane of the intestine leads to various associated nutritional problems such as anorexia, nutritional edema, anemia, avitaminosis, protein losses, negative nitrogen balance, dehydration, and electrolyte disturbances. Clinicians have observed evidence of specific deficiencies of zinc and vitamin E, with improvement occurring when supplements of the particular nutrients involved are taken. There is general weight loss, often general malnutrition, fever, skin lesions, and arthritic joint involvement. In Crohn's disease, the overall malnutrition resembles kwashiorkor and is an important cause of abnormal immunologic function.[39]

Medical Management

The medical management of IBD centers on drug therapy to control the inflammatory process and promote healing. Ongoing development of new agents in addition to mainstays of the past hold even greater promise for future therapy.[36,40] Currently the physician has available three types of drugs to use in developing individual therapy for IBD: (1) a corticosteroid—prednisone, (2) an antiinflammatory agent—sulfasalazine, which is a combination of sulfapyridine and 5-aminosalicylic acid, and (3) an immunosuppressant agent especially for Crohn's disease—mercaptopurine.[36,41] Effects of these drugs become important aspects of planning supportive nutritional care.

Nutritional Management

Nutritional therapy centers on supporting the healing process and avoiding nutritional deficiency states. In serious conditions, enteral nutrition support includes elemental formulas of absorbable isotonic preparations of amino acids, glucose, fat, minerals, and vitamins. In patients who tolerate these feedings, there is diminished gastrointestinal protein loss and improved nutrition, accompanied by clinical remission. In cases where the small bowel has been shortened or the disease process is extensive, as in Crohn's disease, parenteral nutrition support (TPN) is most effective (see Chapter 18). Such vigorous nutritional therapy is particularly important in childhood to prevent severe growth retardation. Nutritional repletion improves symptoms dramatically. There is diminished gastrointestinal secretion and motility, decreased disease activity, relief of partial intestinal obstruction, occasional closure of enteric fistulas, and renewed immunocompetence. Nutritional supplements are usually necessary to avoid deficiencies in agents such as zinc, copper, chromium, selenium, and other nutrients.

General Continuing Nutritional Management

The emphasis of continuing treatment is to restore optimal nutrient intake, remove deficits, prevent local trauma to inflamed areas, and control less easily absorbed material such as fats. To help secure additional kcalories, medium-chain triglycerides (MCT), as in the commercial preparation MCT oil, may be used instead of regular fats. The focus of the diet centers on protein and energy, minerals and vitamins, and texture, with supplemental feedings as needed.

High protein. There are large losses of protein from the intestinal mucosal tissue by exudation and bleeding, as well as losses associated with impaired intestinal absorption. Healing can occur only if adequate protein is provided. The total diet must supply adequate protein, about 100 g/day in highly malnourished patients, for essential tissue synthesis and healing. Tasteful ways of including protein foods of high biologic value (eggs, meat, and cheese) can be devised to tempt poor appetites. Milk often causes difficulty with many patients, so it is usually omitted at first, then added as tolerated.

High energy. About 2500 to 3000 kcal/day are needed to restore nutritional deficits from daily losses in stools and consequent weight loss. Also, the negative nitrogen balance can be overcome only if sufficient kcalories are present to spare protein for tissue building.

Increased minerals and vitamins. When anemia is present, iron therapy is used. Extra vitamins needed for healing and the increased protein and energy metabolism should be added. These are the B vitamins, including thiamin, riboflavin, and niacin, and ascorbic acid. Trace minerals such as zinc, which participates in tissue synthesis, are needed along with vitamin E, which contributes to tissue integrity. Usually supplements of these vitamins and minerals are routine. Potassium therapy may be indicated if undue losses from diarrhea and tissue destruction occur, causing hypokalemia.

Dietary fiber control. Over the past years, on the belief that dietary fiber or residue would irritate the mucosal lining, a diet low in dietary fiber or residue has sometimes been used until healing is well established. However, the bland, low-residue diets are based on old literature, tradition, and studies on laboratory animals, inappropriately applied to humans, which some investigators even then seemed to suggest.[42,43] These unappetizing and often less than nourishing diets seem to have been based on past anecdotal accounts and beliefs rather than on human scientific study.[44] Current study and clinical practice indicate the benefit of a regular highly nourishing diet, respecting individual tolerances and disease status.[45]

Perhaps no other condition better illustrates the need for a close working relationship among the team of physician, clinical dietitian, nurse, and patient than does inflammatory bowel disease. The appetite is poor, but adequate nutritional intake is imperative. In many creative ways, individually explored and implemented, the fundamental therapeutic needs must be met. This is done through vigorous nutritional care using a range of feeding modes, including enteral or parenteral nutrition support as needed, always with personal supportive warmth and encouragement.[46-48]

Short Bowel Syndrome
Etiology

Short bowel syndrome is a pattern of varying metabolic and physiologic consequences of surgical removal of parts of the intestine with extensive dysfunction of the remaining portion of the organ.[49] The resections result from intrinsic disease such as Crohn's disease or radiation enteritis, surgical bypass, or massive abdominal injury and trauma. They may also be required for vascular problems such as blood clots leading to death of involved tissue, or for extensive fistulas, radiation injury, congenital abnormalities, or cancer.

Clinical Symptoms

Clearly, severity of the clinical problem remaining and the clinical symptoms vary with length and location of the remaining intestine and its mucosal integrity and function. Other factors include whether or not the ileocecal valve remains, and any disease of the colon. Consider the complex nature and functions of the

small intestine, for example (see Chapter 5). Its estimated length is between 12 and 20 ft (about 365 to 600 cm) and it receives every day about 7 to 10 L of nutrient-filled fluid. So efficiently does it do its specialized jobs along the way that only 100 to 200 cc of feces remains to be excreted. Now think of the metabolic impact if 80% or more of the ileum, which has a functional length of about 400 cm, is surgically removed. Among numerous other results, hepatic synthesis of bile cannot maintain the normal circulating bile pool to sustain normal fat digestion. Steatorrhea and a chain of metabolic events follow.[49] Also, without this normal enterohepatic circulation that occurs in the distal part of the ileum, the liver's usually efficient regulation of cholesterol is affected.[50]

Nutritional Management

Degrees of surgical resection create different problems. Thus the nutritional management of each short bowel syndrome patient must be tailored to individual functional capacity remaining. Early enteral or parenteral nutrition support usually supplies initial needs (see Chapter 18). Frequent monitoring of nutritional responses, especially fluid and electrolyte balances and malnutrition signs, is essential. Later weaning to an oral diet with vitamin and mineral supplementation follows as tolerated, with continued nutrition assessment. The common deficit of vitamin D (cholecalciferol) can be more easily met with its intermediate metabolic product, oral 25-hydroxycholecalciferol (see Chapter 7).[51] As adaptation progresses, the early restriction of fat may be liberalized somewhat with moderate use of the more easily absorbed medium-chain triglycerides (MCT oil) to obtain needed kcalories.

Large Intestine Diseases
Diverticular Disease
Nature and Etiology

A diverticulum is a small tubular sac protruding off from a main canal or cavity in the body. The formation and presence of these small diverticula protruding from the intestinal lumen, usually the colon, produces the condition diverticulosis. More often diverticulosis occurs in older adults. It develops at points of weakened musculature in the bowel wall, along the track of blood vessels entering the bowel from without. The direct cause is a progressive increase in pressure within the bowel from segmental circular muscle contractions that normally move the remaining food mass along and form the feces for elimination. When pressures become sufficiently high in one of these segments, and dietary fiber is insufficient to maintain the necessary bulk for preventing high internal pressures within the colon, diverticula, small protrusions of the muscle layer, develop at that point. The condition causes no problem unless the small diverticula become infected and inflamed from fecal irritation and colon bacteria. This diseased state is called **diverticulitis.** The commonly used collective term covering diverticulosis and diverticulitis is *diverticular disease.*

Clinical Symptoms

As the inflammatory process grows, increased hypermotility and pressures from luminal segmentation cause pain. The pain and tenderness are usually localized in the lower left side of the abdomen and are accompanied by nausea, vomiting, distention, diarrhea, intestinal spasm, and fever. If the process continues, intestinal obstruction or perforation may necessitate surgical intervention.

Nutritional Management

Diverticular disease is a common gastrointestinal disorder among middle-age and elderly persons. It may often be accompanied by malnutrition. Sensitive laboratory tests, such as prealbumin with a short half-life of only 2 days, should be included in initial and ongoing assessment of nutritional status to detect any degree of malnutrition (see Chapter 16). Aggressive nutritional therapy hastens recovery from an attack, shortens the hospital stay, and reduces costs.[52] Current studies and clinical practice have demonstrated better management of chronic diverticular disease with an increased amount of dietary fiber than with old practices of restricting fiber. In acute episodes of active disease, however, the amount of dietary fiber may need to be moderately reduced. The relationship of dietary fiber and diverticular disease has been further reinforced by studies of populations, such as those in Japan since the current westernizing of its culture. Chapter 3 provides an extended discussion of dietary fiber and its relation to health and disease.

Irritable Bowel Syndrome
Incidence and Etiology

Data from the second National Health and Nutrition Examination Survey (NHANES II, 1976-1980) indicated that almost 5 million Americans, about 3% of the population, self-reported problems consistent with the condition now called irritable bowel syndrome (IBS). The rates reported for women were 3.2 times those for men, 5.3 times higher for whites than for blacks, and highest among those ages 45 to 64 years.[53,54] Follow-up national surveys in the mid-1980s documented between 2.4 and 3.5 yearly visits to physicians for IBS and more than 2.2 million medications prescribed.[54] Currently, gastroenterologists estimate that 15% to 20% of the general U.S. population have symptoms of IBS, about 5% of whom seek medical help and become patients.[55] Although IBS is one of the most common of all gastrointestinal disorders, its precise nature and cause continue to puzzle practitioners.

Clinical Symptoms

A recent international working team report has more clearly defined IBS for medical diagnosis guidance as a functional, nonorganic disorder and has outlined its characteristic symptoms for general care.[56] The three major types of symptoms of IBS have been classified as (1) pain, chronic and recurrent, in any area of the abdomen; (2) bowel dysfunction, small volume, varying from constipation or diarrhea to an intermittent combination of both; and (3) flatulence, excess gas formation with increased distention and bloating, accompanied by rumbling abdominal sounds (borborygmi), belching, and passing of gas (see Chapter 5). Patients appear tense and anxious, and stress is a major triggering factor. Somatization, the transference of anxiety to body symptoms, is common in patients with IBS.[57]

Nutritional Management

A highly individual and personal approach to nutritional care of persons with IBS is essential. Initial nutrition assessment must include detailed personal history in relation to IBS attacks, the role of stress and any particular food associations, as well as living situation, personal concerns, and experiences related to attacks. Baseline measures for nutritional status should include the usual ABCD pattern (see Chapter 16). With this careful assessment and history as a base, a reasonable and appropriate food plan may be developed with the patient. Periodic food records and related symptoms can follow for continued counseling and adjustments. In general, the food plan gives attention to the following basic principles:

- *Increase dietary fiber:* A regular diet with optimal energy-nutrient composition and dietary fiber food sources—whole grains, legumes, fruits, and vegetables provides basic therapy (Table 19-7). Moderate supplemental dietary fiber may be used if needed, such as controlled amounts of bran or more soluble forms of bulking agents such as psyllium seed products (Metamucil).
- *Recognize gas formers:* Some foods are recognized gas formers for many people because of known constituents, such as certain oligosaccharides as in the case of legumes (see Chapter 2).[58] Others provide gaseous discomfort on an individual basis.
- *Respect food intolerances:* Lactose intolerance in persons lacking the enzyme lactase, for example, causes intestinal cramping, bloating, and diarrhea after drinking milk or eating dairy products made with milk.
- *Reduce total fat content:* Excess fat delays gastric emptying and contributes to malabsorption problems.
- *Avoid large meals:* Large amounts of food in one meal create discomfort from gastric distention and gas generated in the stomach. Smaller, more frequent meals usually reduce these symptoms.
- *Decrease air-swallowing habits:* Certain habits of eat-

TABLE 19-7
Dietary Fiber and Kilocalorie Values for Selected Foods

Foods	Serving	Dietary fiber (g)	Kcalories
Breads and cereals			
All Bran	⅓ cup	8.5	70
Bran (100%)	½ cup	8.4	75
Bran Buds	⅓ cup	7.9	75
Corn Bran	⅔ cup	5.4	100
Bran Chex	⅔ cup	4.6	90
Cracklin' Oat Bran	⅓ cup	4.3	110
Bran Flakes	¾ cup	4.0	90
Air-popped popcorn	1 cup	2.5	25
Oatmeal	1 cup	2.2	144
Grapenuts	¼ cup	1.4	100
Whole-wheat bread	1 slice	1.4	60
Legumes, cooked			
Kidney beans	½ cup	7.3	110
Lima beans	½ cup	4.5	130
Vegetables, cooked			
Green peas	½ cup	3.6	55
Corn	½ cup	2.9	70
Parsnip	½ cup	2.7	50
Potato, with skin	1 medium	2.5	95
Brussels sprouts	½ cup	2.3	30
Carrots	½ cup	2.3	25
Broccoli	½ cup	2.2	20
Beans, green	½ cup	1.6	15
Tomato, chopped	½ cup	1.5	17
Cabbage, red and white	½ cup	1.4	15
Kale	½ cup	1.4	20
Cauliflower	½ cup	1.1	15
Lettuce (fresh)	1 cup	0.8	7
Fruits			
Apple	1 medium	3.5	80
Raisins	¼ cup	3.1	110
Prunes, dried	3	3.0	60
Strawberries	1 cup	3.0	45
Orange	1 medium	2.6	60
Banana	1 medium	2.4	105
Blueberries	½ cup	2.0	40
Dates, dried	3	1.9	70
Peach	1 medium	1.9	35
Apricot, fresh	3 medium	1.8	50
Grapefruit	½ cup	1.6	40
Apricot, dried	5 halves	1.4	40
Cherries	10	1.2	50
Pineapple	½ cup	1.1	40

Adapted from Lanza E, Butrum RR: A critical review of food fiber analysis and data, *J Am Diet Assoc* 86:732, 1986.

ing contribute to air swallowed or gas generated in the stomach. These include eating rapidly, in addition to eating large amounts, and excessive fluid intake, especially carbonated beverages, and gum-chewing.

Experienced practitioners have learned that in helping a patient to manage IBS an honest and creative re-

lationship is basic.[59] Two such approaches include avoiding dogma and helping the patient to cope. Lifestyle and diet are highly personal and individual. Thus wise nutrition management involves both in realistic counseling toward a healthier life.

Constipation

A common disorder, usually of short duration, constipation is characterized by retention of feces in the colon beyond the normal emptying time. It is a problem for which Americans spend a quarter of a billion dollars for laxatives each year but hardly ever discuss. However, the regularity of elimination is highly individual, and it is not necessary for health to have a bowel movement every day. Usually this common short-term problem results from various sources of nervous tension and worry and changes in social setting. Such situations include vacations and travel, with alterations in usual routines. Also, it may be caused by prolonged use of laxatives or cathartics, low-fiber diets, or lack of exercise, all of which can contribute to a decreased intestinal muscle tone. Improved exercise, dietary, and bowel habits are usually sufficient to remedy the situation. The diet should include increased dietary fiber and naturally laxative fruits, such as dried prunes and figs, as well as increased fluid. If chronic constipation persists, however, agents that increase stool bulk may be necessary. These bulking agents include bran or more soluble forms (see Chapter 2). Taking laxatives or enemas on a regular basis should be avoided. The problem of constipation occurs in all age groups, but is almost epidemic in elderly people. In all cases a personalized approach to management of constipation is fundamental.[60]

Food Allergies and Sensitivities
Underlying Etiology

The word *allergy* comes from the Greek *allos* (other) and *ergon* (work). Thus the name implies an unusual or inappropriate response to a stimulus, usually an environmental factor. An allergic condition results from a disorder of the immune system (see Chapter 25). It is immunity gone wrong.

The term *food allergy* should be used only for hypersensitivity that is caused by an immunoglobulin E–mediated food reaction to specific food constituents or their digestive products.[61] The term *food sensitivity* is a general nonspecific term often used incorrectly as synonymous with food allergies. However, in tests many of these claimed sensitivities are unconfirmed.[61] Food al-

diverticulitis • Inflammation of pockets of tissue (diverticuli) in the lining of the mucous membrane of the colon.

lergy is distinct from food intolerances, which are caused by nonimmunologic mechanisms, for example, cow's milk intolerance resulting from lactase deficiency. In general, the process of diagnosis and treatment of adverse reactions to foods includes clinical assessment, dietary manipulation, and laboratory tests. Appropriate dietary counseling is essential.

Common Food Allergens

The care of an allergic child presents many problems. A wide variety of environmental, emotional, and physical factors influence reaction, and a suitable regimen is sometimes difficult to find. Since sensitivity to protein substances is a common basis for food allergy, the early foods of infants and children are frequent offenders. Fortunately, however, children tend to become less allergic to food sources as they become older.

Milk

Cow's milk has long been a common cause of allergic response in infants.[62] In sensitive children it causes gastrointestinal difficulties such as vomiting, diarrhea, and colic, or respiratory and skin problems. The problem is generally identified by clinical symptoms, family history, and a trial on a milk-free diet, using an appropriate substitute hypoallergenic formula such as the casein hydrolysate formulas Nutramigen and Pregestimil (both from Mead Johnson) or the special hydrolysate formula Alimentum (Ross).[63] Freedom from symptoms on a milk-free diet is then followed by a retrial on milk to determine if it causes the symptoms to reappear. Only then is the diagnosis of milk allergy established. Often symptoms appear and disappear spontaneously, regardless of dietary changes. But they tend to be more often caused by food if gastrointestinal problems are present.

Eggs, Wheat, and Other Foods

Among the dominant food allergens in infants are chicken eggs, cow's milk, and wheat. The specific biochemical sensitivity to gluten (a protein found in wheat) in the child with gluten-induced celiac sprue is caused by a specific biochemical defect in the mucosal cells in celiac disease and represents a different sensitivity mechanism from the immunophysiology causing a true food allergy. Other true food allergens among children, some continuing through adulthood, include peanuts, soy, tree nuts, other cereal grains, and shellfish.[64]

Nutritional Management

In an allergic child's diet solid foods are usually added slowly to the original formula, with common offenders excluded in early feedings. The following basic list of most frequently offending food allergens must be avoided[64,65]:

- Chicken eggs
- Cow's milk
- Wheat
- Peanuts
- Tree nuts
- Soy products
- Shellfish, fish

Citrus fruits, berries, and tomatoes may cause skin rash, but this is a local reaction. It is not the immunologic response that identifies true allergy.[64]

In some cases a series of diagnostic food elimination diets may be used to identify offending food allergens. A core of less-often offending foods is used initially, with gradual addition of other single foods one at a time to test the response. If a given food causes return of the allergy, the food is then identified as an allergen and eliminated from use. It may be retested later to determine if it is still an allergen. Guidance in the substitution of special food products and in the use of special recipes can be provided for the child's parents. Most food allergies tend to weaken as the child grows older. However, serious allergy to a few key foods, especially peanuts, may continue into adulthood and require constant monitoring of food products and dishes to avoid severe attacks.[65] These attacks of severe anaphylactic shock are marked by sudden bronchial spasms, vomiting, dropping blood pressure, and irregular heart rhythm.

Family Education and Counseling

The education of the parents and family of an allergic child must include a knowledge and understanding of the allergic state and the many factors that may influence it. If specific foods have been definitely identified as offenders, careful guidance to eliminate these from the diet is needed. Common uses of the offending food in daily meal patterns and its occurrence in a number of commercial products and other hidden sources should be discussed. Label reading and recipe adaptation are important. As an allergic child grows older, reaction to a given food may wane, and it can gradually be added to the diet.

Food Intolerances from Genetic-Metabolic Disease

Certain food intolerances may also stem from underlying genetic disease that affects the metabolism of one or more specific nutrients. Genetic disease results from the individual's specific gene inheritance. Genes in each cell control the metabolic functions of the cell. They regulate the synthesis of some 1000 or more specific cell enzymes that control metabolism within the cell. When a specific gene is abnormal (mutant), the enzyme whose synthesis that gene controls cannot be made. In turn, then, the specific metabolic reaction controlled by that specific missing enzyme cannot take place. The specific genetic disease caused by this metabolic block then manifests clinical symptoms connected with resulting abnormal metabolic products. As primary examples here, we look briefly at two such genetic diseases affecting food-nutrient intolerances: (1) phenylketonuria, which affects amino acid metabolism and hence protein foods, and (2) galactosemia, which affects carbohydrate metabolism, specifically food sources of lactose. Both are detected by newborn screening procedures, mandatory now by law.

Phenylketonuria (PKU)

Metabolic Defect and Clinical Symptoms

PKU results from the missing cell enzyme, phenylalanine hydroxylase, which metabolizes one of the essential amino acids, phenylalanine, to tyrosine, another nonessential amino acid (see Chapter 4). Phenylalanine then accumulates in the blood, and its alternate metabolites, the phenyl acids, are excreted in the urine. One of these urinary acids, phenylpyruvic acid, is a phenylketone; hence the name of the disease. Untreated PKU can produce devastating effects, but present nutritional therapy can prevent these results.[66] In past years, before current newborn screening laws and dietary treatment practices from birth, the most profound effect observed in persons with untreated PKU was severe mental retardation. The IQ of affected persons was usually below 50 and frequently less than 20. Central nervous system damage caused irritability, hyperactivity, convulsive seizures, and bizarre behavior.

Nutritional Therapy

PKU can now be well controlled by special diet therapy. After screening at birth, a special low-phenylalanine diet effectively controls the serum phenylalanine levels so they are maintained at appropriate amounts to prevent clinical symptoms and promote normal growth and development.[66] Since phenylalanine is an essential amino acid necessary for growth, it cannot be totally removed from the diet. Blood levels of phenylalanine are constantly monitored, and the metabolic team nutritionist calculates the special diet for each infant and child to allow only the limited amount of phenylalanine tolerated. Based on extensive studies, guidelines for dietary management of PKU are currently being used effectively to build lifetime habits, since research now indicates that there is no safe age at which a child may discontinue the diet.[66] This dietary management is built on two basic components: (1) a substitute for milk, a special medical food continued past infancy and childhood into adolescence and adulthood, and (2) guidelines for adding solid foods, both regular and special low-protein products, and then building continuing food habits.

Family Education and Counseling

Initial education and continuing support of parents is essential, since dietary management of PKU is the only known effective method of treatment, and maintaining the diet becomes more difficult as the child grows older.[67] But parents must understand and accept the necessity of the diet, and this requires patience, understanding, and continued reinforcement. The PKU team, together with wise parents, provides initial and continuing care so that the PKU child will grow and develop normally (Fig. 19-3). Such a child, diagnosed at birth by widespread screening programs, can have a healthy and happy life, instead of the profound disease consequences experienced in the past. This current practice of long-term dietary management is especially critical for young women who are reaching the age of potential high-risk pregnancies with maternal PKU (Chapter 11).

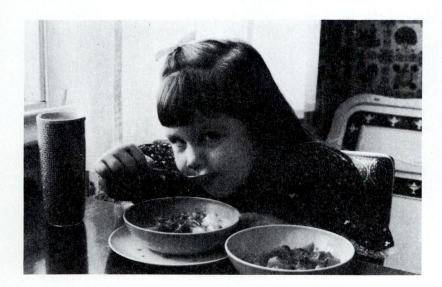

FIG. 19-3 PKU. This child is a delightful, perfectly developed 3-year-old. With her condition screened and diagnosed at birth, she has eaten a carefully controlled low-phenylalanine diet and is growing normally.

Galactosemia

Metabolic Defect and Clinical Symptoms

This genetic disease, also caused by a missing cell enzyme, affects carbohydrate metabolism. The missing enzyme controls the conversion of galactose, which is derived from lactose, to glucose (see Chapter 2). Milk, the infant's first food, contains a large amount of the precursor lactose (milk sugar). After galactose is initially combined with phosphate to begin the metabolic conversion to glucose, it cannot proceed further in the galactosemic infant. Galactose rapidly accumulates in the blood and in various body tissues. In the past the excess tissue accumulations of galactose caused rapid damage to the untreated infant. The child failed to thrive, and clinical symptoms appeared soon after birth. Continued liver damage brought jaundice, an enlarged liver with cirrhosis, enlarged spleen, and ascites. Without treatment, death usually resulted from liver failure. If the infant survived, continuing tissue damage and hypoglycemia in the optic lens and the brain caused cataracts and mental retardation. Now, however, with newborn screening programs, these infants are diagnosed at birth and started on special dietary management. With this vital nutritional therapy, they continue to grow and develop normally.

Nutritional Therapy

The main indirect source of dietary galactose is the lactose in milk. Therefore, all forms of milk and lactose must be removed from the diet. In this instance a galactose-free diet is used. Any needed amount of galactose for certain body structures can be synthesized by the body. A soy-base formula is used. Breast-feeding, of course, cannot be used. Later, as solid foods are added to the infant's diet at about 6 months of age, careful attention must be given to avoiding lactose from other food sources. Parents quickly learn to check labels carefully on all commercial products to detect any lactose or lactose-containing substances.

Diseases of the Gastrointestinal Accessory Organs

Three major accessory organs lie adjacent to the gastrointestinal tract and produce important digestive agents that enter the intestine and aid in the handling of food substances. Specific enzymes are produced for each of the major nutrients, and bile is added to assist in the enzyme digestion of fats. These three major organs are the liver, gallbladder, and pancreas. Diseases of these organs can easily affect gastrointestinal function and cause problems in the normal handling of specific types of food.

Viral Hepatitis

Structural Scheme of the Liver Lobules

The unique structural design of these basic functional units of the liver enable this vital organ to do its life-sustaining work. Each liver lobule is constructed around a central vein that empties into the hepatic veins and flows into the vena cava. From this central vein many hepatic cellular plates radiate outward like spokes in a wheel (Fig. 19-4).

Etiology

Viral hepatitis, inflammation of the liver, is a major public health problem throughout the world affecting hundreds of millions of people. It causes considerable

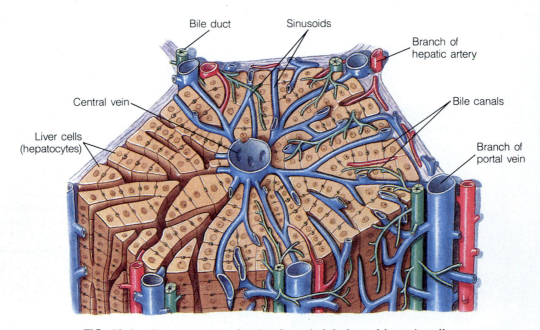

FIG. 19-4   Liver structure showing hepatic lobule and hepatic cell.

illness and death in human populations from the acute infection or its effects, which may include chronic active hepatitis, cirrhosis, and primary liver cancer. During the past few years, knowledge of the viruses causing different types of hepatitis has grown rapidly. Currently, five totally unrelated and often unusual human hepatitis viruses, named by the letters A through E as they have become known, have now been discovered and described.[68] The two most common and well known are A and B, which serve as examples.

Hepatitis A virus (HAV). HAV, the infectious agent of hepatitis type A, was formerly called infectious hepatitis. It was discovered in the early 1970s in the feces of infected patients and is transmitted by the classic oral-fecal route by contaminated food and water. It is a prevalent infection worldwide, especially where there is overcrowding and poor hygiene and sanitation. A new HAV vaccine has recently been developed that is far more effective than the former large and painful injection of gamma globulins, antibodies isolated from the blood.[69] This new vaccine protects travelers to developing countries, where the virus is **endemic** and may easily contaminate water and food.

Hepatitis B virus (HBV). HBV, the infectious agent of hepatitis type B, was formerly called serum hepatitis. It was discovered in the late 1960s, mainly spread sexually and by sharing of contaminated needles among drug users. It has now been implicated worldwide as the major causative factor in chronic liver disease and associated liver cancer. The HBV infection is closely related to the body's immune system. The estimate of carriers is about 300 million worldwide, 75% of whom are Asians. The WHO indicates that about 40% of these infected persons will die of chronic active hepatitis or liver cancer.[70] An improved vaccine was developed in 1986 and is now being used with high-risk groups such as health care personnel and babies of antibody-carrier mothers in most developed countries. In some endemic areas, all newborns are routinely vaccinated.

Clinical Symptoms

The viral agents of hepatitis produce diffuse injury to liver cells, especially the **parenchymal cells.** In milder cases the liver injury is largely reversible, but with increasing severity more extensive **necrosis** occurs. In some cases massive necrosis may lead to liver failure and death. A cardinal symptom of hepatitis is anorexia, contributing to the risk of malnutrition. Varying clinical symptoms appear depending on the degree of liver injury. **Jaundice,** a major symptom, may be obvious or not, depending on the severity of the disease, and can have both nutritional and psychologic effects (see Clinical Application, p. 372). In an outbreak of hepatitis, many infected persons may be **nonicteric** and thus go undiagnosed and untreated because jaundice has not developed enough to be seen. Malnutrition and im-

paired **immunocompetence** contribute to spontaneous infections and continuing liver disease. General symptoms, in addition to the main sign of anorexia, include malaise, weakness, nausea and vomiting, diarrhea, headache, fever, enlarged and tender liver, and enlarged spleen. When jaundice develops, it usually occurs for a **preicteric** period of 5 to 10 days, deepens for 1 to 2 weeks, then levels off and decreases. After this crisis point there is a sufficient recovery of injured cells, and convalescence of 3 weeks to 3 months follows. Optimal care during this time is essential to prevent relapse.

General Treatment

Bed rest is essential. Physical exercise increases both severity and duration of the disease. A daily intake of 3000 to 3500 ml of fluid guards against dehydration and gives a general sense of well-being and improved appetite. However, optimal nutrition is the major therapy.[71] It provides the essential foundation for recovery of the injured liver cells and overall return of strength.

Nutritional Therapy

Full nutrition assessment and initial personal histories provide the basis for planning care. Nutritional therapy principles relate to the liver's function in metabolizing each of the nutrients:

Adequate protein.   Protein is essential for liver cell regeneration, as well as for maintaining all of the body's essential functions.. It also provides lipotropic agents such as methionine and choline (see Chapters 4 and 5) for the conversion of fats to lipoproteins and re-

---

endemic • Characterizing a disease of low morbidity that remains constantly in a human community but is clinically recognizable in only a few.

icterus • Alternate term for jaundice: **nonicteric** indicates absence of jaundice; **preicteric** indicates a state prior to development of icterus, or jaundice.

immunocompetence • The ability or capacity to develop an immune response, that is, antibody production and/or cell-mediated immunity, following exposure to antigen.

jaundice • A syndrome characterized by hyperbilirubinemia and deposits of bile pigment in the skin, mucous membranes, and sclera giving a yellow appearance to the patient.

necrosis • Cell death caused by progressive enzyme breakdown.

parenchymal cells • Functional cells of an organ as distinguished from the cells comprising its structure or framework.

CLINICAL APPLICATION

Jaundice: When to Expect It and What to Do About It

Since jaundice is not usually a life-threatening condition, it is easy for the health care professional to take it lightly. The resulting yellow to orange skin color seems harmless, only reflecting an accumulation of excessive bile pigments in the blood that results from a rise in bilirubin, a product of heme released when red blood cells are destroyed. Certainly the underlying condition resulting in hemolysis is the major issue.

This may be true in a biologic sense. However, in a psychologic sense it can be devastating. The embarrassment of an altered body image, with accompanying depression and withdrawal, can affect the appetite and willingness to comply with the therapy that is recommended for the illness. To promote a healthy recovery, health workers must treat jaundice as seriously as these effects dictate. Several actions would be helpful:

1. Explain to the patient the reason for jaundice.
   - *Prehepatic jaundice:* Prehepatic jaundice most often is caused by a massive breakdown in red blood cells. It is seen most often in Rh factor sensitization, hemolytic anemias, sickle cell anemia, massive lung infarctions, transfusion reactions, and septicemia. The result is an excessive amount of bilirubin in a form that cannot be excreted, that is, fat soluble. The body's bilirubin transport system, based on albumin, then deposits the excess in the patient's skin and in a few other tissues.
   - *Hepatic jaundice:* In hepatic jaundice the liver cannot convert fat-soluble bilirubin into the water-soluble form required for its removal from the blood. This condition is seen in hepatitis, cirrhosis, metastatic cancer, and prolonged drug use, especially of drugs broken down by the liver.
   - *Posthepatic jaundice:* Posthepatic jaundice occurs when the flow of bile into the duodenum is blocked. Since bile carries water-soluble excretable bilirubin, this blockage backs up the bile, resulting in a backlog of bilirubin in the blood. Blockage often occurs with inflammation, scar tissue, stones, or tumors in the liver, bile, or pancreatic systems.
2. Explain to the patient assessment procedures and tests. A careful and comprehensive assessment process involving members of the health care team provides vital information for medical, nutritional, and nursing care plans.
   - *Include a careful history and anthropometry:* A full personal, family, psychosocial, medical, and nutritional history will help detect any possible hepatic virus sources and current nutritional status and needs.
   - *Check anthropometric data:* Routine body measures including skin fold thicknesses help determine nutritional status.
   - *Evaluate results of routine biochemical tests:* Relate these tests to medical diagnosis and nutritional status and needs.
   - *Explain each procedure:* A clear explanation of each procedure will help the patient participate more meaningfully in diagnostic and care-planning processes and will allay anxieties about the jaundice.
3. Identify nutrition-related problems. Jaundice is often associated with anorexia, indigestion, nausea, and vomiting.
   - *Help resolve nutrition-related problems:* To overcome indigestion or anorexia, recommend small meals that offer some of the patient's favorite foods. To overcome nausea or vomiting, simple foods may be necessary. Also, foods rich in fat and caffeine should also be avoided.
   - *Encourage the patient to discuss personal feelings and concerns:* Such information is essential for the nurse and nutritionist to develop a treatment plan. Also, this counseling may help the patient feel psychologically stronger and ready to contribute to the health care process.
   - *Discuss pertinent needs with the patient's family and friends:* Often other significant persons avoid the patient out of embarrassment or lack of understanding. A discussion of the patient's need for support may help other persons accept the patient socially and support any other efforts made to resolve the underlying health problem.
   - *Make appropriate referrals as needed:* If jaundice was caused by alcohol or drug abuse, the patient and possibly the patient's family may require special counseling. Referral to community programs after hospital discharge may help provide needed follow-up therapy.

REFERENCE

Sherlock S: *Diseases of the liver and biliary system,* ed 8, Cambridge, Mass, 1989, Blackwell Scientific Publications. ◆

TABLE 19-8

High-Protein, High-Kilocalorie Formula for Patient with Hepatitis

Ingredients	Amount	Approximate food value	
Milk	1 cup	Protein	40 g
Egg substitute	Equivalent of 2 eggs	Fat	30 g
Skimmed milk powder or Casec	6 to 8 tbsp 2 tbsp	Carbohydrates	70 g
Sugar	2 tbsp	Kilocalories	710
Ice cream	2.5 cm (1 in) slice or 1 scoop		
Cocoa or other flavoring	2 tbsp		
Vanilla	Few drops, as desired		

TABLE 19-9

High-Protein, High-Carbohydrate, Moderate-Fat Daily Diet

Food	Amount
Milk	1 L (1 qt)
Egg substitute	Equal to 1-2 eggs
Lean meat, fish, or poultry	224 g (8 oz)
Vegetables (4 servings)	
Potato or substitute	2 servings
Green leafy or yellow	1 serving
Other vegetables (including 1 raw)	1-2 servings
Fruit (3-4 servings, includes juices often)	
Citrus (or other good source of ascorbic acid)	1-2
Other fruit	2 servings
Bread and cereal (whole grain or enriched)	6-8 servings
Cereal	1 serving
Sliced bread or crackers	5-6
Butter or fortified margarine	2-4 tbsp
Jam, jelly, honey, and other carbohydrates	As patient desires and is able to eat them
Sweetened fruit juices	To increase carbohydrates and fluids

moval from the liver, thus preventing fatty infiltration. The daily diet should supply 1.5 to 2.0 g/kg actual body weight, or about 100 to 150 g, of high-quality protein. This amount is usually enough to achieve a positive nitrogen balance.

High carbohydrate. Sufficient available glucose must be provided to restore protective glycogen reserves and meet the energy demands of the disease process. Also, adequate glucose for energy ensures the use of protein for vital tissue regeneration. The diet should supply about 50% to 55% of the total kcalories as carbohydrates, or about 300 to 400 g/day.

Moderate fat. A moderate amount of fat makes the food more palatable and therefore encourages the anorexic patient to eat. If steatorrhea is present, a more easily absorbed medium-chain triglyceride product such as MCT oil may be used for a brief time. Then regular vegetable oil products and small amounts of butterfat may be resumed to ensure adequate amounts of essential linoleic acid. The diet should supply about 30% to 35% of the total kcalories as fat, or about 80 to 100 g/day.

Increased energy. The classic Harris-Benedict equations (see Chapter 16) are used to estimate basal energy expenditure (BEE). For total energy needs, malnourished patients should receive 150% of these calculated BEE values. Ambulatory patients require more energy intake to cover any physical activity, or a total of about 2500 to 3000 kcal/day. This increased energy intake is needed to furnish energy demands of the tissue regeneration process, to compensate for losses from fever and general debilitation, and to renew strength and recuperative powers.

Micronutrients. Fat-soluble vitamins in water-soluble form should be provided in amounts twice the

normal RDAs. Other water-soluble vitamins also require supplementation.

Meals and Feedings

The problem of supplying a diet adequate to meet the increased nutritive demands for a patient whose illness makes food almost repellent calls for creativity and supportive encouragement. The food may need to be in liquid form at first, using concentrated commercial or blended formulas for frequent feedings (Table 19-8). As the patient improves, appetizing and attractive food is needed. Since nutritional therapy is the key to recovery, a major nutrition and nursing responsibility requires devising ways to encourage the increased amounts of food intake needed, as suggested in Table 19-9. The clinical dietitian and the nurse will work together closely to achieve this goal. All staff attendants follow appropriate precautions in handling the patient's tray to prevent spread of the infection.

Cirrhosis

Cirrhosis is the general term used for advanced stages of liver disease, whatever the initial cause of the disease

> **cirrhosis** • Chronic liver disease, characterized by loss of functional cells, with fibrous and nodular regeneration.

may be. Among all digestive diseases, cirrhosis of the liver is the leading nonmalignant cause of death in the United States and most of the developed world.[72] These deaths occur largely among young and middle-age adults. In 1989, for example, three fifths of the 26,694 deaths caused by chronic liver disease and cirrhosis occurred in persons between the ages of 25 and 64 years. The French physician René Laënnec (1781-1826) first used the term *cirrhosis* (from the Greek word *kirrhos*, meaning "orange-yellow") to describe the diseased liver's abnormal color and rough surface. The cirrhotic liver is a firm, fibrous, dull yellowish mass with orange nodules projecting from its surface (Fig. 19-5).

Etiology

Some forms of cirrhosis result from biliary obstruction, with blockage of the biliary ducts and accumulation of

bile in the liver.[74] Other cases may result from liver necrosis from undetermined causes or in some cases from previous viral hepatitis. A common problem is fatty cirrhosis, associated with the complicating factor of malnutrition. Continuing fatty infiltration causes cellular destruction and fibrotic tissue changes.

Clinical Symptoms

Early signs of cirrhosis include gastrointestinal disturbances such as nausea, vomiting, loss of appetite, distention, and epigastric pain. In time jaundice may appear, with increasing weakness, edema, ascites, and anemia from gastrointestinal bleeding, iron deficiency, or hemorrhage. A specific **macrocytic anemia** from folic acid deficiency is also frequently observed. Steatorrhea is a common symptom. Essentially, the major symptoms are caused by a basic protein deficiency and its mul-

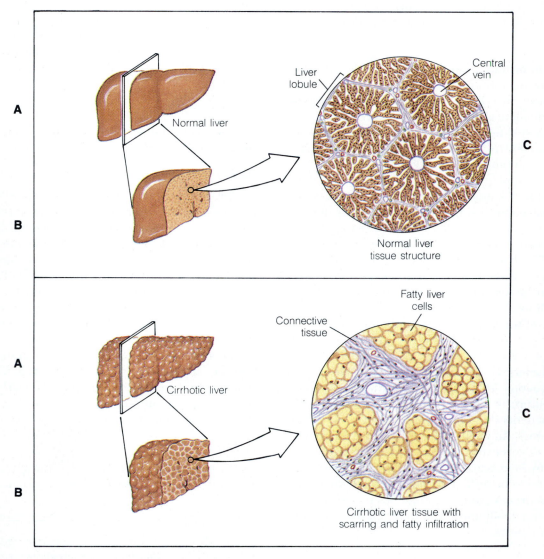

FIG. 19-5   Comparison of normal liver and liver with cirrhotic tissue changes.
A, Anterior view of organ; **B,** cross-section; **C,** tissue structure.

tiple metabolic problems: (1) plasma protein levels fall, leading to failure of the capillary fluid shift mechanism (see Chapter 8), causing ascites; (2) lipotropic agents are not supplied for fat conversion to lipoproteins, and damaging fat accumulates in the liver tissue; (3) blood clotting mechanisms are impaired since factors such as prothrombin and fibrinogen are not adequately produced; and (4) general tissue catabolism and negative nitrogen balance continue the overall degenerative process.

As the disease progresses, the increasing fibrotic scar tissue impairs blood circulation through the liver, and portal hypertension follows.[75] Contributing further to the problem is the continuing ascites. The impaired portal circulation with increasing venous pressure may lead to esophageal **varices,** with danger of rupture and fatal massive hemorrhage.

Nutritional Therapy

When alcoholism is an added underlying problem, treatment is difficult. Each patient requires supportive care. Therapy is usually aimed at correcting fluid and electrolyte problems and providing nutritional support for hepatic repair as much as possible. In any case, guidelines for nutritional therapy for cirrhosis of the liver should include the following principles:

1. *Protein according to tolerance.* In the absence of impending hepatic encephalopathy (see the following discussion), the protein intake should be continued at the level indicated for hepatitis, about 1.5 to 2.0 g/kg actual body weight, or about 100 to 150 g/day. The protein is needed to correct severe undernutrition, regenerate functional liver tissue, and replenish plasma protein. However, if signs of hepatic encephalopathy appear, protein must be decreased to individual tolerance.
2. *Low sodium.* Sodium is usually restricted to about 1000 mg/day (see Chapter 20) to help reduce fluid retention.
3. *Texture.* If esophageal varices develop, it may be necessary to give soft foods that are smooth in texture to prevent danger of rupture and hemorrhage.
4. *Optimal general nutrition.* The remaining overall diet principles outlined for hepatitis are continued for cirrhosis for the same reasons. Kcalories, carbohydrates, and vitamins are supplied according to individual need and deficiency. Moderate fat is used. Alcohol is strictly forbidden.

Hepatic Encephalopathy

The term **encephalopathy** refers to any disease or disorder that affects the brain, especially chronic degenerative conditions. The brain effect in hepatic encephalopathy is a serious complication of end-stage liver disease. The accumulation of toxic substances in the blood as a result of liver failure impairs consciousness and contributes to memory loss, personality change, tremors, seizures, stupor, and coma.

Etiology

As cirrhotic changes continue in the liver, the portal blood circulation diminishes and liver functions begin to fail. The normal liver has a major function of removing ammonia from the blood by converting it to urea for excretion. The failing liver can no longer inactivate or detoxify substances or metabolize others. A key factor involved in the progressive disease process is an elevated blood level of ammonia, though it is by no means the sole agent. The resulting hepatic encephalopathy brings changes in consciousness, behavior, and neurologic status.

Clinical Symptoms

Typical response involves disorders of consciousness and alterations in motor function. There is apathy, confusion, inappropriate behavior, and drowsiness, progressing to coma. The speech may be slurred or monotonous. A coarse, flapping tremor known as **asterixis,** is observed in the outstretched hands, caused by a sustained contraction of a group of muscles. The breath may have a fecal odor, **fetor hepaticus.**

Basic Treatment Objectives

The fundamental objective of treatment is twofold: (1) removal of the sources of excess ammonia and (2) provision of nutritional support. Medical and nutritional therapy are involved. Parenteral fluid and electrolytes are used to restore normal balances. Two drugs may be used to control ammonia—lactulose and neomycin. Lactulose is a nonabsorbable synthetic disaccharide that reduces the absorption of intestinal ammonia. Neomycin is an antibiotic that reduces the population of urea-splitting organisms within the bowel that produce ammonia. To stop bleeding into the intestine as another source of intestinal ammonia, a Sengstaken-Blakemore tube may be used.

---

asterixis • Neuromotor disturbance marked by an inability to hold outstretched hands in a steady position, resulting in an intermittent flapping of the hands, characteristic of hepatic coma.

encephalopathy • Any degenerative disease of the brain.

fetor hepaticas • The peculiar odor of the breath that is characteristic of advanced liver disease.

macrocytic anemia • An anemia (deficiency of normal red cells) characterized by abnormally large red cells.

varices (plural) • Varicose veins; enlarged and tortuous veins, full of twists, curves, or windings.

Nutritional Therapy

General nutritional support for hepatic encephalopathy is based on the following principles of dietary management.

Low protein.   General protein intake is reduced individually as necessary to restrict the dietary sources of nitrogen in amino acids. The amount of restriction varies with the circumstances, but the usual amounts range from 30 to 50 g/day, depending on whether symptoms are severe or mild. A simple method for controlling dietary protein uses a base meal pattern containing approximately 15 g protein and then adds small items of protein foods according to the level of protein desired (Table 19-10).

Branched-chain amino acids.   The three branched-chain amino acids (BCAAs)—leucine, isoleucine, and valine (see Chapter 4)—are not catabolized by the liver but are taken up by other tissues. Thus they can be metabolized without depending on healthy liver tissue, as is the case with the other amino acids. They provide a useful energy source, as well as a better tolerated source of needed protein that may be utilized directly by the muscles, heart, liver, and brain.[76] Oral BCAA formula has been used, with the patients becoming neurologically normal. The clinical use of BCAA supplementation in enteral and parenteral nutrition support formulas is an important part of standard therapy in liver failure and may improve chance of survival.

Kilocalories and vitamins.   Adequate energy intake is crucial to the patient's recovery, especially through the impact of kcaloric intake on liver glycogen reserves and their protective role in the healing process. The amounts of kcalories and vitamins are prescribed according to need. About 2000 kcal/day is needed to prevent tissue catabolism, with sufficient carbohydrate as the primary energy source and some fat as tolerated. Vitamin K is usually given parenterally, along with other vitamins and minerals, especially zinc, that may be deficient.

Fluid Intake

Fluid intake-output balance is carefully controlled.

Liver Transplantation

The development of liver transplantation as an acceptable therapy for end-stage liver disease has been an important recent medical advance. Candidates for trans-

---

TABLE 19-10

Low-Protein Diets (15 g, 30 g, 40 g, and 50 g Protein)

General description

- The following diets are used when dietary protein is to be restricted.
- The patterns limit foods containing a large percentage of protein, such as milk, eggs, cheese, meat, fish, fowl, and legumes.
- Avoid meat extractives, soups, broth, bouillon, gravies, and gelatin desserts.

Basic meal patterns (contains approximately 15 g of protein)

Breakfast	Lunch	Dinner
½ cup fruit or fruit juice	1 small potato	1 small potato
½ cup cereal	½ cup vegetable	½ cup vegetable
1 slice toast	Salad (vegetable or fruit)	Salad (vegetable or fruit)
Butter	1 slice bread	1 slice bread
Jelly	Butter	Butter
Sugar	1 serving fruit	1 serving fruit
2 tbsp cream	Sugar	Sugar
Coffee	Coffee or tea	Coffee or tea

For 30 g protein

Add: 1 cup milk
    28 g (1 oz) meat, 1 egg, or equivalent

For 40 g protein

Add: 1 cup milk
    70 g (2½ oz) meat, or 1 egg and 42 g (1½ oz) meat

For 50 g protein

Add: 1 cup milk
    112 g (4 oz) meat, or 2 eggs and 56 g (2 oz) meat

Examples of meat portions

28 g (1 oz) meat = 1 thin slice roast, 4 × 5 cm (1½ × 2 in)
                1 rounded tbsp cottage cheese
                1 slice American cheese

70 g (2½ oz) meat = Ground beef patty (5 can be made from 448 g [1 lb])
                  1 slice roast

112 g (4 oz) meat = 2 lamb chops
                  1 average steak

plant include patients with end-stage chronic liver disease or acute liver failure, progressive liver disease for which conventional treatment has failed, and the prognosis of which indicates a survival of less than 10%. In such cases, **orthotopic** (normal placement) liver transplantation remains the best chance of prolonged survival. Less suitable cases include problems such as alcoholic cirrhosis and malignant tumors, and those complicated by sepsis or advanced lung and kidney disease.[77] As with all major surgery, aggressive nutritional support reduces risks. Careful pretransplant nutritional assessment and support helps prepare the patient for the major surgery. Enteral or parenteral nutritional support may be required for optimal postoperative nutritional status. A number of posttransplant young women, after return of fertility with the new healthy liver and good nutrition support, have been able to conceive and maintain the high-risk pregnancy to a successful conclusion with closely monitored medical and nutritional management.[78] In such cases, immediate follow-up contraception with a barrier method is recommended because birth control pills may interfere with accurate **cyclosporine** dosing for maintaining the transplant.

Gallbladder Disease
Metabolic Function

The basic function of the gallbladder is to concentrate and store the bile produced in its initial watery solution by the liver. The liver secretes about 600 to 800 ml/day of bile, which the gallbladder normally concentrates fivefold to tenfold to accommodate this daily bile in its small capacity of 40 to 70 ml. Through the cholecystokinin (CCK) mechanism (see Chapter 5), the presence of fat in the duodenum stimulates contraction of the gallbladder with the release of concentrated bile into the common duct and then into the small intestine.

Cholecystitis and Cholelithiasis

The prefix *chole-* of the two terms *cholecystitis* and *cholelithiasis* comes from the Greek word *cholē,* which means "bile." Thus cholecystitis is an inflammation of the gallbladder, and cholelithiasis is the formation of gallstones.

Inflammation of the gallbladder usually results from a low-grade chronic infection and may occur with or without gallstones. However, in 90% to 95% of patients, acute cholecystitis is associated with gallstones and is due to the obstruction of the cystic duct by stones, resulting in acute inflammation of the organ. Gallstones can be classified into two main groups: cholesterol and pigment stones.

Cholesterol stones.   In the United States and most Western countries, more than 75% of the gallstones are cholesterol stones. The infectious process produces changes in the gallbladder mucosa, which affect its absorptive powers. Normally bile's main ingredient cholesterol, which is insoluble in water, is kept in solution by the other bile ingredients. However, when the absorbing mucosal tissue of the gallbladder is inflamed or infected, changes occur in the tissue. The absorptive powers of the gallbladder may be altered, affecting the solubility of the bile ingredients. Excess water or excess bile acid may be absorbed. Under these abnormal absorptive conditions cholesterol may precipitate, forming gallstones of almost pure cholesterol. Excessive use of dietary fat over a long period of time predisposes persons to gallstone formation because of the constant stimulus to produce more cholesterol as a necessary bile ingredient to metabolize fat.

Pigment stones.   Both black and brown pigment gallstones, although they differ in chemical composition and clinical features, are colored by the presence of bilirubin, the pigment in red blood cells. They are associated with chronic hemolysis in conditions such as sickle cell disease, thalassemia, cirrhosis, long term TPN, and advancing age.[79] Pigment stones are often found in the bile ducts and may be related to a bacterial infection with *Escherichia coli.*

Clinical Symptoms

When inflammation, stones, or both are present in the gallbladder, contraction from the cholecystokinin-pancreozymin (CCK-PZ) mechanism (see Chapter 5) causes pain. Sometimes the pain is severe. There is fullness and distention after eating and particular difficulty with fatty foods.

General Treatment

Surgical removal of the gallbladder, a cholecystectomy, is usually indicated (see Chapter 23). If the patient is obese, some weight loss before surgery is advisable if surgery can be delayed. Supportive therapy is largely nutritional. Several new nonsurgical treatments for removing the stones, using chemical dissolution or mechanical stone fragmentation, have been developed (see To Probe Further, p. 378). These methods provide effective alternatives to surgery in some cases.

cyclosporine • An immunosuppressant drug widely used following organ transplants to control the immune system and prevent rejection of the new tissue.

orthotopic • Occurring at the normal place in the body; placement of a transplanted organ in the position formerly occupied by tissue of the same kind.

Dissolution and Fragmentation: Alternate Solutions to the Problem of Gallstones

The 25 million Americans with gallstones may be able to have relief without surgery. Chemical dissolution by use of a drug, alone or combined with mechanical fragmentation by ultrasound waves, offers possible alternatives.

Chenodiol (chenodeoxycholic acid), and its companion ursodiol (ursodeoxycholic acid) are two natural bile acids that reduce the concentration of cholesterol in bile and dissolve cholesterol stones harmlessly, thus sparing many persons the discomfort, risk, and cost of major surgery. Their biologic activity prevents excessive cholesterol from separating out of bile to form the most common type of gallstone. Other stones consisting of combinations of calcium carbonate, bilirubin, and other compounds make up only 15% to 20% of all gallstones.

These two naturally occurring bile acids, CDCA and UDCA, have been studied for a number of years and are now used to treat gallstones in more than 40 countries. Clinically, they appear to be effective at dissolving "floating" gallstones less than 1.25 cm (½ inch) in diameter with few side effects (such as diarrhea) and only temporary reversible changes in some liver enzymes. This makes it potentially beneficial to patients who are surgical risks because of other medical problems.

Other nonsurgical methods of removing gallstones are also now in experimental stages of development and may

TO PROBE FURTHER

expand these alternatives still further. An additional chemical dissolution method is the instillation of liquid solvents such as methyl tert-butyl ether (MTBE) directly into the gallbladder or the common bile duct. Additional mechanical fragmentation by pulsed lasers is being studied.

These alternate means may help patients avoid gallbladder surgery, but they do not eliminate the need for a diet emphasizing carbohydrates and fiber and controlling fat with an eye to weight management. Further, most of these alternatives work mainly on small stones rather than on larger clumps of cholesterol. Also, they are not recommended for everyone. Chronic liver disease or a bile duct obstruction may rule them out, as does pregnancy. For many persons however, these alternatives may provide long-sought, successful treatments. Those who suffer from gallstones may be able to say goodbye to pain, indigestion, nausea, and jaundice without fear of surgery.

REFERENCES

Albert MB, Fromm H: Nonsurgical alternatives in the management of gallstones, *J Intensive Care Med* 4(1):3, 1989.
Bile acid therapy in the 1990s, *Lancet* 340:1260, Nov 21, 1992 (editorial).
Hochberger J and others: Lithotripsy of gallstones by means of a quality-switched giant-pulse neodymium:yttrium-aluminum-garnet laser, *Gastroenterology* 101(5):1391, 1991.

Nutritional Therapy

Basic principles of nutritional therapy for gallbladder disease include the following.

Fat. Because dietary fat is the principal cause of contraction of the diseased organ and subsequent pain, it is poorly tolerated. Energy should come primarily from carbohydrate foods, especially during acute phases. Control of fat will also contribute to weight control, a primary goal because obesity and excess food intake have been repeatedly associated with the development of gallstones.

Kilocalories. If weight loss is indicated, kcalories will be reduced according to need. Principles of weight management are discussed in Chapter 6. Usually such a diet will have a relatively low fat ratio and meet the needs of the patient for fat moderation.

Cholesterol and "gas formers." Two additional modifications usually found in traditional diets for gallbladder disease concern restriction of foods containing cholesterol and foods labeled "gas formers." Neither modification has a valid rationale. The body synthesizes

daily several times more cholesterol than is present in an average diet. Thus restriction of dietary cholesterol has little effect in reducing gallstone formation. Total dietary fat reduction is more to the point. As for the use of so-called gas-formers, such as legumes, cabbage, or fiber, blanket restriction seems unwarranted, since food tolerances in any circumstances are highly individual.

Diseases of the Pancreas
Pancreatitis

Acute inflammation of the pancreas, pancreatitis, is caused by the digestion of the organ tissues by the very enzymes it produces, principally trypsin. Normally enzymes remain in the inactive form until the pancreatic secretions reach the duodenum through the common duct. However, gallbladder disease may cause a gallstone to enter the common bile duct and obstruct the flow from the pancreas or cause a reflux of these secretions and bile from the common duct back into the pancreatic duct. This mixing of digestive materials activates the powerful pancreatic enzymes within the gland. In such activated form, they begin their damaging effects on the pancreatic tissue itself, causing acute pain. Sometimes infectious pancreatitis may occur as a complication of mumps or a bacterial disease. Mild or moderate pancreatitis may subside completely, but it has a tendency to recur.

General Treatment

Initial care consists of measures recommended for acute disease involving shock. These measures include intravenous feeding at first, replacement therapy of fluid and electrolytes, blood transfusions, antibiotics and pain medications, and gastric suction.

Nutritional Therapy

In early stages nutritional support is maintained by parenteral feeding, and oral feedings are withheld because entry of food into the intestines stimulates pancreatic secretions. As healing progresses and oral feedings are resumed, a light diet is used to avoid excessive stimulation of pancreatic secretions. Alcohol and caffeine should be avoided to decrease pancreatic stimulation. Alcohol in Western societies and malnutrition worldwide are the major causes of chronic pancreatitis.[80]

To Sum Up

The nutritional management of gastrointestinal disease is based on careful consideration of four major factors: (1) secretory functions, providing the chemical agents and environment necessary for digestion; (2) neuromuscular functions, required for motility and mechanical digestion; (3) absorptive functions, transporting nutrients into the circulatory system; and (4) psychologic factors, reflected by changes in gastrointestinal function.

Esophageal problems vary widely from simple dysphagia to serious disease or obstruction. Nutritional therapy and mode of intake vary according to degree of dysfunction.

Peptic ulcer disease is a common gastrointestinal problem affecting millions of Americans. It is an erosion of the mucosal lining, mainly the duodenal bulb and less commonly the lower stomach. It results in such nutritional problems as low plasma protein levels, anemia, and weight loss. Current medical management consists of acid and infection control with a coordinated system of new drugs, rest, and a regular diet with few food and drink considerations to supply the essential nutritional support for tissue healing.

Intestinal diseases include conditions of malabsorption and diarrhea such as celiac sprue, a gluten-induced enteropathy; cystic fibrosis, a genetic pancreatic insufficiency; and inflammatory bowel disease, Crohn's disease and ulcerative colitis. Further lower intestinal diseases include conditions such as diverticular disease, with anatomic changes and infection risks, and irritable bowel syndrome, with intermittent diarrhea and consti-

pation with large somatic overlay requiring individual support. Nutritional therapy involves various modifications of energy-nutrient content and food texture, with continuous dietary adjustment according to need. Allergic responses to common food allergens, as well as missing cell enzymes in genetic disease, may also contribute to gastrointestinal and metabolic problems from related food intolerances.

Accessory organs to the gastrointestinal tract—liver, gallbladder, and pancreas—have important functions related to nutrient digestion, absorption, and metabolism, and their diseases interfere with these normal functions. Common liver disorders include hepatitis, usually caused by viral infection, and cirrhosis, advanced liver disease, leading to hepatic encephalopathy and progressive liver failure. Nutrient and energy levels required vary with each condition.

Diseases of the gallbladder include cholecystitis, inflammation that interferes with the absorption of water and bile acids, and cholelithiasis, or gallstone formation. Treatment involves a generally reduced fat diet and surgical removal of the gallbladder. Diseases of the pancreas include acute and chronic forms of pancreatitis, in which alcohol abuse can be a primary cause. Other causes include biliary disease, malnutrition, drug reactions, abdominal injury, and genetic predisposition. In acute pancreatitis, pain is severe because of pancreatic enzyme reflux with self-digestion of pancreatic tissue by its own enzymes, and parenteral nutrition support is used to avoid enzyme stimulus, with gradual return to small, frequent meals as the attack subsides. In chronic pancreatitis, which is caused by alcoholism in Western societies and malnutrition worldwide, maldigestion from lack of enzymes because of pancreatic insufficiency creates nutritional problems. Nutritional care focuses on a nourishing diet with enzyme replacement and vitamin-mineral supplementation.

QUESTIONS FOR REVIEW

1. What is the basic principle of diet planning for patients with esophageal problems? Outline a general nutritional care plan for a patient with gastroesophageal reflux disease (GERD) complicated by a hiatal hernia.

2. In current practice, what are the basic principles of diet planning for patients with peptic ulcer disease? How do these principles differ from former traditional therapy?

3. Outline a course of nutritional management for a person with peptic ulcer disease, based on the current approaches to medical management. How would you plan nutrition education for continuing self-care and avoidance of recurrence?

4. Describe the etiology, clinical signs, and treatment of each of the following intestinal diseases: malabsorption and diarrhea, inflammatory bowel disease, diverticular disease, irritable bowel disease, constipation.

5. Compare the basis of food intolerances due to food allergy and a specific genetic disease such as PKU.

6. How are the major metabolic functions of the liver affected in liver disease? Give some examples.

7. What is the rationale for treatment in the spectrum of liver disease—hepatitis, cirrhosis, and hepatic encephalopathy?

8. Develop a 1-day food plan for a 45-year-old man, 183 cm (6 ft, 1 in) tall, weighing 90 kg (200 lb), with infectious hepatitis; another plan for a similar patient with cirrhosis of the liver; and another for a patient with hepatic encephalopathy. What principles of diet therapy apply for each?

9. What are the principles of nutritional therapy for gallbladder disease? Write a 1-day meal plan for a 30-year-old woman, 165 cm (5 ft, 6 in) tall, weighing 81 kg (180 lb), who has an inflamed gallbladder with stones and is awaiting a cholestectomy.

10. Compare acute and chronic forms of pancreatitis in terms of etiology, symptoms, and nutritional therapy. What role does special enteral and parenteral nutrition support play in this therapy?

REFERENCES

1. Yankelson S and others: Dysphagia: a unique interdisciplinary treatment approach, *Top Clin Nutr* 4:43, 1989.

2. Loughlin GM: Respiratory consequences of dysfunctional swallowing and aspiration, *Dysphagia* 3:126, 1989.

3. Tuchman DN: Cough, choke, sputter: the evaluation of the child with dysfunctional swallowing, *Dysphagia* 3:111, 1989.

4. Dantas RD and others: Effects of swallowed bolus variables on oral and pharyngeal phases of swallowing, *Am J Physiol* 258:G675, 1990.

5. Stanek K and others: Factors affecting use of food and commercial agents to thicken liquids for individuals with swallowing disorders, *J Am Diet Assoc* 92(4):488, 1992.

6. Gelfans MD: Gastroesophageal reflux disease, *Med Clin North Am* 75(4):923, 1991.

7. Kitchin LI, Castell DO: Rationale and efficiency of conservative therapy for gastroesophageal reflux disease, *Arch Intern Med* 151:448, 1991.

8. Katz J: The course of peptic ulcer disease, *Med Clin North Am* 75(4):1013, 1991.

9. Gryboski JD: Peptic ulcer disease in children, *Med Clin North Am* 75(4):889, 1991.

10. Miller TA and others: Stress erosive gastritis, *Curr Probl Surg* 28:458, 1991.

11. Pilchman J and others: Cytoprotection and stress ulceration, *Med Clin North Am* 75(4):853, 1991.

12. Schindler BA, Ramchandani D: Psychologic factors associated with peptic ulcer disease, *Med Clin North Am* 75(4):865, 1991.

13. Rubin W: Medical treatment of peptic ulcer disease, *Med Clin North Am* 75(4):981, 1991.

14. Isenberg JI and others: Acid-peptic disorders. In Yamada T, ed: *Textbook of gastroenterology*, Philadelphia, 1991, JB Lippincott.

15. Mertz HR, Walsh JH: Peptic ulcer pathophysiology, *Med Clin North Am* 75(4):799, 1991.

16. McCarthy DM: Sucralfate, *N Engl J Med* 325(14):1017, 1991.

17. Bauerfeind P and others: Fate of antacid gel in the stomach, site of action and interaction with food, *Dig Dis Sci* 35(5):553, 1990.

18. Earnest DL: Maintenance therapy in peptic ulcer disease, *Med Clin North Am* 75(4):1013, 1991.

19. Marotta RB, Floch MH: Diet and nutrition in ulcer disease, *Med Clin North Am* 75(4):967, 1991.

20. Food and Nutrition Board, Committee on Diet and Health, National Academy of Science-National Research Council: *Diet and health: implications for reducing chronic disease risk*, Washington, DC, 1989, National Academy Press.

21. Kruis W and others: Effects of diets high and low in refined sugars on gut transit, bile acid metabolism, and bacterial fermentation, *Gut* 32:367, 1991.

22. Banwell JG: Pathophysiology of diarrheal disorders, *Rev Infect Dis* 12(supp 11):530, 1990.

23. Caspary WF: Physiology and pathophysiology of intestinal absorption, *Am J Clin Nutr* 55(suppl):299S, 1992.

24. Trier JS: Celiac sprue, *N Engl J Med* 325(24):1709, 1991.

25. Anson O and others: Celiac disease: parental knowledge and attitudes of dietary compliance, *Pediatrics* 85:98, 1990.

26. Skerritt JH, Hill AS: Self-management of dietary compliance in coeliac disease by means of ELISA "home test" to detect gluten, *Lancet* 337:379, 1991.

27. Roberts L: CF screening delayed for awhile, perhaps forever, *Science* 247:1296, 1990.

28. Marcus MS and others: Nutritional status of infants with cystic fibrosis associated with early diagnosis and intervention, *Am J Clin Nutr* 54:578, 1991.

29. Roberts L: The race for the cystic fibrosis gene, *Science* 240:141, 1988.

30. Thomas PJ and others: Cystic fibrosis transmembrane conductance regulator: nucleotide binding to a synthetic peptide, *Science* 251:553, 1991.

31. Cystic Fibrosis Foundation: Guidelines for patient services, evaluation, and monitoring in cystic fibrosis centers, *Am J Dis Child* 144:1311, 1990.

32. Moran A and others: Pancreatic endocrine function in cystic fibrosis, *J Pediatr* 118:715, 1991.

33. Brady MS and others: Effectiveness of enteric coated pancreatic enzymes given before meals in reducing steatorrhea in children with cystic fibrosis, *J Am Diet Assoc* 92(7):813, 1992.

34. Ramsey BW and others: Nutritional assessment and management in cystic fibrosis, *Am J Clin Nutr* 55:108, 1992.

35. Podolsky DK: Inflammatory bowel disease. Part I, *N Engl J Med* 325(13):928, 1991.

36. Podolsky DK: Inflammatory bowel disease. Part II, *N Engl J Med* 325(14):1008, 1991.

37. Bennett RA and others: Frequency of inflammatory bowel disease in offspring of couples both presenting with IBD, *Gastroenterology* 100:1638, 1991.

38. Tysk C and others: Ulcerative colitis and Crohn's disease in unselected populations of monozygotic and dizygotic twins: a study of heritability and the influence of smoking, *Gut* 29:990, 1988.

39. Ainley C and others: The influence of zinc status and malnutrition on immunological function in Crohn's disease, *Gastroenterology* 100:1616, 1991.

40. Peppercorn MA: Advances in drug therapy for inflammatory bowel disease, *Ann Intern Med* 112:50, 1990.

41. O'Brien JJ and others: Use of azathioprine or 6-mercaptopurine in the treatment of Crohn's disease, *Gastroenterology* 101:39, 1991.

42. Donaldson RM: The muddle of diets for gastrointestinal disorders, *JAMA* 225:1243, 1973.

43. Bingham S: Low residue diets: a reappraisal of their meaning and content, *J Hum Nutr* 33:5, 1979.

44. Christian GM and others: Milk and milk products in low residue diets: current hospital practices do not match dietitians' beliefs, *J Am Diet Assoc* 91(3):341, 1991.

45. Rosenburg IH, Jenkins DJA: Intestinal disorders: (A) Short bowel syndrome; (B) Inflammatory bowel disease; (C) Diseases of the small bowel. In Shils ME, Olson JA, Shike M, eds: *Modern nutrition in health and disease*, ed 8, Philadelphia, 1993, Lea & Febiger.

46. Polk DB and others: Improved growth and disease activity after intermittent administration of a defined formula diet in children with Crohn's disease, *J Parenter Enteral Nutr* 16(6):499, 1992.

47. Teahon K and others: Ten years' experience with an elemental diet in the management of Crohn's disease, *Gut* 31:1133, 1990.

48. Christie PM, Hill GL: Effect of intravenous nutrition on nutrition and function in acute attacks of inflammatory bowel disease, *Gastroenterology* 99:730, 1990.

49. Purdum PP, Kirby DF: Short-bowel syndrome: a review of the role of nutrition support, *J Parenter Enteral Nutr* 15(1):93, 1991.

50. Åkerlund J-E and others: Hepatic metabolism of cholesterol in Crohn's disease: effect of partial resection of ileum, *Gastroenterology* 100:1046, 1991.

51. Leichtmann GA and others: Intestinal absorption of cholecalciferol and 25-hydroxycholecalciferol in patients with both Crohn's disease and intestinal resection, *Am J Clin Nutr* 54:548, 1991.

52. Wunderlich SM, Tobias A: Relationship between nutritional status indicators and length of hospital stay for patients with diverticular disease, *J Am Diet Assoc* 92(4):430, 1992.

53. Sandler RS: Epidemiology of inflammatory bowel disease in the United States, *Gastroenterology* 99:409, 1990.

54. Schuster MM: Diagnostic evaluation of the irritable bowel syndrome, *Gastroenterol Clin North Am* 20(2):269, 1991.

55. Thompson WC: Symptomatic presentations of the irritable bowel syndrome, *Gastroenterol Clin North Am* 20(2):235, 1991.

56. Drossman DA and others: Identification of the subgroups of functional gastrointestinal disorders, *Gastroentrol Int* 3:159, 1990.

57. Whitehead WE, Crowell MD: Psychologic considerations in the irritable bowel syndrome, *Gastroenterol Clin North Am* 20(2):249, 1991.

58. Friedman G: Treatment of the irritable bowel syndrome, *Gastroenterol Clin North Am* 20(2):325, 1991.

59. Wingate DL: Irritable bowel syndrome, *Gastroenterol Clin North Am* 20(2):351, 1991.

60. Donatelle EP: Constipation: pathophysiology and treatment, *Am Fam Physician* 42(5):1335, 1990.

61. Parker SL and others: Foods perceived by adults as causing adverse reactions, *J Am Diet Assoc* 93(1):40, 1993.

62. Bishop JM and others: Natural history of cow milk allergy: clinical outcome, *J Pediatr* 116:862, 1990.

63. Sampson HA and others: Safety of casein hydrolysate formula in children with cow milk allergy, *J Pediatr* 118:520, 1991.

64. Björkstén B: Dietary management of food allergy, *Semin Pediatr Gastroenterol Nutr* 3(2):13, 1992.

65. Nash JM and others: Allergies, *Time* 139(25):54, 1992.

66. Elsas LJ II, Acosta PB: Nutritional support of inherited metabolic disease. In Shils ME, Olson JA, Shike M, eds: *Modern nutrition in health and disease*, ed 8, Philadelphia, 1993, Lea & Febiger.

67. Jahn D: Inside, looking out: one mother's view on phenylketonuria, *Top Clin Nutr* 2(3):40, July 1987.

68. Lau JYN and others: Viral hepatitis, *Gut* 32(suppl 9):47, 1991.

69. Hoffman M: Hepatitis A vaccine shows promise, *Science* 254:1581, 1991.

70. *Bull World Health Organ* 66:443, 1988.

71. Silk DBA and others: Nutritional support in liver disease, *Gut* 32(suppl 9):29, 1991.

72. Everhart JE, Hoofnagle JH: Hepatitis B–related end-stage liver disease, *Gastroenterology* 103(5):1692, 1992.

73. National Center for Health Statistics: Advance report of the final mortality statistics, 1989, *Monthly Vital Statistics Report* 40(suppl 8):1, Hyattsville, Md, 1992, Public Health Service.

74. Neuberger J and others: Primary biliary cirrhosis, *Gut* 32(suppl 9):573, 1991.

75. MacDougall BRD and others: Portal hypertension—25 years of progress, *Gut* 32(suppl 9):18, 1991.

76. Fischer JE: Branched-chain-enriched amino acid solutions in patients with liver failure: an early example of nutritional pharmacology, *J Parenter Enteral Nutr* 14(suppl 5):29, 1990.

77. O'Grady JG, Portman B: Liver transplantation, *Gut* 32(suppl 9):79, 1991.

78. Laifer SA and others: Pregnancy in liver transplant patients—and vice versa, *Gastroenterology* 10(5):1443, 1991.

79. Lee SP, Sekijima J: Gallstones. In Yamada T, ed: *Textbook of gasteroenterology*, vol 2, New York, 1991, JB Lippincott.

80. Owyang C, Levitt M: Chronic pancreatitis. In Yamada T, ed: *Textbook of gastroenterology*, vol 2, New York, 1991, JB Lippincott.

FURTHER READING

Albert MB, Fromm H: Nonsurgical alternatives in the management of gallstones, *Intensive Care Med* 4(1):3, 1989.

This article reviews the status of nonsurgical procedures for removing gallstones and avoiding surgical removal of the gallbladder.

Donatelle EP: Constipation: pathophysiology and treatment, *Am Fam Physician* 42(5):1335, 1990.

This family physician provides an excellent review of this common problem, especially among elderly hospitalized patients, and includes a full-page table of laxative products with evaluations and comments.

Marotta RB, Floch MH: Diet and nutrition in ulcer disease, *Med Clin North Am* 75(4):967, 1991.

This clinical dietitian-physician team reviews the new directions for treatment of peptic ulcer disease and the use of regular diets for nutritional support rather than the various old bland diet therapies.

Thompson WG: *Gut reactions*, New York, 1989, Plenum Press.

This little book, written by a well-known gastroenterologist especially for persons with irritable bowel syndrome, provides much helpful information for patients with this difficult chronic disorder.

CASE STUDY

The Patient with Peptic Ulcer Disease

Lowell Randolph is a 40-year-old businessman who was admitted to the city hospital 3 weeks ago after an incidence of vomiting bright-red blood. A medical history revealed that a dull, gnawing pain in the upper abdomen began several months ago and has increased in severity during that time. It became more severe after his most recent out-of-state trip to one of his stores. Because the pain was usually accompanied by headaches, he took aspirin to help relieve it.

Initial hospital treatment consisted of blood transfusions, intravenous fluids and electrolytes, and vitamin C. Mr. Randolph continued to feel nauseated and weak but stopped vomiting. However, he passed several large, tarry stools during the first 24 hours. His initial nutritional assessment results included: weight 68 kg (150 lb); height 179 cm (70 in); albumin 2.8 g/dl; prealbumin 14 mg/dl; transferrin 18% saturation value; hemoglobin 11 g/dl; and hematocrit 35%. His medications included cimetidine, sucralfate, magnesium-aluminum hydroxide, and triple antibiotic therapy.

The patient began slowly to tolerate sips of clear liquids, then advanced to a regular diet as tolerated, showing continued improvement. Before he was discharged at the end of the second week, the nutritionist and the nurse discussed general nutritional needs with Mr. Randolph and his wife. They advised him to eat his meals regularly in as relaxed a setting and manner as possible, eliminate his frequent between-meal snacks, and take his multivitamin supplement daily with his meals. Also, they reviewed his general guidelines sheet, listing a few food-related items or habits to avoid. They also advised him to stop smoking and to rest as much as possible before returning to work. His physician had also advised him to reduce his work load and scheduled a follow-up appointment in 1 week.

Mrs. Randolph accompanied her husband to the next appointment and reported that she was pleased with his ability to put aside business duties and take more time to enjoy his family. Mr. Randolph stated that his two teenage sons had been surprisingly supportive in assisting him in following the prescribed regimen and that he plans to make it his general habit.

Questions for Analysis

1. The x-ray diagnosis of Mr. Randolph's illness was a gastric ulcer in the antrum lesser curvature. What does this mean? Where do most ulcers occur? Why?
2. What factors contributed to Mr. Randolph's ulcer? What effect did each of them have?
3. Evaluate the results of Mr. Randolph's initial nutritional assessment data. How would you use this information in nutrition counseling?
4. Identify Mr. Randolph's basic nutritional needs. Outline a teaching plan based on these needs that you would use to help him with his new diet plan. How would you include his wife in formulating and implementing his nutritional care plan?
5. What role does vitamin C play in Mr. Randolph's therapy? What other vitamins and minerals play a significant role in his care? Describe each role.
6. Why should Mr. Randolph give up coffee, cigarettes, and alcohol? What problems do you think he may encounter in trying to change these habits?

ISSUES · AND · ANSWERS

Nutritional Aspects of Diarrhea

Gastrointestinal disease so often presents barriers to efficient nutrient absorption that nutritional deficiencies are planned for automatically. Ironically these conditions also lead frequently to diarrhea, all of which result in loss of fluids and electrolytes. As expected, their replacement is the initial and primary concern of therapy. However, different types of diarrhea also present other differences; the control of type-specific problems requires different modes of treatment coordinated with the treatment of the disease it accompanies. Before looking into possible treatment modes, examine first three of the most common types of diarrhea: watery, fatty, and small volume.

Watery diarrhea occurs when the amount of water and electrolytes moving into the intestinal mucosa exceeds that amount absorbed into the blood stream. This movement of water and electrolytes into the mucosa may be secretive or osmotic.

If this movement of water and electrolytes into the mucosa is secretive, it may be active or passive. Active movement occurs with excessive gastric hydrochloric acid secretion or enterotoxin-induced infections such as cholera. Passive movement occurs with a rise in hydrostatic pressure that accompanies such infectious diseases as salmonellosis or tuberculosis, nonbacterial infections, fungal infections, renal failure, irradiation enteritis, and inflammatory bowel disease. Other conditions associated with watery diarrhea include hyperthyroidism, thyroid carcinoma, and hypermotility of the gastrointestinal tract.

If this movement of water and electrolytes into the mucosa is osmotic, it will occur when these nutrients are not absorbed because of intolerable levels of nonabsorbable particles present in the intestinal chyme. Such particles include lactose (milk sugar) in lactase-deficient individuals and gluten (grain protein) in persons with a reduced gastrointestinal transit time caused by the removal of part of the intestinal tract.

Fatty diarrhea, or steatorrhea, occurs with maldigestion or malabsorption. Maldigestion involves a lack of enzymatic activity required to completely digest food, such as reduced pancreatic exocrine activity (release of intestinal enzymes from the pancreas) caused by pancreatic insufficiency. Malabsorption means that digested materials do not make it across the intestinal mucosa to enter the blood stream. This failure occurs in conditions in which the intestinal villi are destroyed, such as celiac disease.

Small-volume diarrhea occurs mainly when the rectosigmoid area of the colon is irritated, such as in inflammatory bowel disease (Crohn's disease or ulcerative colitis). It also occurs when inflammatory conditions affect areas adjacent to the colon, as in pelvic inflammatory disease, diverticulitis, appendicitis, and hemorrhagic ovarian cysts.

The metabolic consequences of each type of diarrhea are similar. Uncontrolled, they result in syncope, hypokalemia, acid-base imbalances, and hypovolemia, with resulting renal failure. They may also be accompanied by low levels of fat-soluble vitamins, B_{12}, or folic acid, or eventually lead to protein-energy malnutrition. In addition to these conditions, each type also manifests problems associated with the disorder they accompany. Workers with the Memorial Sloan-Kettering Cancer Center in New York and the Department of Medicine at Brooke Army Medical Center in Texas have developed recommendations for treating gastrointestinal diseases associated with each type of diarrhea. These are summarized here, with the focus on the diarrheal aspects of disease.

Watery diarrhea often accompanies inflammatory bowel conditions, such as Crohn's disease, for which diet therapy involves (1) increased protein and kcalories, (2) low fats and lactose, and (3) avoidance of foods that stimulate peristalsis. Thus secretive diarrhea is reduced by eliminating foods that may stimulate gastric acid secretion, and all types of watery diarrhea are avoided by reducing the motility of the gastrointestinal tract. In other conditions in which osmotic diarrhea occurs, such as dumping syndrome, this problem is avoided by giving fluids *between* meals to avoid any extreme difference in osmotic pressures on either side of the intestinal wall. Small, frequent meals also help prevent this problem, as well as painful distention.

Fatty diarrhea frequently accompanies conditions associated with maldigestion, such as chronic pancreatitis. The dietary management of this disease involves (1) frequent meals, high in protein and carbohydrates and low in fat; (2) use of medium-chain triglycerides, which are more easily absorbed under adverse conditions; and (3) avoiding gastric stimulants, especially caffeine and alcohol. Fatty diarrhea also accompanies conditions of malabsorption, such as gluten-sensitive enteropathy. In addition to diet management strategies listed, treating this type of diarrhea also requires the removal of products that damage the mucosal villi, including lactose and gluten, which are found in wheat, rye, barley, and oats, and food products and fillers such as hydrolyzed vegetable protein products. It sometimes requires restricting fat as well. In both cases the primary concern is to monitor fats that would otherwise appear in the feces. As the therapy progresses, the fat content of the meal can be increased as tolerated to normal levels to improve palatability.

Small-volume diarrhea may accompany diverticulosis of the colon. A high-residue diet is recommended to increase fecal bulk, thereby preventing diarrhea. To prevent flatulence and distention, however, the fiber—such as wheat bran, fruits, and vegetables—should be added to the diet gradually.

All types of diarrhea can result in malnutrition, primarily because of electrolyte and fluid losses. It is important to identify the type of diarrhea occurring with each patient. Only then can an effective nutritional management strategy be designed to replace those losses, as well as to eliminate or prevent other nutrition-related problems that are possible for each case.

REFERENCES

Banwell JG: Pathophysiology of diarrheal disorders, *Rev Infect Dis* 12(suppl 1):30, 1990.

Barrett KE, Dharmsathaphorn K: Secretion and absorption: small intestine and colon. In Yamada T, ed: *Textbook of gastroenterology,* Philadelphia, 1991, JB Lippincott.

CHAPTER 20

Diseases of the Heart, Blood Vessels, and Lungs

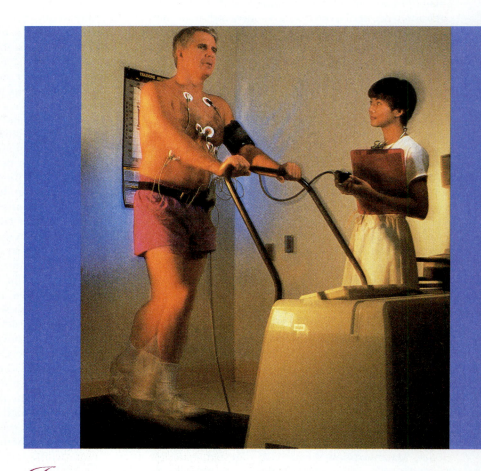

In this chapter, we consider interrelated diseases of the circulatory system—the heart, blood vessels, and lungs. In recent decades these diseases of modern civilization have become the major causes of death in the United States and most other Western societies. The magnitude of this overall health care problem is enormous.

Here we examine the health problems relating to blood circulation and the vital organs that maintain it. We see how nutrition therapy focuses on modification of key nutrients involved.

Interactions of the Circulatory System

Efficient interaction of three major organ systems is essential for normal operation of the body's life-sustaining blood circulation to service cell metabolism. First, a healthy heart muscle must provide a never-ceasing pump to keep the life-blood constantly flowing. Second, a vast network of healthy blood vessels, from large arteries to minute capillaries, must transport multiple nutrients and metabolites to nourish every single microscopic body cell. And third, healthy lungs must provide the necessary oxygen–carbon dioxide gas exchange to sustain continuing metabolic life.

Heart: The Central Pump

The heart lies in the center of the chest with its right edge directly underneath the right side of the *sternum* (breastbone). The remaining body of the heart leans to the left, and its lowest point—the apex—lies directly underneath the left nipple. Throughout life, this muscular pump beats rhythmically and continuously to send blood to the lungs and the rest of the body. At an average rate of 75 heartbeats per minute, your heart beats about 108,000 times every 24 hours. During an average lifetime, it contracts (beats) more than 2.5 billion times.

Structure and Function

The heart muscle, the *myocardium,* is a thick interconnecting network of muscle fibers. A smooth inner membrane, the *endocardium,* lines its interior surface. A

> **atrium** • An anatomic chamber; usually used alone to designate one of the pair of smaller upper chambers of the heart, with thin muscular walls, which receives blood from the body's inflowing circulation via the superior and inferior vena cava and delivers it to the thicker-walled ventricles.
>
> **ventricle** • A small cavity; one of the pair of lower chambers of the heart, with thick muscular walls, that make up the bulk of the heart. The ventricles receive blood from the atria and in turn force blood out into body circulation to the lungs for oxygenation and then into systemic body circulation to service the cells.

tough outer membrane, the *epicardium,* covers and protects its exterior surface. Together these three layers compose the strong wall of the heart. In its interior layout, the heart is actually two separate pumps. The *right side of the heart* pumps blood through the lungs to get rid of carbon dioxide and take on needed oxygen, and the *left side of the heart* pumps the returning freshly oxygenated blood through the body—indeed a brilliant functional design. A thick central muscular wall, the *septum,* divides the heart's interior into these two separate halves. The separate pump in each half has an upper chamber, the **atrium,** and a lower larger one, the **ventricle,** joined by special one-way valves to prevent backflow. In both of the separate pumps, the atrium serves mainly as a receiving blood reservoir and a primer

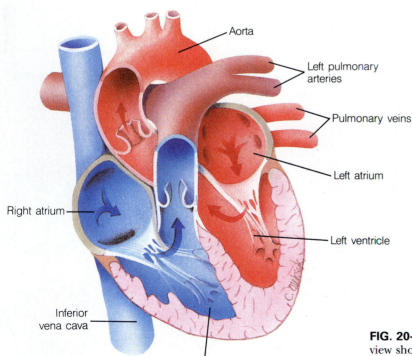

Aorta

Left pulmonary arteries

Pulmonary veins

Left atrium

Left ventricle

Right atrium

Inferior vena cava

Right ventricle

FIG. 20-1   The normal human heart. Anterior internal view showing cardiac circulation. *(From Seeley RR, Stephens TD, Tate P:* Anatomy and physiology, *ed 2, St Louis, 1992, Mosby.)*

FIG. 20-2   General scheme of the human circulatory system showing relative arrangement of heart, blood vessels, and lungs.

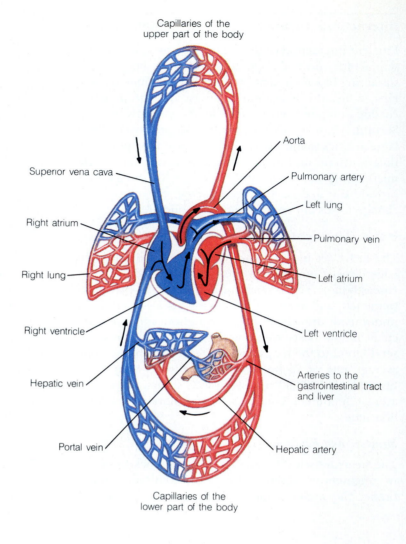

Capillaries of the
upper part of the body

Aorta

Superior vena cava

Pulmonary artery

Left lung

Right atrium

Pulmonary vein

Right lung

Left atrium

Right ventricle

Left ventricle

Hepatic vein

Arteries to the
gastrointestinal tract
and liver

Portal vein

Hepatic artery

Capillaries of the
lower part of the body

FIG. 20-3   Three phases of one heart beat that comprise the cardiac cycle. **A,** Heart action and blood flow at each phase as incoming blood is received and efficiently pumped out with heart muscle contraction. **B,** Electrocardiogram tracing of each phase. **C,** Action of the heart's own pacemaker, the sinoatrial node, sending electric waves that are picked up by the atrioventricular node and passed on to both ventricles, the major strong muscular pumps, signaling strong contractions that empty the heart.

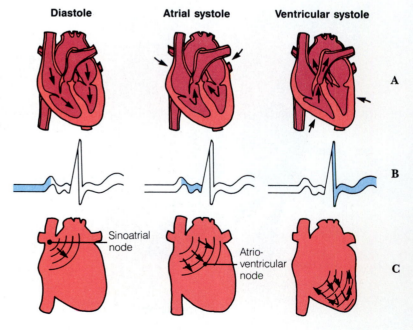

Diastole   Atrial systole   Ventricular systole

A

B

C

Sinoatrial
node

Atrio-
ventricular
node

pump. The larger ventricle supplies the major force that drives the blood forward into circulation. This functional design that routes blood through the heart can be traced in Fig. 20-1. The broad overall scheme of the body's blood circulation and the central control position of the heart is outlined in Fig. 20-2.

Cardiac Cycle

The period from the beginning of one heartbeat to the beginning of the next is called the *cardiac cycle*. The pumping action of the heart in one beat has three phases regulated by electrical waves that spread from the heart's own pacemaker, the *sinoatrial node,* and are clearly seen in an electrocardiogram tracing (Fig. 20-3).[1]

1. *Diastole.* In diastole, the resting phase, the heart fills with blood as deoxygenated blood from the body flows into the right side and at the same time oxy-

genated blood from the lungs flows into the left side. The heart muscle is at rest, and the electrical impulse begins to spread from the sinoatrial node (Fig. 20-3).

2. *Atrial systole.* In the second phase, atrial systole, both atriums (upper heart chambers) contract simultaneously and squeeze more blood into the ventricles (lower heart chambers), completely filling them. The electrical impulse reaches the atrioventricular node (see Fig. 20-3).

3. *Ventricular systole.* In the final phase, ventricular systole, both ventricles contract producing two simultaneous actions: (1) *deoxygenated blood* from the right ventricle is pumped into the pulmonary artery going to the lungs for more oxygen, and (2) *oxygenated blood* from the left ventricle is pumped into the *aorta,* the body's major central artery that serves the network of smaller branching blood vessels through-

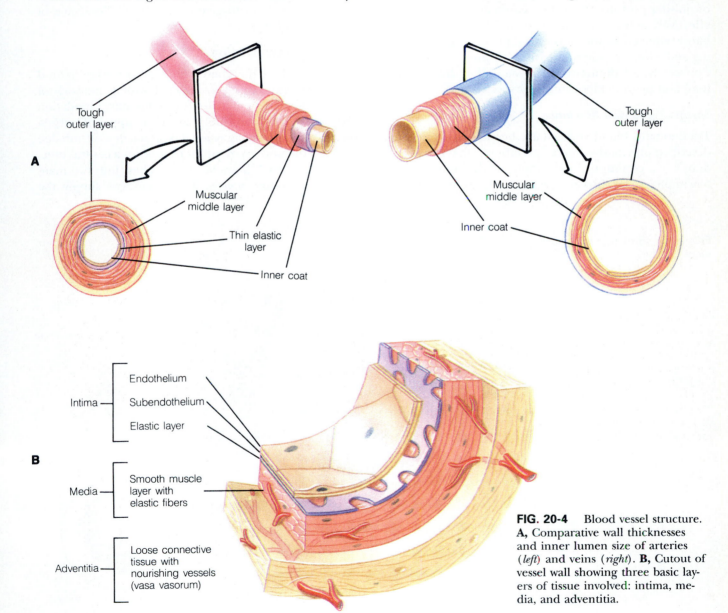

FIG. 20-4 Blood vessel structure. **A,** Comparative wall thicknesses and inner lumen size of arteries (*left*) and veins (*right*). **B,** Cutout of vessel wall showing three basic layers of tissue involved: intima, media, and adventitia.

out body tissues. By these two simultaneous actions, both lower heart chambers are emptied. During this final phase, waves of electrical activity cover the ventricles and stimulate this forceful emptying, and then the cycle begins again (see Fig. 20-3).

Blood Vessels: Transport and Regulatory Systems

General Structure and Function

Blood vessels are uniquely structured to meet their functional needs as a transport system to convey a smooth, steady blood supply to working body cells. Basically the arteries and veins are pliable tubes with relatively thick walls composed of three layers: (1) a smooth inner lining, (2) a muscular elastic middle layer, and (3) a fibrous outer layer (Fig. 20-4). The arteries have a thicker muscle layer, a tough outer layer, and an extra thin elastic layer, enabling them to control surges of pulsing pressure from the heartbeat. Thus they are effectively able to provide a tissue blood flow that is hardly affected by the pulsating nature of heart pumping and allows the blood to efficiently nourish the cells. Conversely, the thinner walls of veins allow them to distend and provide blood reservoirs as needed.

Specific Endothelial Regulation

Traditionally, blood vessels have been viewed solely as described previously—mere "plumbing," that is, as conduits for a constant blood supply, as the term *circulation* implies. Now, however, researchers are discovering

that blood vessels play a far more dynamic role in regulating blood pressure and blood clotting, as well as their own growth.[2] The key to these regulatory functions, according to the new research findings, lies in the *endothelial cells*. These thin, flat, elongated cells form the inner cell layer of blood vessels and provide an essential interface between the vessel and the blood. They constitute a major line of defense for the cardiovascular system. Endothelial injury is now recognized as a major underlying link to cardiovascular disease and hypertension.[2,3] A functionally intact **endothelium** and the release of its key substance, now known to be *nitrous oxide (NO)*—which affects vascular tone and can dilate blood vessels—is necessary to maintain appropriate blood pressure,. Although scientists are just now beginning to discover some of the extraordinarily beneficial roles that NO has in human physiology and health, this clearly demonstrated role in cardiovascular health was sufficient for them to give it their 1992 "Molecule of the Year" award.[4,5]

Lungs: Oxygen Station

The lungs lie in the chest within the rib cage behind the heart immediately connected with a network of blood vessels that comprise the pulmonary circulation (Fig. 20-5). They provide a constant supply of oxygen through the *respiratory system*. Oxygen-laden air inhaled through the nose or mouth travels down a central tube, the *trachea*, which branches in the chest into two main air passages—the *bronchi*. These passages supply the

FIG. 20-5   Structure and placement of lungs.

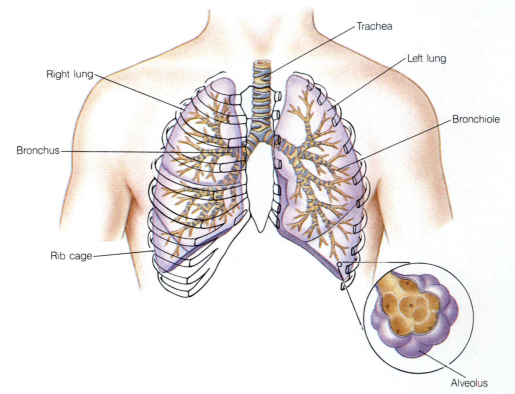

Trachea

Left lung

Right lung

Bronchiole

Bronchus

Rib cage

Alveolus

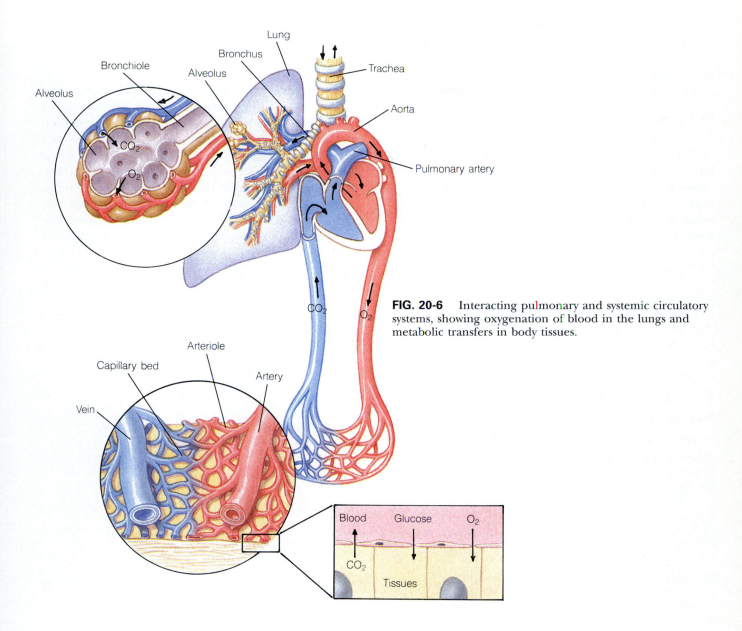

FIG. 20-6 Interacting pulmonary and systemic circulatory systems, showing oxygenation of blood in the lungs and metabolic transfers in body tissues.

right and left lungs. Each of the bronchi in turn forms a bronchial tree, branching out into smaller bronchi and then into still smaller *bronchioles,* which open out into tiny grapelike clusters of air sacs—the *alveoli.* Through the thin walls of the tiny alveoli, the blood gases oxygen (O_2) and carbon dioxide (CO_2) diffuse into and out of the blood. An extensive capillary network, often called a capillary bed, fans out through each lung and surrounds each tiny twig of the bronchial tree. Here the oxygen is absorbed, and carbon dioxide is released and exhaled into the air (Fig. 20-6). To facilitate this task of respiration, each lung is covered with a double membrane called the *pleura.* This unique membrane allows the lungs to slide freely as they expand and contract during breathing.

Oxygen Uptake

Oxygen diffuses from the alveoli into the pulmonary blood, where it combines with hemoglobin in red blood cells to form oxyhemoglobin as a carrier. The oxygenated blood then returns through the pulmonary circulation to the heart. Here the heart pumps the oxygenated blood throughout the body network of main

endothelium · Layer of epithelial cells that line the cavities of the heart, the blood and lymph vessels, and the serous cavities of the body, originating from the mesoderm.

arteries and smaller branching arterioles. Finally it reaches the feathery network of tissue capillaries, whose thin membrane is a single layer of thin, elongated epithelial cells to facilitate passage of blood gases, fluids and electrolytes, and nutrients. Here the oxygen is released to the cells for use in cell metabolism of the nutrients. These metabolic cell actions form large quantities of carbon dioxide, which in turn enters the tissue capillaries and is transported back via the heart to the lungs for expiration and exchange for more oxygen.

Diseases in any of the vital organs that form the body's circulatory system—heart, blood vessels, and lungs—have devastating effects. We consider now such disorders in each of the organ systems involved.

Coronary Heart Disease: The Problem of Atherosclerosis

The Underlying Disease Process

Atherosclerosis, the major **arteriosclerosis** disease and the underlying pathologic process in coronary heart disease, is paramount in ongoing study in modern medicine. The characteristic lesions involved, as they have been observed at autopsy, are raised fibrous **plaques** (Fig. 20-7). They appear on the interior surface of the blood vessel, the **intima,** as discrete lumps, elevated above the unaffected surrounding tissue and ranging in color from pearly gray to yellowish gray. The main cellular component of the plaque is a smooth

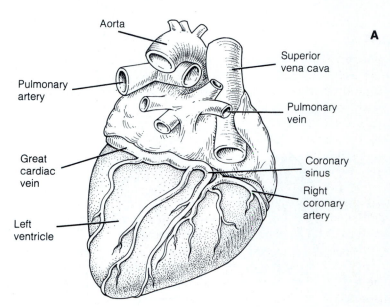

A

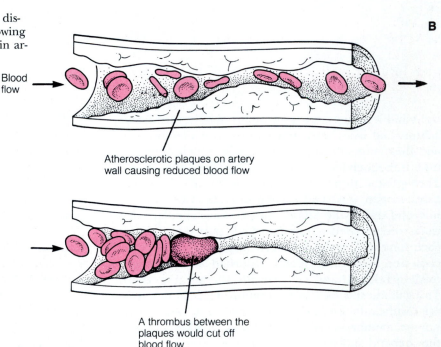

B

FIG. 20-7   Coronary blood circulation and diseased arteries. **A,** Posterior external view showing coronary arteries. **B,** Atherosclerotic plaque in artery.

TABLE 20-1

Multiple Risk Factors in Cardiovascular Disease

Personal characteristics (no control)	Learned behaviors (intervene and change)	Background conditions (screen and treat)
Gender	Stress and coping	Hypertension
Age	Smoking cigarettes	Diabetes mellitus
Family history	Sendentary life-style	Hyperlipidemia (especially
	Obesity	hypercholesterolemia)
	Food habits	
	Excess fat	
	Excess sugar	
	Excess salt	

muscle cell similar to the major cell of the normal artery wall. The plaque usually contains fatty material, such as lipoproteins, the carriers of cholesterol in the blood, which are found both inside and outside the cells. Deep in the lesions is debris from dead and dying cells, as well as various amounts of lipids. Crystals of cholesterol can be seen with the unaided eye in the softened cheesy debris of advanced lesions.

It is this fatty debris that suggested the original name **atherosclerosis,** from the Greek words *athera* (gruel) and *sclerosis* (hardening). This fatty degeneration and thickening narrow the vessel lumen and may allow a blood clot, an *embolus*, to develop from its irritating presence. Eventually the clot may cut off blood flow in the involved artery. If the artery is a critical one, such as a major coronary vessel, a heart attack occurs. The tissue area serviced by the involved artery is deprived of its vital oxygen and nutrient supply, a condition called **ischemia,** and the cells die. The localized area of dying or dead tissue is called an **infarct.** Because the artery involved supplies the cardiac muscle, the *myocardium,* the result is called an acute *myocardial infarction (MI).* The two major *coronary arteries,* with their many branches, are so named because they lie across the brow of the heart muscle and resemble a crown (see Fig. 20-7).

Thus the focus of the problem in coronary heart disease is the development of these characteristic fatty plaques called **atheromas.** Injury to the important inner *endothelial lining* of the blood vessel wall leads to a thickening thrombosis and lipid deposits, with the development of *atherosclerosis.* Analysis of the fatty plaques involved has shown considerable content of lipid materials, especially cholesterol crystals. A growing mass of evidence from large clinical trials relates these lipids, especially cholesterol, and other life-style risk factors to incidence of the disease process in numerous population groups (Table 20-1).

Causation: Relationship to General Lipid Metabolism

Over the past few years, large-scale studies have demonstrated a definite association between types of dietary fat and elevated blood lipid levels, especially cholesterol.[6] This key relationship has been demonstrated repeatedly. Dietary substitution of plant foods high in *polyunsaturated* fatty acids for animal foods high in *saturated* fatty acids, as well as total dietary fat reduction, has produced a lowering of blood cholesterol levels. The work of many investigators has provided an increasing understanding about the mechanisms, transport, and catabolism of cholesterol, and thus the control of blood cholesterol levels. This knowledge has paved the way for present practice and future directions.[7,8]

A broad international consensus has emerged, which the cholesterol-lowering guidelines of the U.S. Consensus Conference and the follow-up National Cholesterol Education Program reflect.[9-11] A concerted effort has been made to control cholesterol levels as a major means of controlling heart disease. Advancing research knowledge indicates two things about atherosclerosis:

- *Elevated serum cholesterol* is a major contributor to the heart disease process.

---

arteriosclerosis • Blood vessel disease characterized by thickening and hardening of artery walls, with loss of functional elasticity, mainly affecting the intima (inner lining) of the arteries.

atheroma • A mass of fatty plaque formed in inner arterial walls in atherosclerosis.

atherosclerosis • Common form of arteriosclerosis, characterized by the gradual formation—beginning in childhood in genetically predisposed individuals—of yellow cheeselike streaks of cholesterol and fatty material that develop into hardened plaques in the intima or inner lining of major blood vessels, such as coronary arteries, eventually in adulthood cutting off blood supply to the tissue served by the vessels; the underlying pathology of coronary heart disease.

infarct • An area of tissue necrosis due to local ischemia, resulting from obstruction of blood circulation to that area.

intima • General term indicating an innermost part of a structure or vessel; inner layer of the blood vessel wall.

ischemia • Deficiency of blood to a particular tissue, due to functional blood vessel constriction or actual obstruction.

plaque • Thickened deposits of fatty material, largely cholesterol, within the arterial wall that eventually may fill the lumen and cut off blood supply to the tissue served by the damaged vessel.

- *Dietary fat intake,* especially saturated fat, affects serum cholesterol levels.

These major strides, incorporated in the National Research Council's recent review, *Diet and Health: Implications for Reducing Chronic Disease Risks,* have given impetus to our nutrition intervention efforts.[12]

Lipoproteinemia

Increased blood concentrations of certain cholesterol-carrying *lipoproteins,* the low-density lipoproteins (LDLs) and the very–low-density lipoproteins (VLDLs), which are derived from chylomicrons by the action of lipoprotein lipase, are without question atherogenic.[13] Lipoproteins are the major transport form of lipids, especially cholesterol, in the blood (see Chapter 3). An increase in one or more of these plasma lipoproteins creates the condition called **hyperlipoproteinemia.** A more general term referring to elevated blood lipid levels is *hyperlipidemia.*

Classes of Lipoproteins

The lipoproteins in the blood are produced mainly in two places: (1) the intestinal wall after initial ingestion, digestion, and absorption of exogenous fat from a meal, and (2) the liver, from endogenous fat sources in the body. These endogenous lipoproteins carry fat and cholesterol to the tissues for use in energy production and for interchange with other products in cell metabolism. The five types of lipoproteins are classified according to their fat content and thus their density, with those having the highest fat content possessing the lowest density:

1. **Chylomicrons.** Of the lipoproteins, chylomicrons have the highest lipid content and lowest density and are composed mostly of dietary triglycerides

(TGs), with a small amount of carrier protein. They accumulate in portal blood after a meal and are efficiently cleared from the blood by the specific enzyme *lipoprotein lipase.*

2. **Very–low-density lipoproteins (VLDLs).** VLDLs still carry a large lipid (TG) content but include about 10% to 15% cholesterol. These lipoproteins are formed in the liver from endogenous fat sources.

3. **Intermediate-density lipoproteins (IDLs).** IDLs continue the delivery of endogenous TGs to cells and carry about 30% cholesterol.

4. **Low-density lipoproteins (LDLs).** In addition to other lipids LDLs carry about two thirds or more of the total plasma cholesterol; they are formed in the serum from catabolism of VLDLs. Because LDLs carry cholesterol to the cells for deposit in the tissues, they are considered the main agent in elevated serum cholesterol levels, the so-called "bad" cholesterol.

5. **High-density lipoproteins (HDLs).** HDLs carry less total lipid and more carrier protein. They are formed in the liver from endogenous fat sources. Because HDLs carry cholesterol from the tissues to the liver for catabolism and excretion, higher serum levels of this so-called "good" cholesterol form are considered protective against cardiovascular disease. The "normal" (statistical) range for HDL-cholesterol is 30 to 80 mg/dL, and a value of 75 mg/dL or above contributes definite protection and decreased risk.

The characteristics of these classes of lipoproteins are summarized in Table 20-2. Note the comparative functions of LDL and HDL. Because LDL carries cholesterol to the peripheral cells, for example, it contributes the "cholesterol of concern" in *familial hypercholester-*

TABLE 20-2

Characteristics of the Classes of Lipoproteins

Characteristic	Chylomicrons	Very–low-density (VLDL)	Intermediate-density (IDL)	Low-density (LDL)	High-density (HDL)
Composition					
Triglycerides (TGs)	80%-95%; diet, exogenous	60%-80%; endogenous	40%; endogenous	10%-13%; endogenous	5%-10%; endogenous
Cholesterol	2%-7%	10%-15%	30%	45%-50%	20%
Phospholipid	3%-6%	15%-20%	20%	15%-22%	25%-30%
Protein	1%-2%	5%-10%	10%	20%-25%	45%-50%
Function	Transport dietary TGs to plasma and tissues, cells	Transport endogenous TGs to cells	Continue transport of endogenous TGs to cells	Transport cholesterol to peripheral cells	Transport free cholesterol from membranes to liver for catabolism
Place of synthesis	Intestinal wall	Liver	Liver	Liver	Liver
Size, density					
Description	Largest, lightest	Next largest, next lightest	Intermediate size, lighter	Smaller, heavier	Smallest, densest, heaviest
Density	0.095	0.095-1.006	1.00-1.03	1.019-1.063	1.063-1.210
Size in nanometers (nm)	75-100	30-80	25-40	10-20	7.5-10

TABLE 20-3

Apoproteins in the Structure of Human Plasma Lipoproteins

Apoprotein	Related lipoprotein	Tissue origin	Function
A-I	CM, VLDL, HDL	Intestine, liver	Activates LCAT
A-II	CM, VLDL, HDL	Intestine, liver	Unclear
A-III	Subfraction of HDL		Catalyzes transfer of cholesterol esters among lipoproteins
A-IV	CM, VLDL, HDL, free in plasma	Intestine, liver	May activate LCAT
B-48	CM	Intestine	Secretes CM; transports cholesterol and TGs
B-100	VLDL, IDL, LDL	Liver	Secretes VLDL; recognizes LDL receptor
C-I	CM, VLDL, HDL	Liver	Inhibits hepatic uptake of lipoproteins
C-II	CM, VLDL, HDL	Liver	Activates lipoprotein lipase
C-III	CM, VLDL, HDL	Liver	Inhibits lipoprotein lipase and premature remnant clearance
D	HDL	Spleen, liver, intestine, and adrenal glands	Functions in cholesterol ester transfer complex
E	CM, VLDL, IDL, trace amounts in LDL and HDL	Liver, macrophages, and body tissues except the intestine	Recognizes remnant and LDL receptor; acts as regulator in immune system; modulates cell growth

CM, chylomicron; HDL, high-density lipoprotein; IDL, intermediate-density lipoprotein; LDL, low-density lipoprotein; VLDL, very–low-density lipoprotein; LCAT, lecithin-cholesterol acyltransferase; TG, triglyceride.

olemia and is a more valid measure of risk status than is the total cholesterol value.[14] The LDL value may be calculated by the following formula:

$$LDL = Total\ cholesterol - (20\%\ TG + HDL)$$

Functional Classification of Lipid Disorders

Current clinical practice is based on a functional classification system that reveals two important factors: (1) recognition of the genetic factors involved, and (2) focus on the role of *apoproteins* in the course of lipoprotein formation, transport, or destruction. Both of these factors will be encountered in readings and in clinical work with patients. Thus the outline provided in this discussion and the summaries in Table 20-3 of apoproteins and in Table 20-4 of the functional classification of lipid disorders are useful in understanding the clinical problems involved and in counseling patients.

Apoproteins

The term **apoprotein** refers to a major protein part of a combined metabolic product—in this case, a specific protein part of a combined lipid-protein molecule (Fig. 20-8). These apoproteins are increasingly recognized as important parts of the lipoprotein molecule as more of them are identified, analyzed, and classified by letter and number. For example, apoprotein B is a common attachment to LDLs and serves two basic functions: (1) it aids transport of lipids in a water medium, the blood, and (2) it transports lipids into cells for metabolic purposes. When apoprotein B-100, a single large protein molecule, attaches to one pole of the LDL (see Fig. 20-8), it provides a recognition site for the LDL receptors on the cell, causing the entire LDL to be transported by pinocytosis into the cell for use in cell metabolism.[1]

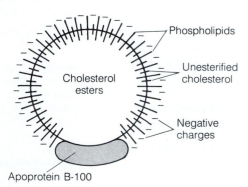

FIG. 20-8 Composition and structure of low-density lipoprotein (LDL), primary transporter of cholesterol in human plasma. Apoprotein B-100 binds to LDL and provides recognition site for transport into cells. (*Modified from Guyton AC: Textbook of medical physiology, ed 8, Philadelphia, 1991, WB Saunders.*)

apoprotein • A separate protein compound that attaches to its specific receptor site on a particular lipoprotein and activates certain functions, such as synthesis of a related enzyme. For example, apoprotein C II is an apoprotein of HDL and VLDL that functions to activate the enzyme lipoprotein lipase.

hyperlipoproteinemia • Elevated level of lipoproteins in the blood.

TABLE 20-4

Functional Classification of Lipid Disorders

Type of defect or lipid disorder	Abnormal lipid pattern	Clinical characteristics	Nutritional therapy
Defective synthesis of apolipoproteins			
Apolipoprotein A deficiency	Decreased HDL level Increased tissue cholesterol level Decreased serum cholesterol level Increased serum TG level	Rare Genetic Tangier disease	Low cholesterol Low fat
Apolipoprotein B deficiency	High mucosal tissue fat No lipoprotein synthesis possible	Rare Genetic Serious prognosis for child Malabsorption Steatorrhea	Very low fat
Apolipoprotein C deficiency	Increased TG level Increased chylomicron level	Rare Genetic Early childhood Abdominal pain (pancreatitis) Lipemia, retinalis Xanthomas Hepatosplenomegaly	Very low fat (20 g) High carbohydrate Medium-chain triglycerides (MCTs)
Apolipoprotein E deficiency	Increased chylomicron remnants Decreased serum LDL level Increased cholesterol level Increased TG level	Relatively uncommon Genetic Xanthomas Premature atherosclerosis	Low cholesterol (<300 mg) Low saturated fat Increased substitution of polyunsaturated fat Weight reduction
Enzyme deficiency			
Lipoprotein lipase deficiency	Increased chylomicron level	Rare Genetic Early childhood Abdominal pain (pancreatitis) Lipemia, retinalis Xanthomas Hepatosplenomegaly	Very low fat (20 g) High carbohydrate MCTs
Lecithin-cholesterol acyltransferase deficiency	Overall abnormal lipid pattern: all lipoproteins have low amounts of cholesterol esters and high concentrations of free cholesterol and lecithin Accumulation of large LDL particles rich in unesterified cholesterol	Rare Genetic Abnormal cornea Anemia Kidney damage	Low cholesterol Low fat
LDL-receptor deficiency			
Familial hypercholesterolemia	Increased LDL level Increased total cholesterol level Increased VLDL level	Common Genetic Increased atherosclerosis All ages Xanthomas	Low cholesterol (<300 mg) Low saturated fat Substitution of polyunsaturated fat
Other inherited hyperlipidemias			
Familial hypertriglyceridemia	Increased VLDL level Increased TG level Increased cholesterol level Sometimes increased blood sugar	Common Genetic Glucose intolerance Possible type II (non–insulin-dependent) diabetes mellitus Obesity Accelerated atherosclerosis	Weight reduction Low simple carbohydrates Low saturated fat Low cholesterol
Familial multiple hyperlipoproteinemia	Increased VLDL level Increased LDL level	Fairly common Genetic Adult Xanthomas; vascular disease	Low cholesterol (<300 mg) Low saturated fat Substitution of polyunsaturated fat Weight reduction
Familial type V hyperlipoproteinemia	Increased chylomicron level Increased VLDL level Increased cholesterol level Increased TG level	Rare Glucose intolerance Obesity Abdominal pain (pancreatitis) Hepatosplenomegaly	Weight reduction Controlled carbohydrate and fat intake High protein

Various types of LDLs have specific receptor sites for particular apoproteins to which the apoprotein is attracted and which in large measure determine function.

Function

When lipoproteins are synthesized in the intestinal wall, liver, and serum, the protein component is made up of varying kinds of apoprotein parts. These genetically determined components influence the structure, receptor binding, and metabolism of lipoproteins. It is an apoprotein component that helps to form the special spherical droplets of lipid material for transport in the bloodstream (see Chapter 5). Apoprotein determination is currently a useful laboratory tool for identifying persons at high risk for coronary heart disease.[13,15]

Classes

A number of apoproteins and their corresponding *apolipoproteins* have been identified. The class designations in common use are apoprotein A, B, C, and E. In turn, each class consists of several different proteins—for example, A-I, A-II, A-III, and A-IV. All of these classes of apoproteins are made by the liver, and the intestinal mucosa makes A and B apoproteins. Table 20-3 lists these various classes of apoproteins with their related lipoproteins and functions.

Defects in Synthesis of Apolipoproteins

The current functional approach classifies lipid disorders in four major groups based on the underlying functional problem: (1) defects in apoprotein synthesis, (2) enzyme deficiencies, (3) LDL-receptor deficiency, and (4) other inherited hyperlipidemias. The summary of these lipid disorders in Table 20-4 provides a review of these basic related conditions and nutritional therapies.

General Principles of Nutritional Therapy: Fat-Modified Diets

Basic Guidelines

The two major lipid factors of concern in a fat-controlled diet are (1) the total amount of fat in the diet and (2) the kind of fat used in terms of cholesterol and saturated fats. These two principles were first applied in the generally used approach of the "prudent" food pattern, as originally proposed a decade ago by the American Heart Association (AHA) and compared with the usual American diet still followed by too many persons (Table 20-5).[16] The initial AHA prudent diet has been revised to meet current lipid-lowering recommendations (Table 20-6). The reports of the Expert Panel on Detection, Evaluation, and Treatment of High Blood Cholesterol in Adults issued in 1988 and the Expert Panel on Population Strategies issued in 1990 further refined these dietary principles with spe-

---

TABLE 20-5

The Prudent Diet as Compared with the Usual American Diet

	Prudent diet	Usual American diet
Total kcalories	Sufficient to maintain ideal body weight	Often excessive for need
Cholesterol	300 mg	600-800 mg
Total fats (% of kcalories)	30%-35%	40%-45%
Saturated	10% or less	15%-20%
Monounsaturated	15%	15%-20%
Polyunsaturated	10%	5%-6%
P/S ratio (polyunsaturated/saturated fat in the diet)	1-1.5:1	0.3:1
Carbohydrates (% of kcalories)	50%-55%	40%-45%
Starch (complex CHO)	30%-35%	20%-25%
Simple sugars	10%	15%-20%
Proteins (% of total kcalories)	12%-20%	12%-15%
Sodium	130 mEq	200-250 mEq

TABLE 20-6

American Heart Association Revised Prudent Diet Guidelines for Lowering Elevated Blood Lipid Levels

	Step 1 % total kcalories	Step 2 % total kcalories
Total fat	<30	<30
Saturated	<10	<7
Monounsaturated	10-15	10-15
Polyunsaturated	10	10
Carbohydrates	50-60	50-60
Protein	15-20	15-20
Cholesterol	<300 mg/day	<200 mg/day

TABLE 20-7

Step 1 and Step 2 Diets for Treating High Plasma Cholesterol Levels in Adults (NCEP)*

Nutrient	Step 1 % total kcalories	Step 2 % total kcalories
Total fat	30	30
Saturated	10	7
Monounsaturated	10-15	10-15
Polyunsaturated	10	10
Carbohydrates	50-60	50-60
Protein	10-20	10-20
Cholesterol	300	200
Total kcalories	Sufficient to achieve and maintain desirable weight	Sufficient to achieve and maintain desirable weight

*National Cholesterol Education Program, adult treatment panel guidelines.

TABLE 20-8

Step 1 Diet Guide: Modifications to Lower Plasma Cholesterol Levels in Adults (NCEP)*

Food groups	Choose	Decrease
Fish, chicken, turkey, and lean meats (3-oz cooked portions)	Fish; poultry without skin; lean cuts of beef, lamb, pork, or veal; shellfish	Fatty cuts of beef, lamb, or pork; spare ribs; organ meats; regular cold cuts; sausages; hot dogs; bacon; sardines; roe
Skimmed and low-fat milk, cheese, yogurt, and dairy substitutes	Skimmed or 1%-fat milk (liquid, powdered, evaporated), buttermilk	Whole milk: (4% fat) regular, evaporated, condensed; cream, half & half, 2% milk, imitation milk products, most nondairy creamers, whipped toppings
	Nonfat (0% fat) or low-fat yogurt	Whole milk yogurt
	Low-fat cottage cheese (1% or 2% fat)	Whole milk cottage cheese (4% fat)
	Low-fat cheeses, farmer or pot cheeses (all of these should be labeled no more than 2 to 6 g fat per oz)	All natural cheeses (e.g., blue, Roquefort, Camembert, cheddar, Swiss)
		Low-fat or "light" cream cheese, low-fat or "light" sour cream
		Cream cheeses, sour cream
	Sherbet, sorbet	Ice cream
Eggs	Egg whites (2 whites = 1 whole egg in recipes), cholesterol-free egg substitutes	Egg yolks
Fruits and vegetables	Fresh, frozen, canned, or dried fruits and vegetables	Vegetables prepared in butter, cream, or other sauces
Breads and cereals	Homemade baked goods using unsaturated oils sparingly, angel food cake, low-fat crackers, low-fat cookies	Commercially baked goods: pies, cakes, doughnuts, croissants, pastries, muffins, biscuits, high-fat crackers, high-fat cookies
	Rice, pasta	Egg noodles
	Whole-grain breads and cereals (e.g., oatmeal, whole wheat, rye, bran, multigrain)	Breads in which eggs are major ingredient
Fats and oils	Baking cocoa	Chocolate
	Unsaturated vegetable oils: corn, olive, rapeseed, safflower, sesame, soybean, sunflower	Butter, coconut oil, palm oil, palm kernel oil, lard, bacon fat
	Margarine or shortenings made from one of the unsaturated oils listed above	
	Diet margarine	
	Mayonnaise, salad dressings made with unsaturated oils listed above	Dressings made with egg yolk
	Low-fat dressings	
	Seeds and nuts	Coconut

*National Cholesterol Education Program.

cific guidelines for practitioners.[10,11] These current dietary recommendations for adults are shown in Table 20-7, and the related food guide for adults is given in Table 20-8. The related National Cholesterol Education Program treatment criteria for adults is shown in Table 20-9 and Fig. 20-9. This stepwise approach calls first for a vigorous dietary effort to lower the serum cholesterol level before drugs are added.

Recent recommendations have also been made for children and adolescents, especially for those in high-risk families. These similar guides focus on helping children and adolescents develop early food habits on a healthful, less rich, and excessive basis. These recommendations have been made for public health (population) needs, especially for children from high-risk families, and for individual needs of children and adolescents with identified high serum levels of total cholesterol and LDL-cholesterol (Tables 20-10 through 20-

12).[17] A general population (Steps 1 and 2 diets) food guide for children and adolescents is provided in Table 20-13.

Amount of Fat

Almost half of the kilocalories of the average American's diet is contributed by fat. It is recommended that this excess be moderated to at most 30% of the total kilocalories or lowered further to 20% for higher levels of serum cholesterol. Limiting the total amount of fat is, of course, especially indicated when weight management is needed.

Kind of Fat

Largely because of the high status of meat and dairy products in the traditional American diet, about two thirds of the total fat in the American diet has been of animal origin and therefore mainly saturated fat. The

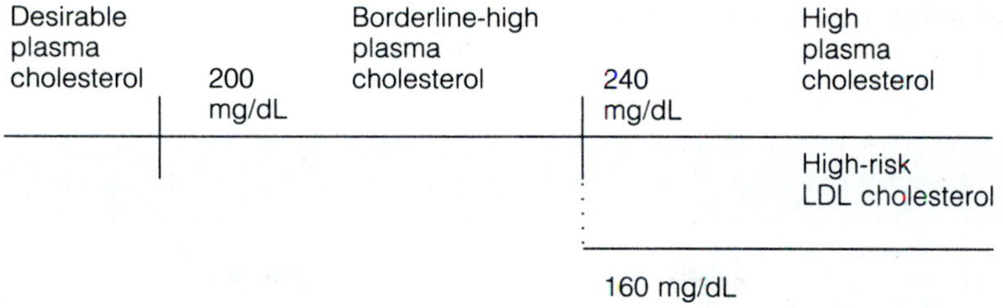

FIG. 20-9 Classification spectrum by total and low-density lipoprotein (LDL) cholesterol levels. Initial classification by plasma total cholesterol followed by LDL cholesterol evaluation for persons with high levels. (*National Cholesterol Education Program, adult treatment panel guidelines.*)

TABLE 20-9

Evaluation Criteria for Screening and Monitoring Adults for Treatment of Elevated Blood Cholesterol (NCEP)*

Type of test	Blood level classifications (mg/dl)
Total plasma cholesterol	
Desirable level	<200
Borderline high level	200-239
High level	≥240
LDL-cholesterol	
Borderline high risk	130-159
High risk	≥160

*National Cholesterol Education Program, adult treatment panel guidelines.

TABLE 20-10

Current vs Recommended Nutrient Intake in Children and Adolescents

	Current	Recommended
Saturated fatty acids (% of kcalories)	14	<10
Total fat (% of kcalories)	35-36	Average no more than 30
Polyunsaturated	6	Up to 10
Monounsaturated	13-14	10-15
Cholesterol (mg/day)	193-296	<300

From preliminary data from USDA's 1987-1988 Nationwide Food Consumption Survey and National Cholesterol Education Program: Recommendations for children and adolescents.

TABLE 20-11

Cutpoints of Total and LDL-Cholesterol for Dietary Intervention in Children and Adolescents with a Family History of Hypercholesterolemia or Premature Cardiovascular Disease

Category	Total cholesterol (mg/dl)	LDL-C (mg/dl)	Dietary intervention
Acceptable	<170	<110	Recommended population eating pattern
Borderline	170-199	110-129	Step 1 Diet prescribed, other risk factor intervention
High	≥200	≥130	Step 1 Diet prescribed, then Step 2 Diet if necessary

From National Cholesterol Education Program, *Report of the expert panel on blood cholesterol levels in children and adolescents,* USDHHS (PHS), National Institutes of Health, Washington, DC, 1991, US Government Printing Office.

TABLE 20-12

Characteristics of Step 1 and Step 2 Diets for Lowering Blood Cholesterol in Children and Adolescents

Nutrient	Recommended intake Step 1 diet	Step 2 diet
Total fat	Average of no more than 30% of total kcalories	Same
Saturated fatty acids	Less than 10% of total kcalories	Less than 7% of total kcalories
Polyunsaturated fatty acids	Up to 10% of total kcalories	Same
Monounsaturated fatty acids	Remaining total fat kcalories	Same
Cholesterol	Less than 300 mg/day	Less than 200 mg/day
Carbohydrates	About 55% of total kcalories	Same
Protein	About 15%-20% of total kcalories	Same
Kcalories	To promote normal growth and development and to reach or maintain desirable body weight	Same

From National Cholesterol Education Program, *Report of the expert panel on blood cholesterol levels in children and adolescents,* USDHHS (PHS), National Institutes of Health, Washington, DC, 1991, US Government Printing Office.

TABLE 20-13

Foods to Choose and Decrease for the Step 1* and Step 2 Diets for Children and Adolescents

Food group	Choose	Decrease
Meat, poultry, fish	Beef, pork, lamb; lean cuts trimmed well before cooking	Beef, pork, lamb, regular ground beef, fatty cuts, spare ribs, organ meats, sausage, regular luncheon meats, wieners, bacon
	Poultry without skin	Poultry with skin, fried chicken
	Fish, shellfish	Fried fish, fried shellfish
	Processed meat prepared from lean meat (e.g., turkey ham, tuna, wieners)	Regular luncheon meat (e.g., bologna, salami, sausage, wieners)
Eggs	Egg whites (2 whites = 1 whole egg in recipes), cholesterol-free egg substitute	Egg yolks (if more than 4 per week on Step 1 or if more than 2 per week on Step 2; includes egg used in cooking
Dairy products	Milk: skim or 1% fat (fluid, powdered, evaporated), buttermilk	Whole milk (fluid, evaporated, condensed), 2% low-fat milk, imitation milk
	Yogurt: nonfat or low-fat yogurt or yogurt beverages	Whole milk yogurt, whole milk yogurt beverages
	Cheese: low-fat natural or processed cheese (part-skim mozzarella, ricotta) with no more than 6 g fat per oz on Step 1, or 2 g fat per oz on Step 2	Regular cheeses (American, blue, Brie, cheddar, Colby, Edam, Monterey Jack, whole milk mozzarella, Parmesan, Swiss), cream cheese, Neufchâtel cheese
	Cottage cheese: low-fat, nonfat, or dry curd (0 to 2% fat)	Cottage cheese (4% fat)
	Frozen dairy dessert: ice milk, frozen yogurt (low-fat or nonfat)	Ice cream
		Cream, half & half, whipping cream, nondairy creamer, whipped topping, sour cream
Fats and oils	Unsaturated oils: safflower, sunflower, corn, soybean, cottonseed, canola, olive, peanut	Coconut oil, palm kernel oil, palm oil
	Margarine made from unsaturated oils listed above, light or diet margarine	Butter, lard, shortening, bacon fat
	Salad dressings made with unsaturated oils listed above, low-fat or oil-free	Dressings made with egg yolk, cheese, sour cream, whole milk
	Seeds and nuts: peanut butter, other nut butters	Coconut
	Cocoa powder	Chocolate
Breads and cereals	Breads: whole-grain bread, hamburger and hot dog bun, corn tortilla	Bread in which eggs are a major ingredient, croissants
	Cereals: oat, wheat, corn, multigrain	Granola made with coconut
	Pasta	Egg noodles and pasta containing egg yolk
	Rice	
	Dry beans and peas	
	Crackers, low-fat: animal-type, graham, saltine-type	High-fat crackers
	Homemade baked goods using unsaturated oil, skim or 1% milk, and egg substitute: quick breads, biscuits, cornbread muffins, bran muffins, pancakes, waffles	Commercial baked pastries, muffins, biscuits
	Soup: chicken or beef noodle, minestrone, tomato, vegetarian, potato	Soup containing whole milk, cream, meat fat, poultry fat, or poultry skin
Vegetables	Fresh, frozen, or canned	Vegetables prepared with butter, cheese, or cream sauce
Fruits	Fruit: fresh, frozen, canned, or dried	Fried fruit or fruit served with butter or cream sauce
	Fruit juice: fresh, frozen, or canned	
Sweets and modified fat desserts	Beverages: fruit-flavored drinks, lemonade, fruit punch	
	Sweets: sugar, syrup, honey, jam, preserves, candy made without fat (candy corn, gumdrops, hard candy), fruit-flavored gelatin	Candy made with chocolate, coconut oil, palm kernel oil, palm oil
	Frozen desserts: sherbet, sorbet, fruit ice, popsicles	Ice cream and frozen treats made with ice cream
	Cookies, cake, pie, pudding prepared with egg whites, egg substitute, skim milk or 1% milk, and unsaturated oil or margarine; gingersnaps; fig bar cookies; angel food cake	Commercial baked pies, cakes, doughnuts, high-fat cookies, cream pies

From the National Cholesterol Education Program: *Report of the expert panel on blood cholesterol levels in children and adolescents,* USDHHS (PHS), National Institutes of Health, Washington, DC, 1991, US Government Printing Office.

*The Step 1 Diet has the same nutrient recommendations as the eating pattern recommended for the general population.

Added Food Factors in CHD Therapy

TO PROBE FURTHER

The primary focus of nutritional therapy for coronary heart disease (CHD) is the control of lipid factors, including cholesterol and saturated fats. Two other food factors, however, play a different role. In varying ways they help to protect us from CHD development.

Dietary fiber

Studies indicate that water-soluble types of dietary fiber have significant cholesterol-lowering effect. Soluble fiber includes gums, pectin, certain hemicelluloses, and storage polysaccharides. Foods rich in soluble fiber include oat bran and dried beans, with additional amounts in barley and fruits. Oat bran, for example, contains a primary water-soluble gum, beta-glucan, which is a lipid-lowering agent. Soluble dietary fiber (1) delays gastric emptying, (2) increases intestinal transit time, (3) slows glucose absorption, and (4) is fermented in the colon into short-chain fatty acids that may inhibit liver cholesterol synthesis and help clear LDL-cholesterol.

On the other hand, insoluble dietary fiber—cellulose, lignin, and many hemicelluloses—found in vegetables, wheat, and most other grains does not have these lipid-lowering effects. Thus an increased use of soluble fiber food sources, especially oat bran and legumes, would have beneficial effects.

Omega-3 fatty acids

Studies indicate that the omega-3 fatty acids, *eicosapentaenoic acid (EPA)* and *docosahexaenoic acid (DHA)* (see Chapter 3), which are found mostly in seafood and marine oils, also have protective functions. They can (1) change the pattern of plasma fatty acids to alter platelet activity and reduce platelet aggregation that causes blood clotting, thus lowering risk of coronary thrombosis, (2) decrease synthesis of very–low-density lipoproteins (VLDLs), and (3) increase antiinflammatory effects.

It would seem, then, that factors in foods such as oats, dried beans, and fatty fish would provide valuable lipid-lowering additions to our diets.

REFERENCES

Anderson JW, Gustafson NJ: Dietary fiber and heart disease: current management concepts and recommendations, *Top Clin Nutr* 3(2):21, 1988.
Simopoulos AP: Omega-3 fatty acids in growth and development. II. The role of omega-3 fatty acids in health and disease: dietary implications, *Nutr Today* 23(3):12, 1988.

remaining one third has come from vegetable sources and is mainly unsaturated fat. However, this ratio has gradually been changing over the past few years with the use of less animal and more plant fat. This has been the general goal of the prudent diet (see Table 20-5), illustrated by its breakdown of total fat according to degree of saturation with emphasis on unsaturated fats reflected in the **polyunsaturated/saturated (P/S) ratio.**

Cholesterol

The current stepwise guidelines place greater emphasis on the control of cholesterol and total fat and its degrees of saturation, according to serum levels of LDL-cholesterol and presence of heart disease history and other risk factors (see Table 20-7). Serum cholesterol values used in the program as guidelines for testing and monitoring are shown in Table 20-9 for adults and Table 20-11 for children.

Additional Dietary Factors

Several additional dietary factors are involved in nutritional therapy for heart disease. These include dietary fiber, omega-3 fatty acids (see box above), and sodium. Each of these factors may need consideration, along with the primary focus on fat and cholesterol.

Acute Cardiovascular Disease: Myocardial Infarction

Medical Management

Initial medical treatment of myocardial infarction (MI), or heart attack, usually includes strong analgesics for the severe unremitting pain, oxygen therapy, and intravenous fluids for shock. Drugs may include lidocaine, an antiarrhythmic drug to reduce risk of ventricular fibrillation (irregular heartbeat); diuretics for heart failure to avoid accumulation of fluid in the lungs; and beta-blockers, which occupy the beta-receptors and prevent norepinephrine from stimulating the muscles. In some hospitals, patients who arrive shortly after the heart attack are treated with a fast-acting thrombolytic drug, *streptokinase,* an enzyme that dissolves blood clots, followed by an *angioplasty,* a procedure used to widen the narrowed coronary arteries. In this procedure, done with a local anesthestic and guided by x-ray imaging, a balloon at the tip of a cath-

P/S ratio • Ratio of polyunsaturated to saturated fats in the diet.

eter is inserted into the artery and positioned at the narrowed point. The balloon is then inflated and deflated a few times to widen the vessel and then withdrawn.

Nutritional Management

In the initial acute phase of cardiovascular disease, a myocardial infarction requires close attention to dietary modifications. The basic clinical objective is cardiac rest to allow the healing process to begin. All care is directed toward this basic need for cardiac rest, so that the damaged heart can be restored to normal functioning. The diet is therefore modified in energy value and texture, as well as in fat and sodium.

1. **Energy—kilocalories.** A brief period of undernutrition during the first few days after the attack is advisable. The metabolic demands for digestion, absorption, and metabolism of food require a generous cardiac output volume. Small intakes of food at a time, spread over the day, decrease the metabolic work load to a level that the weakened heart can accommodate. The patient progresses to more food as healing occurs. During the initial recovery stages, the diet may be limited to about 1200 to 1500 kilocalories to continue cardiac rest from metabolic work loads. If the patient is obese, as is frequently the case, this kilocalorie level may be continued for a longer period to help the patient begin very gradually to lose some of the excess weight.
2. **Texture.** Early feedings generally include foods soft in texture or easily digested to avoid excess effort in eating. Smaller meals served more frequently may give needed nutrition without undue strain or pressure. Avoid temperature extremes in solid and liquid foods.
3. **Lipids.** The general prudent diet (see Table 20-6) controls the amount and kind of fat, as well as cholesterol, for most patient needs. Individual modifications may be used to meet any additional needs.
4. **Sodium.** A moderately reduced sodium content in the foods selected is also emphasized. This will help control any tendency for fluid to accumulate in the body tissues. Added tissue fluid causes more work for the heart to maintain an increased blood volume circulation.

Additional Risk Factors

Heavy coffee drinking has an effect on blood cholesterol levels and also disrupts heart rhythms. An abnormal heart rhythm is seen after only one or two cups of coffee in patients with a history of irregular heart rate. The bast practice is to avoid caffeine, or limit regular coffee to two cups per day.[18] Heavy use of alcohol also increases triglyceride levels and atherosclerotic risk. If alcohol is used, the amount should be moderate.

Chronic Coronary Heart Disease: Congestive Heart Failure

In chronic coronary heart disease, a condition of congestive heart failure may develop over time. The progressively weakened heart muscle, the myocardium, is unable to maintain an adequate cardiac output to sustain normal blood circulation. The resulting fluid imbalances cause edema, especially **pulmonary edema,** to develop. This condition brings added problems in breathing called respiratory distress or *dyspnea,* which places added stress on the laboring heart. Thus heart failure is now considered a disorder of circulation, not merely a disease of the heart.[19]

Causation: Relationship to Sodium and Water

The fluid congestion of chronic heart disease relates to imbalances in the body's capillary fluid shift mechanism and its resulting hormonal effects.

1. **Imbalance in capillary fluid shift mechanism.** As the heart fails to pump out the returning blood fast enough, the venous return is retarded. This causes a disproportionate amount of blood to accumulate in the vascular system working with the right side of the heart. The venous pressure rises, a sort of "backup" pressure effect, and overcomes the balance of filtration pressures necessary to maintain the normal capillary fluid shift mechanism (see Chapter 8). Fluid that would normally flow between interstitial spaces and blood vessels is held in the tissue spaces, rather than recirculated.
2. **Hormonal mechanisms.** Two hormonal mechanisms are involved in fluid balance in the normal circulation. In this instance, both contribute to cardiac edema.
   - *Aldosterone mechanism.* This mechanism, described more completely by its full name *renin-angiotensin-aldosterone* mechanism, is normally a life-saving sodium-conserving, and hence water-conserving, mechanism to ensure essential fluid balances. In this case, however, it only compounds the edema problem. As the heart fails to propel the blood circulation forward, the deficient cardiac output effectively reduces the blood flow through the kidney nephrons. The decreased renal blood pressure triggers the renin-angiotensin-aldosterone system. Renin is an enzyme from the renal cortex that combines in the blood with its substrate, *angiotensinogen,* which is produced in the liver, to produce in turn *angiotensin I* and *II.* Angiotensin II acts as a stimulant to the adrenal glands to produce aldosterone. This hormone in turn effects a resorption of sodium in an ion exchange with potassium in the distal tubules of the nephrons, and water resorption follows. Ordinarily this is a life-saving mechanism to protect the body's vital water sup-

ply. In congestive heart failure, however, it only adds to the edema problem. The mechanism reacts as if the body's total fluid volume is reduced, when in truth the fluid is excessive. It simply is not in normal circulation but is being retained in the body's tissues.

- *ADH mechanism.* This water-conserving hormonal mechanism also adds to the edema. The cardiac stress and reduced renal flow cause the release of the **antidiuretic hormone (ADH),** also known as **vasopressin,** from the pituitary gland. ADH then stimulates still more water resorption in the nephrons of the kidney, further increasing the problem of edema.

Increased Cellular Free Potassium

As the reduced blood circulation depresses cell metabolism, cell protein is broken down and releases its bound potassium in the cell. As a result, the amount of free potassium inside the cell is increased, which increases intracellular osmotic pressure. Sodium ions in the fluid surrounding the cell then also increase in number to balance the increased osmotic pressure within the cell and prevent cell dehydration. In time the increased sodium outside the cell causes still more water retention.

Nutritional Management

The basis for all care of the person with congestive heart disease is reduction of the work load of the heart. Medical treatment involves oxygen therapy, decreased physical activity, and drug therapy with (1) diuretic agents to control fluid congestion in the lungs and (2) digitalis drugs to strengthen contractions of the heart muscle. Nutritional support involves the following:

- *Low sodium.* Sodium should be restricted to 500 to 1000 mg/day, with individual fluid restriction as needed to help reduce fluid retention, and amounts depending on the severity of the heart failure and tissue fluid accumulation.
- *Food texture and meal pattern.* Food should have relatively soft texture, require little physical effort to eat, and be divided into small feedings eaten slowly.
- *Kilocalories.* Kilocalories should be decreased to reduce any obesity, as well as to decrease the work of the heart, to meet circulatory demands for digestion and absorption.
- *Vitamins and minerals.* The person with congestive heart disease should receive a full allowance of vitamins and minerals, with special attention to any drug-nutrient interactions causing losses. For example, potassium replacement is needed when potassium-losing diuretics are used, and added vitamin B_6 may be needed when the vasodilator *hydralazine* is used for hypertension control. This drug binds vitamin B_6 and increases its excretion.

Cardiac Cachexia
Cause

Sometimes with prolonged myocardial insufficiency and heart failure, an extreme clinical condition of *cardiac cachexia* develops. Progressive and profound malnutrition results from an insufficient oxygen supply that cannot meet the demands of red blood cell formation by the bone marrow or energy needs for basic breathing. The enlarged laboring heart is unable to maintain a sufficient blood supply to the body tissues, and nutrient delivery to cells is impaired. The edema, unpalatable sodium-restricted diets, drug reactions, and postoperative complications of cardiac surgery all deepen the anorexia and reduce food intake. It should be no surprise that the incidence of *nosocomial* (hospital-induced) cardiac cachexia is not an uncommon occurrence.

Nutritional Therapy

The goal is to help restore heart-lung function as much as possible and rebuild body tissue. Team care involving the physician, clinical dietitian, nurse, patient, and family is essential. Nutrition support focuses on energy, nutrients, supplements, and feeding plan:

- *Energy.* Sufficient kilocalories are needed to cover basal energy needs, as well as energy for minimal activity; the hypermetabolism of severe congestive heart failure; and more if major surgery is planned. Depending on the extent of malnutrition indicated by the nutritional assessment, an increase of 30% to 50% of basal needs may be indicated.
- *Fluids.* Sufficient but not excessive fluid intake is needed, at a rate of about 0.5 ml/kcal/day or 1000 to 1500 ml/day.
- *Protein.* Approximately 0.8 to 1.0 g/kg body weight is needed to replace tissue losses and cover malabsorption.
- *Fat.* Using a medium-chain triglyceride (MCT) oil for part of the fat allowance modifies losses from malabsorption.
- *Sodium.* Sodium restriction varies with individual status, usually in a range of 500 to 2000 mg/day, with attention to multiple alternate seasonings to enhance palatability of food (see Appendix F).

---

antidiuretic hormone (ADH) • Water-conserving hormone from posterior lobe of pituitary gland; causes resorption of water by kidney nephrons according to body need.

pulmonary edema • Accumulation of fluid in tissues of the lung.

vasopressin • Alternate name of ADH.

- *Mineral-vitamin supplementation.* General supplementation at 1.5 to 2.0 times the RDAs, with follow-up monitoring of blood concentrations, is usually provided to meet needs for tissue rebuilding, malabsorption losses, and hypermetabolic state.
- *Feeding plan.* Small, frequent feedings are better tolerated. Large meals add to the risk of carbon dioxide accumulation and respiratory failure.
- *Enteral and parenteral nutrition support.* Enteral feeding of high-density formula is needed if regular intake is less than 1500 kcal/day, and carefully monitored parenteral nutrition support is required if intake drops to less than 500 kcal/day (see Chapter 18).

Essential Hypertension and Vascular Disease

The Problem of Hypertension

Incidence

High blood pressure is one of the most prevalent vascular diseases worldwide.[22] It presents a problem in the lives of some 62 million Americans and is a major factor in the half million strokes and 1.25 million heart attacks that occur each year.[23,24] At least 95% of these persons have **essential hypertension,** meaning that its cause is unknown, although there is apparently a strong familial predisposition with its onset in young teen years. It has become the fourth largest public health problem in America. It has often been called the "silent disease" because it carries no overt signs, but it can have serious implications if not treated and controlled. Improved control can be achieved with individual treatment, using the current antihypertensive drugs available today as needed. However, other sociocultural factors—such as access to medical care, health education, and life-style—influence mass *population* hypertension and stroke risk in the "high normal blood pressure and mild hypertensive" groups.[22,25,26]

Public Awareness

During the past decade, the U.S. National Heart, Lung, and Blood Pressure Institute of the National Institutes of Health (NIH) has initiated a public education campaign about the serious problem of hypertension and the value of preventive care. As a result, public awareness of the successful treatment of hypertension with new drugs, as well as nondrug programs for mild elevations, has grown widely.[27,28]

Nondrug Approaches

Within the broader current preventive move in health care, there is a renewed focus on nondrug approaches, which have proved to be effective treatment for mild hypertension and an important adjunct in more severe cases. In any case, the goal of all treatment is to reduce the quantity of drugs required as much as possible. Numerous continuing studies have shown the value of nondrug nutritional therapy.[29-31] These therapies have included weight reduction, regular physical exercise, reduction of salt intake, reduction of dietary fat and cholesterol, and relaxation and stress management. Such nutrition and health therapies help to avoid some unwanted side effects and the considerable cost of lifetime drug treatment.[32]

Blood Pressure Controls

Arterial Pressure

As commonly measured, blood pressure is an indication of the arterial pressure in the vessels of the upper arm. This measure is obtained by an instrument for determining the force of the pulse (Fig. 20-10). This instrument is called a *sphygmomanometer,* from the Greek words *sphygmos* (pulse), *manos* (thin), and *metron* (measure). The pulse pressure is measured in millimeters of mercury (mm Hg) rise in thin contained tubes, or in equivalent values read on gauges or digital indicators. The higher or upper value recorded is the *systolic* pressure from the contraction of the heart muscle. The lower value recorded is the *diastolic* pressure, produced during the relaxation phase of the cardiac cycle. Thus the upper limit of a normal adult blood pressure would be recorded 150/89 mm Hg.

Several factors contribute to maintaining the fluid dy-

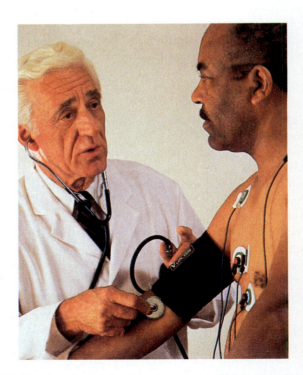

FIG. 20-10 Monitoring blood pressure. This patient has successfully used nonpharmacologic therapy to control her hypertension.

namics of normal blood pressure: (1) increased pressure on the forward blood flow, (2) increased resistance from the containing blood vessels, and (3) increased viscosity of the blood itself, making movement through the vessels more difficult. Of these factors, increased viscosity is a rare event. Thus, in discussing high blood pressure in general terms, we are dealing with the first two factors—the pumping pressure of the heart muscle propelling the blood forward and the resistance to this forward flow presented by the blood vessel walls normally or by any abnormal added constriction or thickening.

Muscle Tone of Blood Vessel Walls

In hypertension the body's finely tuned mechanisms designed to maintain fluid dynamics are not operating effectively. Normally, these systems include several agents that act to variously dilate and constrict the blood vessels to meet whatever need is present at a given time. In a hypertensive person, however, the dilation or constriction of blood vessels does not occur in the normal manner. If not effectively treated, uncontrolled elevated blood pressure results. The body systems that operate to help maintain normal blood pressure include (1) neuroendocrine functions of the sympathetic nervous system, mainly mediated by chemical neurotransmitters, such as *norepinephrine* (see Chapter 15), (2) hormonal systems, such as the renin-angiotensin-aldosterone mechanism and its *vasopressor* effect, and (3) enzyme systems such as the *kallikrein-kinin* mechanism (sometimes operating with *prostaglandins*), which controls substances that act to dilate or constrict smooth muscle as needed.

Step-Care Treatment Approach

Based on national studies and widespread community screening programs, current medical treatment centers on an improved "step-care" method of identifying types of blood pressure levels and matching standard treatment programs to these diagnosed types. Increased emphasis is given to nondrug therapies, limited use of drugs, and "step-down" weaning from drugs as life-style habits improve.[32] The identification of persons with hypertension according to degree of severity has improved the basic approach to care. These steps of care are termed mild, moderate, or severe.

Mild Hypertension

Diastolic pressure (relaxed phase of the cardiac cycle; the lower value) is 90 to 104 mm Hg. Initial consideration is given to other risk factors, such as excess weight, lack of exercise, and stress. Individual treatment is started with nondrug approaches and centers on nutritional therapies of weight control, fat and sodium modification, regular physical activity, relaxation exercises, and behavioral techniques for habit changes.

Moderate Hypertension

Diastolic pressure is 105 to 119 mm Hg. Prompt evaluation and treatment is indicated. A combination of drugs may be used: a diuretic agent to decrease the blood volume and a blocking agent to decrease muscle constriction of blood vessel walls. The basic nutritional therapy, exercise, and relaxation modes described previously continue as vital support, with the goal of reducing the amount of medication required.

Severe Hypertension

Diastolic pressure is 120 mm Hg and above. Immediate evaluation and vigorous drug therapy are demanded. Diuretic and blocking agents are continued, and a third drug may be added—a peripheral vasodilator to assist in reducing arterial resistance to blood flow. In all cases, the implications for diet therapy revolve around potassium replacement, the use of diuretics, and nutritional support for weight management, sodium modification, as well as physical exercise, stress-reduction activities, and nonsmoking.

Cerebrovascular Accident
Incidence

Arteriosclerotic vascular injury and hypertension may also affect blood vessels in the brain. In small vessels the result may be brief passing *transient ischemic attacks (TIAs)*. But in larger vessels serving more tissue, the result is a *cerebrovascular accident (CVA)*. A CVA may vary in degree from a disabling stroke to major artery involvement causing massive hemorrhage and a fatal stroke. Over the past two decades, with the declining U.S. early death rate from heart disease, stroke stands in fourth place—following cancer, heart disease, and injuries—in the leading causes of death of adults aged 25 to 65.[33] Of the nearly 150,000 Americans who die annually of stroke, approximately 13% are aged 25 to 65. However, the large majority of stroke victims are older adults. Among all U.S. population groups, black men have the highest rate of stroke. Their resulting death rate is about twice that of white men and substantially higher than for black women.[34,35]

Treatment

Treatment of TIAs includes an absolute ban on smoking, drug therapy for hypertension, and moderate di-

> **essential hypertension** • An inherent form of hypertension with no specific discoverable cause and considered to be familial; also called primary hypertension.

etary control of sodium, with the fat and cholesterol modification indicated for a prudent healthful diet. The proportion of elderly persons in the American population has been progressively increasing, and age appears to be the most important risk factor for stroke. Thus the number of elderly stroke patients is gradually increasing, and their evaluation and management requires particular attention.[36] In the case of a CVA, a permanent disability requiring rehabilitation care may result (see Chapter 26).

Peripheral Vascular Disease
Cause

Peripheral vascular disease (PVD) is characterized by narrowing of blood vessels in the legs and sometimes in the arms. The blood flow is restricted and causes pain in the affected area. Contributory risk factors include hypertension and diabetes mellitus. However, the greatest risk factor is cigarette smoking, which constricts blood vessels. More than 90% of patients with PVD are or were moderate to heavy smokers.

Symptoms and Complications

As the arteries gradually narrow because of atherosclerosis (the most common cause), an aching, tired feeling occurs in the leg muscles when walking. Resting the leg for a few minutes relieves the pain, but it recurs shortly when walking is resumed. For this reason the symptom is called **intermittent claudication.** Sometimes, a sudden arterial blockage occurs when a blood clot develops on the top of a plaque or a clot formed in the heart is carried to a peripheral artery and blocks it. The blockage causes sudden severe pain in the affected area, which becomes cold and either pale and blue and has no pulse. Movement and sensation are lost.

Treatment

By far the most important treatment for the patient is to stop smoking. As with coronary vessels, surgery on the diseased vessels is sometimes required: (1) *arterial reconstructive surgery* to bypass them, (2) *endarterectomy* to remove the obstructing fatty deposits on the inner linings, or (3) *balloon angioplasty* to widen them. Drug therapy may include antiplatelet or anticoagulant agents to prevent blood clotting. Nutritional therapy consists of the regular fat and cholesterol modifications described for coronary heart disease. Exercise is also important. The person should walk every day, gradually increasing to about an hour, stopping whenever intermittent pain occurs and resuming when it stops. Regular inspection of the feet, daily washing and stocking change, good-fitting shoes to avoid pressure, and scrupulous foot care (ideally by a *podiatrist*) are essential to prevent infection.

Chronic Obstructive Pulmonary Disease
Clinical Characteristics

Progressive congestive heart failure, as well as other respiratory problems, contributes to lung disease and the risk of respiratory failure. Malnutrition is common with the debilitating condition of *chronic obstructive pulmonary disease (COPD)*. This term describes a group of disorders in which the airflow in the lungs is limited and respiratory failure develops. The two main interrelated COPD conditions are chronic bronchitis and emphysema. Malnutrition usually accompanies COPD, and its presence increases the illness and death rates associated with the disease process. Anorexia and significant weight loss reflect a growing inability to maintain adequate nutritional status, which in turn severely compromises pulmonary function.[37] Progression of the disease process, with its increasing shortness of breath, prevents the person from living a normal life. Eventually, in progressive respiratory failure, the patient becomes dependent on a mechanical respirator and controlled oxygen supply.

Nutritional Management
Ratio of Fuel Macronutrients

Respiratory failure is actually a failure of the pulmonary exchange of oxygen and carbon dioxide. Thus its common manifestations are **hypoxemia,** deficient oxygenation of the blood, and **hypercapnia,** excess carbon dioxide in the blood. Nutritional therapy is guided by the *respiratory quotient (RQ),* the ratio of carbon dioxide produced and oxygen consumed, per unit of time, by each of the fuel nutrients. This becomes apparent in the special diet nutrient proportions used[38]:

- *Fat.* Contrary to generally recommended diets, fat is the favored fuel source in COPD because of its lower oxidative RQ value (0.7, compared with 1.0 for carbohydrate). Also, fat is a concentrated source of needed kilocalories. It is lower in osmolality than carbohydrate, and it does not contribute to the hyperglycemia often seen in critically ill patients fed formulas largely composed of dextrose and amino acids. Fat should provide about 30% to 50% of the nonprotein kilocalories in the diet.
- *Carbohydrate.* Conversely, a lower-than-usual amount of carbohydrate is recommended because of its less favorable RQ value. The metabolic effect of larger amounts of carbohydrate is to increase oxygen consumption and carbon dioxide production and retention. This is a critical imbalance for a patient with failing respiratory function. Carbohydrate should provide no more than about 50% of the nonprotein kilocalories in the diet.
- *Protein.* The need for protein in ill persons' diets to counteract the catabolic stress on body tissue is well

understood. The recommended amount for this person ranges from 1.0 to 2.5 g protein/kg/day. This amount is adjusted according to the degree of malnutrition and stress. However, in respiratory failure more is not better, and protein allowances must be carefully prescribed. In a prudent diet for failing pulmonary function, protein should provide about 15% of the total kilocalories.

Energy Needs

Adequate energy intake is based on extent of protein-kilocalorie malnutrition and loss of lean body mass. However, as with protein, kilocalorie increases are approached with caution to avoid the dangers of hypercaloric feeding in a patient with limited respiratory reserve.[39,40] Individual needs are calculated to cover basal energy expenditure, with added amounts of metabolic activity factors according to the degree of disease activity and its physiologic stress. Based on body weight, energy needs are about 25 to 35 kcal/kg/day for maintenance and 45 kcal/kg/day for anabolic needs to restore lean body mass.[37,41]

Special Enteral Feeding

Enteral feeding is the preferred mode of feeding, orally for dietary supplementation if possible or by nasoenteric tube if needed (see Chapter 18). Appropriate commercial formulas based on the recommended nutrient ratios indicated, such as Pulmocare (Ross), are available.

General guidelines for dietary modification in chronic pulmonary disease for professional use based on these nutritional support principles are available.[42] Suggestions for use in counseling COPD clinical patients in menu planning and food preparation are included.

Education and Prevention
Practical Guidance: "Why" and "How"

Personal life-style habits, especially rich food and limited exercise, create risks for heart disease and hypertension problems. Thus a large part of the health team's work is to help individuals change long-standing habits rooted in the larger society's way of life. These life-style changes are important both in treating present disease and in preventing disease development. This is not an easy task, but it is a primary task. Persons want to know *why* such personal habit change is important, which requires a sound knowledge base for motivation. And they want to know *how* to achieve these desired changes in practical ways in their life situation. All the while, they need to feel a sense of being in control of their own lives and their own decision making. So a basic part of the healing process is a partnership with pa-

tients that empowers each one to achieve that degree of self-care to the best of his or her ability, with constant encouragement and support. This is the primary goal of our therapy.

In this final section, we look at this important area of patient education and disease prevention in relation to our society's major health problems of cardiovascular disease and hypertension. Nutrient management focuses, for the most part, on fat, cholesterol, and sodium. The larger background and guidelines for fat and cholesterol control have been detailed in previous sections of this chapter. In this final section we provide general guides for sodium-restricted diets and practical approaches to planning nutritional and disease prevention.

Sodium in General Diets

The taste for a given amount of salt with food is an acquired one, not a physiologic necessity. Sufficient sodium for the body's need is provided as a natural mineral in foods. Some persons salt their foods heavily and thus form high salt taste levels. Others form lighter tastes and use smaller amounts. Common daily adult intakes of sodium range widely, from about 2 to 4 g with lighter tastes to as high as 10 to 12 g with heavier use. Salt (sodium chloride—NaCl) intakes are about twice these amounts, because sodium (Na) makes up about 40% of the NaCl molecule. The large amount of salt in the American diet, estimated to be about 6 to 15 g sodium/day (260 to 656 mEq), is largely due to the increased use of many processed food products.

Sodium-Restricted Diets

The main source of dietary sodium is common table salt. Sodium compounds that are used less often, such as baking powder and baking soda, contribute small amounts. Otherwise, the remaining dietary source is sodium occurring in some foods as a natural mineral. In general, three levels of dietary sodium restriction are

---

hypercapnia • Excess carbon dioxide in the blood.

hypoxemia • Deficient oxygenation of the blood, resulting in hypoxia, reduced oxygen supply to tissue.

intermittent claudication • A symptomatic pattern of peripheral vascular disease, characterized by absence of pain or discomfort in a limb, usually the legs, when at rest, which is followed by pain and weakness when walking, intensifying until walking becomes impossible, and then disappearing again after a rest period; seen in occlusive arterial disease.

used, as initially outlined by the American Heart Association—mild, moderate, and strict. For practical purposes, each of these levels of restriction can be achieved by a regular diet with the following basic food guides for deletion of higher salt/sodium foods:

- *Mild sodium restriction: 2 to 3 g sodium (70 to 130 mEq).* Salt may be used *lightly* in cooking, but *none* is added at the table. Salty processed foods—for example, pickles, olives, bacon, ham, and chips—are avoided.
- *Moderate sodium restriction: 1 g sodium (43.5 mEq).* No salt is used in cooking, no salt is added at the table, and no salty foods are used. Some control of natural sodium foods begins at this level. Vegetables with higher sodium levels are somewhat limited in use (see the following list under strict guide). Salt-free canned vegetables are substituted for regular canned ones, salt-free baked products are used, and meat and milk are used in moderate portions.
- *Strict sodium restriction: 0.5 g sodium (22 mEq).* This strict level is used occasionally in more severe cases. In addition to the deletions thus far, foods with higher natural sodium content—meat, milk, and eggs—are allowed only in small portions, and higher sodium vegetables (artichoke, beet greens, beets, carrots, celery, kale, mustard greens, spinach, Swiss chard, and turnips) are generally avoided.

Nutritional Management of Hypertension

There is no question that nutritional therapy, including sodium restriction, plays a large role in the treatment of hypertension. Widespread studies conducted throughout the world in a variety of communities indicate that hypertensive persons respond to some degree of sodium restriction.[43,44] Adequate potassium relates to its electrolyte balance with sodium and its replacement need when potassium-losing diuretics are used. Studies of the influence of calcium on hypertension have shown variable results, and the mechanism involved remains unclear (see box below).

In general, the current focus of nutritional therapy is on (1) sodium restriction, (2) weight management following NCEP guidelines for fat and cholesterol control, and (3) an individualized food plan. A moderately reduced daily sodium intake of about 2 to 3 g (90 to 120 mEq) is a reasonable goal. Persons in a high-risk category for the development of hypertension should certainly reduce their sodium intake as a preventive measure.

◆ **CLINICAL APPLICATION**   *The Spice of Life: Breaking Up the Salt Monopoly*

If you counsel persons on sodium-restricted diets, you probably spend a lot of time answering the question "Is there life without salt?" The standard reply is something like, "Of course there is. You'll just have to get used to the natural flavor of foods." This answer usually falls flat.

We learn to like the taste of salt; it's a taste that "accumulates" over the years. That's why it's unreasonable, for example, to expect a middle-aged man who has just discovered he has hypertension to suddenly give up his lifetime seasoning habits. It's overly optimistic to expect anyone raised on hot dogs, potato chips, and TV dinners to fall in love with the flavor of fresh broccoli overnight if it has never been a favorite food.

There is hope, however. Subjects in one study developed a lower tolerance for salty foods after following a low-sodium diet for 5 months. So if you can convince clients to reduce their salt intake for a significant period, you might get them to fall out of love with the taste of salt.

There's still the problem of getting clients to use less salt to begin with. The solution is to introduce them to the world of salt-free seasonings. Some persons are already familiar with a variety of alternate seasonings and only need some recipes that show how to use them creatively. Those who think that gourmet cooking means just using pepper instead of salt need a little extra help in selecting and using salt-free seasonings successfully. The following are some suggestions for guidelines:

- Stop adding salt at the table; it's pure habit. Get rid of the shaker—throw it away, hide it, or get it out of sight—anything to remove the reminder.
- If foods taste too bland without added salt, sprinkle them with fresh lemon juice, not salt.
- When cooking, cut the amount of salt in the recipe in half and avoid other sodium-rich seasonings.
- If you're already a good cook, or even if you're not, refer to guides for hints on spicing up old favorites without salt.

- If you're not the world's greatest chef, enroll in a basic cooking class at a local adult education center or community college and use these guidelines when preparing meals at home. You may also want to check the foods section of your local newspaper for listings of special low-sodium cooking classes offered by local health organizations.
- Relax for a moment while dinner is simmering on the stove and enjoy the wonderful new aromas filling your kitchen. Sodium reduction introduces you to a flavorful new adventure with food.

REFERENCES

Bertino M and others: Long-term reduction in dietary sodium alters the taste of salt, *Am J Clin Nutr* 36:1134, 1982.

Wylie-Rossett J: Spices to the rescue, *Prof Nutr* 14:4, 1982. ◆

Low-Sodium Food Plan

Food Preparation

Public awareness of healthful diets is creating a new market for popular guides in cookbooks and magazines for preparation of primary foods with alternative seasonings to salt and fat. Many are available, full of good ideas. A variety of alternate seasonings can be used, such as herbs and spices, onions and garlic, and whole fruit and juices, especially lemon and lime juice. Such substitute seasonings create appetizing dishes and help train the taste for less salt (see box, p. 406). References related to sodium values of foods and a salt-free seasoning guide are provided in Appendixes D to F.

Food Products

Close attention to the new food product labeling system is important. The new labeling regulations and format (see Chapters 9 and 10) provide additional information about product ingredients so that consumers can make wise choices for controlled use of or eliminating altogether salt, fat, and cholesterol, or other food additives of concern.

Special Needs

Individual adaptation is fundamental in all nutrition counseling. In this case, special attention needs to be given to those types of ethnic diets, such as Chinese, that are traditionally high in sodium. Some reduced-sodium products, such as soy sauce, are now being marketed. Also, a number of alternate, nonsalty condiments are used in Chinese dishes.

Planning Nutrition Intervention and Education

Coronary heart disease and hypertension and their related vascular problems are chronic in nature. Thus an important responsibility of the health care team is educating the patient and family about self-care needs for maintaining health.

Start Early for the Hospitalized Patient (Phase I)

Current hospital stays after a heart attack, as well as coronary bypass graft or coronary angioplasty, are brief. Opportunity for preparing patients and families, especially the spouse, for convalescence and recovery at home is limited.[45] During this period of hospitalization, or Phase I, the main concern of patient and family is survival. Attention span and information retention are limited. Forget about the old involved so-called "discharge instructions" during the anxious preparation for departure. Instead, the clinical dietitian meets with the patient and family a day or so before discharge for brief follow-up planning:

- Provide a firm connection for continuing personal support.
- Supply written names and telephone numbers for communication.
- Briefly describe individual or group resources and programs.
- Plan appointment for initial follow-up contact at home, office, or clinic to provide counseling and education services.
- Respond to any immediate needs expressed.

Use a Variety of Resources (Phase II)

After the patient returns home, Phase II rehabilitation begins. Many excellent resources are available for patient and family education. Practical discussions need to center on self-management development, spouse involvement, life-style risk factor changes, and food buying and preparation to make diets palatable and enjoyable.[46-49] Many helpful suggestions and recipes are included in the American Heart Association cookbook (one of our family favorites is Apricot Chicken). A survey trip to local markets helps identify commercial products and label information. Guidelines and food plans for general weight management (see Chapter 6) can be modified as needed to control sodium, fat, and cholesterol.

Build Family Health Habits

The wisest control of coronary heart disease and hypertension lies in prevention and positive health promotion. Real contributions begin in childhood, especially in families with strong histories of heart disease and hypertension. Sound health habits learned and practiced early within the family focus on good nutrition—including food behaviors related to fat, sugar, and salt—and a physically active life.

Target High-Risk Groups

The medical community is giving increased attention to preventing elevated blood cholesterol levels and hypertension in children of high-risk families. Along with meeting general growth needs, some preventive measures related to weight management through physical exercise and healthful food habits without excess fat and salt should be included.[50,51] Prevention in childhood is easier than trying to change strong adult habits. Also, certain high-risk groups for hypertension, including black Americans, should have access to family educational activities, counseling, and materials concerning the risks of hypertension.

Use Community Resources

A number of community agencies, programs, and materials provide resources on hypertension and heart disease.

- *Community health agencies.* In addition to local chapters of the American Heart Association, hypertension councils have been formed in many areas. A number of materials and active educational programs are available.

- *Nutrition resources.* A number of resource persons and programs may be found in most communities to assist clients and their families in planning self-care. These include various weight-management programs, registered dietitians in private practice or in local health centers who provide nutritional counseling, or public health nutritionists and nurses in city and county Public Health Departments. Other outreach programs of the Cooperative Extension Service, such as the highly successful course "Eating Today for a Healthier Tomorrow," reach rural and urban communities through county-city networks.[52]
- *Educational materials.* Cooking guides and informational material for diets low in fat, cholesterol, and salt may also be found in public bookstores and libraries. Community screening programs sponsored by industry and community agencies are other sources for additional guidance. Through community health agencies, persons with heart disease or hypertension and their families may learn to make decisions about their own health, change food habits to reduce health risks, and take more control in managing their own health needs.

To Sum Up

Coronary heart disease remains the leading cause of death in the United States. *Atherosclerosis,* its underlying pathology, involves the formation of plaque, a fatty substance that builds up along the interior surfaces of blood vessels, interfering with blood flow and damaging blood vessels. If this buildup becomes severe, it cuts off blood supplies of oxygen and nutrients to tissue cells, which in turn begin to die. When this occurs in a coronary artery, the result is a *myocardial infarction,* or heart attack. When it occurs in a brain vessel, the result is a *cerebrovascular accident,* or stroke.

The risk for atherosclerosis increases with the amount and type of blood lipids (lipoproteins) available. The *apoprotein* portion of lipoproteins is an important genetically determined part of the disease process. An elevated *serum cholesterol level* is a primary factor in atherosclerosis development.

Initial dietary recommendations for *acute cardiovascular disease* (heart attack) include caloric restriction, soft-textured foods, and small, frequent meals to reduce the metabolic demands of digestion, absorption, and metabolism of foods and their nutrients. Maintenance of a lean body weight is important. In addition, fat, saturated fat, cholesterol, and sodium should be restricted. Persons with *chronic coronary disease* (congestive heart failure) and those with *essential hypertension* benefit from weight management, exercise, and sodium restriction to overcome cardiac edema and help control elevated blood pressure.

Current dietary recommendations to help prevent coronary heart disease involve maintaining a healthy weight, limiting fats to 25% to 30% of all kilocalories with the majority being unsaturated food forms; limiting sodium intake to 2 to 3 g/day; and increasing exercise.

Concerted efforts are needed to combat the development of *cardiac cachexia* in progressive heart failure. Also, atherosclerotic plaques may occur in the extremities, usually the legs, causing *peripheral vascular disease* and the pain of *intermittent claudication* when walking. Progressive respiratory failure interferes with normal exchange of blood gases, oxygen and carbon dioxide, and results in *chronic obstructive pulmonary disease (COPD),* for which changed ratios of the fuel macronutrients are required.

QUESTIONS FOR REVIEW

1. Which types of hyperlipoproteinemia occur most often? Identify the lipids that are elevated in each case, as well as predisposing factors. Describe the types of diet recommended for each.
2. Identify four dietary recommendations that should be made for the person who has had a heart attack. Describe how each recommendation helps recovery.
3. Discuss the three levels of sodium restriction, describing general food choices and preparation methods.
4. What dietary changes could the average American make to reduce saturated fats and to substitute polyunsaturated fats?
5. What does the term *essential hypertension* mean? Why would weight management and sodium restriction contribute to its control?
6. Outline the nutritional therapy for cardia cachexia, and discuss the rationale for each aspect of the feeding plan.
7. Discuss the cause and treatment of peripheral vascular disease.
8. Outline the nutritional therapy for chronic obstructive pulmonary disease (COPD) and discuss the rationale for the fuel macronutrient adjustments.

REFERENCES

1. Guyton AC: *Textbook of medical physical physiology,* ed 8, Philadelphia, 1991, WB Saunders.
2. Marx J: Holding the line against heart disease, *Science* 248:1491, 1990.
3. Rau L: Hypertension, endothelium, and cardiovascular risk factors, *Am J Med* 90(suppl 2A):13S, 1991.
4. Culotta E, Koshland DE: NO news is good news, *Science* 258:1862, 1992.
5. Koshland DE: The molecule of the year, *Science* 258:1861, 1992.
6. Gotto AM and others: The cholesterol facts: a joint statement of the American Heart Association and the National Heart, Lung, and Blood Institute, *Circulation* 81(5):1721, 1990.

7. Grundy SM: Cholesterol and coronary heart disease: a new era, *JAMA* 256:2849, 1986.

8. Grundy SM: Cholesterol and coronary heart disease: future directions, *JAMA* 264(23):305, 1990.

9. Lowering blood cholesterol to prevent heart disease, Consensus Conference, *JAMA* 253:2080, 1985.

10. National Cholesterol Education Program: *Report of the Expert Panel on Detection, Evaluation, and Treatment of High Blood Cholesterol in adults*, USDHHS (PHS), National Institutes of Health, National Heart, Lung, and Blood Institute, Pub No 88-2925, Washington, DC, 1988, US Government Printing Office.

11. National Cholesterol Education Program: *Report of the Expert Panel on Population Strategies for Blood Cholesterol Reduction*, USDHHS (PHS), National Institutes of Health, National Heart, Lung, and Blood Institute, Pub No 90-3046, Washington, DC, 1990, US Government Printing Office.

12. Food and Nutrition Board, Committee on Diet and Health, National Academy of Science—National Research Council: *Diet and health: implications for reducing chronic disease risk*, Washington, DC, 1989, National Academy Press.

13. Steinberg D, Witztum JL: Lipoproteins and atherogenesis: current concepts, *JAMA* 264(23):3047, 1990.

14. Kane JP and others: Regression of coronary atherosclerosis during treatment of familial hypercholesterolemia with combined drug regimens, *JAMA* 264(23):3007, 1990.

15. Young SG: Recent progress in understanding apolipoprotein B, *Circulation* 82(5):1574, 1990.

16. American Heart Association Nutrition Committee: Rationale for the diet-heart statement of the American Heart Association, *Arterioscler Thromb* 4:177, 1982.

17. National Cholesterol Education Program: *Report of the Expert Panel on Blood Cholesterol Levels in Children and Adolescents*, USDHHS (PHS), National Institutes of Health, National Heart, Lung, and Blood Institute, Pub No 91-2732, Washington, DC, 1991, US Government Printing Office.

18. Chelsky LB and others: Caffeine and ventricular arrhythmias, *JAMA* 265(17):2236, 1990.

19. Packer M: Pathophysiology of chronic heart failure, *Lancet* 340:88, 1992.

20. Heymfield S and others: Nutritional support in cardiac cachexia, *Surg Clin North Am* 61:635, 1981.

21. Ney SM: The cardiovascular system. In Zeman FJ: *Clinical nutrition and diet therapy*, ed 2, New York, 1991, Macmillan.

22. Kannel WB, Wolf PA: Inferences from secular trend analysis of hypertension control, *Am J Public Health* 82(12):1593, 1992.

23. National Center for Health Statistics: *Health, United States, 1990*, USDHHS (PHS) Pub No 91-1232, Washington, DC, 1990, US Government Printing Office.

24. National Institutes of Health, National Heart, Lung, and Blood Institute: *Morbidity and mortality chartbook on cardiovascular, lung, and blood diseases—1990*, Washington, DC, 1990, US Government Printing Office.

25. Casper M and others: Antihypertensive treatment and U.S. trends in stroke mortality, 1962 to 1980, *Am J Public Health* 82(12):1600, 1992.

26. Jacobs DR and others: The United States decline in stroke mortality: what does the ecological analysis tell us? *Am J Public Health* 82(12):1596, 1992.

27. Dustan HP and others: The 1984 report of the Joint National Committee on Detection, Evaluation, and Treatment of High Blood Pressure, *Arch Intern Med* 144:1045, 1984.

28. National Institutes of Health, National Heart, Lung, and Blood Institute: *Nonpharmacological approaches to the control of high blood pressure, final report of the Subcommittee on Nonpharmacological Therapy of the 1984 Joint National Committee on Detection, Evaluation, and Treatment of High Blood Pressure*, USDHHS (PHS) Pub No 1986-491-292:41147, Washington, DC, 1986, US Government Printing Office.

29. Fedor JG, Chockalingam A: The Canadian Consensus Report on Non-pharmacological Approaches to the Management of High Blood Pressure, *Clin Exp Hypertens* 12(5):729, 1990.

30. Scherrer U and others: Effects of weight reduction in moderately overweight patients on recorded ambulatory blood pressure and free systolic platelet calcium, *Circulation* 83(2):552, 1991.

31. Wylie-Rosett J and others: Trial of antihypertensive intervention and management: greater efficacy with weight reduction than with a sodium-potassium intervention, *J Am Diet Assoc* 93(4):408, 1993.

32. Schieder RE and others: Antihypertensive therapy: to stop or not to stop? *JAMA* 265(12):1566, 1991.

33. US Department of Health and Human Services, Public Health Service: *Healthy people 2000: national health promotion and disease prevention objectives*, Pub No 91-50212, Washington, DC, 1990, US Government Printing Office.

34. National Center for Health Statistics: *United States, 1989, and preventive profile*, USDHHS (PHS) Pub No 90-1232, Washington, DC, 1990, US Government Printing Office.

35. Saunders E: Hypertension in blacks, *Prim Care* 18(3):607, 1991.

36. Shuaib A, Hachinski VC: Mechanisms and management in the elderly, *Can Med Assoc J* 145(5):433, 1991.

37. Armstrong JN: Nutrition and the respiratory patient, *Nutr Support Serv* 6(3):8, 1986.

38. Miller MA: A practical approach to eating and breathing in respiratory failure, *Top Clin Nutr* 1(4):61, 1986.

39. DeMeo MT and others: The hazards of hypercaloric nutritional support in respiratory disease, *Nutr Rev* 49(4):112, 1991.

40. Schols A and others: Resting energy expenditure in patients with chronic obstructive pulmonary disease, *Am J Clin Nutr* 54:983, 1991.

41. Pingleton SK, Harmon GS: Nutritional management in acute respiratory failure, *JAMA* 257:3094, 1987.

42. Monograph: *Dietary modification in chronic pulmonary disease,* Columbus, Ohio, 1986, Ross Laboratories.

43. Kaplan NM: New evidence on the role of sodium in hypertension: The Intersalt Study, *Am J Hypertens* 3:168, 1990.

44. Law MR and others: By how much does dietary salt reduction lower blood pressure? *BMJ* 302:811, 1991.

45. Montgomery DA, Amos RJ: Nutrition information needs during cardiac rehabilitation: perceptions of the cardiac patient and spouse, *J Am Diet Assoc* 91(9):1078, 1991.

46. Barnes MS, Terry RD: Adherence to the cardiac diet: attitudes of patients after myocardial infarction, *J Am Diet Assoc* 91(11):1435, 1991.

47. McCann BS and others: Promoting adherence to low-fat, low-cholesterol diets: review and recommendations, *J Am Diet Assoc* 90(10):1408, 1990.

48. Sharlin J and others: Nutrition and behavioral characteristics and determinants of plasma cholesterol levels in men and women, *J Am Diet Assoc* 92(4):434, 1992.

49. Shenberger DM and others: Intense dietary counseling lowers LDL cholesterol in the recruitment phase of a clinical trial of men who had coronary artery bypass graft, *J Am Diet Assoc* 92(4):441, 1992.

50. McMurray MP and others: Family-oriented nutrition intervention for the lipid population, *J Am Diet Assoc* 91(1):57, 1991.

51. Shannon B and others: A dietary education program for hypercholesterolemic children and their parents, *J Am Diet Assoc* 91(2):208, 1991.

52. Boeckner LS and others: A risk-reduction nutrition course for adults, *J Am Diet Assoc* 90(2):260, 1990.

FURTHER READING

Fortmann SP and others: Effect of long-term community health education on blood pressure and hypertension control: The Stanford Five-City Project, *Am J Epidemiol* 132(4):629, 1990.

This report provides ample evidence of the strong relation between elevated blood pressure and sodium, and the values of community health education in preventing and controlling essential hypertension.

Owen AL: Dietary trends in fat and cholesterol consumption, *Top Clin Nutr* 5(3):48, 1990.

This article reviews changing consumer attitudes and practices in fat- and cholesterol-modified food product purchases and uses.

CASE STUDY

The Patient with Myocardial Infarction

Edward Bennett is a 37-year-old sedentary executive seen for an annual physical examination 6 months ago. He had no complaints, other than feeling the "everyday pressures" of his job as a corporate attorney and head of the legal division. He admitted smoking two packs of cigarettes a day as a means of relieving stress.

Mr. Bennett is 175 cm (5 ft 10 in) tall and at the time of his examination weighed 83 kg (185 lb). His blood pressure was 148/90, and his serum cholesterol level was 285 mg/dl. He was advised to quit smoking, exercise daily at a moderate pace, and lose 9 kg (20 lb).

He arrived in the hospital emergency room 3 months later complaining of severe chest pains and difficulty breathing. His wife reported that he had appeared pale that evening, had broken out into a cold sweat, and had vomited shortly after arriving home from work. Once regular breathing was restored by the emergency medical team and his pain subsided, a number of laboratory tests were ordered. These tests included serum glutamic-oxaloacetic transaminase (SGOT), lactate dehydrogenase (LDH), prothrombin time, lipid panel plus HDL-cholesterol, sedimentation rate, coagulation times, fasting blood sugar (FBS), blood urea nitrogen (BUN), and complete blood count (CBC). An electrocardiogram (ECG) was also ordered. The patient was then transferred to the coronary care unit for closer monitoring.

The tests results were elevated: SGOT, LDH, LDL and total cholesterol, triglycerides, glucose, prothrombin time, white blood cell count, and sedimentation rate. The HDL level was low. The ECG revealed an infarction of the posterior wall of the myocardium. The diagnosis was myocardial infarction, with underlying familial hypercholesterolemia.

In consultation with the clinical nutritionist, the cardiologist ordered a liquid diet, increasing it to an 800-kilocalorie soft diet with low saturated fats 2 days later. The nutritionist noted continued improvement in the patient's appetite accompanying recovery and recommended a full diet. A 1200-kilocalorie low-saturated fat, low-cholesterol full diet was ordered by the end of the week. The nutritionist specified that the cholesterol be limited to 300 mg or less and that the total dietary fat content be limited to 25% of total kilocalories with emphasis on use of unsaturated fats.

Mr. Bennett was discharged 2 weeks later. During his convalescence the nutritionist and the nurse met with him and his wife several times to discuss his continuing care at home. At each follow-up clinic visit with the physician and with the nutritionist, Mr. Bennett showed good general recovery and enjoyment of his new modified fat and cholesterol food habits.

Questions for Analysis

1. What predisposing factors in Mr. Bennett's life-style place him in the high-risk category for coronary heart disease?
2. Why was moderate, consistent exercise originally recommended?
3. Explain the causes for Mr. Bennett's initial symptoms.
4. How does each laboratory test ordered in the emergency room relate to cell metabolism? Why were the results elevated?
5. What were the reasons for modifications in texture, fat, and total caloric levels in each diet prescribed for Mr. Bennett? Explain the association between the final diet order and his lipid disorder.
6. Outline a 1-day menu for Mr. Bennett that complies with the final hospital diet order.
7. What nondietary needs might Mr. Bennett have while convalescing at home? What community agencies might be of assistance?

Is Calcium a New Risk Factor in Hypertension Control?

If you had high blood pressure, what would you do—give up salt or drink more milk? This question may sound absurd to anyone familiar with traditional methods of hypertension control, which include a low-sodium diet. To them, giving up salt is the obvious reply. However, in the general public the question is being taken seriously, because a growing number of popular news articles state that persons with high blood pressure may need more calcium.

These reports are based on a number of studies showing that persons with hypertension drink less milk than those with normal blood pressure levels and also have lower serum calcium levels. These studies contradict the findings of earlier studies in which high serum calcium levels were observed in persons with high blood pressure. The latter results are to be expected because of calcium's known contractive effect on smooth muscle tissue, such as blood vessels. Large amounts of calcium should cause blood vessels to contract, thus squeezing on the blood flow and bringing a buildup of pressure against arterial walls. The "new" research claims that persons with hypertension don't handle calcium normally. Some of these researchers believe that the sodium-calcium exchange system through which the calcium enters the cell when the sodium leaves it is defective. They tend to discredit the sodium theory, because sodium reduction doesn't work for everyone with hypertension; even traditionalists realize that only about half of those with high blood pressure can control it through sodium reduction alone. Nonetheless there are problems with the calcium research:

- Most of the studies are based on a small number of subjects. For example, McCarron's study at the University of Oregon was based on only 23 subjects. Another study that found a different correlation of high blood pressure with high serum calcium was based on 9321 subjects.
- Although calcium researchers found low serum cal-

cium levels in subjects with hypertension, total blood calcium levels did not vary with variable blood pressure readings in their study.
- In conditions characterized by high calcium levels, such as hyperparathyroidism, blood pressure levels are also high. As the condition improves and the serum calcium levels fall, blood pressure readings also fall.
- The calcium intake of subjects in the studies was based on oral 24-hour recall information on diet, which is not generally considered the most accurate method of determining nutrient intake.
- Assuming that the dietary information obtained is accurate, it indicated that subjects with hypertension may have consumed less milk but still obtained *adequate* amounts of calcium.

Another important point to remember is that most calcium-rich foods have higher-than-average sodium levels per serving. For example, 1½ oz of American cheese may provide 250 to 300 mg calcium, but it also provides more than 400 mg of sodium.

Newer studies in many parts of the world, modern and primitive, have demonstrated a strong relationship between sodium and blood pressure. Unanswered questions remain about the effects of calcium, potassium, and many other factors on blood pressure. In any event the American Heart Association and other health organizations strongly advise the general public (1) to limit sodium intake, and (2) to take in enough calcium to meet various needs for growth, bone and tooth maintenance, and muscle function.

REFERENCES

Kaplan NM: New evidence on the role of sodium in hypertension: The Intersalt Study, *Am J Hypertens* 3:168, 1990.

Law MR and others: By how much does dietary salt reduction lower blood pressure? *BMJ* 302:811, 1991.

McCarron DA, Morris CD: Blood pressure response to oral calcium in persons with mild to moderate hypertension, *Ann Intern Med* 103:825, 1985.

McCarron DA and others: Dietary calcium and blood pressure: modifying factors in specific populations, *Am J Clin Nutr* 54:215S, 1991.

McGregor GA: Sodium is more important than calcium in essential hypertension, *Hypertension* 7:628, 1985.

CHAPTER 21

Diabetes Mellitus

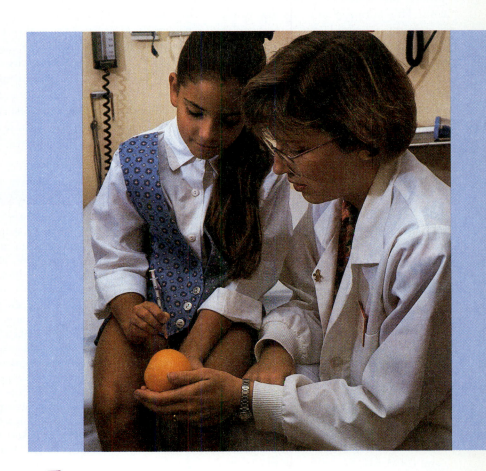

CHAPTER OUTLINE

In this continuing chapter in our clinical nutrition series, we look at the problem of diabetes. We seek to understand its nature and how it can be managed to maintain good health and to avoid complications.

About 11 million Americans have diabetes, one in 20 persons. Of this total, 15% are insulin-dependent and 85% are non–insulin-dependent. In the North American population, diabetes complications have become the fifth ranking cause of death from disease.

Here, we see that sound nutritional therapy remains the fundamental base of management for all persons with diabetes. This nutritional base; newer forms of insulin, if necessary; and self-monitoring of blood glucose have become indispensible tools of daily self-management.

Nature of Diabetes

History

The metabolic disease we know today as *diabetes mellitus* has been with us for a long time. Ancient records describe its devastating effects as observed by early healers. In the first century AD, the Greek physician Aretaeus wrote of a malady in which the body "ate its own flesh" and gave off large quantities of urine. He gave it the name *diabetes,* from the Greek word meaning "siphon" or "to pass through." Much later, in the seventeenth century, the word *mellitus,* from the Latin word for "honey," was added because of the sweet nature of the urine. This addition also distinguished it from **diabetes insipidus** ("insipid," meaning tasteless, or *not* sweet), another disorder, uncommon, in which the passage of copious amounts of urine had been observed. Today, use of the single name diabetes always means diabetes mellitus.

As medical knowledge began to grow, early clinicians—such as Rollo in England and Boushardat in France—observed that diabetes became less severe in overweight patients who lost weight. Later another French physician, Lancereaux, and his students described two kinds of diabetes: *diabete gras*—"fat diabetes" and *diabete maigre*—"thin diabetes."[1] All these observations preceded any knowledge about insulin or any relation to the pancreas. Throughout these times, which have aptly been called the "diabetic dark ages," persons with diabetes had short lives and were maintained on a variety of semistarvation diets.[2]

Later evidence began to point to the pancreas as a primary organ involved in the disease process. Paul Langerhans (1847-1888), a young German medical student, found special clusters—or islets—of cells scattered about the human pancreas that were different from the rest of the tissue. Although their function was still unknown, these special islet cells were named for their young discoverer: the islets of Langerhans. Research focus then centered on the pancreas. Finally, from 1921 to 1922, a University of Toronto team discovered and successfully used the controlling agent from the "island cells," naming it **insulin** for its source (see box below).[3]

Insulin: Saga of a Success Story

On first glance, looking at numbers only, it would appear that the development of insulin was a causal factor in changing the status of diabetes mellitus from a rare disease to one that affects over 10 million Americans. Closer inspection of the facts, however, reveals that the disease was thought to be rare only because its victims died young—fewer persons were around who had the disease. Today, insulin enables over 2 million insulin-dependent individuals to live longer and enjoy productive lives.

The success story behind insulin lies not only in its ability to extend the life span of the person with diabetes, but also in its own resilience. Insulin was discovered during the summer of 1921 at the University of Toronto by Frederick Banting, a surgeon who according to newspaper accounts of the day solved the mystery of insulin in his sleep, and Charles Best, a college graduate who was not yet enrolled in medical school. Their insulin was derived from the pancreas of dogs by tying off pancreatic ducts, waiting for the organ to "die," and then making an extract of the remaining tissue.

The extract worked fairly well in their tests with dogs. An extract that worked in humans was not developed for another 6 months, partly because their extract was originally given by mouth. Even when injected their formula failed, which indicated that faulty purification methods may have been involved.

Finally, in January of 1922, a successful extract was developed by a new member who joined the research team, James B. Collip. Its effect on one patient's diabetic condition was not enough to counteract the effect of the treatment of the day—a diet that derived almost 71% of its kilocalories from fat. The patient died at age 27 with atherosclerosis and coronary heart disease. However, the team was successful with their third patient. The young girl, who was first diagnosed as having diabetes when she was 11 years old, lived to be 73 years of age. After insulin therapy was initiated, she was taken off the popular "starvation" diet of the day, gained weight, and led a normal life.

Ironically, despite Collip's successful extraction procedure, his subsequent actions almost stopped the project. Jealousies developed and, with the permission of the head of the university's physiology department, Collip refused to share his purification methods with Banting. Then, after his extraction product was a success, Collip conveniently "forgot" how to make it! As a result of this foolish battle, at least one patient died because the researchers ran out of the original extract.

Fortunately, Collip miraculously "remembered" how to make his extract the following May. Soon after, insulin was being mass-produced and made available to the growing number of persons who depended on it for their very survival.

TO PROBE FURTHER

REFERENCES

Altman LK: The tumultuous discovery of insulin: finally, hidden story is told, *New York Times,* pp C-1, C-6, Sept 14, 1982.

Bliss M: *The discovery of insulin,* Chicago, 1982, University of Chicago Press.

Nestle M and others: A case of diabetes mellitus, *N Engl J Med* 81:127, 1982.

Contributing Causes

Genetics: Insulin Activity

For some time, insulin assay tests developed to measure the level of insulin activity in the blood found insulin-like activity in early diabetes to be two to three times the normal insulin levels. Investigators postulated that the insulin was present but bound with a protein, making it unavailable. It is now evident that diabetes is a syndrome with multiple forms, resulting from (1) lack of insulin, as in *insulin-dependent diabetes mellitus (IDDM)*, or (2) insulin resistance and subsequent beta cell dysfunction, as in *non–insulin-dependent diabetes mellitus (NIDDM)*.[4,5]

Weight

Diabetes has long been associated with weight, since early observations of differences in "fat diabetes" and "thin diabetes."[1] Current research has reinforced the relation of the overweight state to NIDDM. Apparently, the obesity interacts with an underlying genetic predisposition to trigger the non–insulin-dependent form of diabetes.

Heredity

Diabetes has usually been defined in terms of heredity. But increasing evidence indicates that there is considerable *genetic* variation between the two main types of diabetes, IDDM and NIDDM. Studies have shown that an autoimmune attack of the body's insulin-producing cells is at fault, and scientists express growing confidence that within this decade continuing research will lead to safe preventive therapies.[6]

Environmental Role: "Thrifty Gene"

Environmental factors apparently play a role in unmasking the underlying genetic susceptibility, a "thrifty" diabetic genotype that probably developed from primitive times for survival. This theory indicates that diabetes may be associated with past genetic modifications for survival during varying periods of food availability. In the past, this state of diabetes was a saving—or "thrifty"—trait that provided better storage and metabolism of food during times when our ancestors lived under more primitive and difficult survival conditions. As food supplies became more plentiful, the negative aspects of the diabetic trait began to appear. Such is indeed the case, for example, with the experience of the Pima Indians in Arizona, as earlier studies and recent archeologic excavations there have indicated.[7,8] In earlier times this group ate a limited diet, mainly of carbohydrate foods harvested by heavy physical labor in a primitive agriculture. Now, however, with the "progress" of civilization, the Pimas have become obese, and half of the adults have NIDDM, the highest reported rate of this type of diabetes in the world. This same pattern is seen among populations of now-urbanized Pacific Islanders, South Asians, Asian Indians, and Creole.[10,11] Thus evidence suggests that groups such as these have a genetic susceptibility to NIDDM (diabetic genotype) and that the disease is triggered by environmental factors, including obesity. Just as obesity may result from more than one genetic error, so too may diabetes.[8] As we commonly observe, diet can indeed interact with genetics to cause adult-onset diabetes.

Classification

Increasing evidence indicates differences between insulin-dependent and non–insulin-dependent diabetes, and epidemiologic studies in various population groups have provided newer clinical and pathogenic information. With this growing evidence, an international work group sponsored by the National Institutes of Health (NIH) proposed a basic classification for the diabetes syndrome according to the need of insulin for control. This basis is now used to designate the two main types—IDDM and NIDDM (Table 21-1).

Insulin-Dependent Diabetes Mellitus (IDDM)

In its insulin-dependent form, diabetes develops very rapidly and is more severe and unstable. This form occurs mainly in children, and the child is usually underweight. Acidosis is fairly common. Peak ages of onset are between 6 and 11 years of age, affecting about 1 in every 600 school-aged children.[9]

diabetes insipidus · A condition of the pituitary gland and insufficiency of one of its hormones, vasopressin or antidiuretic hormone; characterized by a copious output of a nonsweet urine, great thirst, and sometimes a large appetite. However, in diabetes insipidus these symptoms result from a specific injury to the pituitary gland, not a collection of metabolic disorders as in diabetes mellitus. The injured pituitary gland produces less vasopressin, a hormone that normally helps the kidneys resorb adequate water.

insulin · Hormone formed in the B cells of the islets of Langerhans in the pancreas. It is secreted when blood glucose and amino acid levels rise and assists their entry into body cells. It also promotes glycogenesis and conversion of glucose into fat and inhibits lipolysis and gluconeogenesis (protein breakdown). Commercial insulin is manufactured from pigs and cows; new "artificial" human insulin products have recently been made available.

TABLE 21-1

Comparison of IDDM and NIDDM

	IDDM	NIDDM
Other names	Type I Juvenile-onset Brittle diabetes Ketosis-prone	Type II Adult-onset Stable diabetes Ketosis-resistant Maturity-onset
Prevalence	5%-10%	80%-95%
Age of onset	Any age; usually less than 40 years	Any age; usually more than 40 years
Cause	Deficient or no insulin production, autoim- mune disorder, viral infection	Insulin resistance, hyper- insulinemia, obesity
Symptoms at onset	Polydipsia, polyuria, polyphagia, weight loss	Often none; can have polydipsia, fatigue, blurred vision, symp- toms of vascular or neural complications
Usual medical treatment:		
Medication	Insulin	Sulfonylureas (insulin required by some)
Diet	Required (timing and consistency critical)	Required (may be the only form of treatment for some)
Exercise	Recommended (to be integrated with other treatments)	Recommended (to be integrated with other treatments)

Non–Insulin-Dependent Diabetes Mellitus (NIDDM)

In this non–insulin-dependent form, diabetes develops more slowly and is usually milder and more stable. This form occurs mainly in adults. The obesity-diabetes genetic base plays a strong role—80% to 90% of these adults are obese. Thus obesity and physical inactivity in adults are strong risk factors.[10-12] Because NIDDM is a milder metabolic form, acidosis is infrequent. The majority of patients improve with weight loss and are maintained on diet therapy alone. Sometimes there is a need for an oral hypoglycemic medication.

Symptoms

Initial Observations

Early signs of diabetes, or its uncontrolled state, include the following:

- Increased thirst (polydipsia)
- Increased urination (polyuria)
- Increased hunger (polyphagia)
- Weight loss with IDDM or obesity with NIDDM

Laboratory Test Results

Various clinical laboratory tests taken at this time reveal the following:

- Glycosuria (sugar in the urine)
- Hyperglycemia (elevated blood sugar level)
- Abnormal glucose tolerance tests

Other Possible Symptoms

Additional signs may appear as the uncontrolled condition becomes more serious:

- Blurred vision
- Skin irritation or infection
- Weakness and loss of strength

Results of Uncontrolled Diabetes

Continued metabolic consequences may occur as the uncontrolled condition progresses:

- Fluid and electrolyte imbalance
- Acidosis (ketoacidosis)
- Coma

The Metabolic Pattern of Diabetes

Overall Energy Balance and the Energy Nutrients

Because the initial symptoms of glycosuria and hyperglycemia are related to excess glucose, diabetes has been called a disease of carbohydrate metabolism. However, as more becomes known about the intimate interrelationships of carbohydrate, fat, and protein metabolism, we now view it in more general terms. It is a metabolic disorder resulting from a lack of insulin (absolute, partial, or unavailable) affecting more or less each of the basic energy nutrients. It is especially related to the metabolism of the two fuels, carbohydrate and fat, in the body's overall energy system.

Normal Blood Glucose Controls

Control of the blood glucose level within its normal range of 70 to 120 mg/dL (3.9 to 6.7 mmol/L) is vital to life. A knowledge of these controls in maintaining a normal blood glucose level is essential to understanding the impairment of these controls in diabetes (see Chapters 2 and 3). An overview of these normal balancing controls is given in Fig. 21-1.

Sources of Blood Glucose

Two sources of blood glucose ensure a constant supply of this primary body fuel: (1) *diet*—the energy nutrients in our food—dietary carbohydrate, protein, and fat, and (2) *glycogen*—the backup source from constant turnover of "stored" liver glycogen by a process called **glycogenolysis.**

Uses of Blood Glucose

To prevent a continued rise of the blood glucose level above normal limits, several basic uses for blood glucose are constantly available according to need. These include the following: (1) **glycogenesis**—conversion of glucose to glycogen for "storage" in liver and muscle, (2) **lipogenesis**—conversion of glucose to fat and stor-

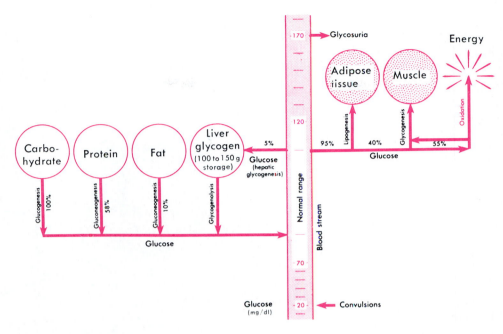

FIG. 21-1   Sources of blood glucose (food and stored glycogen) and normal routes of control.

age in adipose tissue, and (3) **glycolysis**—cell oxidation of glucose for energy.

Pancreatic Hormonal Controls

Three types of islet cells scattered in clusters throughout the pancreas (Islets of Langerhans) provide hormones closely interbalanced in regulating blood glucose levels. This specific arrangement of human islet cells is illustrated in Fig. 21-2:

1. **B cells.** The largest portion of the islets is occupied by B cells filling the central zone or about 60% of the gland. These primary cells synthesize *insulin.*
2. **A cells.** Arranged around the outer rim of the islets are the A cells, one to two cells thick, making up about 30% of the total cells. These cells synthesize *glucagon.*
3. **D cells.** Interspersed between the A and B cells—or occasionally between A cells alone—are the D cells, the remaining 10% of the total cells. These cells synthesize *somatostatin.*

Interrelated Hormone Functions

Juncture points of the three types of islet cells act as sensors of the blood glucose concentration and its rate of change. They constantly adjust and balance the rate of secretion of insulin, glucagon, and somatostatin to match whatever conditions prevail at any time. Each one of the three hormones has specific interbalanced functions.

1. **Insulin.** Although the precise mechanisms are not entirely clear in every case, insulin has a profound

effect on glucose control. It functions extensively in the metabolism of all three of the energy nutrients:

- Insulin facilitates transport of glucose through cell membranes by way of special insulin receptors. These receptors are located on the membrane of insulin-sensitive cells, including those in adipose tissue, muscle tissue, and monocytes. Researchers are reaching a better understanding of these special receptors and how to treat the disease by studying insulin receptors.[13] These insulin receptors mediate all the metabolic effects of insulin. Research has shown that the cells of obese persons with diabetes have fewer than the normal number of insulin receptors. Weight loss in obese individuals and physical exercise increase the number of these receptors.
- Insulin enhances the conversion of glucose to glycogen and its consequent storage in the liver (glycogenesis).
- Insulin stimulates conversion of glucose to fat (lipogenesis) for storage as adipose tissue.

glycogenesis • Synthesis of glycogen from blood glucose.

glycogenolysis • Production of blood glucose from liver glycogen.

glycolysis • Cell oxidation of glucose for energy.

lipogenesis • Synthesis of fat from blood glucose.

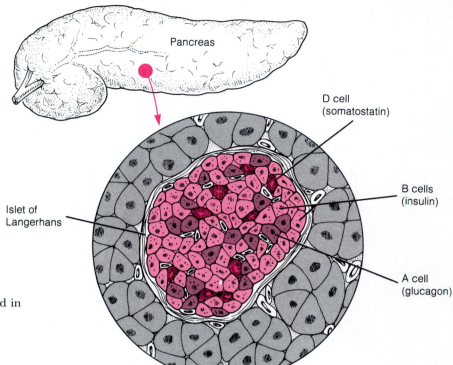

FIG. 21-2.   Islets of Langerhans, located in the pancreas.

- Insulin inhibits fat breakdown (lipolysis) and the breakdown of protein.
- Insulin promotes the uptake of amino acids by skeletal muscles, thus increasing protein synthesis.
- Insulin influences glucose oxidation through the main glycolytic pathway.

2. **Glucagon.** The hormone **glucagon** functions as a balancing antagonist to insulin. It rapidly breaks down liver glycogen, and—to a lesser extent—fatty acids from adipose tissue, to serve as body fuel. This action raises blood glucose levels to protect the brain and other body tissues. It helps maintain normal blood glucose levels during fasting hours of sleep. A lowering of the blood glucose concentration, increased amino acid concentrations, or sympathetic nervous system stimulation triggers glucagon secretion.

3. **Somatostatin.** Although the pancreatic islet D cells are the major source of **somatostatin,** this hormone is also synthesized and secreted in different regions of the body, including the hypothalamus. It acts in balance with insulin and glucose to inhibit their interactions as needed to maintain normal blood glucose levels. It also helps regulate blood glucose levels by inhibiting the release of a number of other hormones as needed.

Metabolic Changes in Diabetes

In uncontrolled diabetes, insulin is lacking to facilitate the operation of normal blood glucose controls. Abnor-

mal metabolic changes occur that affect glucose, fat, and protein and cause the symptoms of diabetes.

Glucose

The blood glucose cannot be oxidized properly through the main glycolytic pathway in the cell to furnish energy. Therefore it builds up in the blood.

Fat

The formation of fat is curtailed, and fat breakdown increases. This leads to excess formation and accumulation of ketones, causing ketoacidosis. The appearance of one of these ketones, **acetone,** in the urine indicates the development of ketoacidosis.

Protein

Tissue protein is also broken down in an effort to secure energy. This causes weight loss and nitrogen excretion in the urine.

General Management of Diabetes

Diagnosis

Glucose-Tolerance Testing

The guiding principles for treating diabetes are early detection and prevention of complications. The former traditional glucose tolerance test is no longer used in regular practice. Instead, in the current procedure, a 75 g dose of glucose is used and two blood tests are taken: fasting and a 2-hour plasma glucose. A 2-hour plasma glucose value of 200 mg/dL (11.0 mmol/L) or above indicates diabetes, and 140 mg/dL (7.8 mmol/L) is the upper level of normal. Those values falling between 140 and 200 mg/dL are labeled *impaired* glucose tolerance. Clinical experience indicates that persons in this latter group tend to progress toward diabetes at a rate about four times that of normal persons. Thus those diagnosed as diabetic and those with impaired glucose tolerance should have follow-up diet therapy and monitoring for glucose management.

Glycosylated Hemoglobin A_{1c}

This additional test, Hb A_{1c}, is used in diabetes screening and monitoring. Glycohemoglobins are relatively stable molecules within the red blood cell. During the life of the cell, about 120 days, glucose molecules attach themselves to the hemoglobin. This irreversible glycosylation of hemoglobin depends on the concentration of blood glucose. The higher the level of circulating glucose over the life of the red blood cells, the higher the concentration of glycohemoglobin. Thus the measurement of hemoglobin A_{1c} relates to the level of blood glucose over a longer time. It provides an effective tool for evaluating long-term management of diabetes and degree of control.

Treatment Goals
Basic Objectives

The health team is guided by three basic objectives in the care of a person with diabetes.

1. **Maintenance of optimal nutrition.** The first objective is to fulfill the basic nutritional requirement for health, growth and development, and a desirable body weight.
2. **Avoidance of symptoms.** This objective is designed to keep the person relatively free of hypoglycemia or insulin reaction, which requires immediate countermeasures, or hyperglycemia, which if untreated contributes to more serious ketoacidosis or diabetic coma.
3. **Prevention of complications.** The third objective recognizes the increased risk a person with diabetes faces for developing complicating problems that reflect the tissue-damaging effects of chronic diabetes. These damages may occur in tissues such as eyes—**retinopathy;** nerve tissues—**neuropathy;** and renal tissues—**nephropathy.** In addition, coronary artery disease occurs in persons with diabetes about four times as often as in the general population. Peripheral vascular disease occurs about 40 times as often.

In all of these areas there is evidence that consistent well-planned food habits and exercise, balanced as needed with early aggressive insulin therapy—through multiple daily injections or continuous subcutaneous infusion by pump and constantly guided by self-monitoring of blood glucose levels—can significantly reduce risks of these potentially serious complications.[14] Current nutritional recommendations of the American Diabetes Association recognize the added risk of vascular disease for persons with diabetes and include revised lipid-lowering diet guidelines.

Self-Care Role of the Person with Diabetes

To control diabetes effectively, the person with diabetes must of necessity have a central position. Daily self-discipline and informed self-care, supported by a skilled and sensitive health care team, are required for sound diabetes management. Ultimately, in the final analysis all persons with diabetes must treat themselves. This is especially true with the tighter normal blood sugar control currently being used with frequent self-monitoring of blood glucose levels and multiple insulin injections. Thus there is even greater need now for comprehensive diabetes education programs that encourage self-monitoring and self-care responsibility.

---

glucagon • A polypeptide hormone secreted by the A cells of the pancreatic islets of Langerhans in response to hypoglycemia; has an opposite balancing effect to that of insulin, raising the blood sugar, and thus is used as a quick-acting antidote for the hypoglycemic reaction of insulin. It stimulates the breakdown of glycogen (glycogenolysis) in the liver by activating the liver enzyme phosphorylase, and thus raises blood sugar levels during fasting states to ensure adequate levels for normal nerve and brain function.

nephropathy • Disease of the kidneys; in diabetes, renal damage associated with functional and pathologic changes in the nephrons, which can lead to glomerulosclerosis and chronic renal failure.

neuropathy • General term for functional and pathologic changes in the peripheral nervous system; in diabetes, a chronic sensory condition affecting mainly the nerves of the legs, marked by numbness from sensory impairment, loss of tendon reflexes, severe pain, weakness, and wasting of muscles involved.

retinopathy • Noninflammatory disease of the retina—the visual tissue of the eye—characterized by microaneurysms, intraretinal hemorrhages, waxy yellow exudates, "cotton wool" patches, and macular edema; a complication of diabetes that may lead to proliferation of fibrous tissue, retinal detachment, and blindness.

somatostatin • A hormone formed in the D cells of the pancreatic islets of Langerhans and the hypothalamus. It is a balancing factor in maintaining normal blood glucose levels by inhibiting insulin and glucagon production in the pancreas as needed.

Principles of Nutritional Therapy: The Balance Concept

The Core Problem

The core problem in diabetes is energy balance, the regulation of the body's primary fuel, blood glucose. Based on this concept of balance, three main principles of nutritional therapy emerge: (1) total energy balance, (2) nutrient balance, and (3) food distribution balance. The fundamental underlying principle may be stated simply: *The diet for any person with diabetes is always based on the normal nutritional needs of that individual.* The personal diet, then, is expressed in terms of (1) total requirement of kilocalories for energy needs, (2) a balanced ratio of these kilocalories in grams of carbohydrate, protein, and fat, and (3) a general food distribution pattern for the day.

Total Energy Balance

Weight Management

Because insulin-dependent diabetes mellitus (IDDM) usually begins during childhood (average age is 11), the weight-height measure for children is an index to adequate growth. In adult years, maintaining a desirable lean weight is a continuing goal (see Chapter 6). Because non–insulin-dependent diabetes mellitus (NIDDM) usually occurs in overweight adults, the major goal is losing excess weight with a sound diet and maintaining a healthy body weight.

Kilocalories

The energy value of a diabetic diet should be expressed in terms of kilocalories sufficient to meet individual needs for normal growth and development, physical activity, and maintenance of a desirable lean weight.

Nutrient Balance

The ratio of carbohydrate, protein, and fat in the diet is based on current recommendations of the American Diabetes Association and the American Dietetic Association for ideal glucose regulation and lower fat intake to reduce risks of cardiovascular complications.[9,15]

Carbohydrate

A more liberal use of carbohydrates, mainly in complex forms, is needed for smoother blood sugar control. About 50% to 55% of the total kilocalories of the diet is assigned to carbohydrates. Several characteristics of carbohydrate foods need to be examined:

1. **Complex carbohydrates.** The majority of the carbohydrate kilocalories, about 40% to 50% of the total diet kilocalories, should be used as complex carbohydrates—starches. In most cases, these complex carbohydrates break down more slowly than simple sugars and release their available glucose over time.

2. **Glycemic index.** Modification of carbohydrate food to take into account the glycemic index of single foods and food combinations, at least in the light of our current knowledge, provides little clinical assistance in designing meals for diabetic patients.[16] In comparison with the Diabetes Food Exchange Lists, it less accurately predicts postprandial responses to carbohydrate foods in mixed meals. However, most persons with IDDM have developed their own personal "glycemic index" list based on their individual experience of blood glucose response to specific foods and make insulin adjustments accordingly.

3. **Dietary fiber.** The degree to which dietary fiber is present in complex carbohydrates—such as grains, legumes, vegetables, fruits, and other starches—will influence the rate of absorption of the food mix components and alter their effect on the blood glucose level. An increased dietary fiber content—especially of soluble dietary fiber forms, such as those found in oats, barley, legumes, and fruits—appears to have beneficial effects, particularly in lowering plasma lipids.[17] A dietary fiber intake of about 40 g/day of dietary fiber or 25 g/1000 kcal is a reasonable goal.

4. **Simple carbohydrates.** The small remainder of the carbohydrate kilocalories, about 5% or less of the total dietary kilocalories, may be used as simple carbohydrates. In general, simple carbohydrates (single or double sugars found in fruits, milk, and sucrose-sweetened food items) should be controlled in the diabetic diet, placing greater emphasis on the complex forms. Research has indicated that small amounts of sucrose or fructose in special food items is not necessarily detrimental, but it needs to be carefully controlled and used in mixed forms with other foods. Honey is a form of sugar (mainly fructose) and is not a sugar substitute, as some persons may believe.

5. **Sugar substitute sweeteners.** A variety of sugar substitutes are available. Noncaloric sweeteners, such as saccharin and aspartame, are acceptable. Aspartame is a recently marketed nutritive sweetener made from two amino acids, phenylalanine and aspartic acid, and is metabolized as such.[18] Caloric sweeteners, such as fructose and sorbitol, must be accounted for in the meal. However, many persons with diabetes do not tolerate sorbitol and experience significant diarrhea from its use.[19] A summary of dietary sweeteners is given in Table 21-2.

Protein

Normal age requirements for protein govern the amount indicated for persons with diabetes. In general,

TABLE 21-2

A Summary of Dietary Sweeteners

Sweetener	Commercial use	Comparative sweetness*	Effectiveness in carbohydrate metabolism and diabetes control	Problems
Nutritive sweeteners (provide 4 kcal/g)				
Aspartame Combination of two amino acids: aspartic acid and a methyl ester of phenylalanine	Soft drinks Chewing gum Powdered beverages Whipped toppings Puddings Gelatin Tabletop sweetener	180-200	Does not contribute significant amount of kcalories or carbohydrates	Possibly tumorigenic† Possible source of excess phenylalanine for children with PKU
Fructose Naturally-occurring monosaccharide found in honey, fruits, high-fructose corn syrup	Baked products Frosting mixes Tabletop sweetener Home food preparation	1.4 Enhanced by Use in liquids Low temperature Acidity Dilution	Absorbed more slowly than sucrose Does not require insulin for entry into cells Achieves similar level of sweetness with smaller amounts Contributes moderate amounts of kcalories and carbohydrates to prevent hypoglycemia Should not be used by poorly-controlled, obese diabetics	Caloric, carbohydrate values must be considered in calculating diets and recipes Intake of more than 75 g/day increases risk of hyperglycemia
Sorbitol Sugar alcohol naturally occurring in fruits and vegetables	Baked products Sugar-free gum	0.67	Not generally recommended for diabetes control, because large amounts are needed to sweeten foods Lack of insulin results in increased conversion to glucose‡	Doses of more than 50-60 g/day result in diarrhea
Xylitol "Wood sugar" found in straw, fruits, corncobs	Banned for commercial use in the United States in 1982	1.22		Tumorigenic
L-Glucose, L-fructose: mirror images (isomers) of D-glucose and D-fructose	Currently under study for possible commercial use	Same as D-glucose (0.72) and D-fructose (1.4)	Contributes no kcalories or carbohydrates because isomeric configuration prevents absorption	
Nonnutritive sweeteners (noncaloric)				
Saccharin	Baked products Soft drinks Tabletop sweetener	300-600	Contributes no kcalories or carbohydrates to the diet	Bladder cancer in test animals§
Cyclamate	Banned for commercial use in the United States in 1970			Bladder cancer in test animals

*The sweetness of sucrose is assigned the value of 1.
†A breakdown product of aspartame, diketopiperazine, is considered tumorigenic by some researchers.
‡Sorbitol is metabolized to fructose, then glucose.
§FDA plan to ban saccharin in 1977 failed because of saccharin's popularity.

protein intake among Americans is excessive and may accelerate the development of nephropathy in persons with diabetes.[20] Thus the intake recommended is restricted to the adult RDA 0.8 g/kg body weight—approximately 12% to 20% of the total kilocalories—for all persons with diabetes, other than children and pregnant or lactating women.

Fat

Fat should always be used in limited amounts, with greater attention given to the control of saturated fats and cholesterol. Total fat intake is lowered to 30% or less of the day's total kilocalories. With this reduction of total fat, all fat components according to degree of saturation should be reduced proportionately. Of the total kilocalories, the recommended proportion is less than 10% polyunsaturated, less than 10% saturated, and 10% to 15% monounsaturated fat. The daily intake of cholesterol is limited to 300 mg/day. These current recommendations are summarized in Table 21-3.

In addition, it is recommended that sodium intake should not exceed 3000 mg/day. Alcohol should also be limited to occasional use or no use. If used, it should be limited to one or two alcohol equivalents one to two times per week (see p. 431).

Food Distribution Balance

General Rule

In general, fairly even amounts of food should be eaten throughout the day, adjusted to blood glucose self-monitoring. This will avoid excessive intakes at some points and longer fasting periods between, eliminating the "peaks and valleys" in food intake and consequent blood sugar swings. This means that a basic pattern is a regular schedule of meals at fairly consistent times through the day, with interval snacks as needed.

Daily Activity Pattern

Food distribution needs to be planned ahead and adjusted according to each day's scheduled activities.

Practical consideration needs to be given to work, school, social events, and stress periods.

Exercise

For persons with insulin-dependent diabetes mellitus (IDDM), it is especially important that any exercise period or additional physical activity be accommodated in the food distribution plan. For obese adults with diabetes, regular exercise is an essential part of a successful weight-management program.

Drug Therapy

The food pattern will also be influenced by any form of drug therapy required for control. As indicated, the current management goal for persons with IDDM is to maintain a normal blood glucose level as much as possible, because there is strong evidence that such tight control prevents the chronic complications of long-term uncontrolled hyperglycemia.[14] To achieve this goal, more aggressive insulin therapy with different types of insulins now available is being used. Oral antidiabetic agents may be used also.

Types of Insulin

A number of insulin preparations are available for therapeutic use. According to the time of action, they are rapid-, intermediate-, and long-acting, although individual responses are highly variable.

1. **Rapid-acting insulins.** These insulins have various names, depending on the manufacturer: for example, Humulin R, Regular, Semilente, and Velosulin R. A number of variables influence absorption rate, such as site of injection, physical activity, skin temperature, and any circulating antiinsulin antibodies. The effect on the blood glucose level can be detected in about an hour, peaks at 4 to 6 hours, and lasts about 12 to 16 hours.
2. **Intermediate-acting insulins.** These insulins include Humulin L, Lente, NPH, Insulatard N, and Insulatard. The effect is detected in about 2 hours, peaks at about 11 hours, and lasts about 20 to 29 hours.
3. **Long-acting insulins.** These insulins include Humulin U and Ultralente. Their duration is somewhat longer than that of the intermediate-acting insulins. They are seldom used, except for special needs, because their slow onset and extended action are more difficult to predict or control. Also, the tighter control being used today requires shorter-acting insulins, with multiple injections according to self-monitoring of blood glucose levels, to meet variations in need during the day. This is especially true of the more labile or "brittle" forms of IDDM.

Sources of Insulin

The commercial source of insulins has been beef and pork pancreases, which had been the main U.S. source

---

TABLE 21-3

Comparison of AHA and ADA Diet Recommendations*

	AHA Step 1 (% total kcal)	AHA Step 2 (% total kcal)	ADA/ADA (% total kcal)
Total fat	30	30	30
Monounsaturated	10-15	10-15	12-14
Saturated	10	7	10
Polyunsaturated	Up to 10	Up to 10	6-8
Carbohydrate	50-60	50-60	55-60
Protein	15-20	15-20	0.8 g/kg
Cholesterol	300 mg/day	200 mg/day	300 mg/day

*AHA, American Heart Association; ADA, American Diabetes Association and American Dietetic Association.

until recently. But these animal-derived insulins are immunogenic to humans, beef more so than pork. In time they induce antiinsulin antibodies that delay or blunt their action. Now, however, human insulin is available from two sources: (1) biosynthesis by recombinant DNA technology through rapidly reproducing bacteria that have been given the human gene, and (2) chemical substitution of the terminal amino acid on the beta-chain of pork insulin. Because they carry the human insulin structure, these newer insulins are almost nonimmunogenic.

Insulin and Exercise

Exercise benefits all persons with diabetes through its action in increasing the number of insulin receptors on muscle cells, thus increasing insulin efficiency. However, physical activity must be regular to be effective. A detailed history of personal activity and exercise habits provides the information needed to help a client plan a wise program of regular moderate exercise. Guidelines for extra food to cover periods of heavier exercise, or athletic practice and competition, can be included (Table 21-4). In general, exercise programs make persons feel better, both physically and psychologically.[23] This improved sense of well-being should not be underestimated in persons facing a chronic disease. Also, blood glucose self-monitoring is a simple procedure that can help determine the balance needed at any point between exercise, insulin, and food.

Oral Hypoglycemic Agents

For some persons with non–insulin-dependent diabetes mellitus (NIDDM), an oral hypoglycemic drug may be used. These drugs act to lower the elevated blood glucose level by stimulating the pancreas to produce more endogenous insulin. They belong to a group of sulfonylurea compounds and include agents such as tolbutamide and the newer glipizide. Because their action

induces increased insulin activity, their use must be balanced with food and exercise just as insulin injections would be.

Diet Management

Many of the basic diet therapy principles carry over for both types of diabetes. The nutrient ratios are approximately the same. But energy balance needs will vary widely, depending on individual needs, such as growth requirements for children or weight reduction for overweight adults. A summary of the comparative diet planning needs for both types of diabetes is provided in Table 21-5.

TABLE 21-4

Meal-Planning Guide for Active People with Type I Diabetes Mellitus

Exchange needs for	Sample menus
Moderate activity	
30 minutes	
1 bread *or*	1 bran muffin *or*
1 fruit	1 small orange
1 hour	
2 bread + 1 meat *or*	Tuna sandwich *or*
2 fruit + 1 milk	½ cup fruit salad + 1 cup milk
Strenuous activity	
30 minutes	
2 fruit *or*	1 small banana *or*
1 bread + 1 fat	½ bagel + 1 tsp cream cheese
1 hour	
2 bread + 1 meat +	Meat and cheese sandwich +
1 milk *or*	1 cup milk *or*
2 bread + 2 meat +	hamburger +
2 fruit	1 cup orange juice

TABLE 21-5

Dietary Strategies for the Two Main Types of Diabetes Mellitus

Dietary strategy	IDDM (nonobese)	NIDDM (usually obese)
Decrease energy intake (kcalories)	No	Yes
Increase frequency and number of feedings	Yes	Usually no
Have regular daily intake of kcalories, carbohydrates, protein, and fat	Very important	Not important if average kcaloric intake remains in low range
Plan consistent daily ratio of protein, carbohydrates, and fat for each feeding	Desirable	Not necessary
Use extra or planned-ahead food to treat or prevent hypoglycemia	Very important	Not necessary
Plan regular times for meals/snacks	Very important	Not important
Use extra food for unusual exercise	Yes	Usually not necessary
During illness use small, frequent feedings of carbohydrates to prevent starvation ketosis	Important	Usually not necessary because of resistance to ketosis

Individual Needs

A comprehensive nutrition assessment and history will provide the necessary information to develop a personal food plan (see Chapters 10 and 16). A wide range of areas should be included, such as personal and family needs, living situation, social activities, work and school commitments, and food and exercise habits. Also, a full medical history will review the course of the person's diabetes and his or her personal experiences with it. Then, based on this assessment of status and needs, the clinical dietitian determines the appropriate diet prescription for the individual and calculates the nutritional needs according to the balance concept of nutritional therapy, which was previously described.

Diet Planning With Food Exchanges
Personal Diet Planning

Personal adaptations and approaches are important in planning nutritional therapy for any patient. But this basic principle is especially important for the person with diabetes who must eventually carry the responsibility for long-term self-care. There are numerous planning approaches used by skilled and sensitive clinical dietitians who tailor their actions to the person's learning needs and abilities, nutritional needs, personal needs, and life-style. Members of the diabetes care and education practice group of the American Dietetic Association, for example, have published a helpful monograph in which they discuss no less than 11 meal-planning approaches according to individual needs,

such as degree of literacy, structure, complexity, and area of emphasis on weight loss and glucose control.[24] However, because the Food Exchange System is the most widely used method of meal planning, it is the approach discussed here.

The Food Exchange System

This system of diet planning is based on the concept of food equivalents and their exchange to maintain both diet control and food choice variety. It was developed jointly by the American Dietetic Association and the American Diabetes Association and has been used successfully for a number of years with periodic revisions. It is designed for use by a professional diet counselor, usually a registered dietitian (RD) with extensive clinical experience, who can adapt it to meet many needs. With such personalized initial instruction and continued counseling, the person with diabetes will find the well-written and colorfully illustrated booklet, *Exchange Lists for Meal Planning*, a helpful guide and tool for planning meals and snacks.[25] It can be a sound means of dietary regulation that is flexible enough to meet a wide variety of situations.

Six food groups are used: starch/bread, meat, vegetable, fruit, milk, and fat. The revised food lists incorporate the low saturated fat modification in subgroups and highlight fiber and sodium content of foods. These revised food lists are provided here in Appendix K for reference. A general description of nutrient composition and characteristics is given in Table 21-6. In using

---

TABLE 21-6

Food Exchange Groups

Food group	Unit of exchange	Composition Carbohydrate (g)	Protein (g)	Fat (g)	kcalories	Characteristic items
Milk	1 cup					
Skim		12	8	—	80	Skim or very low fat
Low fat		12	8	5	120	
Whole		12	8	8	150	
Vegetables	½ cup	5	2	—	35	Medium carbohydrate
Fruit	Varies	15	—	—	40	Portion size varies with carbohydrate value of item
Bread	Varies; 1 slice bread	15	3	—	70	Variety of starch items, breads, cereals, vegetables; portions equal in carbohydrate value to 1 slice bread
Meat	28 g (1 oz)	—				Protein foods; exchange units equal to protein value of 28 g lean meat
Lean		—	7	3	50.5	
Medium fat		—	7	5	75	
Higher fat		—	7	8	100	
Fat	1 tsp					Fat food items equal to 1 tsp margarine (oil, mayonnaise, olives, avocados)
Polyunsaturated		—	—	5	45	
Monounsaturated		—	—	5	45	
Saturated		—	—	5	45	

the food groups as a guide, food items in any one group may be freely exchanged within that group, because all foods in a particular group have approximately the same food value. These food groups form the basis for calculating diet needs and for helping clients learn to make wide food selections and substitutions. A guide for estimating daily energy needs, the first step, is given in Table 21-7. Then calculations of energy nutrient needs follow, based on the dietary principles previously discussed (see Table 21-3).

Personal Meal/Snack Plan

On the basis of the individual's calculated diet prescription and food pattern, the clinical dietitian and the client should work out a personal food plan. The client will learn how to plan a menu by using the meal/snack food distribution pattern. A variety of foods from the food lists are chosen in the amounts indicated to meet the overall food plan. A sample menu based on the 2200-kilocalorie diet calculated in Table 21-8 is given in Table 21-9.

Special Concerns

In the course of daily living, a number of special concerns arise and become part of ongoing diet counseling:

1. **Special diet items.** The diet of the person with diabetes is planned using regular foods. No special foods are required. As with any consumer, the person with diabetes should read the labels on processed foods to make wise selections.
2. **Alcohol.** Occasional use of small amounts of alcohol in the diet for persons with diabetes can be planned, but caution must be used. Not only must the amount, timing, frequency, and kind of drink be considered, but also the nature of the diabetes and any medications of any kind being used.

TABLE 21-7

Guidelines for Estimating Approximate Daily Energy Need for Persons with Diabetes Mellitus According to Age, Gender, and General Physical Activity

	Daily energy intake	
Persons with diabetes	kcal/lb	kcal/kg
Children		
1 year	55	120
1-10 years (gradual decline with age)	45-36	100-80
Males		
11-15 years	20-36 (average, 30)	50-80 (average, 65)
16-20 years		
Very active	20-22	50
Average activity	18	30
Sedentary	15	30
Females		
11-15 years	17	35
15 years	15	30
Adults		
Men, active women	15 × DWB* (lb)	30
Sedentary men, most women, adults over age 55	13 × DBW (lb)	28
Sedentary women, obese persons, sedentary adults over age 55	10 × DBW (lb)	20
Pregnant women		
First trimester	13-15	28-32
Second and third trimesters; lactation	16-17	36-38

From Franz MJ: Diabetes and nutrition: state of the science and the art, *Top Clin Nutr* 3(1):1, 1988.
*DBW, desirable body weight (reasonable body weight).

TABLE 21-8

Calculation of Diabetic Diet: Short Method Using Exchange System (2200 kcal)

								Snacks	
Food group	Total day's exchanges	Carbohydrates: 275 g (50% kcal)	Protein: 110 g (20% kcal)	Fat: 75 g (30% kcal)	Breakfast	Lunch	Dinner	PM	hs
Milk (skimmed)	2	24	10		1				1
Vegetable	4	20	8			2	2		
Fruit	3	45			1	1	1		
		89							
Bread	12.5	187	37		3	3	3	2	1.5
		27.6	55						
Meat	8		56	40	1	2	4		1
			111						
Fat	7			35	2	2	3		
				75					

TABLE 21-9

Sample Menu Prescription:
2200 kcal:
275 g carbohydrates (50% kcal)
        +
110 g protein (20% kcal)
        +
75 g fat (30% kcal)

Meal	Food item

Breakfast

1 medium, sliced fresh peach
Shredded Wheat cereal
1 poached egg on whole-grain
   toast
1 bran muffin
1 tsp margarine
1 cup low-fat milk
Coffee or tea

Lunch	**Afternoon snack**

Lunch

Vegetable soup with wheat
   crackers
Tuna sandwich on whole wheat
   bread
   Filling: Tuna (drained ½ cup)
           Mayonnaise (2 tsp)
           Chopped dill pickle
           Chopped celery
Fresh pear

Afternoon snack

10 crackers with 2 tbsp peanut
   butter
Orange

Dinner

Pan-broiled pork chop (trimmed
   well)
1 cup brown rice
½-1 cup green beans
Tossed green salad Italian
   dressing (1-2 tbsp)
½ cup applesauce
1 bran muffin

Evening snack

3 cups popped, plain popcorn
1 oz cheese
1 cup low-fat milk

TABLE 21-10

How to Modify a Diabetic Meal Plan for Sick Days

Usual food intake	Exchange	Carbohydrates (g)
½ chicken breast, roasted	3 meat	0
1 tsp margarine	1 fat	0
½ cup rice	1 bread	15
Tossed green salad, lemon wedge	Free food	0
¾ cup strawberries	1 fruit	15
1 cup skim milk	1 milk	12
		TOTAL 42

Sick day intake*	Exchange	Carbohydrates (g)
2 cups broth	Free food	0
½ cup gelatin	1 fruit	15
1 cup ginger ale (regular)	2 fruit	30
2 cups herbal tea	Free food	0
		TOTAL 45

*The objective is to provide required amounts of carbohydrates for times when the person with diabetes just does not feel like eating much.

3. **Physical activity.** For any unusual physical activity, moderate or strenuous, the person with insulin-dependent diabetes mellitus (IDDM) needs to plan ahead for added food allowances to balance the exercise. This is particularly true for the young person with "brittle" diabetes engaging in strenuous athletic practice or competition. You can review the energy demands of exercise in Chapter 14.

4. **Illness.** When general illness occurs, food and insulin need to be adjusted (see box, p. 427). As needed, the texture of the food can be modified to incorporate easily digested and absorbed liquid foods with similar glucose equivalents of the usual food plan. This same procedure may be followed for glucose equivalent replacement of meals not eaten, as shown in Table 21-10.

5. **Travel.** When a trip is planned, the diet counselor and the client should confer to guide food choices according to what will be available. Both self-monitoring of blood glucose and insulin therapy equipment, as well as food plans, are as important on vacation or business trips as they are at home.[26] The traveler always needs to plan ahead with members of the health care team (see box, p. 427).

6. **Eating out.** Similar guidelines and suggestions can be provided for eating away from home. As a general rule, the plan should be made ahead of time so that accommodations for what is eaten at home before and after the outside meal can balance with needs for the day. Practice with restaurant menus is a helpful teaching tool.

7. **Stress.** Any form of physiologic or psychosocial stress affects blood glucose levels and will be reflected in varying changes in diabetes control. These variations are caused by hormonal stress responses antagonistic to insulin. Persons with diabetes can learn useful stress-reduction and relaxation exercises and activities to help handle stress in their lives (see Chapter 15).

Diabetes Education Program

Goal: Person-Centered Self-Care

Changing Roles

The respective roles of patient or client and their professional therapists are changing in modern health care. In past years a traditional medical model has guided diabetes education in its methods, language, and assumed roles. The professionals viewed themselves as having major authoritative roles and assigned

---

◆   **CLINICAL APPLICATION**   *Travel and Illness: "Real-life" Diabetic Situations*

Routine meal-planning tips are all well and good. But what do you do when your client with diabetes wants to travel or catches cold? In both cases, the client has too many distractions to concentrate fully on planning the most ideal menu. The fact remains, however, that diabetes management relies heavily on the food plan and, in the case of IDDM, on a flexible meal and snack pattern that can be adjusted to meet changing demands.

The following are a few helpful hints you may want to offer clients for those all too common situations.

Travel

Promote confidence about meal-planning skills. Review the number and type of exchanges allowed at each meal. Encourage the client to practice measuring portion sizes. Review tips on eating out.

Learn about the foods that will be available. For a cruise, the client should get a copy of the menu in advance. For air travel, advise the client to order diabetic meals in advance. If foreign travel is involved, the client should ask the travel agent for information about foods commonly served to tourists.

Select appropriate snacks. Extra carbohydrate and caloric needs must be met during extra physical activities, such as hiking, swimming, skiing, and mountain climbing.

Plan for time. Extended driving time should be avoided. The client should

plan to include about 20 g of carbohydrates for every 2 hours of travel. For emergencies and unexpected delays, food for two meals and two snacks, including nonperishable items and liquids, should be on hand.

Plan for time zone changes. The schedule may need to be changed. If so, discuss any necessary meal schedule revisions to balance with insulin activity pattern.

Prepare companions. The client's companions must be able to recognize signs and symptoms of hypoglycemia and hyperglycemia and know their treatment. Remind the client to carry quick-acting carbohydrates at all times.

To support the medical regimen of insulin-dependent clients, remind them (1) to carry an identification bracelet, pendant, or card at all times, (2) to ask their physician for a letter explaining the need for syringes, (3) to carry adequate supplies and equipment for maintaining a schedule for self-testing blood, and (4) to take a prescription for insulin and secure brand names used for insulin in the country to which they are traveling.

Sick-day survival

Nausea and diarrhea. Fluid and electrolyte replacement is crucial with nausea and diarrhea. Advise the client to use salted crackers, broth, or soups as tolerated to replace sodium. The client should use a cola drink, such as Coca

Cola (small amounts of high-sugar foods may be tolerated as replacement for short periods, such as during illness), tea, broth, or orange juice to replace potassium. The client should drink something at least every 2 to 3 hours to replace liquids.

Gastrointestinal disturbances. The insulin dosage may have to be decreased. A clear liquid diet—including fruit juices, fruit ices, and soups—for adequate amounts of carbohydrates is recommended. Protein supplementation through elemental nutrition may be necessary if symptoms last longer than 72 hours. As food tolerance improves, the client should progress to a soft diet that includes milk drinks, custards, and eggs.

Colds and fever. These conditions are often treated with aspirin, which tends to lower the sugar level. The client must not skip meals. If necessary, regular meals may be subdivided into small, frequent snacks. Insulin must not be omitted. If the client is completely unable to eat, the physician should be contacted for advice about insulin dosage.

In summary, in all cases the client must be advised (1) to maintain a steady intake of food every day, (2) to replace the carbohydrate value of solid foods with that of liquid or soft foods as needed, (3) to monitor blood and urine frequently for sugar and acetone levels, and (4) to contact the physician if the illness lasts for more than a day or so. ◆

---

the passive role of "patient" to the person with diabetes. With notable exceptions, this model has been followed in most cases. However, with the increasing movement toward changing roles of practitioners and consumers in the health care system, persons with diabetes are assuming a more active voice in planning and conducting their own care. Barriers in our traditional system stem from three sources: (1) our culture, (2) our health care delivery system, and (3) our professional training and habits.

Communication Needs

Essentially, much of the core problem centers on *communication.* For example, here is a list of words we of-

ten use that are objectionable to persons with diabetes, along with suggestions for preferred language we might use instead:

1. *"Diabetic" used as a noun.* The word "diabetic" is an adjective and should not be used alone as an impersonal noun. Use instead the phrase "person with diabetes."

2. *Compliance.* The word "compliance" raises red flags in the minds of persons with diabetes. It is purely a medical term and connotes an authoritative physician position. Instead use the word "adherence." This word has been adopted by national committees and associations working in the field of diabetes. The word "adherence" indicates that the decision-

making responsibility rests with the person who has diabetes to determine courses of action in varying life situations—which is the actual fact.

3. *Patient.* In general use, the phrase "person with diabetes" is the correct reference. Persons with diabetes are patients *only* when they are in the hospital or are seeing a physician for an illness, just like anybody else.

4. *Cheating.* A particularly abusive word to many persons with diabetes, especially to parents of children and young people with diabetes, is the word "cheating." This flagrant language abuse suggests dishonesty or failure to live up to an external code. By and large, persons with diabetes do not "cheat." They may kid themselves or they may be inaccurate in their reporting, but they do not cheat. Use instead such phrases as "having difficulty" or "having a problem with."

Content: Tools for Self-Care

A plan for diabetes education must recognize the need for building self-sufficiency and responsibility within persons with diabetes and their families. It should involve the necessary skills a person with diabetes must have for the best possible control. It should relate to factors related to life situation and psychosocial needs. Content areas include needs associated with the nature of diabetes; nutrition and basic meal planning; insulin (or oral medication) effects and how to regulate them; monitoring of blood glucose, urine, and acetone levels; hypoglycemia control; and how to deal with illness. These educational needs may be organized on three levels: survival, home and work management, and lifestyle. The Diabetes Care and Education dietetic practice group has provided two such management guidelines, one for children and adolescents and one for adults.[9,15]

Educational Materials: Person-Centered Standards

A broad, often confusing array of diabetes education materials is available. Some are excellent, and some should be discarded. We are wisely reminded, especially by parents of some of our young adolescent clients, that whatever we use should measure up to several basic person-centered requirements. As health care providers, we should do the following:

1. Give the client credit for having some intelligence and wanting new information.
2. Inform persons fully and completely of health care information, giving both sides of an issue when experts disagree—as surely they will on occasion.
3. Appeal to various levels of understanding, ranging from basic to sophisticated.
4. *Never* be patronizing, dehumanizing, or childish.

In the last analysis, whatever methods or materials we use, one central fact remains: the person who has diabetes is the *most* important and *fully equal* member of the diabetes care team. Interdisciplinary approaches and strategies that involve this recognition can be developed and are the most likely ones to succeed.

To Sum Up

Diabetes mellitus is a syndrome composed of many metabolic disorders collectively characterized by hyperglycemia and other symptoms. The treatment relies heavily on a basic type of therapy—a carefully controlled diet. Diabetes is classified in two main types: insulin-dependent diabetes mellitus (IDDM) and non–insulin-dependent diabetes mellitus (NIDDM).

Blood glucose levels are controlled primarily by the hormones of the pancreatic islet cells: *insulin,* which facilitates passage of glucose through cell membranes via special membrane receptors; *glucagon,* which ensures adequate levels of glucose to pervent hypoglycemia; and *somatostatin,* which controls the actions of insulin and glucagon to maintain normal blood glucose levels. The diabetic state results from inadequate insulin secretion or insulin resistance from too few receptor sites. Symptoms range from polydipsia, polyuria, polyphagia, and signs of abnormal energy metabolism to fluid and electrolyte imbalances, acidosis, and coma in seriously uncontrolled conditions.

IDDM affects about 15% of all persons with diabetes. It occurs more often in children and is more severe and unstable. Its treatment involves blood glucose self-monitoring, insulin administration, and regular meals and exercise to balance insulin activity. NIDDM occurs mostly in adults, particularly those who are overweight. Acidosis is rare. Its treatment consists of weight management and exercise. The food plan for both types of diabetes should be rich in complex carbohydrates and fiber; low in simple sugars and fats, especially saturated fats and cholesterol; and moderate in protein. Moderate regular exercise increases the number of insulin receptor sites on cell membranes and aids in weight control.

QUESTIONS FOR REVIEW

1. Describe the major characteristics of the two types of diabetes mellitus. Explain how these characteristics influence differences in nutritional therapy. List and describe medications used to control these conditions.

2. Identify and explain symptoms of uncontrolled diabetes mellitus.

3. Describe the three major complications of uncontrolled chronic diabetes and the current program of intensive individual therapy designed to maintain normal blood glucose levels and help to avoid these complications.

4. Mr. Smith just found out that he has diabetes mellitus. He is a sedentary, 45-year-old man who is 170 cm (5 ft, 8 in) tall and weighs 94 kg (210 lb). No medications were prescribed for him. What is his desirable lean body weight? If a 1500-kilocalorie diet is prescribed, how

many grams of carbohydrate, protein, and fat should be included? If he decides to drink, how much alcohol could be allowed and how should he fit it into his diet? Should he purchase sugar substitutes or diet foods? Defend your answer. Mr. Smith wants to help his children reduce their chances of developing diabetes. What advice would you offer?

REFERENCES

1. Whitehouse FW: Classification and pathogenesis of the diabetes syndrome: a historical perspective, *J Am Diet Assoc* 81(3):243, 1982.

2. Nestle M and others: A case of diabetes mellitus, *N Engl J Med* 81:127, 1982.

3. Bliss M: *The discovery of insulin,* Chicago, 1982, University of Chicago Press.

4. McNabb WL and others: Weight loss program for inner-city black women with non–insulin-dependent diabetes mellitus: PATHWAYS, *J Am Diet Assoc* 93(1):75, 1993.

5. Moller DE, Flier JS: Insulin resistance—mechanisms, syndromes, and implications, *N Engl J Med* 325(13):938, 1991.

6. Atkinson MA, Maclaren NK: What causes diabetes? *Sci Am* 263(1):62, 1990.

7. Knowler WC and others: Diabetes incidence in Pima Indians: contribution of obesity and parental diabetes, *Am J Epidemiol* 113:144, 1981.

8. Wendorf M, Goldfine ID: Archeology of NIDDM—excavation of the thrifty genotype, *Diabetes* 40:161, 1991.

9. Connell JE, Thomas-Doberson D: Nutritional management of children with insulin-dependent diabetes mellitus: a review by the Diabetes Care and Education dietetic practice group, *J Am Diet Assoc* 9(12):1556, 1991.

10. McKeigue PM and others: Relation of central obesity and insulin resistance with high diabetes prevalence and cardiovascular risk in South Asians, *Lancet* 337:382, 1991.

11. Dowse GK and others: Abdominal obesity and physical inactivity as risk factors for NIDDM and impaired glucose tolerance in Indian, Creole, and Chinese Mauritians, *Diabetes Care* 14(4):271, 1991.

12. Horton ES: Exercise and decreased risk of NIDDM, *N Engl J Med* 325(3):196, 1991.

13. Bell GI: Molecular defects in diabetes mellitus, *Diabetes* 40:413, 1991.

14. Dahl-Jorgensen K and others: Effect of near normoglycemia for two years on progression of early diabetic retinopathy, nephropathy, and neuropathy: the Oslo study, *Diabetes Spectrum* 1(2):98, 1988.

15. Beebe CA and others: Nutrition management for individuals with non–insulin-dependent diabetes mellitus in the 1990s: a review of the Diabetes Care and Education dietetic practice group, *J Am Diet Assoc* 91(2):196, 1991.

16. Coulston AM, Hollenbeck CB: Source and amount of dietary carbohydrate in patients with NIDDM, *Top Clin Nutr* 3(1):17, 1988.

17. Anderson JW and others: Metabolic effects of high-carbohydrate, high-fiber diets for insulin-dependent diabetic individuals, *Am J Clin Nutr* 54:936, 1991.

18. Butchko HH, Kotsonia FN: Acceptable daily intake vs actual intake: the aspartame example, *J Am Coll Nutr* 10(3):258, 1991.

19. Badiga MS and others: Diarrhea in diabetics: the role of sorbitol, *J Am Coll Nutr* 9(6):578, 1990.

20. Narins RG: Diabetic neuropathy: can the natural history be modified? *Am J Med* 90(suppl 2A):70, 1991.

21. Chitwood M, Wetch CB: Alcohol, alcohol, everywhere—but not a drop to drink? *Diabetes Forecast* 46(11):38, 1992.

22. Franz MJ: Exercise and the management of diabetes mellitus, *J Am Diet Assoc* 87(7):872, 1987.

23. Gill G: Psychological aspects of diabetes, *Br J Hosp Med* 46:301, 1991.

24. Green J, Holler H: *Meal planning approaches in the management of the person with diabetes,* Chicago, 1987, American Dietetic Association.

25. American Diabetes Association, American Dietetic Association: *Exchange lists for meal planning,* Chicago, 1986, The Associations.

26. Joursay DL, Lorber DL: Diabetes and the traveler, *Clin Diabetes* 6(3):49, 1988.

FURTHER READING

Beebe CA and others: Nutrition management for individuals with non–insulin-dependent diabetes mellitus in the 1990s: a review by the Diabetes Care and Education dietetic practice group, *J Am Diet Assoc* 91(2):196, 1991.

Connell JE, Thomas-Dobersen D: Nutrition management of children and adolescents with insulin-dependent diabetes mellitus: a review by the Diabetes Care and Education dietetic practice group, *J Am Diet Assoc* 91(12):1556, 1991.

Gallagher AM, Crawley C, editors: Applying new technology in diabetes management to nutrition counseling: meters, insulin, and insulin delivery systems, *On the Cutting Edge* 13(4):1-33, 1992.

These three resources from the Diabetes Care and Education (DCE) dietetic practice group of the American Dietetic Association provide excellent references for the current care of persons with diabetes. The first two articles from the journal review curent practice guidelines. In the third reference the Diabetes Care and Education practice group devotes an entire issue of its bimonthly newsletter, *On the Cutting Edge,* to new technologies used in the care of diabetes. Copies of this excellent resource are available from the DCE group (Joanne Gibbons, DCE Administrative Assistant, 9212 Delphi Road, S.W., Olympia, WA 98512; $5.00 plus $0.75 shipping/handling; make check payable to The American Dietetic Association/DCE).

Helmrich SP and others: Physical activity and reduced occurrence of non–insulin-dependent diabetes mellitus, *N Engl J Med* 325(3):147, 1991.

Horton ES: Exercise and decreased risk of NIDDM, *N Engl J Med* 325(3):196, 1991.

These references provide current information for the important role of exercise in managing NIDDM and in the balanced care of IDDM.

CASE STUDY

The Patient with Insulin-Dependent Diabetes Mellitus

Angela Delano is a 45-year-old woman diagnosed 2 years ago with insulin-dependent diabetes mellitus (IDDM). She has three children whose birth weights were in the range of 4.5 to 5.0 kg (10 to 11 lb). The children—now teenagers—show no signs of diabetes, and their weights are reported to be within normal limits, despite their mother's fondness for cooking. Her husband, an underpaid construction worker, is slightly overweight.

Six months ago, Mrs. Delano was seen with a complaint of a series of infections during the past 2 months that lasted longer than usual. At that time she was measured as 165 cm (5 ft 5 in) and 93 kg (205 lb). Her glucose tolerance test was positive. She was seen for follow-up twice during the following month, each time showing hyperglycemia and glycosuria. At the second follow-up, an oral hypoglycemic agent was prescribed, and she was referred to the Nutrition Clinic for weight-management counseling.

Mrs. Delano did not keep this appointment or her subsequent medical appointment. She was not seen again until a month ago, when she was admitted with ketoacidosis. She responded well to treatment and was placed on a 1200-kilocalorie diet and a mixture of intermediate- and rapid-acting insulin given in two injections a day. On discharge, she was again referred to the Nutrition Clinic for individual counseling and diabetes education classes.

Questions for Analysis

1. What factors do you think contributed to the ketoacidosis? Why? What relation do these factors have to diabetes control?
2. What additional information about Mrs. Delano is necessary to understand her major nutritional problems? Why? How could this information be obtained?
3. Based on the information provided, what nutritional problems can be identified? What is the scientific basis for each problem?
4. Determine an appropriate diet prescription for Mrs. Delano, and calculate her diet using the exchange system and short method. Using this diet calculation as a guide, outline a meal plan and a schedule of self-monitoring of blood glucose for Mrs. Delano. Assume that she administers the insulin before breakfast and before the evening meal.
5. Identify any personal factors that may affect Mrs. Delano's follow-through with her treatment plan. Do you anticipate any problems? If so, how would you attempt to help her solve them? Outline a diabetes education plan for Mrs. Delano.

ISSUES·AND·ANSWERS

Persons with diabetes have many questions about their diets, especially when they are newly diagnosed and anxieties are high. They don't want just a "yes" or "no" answer. For any item of concern, they want to know whether it can be used at all or whether use is limited, why, and how much. Questions about alcohol and various sweeteners are common.

Alcohol and diabetes: do they mix?

Two shots of whiskey on an empty stomach lowers the blood sugar level dramatically. For this reason, alcohol has been a taboo for years for persons with diabetes. It definitely has some negative effects because of the following:

- Alcohol interferes with the body's ability to regulate insulin-induced hypoglycemia (persons with poorly-controlled diabetes are most susceptible to this effect).
- It increases serum cholesterol levels, although this effect is transient.
- Alcohol consumption leads to hyperlipoproteinemia in susceptible persons, including persons with diabetes, when it is excessive.
- Alcohol consumption leads to hyperglycemia when it is excessive, although this is a transient effect usually lasting only a few hours.
- Alcohol induces a diabetic condition when used in excess by a prediabetic individual (in such persons, however, the blood sugar level returns to normal after total abstinence, without the patient's having to resort to the use of insulin or an oral hypoglycemic agent).

But alcohol may not be quite as bad as most people think for the person with diabetes, because it does the following:

- Alcohol does not require insulin for its metabolism.
- It enhances the glucose-lowering effect of hypoglycemic agents, including insulin, when used in *moderate* amounts.
- It raises the high-density lipoprotein-cholesterol (HDL-C) levels when used in *moderate* amounts, thus possibly providing some protection against cardiovascular disease.

In light of this information, it appears that diabetes and alcohol can mix—*if* shaken gently. For your clients who choose to use alcohol, you will want to discuss the following items with them:

1. Carry personal diabetes identification at all times in case of a hypoglycemic attack induced by alcohol.
2. Ask the physician whether there are any contraindications to using alcohol, such as hypertriglycerides, gastritis, pancreatitis, some types of cardiac and renal disease, and any drug interactions (such as that occurring with the use of barbiturates or tranquilizers).

3. Always sip alcoholic drinks slowly.
4. Never drink alcohol on an empty stomach.
5. Limit alcohol use to no more than one or two alcohol equivalents per day about 2 or 3 days a week. One equivalent is found in the following:
   - 1½ oz (a shot glass) of distilled alcoholic beverage (whiskey, Scotch, rye, vodka, brandy, cognac, rum)
   - 4 oz dry wine
   - 2 oz dry sherry
   - 12 oz beer (preferably "light" or reduced-kilocalorie)
6. Avoid sweet drinks (for example, liqueurs; sweet wines; drinks mixed with tonic, soda, or fruit juice; and other liquids that have a high concentration of sugar).

In addition, warn any clients taking oral hypoglycemic agents about some of the problems that may occur when they drink alcohol (for example, nausea, deep flushing, tachycardia, and impaired speech). The effect is slightly delayed, beginning 3 to 10 minutes after taking a drink and lasting up to an hour or longer.

Warn clients receiving insulin they should *not* reduce their food intake. Persons with NIDDM must consider the kcaloric value of the alcohol and omit 2 fat exchanges for each drink. In contrast, persons with IDDM should continue to eat their full diet as prescribed, because of their susceptibility to hypoglycemia induced by alcohol.

Can I use fructose in my diabetic diet?

How would you answer this question from your diabetic client? Fructose has been touted as a sweetener for persons with diabetes, because it is a naturally-occurring sugar that is as much as one to one and one-half times as sweet as sucrose. But can the person with diabetes use it safely?

Although fructose as a sweetener is not for all persons with diabetes, generally you can reply, "Yes, but with qualifications."

Fructose must be calculated in the diabetic diet. Advertising claims promoting fructose are sometimes so misleading that many consumers mistakenly believe that it can be used as a "free" food. However, fructose has the same nutritive value as other sugars—4 kcal/g. Especially those persons with IDDM should be instructed to use fructose as carefully as they use any other food with a kcaloric and carbohydrate value.

The quantity must be limited. If used, the maximal amount is 75 g a day.

Fructose should be used under specific conditions. Its sweetness varies with temperature, acidity, and dilution. It has been used satisfactorily in some cooked desserts. However, with high temperatures, a rise in the pH level, and increased concentration of solution, its sweetness is reduced. This leads to overconsumption, which affects blood sugar levels.

Refined fructose should be used. Natural sources of fructose, such as honey, also contain considerable amounts of glucose. Thus in comparison, if it is used at all, the person with diabetes is better off using a measured amount of refined fructose.

The American Diabetes Association emphasizes that until further studies show any clinical advantages for using fructose instead of sucrose, fructose should be used only in its pure form, in small amounts, and only by those persons with well-controlled diabetes who are not overweight.

REFERENCES

Chitwood M, Welch CB: Alcohol, alcohol, everywhere—but not a drop to drink? *Diabetes Forecast* 46(11):38, 1992.

Franz MJ: Diabetes mellitus: considerations in the development of guidelines for the occasional use of alcohol, *J Am Diet Assoc* 83(2):147, 1983.

Laine DC: Are sucrose and fructose compatible with a diabetic diet? *Top Clin Nutr* 3(1):46, 1988.

Powers MA, Laine DC: Sweeteners. In Powers MA, editor: *Handbook of diabetes nutritional management,* Rockville, Md, 1987, Aspen.

CHAPTER 22

Renal Disease

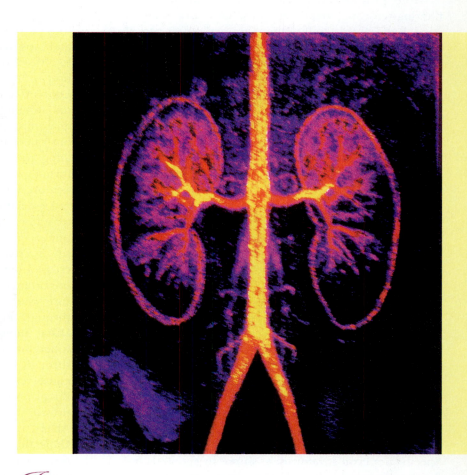

In this chapter we look at the problems of renal disease. First, we examine the vital structure and function of the kidney and its vast array of minute functional units, the nephrons. Then we see how serious functional problems develop when disease attacks these tissues.

Kidney diseases affect the lives of more than 8 million Americans and kill 60,000 a year. The recent advent of renal dialysis technology and kidney transplant techniques prolong life, but this survival is not without great human and monetary cost.

Here, we consider problems of infection, tissue breakdown, renal failure, and stone formation. In each case we relate nutritional therapy to the nature of the illness and the renal functions impaired.

Physiology of the Kidney

Renal Functions

Basic Functional Unit—The Nephron

Knowledge of the normal functions of the kidney forms the essential background for understanding therapy in renal disorders based on the organ's impaired functioning in disease. The basic anatomic and functional unit of the kidney is the **nephron.** Major advances today in treating kidney disease are based on providing maximal support for these vital functions of the nephron (Fig. 22-1).

We are provided at birth with about 2 million of these filtering-resorbing nephron units, far more than we need. But we begin to lose them gradually after age 30. Each nephron is an exquisite example of a highly complex, minute tissue unit. It is adapted in fine detail to its vital function—maintaining an internal fluid environment compatible with life. These small vital units of the kidney are the master chemists of our bodies. We have the kind of body fluids and tissues that we have not merely because of what the mouth takes in but because of what the kidneys keep. Only because they work in the way they do has it become possible for us to have specific tissues of a specific nature to do specific tasks.

Specific Integrated Nephron Functions

Each kidney contains some 1 million nephrons. As the body fluid flows through these finely structured units, the nephrons perform four significant functions to support life:

1. **Filtering** most constituents to prevent them from the entering blood, except red cells and proteins
2. **Resorbing** needed substances as the filtrate continues along the winding tubules
3. **Secreting** additional ions to maintain acid-base balance
4. **Excreting** unneeded materials in a concentrated urine

Nephron Structures

Specific nephron structures, as shown in Fig. 22-1, perform unique metabolic tasks to maintain body balances. These key structures include the glomerulus and the tubules.

Glomerulus

At the head of each nephron, blood enters in a single capillary and then branches into a group of collateral capillaries. This tuft of collateral capillaries is held closely together in a cup-shaped membrane. This cup-shaped capsule is named **Bowman's capsule,** for the young English physician, Sir William Bowman, who in 1843 first clearly established the basis of plasma filtration and consequent urine secretion based on this intimate relationship of the blood-filled glomeruli and the enveloping membrane. The filtrate formed here is cell free and virtually protein free. Otherwise, it carries the same constituents as does the entering blood.

Tubules

Continuous with the base of Bowman's capsule, the nephron tubules wind in a series of convolutions toward their terminal in the renal pelvis. Specific resorption functions are performed by the four sections of the tubule:

1. **Proximal tubule.** In the first section nearest the glomerulus, major nutrient resorption occurs. Essentially 100% of the glucose and amino acids and 80% to 85% of the water, sodium, potassium, chloride, and most other substances are resorbed. Only 15% to 30% of the filtrate remains to enter the next section.
2. **Loop of Henle.** This narrowed midsection of the renal tubule is named for the celebrated German anatomist, Friedrich Henle, who in 1845 first demonstrated its unique structure and function in creating the necessary fluid pressures for ultimately forming a concentrated urine. At this narrowed midsection, the thin loop of tubule dips into the central renal medulla. Here, through a balanced system of water and sodium exchange through sodium pumps in the limbs of the loop, important fluid density is created around the loop. This area of increased density in the central part of the kidney is important to concentrate the urine by osmotic pressure when the lower collecting tubule later passes through this same area of the kidney.
3. **Distal tubule.** This latter portion of the tubule functions primarily in providing acid-base balance through the secretion of ionized hydrogen. It also conserves sodium by resorbing it under the influence of the hormones aldosterone and vasopressin (also called antidiuretic hormone, or ADH).
4. **Collecting tubule.** In the final widened section of the tubule the filtrate is concentrated to save water and form urine for excretion. Water is absorbed under the influence of the pituitary hormone ADH and the osmotic pressure of the more dense surrounding fluid in this central part of the kidney. The resulting volume of urine, now concentrated and excreted, is only 0.5% to 1.0% of the original water and solutes filtered at the beginning in Bowman's capsule.

General Causes of Renal Disease

A number of agents or conditions may interfere with the normal functioning of the nephrons and cause renal disease.

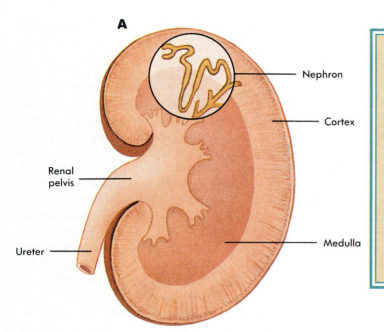

A

Nephron

Cortex

Renal pelvis

Medulla

Ureter

nephron • Microscopic anatomic and functional unit of the kidney that selectively filters and resorbs essential blood factors, secretes hydrogen ions as needed for maintaining acid-base balance, then resorbs water to protect body fluids, and forms and excretes a concentrated urine for elimination of wastes. The nephron includes the renal corpuscle (glomerulus), the proximal convoluted tubule, the loop of Henle, the distal convoluted tubule, and the collecting tubule, which empties the urine into the renal medulla. The urine passes into the papilla and then to the pelvis of the kidney. Urine is formed by filtration of blood in the glomerulus and by the selective reabsorption and secretion of solutes by cells that comprise the walls of the renal tubules. There are approximately 1 million nephrons in each kidney.

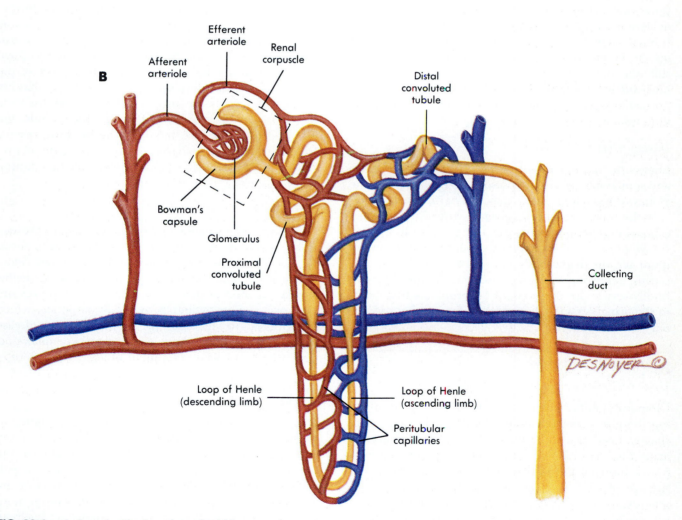

B

Efferent arteriole

Afferent arteriole

Renal corpuscle

Distal convoluted tubule

Bowman's capsule

Glomerulus

Proximal convoluted tubule

Collecting duct

Loop of Henle (descending limb)

Loop of Henle (ascending limb)

Peritubular capillaries

DESNOYER ©

FIG. 22-1 **A,** Longitudinal section of a kidney, showing the location of a nephron in the kidney. **B,** The nephron—functional unit of the kidney.

Inflammatory and Degenerative Disease

Inflammation of the small blood vessels and membranes in the nephrons may be short term, as in acute forms of glomerulonephritis. In other cases it may diffusely involve entire nephrons or nephron segments, disrupting normal function. Nephrotic lesions develop, leading to progressive chronic renal failure. Nutritional disturbances in the metabolism of protein, electrolytes, and water follow.

Infection and Obstruction

Bacterial infection of the urinary tract may range from occasional mild, uncomfortable bladder infection to more-involved chronic recurrent disease and obstruction from kidney stones. This obstruction anywhere in the urinary tract blocks drainage, causing further infection and tissue damage.

Damage from Other Diseases

Circulatory disorders—such as prolonged hypertension, often associated with the vasopressor effect of the renin-angiotensin-aldosterone mechanism—can cause degeneration of the small renal arteries and curtail efficient function.[1,2] A vicious cycle ensues as the demand on the kidney in turn causes more hypertension and still more damage. Other diseases, such as diabetes mellitus and gout, may also damage kidney function.[3,4] Abnormalities present from birth may lead to poor function, infection, or obstruction.

Damage from Other Agents

Environmental agents—such as insecticides, solvents, and similar materials—are poisons that can damage the kidneys.[5] Some toxic drugs may also harm renal tissue.[6]

In the treatment of renal disease, nutritional therapy is based on impaired renal function and resulting clinical symptoms. In this chapter we focus primarily on the more serious degenerative processes of glomerulonephritis, nephrotic syndrome, and renal failure. Then we briefly review the more common problems that occur in the urinary tract—obstructive kidney stones and urinary tract infection.

Glomerulonephritis

Disease Process

Glomerulonephritis is an inflammatory process affecting the glomeruli, the small blood vessels in the cup-shaped head of the nephron. It is most common in acute form in children 3 to 10 years of age, although 5% or more of the initial attacks occur in adults past the age of 50. The most common cause is a previous streptococcal infection. It has a more or less sudden onset, a brief course in its acute form, and is usually completely cleared in a year or two. In some cases it progresses to a chronic form, involving an increased amount of renal tissue and eventually requiring dialysis and other support treatments.

Immune Complex Disease

Immunologic studies and electron microscopy have demonstrated the underlying process as an immune complex disease. An *antigen* or "foreign invader" in the body excites responses from the defense system to combat potentially harmful effects. In glomerular disease the antigens are usually substances attacking the body from the outside: bacteria, viruses, and chemicals, including antibiotics and other drugs. In response, *antibodies* are produced by the body to ward off or neutralize the effect of the antigen. An excess of antigen and antibodies leads to the the formation of *antigen-antibody complexes* in the circulation, which become trapped in the glomeruli. These complexes bind components of **complement,** a complex series of enzymatic proteins in the blood that serve as part of the body's immune system. The activated complement in turn provides active chemical factors that attract white blood cells, whose lysosomal enzymes incite the resulting injury to the glomerulus.

These antigen-antibody complexes appear as lumpy deposits between the epithelial cells of the cupped nephron capsule and the basement membrane of the glomeruli. Lesions develop, leaving scar tissue that obstructs the circulation through the glomerulus. Fatty degeneration and necrosis of the conjoined tubules follow, and ultimate destruction of the nephron results. In time, if the disease becomes progressive, the net result is a reduction in the number of functioning nephrons available in the kidneys.[7]

Clinical Symptoms

Classic symptoms include gross **hematuria** and **proteinuria.** Varying degrees of edema may occur, with shortness of breath resulting from sodium and water retention and circulatory congestion. Also, moderate **tachycardia** and mild or marked elevation of blood pressure may occur. The patient is generally anorexic, which contributes to feeding problems. If the disease progresses to renal insufficiency, **oliguria** or *anuria* occurs, which signals development of acute renal failure.

Nutritional Therapy

General Care in Uncomplicated Disease

The general treatment is symptomatic and designed to provide optimal nutritional support. In short-term acute cases in children, pediatricians and clinical nutritionists generally favor overall optimal nutrition with adequate protein, unless symptoms of oliguria or anuria develop. These complications usually last no more than 2 or 3 days and are managed by conservative treatment. Salt is usually not restricted unless complications of edema, hypertension, or oliguria become dangerous.

Thus in most patients with acute uncomplicated disease, especially in children with poststreptococcal glomerulonephritis, diet modifications are not crucial. The main treatment centers on bed rest and antibiotic drug therapy. The fluid intake will be adjusted to output as a rule, including losses in vomiting and diarrhea.

Specific Therapy in Progressive Disease

If the disease process advances, however, more specific nutritional therapy measures are indicated. The nutrient factors most involved are protein, carbohydrate, sodium, potassium, and water:

1. **Protein.** If the level of **blood urea nitrogen (BUN)** is elevated and oliguria is present, dietary protein must be restricted. Usually the diet contains 0.5 g of protein/kg of ideal body weight. Some patients may use 1 g/kg as long as renal function is adequate to maintain a normal BUN level.
2. **Carbohydrate.** To provide sufficient kilocalories to meet energy needs, carbohydrate should be given liberally. This will also reduce the catabolism of tissue protein and prevent starvation ketosis.
3. **Sodium.** The restriction of sodium varies with the degree of oliguria. If renal function is impaired, the sodium is restricted to 500 to 1000 mg/day. As recovery occurs, sodium intake can be increased.
4. **Potassium.** With severe oliguria, renal clearance of potassium is impaired. Potassium intoxication may occur, requiring dialysis. Thus potassium intake is monitored carefully according to disease progression.
5. **Water.** Fluids are restricted according to the kidney's ability to excrete urine. If restriction is not indicated, fluids can be consumed as desired.

Nephrotic Syndrome
Disease Process

Nephrotic syndrome, or **nephrosis,** is characterized by a group of symptoms resulting from kidney tissue damage and impaired nephron function. The most evident symptoms are massive *edema* and *proteinuria*. This condition may be caused by progressive glomerulonephritis. It may also be associated with other diseases, such as diabetes or connective tissue disorders (**collagen disease**). In some cases, it may result from drug reactions, especially exposure to heavy metals, or even from reaction to toxic venom after a bee sting. The primary degenerative lesion is in the capillary basement membrane of the glomerulus, permitting escape of large amounts of protein into the filtrate. The tubular changes that occur are due to the high protein concentration in the filtrate, with some protein uptake from the tubular lumen. Both filtration and resorption functions are disrupted.

Clinical Symptoms

The cardinal symptom of massive edema is evident. *Ascites* is common. The abdomen becomes increasingly distended as fluid collects in the serous cavities. Often *striae* (stretch marks) appear on the stretched skin of the abdomen and extremities. The massive edema is largely caused by the gross loss of protein—principally albumin—in the urine, some 4 to 10 g/day. This means that the plasma protein is greatly reduced. The albumin fraction is largely responsibile for maintaining the capillary fluid shift mechanism (see Chapter 8). Thus fluid balance between tissue fluid and circulating fluid is decreased to less than 4 g/dL. Free fat, oval fat bodies, or fatty droplets are found in the urine. Protein losses are also indicated by the presence of urinary globulins and specialized binding proteins for thyroxine and iron, producing signs of hypothyroidism and

blood urea nitrogen (BUN) • The nitrogen component of urea in the blood; a measure of kidney function; elevated levels of BUN indicate a disorder of kidney function.

collagen disease • Diseases attacking collagen tissues, the protein substance of the white fibers (collagenous fibers) of skin, tendon, bone, cartilage, and other connective tissue; any of a group of diseases that are clinically distinct but have in common widespread pathologic changes in the connective tissue, such as rheumatoid arthritis, lupus erythematosis, scleroderma, and rheumatic fever.

complement • A complex series of enzymatic proteins occurring in normal serum that interact to combine with and augment (fill out, complete) the antigen-antibody complex of the body's immune system, producing lysis when the antigen is an intact cell; composed of 11 discrete proteins or functioning components, activated by the immunoglobulin factors IgG and IgM.

hematuria • The abnormal presence of blood in the urine.

nephrosis • Nephrotic syndrome caused by degenerative epithelial lesions of the renal tubules of the nephrons, especially the *mesangium,* the thin basement membrane that helps support the capillary loops in a renal glomerulus; marked by edema, albuminuria, and a decreased serum albumin level.

oliguria • Secretion of a very small amount of urine in relation to fluid intake.

proteinuria • The presence of an excess of serum proteins, such as albumin, in the urine.

tachycardia • Excessively rapid action of the heart; usually applied to a heart rate above 100 beats per minute.

anemia. As serum protein loss continues, tissue proteins are broken down and general malnutrition ensues. Fatty tissue changes in the liver and general sodium retention further contribute to the edema. Severe ascites and *pedal edema* mask the gross tissue-wasting.

Nutritional Therapy

Nutritional therapy is directed toward control of the major symptoms, edema and malnutrition, resulting from the massive protein losses.

Protein

In the past the standard recommendation for patients with nephrotic syndrome was a high-protein diet, sometimes as high as 3 to 4 g/kg body weight/day, to restore the serum protein pool and prevent malnutrition. However, evidence has grown that high-protein diets may accually accelerate loss of renal function.[8,9] Because investigators and clinicians are increasingly concerned that high-protein diets may accelerate progression of renal disease, patients with nephrotic syndrome are now being individually treated with a moderately restricted protein diet. Commonly used protein intakes are 0.6 to 0.8 g/kg body weight/day (the adult RDA is 0.8 g/kg/day), plus 1.0 g/day of high biologic protein for each gram of urinary protein lost daily.[8,10]

Kilocalories

Sufficient kilocalories must always be provided to ensure protein use for tissue synthesis. High daily intakes of 35 to 60 kcal/kg are essential. Because appetite is usually poor, much encouragement and support are needed. The food must be as appetizing as possible and in a form most easily tolerated.

Sodium

With diuretic drugs to help reduce the edema, the use of moderate sodium restriction in the diet supports this tissue fluid management. Usually a 500- to 1000-mg sodium diet (see Chapter 20) is sufficient to help initiate *diuresis.*

The general dietary management is similar to that given for hepatitis (see Chapter 19), with the additional need for sodium restriction. There is no need to restrict potassium. Iron and vitamin supplements may be indicated.

Renal Failure

The two types of renal failure—acute and chronic—are characterized by a number of symptoms, reflecting interference with normal nephron functions in nutrient metabolism. Both forms have similar nutritional therapy, depending on the extent of renal tissue damage.

Acute Renal Failure
Disease Process

Renal failure may occur as an acute phase, with sudden shutdown of renal function after some metabolic insult or traumatic injury to normal kidneys. The situation is often life-threatening and is a medical emergency in which the nutritionist and nurse play important supportive roles. *Acute renal failure* may have various causes: (1) severe injury, such as extensive burns or crushing injuries that cause widespread tissue destruction, (2) infectious diseases, such as peritonitis, (3) traumatic shock after surgery on the abdominal aorta, (4) toxic agents in the environment, such as carbon tetrachloride or poisonous mushrooms, or (5) immunologic drug reactions in allergic or sensitive persons, such as penicillin reaction.

Clinical Symptoms

The major sign of such an acute renal failure is *oliguria,* which is diminished urine output, often accompanied by proteinuria or hematuria. This diminished urine output is brought on by the underlying tissue problems that characterize acute renal failure. Usually there is blockage of the tubules caused by cellular debris from tissue trauma or urinary failure with back-up retention of filtrate materials. Water balance becomes a crucial factor. The course of the disease is usually divided into an oliguric phase, followed by a diuretic phase. The urinary output during the oliguric phase varies from as little as 20 to 200 ml/day.

During this initial phase of acute renal failure, the patient may be lethargic and anorectic and may suffer from nausea and vomiting. Blood pressure elevation and signs of *uremia* may be present. Oral intake is usually difficult in this catabolic period. The serum urea nitrogen (SUN) level increases along with the creatinine level, which results from the tissue breakdown of muscle mass. Usually after an initial conservative treatment, recovery occurs in a few days to 6 weeks. However, in more complicated cases in which the oliguria continues 4 or 5 days, more aggressive therapy—including **hemodialysis** and total parenteral nutrition (TPN)—is used.

Nutritional Therapy

The major challenge for nutritional therapy is the improvement of nutritional status, especially in patients with marked catabolism. Depending on the patient's condition, nutrient intake may be oral or intravenous. In this early acute phase no protein should be given, so as to limit nitrogen sources and potassium, phosphate, and sulfate levels. Carbohydrate is increased to supply energy, with additional kilocalories from fat, either through oral feedings or continuous peripheral vein feedings. During dialysis, TPN may be used as a feeding method (see Chapter 18). In these cases, a mix-

The Aging Western Kidney

TO PROBE FURTHER

Renal disease typically follows a progressive downhill course. Why should this be? The work of Brenner's group at Harvard indicates that the stage may well have been set in our distant evolutionary past as an adaptation of the kidney to meet the nitrogenous excretion needs of our hunter/scavenger, meat-eating ancestors.

Because our ancestors were carnivores, their protein intake was transient and intermittent; they could eat only after a successful hunting expedition. Thus at these times of surfeit a large number of extra nephrons had to be available to meet their needs for the prompt excretion of waste products, largely urea, and the conservation of fluid and electrolytes until the next meal became available. They achieved this metabolic task mainly by *hyperfiltration* through increased use of their many extra superficial glomeruli, largely in the outer part (cortex) of the kidney, which normally maintains a resting state. It was only in the past 500 to 10,000 years, when population groups developed agriculture and herding, that a more continuous food intake pattern became possible. Now in many Western countries our adult diet averages approximately 3000 kcal and more than 100 g of protein, largely meat, *daily*.

Thus the answers to our initial questions—Why do we have far more nephrons than we seem to need? Why do we begin losing some of these nephrons through a "normal aging process" of glomerular sclerosis after age 30? Why is renal disease so inexorably progressive?—lie in a fundamental mismatch between the evolutionary design of our kidneys and the functional burden we place on them by our modern eating habits. Our sustained excessive protein levels in the blood, along with other solutes, impose demands for sustained increases in renal blood flow and glomerular filtration rates. This requires that our reserve glomeruli of the outer renal cortex be in more or less continuous use and predisposes even healthy persons to the observed progressive glomerular sclerosis over time, with deterioration of normal kidney function. In health this deterioration poses no problem because we have so many extra nephrons. But when renal disease occurs, the burden is compounded. The disease accelerates the deterioration process and makes coping impossible. The downhill course inevitably ensues. The aging and vulnerable kidney of people living in the Western countries thus seems to be related inevitably to our lifetime of large protein meals.

REFERENCES

Brenner BM, and others: Dietary protein intake and the progressive nature of kidney disease, *N Engl J Med* 307(11):652, 1982.

Klahr S and others: The progression of renal disease, *N Engl J Med* 318(25):1657, 1988.

Mitch WE and others: *The progressive nature of renal disease*, New York, 1986, Churchill Livingstone.

---

ture of essential and nonessential amino acids as tolerated—especially those which are partially synthesized in the kidney, glucose, lipid emulsions, supplemented by needed B-complex and C vitamins—is given to support healing and recovery of renal function.[11,12] Electrolytes are monitored carefully and provided only for observed deficits. Children with acute renal failure especially require prompt, carefully monitored fluid resuscitation.[13] After successful initial therapy, the following diuretic phase signals improved renal function. Fluid and dietary intake is increased as the diuresis progresses, until a normal intake is reached. If sodium retention accompanies the diuresis, dietary sodium is restricted as needed. Sufficient quantities of water and glucose also are needed to correct **hypernatremia.**

Chronic Renal Failure

Disease Process

The course of renal failure may become chronic with progressive degenerative changes in renal tissues and marked depression of all renal functions.[7] At this stage, few functioning nephrons remain and these gradually deteriorate (see box above). The symptom complex of advanced renal insufficiency is commonly, though imprecisely, called by its old term *uremia*.

Chronic renal insufficiency may result from a variety of diseases that involve the nephrons: (1) primary glomerular disease, (2) metabolic disease with renal involvement, such as insulin-dependent diabetes mellitus (IDDM), (3) exposure to toxic substances, (4) infections, (5) renal vascular disease, (6) renal tubular disease, (7) chronic pyelonephritis, or (8) congenital abnormality of both kidneys. Depending on the nature of the predisposing renal disease, there is extensive scarring of renal tissue. This distorts the kidney structure and brings vascular changes from the prolonged hypertension involved.

hemodialysis • Removal of certain elements from the blood according to their rates of diffusion through a semipermeable membrane—e.g., by a hemodialysis machine.

hypernatremia • Excessive levels of sodium in the blood.

Clinical Symptoms

Symptoms result from the progressive loss of nephrons and the consequent decreased renal blood flow and glomerular filtration. As the nephrons are lost one by one, the remaining nephrons gradually lose their ability to maintain body water balance, concentration of solutes in body fluids (osmolality), and electrolyte and acid-base balance. This continuing loss of nephrons brings many metabolic insults.

1. **Water balance.** The increased load of solutes causes an osmotic diuresis. Increasingly, the kidney cannot excrete a normal concentrated urine. Dehydration follows and may become critical. On the other hand, water intoxication may occur if there is excess fluid intake.

2. **Electrolyte balance.** A number of imbalances among electrolytes result from the decreasing nephron function:
   - *Sodium.* With the osmotic diuresis, sodium loss contributes to a decreasing extracellular fluid volume. As the plasma volume decreases, renal filtration declines further, worsening the renal failure. In this state the kidney cannot respond appropriately to maintain sodium balance. Any sudden increase in sodium intake cannot be excreted readily and causes more edema.
   - *Potassium.* The balance of potassium is usually not impaired as readily until the oliguria becomes severe or acidosis increases.
   - *Phosphate, sulfate, and organic acids.* With reduced nephron function there is reduced filtration and excretion of these materials produced by the metabolism of food nutrients. Thus these anions become concentrated in body fluids, with subsequent displacement of bicarbonate, causing metabolic acidosis.
   - *Calcium and phosphate.* Metabolism of these electrolytes is greatly disturbed as a consequence of renal tissue loss. Two metabolic functions of the kidney—(1) activation of vitamin D hormone and (2) parathyroid hormone control of serum calcium-phosphorus levels—cannot proceed at normal levels. The impaired vitamin D hormone activation results in a bone disease called **osteodystrophy.** This disturbance causes bone pain, various bone deformities, awkward gait, and in children impaired growth. Also, there may be calcification of soft tissues, which further hinders renal function.

3. **Nitrogen retention.** Increasing loss of nephron function brings elevated amounts of nitrogenous metabolites, such as urea and creatinine. The urea load results from dietary protein metabolism; the creatinine load, from increasing catabolism of muscle mass.

4. **Anemia.** The normal kidney participates in the production of red blood cells, through action of a specific enzyme. The damaged kidney cannot accomplish this task, and there is depressed red blood cell production. The red blood cells that are produced survive a shorter time but have a usual size and hemoglobin content.

5. **Hypertension.** When blood flow to renal tissue is increasingly impaired, the resulting *ischemia* brings increasing hypertension through the nephrons' close relationship to the renin-angiotensin-aldosterone mechanism. In turn hypertension causes cardiovascular damage and further deterioration of the kidney.

6. **Azotemia.** The elevated blood urea nitrogen (BUN), serum creatinine, and serum uric acid levels are reflected in the characteristic laboratory finding of **azotemia.**

General Signs and Symptoms

The increasing loss of renal function brings progressive weakness, shortness of breath, general lethargy, and fatigue. Thirst, anorexia, weight loss, and gastrointestinal irritability with diarrhea or vomiting result. Increased capillary fragility brings skin, nose, oral, and gastrointestinal bleeding. Nervous system involvement brings muscular twitching, burning sensations in the extremities, or uremic convulsions. Cheyne-Stokes respiration (irregular, cyclic type of breathing) indicates acidosis. There is ulceration of the mouth, a persistent bad or metallic taste, and fetid breath. Malnutrition lowers resistence to infection. Osteodystrophy continues with aching and pain in bone and joints.

Nutritional Therapy Goals

Treatment must be individual, adjusted according to progression of the illness, type of treatment being used, and the patient's response. In general, however, basic therapy objectives are as follows:
- Reduce and minimize protein breakdown
- Avoid dehydration or overhydration
- Correct acidosis carefully
- Correct electrolyte depletions and avoid excesses
- Control fluid and electrolyte losses from vomiting and diarrhea
- Maintain optimal nutritional status
- Maintain appetite, general morale, and sense of well-being
- Control complications—hypertension, bone pain, nervous system problems
- Retard progression of renal failure, postponing ultimate dialysis

Nutritional care plays a major role in many of these treatment objectives. The clinical nutritionist becomes an indispensable member of the renal care team. Principles of therapeutic nutrition for chronic renal failure include nutrient adjustments according to individual need.

1. **Protein.** The crucial problem is to provide sufficient protein to prevent protein breakdown, yet avoid an excess that would elevate urea levels. In general, limitation of protein to 0.5 g/kg body weight/day helps reduce azotemia and hyperkalemia and control acidosis. Protein is usually adjusted according to creatinine clearance. Restriction of protein intake is not needed until the creatinine clearance falls below 40 ml/minute. Thereafter the dietary protein must be regulated according to declining renal function (see Table 22-1).

   If caloric requirements are liberally met, patients may be maintained in nitrogen balance for prolonged periods on as little as 35 to 40 g protein/day. However, when blood urea levels rise, protein intake must be reduced to 20 g/day. Only essential amino acids are supplied by small amounts of milk and egg protein. Thus the patient is not burdened with nonessential amino acids that make demands on the body for the disposal of their nitrogenous waste products and do little to counteract the tissue protein catabolism. In any event, protein must be closely controlled according to individual need, ranging in quantity from 20 to 70 g/day and having a high biologic value to supply essential amino acids.

2. **Amino acid supplements.** Promising approaches to protein replacement have been developed using mixtures of essential amino acids or of amino acid precursors, such as alpha-keto-acid and alpha-hydroxy-acid analogs. Supplements have been developed containing nitrogen-free analogs of the branched-chain amino acids phenylalanine and methionine, which are metabolized in the liver, plus the remaining amino acids.

3. **Kilocalories.** Adequate kilocalories are mandatory. Carbohydrate and fat must supply sufficient nonprotein kilocalories to spare dietary protein for tissue protein synthesis and energy supply. About 300 to 400 g carbohydrate is the average daily need. Sufficient fat, 75 to 90 g, is added to give the patient 2000 to 2500 total kcal daily. Patients are encouraged to consume all the carbohydrates and fats they can, because the end products of their metabolism—carbon dioxide and water—do not impose a burden on the progressive renal failure. If the kilocalorie intake is inadequate, body protein tissue catabolism to supply energy further aggravates the renal failure.

4. **Water.** Total fluid intake must be guarded to avoid water intoxication from overloading or dehydration from too little water. The capacity of the damaged kidney to handle water is limited, and in many cases solids are excreted better with a controlled amount of water. With predialysis patients, the fluid intake should be sufficient to maintain adequate urine volume. Sometimes the obligatory water loss may be high because of the large solute load in sodium and urea that must be excreted by an increasingly smaller number of nephrons.

5. **Sodium.** The need for sodium intake varies. Both severe restriction and excess are to be avoided. The dietary need is closely related to the patient's handling of water. If hypertension and edema are present, sodium intake needs to be restricted. Usually, sodium intake will vary between 500 to 2000 mg/day.

6. **Potassium.** Serum potassium levels may be depressed or elevated. Adjustment of intake is made accordingly to maintain normal levels. If significant losses occur with severe vomiting or diarrhea, *careful* supplementation may be needed. In general the damaged kidney cannot clear potassium adequately. Thus the dietary intake is kept at about 1500 mg/day.

7. **Phosphate and calcium.** Abnormal serum electrolyte levels of phosphate and calcium result from the secondary **hyperparathyroidism** caused by the damaged kidney function. Phosphate intake should be restricted early to retard or prevent this developing imbalance, which leads to the complicating bone disease *osteodystrophy*, before symptoms of bone pain or deformity occur.[12] Further control of phosphate levels is ensured by use of aluminum hydroxide gel to bind phosphate and prevent its intestinal absorption. A calcium supplement, such as calcium lactate tablets, relieves the hypocalcemia and its resulting tetany. In some cases, calcium carbonate is used because it also buffers the accompanying metabolic acidosis.

8. **Vitamins.** In more restricted protein diets, supplementary vitamins are usually advisable, because a diet supplying 40 g protein or less does not contribute the full daily spectrum of all vitamins. A multivitamin tablet or capsule is usually added to the diet of renal patients on protein restriction. To help correct the bone disease present, an activated form of vitamin D hormone may be used with caution.

---

azotemia • An excess of urea or other nitrogenous substances in the blood.

hyperparathyroidism • Abnormally increased activity of the parathyroid gland, resulting in excessive secretion of parathyroid hormone, which normally helps regulate serum calcium levels in balance with vitamin D hormone; excess secretion occurs when the serum calcium level falls below normal, as in chronic renal disease or in vitamin D deficiency.

osteodystrophy • Defective bone formation.

Maintenance Kidney Dialysis

Since the advent of the artificial kidney machine, a number of kidney **dialysis** centers have been established for the treatment of progressive chronic renal insufficiency (Fig. 22-2). Home units are also available, although considerable skill is required to operate them. These treatments, however, are expensive. The combined costs of the dialysis machine, replacement materials, various drugs, and trained personnel in dialysis centers is from $20,000 to $35,000 per year or more. The home treatment runs between $5,000 to $15,000 per year. Much of the cost is now paid under a provision of Medicare. Some 18,000 to 20,000 patients receive this needed artificial kidney care, usually at dialysis centers. A patient with chronic renal failure usually requires two or three treatments per week, each treatment lasting 4 to 8 hours.

During each treatment the patient's blood makes a number of round-trips through the dialysis solution in the artificial kidney, "laundering" it to maintain normal blood levels of life-sustaining substances that the patient's own kidneys can no longer accomplish. In some selected cases, an alternative form of **peritoneal dialysis** is practical for long-term ambulatory therapy at home (see box, p. 443).

The diet of a patient on kidney dialysis is a very important aspect of maintaining biochemical control. Several basic objectives govern each individually tailored diet, which are designed to (1) maintain protein and kilocalorie balance, (2) prevent dehydration or fluid overload, (3) maintain normal serum potassium and sodium blood levels, and (4) maintain acceptable phosphate and calcium levels. Control of infection is an underlying goal. In most cases, nutritional therapy can be planned with more liberal nutrient allowances. An underlying zinc deficiency, shown in impaired taste acuity, is often reported in chronic dialysis patients and improved with a supplement of 25 mg of zinc/day, thus enabling them to eat a better diet.[14]

Protein

For most adult dialysis patients, a standard protein allowance of 1 g/kg lean body weight provides for nutritional needs, maintains positive nitrogen balance, does not produce excessive nitrogenous waste, and replaces the amino acids lost during each dialysis treatment. At

---

dialysis • Process of separating crystalloids and colloids in solution by the difference in their rates of diffusion through a semipermeable membrane; crystalloids pass through readily and colloids very slowly or not at all.

peritoneal dialysis • Dialysis through the peritoneum into and out of the peritoneal cavity.

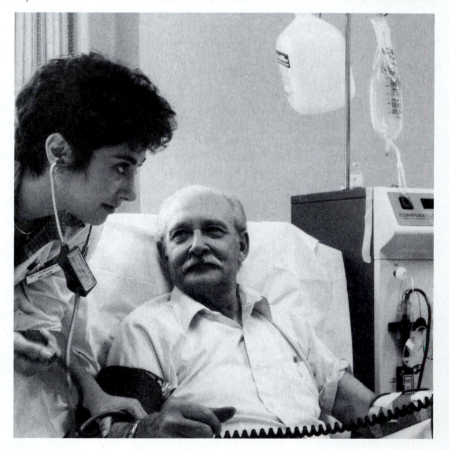

FIG. 22-2   The patient undergoing maintenance kidney dialysis must carefully follow an individualized diet plan.

Continuous Ambulatory Peritoneal Dialysis: Nutritional Needs of Clients on Portable Dialysis Machines

Persons with end-stage renal disease used to spend up to 18 hours a week on hemodialysis machines in a hospital or dialysis center. Now approximately 2800 Americans undergo dialysis 24 hours a day, 7 days a week, without spending 1 minute in a hospital room.

These individuals use continuous ambulatory peritoneal dialysis (CAPD), a home dialysis process that introduces dialysate directly into the peritoneal cavity, where it is exchanged for fluids that contain the metabolic waste products. This is done by attaching a disposable bag containing the dialysate to a catheter permanently inserted into the peritoneal cavity, waiting 20 to 30 minutes for the solution exchange, and then lowering the bag to allow the force of gravity to cause the waste-containing fluid to drain into it. When the bag is empty, it can be folded around the waist or tucked into a pocket, allowing the user mobility.

The exchange takes place by osmosis and diffusion, the rate being determined by the amount of dextrose in the solution. The most common dialysates are 1.5%, 2.5%, or 4.25%, dextrose in 1.5 to 2.0 L of solution. Most CAPD users require three to five exchanges each day. They are not only free to move, but with good self-care they are also free from some of the following extensive dietary restrictions placed on hemodialysis patients:

- **Protein and amino acid** losses are usually minimal and easily replaced by diet. High losses were more common in early CAPD systems because of peritonitis, a common problem associated with the need to replace bags frequently.
- **Potassium** requirements depend on the number of solution exchanges that take place each day. The fewer the number of exchanges, the greater

the chance of developing high serum potassium levels. Also, patients who stop using CAPD must immediately reduce their potassium intake, because serum levels rise rapidly.

- **Phosphorus**-binding antacids are not needed as much because of improved control of phosphorus blood levels with CAPD use.
- **Sodium** restriction is not necessary. In patients susceptible to hypotension, high-sodium diets have even been recommended.
- **Fluid** restriction is unnecessary, because 2000 to 2200 ml fluid may be removed with two 1.5% plus two 4.25% dextrose solutions used in 1 day. Some CAPD users even become dehydrated easily.

CAPD does pose a few nutrition-related problems, mainly because of the amount of dextrose in the dialysate. A study of patients given three 1.5% and two 4.25% dextrose solutions in 1 day revealed an intake of more than 800 kcal above the energy value of their regular diets. In addition to posing possible weight-management problems, the extra dextrose can lead to elevated triglyceride and low-density lipoprotein (LDL) levels and depressed levels of protective high-density lipoprotein (HDL), thus increasing the risk of coronary heart disease in long-term users.

Nutritionists and nurses who counsel patients being transferred from hemodialysis to the CAPD regimen are faced with a special problem: patients are often reluctant to give up their special diets. To help the individual with end-stage renal disease make the transition to CAPD as trouble free as possible, you may find it useful to explain clearly some of the possible effects of a restricted diet while on CAPD: (1) **hypotension** and dizziness from sodium depletion, (2) **potassium depletion,**

resulting in nausea, vomiting, muscle weakness, irregular heartbeat, or listlessness, and (3) **dehydration** caused by rapid fluid removal.

As a guide for patient counseling, you may find it helpful to use the dietary regimen followed by nutritionists at a number of clinics:

- Increase protein intake to provide 1.2 to 1.5 g/kg body weight.
- Limit phosphorus intake to 1200 mg/day by restricting phosphorus-rich foods—such as nuts and legumes—to one serving a week, and dairy products—including eggs—to a half-cup portion or one egg or its equivalent each day.
- Increase potassium intake by eating a wide variety of fruits and vegetables each day.
- Encourage liberal fluid intake to prevent dehydration.
- Avoid sweets and fats to control triglyceride and HDL levels.
- Maintain lean body weight by incorporating the kilocalories provided by the dialysate into the total meal plan.

Another important factor to keep in mind is that hemodialysis patients often lose their appetite. Thus the most basic aspect of your efforts to help CAPD clients adjust to this new system is to encourage them to eat.

REFERENCES

Bannister DK and others: Nutritional effects of peritonitis in continuous ambulatory peritoneal dialysis (CAPD) patients, *J Am Diet Assoc* 87(1):53, 1987.

Blumenkrantz MJ and others: Metabolic balance studies and dietary protein requirements in patients undergoing continuous ambulatory peritoneal dialysis, *Kidney Int* 21(6):849, 1982.

Bodnar DM: Rationale for nutritional requirements for patients on continuous ambulatory peritoneal dialysis, *J Am Diet Assoc* 80(3):247, 1982. ◆

least 75% of this daily protein allowance should consist of protein of high biologic value, such as eggs, meat, fish, and poultry, but little if any milk. Milk is restricted because it adds more fluid and has a high content of sodium, phosphate, and potassium (Table 22-1).

Kilocalories

Carbohydrates and fats, depending on blood lipid levels, are supplied in generous amounts to provide the needed energy for daily activities and to prevent tissue protein breakdown. The usual need is 40 kcal/kg lean body weight. Most of the carbohydrate should be supplied by simple carbohydrate foods, with control of complex carbohydrates. The complex carbohydrate food forms, such as grains and legumes, contribute incomplete protein and should not take up large amounts of the limited protein allowance.

Water Balance

Fluid is usually limited to 400 or 500 ml/day, plus an amount equal to urinary output, if any. The total intake must account for additional fluids in the foods consumed and in water derived from metabolism of the food nutrients, as well as in fecal fluid losses. Even with this restriction, there may be a mild fluid retention between dialysis treatments, with a daily weight gain in that period of about 1 lb (0.45 kg).

Sodium

To control body fluid retention and hypertension, sodium should be limited to 1000 to 2000 mg/day. This restriction helps to prevent pulmonary edema or congestive heart failure from fluid overload.

Potassium

Potassium restriction is imperative to prevent hyperkalemia, which can become a problem. Potassium accumulation can easily cause cardiac arrhythmias or cardiac arrest. Thus a dietary allowance of 1500 to 2000 mg/day of potassium is usually followed.

Vitamins

During the dialysis treatments, water-soluble vitamins from the blood are lost in the dialysate filtered out of the circulating blood. A daily supplement of all the water-soluble vitamins is therefore usually given. However, the fat-soluble vitamins—especially vitamins A and D—may build up. Thus multivitamin preparations used usually exclude these vitamins.

Peritoneal Dialysis

An alternate form of dialysis, peritoneal dialysis, allows dialysate solutions to flow directly through a catheter port established through the abdominal wall into the abdominal cavity. The presence of this concentrated solution causes the waste materials to diffuse across the

TABLE 22-1

Protein and Nitrogen Needs for Those in Chronic Renal Failure

Creatinine clearance (ml/min)	Nitrogen* (g/day)	Protein (g/day)
40 and above	Unrestricted	Unrestricted
10-40	9.6	60
5-20	6.4	40†
2-10	2.5-3.0 (+1.3-2.6)	20 (+EAA/analogs)†
8 and below	Transplantation Dialysis	
5 and below	Dialysis	

From Bergstrom J: *Proceedings of the Twelfth Annual Contractors Conference, Artificial Kidney—Chronic Uremic Program,* NIAMDD, National Institutes of Health, Bethesda, Md, NIH Pub No 81-1979, 1981.

*Total protein: 6.25.

†*EAA,* essential amino acids; alpha-keto-acid and alpha-hydroxy-acid analogs of EAAs.

saclike **peritoneum** lining the abdominal cavity. Then this dialysate collection of waste materials flows back into the dialysate bag for disposal. The peritoneal membrane serves as the filtering mechanism. This procedure may be used in the following cases: (1) for short periods of acute renal failure or brief infections, (2) for preoperative maintenance before a kidney transplant or predialysis maintenance before starting a chronic hemodialysis program, and (3) for longer-term home care, especially for elderly persons, children, and persons with diabetes or systemic diseases.

Any one of three procedures may be used for peritoneal dialysis: (1) *intermittent peritoneal dialysis (IPD),* which is usually given at night, 10 hours each time, four times a week, (2) *continuous ambulatory peritoneal dialysis (CAPD)* in which a dialysis solution in a plastic pouch is infused and drained by gravity each day (24 hours), five times at 4-hour intervals, and (3) *continuous cyclic peritoneal dialysis (CCPD)* in which three or four machine-delivered exchanges are given at night, about 3 hours each, leaving about 2 L of dialysate solution in the peritoneal cavity for 12 to 15 hours during the day. Dietary management in each case is based on nutritional requirements and protein intake sufficient to cover any losses, with individual monitoring of need. An example of peritoneal dialysis is given in the box, p. 443.

Clearly, all of the dietary factors play a role in the progression of renal disease. Although the relative importance of each factor depends on the underlying cause of the disease and its stage of progression, studies do show that nutritional therapy helps decrease the rate of renal function deterioration.[15] For many appropriate candidates, this delayed progression provides the needed time and nutritional status to prepare for the possible alternative of kidney transplant.

Patient Education Materials

The diet for the renal patient is complex and presents a challenge to practitioners and, even more so, to patients. A new resource, the National Renal Diet educational series, provides valuable guides.[16] These standardized guidelines for nutrition intervention and patient education in renal disease have been developed by the collaborative work of renal dietitians from The American Dietetic Association (ADA) Renal Dietitians dietetic practice group and the National Kidney Foundation Council on Renal Nutrition. The new *Professional Guide* can be used in conjunction with the ADA's other guides for care of renal disease patients.[17,18] Because dietary management must be tailored to the stage of the disease and method of treatment, the new series of materials contains a professional guide and six client booklets, each designed with special food lists to meet specific needs of the various renal disease requirements. These excellent resources give the practitioner a comprehensive basis for individualizing dietary instructions. They provide the patient and family with a practical guide for everyday decisions and plans for food choices.

Kidney Transplant

Kidney transplantation has become a widely accepted treatment for chronic renal failure. With refined techniques and development of immunosuppressive drugs to prevent organ rejection, approximately 9000 kidney transplants are performed each year in the United States and about 14,000 persons are awaiting transplants.[19] Nutritional support for the surgical procedures is an important adjunct to therapy. This care is complex and individual and best provided by a clinical dietitian specialist in renal disease. Consideration is given to optimal protein and energy intake, with relative restriction of simple sugars, total fat, cholesterol, and saturated fat.[20] Successful kidney transplantations have given new life to many patients. The quality of this extended life becomes a part of patient and family counseling (see box, p. 452).

Kidney Stone Disease

Disease Process

Kidney stone disease is an ancient medical problem. Since the days of Hippocrates, records of its incidence have appeared in medical documents. It continues to be a prevalent health problem. In North America, some 5% to 10% of the population suffers from kidney stones, 70% to 80% of which are composed of calcium oxalate with or without phosphate.[21] Kidney stone disease appears to be chronic and recurrent. The basic cause is unknown, but many factors contribute directly or indirectly to the stone formation. These factors relate to the nature of the urine itself or to the conditions of the urinary tract environment. According to the concentration of urinary constitutients, the major stones formed are calcium, struvite, uric acid, and cystine stones (Fig. 22-3).

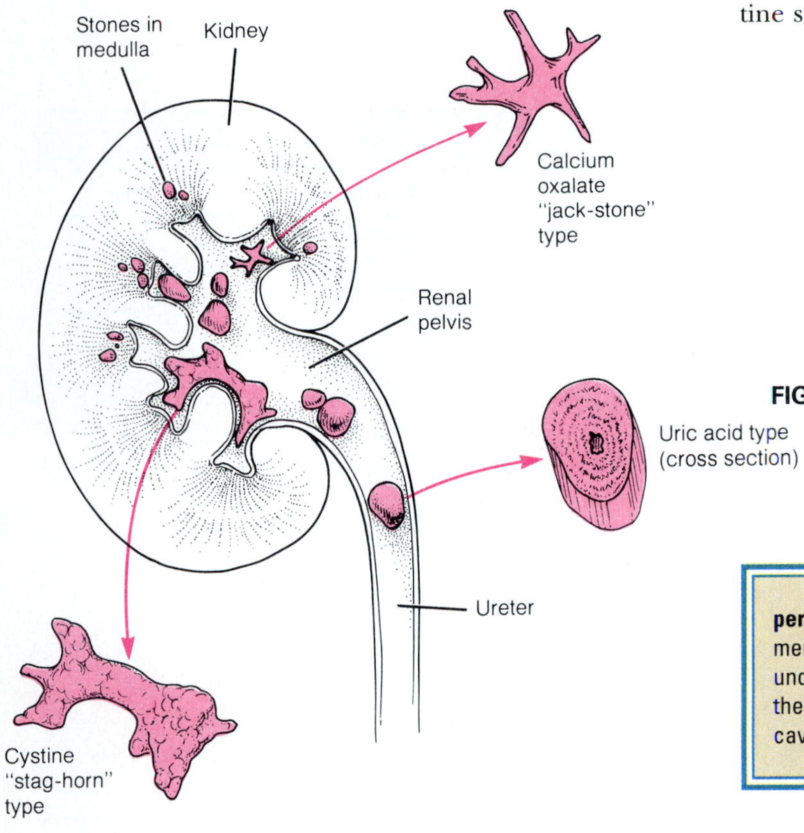

Stones in medulla

Kidney

Calcium oxalate "jack-stone" type

Renal pelvis

Uric acid type (cross section)

Ureter

Cystine "stag-horn" type

FIG. 22-3 Renal stones in kidney, pelvis, and ureter.

peritoneum • A strong smooth surface—a serous membrane—lining the abdominal/pelvic walls and the undersurface of the diaphragm, forming a sac enclosing the body's vital visceral organs within the peritoneal cavity.

Calcium Stones

Most kidney stones are composed of calcium compounds, usually calcium oxalate or calcium oxalate mixed with calcium phosphate. In persons who form stones—which is a familial tendency—the urine produced is supersaturated with these crystalloid elements, and there is a lack of normal urine substances that prevent the crystals from forming stones. Excessive urinary calcium may result from the following:

1. *Excess calcium intake.* Prolonged use of large amounts of milk, alkali therapy for peptic ulcer, and use of a hard water supply contribute to calcium loads.
2. *Excess vitamin D.* Hypervitaminosis D may cause increased calcium absorption from the intestine, as well as increased withdrawal from bone.
3. *Prolonged immobilization.* Body casting or immobilization from illness or disability may lead to withdrawal of bone calcium and increased urinary concentration.
4. *Hyperparathyroidism.* Primary hyperparathyroidism causes excess calcium excretion. About two thirds of the persons with this endocrine disorder have kidney stones, but this disorder accounts for only about 5% of total calcium stones.
5. *Renal tubular acidosis.* Excess excretion of calcium is caused by defective ammonia formation.
6. *Idiopathic calcinuria.* Some persons, even those on a low-calcium diet, for unknown reasons may excrete as much as 500 mg of calcium daily.
7. *Oxalate.* Because of a metabolic error in handling oxalates, about half of the calcium stones are composed with this material. Oxalates occur naturally only in a few food sources (Table 22-2).
8. *Animal protein.* A diet high in animal protein—for example, the typical American diet—has been linked to increased excretions of calcium, oxalate, and urate. A vegetarian-type diet has been recommended by some investigators as a wise choice for stone-forming persons.
9. *Dietary fiber.* Added dietary fiber has been found to reduce risk factors for stone formation, especially calcium stones.[21]

Struvite Stones

Next to calcium stones in frequency are struvite stones, composed of a single compound—magnesium ammonium phosphate ($MgNH_4PO_4$). These are often called "infection stones" because they are associated with urinary tract infections. The offending organism in the infection is *Proteus mirabilis*. This is a urea-splitting bacterium that contains urease, an enzyme that hydrolyzes urea to ammonia. Thus the urinary pH becomes alkaline. In the ammonia-rich environment, struvite precipitates and forms large, "stag-horn" stones. Surgical removal is usually indicated.

Uric Acid Stones

Excess uric acid excretion may be caused by an impairment in the intermediary metabolism of purine, as occurs in gout. It may also result from a rapid tissue breakdown in wasting disease.

TABLE 22-2

Food Sources of Oxalates

Fruits	Vegetables	Nuts	Beverages	Other
Berries, all	Baked beans	Almonds	Chocolate	Grits
Currants	Beans, green and wax	Cashews	Cocoa	Tofu
Concord grapes	Beets	Peanuts	Draft beer	Soy products
Figs	Beet greens	Peanut butter	Tea	Wheat germ
Fruit cocktail	Celery			
Plums	Chard, Swiss			
Rhubarb	Chives			
Tangerines	Collards			
	Eggplant			
	Endive			
	Kale			
	Leeks			
	Mustard greens			
	Okra			
	Peppers, green			
	Rutabagas			
	Spinach			
	Squash, summer			
	Sweet potatoes			
	Tomatoes			
	Tomato soup			
	Vegetable soup			

Cystine Stones

A heredity metabolic defect in renal tubular resorption of the amino acid cystine causes this substance to accumulate in the urine. This condition is called cystinuria. Because this is a genetic disorder, it is characterized by early onset age and a positive family history. This is one of the most common metabolic disorders associated with kidney stones in children.

Urinary Tract Conditions

The physical changes in the urine and the organic stone matrix result in urinary tract conditions that lead to the formation of kidney stones.

Physical Changes in the Urine

Susceptible persons form stones when physical changes in the urine predispose to such formation. Such physical conditions include the following:

1. *Urine concentration.* The concentration of the urine may result from a lower water intake or from excess water loss, as in prolonged sweating, fever, vomiting, or diarrhea.
2. *Urinary pH.* Changes in urinary pH from its mean 5.85 to 6.0 may be influenced by the diet or altered by the ingestion of acid or alkali medications.

Organic Stone Matrix

Formation of an organic stone matrix provides the necessary core or nucleus (nidus) around which crystals may precipitate and form a mucoprotein-carbohydrate complex. In this complex galactose and hexosamine are the principal carbohydrates. Some possible sources of these organic materials include the following: (1) bacteria masses from recurrent urinary tract infections, (2) renal epithelial tissue of the urinary tract that has sloughed off, possibly because of vitamin A deficiency, and (3) calcified plaques (Randall's plaques) formed beneath the renal epithelium in hypercalciuria. Irritation and ulceration of overlying tissue cause the plaques to slough off into the collecting tubules.

Clinical Symptoms

Severe pain and numerous urinary symptoms may result, with general weakness and sometimes fever. Laboratory examination of urine and chemical analysis of any stone that is passed help determine treatment.

General Treatment
Fluid Intake

A large fluid intake produces a more dilute urine and is a foundation of therapy. The dilute urine helps to prevent concentration of stone constituents.

Urinary pH

An attempt to control the solubility factor is made by changing the urinary pH to an increased acidity or alkalinity, depending on the chemical composition of the stone formed. An exception is calcium oxalate stones, because the solubility of calcium oxalate in urine is not pH-dependent. Conversely, however, calcium phosphate is soluble in acid urine.

Stone Composition

When possible, dietary constituents of the stone are controlled to reduce the amount of the substance available for precipitation.

Binding Agents

Materials that bind the stone elements and prevent their absorption in the intestine cause fecal excretion. For example, sodium phytate is used to bind calcium, and aluminum gels are used to bind phosphate. Glycine and calcium have a similar effect on oxalates.

Nutritional Therapy

Nutritional therapy is directly related to the stone chemistry.

Calcium Stones

A low-calcium diet of about 400 mg/day is usually given. This amount is half of an average adult intake of about 800 mg/day. This lower level is achieved mainly by removal of milk and dairy products. Other calcium food sources that can be limited are leafy vegetables and whole grains. If the stone is calcium phosphate, phosphorous foods would also be reduced. This is also accomplished mainly by removal of milk and dairy products. Sometimes a test diet of 200 mg of calcium may be used to rule out hyperparathyroidism as a causative factor.

Because calcium stones have an alkaline chemistry, an acid ash diet may also be used to help create a urinary environment less conducive to the precipitation of the basic stone elements. The classification of food groups is based on the pH of the metabolic ash produced (Table 22-3). An acid ash diet would increase the amount of meat, grains, eggs, and cheese. It limits the amounts of vegetables, milk, and fruits. An alkaline ash diet outlines the opposite use of these foods. The use of cranberry juice has been promoted to assist in the

TABLE 22-3

Acid and Alkaline Ash Food Groups

Acid ash	Alkaline ash	Neutral
Meat	Milk	Beverages (coffee, tea)
Whole grains	Vegetables	
Eggs	Fruits (except cranberries,	
Cheese	prunes, plums)	
Cranberries		
Prunes		
Plums		

acidification of urine. However, the commercially-prepared cranberry juices on the consumer market are too dilute to be effective, because they contain only about 26% cranberry juice. Thus an inordinate volume would be required to achieve any consistent effectiveness as a urinary acidifying agent. Instead, to effect a sustained acidifying of urinary pH, most physicians rely on drugs.

Calcium oxalate stones resulting from *hyperoxaluria* would be treated by dietary avoidance of foods high in oxalates (see Table 22-2). Persons with calcium oxalate stones should avoid taking vitamin C supplements, because about half the ingested ascorbate may be converted to oxalic acid. However, this is not always the case, and more studies of patients with kidney stones are needed before precise conclusions can be reached.

Uric Acid Stones

About 4% of the total incidence of renal calculi are uric acid stones. Because uric acid is a metabolic product of purines, dietary control of this precursor is indicated. Purines are found in active tissue—such as glandular meat, other lean meat, and meat extractives—and in lesser amounts in plant sources, such as whole grains and legumes. An effort to produce an alkaline ash to help increase the urinary pH is indicated.

Cystine Stones

About 1% of the total stones produced are cystine, because the development of cystine stones is a relatively rare genetic disease. Cystine is a nonessential amino acid produced from the essential amino acid methionine. Thus a diet low in methionine is used. This diet is used with high fluid intake and alkaline diet therapy.

The nutritional therapy principles in renal stone disease are outlined in Table 22-4. Dietary guides for each of these kidney stone conditions are provided in Appendix N.

TABLE 22-4

Summary of Dietary Principles in Renal Stone Disease

Stone chemistry	Nutrient modification	Dietary ash (urinary pH)
Calcium	Low calcium (400 mg)	Acid ash
Phosphate	Low phosphorus (1000-1200 mg)	
Oxalate	Low oxalate	
Struvite (MgNH$_4$PO$_4$)	Low phosphorus (1000-1200 mg) (associated with urinary infections)	Acid ash
Uric acid	Low purine	Alkaline ash
Cystine	Low methionine	Alkaline ash

Urinary Tract Infection

Disease Process

The term *urinary tract infection (UTI)* refers to a wide variety of clinical infections in which a significant number of microorganisms are present in any portion of the urinary tract.[22] A common form is **cystitis,** an inflammation of the bladder very prevalent in young women. At least 20% of women experience a UTI during their lifetime, the vast majority of which are cases of uncomplicated cystitis.[23] The condition is called recurrent UTI if three or more bouts are experienced in a year.

The majority of cases are caused by aerobic members of the fecal flora, especially *Escherichia coli*. The presence of these organisms in the urine is termed *bacteriuria*. Urine produced by the normal kidney is sterile and remains so as it travels to the bladder. In UTI, however, the normal urethra has microbial flora, so that any voided urine normally contains many bacteria. Bacteriuria is present when the quantity of organisms is more than 100,000 bacteria per milliliter of urine. The female anatomy is more conducive to entry of these bacteria into the urinary tract. Recurrent cystitis occurs mostly in young and otherwise healthy women who have infections that usually correspond with sexual activity and diaphragm use. In most cases simply having the diaphragm refitted to a smaller size or changing to another birth control method will solve the problem. Cystitis is characterized by frequent voiding and burning on urination. Untreated, it may lead to stone formation.

Treatment

Currently, antibiotic treatment has been cut back a great deal. Clinical experience indicates that a single dose of antibiotic is just as effective as the usual 7- to 10-day course treatment in 90% of all women who have uncomplicated cystitis. General nutritional measures include acidifying the urine by taking vitamin C, because cranberry juice is not effective, and drinking plenty of fluids to produce a dilute urine. Control of UTI is an important measure, because it is a risk factor in stone formation.

To Sum Up

Through its unique functional units—the nephrons—the kidneys act as a filtration system, resorbing substances the body needs, secreting additional hydrogen ions to maintain a proper pH balance in the blood, and excreting unnecessary materials in a concentrated urine.

Renal function may be impaired by a variety of conditions. These include inflammatory and degenerative diseases; infection and obstruction; chronic diseases, such as hypertension and diabetes; environmental agents, such as insecticides, solvents, and other toxic substances; and some medications and trauma. Some clinical conditions affecting structure and function include glomerulonephritis, nephrotic syndrome, acute and chronic renal failure, renal calculi, and urinary tract infection. In many cases, except nephrotic syndrome, dietary protein may need to be reduced as part of the nutritional care plan. Water, electrolytes, and kilocalorie intake should also be closely monitored to match individual needs.

Chronic kidney disease at its end stage, end-stage renal disease (ESRD), is treated by *dialysis*—either hemodialysis or peritoneal dialysis—and *kidney transplant*. Dialysis patients must be monitored closely for protein, water, and electrolyte balance. Nutritional support of transplant patients is needed primarily as support for the surgical procedure. A normal diet is often well tolerated after surgery and convalescence.

Renal diseases have predisposing factors. For example, untreated urinary tract infections may lead to kidney stones, and progressive glomerulonephritis may lead to nephrotic syndrome. The Western diet is suspect as a predisposing factor in the development of chronic renal failure. Excess protein intake may overtax human nephrons, which were not originally designed to handle a steady diet of protein-rich foods.

QUESTIONS FOR REVIEW

1. For each of the following conditions, outline the nutritional components of therapy, explaining the impact of each on kidney function: glomerulonephritis, nephrotic syndrome, acute renal failure (renal insufficiency), and chronic renal failure.
2. Identify four clinical conditions that impair renal function. Give an example of each, describing its effect on various structures in the kidney.
3. List the nutritional factors that must be monitored in individuals undergoing renal dialysis.
4. Outline the medical and nutritional therapy used for patients with various types of kidney stones. Describe each type of stone and explain the rationale for each aspect of therapy.
5. For what condition is a urinary tract infection a predisposing factor? What general nutritional principles are recommended in the treatment of such infections?

REFERENCES

1. Weir MR, Wolfsthal SD: Hypertension and the kidney, *Prim Care* 18(3):525, 1991.
2. Guyton AC: Blood pressure control—special role of the kidneys and body fluids, *Science* 252:1813, 1991.
3. Brouhard BH, La Groue L: Effect of dietary protein restriction on functional renal reserve in diabetic nephropathy, *Am J Med* 89:427, 1990.
4. Baldree LA, Stapelton FB: Uric acid metabolism in children, *Pediatr Clin North Am* 37(2):391, 1990.
5. Abuelo IG: Renal failure caused by chemicals, foods, plants, animal venom, and misuse of drugs: a review, *Arch Intern Med* 150:505, 1990.
6. McDonald BR and others: Acute renal failure associated with the use of intraperitoneal carboplatin: a report of two cases and review of the literature, *Am J Med* 90:386, 1991.
7. Kalahr S and others: The progression of renal disease, *N Engl J Med* 318(25):1657, 1988.
8. Coggins CH, Cornal BF: Nutritional management of nephrotic syndrome. In Mitch WE and Klahr S, editors: *Nutrition and the kidney,* Boston, 1988, Little, Brown & Co.
9. Kopple JD: Nutrition, diet, and the kidney. In Shils ME, Olsen JA, Shike M, editors: *Modern nutrition in health and disease,* ed 8, Philadelphia, 1993, Lea & Febiger.
10. DiChiro J: Can nutritional therapy alter the course of renal disease? *Dietetic Currents* 18(2):1, 1991.
11. Feinstein EI: Total parenteral nutritional support of patients with acute renal failure, *Nutr Clin Prac* 3(1):9, 1988.
12. Hak LJ, Raasch RH: Use of amino acids in patients with acute renal failure, *Nutr Clin Prac* 3(1):19, 1988.
13. Feld LG and others: Fluid need in acute renal failure, *Pediatr Clin North Am* 37(2):337, 1990.
14. Reid DJ and others: Effects of folate and zinc supplementation on patients ungoing chronic hemodialysis, *J Am Diet Assoc* 92(5):574, 1992.
15. Ahmed FE: Effect of diet on progression of chronic renal disease, *J Am Diet Assoc* 91(10):1266, 1991.
16. Report—For Your Information: Meeting the challenge of the renal diet, *J Am Diet Assoc* 93(6):637, 1993.
17. Wilkens KG, Schiro KB, editors: *Suggested guidelines for nutrition care of renal patients,* ed 2, Chicago, 1992, American Dietetic Association.
18. Stover J, editor: *A clinical guide to nutrition care in end-stage renal disease,* ed 2, Chicago, 1993, American Dietetic Association.
19. Schanbacher B: An overview of development on the field of organ transplantation, *Kidney* 6:4, 1989.
20. Edwards MS, Doster S: Renal transplant diet recommendations: results of a survey of renal dietitians in the United States, *J Am Diet Assoc* 90(6):843, 1990.
21. Firth WA, Norman RW: The effects of modified diets on urinary risk factors for kidney stone disease, *J Can Diet Assoc* 51(3):404, 1990.
22. Sobel JD: Bacterial etiologic agents in the pathogenesis of urinary tract infection, *Med Clin North Am* 75(2):253, 1991.
23. Ronald AR, Pattullo ALS: The natural history of urinary infection in adults, *Med Clin North Am* 75(2):299, 1991.

FURTHER READING

Ahmed FE: Effect of diet on progression of chronic renal disease, *J Am Diet Assoc* 91(10):1266, 1991.

Dr. Ahmed of the Food and Nutrition Board, National Reseach Council—National Academy of Sciences, provides a helpful review of the literature concerning the impact of diet on the course of chronic renal disease and how nutritional management is used as therapy for persons with renal insufficiency.

For Your Information: Meeting the challenge of the renal diet, *J Am Diet Assoc* 93(6):637, 1993.

Stover J, editor: *A clinical guide to nutrition care in end-stage renal disease,* ed 2, Chicago, 1993, American Dietetic Association.

Wilkins KG, Schiro KB, editors: *Suggested guidelines for nutrition care of renal patients,* ed 2, Chicago, 1992, American Dietetic Association.

The American Dietetic Association (ADA) has provided definitive guidelines for practitioner and patient in its comprehensive patient education materials. The new National Renal Diet educational series, developed jointly with the National Kidney Foundation Council on Renal Nutrition, contains a professional guide and six client booklets—each with special food lists—to meet the various needs of renal disease patients. Copies of this new series of resource material are available from the ADA; information on how to order can be found in current copies of the Journal of the American Dietetic Association.

CASE STUDY

The Patient with Chronic Renal Failure

Aaron Steinberg is 45 years old, married, and works as a city planner for a large municipal government. He cited a recent history of nausea, anorexia, hematuria, and swollen ankles during an initial physical examination. His wife reported that he had been tiring more easily than usual during the past year. A history of prior illnesses proved negative, except for a severe case of influenza with sore throat 10 years before during an epidemic when he was stationed with the Army overseas. Tests were ordered, and the patient was advised to return in a week for review of the test results and sooner if there were any changes in his symptoms.

Mr. Steinberg did return, with additional symptoms of headaches and occasional blurred vision. At that time, his blood pressure was 160/98 mm Hg, his temperature was 37.5° C (99.6° F), and he had lost 4 kg (8 3/4 lb). The laboratory tests showed albumin and red and white blood cells in the urine, with an elevated BUN level; a phenolsulfonphthalein (PSP) test indicated a reduced filtration rate. The diagnosis was chronic renal failure.

The physician discussed the diagnosis and its serious prognosis with Mr. and Mrs. Steinberg, explaining the benefits and disadvantages of both hemodialysis and kidney transplantation. Antihypertensive medication was prescribed along with other drugs to minimize discomfort.

During the following weeks, Mr. Steinberg continued to lose weight, had increasing joint pain, and became anemic. He found it increasingly difficult to maintain his hectic schedule of frequent meetings, conferences, and public speeches because of gastrointestinal bleeding, increasing nausea, and occasional muscle spasms. Small mouth sores made eating very difficult.

Finally the Steinbergs informed the physician of their decision to accept the kidney transplant as a means of controlling the disease process. They were referred to the clinical nutritionist for renal diet counseling to control protein, sodium, potassium, phosphate, and fluids, as well as to ensure adequate kilocalories. After discussing these needs for nutritional maintenance before surgery, the nutritionist helped them develop a meal plan based on Mr. Steinberg's food preferences. Food selection and preparation were discussed in detail, with many ideas for building in as much variety and taste appeal as possible.

The Steinbergs' follow-up with the food plan was excellent. One month later the laboratory values were almost normal, blood pressures averaged 140/88 mm Hg, the headaches and blurred vision had virtually disappeared, and Mr. Steinberg had gained 3.2 kg (7 lb) of his lost weight. The nutrient supplements, including the amino acid analogs, were taken each day as instructed.

Fortunately a kidney donor was soon found, and with the aid of drug control of immune responses it was apparently a success. Mr. Steinberg convalesced well at home, kept all follow-up visits with the health care team, and has continued to be asymptomatic 1 year after surgery.

Questions for Analysis

1. Identify a metabolic imbalance caused by renal failure that may account for each symptom presented by Mr. Steinberg.
2. What would be the objectives in the care of renal failure, such as Mr. Steinberg was experiencing?
3. What factors affect the amount of protein needed by persons with chronic renal failure? What amounts are usually used? Why? What are the amino acid analogs used with the low-protein diet, and why are they used?
4. What factors affect the amount of sodium needed by persons with chronic renal failure? How much is usually recommended?
5. Why is it important to control potassium levels? How much is recommended? What clinical signs presented by Mr. Steinberg may indicate that he had not been getting enough potassium?
6. Why is control of phosphate important in the diet for chronic renal failure? What additional means may be used to control it?
7. What factors affect fluid balance in chronic renal failure? How much is usually allowed?
8. What is the basic principle of the low-protein dietary regimen? List and explain each factor in the diet and potential problems in its management.
9. Outline a general teaching plan you would use to instruct the Steinbergs about the presurgical and postsurgical dietary needs.

Renal Disease: Technology vs the Quality of Life

Imagine spending up to 18 hours a week hooked up to a machine to which you literally owe your life. Imagine having a 40% chance of never being able to work outside the home again, leading a life of poverty and restricted mobility, all because of that machine.

This is probably hard for most of us to conceive. Yet for approximately 55,000 Americans on maintenance dialysis—and the number of patients with end-stage renal disease (ESRD) requiring hemodialysis is increasing—this is the reality of their everyday lives. The medical-nutrition-nursing renal care team must also deal with this reality daily in work with these persons and their families. This sensitivity is especially needed in nutrition counseling and teaching. Food is tied up with so many personal values that when it must be drastically changed, or when choice is gone altogether, it's as if a part of the self has been diminished.

Researchers, physicians, and patients are becoming increasingly concerned with the *quality* of life rather than merely the *length* of life available to the person on dialysis. The only alternative currently available is kidney transplantation. On the surface this method could be considered preferable to hemodialysis or even peritoneal dialysis, because it frees the individual from any mechanical device. However, researchers are beginning to investigate the quality of life a transplant provides to determine whether either method is preferable to the other.

The first issue of greatest concern is the effect of the treatment on the person's life span. Mortality rates for individuals on dialysis, 8% to 15%, are in the same range as for those receiving their first kidney transplant, 10% to 15%. However, rates among young dialysis patients with no extrarenal disease can drop as low as 2%, in contrast with rates that can soar to 30% among individuals receiving kidneys from cadavers. Still, some persons believe that the benefits of increased mobility outweigh the drawbacks of a possible reduction in life span.

In one study, life quality measures (sleep habits, food habits, energy level, sexual activity, changes in income and employment, satisfaction with marriage, and so on) were examined among individuals undergoing dialysis or with successful and unsuccessful transplant operations. As expected, subjects who had successful operations reported a near-normal quality of life; they were less tired, were less inconvenienced by frequent medical treatments, and had better incomes and/or more full-time employment after renal failure than did other renal patients.

Also as expected, individuals whose transplant operations were not successful indicated that the quality of their lives was the lowest of all subjects. For example, none of these subjects reported full-time employment since renal failure. They were mainly recipients of kidneys from cadavers; thus this process is assumed to be the least desired of all possible alternatives.

A surprising result of this study was that dialysis patients who never received a transplant thought that the quality of their lives was also near normal. Researchers admit that the reason for this probably includes denial or accommodation. However, they also acknowledge that human response to life experiences is an extremely complex issue, one that is difficult to assess with current "immature" research methods available for evaluating the quality of life in general.

The health care team responsible for the patient with renal failure may have their own set of parameters for determining the quality of life each mode of treatment may provide. The results of this study suggest that the patient's own evaluation of life may involve factors much more complex than those to which the professional has been exposed. The study serves as a reminder that professionals must be open to the concerns and viewpoints of the individual faced with such major choices in treatment and must relate care planning in all areas to these personal concerns.

REFERENCES

Collins AJ and others: Changing risk factor demographics in end-stage renal disease patients entering hemodialysis and impact on long-term mortality, *Am J Kidney Dis* 15:422, 1990.

Husbye DG and others: Psychosocial, social, and somatic prognostic indicators in old patients undergoing long-term dialysis, *Arch Int Med* 147:1921, 1987.

Johnson PJ and others: The quality of life of hemodialysis and transplant patients, *Kidney Int* 22(3):286, 1982.

CHAPTER 23

Nutritional Care of Surgery Patients

CHAPTER OUTLINE

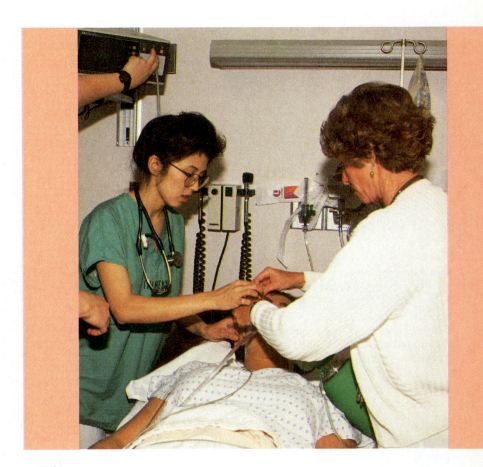

In this chapter, we look at the needs of patients undergoing various surgical procedures for treatment of medical problems or injuries. A major focus is on gastrointestinal surgeries. The type and extent of the surgical procedure, as well as the nature of any preceding injury, influence special nutritional therapy requirements and the mode of feeding needed to meet these nutritional demands.

A primary underlying need is the prevention of malnutrition. Numerous American and European surveys of hospitalized patients indicate that nearly 50% of surgical patients have clinical evidence of protein-energy malnutrition.

Here we see how careful preoperative nutritional preparation, together with vigorous postoperative nutritional support, reduces complications and provides resources for better healing and more rapid recovery.

Nutritional Needs of General Surgery Patients

Preoperative Nutrition

Nutrient Stores

A poor postoperative outcome is often the result of preoperative malnutrition. Thus when surgery is planned, a primary task is immediate attention to nutritional status.[1] Nutritional reserves fortify the patient for the demands of surgery. When time permits, nutritional preparation should correct any nutrient deficiencies. It should also provide resources for the surgery itself and for the immediate postoperative period until regular feedings can be resumed (see Clinical Application below).

Protein. The most common nutritional deficiency of surgery patients is that of protein. Tissue and plasma reserves are imperative to prepare the patient for blood losses during surgery and for tissue breakdown in the immediate postoperative period of catabolism.

Energy. Sufficient kcalories must be provided to build up any deficit. Carbohydrates are needed for glycogen stores and to spare protein for tissue synthesis.

Vitamins and minerals. Normal tissue stores of vitamins are needed for the added metabolism of carbohydrates and protein. Any deficiency state such as anemia should be corrected. Electrolytes and fluids should be in balance and correction made of any dehydration, acidosis, or alkalosis.

Immediate Preoperative Period

In the usual preparation for surgery, nothing is given by mouth for at least 8 hours before surgery. This ensures that the stomach has no retained food at the time of the operation. In case of emergency surgery, if the patient has recently eaten a meal, gastric suction is used. Food in the stomach may be vomited or aspirated during surgery or recovery from anesthesia. Also, any food present may increase the possibility of postoperative gastric retention and dilation. It may also interfere with the procedure itself, especially in abdominal surgery. Before gastrointestinal surgery, a low-residue or residue-free diet may be followed for several days to

---

◆ **C**LINICAL **A**PPLICATION   *Energy and Protein Requirements in General Surgery Patients*

General surgery patients vary in their nutritional needs depending on two basic factors: (1) individual nutritional status and (2) the metabolic stress of the underlying illness or injury and the surgery. For example, compare the following patient situations.

Adequately nourished preoperative patient

For the patient with normal energy and nitrogen balance, approximately 40 kcal/kg/day and 1.5 g of protein/kg/day should maintain these balances for the surgery ahead.

Adequately nourished postoperative patient

After surgery, energy requirements remain about the same—40 kcal/kg/day. However, increased nitrogen losses, from decreased protein synthesis during surgery and the immediate postoperative period, increase protein needs to 1.8 to 1.9 g/kg/day.

Nutritionally depleted, nonstressed patient

The patient requires repletion of body fat stores and lean body mass. Nutrient needs are similar to those of the adequately nourished postoperative patient, with 40 kcal/kg/day and 1.8 to 1.9 g protein/kg/day, producing moderate gains in fat and protein.

Nutritionally depleted, stressed patient

This patient has depleted energy and protein stores. These losses need to be matched, *and* extra protein (2.0 to 2.2 g/kg/day) is required for repletion. Part of the kcalorie load (45 kcal/kg/day) should be given as fat. A 50:50 glucose-fat mix is recommended.

Adequately nourished, stressed patient

This patient has the highest requirements for energy (50 kcal/kg/day) and protein (2.5 g/kg/day), although the aim is to prevent loss, not to replenish.

Glucose is not utilized sufficiently to provide adequate energy intake, so some of the energy needs to be provided as fat (50:50 glucose-fat mix).

An analysis of published reports underscores the importance of nutritional status to surgery outcome. Reviewers conclude that when malnourished patients receive TPN in adequate amounts for 7 to 15 days preoperatively, significant improvements in both nutritional status and postoperative outcome occur.

REFERENCES

Campos ACL, Meguid MM: A critical appraisal of the usefulness of perioperative nutritional support, *Am J Clin Nutr* 55:117, 1992.

Hill GL: The perioperative patient. In Kinney JM and others, editors: *Nutrition and metabolism in patient care*, Philadelphia, 1988, WB Saunders.

Hill GL, Church JM: Energy and protein requirements of general surgical patients requiring intravenous nutrition, *Br J Surg* 71:1, 1984. ◆

clear the operative site of any food residue. Low-residue, chemically defined formulas, or *elemental formulas,* can provide a complete diet in liquid form. Such formulas, if palatable enough, can be taken orally in sufficient amounts to maintain nutritional resources. Otherwise they may be fed by tube (see Chapter 18).

Postoperative Nutrition

Healthy body tissues undergo continuous turnover, with small physiologic losses being constantly replenished by nutrients in the food eaten. In disease, however, especially surgical disease, losses are greatly increased. At the same time, replacement from food is diminished or even absent for a brief or extended period. Nutritional support, therefore, becomes all the more significant as a means of aiding recovery.

Protein

Adequate protein intake in the postoperative recovery period is of primary therapeutic concern to replace losses and supply increased demands. A catabolic period with progressively increasing protein deficiency is common in surgical patients. Negative nitrogen balances of as much as 20 g/day may occur. This amount of nitrogen loss represents an actual loss of tissue protein of more than 1 lb/day. In addition to protein losses from tissue breakdown, added loss of plasma proteins can occur through hemorrhage, wound bleeding, and **exudates.** Increased metabolic losses of protein can also result from extensive tissue destruction and inflammation or from trauma and infection. If any degree of prior malnutrition or chronic infection has existed, the patient's protein deficit may become even more severe and cause serious complications. There are a number of reasons for this increased protein demand.

Tissue synthesis in wound healing. Tissue proteins can be synthesized only by essential amino acids brought to the tissue by the circulating blood. The necessary essential amino acids must come either from the diet protein or by intravenous feeding. Tissue protein deficiencies are best met by oral feeding. When appetite is poor, palatable concentrated liquid drinks or commercial drinks such as Ensure (Ross) may be useful (see Chapter 18). During early feeding periods or with the extremely malnourished patient, only small amounts of protein may be tolerated. However, increased intake is needed as early as possible to achieve the amount of protein required to restore lost protein tissues and to synthesize new tissue at the wound site. Although tissue protein is broken down more rapidly during stress, fortunately it is also built up more rapidly, provided sufficient amino acids are present to supply the anabolic demand.

Avoidance of shock. Reduced blood volume, *hypovolemia,* from a loss of plasma proteins and a decrease

in circulating red blood cell volume contributes to the potential danger of shock. When protein deficiencies exist, this danger is increased.

Control of edema. When the serum protein is low, edema develops as a result of the loss of colloidal osmotic pressure required to maintain the normal shift of fluid between the capillaries and the surrounding interstitial tissue spaces. This general edema may affect heart and lung action. Also, local edema at the surgical site delays closure of the wound and hinders normal healing.

Bone healing. In orthopedic surgery, extensive bone healing is involved. Protein is essential for proper **callus** formation and calcification. A sound protein matrix is mandatory for the anchoring of mineral matter in bone tissue.

Resistance to infection. Amino acids are necessary constituents of the proteins involved in body defense mechanisms. These defense agents include antibodies, special blood cells, hormones, and enzymes. Tissue integrity itself is a first line of defense against infections.

Lipid transport. Proteins are necessary for the transport of lipids in the body's blood circulation. They provide essential material to form lipoproteins, the transport form of fat in the body. Proteins thus protect the liver, a main site of fat metabolism, from danger caused by fatty infiltration.

Multiple clinical problems may easily develop following surgery when protein deficiencies exist. There may be poor wound healing, or **dehiscence;** delayed healing of fractures; anemia; failure of gastrointestinal stomas to function; depressed lung and heart function; reduced resistance to infection; extensive weight loss; liver damage; and increased mortality risks.

Water

Water balance is a vital concern after surgery. Adequate fluid therapy is necessary to prevent dehydration. Large water losses may occur from vomiting, hemorrhage,

---

callus • Unorganized meshwork of newly grown, woven bone developed on pattern of original fibrin clot (formed after fracture or surgery) and normally replaced in the healing process by hard adult bone.

dehiscence • Separation of the layers of a surgical wound

exudate • Various materials (e.g., cells, cellular debris, fluids), usually resulting from inflammation, that have escaped from blood vessels and are deposited in or on surface tissues.

TABLE 23-1

Daily Water Requirements of the Surgical Patient

Type of case and fluid needs	Average fluid required (ml)
Uncomplicated cases	
For vaporization	1000-1500
For urine	1000-1500
TOTAL	2000-3000
Complicated cases (sepsis, elevation of temperature, humid weather, renal damage)	
For vaporization	2000-2500
For urine	1000-1500
TOTAL	3000-4000
Seriously ill patients with drainage	
For vaporization	2000
For urine	1000
For replacement of body fluid losses	
Bile drainage	1000
Wangensteen drainage	3000
TOTAL	7000

exudates, diuresis, or fever. When drainage is involved, as is common in many surgeries, still more fluid loss occurs. Table 23-1 indicates the general magnitude of water requirements for surgical patients. Intravenous therapy will supply initial needs, but oral intake should begin as soon as possible. Water intake must be maintained in sufficient quantity, according to individual needs, to avoid extremes of dehydration and water intoxication. Daily weight measurement of the patient provides a guideline for meeting fluid requirements.

Energy

As is always the case when increased protein is demanded for tissue rebuilding, sufficient nonprotein energy kcalories must be supplied to protect the protein for use in tissue synthesis. Adequate amounts of carbohydrate are essential to ensure the use of protein for building tissue and to supply the energy required for the increased metabolic demands. As protein is increased, the total kcalories must be increased as well, because sufficient caloric intake is often crucial to the successful outcome of the surgical procedure. About 2800 kcal/day must be provided before protein can be used for tissue repair and not be diverted to help provide energy. In acute stress, as in extensive surgery or burns, when protein needs may be as high as 200 g/day, 4000 to 6000 kcal may be required. In addition to its protein-sparing action, carbohydrates also help to avoid liver damage from depletion of glycogen reserves. Fat must be adequate to maintain body tissue fat reserves, but it must not be excessive.

Vitamins

All of the vitamins play important roles in the healing process. Vitamin C is imperative for wound healing. It is necessary for the formation of cementing material in the ground substance of connective tissue, in capillary walls, and in the building up of new tissue. Extensive tissue regeneration such as occurs in burns or radical surgeries may require vitamin C supplements. As kcalorie and protein intake are increased, the B vitamins must also be increased. They provide essential coenzyme factors for protein and energy metabolism. Vitamin K is essential in the blood clotting mechanism.

Minerals

Replacing mineral deficiencies and ensuring continued adequacy is essential. In tissue breakdown, potassium and phosphorus are lost. Electrolyte losses, especially sodium and chloride, accompany fluid losses. Iron-deficiency anemia may develop from blood loss or faulty iron absorption.

General Dietary Management

Oral Feeding

The majority of general surgical patients can and should progress to oral feeding as soon as possible to provide adequate nutrition. Remember that routine postoperative intravenous fluids are intended to supply hydration needs and electrolytes, not to sustain nutritional needs. Routine postoperative intravenous fluids cannot supply full nutrient needs or compete with oral feedings. For example, of a 5% dextrose solution, 1 L contains 50 g of sugar, with an energy value of only 200 kcal. Thus 3 L/day at best supplies only 600 kcal and no protein. The basal energy requirement alone is much more, without taking into consideration the increased metabolic stress demands of surgical illness. Wherever possible, a rapid return to regular eating should be encouraged and maintained.

Parenteral Feeding

In cases of major tissue trauma or damage, or when a patient is unable to obtain sufficient nutrients orally, parenteral feeding may be necessary (see Chapter 18). It provides crucial nutritional support from solutions containing a higher percentage of glucose, as well as amino acids, electrolytes, minerals, vitamins, and lipid admixtures.

Particularly in cases of major surgery, aggressive nutritional support with enteral and parenteral means (see Chapter 18) is often a primary factor determining the outcome. The nutritional status of the patient is a critical focus in avoiding postoperative complications and improving morbidity and mortality rates. Up to 50% or more of patients awaiting or recovering from surgery are malnourished.[2] Studies repeatedly show that malnourished patients have higher postoperative morbidity and mortality than well-nourished ones and that comprehensive nutrition assessment and vigorous therapy support a positive outcome.[2,3] Strong nutritional support is essential for the best outcome after surgery.

Routine Postoperative Diets

As rapidly as possible, as soon as intestinal peristalsis returns, water and clear liquids such as tea, coffee, broth, and juice may be given to help supply important fluids and some sodium and chloride. These initial liquids also help stimulate normal gastrointestinal function and early return to a full diet. Progression to full liquids should soon follow. Milk and milk products—including puddings, cream soups, high-protein beverages, and ice cream—begin to supply vital protein and carbohydrates. Each patient progresses to solid foods in soft to regular diets according to individual tolerances. Oral intake of solid foods should be encouraged and supported as soon as possible to hasten recovery.

Special Nutritional Needs for Head and Neck Surgery Patients

Surgery involving mouth, throat, and neck requires modification in the manner of feeding. The patient usually cannot chew or swallow normally.

Oral Liquid Feedings

Concentrated feedings in liquid form must be planned. These feedings may consist of special enteral formulas of protein hydrolysates or amino acids with added carbohydrates, fat, vitamins, and minerals. As tolerated, milk-based beverages, soups, fruit juices, or special supplemented formulas supply frequent, reinforced oral nourishment.

Tube Feedings

Patients who are comatose or severely debilitated or who have undergone radical neck or facial surgery may require tube-feeding. New developments in small-bore feeding tubes have made this method of feeding easier. In cases of long-term need, rapid development of sophisticated delivery systems and standardized formulas has made continued home enteral nutrition possible for many patients. These advances are discussed in detail in Chapter 18. Whatever type of formula or mode of feeding is used, personal needs require constant sensitive support. Although long-term tube feeding may well meet the patient's physiologic needs, it also contributes to psychologic stress. Personal support for quality of life is an important part of patient care planning.

Special Nutritional Needs for Gastrointestinal Surgery Patients

Gastric Resection

Nutrition Problems

A number of nutrition problems may develop following gastric surgery, depending on the type of surgical procedure (Fig. 23-1) and the patient's response. A partial gastrectomy may create little postoperative difficulty, but a total gastrectomy involves more problems. The normal anatomy is radically changed with complete excision of the stomach and the remaining portion of the esophagus joined to the jejunum *(anastomosis)*. This resectioning may produce serious nutritional deficits and requires careful individual assessment and diet planning. When a **vagotomy** is also performed, there is increased gastric fullness and distention.[3] The

> **vagotomy** • A cutting of the vagus nerve, the tenth cranial nerve, which regulates muscular and secretory actions of the stomach.

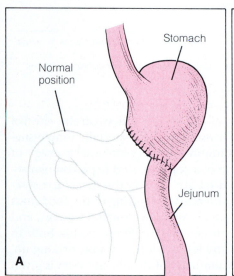
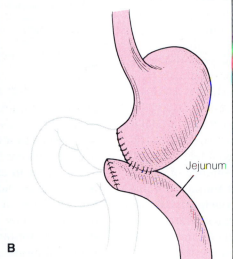
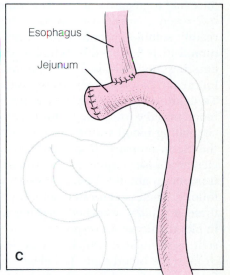

FIG. 23-1 Gastric surgery. **A,** Partial gastrectomy, Bilroth 1. **B,** Partial gastrectomy, Bilroth 1. **C,** Total gastrectomy.

stomach portion remaining becomes atonic and empties poorly, so that food fermentation follows, producing flatus and diarrhea. After gastric surgery, especially with total **gastrectomy,** about 50% of the patients fail to regain weight to optimal levels. The nutritional care of patients who have had gastric surgery primarily falls into two phases: the immediate postoperative period and a later period involving the dumping syndrome.

Immediate Postoperative Period

Generally after surgery, frequent small oral feedings are resumed according to the patient's tolerance. A typical pattern of simple dietary progression may cover about a 2-week period. The basic principles of such a general diet therapy for this immediate postoperative period involve: (1) size of meals—small and frequent, and (2) type of food—simple, easily digested, mild, low in bulk. Increasingly, however, surgeons are using recently developed techniques and equipment, such as a needle-catheter jejunostomy procedure at the time of the gastric surgery, to provide earlier nutritional support with an elemental formula.

Later Dumping Syndrome

After patients have recovered from surgery and begin to eat food in greater volume and variety, they may experience increasing discomfort following meals. About 10 to 15 minutes after eating, cramping and a full feeling occur. The pulse is rapid, and there is a wave of weakness, cold sweating, and dizziness. Frequently nausea and vomiting follow. Such distressing reactions to food intake increase anxiety, so the person eats less and less. Weight loss and increasing malnutrition follow. This postgastrectomy complex of symptoms is commonly called *dumping syndrome.* A more precise term used by some clinicians is *jejunal hyperosmolar syndrome.* This difficulty is more likely to occur in patients who have had total gastrectomy. The symptoms of shock result when a meal containing a high proportion of readily soluble carbohydrate rapidly enters the jejunum, which has been attached to the esophagus. This entering food mass is a concentrated hyperosmolar solution in relation to the surrounding extracellular fluid. To achieve osmotic balance, water is drawn from the blood into the intestine, causing a rapid decrease in the circulating blood volume (see Chapter 8). As a result, the blood pressure drops, and signs of cardiac insufficiency appear: rapid pulse, sweating, weakness, and tremors. In about 2 hours a second sequence of events follows. The concentrated solution of simple carbohydrate is rapidly absorbed, causing a **postprandial** rise in blood glucose. In response, an overproduction of insulin is stimulated, which in turn leads to an eventual drop in the blood sugar to below normal fasting levels. Symptoms of mild hypoglycemia result.

Dramatic relief of these distressing symptoms and

TABLE 23-2

Diet for Postoperative Gastric Dumping Syndrome

General description

- 5 or 6 small meals daily
- Relatively high fat content to retard passage of food and help maintain weight
- High protein content (meat, egg, cheese) to rebuild tissue and maintain weight
- Relatively low carbohydrate content to prevent rapid passage of quickly used foods
- No milk; no sugar, sweets, or desserts; no alcohol or sweet carbonated beverages
- Liquids between meals only; avoid fluids for at least 1 hour before and after meals
- Relatively low-roughage foods; raw foods as tolerated

Meal pattern

Breakfast
  2 scrambled eggs with 1 to 2 tbsp butter or margarine
  ½ to 1 slice bread or small serving cereal with butter or margarine
  2 crisp bacon strips
  1 serving solid fruit*
Midmorning sandwich as follows:
  1 slice bread
  Butter or margarine
  56 g (2 oz) lean meat
Lunch
  112 g (4 oz) lean meat with 1 or 2 tbsp butter or margarine
  Green or colored vegetable† with butter or margarine
  ½ to 1 slice bread with butter or margarine
  ½ banana or other solid fruit*
Midafternoon
  Same snack as midmorning
Dinner
  112 g lean meat with 1 or 2 tbsp butter or margarine
  Green or colored vegetable† with butter or margarine
  ½ to 1 slice bread with butter or margarine (or small serving starchy vegetable substitute)
  1 serving solid fruit*
Bedtime
  56 g meat or 2 eggs or 56 g cheese or cottage cheese
  1 slice bread or 5 crackers
  Butter or margarine

*Fruit choice: applesauce, baked apple, canned fruit (drained), banana, or orange or grapefruit sections.
†Vegetable choice: asparagus, spinach, green beans, squash, beets, carrots, or green peas.

---

gradual regaining of lost weight follow careful control of the diet. Carbohydrate intake, especially simple sugars, is kept to a minimum to prevent rapid passage of food and formation of a concentrated hyperosmolar solution. Protein and fat are increased to provide tissue-building material and retard emptying of the food mass into the large intestine. Meals are small, frequent, and dry, with fluids between meals. There is less bulk to stimulate motility and less water for rapidly forming nutrient solutions. A summary of this dietary plan is given in Table 23-2. Lost weight is usually recovered, and nutritional deficiencies are corrected.

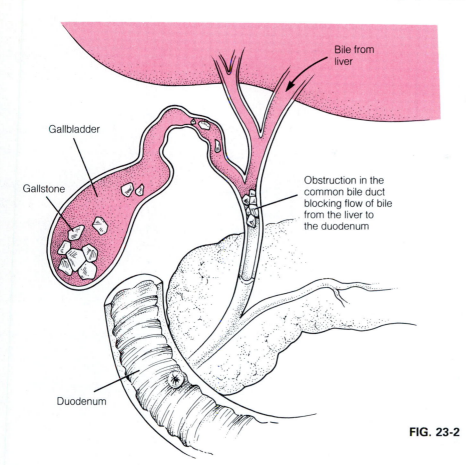

FIG. 23-2   Gallbladder with stones (cholelithiasis).

Gallbladder Surgery

Nutrition Problems

For patients suffering from acute *cholecystitis* or *cholelithiasis* (Fig. 23-2), the treatment is usually surgical removal of the gallbladder—**cholecystectomy.** Following surgery, control of the fat in the diet aids wound healing and comfort. The presence of fat in the duodenum continues to stimulate the *cholecystokinin mechanism* (see Chapter 19), which causes contraction and pain in the surgical area. There is also a period of readjustment to the more aqueous supply of liver bile available to assist fat digestion and absorption.

Dietary Management

Depending on individual tolerance and response, a relatively low-fat diet may need to be followed for a brief time with moderate fat use thereafter, as recommended in the U.S. Dietary Guidelines for all healthy Americans.

Ileostomy and Colostomy

In cases of intestinal lesion or obstruction or when inflammatory bowel disease (see Chapter 19) involves the entire colon, the treatment of choice is usually resection of the intestine to remove the diseased portion. An *ileostomy,* usually permanent but sometimes temporary, may also be established. In this procedure the end

of the remaining small intestine, the ileum, is attached to an opening in the abdominal wall, and a **stoma** is formed to provide for discharge of the intestinal contents (Fig. 23-3, *A*). In other cases a temporary or permanent *colostomy* may be indicated with resection of only the final left side of the colon, and a stoma is made with the remaining sigmoid, or descending, colon (Fig. 23-3, *B*). In other cases a *jejunoileostomy* may be performed (Fig. 23-4).

Nutrition Problems

An ileostomy and a colostomy produce different problems in management. With an ileostomy, the intestinal contents at the point of the ileus are unformed, irritat-

---

cholecystectomy • Surgical removal of the gallbladder.

gastrectomy • Surgical removal of the whole (total gastrectomy) or part (partial gastrectomy) of the stomach.

postprandial • Occurring after a meal.

stoma • The opening established in the abdominal wall, connecting with the ileum or colon, for elimination of intestinal wastes after surgical removal of diseased portions of the intestinal tract.

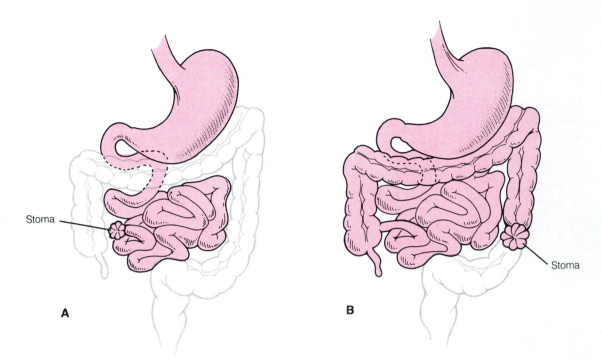

FIG. 23-3   **A,** Ileostomy. **B,** Colostomy.

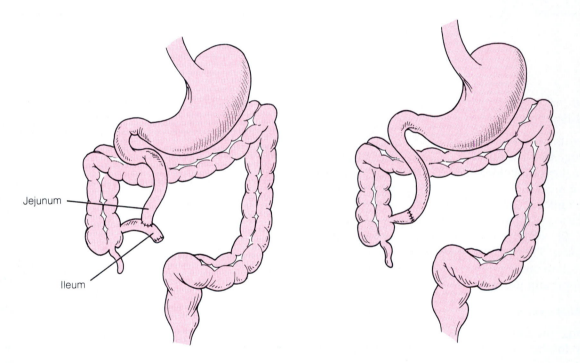

FIG. 23-4   Jejunoileostomy.

ing, and even erosive to the skin. The standard Brooke ileostomy (Fig. 23-3, *A*) with an outside pouch, drains freely, almost continuously.[4] Thus establishment of controlled functioning is difficult. Many patients, however, do develop a reasonable degree of regularity in regard to meals. The modified Koch pouch, an internal abdominal reservoir, has served as an alternative procedure. The surgeon forms a reservoir inside the abdominal cavity out of intestinal tissue, and a one-way valve holds the collection until the patient periodically inserts a catheter to empty it.[4,5] A recently developed, more attractive alternate procedure, the *J-pouch-anal anastomosis,* done in connection with a total colectomy, provides an interior ileoanal reservoir and channel for elimination through the regular anal route.[4,6] The ileoanal reservoir is constructed in two stages. First, a total **proctocolectomy** is done, usually indicated by the progressive inflammatory disease or colon cancer. The ileoanal reservoir is formed from loops of ileum placed in the rectal vault, and a temporary loop ileostomy is created to allow healing of the new ileoanal reservoir.[4,6,7] Second, about 3 months later the loop ileostomy is closed, and the new ileoanal reservoir is used for bowel movements. Stool frequency, although greatly reduced to about eight bowel movements per day, remains a personal concern.

Dietary Management

The diet therapy challenge centers on management of bowel output. In general, patients with ostomies should eat regular diets of foods that agree with them. Their food should be sufficient in quantity and nutritive value to maintain proper weight and energy. Patients with ileoanal reservoirs can best achieve control by (1) consuming no more than three meals a day (every time food is eaten the gastrointestinal tract is stimulated), (2) eating the last meal at least 2 hours before bedtime, and (3) evaluating individual bowel patterns to determine how long after a meal the person can safely leave home. The basis of the diet is a well-balanced regular plan of three meals, including a variety of foods, and noting individual food tolerances. Despite its drawbacks, the ileoanal reservoir is an increasingly popular surgical alternative to stoma formation.[4] However, of the ostomies with external stomas, a colostomy is more manageable. The normal contents of the intestine at

> **proctocolectomy** • Surgical removal of the rectum and colon.

TABLE 23-3

Nonresidue Diet and Postsurgical Nonresidue Diet

General description—nonresidue diet

- This diet includes only those foods free from fiber, seeds, and skins and with the minimal amount of residue.
- Fruits and vegetables are omitted, except for strained fruit juices.
- Milk is omitted.
- The diet is adequate in protein and kcal, containing approximately 75 g protein, 110 g fat, 250 g carbohydrates, and 2260 kcal. It is likely to be inadequate in vitamin A, calcium, and riboflavin.
- If patients remain a long time on this diet, supplementary vitamins and minerals should be given.

	Allowed	Not allowed
Beverages	Carbonated beverages, coffee, tea	Milk and milk drinks
Bread	Crackers, melba, or rusks	Whole grain bread
Cereals	Refined, as Cream of Wheat, farina, fine cornmeal, Malt-o-Meal, pablum, rice, strained oatmeal, corn flakes, puffed rice, Rice Krispies	Whole grain and other cereals
Cheese		None allowed
Desserts	Plain cakes and cookies, gelatin desserts, water ices, angel food cake, arrowroot cookies, tapioca puddings made with fruit juice only	Pastries and all others
Eggs	As desired, preferably hard cooked	Fried eggs
Fats	Butter or substitute, small amount cream	None
Fruits	Strained fruit juices	All others
Meat, fish, poultry	Tender beef, chicken, fish, lamb, liver, veal, and crisp bacon	Fried or tough meat, pork
Potatoes or substitute	Only macaroni, noodles, spaghetti, refined rice	Potatoes, corn, hominy, unrefined rice
Soup	Bouillon and broth only	All others
Sweets	Hard candy, fondant, gumdrops, jelly, marshmallows, sugar, syrup, and honey	Other candy, jam, marmalade
Vegetables	Tomato juice	All others
Miscellaneous	Salt	Pepper

General description—postsurgical nonresidue diet

- This diet is slightly higher in residue but has greater variety, including potatoes, white bread products, processed cheese, sauces, desserts made with milk, and cream for coffee and cereal.
- The average daily menu contains 85 g protein and 2300 kcal and is slightly higher in vitamins and minerals.

Selection of foods

To the list add the following:
- Cheese: processed cheese, mild cream cheeses
- Potatoes: prepared any way, no skin
- Bread: any kind without bran, white bread, rolls, pancakes, waffles
- Fats: 2 oz cream or half-and-half per meal, cream sauce, cream gravy
- Desserts: all desserts, except those containing fruit and nuts
- Condiments: as desired

this point in the lower colon are solid or semisolid, because more water and electrolytes have been absorbed by the first parts of the colon. The consistency of the discharge and its less irritating nature create fewer control problems. Often a sigmoid colostomy can be adequately controlled by simple dietary measures and periodic irrigation, so that in many cases no protective appliance is needed. However, coping with any of these surgical procedures is difficult at best. Patients need much support and practical help, along with resources for learning about self-care.[4,6]

Rectal Surgery
Nutrition Problems

For a brief period following rectal surgery *(hemorrhoidectomy)* there is pain on elimination. Thus bowel movements are delayed until initial healing is begun.

Dietary Management

A clear fluid or nonresidue diet is indicated for initial use. The basic foods used are almost completely digested, and nutrients are absorbed in the small intestine, leaving minimal residue for elimination by the colon. An outline of foods used in such a diet is given in Table 23-3. In some cases a nonresidue commercial for-

mula may be used during the initial postoperative period.

Special Nutritional Needs for Patients with Burns
Nutritional Support Base

A major concern of therapy for the patient with extensive burns is rigorous nutritional support. The clinical dietitian on the burn team is in a most strategic position to assess, plan, implement, and monitor the nutritional care for these patients.[8,9] Strong assistance is needed in nursing care. Three important factors guide this vital nutritional therapy: (1) large catabolic losses, (2) essential anabolic healing demands, and (3) deep personal support needs.

Treatment and Prognosis

The plan of care and its outcome depend on several factors:

1. *Age*—elderly persons and very young children are most vulnerable.
2. *Health condition*—the presence of any preexisting condition, such as diabetes, heart or renal disease,

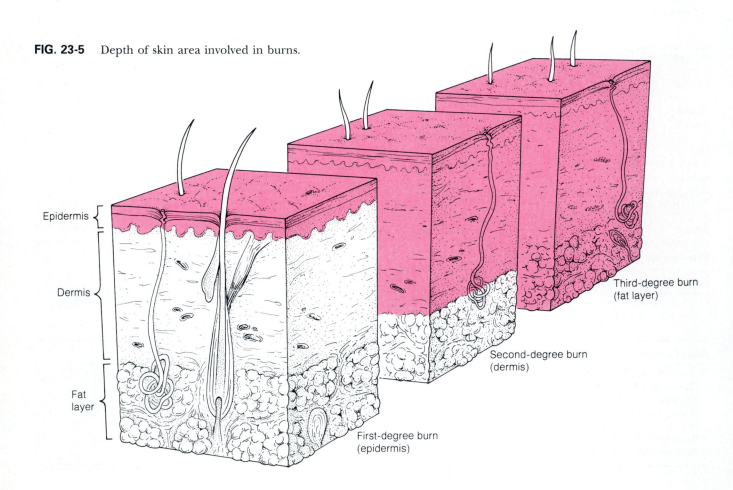

FIG. 23-5   Depth of skin area involved in burns.

Epidermis

Dermis

Fat layer

First-degree burn (epidermis)

Second-degree burn (dermis)

Third-degree burn (fat layer)

Metabolic Response to Injury

Two distinct phases of injury response may be identified: the ebb and the flow. The initial ebb phase occurs immediately after the injury and is associated with shock. It is characterized by the following specific metabolic events:

- Decreased oxygen consumption and cardiac output
- Decreased body temperature
- Increased blood glucose accompanied by normal glucose production
- Increased lactate and free fatty acid production
- Increased catecholamine, glucagon, and cortisol levels
- Decreased insulin production and insulin resistance

If the injured patient survives, the ebb phase evolves into the flow phase. This recovery period is characterized by the following events:

- Increased oxygen consumption and cardiac output

TO PROBE FURTHER

- Increased body temperature
- Increased nitrogen excretion
- Mild elevation of blood glucose accompanied by increased glucose production
- Normal lactate level and mild increase of free fatty acid level
- Increased catecholamine, glucagon, and cortisol levels
- Increased insulin production and insulin resistance

Clinical efforts in the ebb phase are focused on maintaining heart action and blood circulation to pour over and through the tissues. The flow phase is a period of increased metabolism that demands appropriate nutritional support.

REFERENCE

Bessey PQ, Wilmore DW: The burned patient. In Kinney JM and others editors: *Nutrition and metabolism in patient care,* Philadelphia, 1988, WB Saunders.

---

or any other associated injuries, complicates care.

3. *Burn severity*—the location and severity of the burn wounds and the time elapsed before treatment are significant.

Degree and Extent of Burns

The depth of the burn wound affects its healing process (Fig. 23-5). Burns are usually classified by degree:

1. First-degree burns—**erythema** involving cell necrosis above the basal layer of the epidermis
2. Second-degree burns—erythema and blistering, and necrosis within the dermis
3. Third-degree burns—full-thickness skin loss, including the fat layer

First-degree, or partial-thickness, burns regenerate new skin tissue from the epithelial cells lining the skin appendages, such as hair follicles, sweat glands, and **sebaceous** glands. Second- and third-degree, or full-thickness, burns do not leave sufficient skin for healing purposes. Thus they heal only from the skin margins. Small area burns heal in this manner, but extensive burns require skin grafting.

The body surface area injured by the burn is a basic factor in calculating nutritional support needs. Generally the burn team estimates body surface area involved by the so-called rule of nines or by a more accurate calculation using prepared charts. Second- and third-degree burns covering 15% to 20% or more of the total body surface, or even 10% in children and elderly persons, usually cause extensive fluid loss and require intravenous fluid and electrolyte replacement therapy. Burns of severe depth covering more than 50% of the body surface area are often fatal, especially in infants and older persons. Patients with major burn injuries are usually transferred immediately to a specialized burn care facility.

Stages of Nutritional Care

The nutritional care of the patient with massive burns is constantly adjusted to individual responses and needs. At all times attention to amino acid needs is vital, in addition to critical fluid-electrolyte balance and energy (kcalories) support. Generally three stages of care may be identified: (1) immediate "ebb" or shock period and following "flow" or recovery response (see To Probe Further, above); (2) secondary critical recovery phase of vigorous feeding; and (3) the follow-up period of reconstructive surgery and rehabilitation.

Stage 1: Immediate Shock Period

Massive flooding edema occurs at the burn site during the first hours after injury to about the second day. Loss of enveloping skin surface and exposure of tissue fluids lead to immediate loss of water and electrolytes, mainly sodium, and large protein depletion. In an effort to balance this loss, water shifts from the surrounding tissue spaces in the body, only adding to the continuous loss at the burn site. As a result, water circulating in the blood is withdrawn, thus decreasing the overall blood volume *(hypovolemia)* and blood pressure.

---

erythema • Redness of the skin produced by coagulation of the capillaries.

sebaceous • Secreting the fatty lubricating substance *sebum.*

Blood concentration and diminished urine output occur as a result. Cell dehydration follows as cell water is drawn out to balance the tissue fluid losses. Cell potassium is also withdrawn, and circulating serum potassium levels rise.

Immediate intravenous fluid therapy replaces water and electrolytes by use of a balanced salt solution such as **lactated Ringer's solution,** helping to correct the hypovolemia and prevent shock. Acute renal failure is a rare occurrence when resuscitation is started early. During the first part of this initial shock period, the first 12 to 14 hours after the injury, **colloid** solutions such as albumin or plasma are not effective since most of such solutions are lost in fluids at the burn site. Usually vascular endothelial permeability returns to normal after the first day, however, and colloid solutions can then be used to help restore plasma volume. During this initial period, no attempt is made to meet nutritional requirements in protein and kcalories because (1) glucose-free balanced electrolyte solutions are needed, because infusion of glucose at this time may result in hyperglycemia; and (2) an *adynamic ileus* develops after the injury and precludes any use of the gastrointestinal tract at this time.

Stage 1: Recovery Period

After about 48 to 72 hours, tissue fluids and electrolytes are gradually reabsorbed into the general circulation, balance is established, and the pattern of massive tissue loss is reversed. At this point a sudden *diuresis* occurs, indicating successful therapy. The patient returns to preinjury weight by about the end of the first week. A careful check of fluid intake and output is essential, with constant checks for signs of dehydration or overhydration.

Stage 2: Secondary Feeding Period

Toward the end of the first postburn week, adequate bowel function returns, and a vigorous feeding period must begin. At this point, despite the patient's depression and anorexia, life may well depend on rigorous nutritional therapy. Several factors necessitate this increased intake.

Tissue destruction. The massive burn injury has brought large losses of protein and electrolytes that must be replaced.

Tissue catabolism. Tissue protein breakdown has followed the injury, with consequent loss of lean body mass and nitrogen.

Increased metabolism. Increased metabolic demands arise from additional needs. **Sepsis** or fever requires extra kcalories for energy needs. Extra carbohydrates and B vitamins are needed for energy as the body resources mobilize to meet heightened basal metabolic requirements. Tissue regeneration requires extra protein and key vitamins such as ascorbic acid and minerals such as zinc. The success of follow-up skin grafting requires optimal tissue health.

Stage 2: Nutritional Therapy

Successful nutritional therapy during this critical period is based on vigorous energy and protein therapy.

High energy. From 3500 to 5000 kcal, with a high percentage of carbohydrates, is necessary to spare protein for tissue regeneration and to supply the greatly increased metabolic demands for energy. The amount of Kilocalories required depends on the patient's preburn body weight and the percent of body surface area burned. The classic Harris-Benedict equations (see Chapters 16 and 18) may be used to determine basal energy expenditure (BEE) needs. This value is then multiplied by the appropriate metabolic stress activity factor (MAF) involved in such severe illness and trauma (Table 23-4). Adjustment of kcalories is necessary on an individual basis in relation to weight changes or complications such as infection, which change energy requirements.[10]

High protein. Depending on the extent of the burn injury and catabolic losses, individual needs for protein vary from 150 g to as high as 400 g. Children require two to four times the normal RDA of protein for age. In general, most adults require an increased amount of protein, 2 to 3 g/kg body weight, to achieve nitrogen balance.

High vitamins. From 1 to 2 g of vitamin C may be needed for tissue regeneration. Increased thiamin, riboflavin, and niacin are necessary to metabolize the extra carbohydrate and protein.

TABLE 23-4

Added Energy Cost of Metabolic Stress in Illness and Trauma, the Metabolic Activity Factor (MAF)

MAF according to degree of stress	Examples of conditions
BEE × 1.25: minimal stress	Nutritionally sound, little stress
BEE × 1.30: moderate stress	Cancer, inflammatory bowel disease, skeletal trauma, minor surgery
BEE × 1.50: severe stress	Cancer chemotherapy or radiation, burns, major sepsis
BEE × 1.75-2: extreme stress	Acquired immunodeficiency syndrome (AIDS), major trauma or burns

Modified from Konishi CD: Metabolic support teams as nutrition educators: who supports whom? *Top Clin Nutr* 1(4):51, 1986.
MAF, Metabolic activity factor; *BEE,* basal energy expenditure.

Stage 2: Dietary Management

To meet these crucial nutrient demands, either enteral or parenteral modes of feeding may be required.

Enteral feeding. To achieve the necessary intake of increased nutrient density indicated, a careful intake record must be maintained. Oral feedings are desirable if at all tolerated by the patient. Concentrated oral liquids must be given using protein hydrolysates or amino acids to ensure adequate intake. Commercial formulas are usually used to supply large amounts of nourishment. Solid foods, according to individual food preferences, are added by about the second week. Tube feeding may be required by some patients in the beginning. In this case low-bulk defined formula solutions may be given through small-bore feeding tubes (see Chapter 18). In either case, continuous support and encouragement are necessary. Food should be made as attractive and appetizing as possible, supplying items particularly liked and respecting disliked foods.

Parenteral feeding. For some patients, oral intake and tube feedings may be inadequate to meet the accelerated demands, or may be impossible because of associated injuries or complications. In these cases parenteral feeding through a large central vein or peripheral vein is needed to provide the essential nutritional support. Details of this often life-saving procedure are given in Chapter 18.

Stage 3: Follow-up reconstruction. Continued vigorous nutrition support is essential to maintain tissue integrity for successful skin grafting or plastic reconstructive surgery. In addition, the principles of rehabilitative care discussed in Chapter 26 apply in the case of burn patients. Each patient needs not only physical rebuilding of body resources but also much personal support to rebuild the human will and spirit, since there may be disfigurement and disability. Health team members can do much to help instill the courage and confidence the person must have to face the future again. However, whatever the future demands, optimal physical stamina gained through persistent, supportive care—medical, nutritional, and nursing—helps each patient rebuild the personal resources needed to cope.

To Sum Up

The nutritional demands of surgery begin before the patient reaches the operating table. Preoperatively the task is to correct any existing deficiencies and build nutrient reserves to meet surgical demands. Postoperatively it is to replace losses and support recovery. The additional task of encouraging eating is often required during this period.

Presurgical and postsurgical feedings are given in a variety of ways. The oral route is always preferred, but damage to the intestinal tract or a poor appetite may require other enteral or parenteral feedings. Diets are modified according to the surgical procedure performed. For the depleted surgical patient, nutritional support relies heavily on biomedical technology to facilitate enteral and parenteral feedings administeristered by specially trained total parenteral nutrition (TPN) team members.

QUESTIONS FOR REVIEW

1. Describe the general impact of imbalances of the following nutritional factors during the preoperative, immediate postoperative, and postoperative periods: protein, Kilocalories, vitamins, minerals, and fluids.
2. Describe the major surgical effects for which nutrition therapy must be planned following these procedures: mouth, throat, and neck surgery; gastric resection; cholecystectomy; and rectal surgery.
3. Write a 1-day meal plan for a person experiencing the postgastrectomy dumping syndrome. What general dietary guidelines are used? Why?
4. Describe the difference in care between an ileostomy and a colostomy. What are the dietary implications of each?
5. Outline the nutritional care of a burn patient from treatment for immediate shock through recovery and tissue reconstruction.
6. **colloid.** Glutinous, glue-like; a dispersion of matter throughout a liquid.
7. **lactated Ringer's solution.** Sterile solution of calcium chloride, potassium chloride, sodium chloride, and sodium lactate in water given to replenish fluid and electrolytes.
8. **sepis.** Presence in the blood or other tissues of pathogenic microorganisms or their toxins; conditions associated with such pathogens.

REFERENCES

1. Campos ACL, Meguid MM: A critical appraisal of the usefulness of perioperative nutritional support, *Am J Clin Nutr* 55:117, 1992.

---

colloid • Glutinous, glue-like; a dispersion of matter throughout a liquid.

lactated Ringer's solution • Sterile solution of calcium chloride, potassium chloride, sodium chloride, and sodium lactate in water given to replenish fluid and electrolytes.

sepsis • Presence in the blood or other tissues of pathogenic microorganisms or their toxins; conditions associtated with such pathogens.

2. Mughal MM, Meguid MM: The effect of nutritional status on the morbidity after elective surgery for benign gastrointestinal disease, *J Parenter Enteral Nutr* 11(2):140, 1987.

3. Sachdeva AK and others: Surgical treatment of peptic ulcer disease, *Med Clin North Am* 75(4):999, 1991.

4. Tyns FJ and others: Diet tolerance and stool frequency in patients with ileoanal reservoirs, *J Am Diet Assoc* 92(7):861, 1992.

5. Rathgeber MG: Nutrition and ostomies, ADA practice group, *Dietitians in Nutrition Support Newsletter* 8(6):5, 1987.

6. Lerch MM and others: Postoperative adaptation of the small intestine after total colectomy and J-pouch-anal anastomosis, *Dis Colon Rectum* 32:600, 1989.

7. Miedema BW and others: Absorption and motility of the by-passed human ileum, *Dis Colon Rectum* 33:829, 1990.

8. Ireton-Jones CS, Baxter CR: Nutrition for adult burn patients: a review, *Nutr Clin Prac* 6(1):3, 1990.

9. Hutsler DA: Nutrition monitoring of a pediatric burn patient, *Nutr Clin Prac* 6(1):11, 1991.

10. Goran MI and others: Estimating energy requirements in burned children: A new approach derived from measurements for resting energy expenditures, *Am J Clin Nutr* 54:35, 1991.

FURTHER READING

Cerra FB: How nutrition intervention changes what getting sick means, *J Parenter Enteral Nutr* 14(suppl 5):164, 1990.

This article provides a good review of three basic factors that influence what is observed at an ill patient's bedside when considering the effects of nutrition intervention: (1) the disease process inherent in the metabolic response to injury, (2) the presence of starvation, and (3) the presence of the nutritional intervention.

Hutsler DA: Nutritional monitoring of a pediatric burn patient, *Nutr Clin Prac* 6:11, 1991.

This experienced dietitian specialist on a burn-center team provides a case report of a young boy who sustained mostly full-thickness burns over 56% of his total body surface area. She describes in detail the challenge of initial evaluation and therapy, constant close monitoring, and appropriate responses to changing needs.

Tynes JJ and others: Diet tolerance and stool frequency in patients with ileoanal reservoirs, *J Am Diet Assoc* 92(7):861, 1992.

This brief report of a survey of patients with ileoanal reservoirs provides much helpful background information about this recently developed alternative surgical procedure to the ileostomy, with practical guidance for nutritional management and patient counseling.

CASE STUDY

The Patient with a Gastrectomy

Walter Reilly is a 42-year-old male admitted for a total gastrectomy 4 weeks ago. He had a history of repeated episodes of pain and bleeding, for which he had been hospitalized twice during the last 6 months.

Surgery proceeded smoothly, with an anastomosis established between the esophagus and the jejunum. Mr. Reilly received nothing orally for 48 hours postoperatively but received TPN to give nutritional support. He was then given ice chips and water, which he gradually began to tolerate.

Two days later Mr. Reilly was able to tolerate 30 to 60 ml (2 to 4 tbsp; 1 to 2 oz) of milk between sips of water. This amount increased, as did his appetite. He was graduated to servings of a single soft food (eggs, cereal, custards, potato) once or twice a day. By the end of the second week

he was tolerating a full soft diet on six small feedings daily. He was cautioned to use liquids in moderation during a discharge diet session conducted 1 week later.

At a later follow-up visit with his physician, Mr. Reilly complained of general discomfort and cramping following meals. Other symptoms included a rapid heart rate, dizziness, nausea and vomiting, and breaking out in a cold sweat. He had also begun to lose weight, and he appeared slightly emaciated. His physician referred him to the clinical nutritionist to explore any problem with eating habits, and Mr. Reilly seemed to accept most of the recommendations. One week later he telephoned to explain that all symptoms had subsided and that he was tolerating the diet well.

Questions for Analysis

1. Do you think that the surgical procedure performed was warranted? Defend your response.
2. Explain the physiologic rationale for the refeeding program as planned.
3. What nutrient would you emphasize in this patient's diet? Why? What is its significance with surgery?
4. Why was some fluid limitation recommended?
5. Account for the symptoms that followed eating. What dietary recommendations would you make to control them?

ISSUES · AND · ANSWERS

Traditional methods used to assess nutritional status and needs rely heavily on the use of *objective* measures such as anthropometry, clinical criteria, laboratory tests, and in some instances indirect calorimetry. But how does *subjective* evaluation relate? What role does it play in getting the whole picture of the patient's situation and its effect on health and illness?

Canadian researchers seeking some answers to these questions have been studying the relationships between these two basic assessment approaches. Working with hospitalized surgery patients, they demonstrated a subjective clinical assessment of nutritional needs based on a history and physical examination, which they call a subjective global assessment (SGA). They found that this subjective approach is highly correlated with assessments made using the usual objective measures. They also found that with SGA, postoperative infections could be predicted as well or better than with objective measures.

In a follow-up study the investigators applied SGA to 202 patients before gastrointestinal surgery and examined the effect of individual characteristics on the SGA ratings. This study confirmed the validity of SGA as a technique of nutritional assessment. SGA ratings are based on five features of the patient history:

- Weight changes (loss) in the past 6 months and changes in the past 2 weeks
- Changes in dietary intake
- Gastrointestinal symptoms (nausea, vomiting, diarrhea, and anorexia) that have persisted over 2 weeks
- Functional capacity (ambulatory or bedridden)
- Presence of disease and its relation to nutritional needs

Four features of the physical examination are rated as normal, mild, moderate, or severe for five parameters:

- Loss of subcutaneous fat (triceps and chest)
- Muscle wasting (quadriceps and deltoids)
- Ankle and sacral edema
- Ascites

On the basis of these features of the history and physical examination, health team members identify an SGA rank that indicates the person's nutritional status: well nourished, moderate or suspected malnutrition, or severe malnutrition.

The researchers think that a major advantage of SGA is its flexibility in capturing subtle patterns of change in clinical variables and relating them to the effects of disease or surgical stress.

REFERENCE

Detsky AS and others: What is subjective global assessment of nutritional status? *J Parenter Enteral Nutr* 11(1):8, 1987.

Nutrition and AIDS

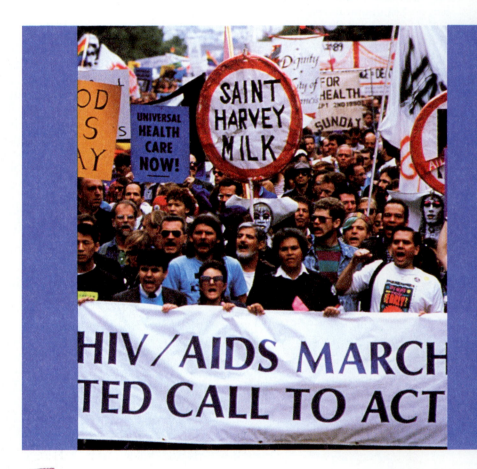

*I*n this chapter of our clinical series we focus on acquired immuno-deficiency syndrome (AIDS). This modern-day plague has eluded modern medical science's search for a cure and left countless numbers of infected and dying young adults and children in its wake.

Here we examine the background of the AIDS epidemic and the nature of the human immunodeficiency virus-1 (HIV-1). We review the current state of medical management, especially the component of nutritional support and its relation to nutritional status and the course of the disease. As knowledge of the disease process has grown over the past decade, it has become increasingly evident that nutritional support plays a vital role in the care of HIV-infected and AIDS patients.

Evolution of HIV and the AIDS Epidemic

In the late 1970s, physicians on the east and west coasts of the United States, centered in New York City and San Francisco, became puzzled about an uncommon medical problem appearing among their patients.[1] No known cause of immune suppression could be found. Nonetheless they were suffering and dying from complications of common infections, largely pneumonia, ordinarily handled easily by the human immune system and the usual antibiotics or other antibacterial drugs.

To add to the puzzle, these and other early patients (June 1991 to January 1993) with the similar immune-suppression condition of unknown cause were coming from quite diverse social and medical backgrounds. They included active homosexual men, intravenous drug users, and recipients of transfused blood and blood products, such as children with **hemophilia.** Still others were heterosexual men and women and their babies. What was this devastating disease? Its **virus** source and **pandemic** effects were soon to become alarmingly evident worldwide.

Early Viral History and Spread
Rapid Pandemic Spread

An alarming decade of frustration and death followed the first reported cases in 1981.[2] Some highlights of that deadly decade include the following events:

- **June 1981.** Reports of an unexplained type of immune system failure among gay men start to surface in the United States; news of similar conditions among heterosexual men and women begins to increase from other parts of the world, especially central Africa.
- **July 1982.** The new disease is found in hemophiliacs; named aquired immune deficiency syndrome (AIDS) by American scientists.
- **January 1983.** Heterosexuals are also declared at risk after several women, whose sexual partners have AIDS, contract the disease.
- **May 1983.** The French scientist Luc Montagnier, a leading pioneer of AIDS research, reports that he and his team at the Pasteur Institute in Paris have isolated the infectious agent now known as human immunodeficiency virus (HIV).
- **September 1984.** First report of HIV infection is found in Thailand, which has subsequently developed one of the world's highest infection rates caused part to its open, thriving sex industry.
- **March 1985.** The first test to detect HIV antibodies in the blood is approved in the United States.
- **March 1987.** The first drug, azidothymidine (AZT), now known as zidovudine, developed to fight the AIDS virus, is approved for experimental use by the U.S. Food and Drug Administration (FDA).
- **April 1990.** The first U.S. Congressional action, named for Ryan White, a young hemophiliac who received HIV-infected blood transfusions as a child and died of AIDS at age 18, provides funds to cities hardest hit by the disease.
- **October 1991.** The second anti-AIDS drug, dideoxyinosine (ddI), is approved by the FDA.
- **June 1992.** British scientists predict a 20% drop over the next decade in the population growth rate of the central African country of Uganda, where AIDS apparently first gained its hold and then spread.
- **June 1992.** The third anti-AIDS drug, dideoxycytosine (ddC), is approved by the FDA.

Evolution of HIV
Social Change

Where did this new deadly virus come from and how did it gain such strength? From studies thus far, scientists are beginning to find some answers. Apparently, HIV represents not a new virus but an old one that has only recently grown deadly in humans as it gained strength during the social upheavals of the 1960s and 1970s.[3] The uprooting effect of this rapid social change and urbanization allowed the virus to spread rapidly through world populations and reproduce aggressively in its human host.

Parasite Nature of Virus

No virus can have a life of its own. All viruses by their structure and nature are the ultimate **parasites.** They are mere shreds of genetic material, a small packet of

---

hemophilia • A hereditary hemorrhagic disease caused by a deficiency of blood coagulation factor VIII, characterized by spontaneous or traumatic bleeding, transmitted as an X-linked (maternal) recesive trait to male children.

pandemic • A widespread epidemic, distributed through a region, continent, or the world.

parasite • An organism that lives on or in an organism of another species, know as the host, from whom all life-cycle nourishment is obtained.

virus • Minute infectious agent, characterized by lack of independent metabolism and by the ability to reproduce with genetic continuity only within living host cells. They range in decreasing size from about 200 nanometers (nm) down to only 15 nanometers (nm). (A nanometer is a linear measure equal to one-billionth of a meter; it is also called a millimicron.) Each particle (virion) consists basically of nucleic acids (genetic material) and a protein shell which protects and contains the genetic material and any enzymes present.

genetic information encased in a protein coat. They contain only a small chromosome of nucleic acids (RNA or DNA), usually with fewer than five genes (see Chapter 25). They can only live through a host, whom they invade and infect. There they hijack the host's cell machinery to run off a multitude of copies of themselves. Their purpose is to make as many self-copies as they can. Today's viruses are those that succeeded in that survival task over time and are, like all plants and animals, simply descendents of earlier forms. Most scientists agree that the human immunoviruses HIV-1 and HIV-2, which are genetically similar to viruses found in African primates (simian immunodeficiency virus [SIV]), were probably transmitted to humans in an earlier age as ancient hunters cut themselves while butchering their kills for food. The rapidly increasing social-sexual changes and world travel of the past few decades have sped HIV-1 transmission and rapid multiplication. Its current deadly strength results from its aggressive growth within an increasing number of hosts.

Extent of Current Problem
Current Spread

Today, more than 12 million people throughout the world are infected with HIV. The great majority live in central Africa, south of the Sahara desert, where the first cases appeared. Now, however, Southeast Asia, with its increasing urbanization, seems poised to become the plague's new epicenter. Currently infected populations are spread in nine main areas of the world[3,4]:

- **Sub-Saharan Africa:** 7.5+ million
- **Southeast Asia:** 1.5 million
- **Latin America (Caribbean):** 1.0 million
- **North America:** 1.0+ million
- **North Africa, Middle East:** 750,000
- **Western Europe:** 500,000
- **Eastern Europe, Central Asia:** 50,000
- **East Asia, China, and Japan:** 25,000
- **Australasia:** 25,000+

These official numbers are horrifying enough, but they tell only part of the story. Some developing world countries report only 5% to 10% of the actual number of cases.[4] Many of these countries simply do not detect or report all of their cases.

Projected Future Course

Epidemiologists and others studying the rapid spread of AIDS project gloomy numbers for the course of the disease during the next decade, before the breakthroughs in curative drugs and population vaccines can eventually take effect. They indicate two new areas of concern: (1) an increasing incidence of AIDS in heterosexual women with the accompanying risk of fetal transmission and (2) the increasing spread of tuberculosis as an opportunistic pathogen in HIV-infected persons.[5] Over the next decade, Southeast Asia is expected

to surpass central Africa in numbers of HIV-infected persons, especially among young women and their babies resulting from the open, expanding sex industry of the region, centered mainly in Thailand.[2] In the United States, by the end of 1994, the Centers for Disease Control in Atlanta estimates that between 415,000 and 535,000 new cases of AIDS will have been diagnosed, and well over a quarter of a million persons will be living with severe HIV disease at that time.[5] Although the course of the worldwide HIV epidemic is difficult to predict, the sobering forecast of the World Health Organization (WHO) is that a minimum of 30 to 40 million people will be infected by the end of the decade.

Disease Progression

The individual clinical course of HIV infection varies substantially. Nonetheless, three distinct stages mark the progression of the disease and are usually referred to as (1) primary HIV infection and extended asymptomatic incubation, (2) AIDS-related complex (ARC), and (3) terminal AIDS.

Primary HIV Infection

About 2 to 4 weeks after initial exposure and infection, a mild flulike syndrome lasting about a week may or may not occur. This brief response corresponds to the process of *seroconversion,* the development of antibodies to the viral infection. Subsequent HIV testing will be positive. Signs of enlarged lymph nodes may occur, and an extended asymptomatic "well" period usually continues for the next 8 to 10 years.

However, this seemingly inactive, relatively well period can be deceiving. New research indicates that it is actually a crucial stage in the underlying growth of the virus.[6,7] This extended period is a critical stage of viral incubation, during which the virus appears to be inactive. In reality, it is hiding in lymphoid tissues such as lymph nodes, spleen, adenoid glands, and tonsils, multiplying constantly in its parasite life-cycle within its host, taking over more and more white blood cells and gaining strength.[8]

In addition, new reports at a spring 1993 U.S. symposium of researchers further reinforced the findings of the virus in lymphoid tissue. Current research reported on the symposium topic "Frontiers in HIV Pathogenesis" added strength to the deception of the inactive period of HIV infection. With a newly developed amplified assay-testing process, the investigators were able to routinely detect the HIV in the special T-helper white blood cells (CD4+) they specifically infect. They found even greater masses of infected cells in lymphoid tissues than had been measured before with standard assays. Thus they issued buttons at the conference aptly summarizing the meeting's major theme with the blunt message: "It's the virus, stupid."[9]

Additional conference reports of HIV in primate studies indicated that as the special CD4+ T-helper white blood cell count drops, it remains high in the lymph nodes, and the immune system crashes only when the CD4+ levels drop sharply in the lymphoid tissue.

Some of the scientists have likened this apparently quiet period before the storm to the active life of a volcano—its inactive period a mountain of still beauty masking its actual interior cauldron developing strength for the inevitable blast. New research findings demonstrate the complexity and strength of this disease and the problems presented in finding a solution to stem the epidemic tide. These researchers underscore the crucial nature of this incubation period and the importance of earlier treatment intervention after HIV-seropositive detection, to slow this viral-strengthening hiatus while drugs and vaccine are being developed to combat its steady progression.

AIDS-Related Complex (ARC)

After the extended asymptomatic HIV-positive stage, which may last as long as 10 years, a period of associated infectious illnesses begins. This AIDS-related complex of opportunistic illnesses is so named because the HIV infection has by now killed enough host-protective white T-cells (mainly T-helper or CD4+ lymphocytes) to severely damage the immune system and lower the body's normal disease resistance, so that even the most common everyday infections have an open opportunity to take root and grow. Common symptoms observed during this pre-AIDS period include persistent fatigue, thrush (oral *Candida albicans*), night sweats, diarrhea, fever over 100° F, unintentional weight loss of 5 kg (11 lbs) or more, remarkable headache, new skin rash, new or unusual cough, sore throat or mouth, unusual bruises or skin discoloration, and shortness of breath.[10]

Final Stage of AIDS

The terminal stage of HIV infection, commonly designated as AIDS, is marked by declining T-helper lymphocyte counts from the normal healthy level of about 1000 such cells in every cubic millimeter of blood ($1000/mm^3$). HIV-infected persons usually experience a decline of these cells by an average of about 40 to $80/mm^3$ every year.[11] Generally, when the falling T-helper lymphocyte counts are roughly between $200/mm^3$ and $500/mm^3$ diseases such as tuberculosis or Kaposi's sarcoma (the most common AIDS-associated malignancy) occur; at counts below $200/mm^3$, *Pneumocystis carinii* pneumonia and *Toxoplasma gondii* (protozoan parasites able to infect a number of body organs) appear; and at counts under $50/mm^3$, cytomegalovirus (CMV) or **lymphoma** can flourish.[1] When the virus finally kills enough white cells to overwhelm the weakened immune-system resistance to the disease complications, death follows.

Public Health Service Responsibilities

In any major epidemic, the Public Health Service and its related agencies have the major task of monitoring and stopping the disease spread. Thus they carry responsibilities in two major areas: (1) surveillance, including testing and counseling and (2) community education and prevention through interrupting its spread, vaccine research, and treatment.

Surveillance

Throughout the AIDS epidemic, as knowledge of this new disease and its nature has grown, the central control agency, the U.S. Centers for Disease Control (CDC) in Atlanta, has worked with state and territorial health departments and has been involved in constant worldwide knowledge exchange, to conduct accurate and comprehensive AIDS surveillance in the United States.[12] Since the mid-1980s, such seroprevalence studies have provided a massive amount of information about the spread of HIV in various population groups and have helped CDC develop early classification guidelines for medical teams caring for HIV-infected patients. The periodic CDC revisions of surveillance criteria reflect advances in the care and understanding of disease caused by HIV infection. In accord with current knowledge and the evolution of the HIV epidemic among demographic groups, CDC has recently expanded the AIDS surveillance definition to include any HIV-seropositive person with a CD4+ (specific T-lymphocyte subset analysis) cell count of less than 200 cells per microliter of blood.[12]

Because of the tremendous life-changing import of a positive HIV-1 test result to the individual and his or her family and loved ones, public health testing programs have developed a coordinated pretest and posttest counseling component, especially in clinics serving high-risk areas.[13] First, a brief pretest interview assesses personal knowledge of HIV infection, provides risk-reduction education, and offers the HIV test. Those who accept the HIV testing are given a 2-week return appointment for a longer follow-up review of test results and counseling concerning health care and personal needs. Also, in addition to regular HIV-1 testing, sentinel testing for the initial African (simian) strain HIV-2 in clinics serving high-risk clients recently arrived from endemic HIV-2 areas has begun to detect the presence of this second form of the virus in the United States.[14]

lymphoma • General term applied to any neoplastic disorder (cancer) of the lymphoid tissue.

Education and Prevention

The U.S. Department of Health and Human Services, through its Public Health Service and FDA divisions, has provided national health promotion and disease prevention objectives for the year 2000 that call for the expansion of HIV education and prevention efforts.[15] Wide community involvement in the community-based process of developing any health promotion/disease prevention program is essential for its successful outcome.[16] This need has been shown, for example, in the mobilizing of community leadership and resources to plan and implement interventions in other health problems such as heart disease or changing life-style habits (such as smoking) that contribute to lung disease. The community-support need is particularly true with HIV infection. Despite its burdening social stigma, it is reaching into all communities in some form, cutting short the lives of children, adolescents, and young adults in ever-increasing numbers. The Harvard Global AIDS Policy Coalition estimates that by the year 2000, between 38 and 110 million adults and more than 10 million children will be infected worldwide.[17] Such a deadly pandemic epidemic warrants mobilizing and coordinating the most realistic and effective preventive strategies possible for all ethnic and socioeconomic community groups to change sexual risk-taking behavior at all levels—local, national, and international.

Nature of the Disease Process

Action of HIV on the Immune System

HIV-1 and HIV-2 are members of a class of viruses called **retrovirus** because of their unique life-cycle, which involves a reverse transcription of RNA into DNA in the cell nucleus; this is then integrated into the host cell DNA.[1] The virus consists of an outer envelope, with attached surface proteins covering the outer protective shell, and an inner shell that contains the small strands of ribonucleic acid (RNA) genetic material and enzymes, including the reverse transcriptase. Of the virus' nine genes, four apparently less essential ones are poorly understood. After entering the body, the virus attaches itself to host cells, mostly the actively replicating T-helper (CD4+) white blood cells, major lymphocytes of the body's immune system. There it integrates itself into the host cell's DNA copying system, infecting and eventually killing the host cell. Rapidly increasing masses of virus particles erupt from the dying cells in small buds to immediately infect new cells.

Methods of Transmission and Groups at Risk

Throughout the world, sexual behavior is central to the epidemic spread of HIV and AIDS. An estimated 71%

of HIV infection worldwide is due to heterosexual behavior, 15% to homosexual behavior, and only a relatively small proportion to intravenous drug use with contaminated needles.[17] In the United States, as of 1992, reported AIDS cases by type of transmission were approximately 58% by homosexual behavior, 29% by intravenous drug use with shared blood-contaminated needles, 6% by heterosexual behavior, and 3% by blood transfusions. About 4% are from other types of transmission, such as health care worker contact with blood of infected patients (a relatively rare event) and vertical transmission from infected mothers to their babies during pregnancy or at birth, which is a growing concern.[2,18,19] Current worldwide studies of HIV-seropositive newborns indicate a maternal-fetal transmission rate of about 30%, with a low rate of 12.9% reported in the European Collaborative Study Group and a high rate of 45% in Nairobi, Kenya.[19] Infection is believed to occur predominately during the intrapartum period of labor and delivery, rather than earlier during pregnancy, and documented records show that such infected newborns require frequent hospitalizations during their first year of life.[19,20] The increase in pediatric cases of HIV infection brings more concern, and care of these children requires special considerations (see Issues and Answers, p. 484). Further, a study of young, sexually active women attending public family planning clinics in New York indicated that the greater disproportionate burden of HIV infection among these potential mothers was carried by non-Hispanic Blacks and Hispanics, whose HIV infection rate was about six times the rate for non-Hispanic Whites.[21]

Overall, current U.S. reports are now in flux, with a rising proportion of cases coming from heterosexual contact. The fastest-growing subgroup of new heterosexual cases is among women, with the proportion among younger women and adolescent girls alarmingly high.[17]

Groups at Risk

Persons at greatest risk of HIV infection, as indicated above, are those who, if sexually active, are not consistently practicing responsible and safe sexual behavior, which consists of (1) consistent and correct condom use for protection (the regular latex male sheath and the new female polyurethane condom, a cervical cap recently approved for use by the Food and Drug Administration)[22-24] and (2) avoidance of sex with multiple partners and persons at risk for HIV. Others at risk are intravenous drug users who share contaminated needles. However, since the public-donated blood supply for transfusions has been thoroughly cleared of HIV infection by a rigorous double-testing program, this route of infection risk by blood units for medical purposes has virtually been eliminated.[1]

TABLE 24-1

Common Infectious Complications of AIDS

Microorganism	Clinical manifestation
Parasites	
Pneumocystis carinii	Pneumonia
Toxoplasma gondii	Focal encephalitis, pneumonia
Cryptosporidium	Malabsorption, diarrhea
Isospora belli	Diarrhea
Microspora	Malabsorption, diarrhea
Entamoeba histolytica	Diarrhea
Giardia lamblia	Diarrhea
Acanthamoeba	Meningoencephalitis
Bacteria	
Campylobacter	Diarrhea, bacteremia
Legionella	Pneumonia
Listeria monocytogenes	Meningitis, bacteremia
Mycobacterium avium-intracellulare	Tuberculosis, diarrhea, other mycobacteria
Norcardia	Pneumonia, encephalitis
Pneumococcus	Pneumonia
Salmonella	Diarrhea, bacteremia
Shigella	Diarrhea, bacteremia
Haemophilus influenzae	Pneumonia
Streptococcus pneumoniae	Pneumonia
Staphylococcus aureus	Pneunomia
Fungi	
Aspergillus	Fungemia, pneumonia
Candida albicans	Thrush, stomatitis, esophagitis, pneumonia
Cryptococcus neoformans	Meningitis, pneumonitis
Histoplasma capsulatum	Pneumonitis, skin lesions
Coccidioides immitis	Pneumonitis
Viruses	
Cytomegalovirus	Esophagitis, pneumonitis, diarrhea
Herpes simplex virus	Ulcerative mucocutaneous lesions, stomatitis, esophagitis, pneumonia
Epstein-Barr	EBV-positive non-Hodgkin's lymphomas, oral hairy leukoplakia
Hepatitis B	Nausea, vomiting, fever, antigenemia
Herpes zoster	Multiple dermatomal zoster
Papillomavirus	Oral hairy leukoplakia

Adapted from Gold, JWM: HIV-1 infection: diagnosis and management, *Med Clin North Am* 76(1):1, 1992; Bernard EM et al: Pneumocystosis, *Med Clin North Am* 76(1):107, 1992; and Ralten, DJ: Nutrition and HIV infection: a review and evaluation of the extent knowledge of the relationship between nutrition and HIV infection, *Nutr Clin Prac* 6(3):1S, 1991.

Diagnosis of HIV Infection

Testing Procedures

HIV infection is diagnosed by detection of the virus or serologic response to the virus. HIV infection can be identified by detection of specific antibodies, as done in the routine screening of blood and blood products for transfusion and in most epidemiologic studies. The recommended procedure for virus detection is a two-step process.[1] The first is *enzyme-linked immunosorbent assay (ELISA)* screening. Second, suspected positive samples from the ELISA screening are followed by *Western blot* testing for confirmation. Both of these tests are highly sensitive and specific, and both are used to confirm the results before informing the individual. Because a positive test is such a personal and life-changing event, most experienced physicians caring for HIV infected patients repeat all positive tests again, even when they have been confirmed by Western blot, before informing the individual. Requirements for the testing procedure include pretest and posttest counseling to cover such issues as[1,25]:

> **retrovirus** • Any of a family of single-strand RNA viruses having an envelope and containing a reverse coding enzyme that allows for a reversal of genetic transcription from RNA to DNA rather than the usual DNA to RNA, the newly transcribed viral DNA then being incorporated into the host cell's DNA strand for the production of new RNA retroviruses.

- **Medical significance** of the test, whether positive or negative
- **Limitations** of the test
- **Information** about HIV-1 and AIDS, how they are spread, and how to prevent their spread
- **Medical, nutritional, and psychosocial care** availability
- **Confidentiality** concept involved with documentation in the medical record; possible social and legal results of testing, personal needs and support system

Clinical Symptoms and Illnesses

The early clinical symptoms that may follow initial exposure to the virus add further confirmation to the HIV-seropositive testing procedures. These initial symptoms, as well as possible associated illnesses and diseases that characterize the later ARC and AIDS stages, have been generally described earlier in discussing the basic disease progression. Some examples of these common infectious complications of AIDS and their clinical problems are listed in Table 24-1.

Basic Role of Nutrition in HIV Disease Process

Nutrition support plays a vital role throughout the HIV disease process in two basic areas. First, it is a vital component of care for the involuntary weight loss and body tissue wasting caused by the disease effects on metabolism, reflected in the severe state of protein-energy malnutrition. Second, and fundamental in all conditions associated with the body's basic immune system (see extended discussion in Chapter 25), nutrition is an intimate and integral component of care through the specific roles of key nutrients in maintaining the body's immunocompetence. Furthermore, for many of the associated diseases, individual nutritional status influences the impact of morbidity and mortality irrespective of the disease process.[26]

Medical Management
Basic Current Goals

The medical management of HIV-1 infection in all its stages is constantly evolving as medical research seeks to eliminate, or at least suppress, the virus. Intensive current research is aimed at preventing the progressive immunodeficiency, stopping HIV-1 transmission to uninfected persons, and restoring depressed immune function to normal to prevent AIDS-associated complications. Thus, present basic medical management objectives are to (1) delay progression of the infection and improve the patient's immune system; (2) prevent opportunistic illnesses; and (3) recognize the infection early and provide rapid treatment for any complications of immune deficiency, including infections and cancers.

Initial Evaluation: AIDS Team

The initial medical evaluation of a newly diagnosed HIV infected patient is critial in beginning and continuing the ongoing comprehensive care by the AIDS team of professional medical, nutritional, nursing, and psychosocial health care specialists. Table 24-2 outlines an initial evaluation guide for beginning the care of a person with newly identified HIV-1 infection. These guidelines emphasize the special coordinated care by all members of the AIDS team, and the importance of personal nutritional and psychosocial support.

Antiretroviral Drug Therapy

After the initial discovery and identification of HIV-1, research began in earnest to develop effective antiretroviral drugs to inhibit replication of the virus. However, the problems involved are complex, and the task has been frustrating. One of the earliest findings in this drug research effort was that certain members of a class of compounds called **dideoxynucleosides** effectively inhibited HIV-1 replication in the laboratory.[27] Subsequent clinical trials with HIV-infected patients have shown that in human cells, dideoxynucleosides act as competitive inhibitors of the virus's necessary enzyme for replicating itself, *HIV reverse transcriptase*, thus effectively preventing viral increase. The first drug in this class to be used in clinical trials, azidothymidine (AZT), or zidovudine, is currently the only antiretroviral drug thus far to be approved by the FDA. Several others, including dideoxyinosine (ddI), dideoxycytidine (ddC),

---

TABLE 24-2

Initial Evaluation of Newly Diagnosed HIV-Infected Patients

Routine history and physical examination include:
  History of exposure to infectious complications of AIDS
  Assessment of baseline mental status
Baseline laboratory studies
  CBC, differential, platelets
  Biochemistry screening profile
  Urinalysis
  Chest x-ray
  Tuberculin test with anergy panel
  Serologic test for syphilis
  Toxoplasma serology
  T-lymphocyte subsets
  Hepatitis B serology (optional)
Nutritional assessment, counseling, support, and follow-up
Psychosocial and financial status assessment
Referral to and involvement in psychosocial support include:
  Social worker, nurse, psychologist or psychiatrist, patient support group, community support group, and agencies
Rehabilitation program for substance abusers
Planning for family members and children, including issues of testing and providing for their care.

Adapted from Gold, JWM: HIV-1 infection: diagnosis and management, *Med Clin North Am* 76(1):1, 1992.

dideoxythymidinene/didehydrothymidine (d4T), and azidodideoxyuridine (AZdU), are in the preliminary stages of clinical trials.[27] However, toxic side effects of these drugs, as shown in Table 24-3, have created problems requiring additional attention. Some side effects, such as nausea, may be helped by diet modifications (see Chapter 25).

AZT's results in patient therapy have been found to diminish over time as the virus, confronted by the drug, readily mutates into slight variations out of the drug's range, making the virus slightly less efficient with each mutation. However, researchers are studying ways of using combinations of these drugs to achieve effective results over longer periods. As knowledge about the biochemistry and molecular biology of HIV-1 and HIV-2 increases, agents are being developed that are targeted at blocking specific steps in the replicating life-cycle of HIV. At the same time, these agents are less suppressive of the bone marrow and create fewer side effects.[27]

Continuing Research and Future Developments

Continuing research for a long-awaited vaccine against HIV is nearing the stage of international trials. Though it has been a bumpy road with some rough spots still ahead, organizations of researchers and policy makers, as well as involved drug companies, indicate that sites are being selected in representative epidemic areas such as central Africa, Southeast Asia, Brazil, and the United States, with clinical trials probably ready to start about 1995.[28,29] The central question seems no longer to be "Can we make a vaccine that works?" but rather "How do we speed up the process?"[29]

Undoubtedly the epidemiology and treatment of HIV-1 infection will change rapidly over the next few years. Patients will live longer and have improved quality of life. Nonetheless, with longer life and treatment for known complications, new complications probably will appear, such as uncommon infections, neurologic disease, or wasting syndromes.[1] The medical management of AIDS will continue to require highly involved health care professionals amd patients.

Nutritional Management

Basic Approach: Individual Status and Needs

Although answers will soon come to many of our puzzling questions, HIV infection is still an elusive, epidemic, terminal disease, and its treatment varies according to individual status and needs—medical, nutritional, and psychosocial. Research breakthroughs will help light the course, but in every case, health care professionals and patients must remain highly involved, seeking the best possible individual care each step of the way.

There are many causes of malnutrition in HIV infection. Thus, at any point, nutritional recommendations and support must be individual and integrated with other therapies. Nutritional care plans must provide a comprehensive view of the disease process through each stage, specific drug use, and the patient's wishes. All patients diagnosed as HIV infected should be considered to be at nutritional risk. Although the patient

---

TABLE 24-3

Toxicities of Dideoxynucleoside Drugs

AZT (azidothymidine, zidovudine, 3'-azido-2', 3'-dideoxythymidline)

Bone marrow suppression. Anemia with increased mean corpuscular volume. Leukopenia and thrombocytopenia often dose-limiting
Nausea and vomiting
Headache
Malaise, fatigue, fever
Myalgias
Seizures (rare, but reported to be fatal)
Confusion, tremulousness
Wernicke's-like encephalopathy
Bluish pigmentation of finger and toenails
Hepatic transaminase elevation
Stevens-Johnson syndrome

ddl (dideoxyinosine,2',3'-dideoxyinosine)

Painful peripheral neuropathy
Sporadic pancreatitis (may be fatal)
Hyperamylasemia, hypertriglyceridemia
Headache
Insomnia, restlessness
Hepatic transaminase elevations (occasional hepatitis)
Hyperuricemia (with high doses)

ddC (dideoxycytidine,2',3'-dideoxycytidine)

Painful peripheral neuropathy
Aphthous stomatitis
Maculopapular rash (occasionally pseudovesicular)
Fevers
Arthralgias, edema
Thrombocytopenia

d4T (2',3'-dideoxythymidinene, 2',3'-dideoxy-2',3'-didehydrothymidine)

Painful peripheral neuropathy
Anemia
Hepatic transaminase elevations

Adapted from Pluda, JM et al: Hematologic effects of AIDS therapies, *Hematology/Oncology Clin North Am* 5(2):229, 1991.

---

dideoxynucleosides • Nucleoside, basic type of chemical compound involved. A class of drugs used to treat HIV-infected persons; a nucleoside is a combination of a sugar (a pentose) with a purine or pyrimidine (two types of compounds that provide the cross-linking "ladders" of the double strands of DNA) base.

may be in an earlier, asymptomatic period, the disease process, its complications, or treatments will begin to take a toll on the person's nutritional status. The nutritional status of any HIV-infected person may be compromised in numerous ways. At all times, each patient must be viewed within the context of his or her own disease and individual life-style.

Wasting Effects of HIV Infection on Nutritional Status

Severe Malnutrition and Weight Loss

A fundamental effect of HIV infection is major weight loss, which eventually leads to extreme cachexia similar to that observed in cancer patients (Chapter 25). Such serious weight loss was recognized in the CDC classification of body weight loss over 10% of usual weight, with more than 30 days of constitutional symptoms in an HIV-positive person, as a primary diagnosis of AIDS.[30] This serious, characteristic body wasting resulting from HIV infection also becomes a cofactor in the development of the full disease syndrome in infected persons, as the malnutrition itself suppresses cellular immune function. So striking is this chronic, relentless body wasting of AIDS, that in Africa it has been named "slim disease."[31] Body wasting in AIDS is characterized by loss of body cell mass, primarily muscle protein; death occurs when body weight reaches two thirds and body cell mass reaches half of normal values.[32] This designation implies that death may be more often due to malnutrition, specifically negative nitrogen balance, than to the direct effects of infection or malignancy.[33] Also, the attendant diseases of the wasting process play a major role in the decreased quality of life, debilitating weakness, and fatigue seen in AIDS patients.

Causes of Body Wasting

The characteristic body wasting of HIV infection may be due to any of the following processes, alone or combined[33]:

- **Inadequate food intake.** Both clinicians and AIDS patients indicate, from their combined clinical observations and personal experience, that an important factor in the profound weight loss is severe *anorexia*. This state is probably related to both the patient's personal life-changing situation and the body's physiologic changes from the disease. Recently, encouraging results have come with the use of the drug megesterol acetate (Megase), a synthetic hormone similar to the natural hormone progesterone, which improves appetite and food intake, leading to weight gain.[34] Anorexia and its resulting decreased food intake, insufficient to meet body needs, clearly contributes to the body wasting.
- **Malabsorption of nutrients.** From early reports, as

well as continuing clinical experience, diarrhea and malabsorption have been common in AIDS patients. These malabsorptive symptoms have been related to both drug-diet interactions and progressive effects of HIV infection. An "AIDS enteropathy" in the early stages of infection has been described, characterized by blunting of the intestinal villi, abnormal intestinal enzymes that cause clinical malabsorption, and HIV infection of infiltrating lymphocytes as well as enterocytes.[35,36] In later stages the intestine is infected more frequently with opportunistic organisms, resulting in severe diarrhea and malabsorption.
- **Disordered metabolism.** In the final stage of weight loss in AIDS patients, changes in metabolism occur, including hypermetabolism and altered energy metabolism, usually associated with end-stage effects of the HIV infection as well as increased spread of opportunistic infections. There is progressive depletion of lean body mass as well as increased resting energy expenditure.

Nutrition Assessment

The initial nutrition assessment must be comprehensive to provide the baseline information necessary for beginning and continuing nutritional care. Table 24-4 provides guidelines for calculating daily kcalories and protein needs, assessing weight changes, and evaluating biochemical data. The calculations and evaluations are required especially for selected patients on special nutritional support therapies, enteral or parenteral.[37] Further person-centered nutritional care required for all HIV-infected patients is evident in the ABCDs of nutrition assessment outlined in the Clinical Application, p. 478. This type of detailed initial nutrition interview includes investigation of the patient's medical history, physical and anthropometric data, biochemical indices, medications, living situation, dietary intake, general socioeconomic status, and assistance needs. All patients, at first contact with a health professional, should be referred to the AIDS team clinical dietitian for screening to evaluate the degree of any nutrition problems. This clinical nutrition specialist, together with the patient, can then develop a continuing plan for ongoing nutritional care and support.

Nutrition Intervention

Experienced clinical dietitians working with AIDS patients build nutrition care plans with each client or patient for appropriate nutrition intervention and guidance.[38] This planning is continually adjusted as needed according to the disease progression and personal needs. It focuses on identifying food-nutrient problems, developing a plan of action for each problem, and outlining the form of nutrition support needed. Suggested guidelines for developing such patient-

TABLE 24-4

Outline of Nutritional Assessment in Persons with HIV Infection and AIDS

I. Estimated daily kcalorie and protein requirements for adults
   A. Kilocalories (total kcal)
                 Male/female: 35-40 kcal/kg
   B. Protein (g)
                 Male/female: 2.0-2.5 g/kg

II. Calculated daily kcalorie and protein requirements for adults
   A. Kilocalories (total kcal) for weight maintenance

$$Male = (66.5 + (13.7 \times wt\ [kg]) + (5 \times ht\ [cm]) - (6.7 \times age\ [yr])) \times AF^* \times IF\dagger + 500\ kcal$$
$$Female = (665.1 + (9.6 \times wt\ [kg]) + (1.8 \times ht\ [cm]) - (4.7 \times age\ [yr])) \times AF^* \times IF\dagger + 500\ kcal$$

   NOTE: Add 500 kcal to the equations above for weight gain.

   B. Protein (g):

$$Male/female = Total\ kcal \times \frac{g\ nitrogen}{150\ kcal} \times \frac{6.25\ g\ protein}{g\ nitrogen}$$

III. Nutritional assessment parameters

	Extent of malnutrition		
	Mild	**Moderate‡**	**Severe‡**
Albumin (g/dL)	2.8-3.2	2.1-2.7	<2.1
Transferrin (mg/dL)	150-200	100-150	<100
Total lymphocyte count (cells/mm³)	1200-2000	800-1200	<800
Creatinine-height index (%) (actual/ideal × 100)	60-80	40-60	<40
Ideal body weight (%)	80-90	70-80	<70
Usual body weight (%)	85-95	75-85	<75
Weight loss/unit time	<5%/mo	<2%/wk	>2%/wk
	<7.5%/3 mo	>5%/mo	
	<10%/6 mo	>7.5%/3 mo	
		>10%/6 mo	
Skin tests (no. reactive/no. placed)	4/4 (Normal)	1-2/4 (Weak)	0/4 (Anergic)
Anthropometry	Normal male	Normal female	
Triceps skinfold (mm)	12.5	16.5	
Mid-arm circumference (cm)	29.3	28.5	

Adapted from Hickey, MS: Nutritional support of patients with AIDS, *Surg Clin North Am* 71(3):645, 1991.
*Activity factors (AF): Confined to bed = 1.2, ambulatory = 1.3, fever factor = 1.13/°C>37.
†Injury factor (IF): Surgery = 1.1-1.2, infection = 1.2-1.6, trauma = 1.1-1.8, sepsis = 1.4-1.8.
‡Nutritional therapy indicated.

centered care plans are outlined in Table 24-5. For persons receiving nutrition support in special enteral or parenteral forms, the dietitian will work with other members of the nutrition support team to develop an appropriate formula and feeding mode, using oral or tube-fed enteral means or intravenous feeding by peripheral or central veins (see Chapter 18).

Nutrition Counseling, Education, and Supportive Strategies

Counseling Principles

An adolescent client once aptly defined a counselor as "someone to talk to while I make up my mind." Client-centered counseling in the care of persons with HIV infection must be just that. Professionals and patients must remain involved throughout the progressive course of the disease because the patient's wishes and needs are ultimately paramount in various treatments and decisions about care. The basic goal of nutrition counseling is to make the fewest possible changes in the person's life-style and food patterns necessary to promote optimal nutritional status while providing maximum comfort and quality of life.[38,39] In this person-centered care process, several counseling principles are particularly pertinent:

- **Motivation.** Changed behavior in any area requires the motivation, desire, and ability to achieve one's goals. Until the patient perceives food patterns and behaviors as appropriate goals, it is best to wait for a better time and begin with establishing a general

CLINICAL APPLICATION

The ABCDs of Nutrition Assessment in AIDS Patients

The initial nutrition assessment visit with an HIV-infected patient is an important beginning point for the continuing nutritional care that is to follow. This encounter serves both informational and relational functions. It provides the necessary baseline information for planning practical individual nutrition support. But more importantly, it establishes the essential provider-patient relationship, the very human context within which this continuing nutritional care and support will be provided as needed. The basic ABCDs of nutrition assessment will provide a practical guide (see Chapter 16), with special EFs added for HIV infection patients.

Anthropometry

- Age, sex, height
- Weight: current, usual, percent of usual, ideal, percent of ideal, weight loss over defined period
- Mid-upper-arm measures: circumference, triceps skinfold thickness; calculated mid-arm muscle circumference

Biochemical indices

- Serum proteins: albumin, prealbumin, transferrin
- Liver function test (evaluate liver function)
- Blood urea nitrogen, serum electrolytes (evaluate renal function)
- Urinary urea nitrogen excretion over 24 hours (nitrogen balance)
- Creatinine height index
- Complete blood count (evaluate for anemia)
- Fasting glucose (evaluate for hyperglycemia or hypoglycemia)

Clinical observations

- General signs of nutritional status (Table 19-2)
- Drug effects

Diet evaluation

- Usual intake, current intake, restrictions, modifications (use 24-hour recall and food diaries)
- Nutrition supplements, vitamin-mineral supplements

- Food allergies, intolerances
- Activity level (average number of kcalories expended per day)
- Support system (caregivers to help with nutrition care plan)

Environmental, behavioral, and psychologic assessment

- Living situation, personal support
- Food environment, types of meals, eating assistance needs

Financial assessment

- Medical insurance
- Income, financial support through caregivers
- Current medical and other expenses
- Ability to afford food, enteral supplements, added vitamins and minerals

REFERENCES

Ghiron L and others: Nutrition support of the HIV-positive, ARC, and AIDS patient, *Clin Nutr* 8(3):103, 1989.

Trujillo EB and others: Assessment of nutritional status, nutrient intake, and nutrition support in AIDS patients, *J Am Diet Assoc* 92(4):477, 1992. ◆

---

supportive climate in which to continue working together. Any specific obstacle raised by the patient, such as time, physical limitations, money, or increased anxiety, can be met with related suggestions to think about. Priorities among needs should be recognized in the care plan, and items should be introduced according to order of importance and immediacy of the patient's nutritional problems.

- **Rationale.** Any diet or food behavior change, with possible benefits and risks, must be clearly explained to the patient. The question "Why?" is always important to everybody.
- **Provider-patient agreement.** In the best interests of all concerned, the patient and health care provider must agree to the change. Any change should be structured around daily routines and should include any caregivers as needed. The nutrition counselor should provide any needed information and encouragement throughout the process.
- **Manageable steps.** All information given and actions agreed upon should proceed in manageable steps, as small as necessary, in order of complexity

and difficulty. Information overload can discourage anyone. But here the particular stress load at any point can be intolerable for the patient. At such points of stress, patients are also more vulnerable to the lure of unproven HIV therapies (see To Probe Further, p. 480).

Personal Food Management Skills

The patient's living situation and general practical skills in planning, purchasing, and preparing food must be considered. Any need for information and guidance in developing skills in any aspect of procuring food, or in sources of needed help, should be provided.

Community Programs

Information may be needed about any available community food programs, such as Meals-on-Wheels, for delivery of prepared meals when the patient is too ill to shop for or prepare food. Also, information may need to be provided about food assistance programs such as Food Stamps or Food Commodities (see Chapter 10), for which the lower income person may qualify.

TABLE 24-5

Planning Nutrition Care for Patients With AIDS

Type of problem	Possible causes	Patient care plan considerations
Food intake		
	Anorexia	Patient, caregiver roles
	Drug, food interaction	Motivation, patient decision making
	HIV, other infection	Education, counseling
	Taste alteration	Resource materials
	Food intolerances, allergies	Nutrition supplements
	Lack of access or ability to prepare food	Vitamin, mineral supplements
	Depression	Drug-food reactions
		Special enteral-parenteral nutrition support
		Monitoring, adjustments as needed
Nutrient absorption		
	HIV-related infections or cancers	Treatment of underlying disease or disorder
	Diminished gastric HCl secretion	Pancreatic enzymes supplement
	Altered mucosal absorbing surface	Drug-nutrient reactions
	Organ involvement; liver, pancreas, gallbladder, kidney	Special enteral-parenteral nutrition support, appropriate formula design
	Drug-nutrient interaction	Monitoring, adjustments as needed
Altered metabolism, excretion		
	HIV infection	Review of drug dosage, schedule
	Associated infections, diseases	Modification of diet, meal pattern
	Drug-nutrient interactions	Treatment of infection, symptoms
	Altered hormonal function	Review of diet nutrients, increase or decrease
	Organ dysfunction	Special enteral-parenteral nutrition support, appropriate formula design
		Monitoring, adjustments as needed

Adapted from Newman CF: *Practical guidelines for improving nutritional status in HIV-related disease,* University of California, Davis Medical School Fifth Annual Conference on Clinical Nutrition, Nutrition in the Treatment of Serious Medical Problems, Feb 28-29, 1992.

Psychosocial Support

In the last analysis, every aspect of care provided should be given within a form and context that also provides genuine psychosocial support. All health care providers working with HIV-infected patients must be particularly sensitive to the special psychologic and social issues that confront persons with AIDS. Major stress areas may include issues relating to autonomy and dependency, a sense of uncertainty and fear of the unknown, grief, change and loss, fear of symptoms, fear of abandonment, and spiritual questions that arise when someone confronts a life-threating illness.[39,40] Common emotions are hostility, denial, withdrawal, depression, anxiety, guilt, and confusion. All of these may significantly influence treatment at some time. Health care providers must always be aware and assess how the patient and caregivers are relating to the disease, using assistance of social workers, clinical psychologists, or psychiatrists as needed.[41,42] Stress-reduction groups, including exercise training, are helpful, as they have proved to be in other life-threatening situations such as cancer and coronary heart disease.[43]

Most of all, however, health care workers must examine their own values and fears regarding sexual orientation, sexual behavior, intravenous drug use, and fears of AIDS transmission. Preconceived judgments are easily picked up by patients and threaten the provider-patient relationship. Before they can be effective with patients, all health care workers must first deal with their own fears and prejudices and learn to let go of such judgmental behavior.

To Sum Up

The viral evolution and current worldwide spread of human immunodeficiency virus (HIV) infection has reached epidemic proportions and is still growing. The overall disease progression follows three distinct stages of HIV infection, ARC with associated opportunistic illnesses, and full-blown AIDS with complicating diseases leading to death. The progression from initial infection to death lasts about 10 to 12 years. The Public Health Service and the CDC have responsibilities for monitoring the disease and providing leadership in research and treatment development, through collaborative information exchange with scientists worldwide.

During the initial decade of the epidemic (the 1980s), scientists learned about the nature and life-cycle of the new mutation of HIV, its transmission modes, and population groups at risk. Development of diagnostic testing procedures has enabled population surveillance and individual detection of disease and personal care to proceed. A fundamental role of nutrition support in this personal care of HIV-infected individuals has become evident.

Medical management of HIV infection, as yet without a vaccine or cure, involves supportive treatment of associated illnesses and complicating diseases. In the terminal HIV stage, as the virus eventually gains sufficient strength to destroy the host's immune system white cells, death follows. New drugs to slow the disease progression are being developed.

Nutritional management centers on providing personal individual nutrition support to counteract the severe body wasting and malnutrition characteristic of the disease. The process of nutritional care involves comprehensive nutrition assessment and evaluation of personal needs, planning care with patients and caregivers, and meeting practical food needs. Throughout the care process, nutrition counseling, education, and strategic services also help provide psychosocial support to each patient.

QUESTIONS FOR REVIEW

1. Describe the evolutionary history of HIV-1 and its current worldwide epidemic spread. How is it transmitted, and why do you think it has spread so rapidly? Identify major population groups at risk.
2. Describe the nature of the AIDS virus and its action in the human body. What is a retrovirus?
3. Describe the progression of HIV infection in terms of its three basic stages of development from initial infection to death.
4. Identify some of the drugs currently used in medical management of HIV infection, and describe any associated actions, side effects, or toxicities that may relate to dietary management.
5. Outline basic parts of a comprehensive initial nutrition assessment of a patient with HIV infection, and describe the reasons for each type of information and its evaluation.
6. Describe the general process of planning nutritional care on the basis of the patient assessment information and the main types of nutrition problems in patients with HIV infection. Devise a related plan of action for each type of problem. Give an example of how you might follow up to see what worked or did not work and make adjustments.

REFERENCES

1. Gold JWM: HIV-1 infection, *Med Clin North Am* 76(1):1, 1992.
2. Gorman C: Invincible AIDS, *Time* 140(5):30, Aug 3, 1992.
3. Cowley G: The future of AIDS, *Newsweek* CXXI(12):46, Mar 22, 1993.
4. Palca, J: The sobering geography of AIDS, *Science* 252:372, Apr 19, 1991.
5. Castro KG and others: Perspectives on HIV/AIDS epidemiology and prevention from the Eighth International Conference on AIDS, *Am J Pub Health* 82(11):1465, 1992.
6. Pantaleo G and others: HIV infection is active and progressive in lymphoid tissue during the clinically latent stage of disease, *Nature* 362(6418):355, Mar 25, 1993.
7. Embretson J and others: Massive covert infection of helper T lymphocytes and macrophages by HIV during the incubation period of AIDS, *Nature* 362(6418):359, Mar 25, 1993.
8. Maddox J: Where the virus hides away, *Nature* 362(6418):287, Mar 25, 1993.
9. Cohen J: Keystone's blunt message: "It's the virus, stupid," *Science* 260(5106):292, Apr 16, 1993.
10. Hoover DR and others: The progression of untreated HIV-1 infection prior to AIDS, *Am J Pub Health* 82(11):1538, 1992.
11. Mills J, Masur H: AIDS-related infections, *Sci Am* 263(2):50, 1990.
12. Buehler JW: The surveillance definition for AIDS, *Am J Pub Health* 82(11):1462, 1992.
13. Otten MW and others: Changes in sexually transmitted disease rates after HIV testing and posttest counseling, Miami, 1988 to 1989, *Am J Pub Health* 83(4):529, 1993.
14. Onorato IM and others: Sentinel surveillance for HIV-2 infection in high-risk US populations, *Am J Pub Health* 83(4):515, 1993.
15. US Department of Health and Human Services, Public Health Service: Healthy People 2000: *National health promotion and disease prevention objectives*, DHHS Pub No (PHS) 91-50212, Washington, DC, 1991, US Government Printing Office.
16. Wickizer TM and others: Activating communities for health promotion: a process evaluation method, *Am J Pub Health* 83(4):561, 1993.
17. Ehrhardt AA: Trends in sexual behavior and the HIV pandemic, *Am J Pub Health* 82(11):1459, 1992.
18. Weiss SH: HIV infection and the health care worker, *Med Clin North Am* 76(1):269, 1992.
19. Pizzo PA, Butler KM: In the vertical transmission of HIV, timing may be everything, *N Engl J Med* 325(9):652, Aug 29, 1991.
20. Glebatis DM and others: Hospitalization of HIV-seropositive newborns with AIDS-related disease within the first year of life, *Am J Pub Health* 81(suppl):46, 1991.
21. Stricof RL and others: HIV seroprevalence in clients of

sentinel family planning clinics, *Am J Pub Health* 81(suppl):41, 1991.

22. Catania JA and others: Condom use in multi-ethnic neighborhoods of San Francisco: the population-based AMEN (AIDS in multi-ethnic neighborhoods) Study, *Am J Pub Health* 82:284, 1992.

23. Roper WL and others: Condoms and HIV/STD prevention: clarifying the message, *Am J Pub Health* 83(4):501, 1993.

24. Gollub EL, Stein ZA: The new female condom: item 1 on a woman's AIDS prevention agenda, *Am J Pub Health* 83(4):498, 1993.

25. New York Statewide Professional Standards Review Council: HIV testing policy. In *Criteria manual for the treatment of AIDS*, New York, 1990, AIDS Intervention Management System.

26. Raiten DJ: Nutrition and HIV infection: a review and evaluation of the extant knowledge of the relationship between nutrition and HIV infection, *Nutr Clin Prac* 6(3 suppl):13S, 1991.

27. Pluda JM and others: Hematologic effects of AIDS therapies, *Hematol Oncol Clin North Am* 5(2):229, 1991.

28. Cohen J: AIDS vaccine trials: bumpy road ahead, *Science* 251(4999):1312, Mar 15, 1991.

29. Cohen J: AIDS vaccine meeting: international trials soon, *Science* 254(5032):647, Nov 1, 1991.

30. Centers for Disease Control: *Acquired immunodeficiency syndrome weekly surveillance report*, US AIDS Program, Centers for Disease Control, Center for Infectious Diseases, Atlanta, Sept 7, 1987.

31. Serwadda D and others: Slim disease: a new disease in Uganda and its association with HTLV-III infection, *Lancet* 2:849, 1985.

32. Kotler DP and others: Magnitude of body-cell mass depletion and the timing of death from wasting in AIDS, *Am J Clin Nutr* 50:444, 1989.

33. Hellerstein MK and others: Current approach to the treatment of human immunodeficiency virus-associated weight loss: pathophysiologic considerations and emerging mamagement strategies, *Semin Oncol* 17(6, suppl 9):17, 1990.

34. Tchekmedyian NS and others: Treatment of anorexia and weight loss with megesterol acetate in patients with cancer or acquired immunodeficiency syndrome, *Semin Oncol* 18(1, suppl 2):35, 1991.

35. Heise C and others: Human immunodeficiency virus infection of enterocytes and mononuclear cells in human jejunal mucosa, *Gastroenterology* 100:1522, 1991.

36. Greenson JK and others: AIDS enteropathy: occult enteric infections and duodenal mucosal alterations in chronic diarrhea, *Ann Intern Med* 114:366, 1991.

37. Hickey MS: Nutritional support of patients with AIDS, *Surg Clin North Am* 71(3):645, 1991.

38. Newman CF, Capazza CM: Home nutrition support in HIV disease, *J Home Health Care Prac* 3(2):25, 1991.

39. Ghiron L and others: Nutrition support of the HIV-positive, ARC, and AIDS patient, *Clin Nutr* 8(3):103, 1989.

40. Cleary PD and others: Depressive symptoms in blood donors notified of HIV infection, *Am J Pub Health* 83(4):534, 1993.

41. Antoni MH and others: Cognitive-behavioral stress management intervention buffers distress responses and immunologic changes following notification of HIV-1 seropositivity, *J Consult Clin Psychol* 59(6):906, 1991.

42. Jacobsberg LB, Perry S: Psychiatric disturbances, *Med Clin North Am* 76(1):99, 1992.

43. LaPerriere A and others: Aerobic exercise training in an AIDS risk group, *Int J Sports Med* 12(suppl 1):S53, 1991.

FURTHER READING

Charny A, Ludman EK: Treating malnutrition in AIDS: comparison of dietitians' practices and nutrition care guidelines, *J Am Diet Assoc* 91(10):1273, 1991.

McCorkindale C and others: Nutritional status of HIV-infected patients during the early disease stages, *J Am Diet Assoc* 90(9):1236, 1990.

Trujillo EB and others: Assessment of nutritional status, nutrient intake, and nutrition support in AIDS patients, *J Am Diet Assoc* 92(4):477, 1992.

Ysseldyke LL: Nutritional complications and incidence of malnutrition among AIDS patients, *J Am Diet Assoc* 91(2):217, 1991.

These four articles from the *Journal of the American Dietetic Association* provide helpful information and nutritional care guidelines for developing nutritional care plans to meet the complicating factors of malnutrition and opportunistic diseases.

Weaver K: Reversible malnutrition in AIDS, *Am J Nurs* 91(9):25, 1991.

From her experiences as a nurse on the nutrition support team of a leading San Francisco Hospital providing care for many AIDS patients, this author gives practical and sensitive attention to quality-of-life problems inherent in progression of disease in the HIV-infected person.

CASE STUDY

HIV Infection in a Young Mother

Theresa Stevens, age 25, is admitted to the hospital with a history of weight loss, weakness, and watery diarrhea. She is married and has a 3-year-old son. Her husband is in a rehabilitation program for intravenous drug abuse. About a year ago she started to notice that she was becoming easily fatigued, but attributed it to taking care of her 2-year-old child. When her appetite began to wane and her weight dropped from 150 to 90 lb, she went to her physician. In addition to the fatigue and weight loss, she reported fever and night sweats. Physical examination revealed swollen lymph glands, tongue lesions of herpes simplex, and perianal ulcers. Her physician admitted her to the hospital; further tests indicated depressed T cells, and bronchial washings showed the presence of *Pneumocystis carinii* pneumonia. She was tested for HIV infection since *P. carinii* is uncommon in persons with healthy immune systems. Her blood test for HIV infection antibodies was positive.

While in the hospital, she developed symptoms of several infections: anorexia, fever, fatigue, nausea, vomiting, watery diarrhea, perianal ulcers, and rectal incontinence. Her temperature frequently registered 39.4° C (103° F) de-

spite therapy with multiple antibiotics. The volume of diarrhea was measured to be 2500 ml/day, and her vomiting necessitated intravenous hydration. She also began to receive treatment for *P. carinii* pneumonia, esophageal candidiasis, oral and lingual herpes, and *Mycobacterium avium intracellulare* infection of the duodenum.

She did not tolerate a soft diet with nutritional supplements; continued to lose weight; and demonstrated severe anorexia, abdominal cramping, and bloating. Results of the nutritional assessment are as follows:

Height	100.1 cm
Weight	40.9 kg
Body weight	65% of ideal
Body weight	70% of usual
Triceps skinfold	40% of standard
Midarm muscle circumference	72% of standard
Serum albumin	2.2 g/dl
Serum total protein	5.6 g/dl
Serum total iron binding capacity (TIBC)	192 µg/dl
Estimated resting energy expenditure	1750

Questions for Analysis

1. Name and describe several major clinical complications of the final stage of AIDS. How can these complicating diseases profoundly compromise a patient's nutritional status?
2. On the basis of the nutritional assessment, what is this patient's nutritional diagnosis?
3. What should be the goal of nutritional therapy based on the baseline nutritional assessment data and the patient's history?

4. By what route of feeding should nutritional support be administered?

REFERENCE

Rago RR, Feurer ID: Acquired immunodeficiency syndrome (AIDS). In Blackburn GL and others, editors: *Nutritional medicine: a case management approach*, Philadelphia, 1989, WB Saunders.

When diseases such as AIDS lack curative therapy and have poor prognosis, many afflicted persons are susceptible to claims of unproven, alternative therapies, that is, nutrition quackery. Some of the alternative therapies and approaches being touted as treatments for HIV infection include the following questionable practices.

Megadoses of nutrients

Large doses of vitamins A, C, E, B_{12}, selenium, and zinc have been recommended to restore cell-mediated immunity by increasing T-cell number and activity. The value of such large doses has not been established by controlled clinical studies. In fact, the opposite is true; megadoses of these nutrients can be dangerous. Chronic intakes of vitamin A in excess of 50,000 IU/day can produce toxicity. Chronic intakes of excess zinc, as little as 25 mg/day, can cause gastrointestinal distress, nausea, and impaired immune function. Selenium is also toxic in high chronic doses, but the level at which this toxicity occurs is uncertain.

Dr. Berger's immune power diet

In his book, Berger (1985) states that poor health is caused by "immune hypersensitivity" to many foods such as milk, wheat, corn, yeast, soy, sugar, and eggs. He suggests a 21-day elimination diet for foods believed to cause allergies, followed by a reintroduction phase, then a maintenance diet to prevent food sensitivities and "revitalize" the immune system. The usefulness of this diet has not been tested or proven by scientific studies. The diet promoted in Berger's book (high in fruits and vegetables, low in fat and calcium) may produce undernutrition, and the suggestion that moldy food be consumed to test for allergy to molds may be dangerous to immunocompromised persons.

AL 721

AL 721, a compound, developed in Israel and approved by the FDA for clinical trials, is composed of "active lipids" (AL) mixed in a ratio of 70% neutral lipid, 20% lecithin, and 10% phosphatidylethanolamine (hence the 721 designation). It has been hypothesized that 721 can reduce or inhibit HIV infection. Clinical trials found little toxicity but no consistent trends in T-cell quantitation or HIV cultures. Increases in body weight, serum total, high- and low-density lipoprotein cholesterol levels were noted. AL 721 can be made at home from soy or egg-yolk lecithin, or obtained already mixed, but it is of unknown purity and can spoil easily if stored improperly.

Butylated hydroxytoluene (BHT)

Claims that butylated hydroxytoluene (BHT) kills HIV by attacking the "coating" on the virus are unfounded and unproven. The safety of its use is also questionable.

Maximum immunity diet

Any value for megadoses of vitamin C to strengthen the immune system has not been established. Rebound scurvy has occurred on cessation of the megadoses.

TO PROBE FURTHER

Laetrile

When used in combination with a strict vegetarian diet and vitamin supplements, laetrile is supposed to destroy a tumor enzyme (B-glucuronidase). In addition to being proven ineffective, this low-energy diet may supply inadequate amounts of calcium, iron, niacin, vitamin B_{12}, and excessive amounts of thiamin, vitamins A and C, and zinc.

Gerson method

The Gerson program restricts all foods other than oatmeal and uncanned fresh fruits and vegetables and advocates regular enemas (especially coffee enemas) to create an internal environment hostile to malignant cells. Efficacy has not been proven, not to mention the inadequacy of the diet.

Kelley regime

The Kelley regime excludes meat, milk in all forms except yogurt, and peanuts from the diet to overcome supposed pancreatic enzyme deficiency. Almonds are substituted for meat, and nutritional supplements including vitamin and minerals are recommended. Deficiencies of protein and calcium and fluid and electrolyte losses are possible, in addition to possible vitamin A toxicity.

Yeast-free diet

The exclusion of high-carbohydrate and yeast-containing foods is supposed to prevent opportunistic yeast infections such as candidiasis. The underlying theory has been characterized as speculative, and undernutrition may result.

Macrobiotic diet

A macrobiotic diet is based on the oriental philosophy that it will restore balance and harmony between yin and yang forces and thereby improve health. However, it is very low in fat and high in fiber: 50% (by volume) whole grain cereals, 20% to 30% vegetables, 10% to 15% cooked beans or seaweed; 5% miso (fermented soy paste) or tamari broth soup. This regimen can produce protein-kilocalorie malnutrition and provides inadequate intake of riboflavin, niacin, calcium in adults, and pyridoxine, vitamins B_{12} and D in children (in addition to those nutrients mentioned for adults).

It is conceivable that some nutrients and other dietary substances may improve some of the symptoms associated with HIV infection. However, it is still too early in our understanding of the disease process to make recommendations about supplementation. Alternative therapies require further study in controlled clinical trials.

REFERENCES

Dwyer JT and others: Unproven nutrition therapies for AIDS: What is the evidence? *Nutr Today* 23:25, 1988.
Raiten, DJ: Nutrition and HIV infection: a review and evaluation of the extant knowledge of the relationship between nutrition and HIV infection. *Nutr Clin Prac* 6(3):S1, 1991.

Special Consideration for Pediatric Patients with AIDS

Although limited, the available information on pediatric AIDS indicates that malnutrition, particularly undernutrition of kcalories, is a recurring problem. In adults, the disease alone impacts nutrition status, but in children, growth and development add to the impact of disease process.

Nutritional assessments should be performed routinely for pediatric patients with AIDS so any problems can be identified and treated as they occur, and nutritional deficits can be minimized. Assessments should include anthropometry, plasma protein evaluation, complete blood counts, and evaluation of appetite and intake. Eating ability should be determined and the social situation evaluated.

Providing enough kcalories to maintain linear growth and weight gain is sometimes difficult. Increasing protein intake 50% to 100% over the RDA has been recommended. However, needs are individual and should be monitored. Suggestions to provide supplemental caloric and nutrient intake are listed below:

- Use a kcalorie-dense formula (24 to 27 kcal/oz) for infants. Add glucose polymers or medium-chain triglycerides to formulas, or reduce the amount of water added to powdered formulas to boost kcalories.
- Try food supplements that are high in kcalories and protein.
- Add fats such as butter, margarine, or mayonnaise to foods to boost kcalories.
- Encourage nutrient-dense snacks such as raisins, peanuts, or peanut butter.
- For the older, lactose-tolerant child, add skim milk powder to whole milk to boost kcalories and proteins.
- Make adjustments in diet consistency and temperatures to overcome eating difficulties associated with disease complications and any other eating problems.

- For lactose intolerance, which occurs frequently in children with AIDS, use lactose-free, soy-based infant formulas instead of milk.
- Add Lactaid, a commercial preparation of lactose, to milk products to permit improved digestion.
- Use low-lactose dairy foods such as yogurt and mild cheddar cheese, if tolerated.

Vitamin and mineral supplements in amounts one or two times the RDA may offset possible deficits and contribute to meeting increased requirements during hypermetabolic states. Attention should also be given to drug-nutrient interactions and other effects of drugs on nutritional status.

Proper procedures and sanitary formula preparation must be followed for infants being bottle fed. Infants should not be put to bed with a bottle of milk or juice, as these are easily contaminated. Unpasteurized milk and milk products should also be avoided, as they may be a source of Salmonella and other microorganisms that can cause intestinal infections.

Children should never be fed any food directly from a jar, to avoid possible bacterial contamination of the remaining food from the child's mouth. Fruits and vegetables should be peeled or cooked, and meats should be well cooked. All utensils and dishes used should be washed in a dishwasher or in hot, sudsy water and air-dried.

REFERENCES

Bentler M, Stanish M: Nutrition support of the pediatric patient with AIDS, *J Am Diet Assoc* 87:488, 1987.

Berry RK: Home care of the child with AIDS, *Pediatr Nurs* 14:341, 1988.

Carrot Top Nutrition Resources: *Nutrition handbook for AIDS*, Aurora, CO, 1988, Carrot Top Nutrition Resources.

Grossman M: Special problems in the child with AIDS. In Sande MA, Volberding PA, editors: *The medical management of AIDS*, ed 2, Philadelphia, 1990, WB Saunders.

Maring Klug R: AIDS beyond the hospital. II. Children with AIDS, *Am J Nurs* 86:1126, 1986.

Raiten DJ: Nutrition and HIV infection: a review and evaluation of the extant knowledge of the relationship between nutrition and HIV infection, *Nutr Clin Prac* 6(3):S1, 1991.

$\mathscr{C}$HAPTER 25

Nutrition and Cancer

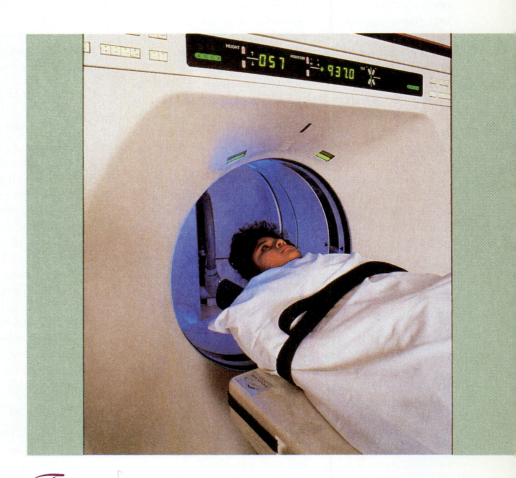

$\mathscr{T}$his chapter focuses on cancer, one of the major diseases in the Western world. We examine the nature of the cancer process and its treatments and seek to relate these processes to the nutritional factors involved.

Here we look at nutrition and cancer in two basic areas: prevention, through the environment and the body's defense system, and therapy, through nutritional support for medical treatment and rehabilitation. To understand these nutritional relationships, we must understand the nature of cancer as a growth process, the physiologic basis of cancer in the structure and function of cells, and the body's defense systems in immunity and in the healing process.

The Process of Cancer Development

Multiple Forms of Cancer

The U.S. Department of Health and Human Services estimates that about 510,000 Americans die of cancer each year, with 30% dying of lung cancer. In its multiple forms, cancer has become one of our major health problems, second only to heart disease, and accounts for about 20% of the total deaths in the United States each year.

Difficulties in the study of cancer have arisen from its varying nature and multiple forms. The word **cancer** is a general term used to designate any one of many malignant tumors or neoplasms (new growths) forming in various body tissue sites. Cancer occurs in many different forms, varying worldwide and changing with population migrations. There are multiple causes and often conflicting research results because of the large number of variables involved. Thus it is clear that we are dealing with a wide range of malignant tumors collectively known as cancer. We would be more correct, then, to use the plural term "cancers" in discussing this great variety of neoplasms.

To better understand cancer development, therefore, we should view it as a growth process that has its physiologic basis in the structure and function of cells. Since nutrition is fundamental to all tissue growth, we need to look briefly at the cancer cell to understand the relationship of nutritional factors to cancer. This "misguided cell" and its tumor tissue represent normal cell growth that has gone wild.

The Cancer Cell

The marvel of human life is that the normal process of cell growth and reproduction goes on almost flawlessly over and over again, guided by the cell's genes. In adult humans some 3 to 4 million cells complete the normal life-sustaining process of cell division every second, largely without mistake, guided by the genetic code. The central question in cell biology has been: How is the process and rate of cell reproduction maintained so precisely in normal cells? The question in cancer research, based on increased knowledge of normal cell physiology, then follows: How and why is this normal, precise regulation of cell reproduction and function lost in cancer cells, and why do cancer cells then remain mutant and malformed, functionally immature and imperfect, incapable of normal cell life?

The first part of the answer lies in the nature of the cell's genetic material and its regulating components. The specific genetic material in the cell's nucleus is arranged as chromosomes and genes, which hold the controlling agent, *deoxyribonucleic acid (DNA)*. Specific sites along the chromosome threads are called genes. Each gene carries specific information that controls synthesis of specific proteins and transmits genetic

heritage. A single chromosome thread is made up of hundreds of genes arranged end to end, and each gene of DNA is made up of some 600 to several thousand smaller subunits called nucleotides. The nucleic acids—DNA and its companion ribonucleic acid (RNA)—compose the controlling system by which both the cell and thus the organism sustain life. The structure of DNA is that of a very large polynucleotide made up of many individual mononucleotides, each one of which has three parts: a sugar (deoxyribose), a phosphate, and a specific nitrogenous base—adenine, cytosine, guanine, or thymine. It is the ladderlike pairing of these nitrogenous bases (Fig. 25-1) that incorporates the genetic code and enables the DNA to transmit messages to guide protein structure. The DNA appears as a twisted ladder or spiral staircase and is thus called a *helix*, the Greek word meaning "coil."

Gene Control of Cell Reproduction and Function

The Normal Cell

Cells arise only from preexisting cells by division and carry the preexisting cell's genetic pattern. Normally the various cell structures and functions operate in an orderly manner under gene control, directing the cell's specific processes of protein synthesis. Gene action, however, may be switched on and off, depending on the position of a cell in the body, the stage of body development, and the external environment. Specific regulator genes control such function by producing a repressor substance as needed to regulate operator genes and structural genes. This orderly regulation of induction and repression in cell activity, however, may be lost with mutation of these regulatory genes. Control also is lost when a specific gene for some reason moves from its position to another location on the chromosome.

The Cancer Cell

A cell may become malignant when one of these potentially cancer-causing genes is translocated and reinserted into a highly active part of the DNA. This has been shown to occur, for example, in patients with Burkitt's lymphoma and the blood cancer, acute nonlymphocytic leukemia. Apparently these root causes of damaged DNA and the cell's impaired ability to repair it are joined by the recently discovered cellular genes called *proto-oncogenes*, which in their developed form of **oncogenes** can cause neoplastic growth. The proliferation of normal cells is regulated by a counter-balance between growth-promoting proto-oncogenes and growth-restraining tumor suppressor genes.[1] This search for genetic damage and the explanation of how that damage affects biochemical function in the cell are key lines of current research that hold much promise for further unfolding the mysteries of cancer.

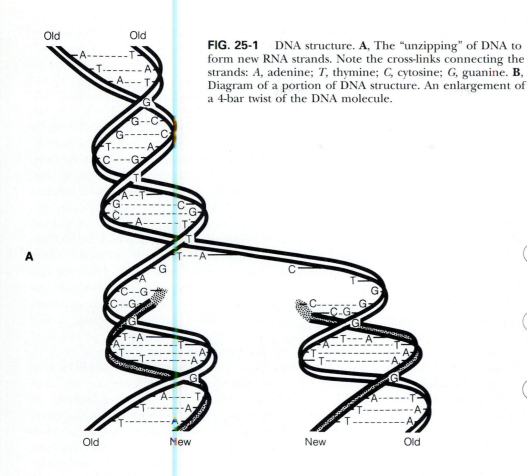

Old   Old

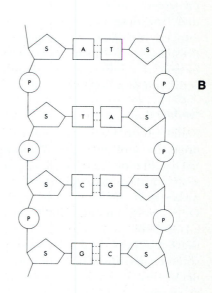

FIG. 25-1   DNA structure. **A,** The "unzipping" of DNA to form new RNA strands. Note the cross-links connecting the strands: *A,* adenine; *T,* thymine; *C,* cytosine; *G,* guanine. **B,** Diagram of a portion of DNA structure. An enlargement of a 4-bar twist of the DNA molecule.

A   B

Old   New   New   Old

Cancer Cell Source

The source of the cancer cell is now clear. It is derived from a normal cell that has lost control over cell reproduction and is thereby transformed from a normal cell into a cancer cell.

Cancer Tumor Types

On this basis of cell nature and differentiation, it is possible to classify cancer tumor types according to (1) the type of originating tissue, with those arising from connective tissues called **sarcomas** and those from epithelial tissues called **carcinomas,** and (2) the extent or degree of cell tissue change, with tumor stages defined in relation to rate of growth, degree of autonomy, and invasiveness.

Relation to the Aging Process

Since the incidence of cancer increases with age, a relationship exists between cancer development and the aging process in cells, tissues, and organ systems.

Causes of Cancer Cell Development

It is thus evident that the basic cause of cancers is the fundamental loss of control over normal cell reproduction. Researchers have discovered several interrelated causes contributing to this loss of cell control.

Mutations

Gene mutations result from loss of one or more regulatory genes in the cell nucleus. Such a mutant gene may be inherited, although some environmental agent may contribute to its expression.

Chemical Carcinogens

A number of chemical carcinogens interfere with the structure or function of regulatory genes. Exposure to such agents may be by individual choice, as in cigarette

---

cancer • A malignant cellular tumor with properties of tissue invasion and spread to other parts of the body.

carcinoma • A malignant new growth made up of epithelial cells, infiltrating the surrounding tissue and spreading to other parts of the body.

oncogene • Any of various genes that, when activated as by radiation or a virus, may cause a normal cell to become cancerous; viral genetic material carrying the potential of cancer and passed from parent to offspring.

sarcoma • A tumor, usually malignant, arising from connective tissue.

smoking, or by exposure to general environmental substances, such as pesticide residues, water and air pollutants, food additives and contaminants, and occupational hazards. However, many of our natural environmental agents can carry more hazards, depending on the dose.[2] For example, a weak carcinogen such as saccharine may be a potential hazard when consumed in relatively large amounts, whereas a potent workplace carcinogen may pose little hazard to a worker who is protected and receives little exposure.[3] The principle that "the dose makes the poison" applies to all substances, including carcinogens, natural or synthetic. Possible cancer-causing actions of such substances may be mutation, effect on regulation of gene function, or activation of a dormant virus.

Radiation

Radiation that is sufficient to damage DNA causes breakage and incorrect rejoining of chromosomes. Such radiation damage may be ionizing, such as from x-rays, radioactive materials, or atomic exhausts or wastes, or it may be nonionizing, such as from sunlight. Our current pursuit of the bronzed-god look has taken a large toll: sun-related skin cancer has risen rapidly in the United States and Europe, afflicting younger and younger persons. The common form on the head and neck is usually basal cell carcinoma and is easily treated by surgical removal. However, a far more lethal form, **malignant melanoma,** occurs in the skin cells that produce the pigment *melanin* and accounts for about 2% of all cancers. In the United States the incidence varies with latitude, from 22,500 cases per year in northern states to 65,000 cases in southern states. The currently rising incidence is probably due to increased exposure to sunlight. The mortality rate is about 45%.

Oncogenic Viruses

Oncogenic, or tumor-producing, viruses that interfere with the function of the regulatory genes have been identified. Oncogenes involved are the focus of much current research related to cell growth factors and possible new therapies for blocking tumor cell growth.[1,4,5] Although oncogenes were first found in viruses, their evolutionary history indicates that they are also present and functioning in normal vertebrate cells. It is their abnormal expression that can lead to cancerous growth. A virus is little more than a packet of genetic information encased in a protein coat (see Chapter 24). It contains a small chromosome, DNA or RNA, with a relatively small number of genes, usually fewer than five and never more than several hundred. In contrast, cells of complex organisms have tens of thousands of genes. Generally, when viruses produce disease, they act as parasites, taking over the cell machinery to replicate themselves. Continuing study indicates that viruses must be thought of as the second most important

risk factor for cancer development, exceeded only by tobacco use.[6]

Epidemiologic Factors

Studies of cancer distribution and occurrence in relation to such factors as race, diet, region, sex, age, heredity, and occupation show variable and conflicting results. It is becoming increasingly clear, for example, that racial differences in cancer incidence between blacks and whites in the United States are great, with more cancer among blacks than whites. However, it is also clear that these differences have nothing to do with race but have much to do with poverty, which has implications for nutritional status, health care, education, and resources.[7,8] The world incidence of cancer varies a great deal from country to country, and specific cancer types vary from sixfold to three hundredfold. Although our cancer rates have not changed markedly over the past few decades, cancer is *endemic* in our population. The U.S. incidence rates are appreciably greater than those in many other countries. Also, racial incidence of cancer seems to change as population groups migrate and aquire the different cancer characteristics of the new population. Although specific dietary factors have been hard to pinpoint in the cause of cancer, worldwide studies do show significant correlation of mortality from breast cancer, for example, with the consumption of fat in the diet. Overall epidemiologic evidence from case-control studies provides a basis for a primary prevention approach for reducing cancer risks (see Issues and Answers, p. 501).[9,10]

Stress Factors

The idea that emotions may play a part in malignancy is not new. Galen, a second century Greek physician, wrote of such relationships, as did many different kinds of "healers" since that time. However, these relationships are difficult to measure. Even with great technologic and scientific advances, Western medicine holds fast to its basic tenet that a thing must be measurable under controlled conditions to be said to exist.

Nonetheless, more observations are being made of relationships between cancer and less measurable factors of stress. Clinicians and researchers have reported that psychic trauma, especially the loss of a central personal relationship, seems to carry with it a strong cancer correlation. The cause of a possible relationship between such trauma and cancer may lie in two physiologic areas: (1) damage to the thymus gland and the immune system, and (2) neuroendocrine effects mediated through the hypothalamus, pituitary, and adrenal cortex. This automatic cascade of physiologic events triggered by stress (see Chapter 15) may well provide the neurologic currency that converts anxiety to malignancy. Such a stressful state may also make a person more vulnerable to other factors present, influencing

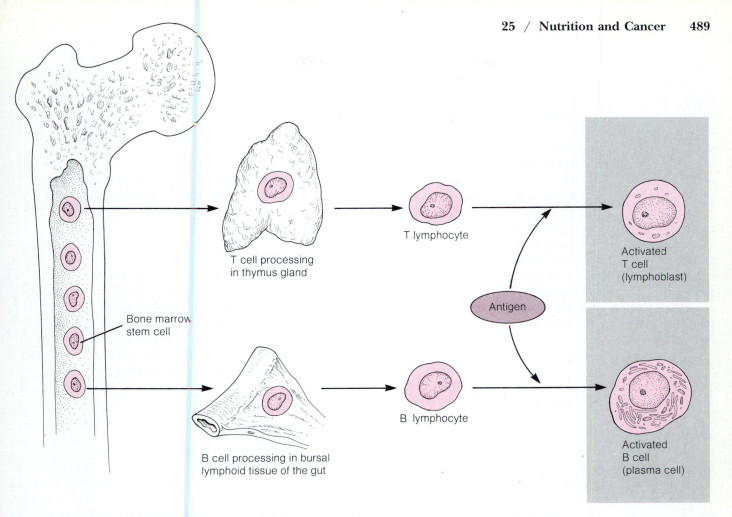

FIG. 25-2   Development of the T and B cells, lymphocyte components of the body's immune system.

the integrity of the immune system, food behaviors, and nutritional status. It may also act as an environmental agent whose physiologic impact stimulates the expression of an underlying mutant or damaged gene.

The Body's Defense System

Components of the Immune System

The human body's defense system is remarkably efficient and complex. Several components of special type cells protect not only against external invaders such as bacteria and viruses but also against internal "aliens" such as malignant tumor cells. These malignant cells from developing tumors in the body can spread invading cells to other body tissues and form secondary tumors, or *metastases*, that become life threatening.[11]

Two major populations of cells provide the immune system's primary line of defense for detecting and destroying malignant cells that arise daily in the body. These cells mediate specific cellular immunity and humoral immunity and provide supportive backup biologic systems. These two populations of lymphoid cells,

or *lymphocytes* (a type of white blood cell), develop early in life from a common stem cell in fetal liver and bone marrow (Fig. 25-2). They then differentiate and populate the peripheral lymphoid organs during the latter stages of gestation. One type are *T cells*, traced from the thymus-derived cells, and the other *B cells*, traced from bursa-derived cells. Both T and B lymphocytes are derived from precursor cells in the bone marrow.

T Cells

After precursor cells migrate to the thymus, the T-cell population is differentiated in this small gland, which lies posterior to the sternum and anterior to the great vessels partly covering the trachea. The majority of the

malignant melanoma · A tumor tending to become progressively worse, composed of melanin (the dark pigment of the skin and other body tissues), usually arising from the skin and aggravated by excessive sun exposure.

circulating small lymphocytes in blood, lymph, and certain areas of the lymph nodes and spleen are T cells. These cells recognize invading antigens by means of specific specialized receptors on their surfaces. When T cells meet an *antigen*—a foreign intruder, a "nonself," or alien substance such as abnormal cancer cells—they proliferate and initiate specific cellular immune responses: (1) They activate the *phagocytes* (special cells that have intracellular killing and degrading mechanisms for destroying invaders), and (2) they cause an inflammatory response through chemical mediators released by the antigen-stimulated T cells. Scientists have now discovered that some T lymphocytes can do even more, not only proliferating in response to an antigen but also attacking it. These special T cells are called "helper cell-independent cytotoxic T lymphocytes," abbreviated more graphically to the name *HIT cells.*

B Cells

The B-cell population matures first in the bone marrow and then, following migration, in the solid peripheral lymphoid tissues of the body: the lymph nodes, spleen, and gut. These cells are responsible for synthesis and secretion of specialized protein known as antibodies. When the B cells contact an antigen, they increase and initiate specific humoral immune responses: (1) They produce specific antibodies or immunoglobulins in the blood, and (2) they produce a particular antibody secretion, immunoglobulin A, in the bowel and upper respiratory mucosa. This combination of antigen and antibody then activates the *complement system,* which attracts phagocytes and initiates the inflammatory response for healing.

Relation to Nutrition
Immune System

Integrity of the body's immune system components requires nutritional support. Severely malnourished persons show changes in the structure and function of the immune system with atrophy of the liver, bowel wall, bone marrow, spleen, and lymphoid tissue.[12,13] Clearly, sound nutrition maintains normal immunity and combats sustained attacks in malignancy.

The Healing Process

Tissue integrity, essential for the healing process, is maintained through protein synthesis. Such strength of tissue is a front line of the body's defense system. This process of healing requires optimal nutritional intake to support (1) cell function and structure of all its parts involving DNA, RNA, amino acids, and proteins, and (2) integrity of all the immune system components. Recent studies in *nutritional immunology* show that wise and early use of vigorous nutritional support for cancer patients provides recovery of normal nutritional status, including immunocompetence, thereby improving

patient response to therapy and prognosis.[12] States of malnutrition, especially alcohol induced, create a high risk of nutritional immunosuppression.[14]

Nutritional Support for Cancer Therapy

Current cancer therapy takes three major forms: surgery, radiation, and chemotherapy. Nutritional support with any form of cancer therapy enhances the potential success of the therapy.

Surgery
Operable Tumors

Early diagnosis of operable tumors has led to successful surgical treatment of many cancer patients. The success of any surgery depends in large measure on the sound nutritional status of the patient (see Chapter 23), but this is especially true of cancer patients because their general condition may be weakened. Optimal nutritional status preoperatively and maximal nutritional support postoperatively are fundamental to the healing process.

Nutrition Relationships

Nutrition has both general and specific relationships: (1) support of the general healing process and overall body metabolism and (2) specific modifications of nutrient factors, texture, or feeding method, according to the surgical site and organ function involved. Prevention of problems through early detection and surgical treatment has significantly increased cancer cure rates. Surgical treatment may also be used with other forms of therapy for removal of single metastases or for prevention and alleviation of symptoms.

Radiation
Treatment Role

Soon after radiation was discovered in the nineteenth century, scientists found that it could damage body tissue. Continued study of its use and control revealed that normal tissue could largely withstand an amount of radiation that would damage and destroy cancer tissue. The subsequent role of radiation in cancer treatment has developed around controlled use with two types of tumor: (1) those responsive to radiation therapy (or radiotherapy) within a dose level tolerable to health of normal tissue, and (2) those that can be targeted without damage to overlying vital organ tissue.

Forms

Radiation used in cancer therapy is produced from three main sources: (1) x-rays (the oldest form of cancer treatment), which are electromagnetic waves similar to heat and light rays, with varying penetration according to the speed at which the electrons strike the target; (2) radioisotopes, such as cobalt 60; and (3) atomic particles, such as neutrons, protons, and electrons, derived from radioactive materials.

Effects

Radiotherapy may be used alone or in conjunction with other therapies both for curative and **palliative** care for some 50% of all cancer patients at some time during the course of their disease. Radiation effects will influence nutritional status and therapy a great deal, depending on the site and intensity of treatment:

1. *Head and neck* radiation will affect the oral mucosa and salivary secretions, as well as the esophagus, influencing taste sensations and sensitivity to food temperature and texture.
2. *Abdomen* radiation may produce denuded bowel mucosa, loss of villi and absorbing surface area, vascular changes from intimal thickening, thrombosis, ulcer formation, or inflammation. Obstruction, fistula formation, or strictures may further contribute to general malabsorption, compounded by curtailment of food intake due to anorexia and nausea.

Chemotherapy
Drug Development

Although chemotherapy has been recognized as a valid cancer therapy over the past few decades, the most effective agents currently in use have largely been developed only within the past few years. Intensive research has resulted in the development of a large number of effective *antineoplastic drugs*. Their therapeutic use is based on two general principles related to rate and mode of action.

Rate of Action

The so-called cell or log (logarithm) kill hypothesis of the action of chemotherapeutic agents on tumors indicates that a single dose can only be as much as 99.9% effective in killing the tumor cells. Thus, if as large a tumor as is compatible with life can be treated with a drug tolerable at a toxicity level that is 99.9% effective, the tumor is gradually reduced with successive doses that cause "fractional killing" with each dose. This process finally brings the tumor within the capability of the body's immune system to take over and make the final kill and cure. The smaller the tumor, either because of early detection or initial treatment by surgery or radiation, the greater the possible effectiveness of the chemotherapeutic agents. Two other principles of dosage rate for greater effectiveness are also important: (1) aggressive use of maximal tolerable dosages in repeated series, and (2) use of several drugs together for a *synergistic* effect.

Mode of Action

Chemotherapeutic agents are effective because they disrupt the normal processes in the cell responsible for cell growth and reproduction. Some agents interfere with DNA synthesis. Others disrupt DNA structure and RNA replication. Still others prevent cell division by mitosis, or cause hormonal imbalances, or make unavailable the specific amino acids necessary for protein synthesis. This diversity in mode of action provides a basis for grouping drugs into six classes of chemotherapeutic agents: alkaloids, alkylating agents, antibiotics, antimetabolites, enzymes, and hormones. These agents are usually used in combined therapy or as adjuvant therapy in conjunction with surgery or radiation.

Toxic Effects

Chemotherapeutic agents have the same effects on rapidly reproducing normal cells as they do on the rapidly reproducing cancer cells. Interference with normal function is most apparent in normal cells of the bone marrow, gastrointestinal tract, and hair follicles, accounting for a number of toxic side effects and problems in nutritional management:

1. **Bone marrow effects** include interference with production of red blood cells (anemia), white cells (infections), and platelets (bleeding).
2. **Gastrointestinal effects** include nausea and vomiting, **stomatitis,** anorexia, ulcers, and diarrhea.
3. **Hair follicle effects** include *alopecia* (baldness) and general hair loss.

Nutritional Therapy
Therapeutic Problems and Goals

Numerous problems present needs for nutritional therapy and care of patients with cancer. In general, nutritional therapy deals with two types of problems: those related to the disease process itself and those related to medical treatment of the disease. Thus the basic objectives of nutritional therapy in cancer are to (1) meet the increased metabolic demands of the disease and prevent catabolism as much as possible, and (2) alleviate symptoms resulting from the disease and its treatment through adaptations of food and the feeding process.

Problems Related to the Disease Process

Feeding problems forming the basic challenge to nutritional therapy are caused by general systemic effects

---

palliative • Care affording relief but not cure; useful for comfort when cure is still unknown or obscure.

stomatitis • Inflammation of the oral mucosa, especially the buccal tissue lining the inside the cheeks but also may involve the tongue, palate, floor of the mouth, and the gums.

of the neoplastic disease process and by specific responses related to the type of cancer.

General Systemic Reactions

The disease process causes three basic systemic effects: (1) *anorexia,* (2) *hypermetabolic state,* and (3) *negative nitrogen balance,* which are often accompanied by a continuing weight loss. Effects may vary widely with individual patients, according to type and stage of the disease. Effects may range from mild, scarcely discernible responses to the extreme forms of debilitating *cachexia* that are seen in advanced disease and are estimated to cause more than 50% of cancer deaths.[15,16] This extreme weight loss and weakness is caused by abnormalities in glucose metabolism; cancer patients with this disorder cannot produce glucose efficiently from carbohydrates and instead "feed" off their own tissue protein and convert it to glucose.[15,17] The "new-old" drug hydrazine sulfate seems to correct this metabolic error, allowing patients to conserve more energy.[18]

Anorexia is frequently accompanied by depression or discomfort during normal eating. This contributes further to a limited nutrient intake at the very time the disease process causes an increased metabolic rate and nutrient demand. Often this imbalance of decreased intake and increased demand creates a negative nitrogen balance, an indication of body-tissue wasting. Sometimes a true tissue loss of protein is masked by outward nitrogen equilibrium as the growing tumor retains nitrogen at the expense of the host, further compounding the problem.

Specific Responses Related to Type of Cancer

Interrelated functional and metabolic problems stem from specific types of cancer and their effects on the body. All these factors contribute to nutritional depletion. In addition to the primary nutritional deficiencies induced by the disease process itself, secondary difficulties in ingestion and use of nutrients relate to specific tumors that cause obstructions or lesions in the gastrointestinal tract or adjacent tissue. Thus these conditions curtail intake or absorption of adequate nutrients.

Problems Related to Cancer Treatment

Medical treatments for cancer entail physiologic stress. Results include toxic tissue effects, often with damage to cell DNA structure and changes in normal body function. Thus the benefit achieved is not without attendant problems. Nutritional support seeks to alleviate these problems.

Problems Related to Surgery

Beyond the regular nutritional needs surrounding any surgical procedure and its healing process, gastrointestinal surgery poses special problems for normal eating and for digesting and absorbing food nutrients. Head and neck surgery, or resections in the oropharyngeal area, are sometimes necessary. In such patients food intake is greatly affected. A creative variety of food forms, semiliquid textures, and feeding modes must be devised. Often the mechanical problems of food ingestion make long-term tube feeding necessary (see Chapter 18).

Gastrectomy may cause numerous postgastrectomy "dumping" problems requiring frequent, small, low-carbohydrate feedings (see Chapter 23). Vagotomy contributes to gastric stasis. Various intestinal resections or tumor excisions may cause steatorrhea due to general malabsorption, fistulas, or stenosis. Pancreatectomy causes loss of digestive enzymes, induced insulin-dependent diabetes mellitus, and general weight loss.

Problems Related to Radiation

Radiation to the oropharyngeal area often produces a loss of taste, with increasing anorexia and nausea. Other means of tempting appetite through food appearance, aroma, and texture must be developed. Abdominal radiation may cause intestinal damage, with tissue edema and congestion, decreased peristalsis, or endarteritis in small blood vessels. Fibrosis, stenosis, necrosis, or ulceration may occur in the intestinal wall. General malabsorption or fistulas may develop, as well as hemorrhage, obstruction, and diarrhea, all contributing to nutritional problems. The liver is somewhat more resistant to damage from radiation in adults, but children are more vulnerable.

Chemotherapy

The major nutritional problems during chemotherapy relate to (1) the gastrointestinal symptoms caused by the effect of the toxic drugs on the rapidly developing mucosal cells, (2) the anemia associated with bone marrow effects, and (3) the general systemic toxicity effect on appetite. Stomatitis, nausea, diarrhea, and malabsorption contribute to many food intolerances. Antiemetic drugs such as prochlorperazine (Compazine) may be used (Table 25-1). Such drugs act on the vomiting center in the brain to prevent the nausea response. Prolonged vomiting seriously affects fluid and electrolyte balance, especially in elderly patients, and needs to be controlled. In breast cancer patients, relief from nausea has been achieved with use of the antiemetic drug megestrol acetate (Megase), a synthetic female sex hormone similar to the natural hormone progesterone. Increased appetites and food intakes were accompanied by weight gains in true body mass rather than fluid retention.[19] In some cases of chronic long-term drug therapy, special nutritional management restricting conditioned (learned) food aversions to odors and colors has been effective. For example, patients receiving periodic treatments of the drug cisplatin (Platinol), who had a special diet of three meals a day of plain, colorless, odorless foods, such as cottage cheese, applesauce, vanilla ice cream, and other predeter-

TABLE 25-1

Medications used to Control Nausea and Vomiting in Patients Receiving Chemotherapy

Antiemetic drug/action	Cancer chemotherapeutic drug counteracted	Dosage used	Side effects	Comments
Phenothiazines Action: blocks CTZ* stimulation by dopamine Examples Compazine (prochlorperazine) Torecan (thiethylperazine) Phenergan (promethazine)	Moderate emetic-potential drugs	5-10 mg, orally or parenterally before chemotherapy; every 4-6 hr after, for 24-48 hr	Sedation Orthostatic hypertension	Less effective when given on "as needed"
Droperidol (Inapsine) Action: sedative and antiemetic	Cisplatin	0.5 mg intravenously 1 hr before chemotherapy; every 4 hr after chemotherapy	Somnolence	Some patients given up to 1.5 mg intravenously developed a tolerance for the drug
Corticosteroids Dexamethasone (Hexadrol, Decadron) Methylprednisolone (Solu-Medrol)	Cyclophosphamide Doxorubicin Nitrogen mustard Mitomycin Methyl-CCNU†	10 mg intramuscularly before chemotherapy 250 mg intravenously every 6 hr for 4 doses beginning 2 hr after chemotherapy	Perianal stinging if given too rapidly Swelling Facial rash Weakness, lethargy	Moderate to high relief in 70% of the patients Effects of methylprednisolone considered disappointing
Tetrahydrocannabinol (THC, marijuana)	Variety of agents studied Methotrexate 5-FU‡ Methyl-CCNU Cyclophosphamide Doxorubicin Nitrosoureas Mechlorethamine Cisplatin	10 mg/m²	Somnolence Visual hallucinations	Patients (usually older) not used to THC refused to continue it because of CNS effects§ Response associated with extent of THC-induced "high" Most effective with fluorouracil, cyclophosphamide, methotrexate, doxorubicin "High" blocked by giving a phenothiazine
Metoclopramide (Reglan)	Cisplatin	Single 20-mg dose, given orally halfway through a 6-hr infusion of cisplatin (100 mg/m²); higher doses might be possible intravenously (1-3 mg/kg/dose)	Sedation	Works well for patients who do not respond to other antiemetic drugs

Data modified from studies reported by Huber SL, Ballentine R: *Nutr Support Serv* 2(10):30, 1982.

*CTZ (chemoreceptor zone; vomiting center in brain).

†Methyl-CCNU [methyl-1-(2-chloroethyl)-3-cyclohexyl-1-nitrosourea].

‡5-FU (5-fluorouracil).

§CNS (central nervous system).

mined foods, experienced little nausea and increased food intake.[20] The potential for developing conditioned food aversions while on long-term chemotherapy is diminished by use of food having little or no odor or color, because the drug-related *dysgeusis* (perverted sense of taste) and *dysosmia* (impaired sense of smell) are correlated with visual olfactory stimulation factors.[20,21]

Certain chemotherapeutic drugs also have special effects. For example, monoaminoxidase (MAO) inhibitors may be used for pretreatment relief of mental and emotional depression or for palliative therapy. These antidepressant drugs cause well-known pressor effects when used with tyramine-rich foods (Table 25-2). Thus these foods should be avoided when using such drugs (see Chapter 18).

Principles of Nutritional Therapy for Cancer Patients

Two important principles of nutritional therapy, vital in any sound nutrition practice but especially essential in care of patients with cancer, provide the basis for planning nutritional care of each patient: (1) personal nutritional assessment and (2) vigorous nutrition

TABLE 25-2

Tyramine-Restricted Diet ·

General directions

- Designed for patients on monoamine oxidase inhibitors, drugs that have been reported to cause hypertensive crises when used with tyramine-rich foods. These include foods in which aging, protein breakdown, and putrefaction are used to increase flavor. Studies indicate that as little as 5 to 6 mg of tyramine may produce a response, and 25 mg is a dangerous dose.
- Food sources of other pressor amines such as histamine, dihydroxyphenylalanine, and hydroxytyramine are also avoided.
- Avoid all foods listed. Limited amounts of foods with a lower amount of tyramine, such as yeast bread, may be included in a specific diet.
- Avoid over-the-counter drugs such as decongestants, cold remedies, and antihistamines.

Foods to Avoid	Representative Tyramine Values in μg/g or ml	Additional Foods to Avoid
Cheeses		Other aged cheeses
New York State cheddar	1416	Blue
Gruyère	516	Boursault
Stilton	466	Brick
Emmentaler	225	Cheddars (other)
Brie	180	Gouda
Camembert	86	Mozzarella
Processed American	50	Parmesan
Wines		Provolone
Chianti	25.4	Romano
Sherry	3.6	Roquefort
Riesling	0.6	Yeast and products made with yeast
Sauternes	0.4	Homemade bread
Beer, ale (varies with brand)		Yeast extracts such as soup cubes, canned meats, and marmite
Highest	4.4	Italian broad beans with pod (fava beans)
Average	2.3	Meat
Least	1.8	Aged game
		Liver
		Canned meats with yeast extracts
		Fish (salted dried)
		Herring, cod, capelin
		Pickled herring
		Other
		Chocolate
		Cream (especially sour cream)
		Salad dressings
		Soy sauce
		Vanilla
		Yogurt

therapy to maintain good nutritional status and support medical treatment.

Nutrition Assessment

It is far more difficult to replenish a nutritionally depleted patient than to maintain a good nutritional status from the outset of the disease process. Therefore a primary goal in nutritional therapy is to prevent a depleted state. Initial assessment for baseline data and regular monitoring thereafter during treatment are necessary. A detailed personal history is essential to determine individual needs, desires, and tolerances. To be valid the interview should be conducted as a conversation, using verbal and nonverbal probes and pauses rather than a cross fire of separate questions and answers.[22] (Review all of these procedures in Chapter 16.)

Nutritional Therapy and Plan of Care

Based on careful individual nutritional assessment, a plan for optimal nutritional therapy may be developed to meet the patient's needs. This nutritional therapy outline is then incorporated into the nursing care plan as the clinical nutritionist works with the nursing staff to carry it out. Primary care provided by the clinical nutritionist and the nurse on a regular basis is a necessary part of the oncology team practice. This early, vigorous care often makes the difference in the success rate of medical therapy. Thus, working closely with the oncology nurse and physician, the clinical nutritionist assesses personal needs, determines nutritional requirements, plans and manages nutritional care, monitors progress and responses to therapy, and makes adjustments in care according to status and tolerances.

Nutritional Needs

Each of the nutrient factors related to tissue protein synthesis and energy metabolism requires careful attention. The increased needs for energy, protein, vitamins and minerals, and fluid are based on the demands of the disease and its treatment. Although individual needs vary, guidelines for nutritional therapy must meet increased nutrient needs.

Energy

Great energy demands are placed on the cancer patient. These demands result from the hypermetabolic state of the disease process and the tissue-healing requirements. Of the total dietary kcaloric value, sufficient carbohydrate to spare protein for vital tissue synthesis is essential. An adult patient with good nutritional status will require about 2000 kcal/day to provide for maintenance needs. A more malnourished patient may require 3000 to 4000 kcal, depending on the degree of malnutrition and body trauma. Carbohydrate should supply most of the energy intake, with fat restricted to 30% or less of the total kcalories. Numerous studies have related excessive dietary fat to cancer metastasis and effectiveness of cancer therapy.[23-25] The practical feasibility of dietary intervention programs to reduce fat intake has been demonstrated by recent studies of the National Cancer Institute, a large multicentered pilot study, and the Women's Health Trial.[26,27] In these studies women with breast cancer and women at high risk of breast cancer reduced their fat intake from a baseline of 40% to 22% of total kcalories while increasing their intakes of all the vitamins and minerals. These results indicate that a nutritionally sound low-fat diet can be successfully implemented in highly motivated, free-living groups of individuals.

Protein

Tissue protein synthesis, a necessary component of healing and rehabilitation, requires essential amino acids and nitrogen. Efficient protein use, which depends on an optimal protein/kcalorie ratio, promotes tissue building, prevents tissue wastage (catabolism), and helps make up tissue deficits. An adult patient with good nutritional status will need about 80 to 100 g of protein per day to meet maintenance needs and ensure anabolism. A malnourished patient will need more to replenish tissue and restore positive nitrogen balance.

Vitamins and Minerals

Key vitamins and minerals control protein and energy metabolism through their roles in cell enzyme systems.

They also play a necessary part in structural development and tissue integrity. The B-complex vitamins in general serve as necessary coenzyme agents in energy and protein metabolism. Vitamins A and C are important tissue-structuring materials. Vitamin A also plays a significant role in protective immunity and cell differentiation; vitamin C has significant antioxidant, enzymatic, and immune biological functions related to cancer.[28,29] Increased dietary consumption of vegetables and fruits is a primary means of obtaining these vitamins.[30] A recent study of nutritional molecular carcinogens suggests also that the expression of certain oncogenes may be reduced by vitamins A, E, and D.[31] Vitamin D hormone ensures proper calcium and phosphorous metabolism in bone and blood serum. Vitamin E protects the integrity of cell wall materials and hence tissue integrity. Many minerals function in structural and enzymatic roles in vital metabolic and tissue-building processes. Thus an optimal intake of vitamins and minerals is indicated, at least to RDA levels but frequently augmented with supplements according to individual patient nutritional status.

Fluids

Adequate fluid intake is important for two reasons: (1) to replace gastrointestinal losses or losses caused by infection and fever, and (2) to help the kidneys dispose of the metabolic breakdown products from the destroyed cancer cells and from the toxic drugs used in treatment. For example, some toxic drugs such as cyclophosphamide (Cytoxan) require as much as 2 to 3 L of forced fluids daily to prevent hemorrhagic cystitis.

Nutritional Management

The specific feeding method used depends on the individual patient's condition. However, the classic dictum of nutritional management should prevail: *"If the gut works, use it."* Details of available enteral and parenteral modes of nutritional support are provided in Chapter 18. If at all possible, an oral diet with supplementation is the most desired form of feeding. A carefully designed personal plan of care based on nutrition assessment data and including adjustments in texture, temperature, food choices, and tolerances, as well as consideration of family food patterns, can often meet needs (see Clinical Application, p. 496). The hospitalized patient's diet can be supplemented with familiar foods from home as the clinical nutritionist plans with the family. Personal food tolerances will vary according to the current treatment and nature of the disease. A number of adjustments in food texture, temperature, amount, timing, taste, appearance, and form can be made to help alleviate symptoms stemming from common problems in successive parts of the gastrointestinal tract. Difficulties in eating may be caused by loss of

CLINICAL APPLICATION

Promoting Oral Intake in Cancer Patients

Encouraging and maintaining adequate oral intake for cancer patients is one of the most difficult aspects of cancer treatment. It is time-consuming and often frustrating, but may be one of the most rewarding experiences in patient care. Identifying feeding problems, initiating appropriate interventions, and providing individual education promotes adequate oral nutrition. The dietitian is the key figure for coordinating the nutritional program, but its success requires the full support and cooperation of the entire health care team, especially the nurse.

The patient interview is one of the most important parts of the nutritional assessment. Information that helps identify adequacy of current nutritional intake and potential nutritional problems is obtained during the interview. The following list of questions may assist in gathering accurate information about the patient's ability to obtain oral nutrition:

- How would you describe your appetite?
- Has it changed recently?
- Are you eating differently from the way you have been eating most of your life?
- Do you usually eat three meals each day? Has this changed recently?
- Are you nauseated? vomiting? Is this food-related or medication-related? How long have you been experiencing this? How often do you vomit or feel nauseated?
- Do you have a bowel movement every day? Has this changed?
- Do you have diarrhea? If so, do you think this may be food-related?
- Do food smells or cooking odors bother you?
- Do you have difficulty chewing?
- Do your dentures (if any) fit? Do you wear them?
- Do you have difficulty swallowing?
- Is your mouth dry? Does your saliva seem different? Is it thicker or decreased?
- Do you find it easier to drink liquids than to eat solid foods?
- What were you able to eat yesterday? (Obtain a brief 24-hour dietary recall.)

- Are you unable to eat certain foods now?
- Do some foods taste different than they did? Can you give an example?
- Have you ever taken any high-kcalorie, high-protein supplements? When? What kind? How often? Were you able to tolerate them?
- Do you take a multivitamin supplement?
- Do you have any food allergies or intolerances? Are these new, or have you always had them?
- Do you prepare your own meals? If so, do you ever feel too tired to prepare something to eat?

The success of the interview depends on the dietitian's professional competence, interviewing skills, and bedside manner. If the dietitian establishes a feeling of comfort and trust with the patient, the opportunity to accomplish successful dietary interventions is great.

REFERENCE

Nahikian-Nelms ML: Encouraging oral intake. In Bloch AS, editor: *Nutrition management of the cancer patient*, Rockville, Md, 1990, Aspen. ◆

---

appetite, problems in the mouth or with swallowing, or various gastrointestinal problems.

Loss of Appetite

Anorexia is a major problem and curtails food intake when it is needed most. It is a general systemic effect of the cancer disease process itself, often further induced by the cancer treatment and progressively enhanced by personal anxiety, depression, and stress of the illness. Such a vicious cycle, if not countered by much effort, can lead to more malnutrition and the well-recognized starvation "cancer cachexia," a syndrome of emaciation, debilitation, and malnutrition. A vigorous program of eating, *not dependent on appetite for stimulus,* must be planned and maintained with the patient and family. The overall goal is to provide food with as much nutrient density as possible so that "every bite will count." If appetite is better in the morning, a good breakfast should be emphasized. Getting some exercise before meals and maintaining surroundings that reduce stress may also help in the eating process.

Mouth Problems

Eating difficulties may stem from sore mouth, **stomatitis,** or taste changes. Sore mouth often results from chemotherapy or from radiation to the head and neck area. It is increased by any state of malnutrition or from infections such as **candidiasis** (thrush), with numerous ulcerations of the oral and throat mucosa. Frequent small meals and snacks that are soft, bland, and cool or cold are often better tolerated. There may also be alterations in the tongue's taste buds, causing taste distortion ("taste blindness") and inability to distinguish the basic tastes of salt, sweet, sour, or bitter, with consequent food aversions. Since the aversion is often toward basic protein foods, a high protein/energy liquid drink supplement may be needed. *Dental problems* may also contribute to mouth difficulties and should be corrected. *Salivary secretions* are also affected by cancer treatment, so foods with a high liquid content should be used. Solid foods may be swallowed more easily with use of sauces, gravies, broth, yogurt, or salad dressings. A food processor or blender can render foods in semisolid or liquid forms and make them easier to swallow. If the swallowing problem is especially severe because of tumor growth or therapy, guides for a special swallowing training program can be followed, including progressive food textures, exercises, and positions.

Gastrointestinal Problems

Eating difficulties may include nausea and vomiting, general indigestion, bloating, or specific surgery responses such as the postgastrectomy "dumping" syndrome (see Chapter 23). Nausea is often enhanced by foods that are hot, sweet, fatty, or spicy, so these can be avoided according to individual tolerance. Other food problems may include general diarrhea, constipation, flatulence, or specific lactose intolerance or surgery responses, such as those that occur with intestinal resections and various ostomies. Patients with colostomies, ileostomies, or ileoanal reservoirs need helpful guidance (see Chapter 23). The effect of chemotherapy or radiation treatment on the mucosal cells secreting lactase contributes to lactose intolerance. In such cases a nutrient supplement formula with a nonmilk protein base may be needed.

A number of commercial nutrient supplement products are available. A comparative review of these products will provide the basis for developing a formulary in the hospital setting for a limited number of such products (see Chapter 18). A food processor or blender can be used at home to produce creative solid and liquid food combinations from regular foods for interval liquid supplementation.

Involving cancer patients in their personal nutritional care plan is necessary for its personal success. They need to feel some sense of personal control. By starting with small amounts, the nutritionist and the patient can then set goals for the quantities that need to be ingested. Individual patients may need to schedule their supplements as medications, which commits the entire health care team to the nutritional care plan. This team involvement helps the patient understand the importance of adequate nutrition.[32]

Feeding in Terminal Illness

Although many advances have been made in the detection and treatment of cancer, mortality rates for patients with some cancers have not declined and for some cancers have actually increased. For example, according to the National Cancer Institute, two decades ago 26.9 women out of every 100,000 died of breast cancer; by the end of the 1980s, the rate had grown to 27.5 per 100,000, and the trend seems to be rising.[33] Cancer is now the leading cause of death for women in the United States, and if trends continue, it will be the leading overall cause of death in the United States by the year 2000.[9]

We feel these results in our work with cancer patients. We see the progressive weight loss and malnutrition that occurs, caused by the primary tumor and its spread, that leads to profound nutritional depletion and is a major cause of morbidity and mortality.[34] For some patients a time comes when the spread of the disease overcomes the body's capacity to combat it. When the patient is no longer able to eat, enteral tube feeding or parenteral feeding may be used. Ultimately, however, ethical questions about continued feeding efforts are faced in many cases (see To Probe Further, p. 500). Answers lie with the patient, as long as possible, and with the family. But sensitive and supportive counseling is needed from the cancer team members, especially from the clinical dietitian responsible for nutritional support and the nurse administering the continued feeding and responsible for personal care. These skilled and sensitive professionals, along with the physician, the patient, and the family, face these decisions together.

To Sum Up

Cancer is a term applied to abnormal, malignant growths in various body-tissue sites. The cancerous cell is derived from a normal cell that loses control over cell reproduction. Cancer cell development occurs via mutation, carcinogens, radiation, and oncogenic viruses. It is also influenced by many epidemiologic factors, such as diet, alcohol, and smoking, as well as by physical and psychologic stress factors. Cell development is mediated by the body's immune system, primarily its T cells, a type of white cell found in blood, lymph, certain parts of the lymph nodes and spleen, and B cells, which manufacture and secrete antibodies.

Cancer therapy consists primarily of surgery, radiation, and chemotherapy. Supportive nutritional therapy for the cancer patient should be highly individualized and depends on the response of each body system to the disease and to the treatment itself. It is based on a thorough nutritional assessment and provided by a number of routes: oral, tube feeding, peripheral vein, TPN. The oral route is preferred if at all possible. Nutrient requirements and feeding mode must be designed for specific physical and psychologic needs of individual patients.

---

candidiasis • Infection with the fungus of the genus *Candida*, generally caused by *C. albicans*, so named for the whitish appearance of its small lesions; usually a superficial infection in moist areas of the skin or inner mucous membranes.

QUESTIONS FOR REVIEW

1. What is cancer? Identify and describe several major causes of cancer cell formation.
2. How does your body attempt to defend itself against cancer? What nutritional factors may diminish this ability?
3. List and describe the rationale and mode of action of the types of therapies used to treat cancer.
4. Differentiate those factors challenging cancer recovery that are associated with the disease versus the type of therapy used.
5. Outline the general procedure for the nutritional management of a cancer patient.

REFERENCES

1. Weinberg RA: Tumor suppressor genes, *Science* 254:1138, 1991.
2. Ames BN and others: Ranking possible carcinogen hazards, *Science* 236:271, Apr 17, 1987.
3. Report: Of interest to you: comparing possible hazards from natural hazards from natural and man-made substances, *J Am Diet Assoc* 92(5):597, 1992.
4. Aaronson SA: Growth factors and cancers, *Science* 254:1146, 1991.
5. Marx J: Oncogenes evoke new cancer therapies, *Science* 249:1376, 1990.
6. Hausen H: Viruses in human cancer, *Science* 254:1167, 1991.
7. Gibbons A: Does war on cancer equal war on poverty? *Science* 253:260, 1991.
8. Coates RJ and others: Race, nutritional status, and survival from breast cancer, *J Natl Cancer Inst* 82(21):1684, 1990.
9. Henderson BE and others: Toward the primary prevention of cancer, *Science* 254:1131, 1991.
10. Wynder EL: Primary prevention of cancer: planning and policy consideration, *J Natl Cancer Inst* 83(7):475, 1991.
11. Liotta LA: Cancer invasion and metatasis, *Sci Am* 266(2):54, 1992.
12. Beisel WP: History of nutritional immunology: introduction and overview, *J Nutr* 122:591, 1992.
13. Chandra RK: Protein-energy malnutrition and immunological responses, *J Nutr* 122:597, 1992.
14. Watzl B, Watson RR: Role of alcohol abuse in nutrition immunosuppression, *J Nutr* 122:733, 1992.
15. Tayek JA, Chlebowski RT: Metabolic response to chemotherapy in colon cancer patients, *J Parenter Enteral Nutr* 16(suppl 6):65, 1992.
16. Shaw JHF and others: Leucine kinetics in patients with benign disease, non-weight-losing cancer and cancer cachexia: studies at the whole body level and the response to nutritional support, *Surgery* 109:37, 1991.

17. Tayck JA: A review of cancer cachexia and abnormal glucose metabolism in humans with cancer, *J Am Coll Nutr* 11:445, 1992.
18. Seligmann J, Witherspoon D: A new, old cancer drug, *Newsweek*, p 95, June 6, 1983.
19. Tchekmedyian NS and others: Nutrition in advanced cancer: anorexia as an outcome variable and target of therapy, *J Parenter Enteral Nutr* 16(suppl 6):88, 1992.
20. Menashian L and others: Improved food intake and reduced nausea and vomiting in patients given a restricted diet while receiving cisplatin chemotherapy, *J Am Diet Assoc* 92(1):58, 1992.
21. Darbinian J, Coulston A: Impact of chemotherapy on the nutritional status of the cancer patient. In Bloch AS, editor: *Nutrition management of the cancer patient*, Rockville, Md, 1990, Aspen.
22. Jain M: Diet history: questionnaire and interview techniques used in some retrospective studies of cancer, *J Am Diet Assoc* 89(11):1647, 1989.
23. Djuric Z and others: Effects of a low-fat diet on levels of oxidative damage to DNA in human peripheral nucleated blood cells, *J Natl Cancer Inst* 83(11):766, 1991.
24. Erikson KL, Hubbard NE: Dietary fat and tumor metastasis, *Nutr Rev* 48(1):6, 1990.
25. Burns CP, Spector AA: Effects of lipids on cancer therapy, *Nutr Rev* 48(6):233, 1990.
26. Buzzard IM and others: Diet intervention methods to reduce fat intake: nutrient and food group composition of self-selected low-fat diets, *J Am Diet Assoc* 90(1):42, 1990.
27. Gorbach SL and others: Changes in food patterns during a low-fat dietary intervention in women, *J Am Diet Assoc* 90(6):802, 1990.
28. Ross C: Vitamin A and protective immunity, *Nutr Today* 27(4):18, 1992.
29. Henson DE and others: Ascorbic acid: Biologic functions and relation to cancer, *J Natl Cancer Inst* 83(8):547, 1991.
30. Negri E and others: Vegetable and fruit consumption and cancer risk, *Int J Cancer* 48:350, 1991.
31. Prasad KN, Edwards-Prasad J: Expressions of some molecular cancer risk factors and their modification by vitamins, *J Am Coll Nutr* 9(1):28, 1990.
32. Nahikian-Nelms ML: Encouraging oral intake. In Bloch AS, editor: *Nutrition management of the cancer patient*, Rockville, Md, 1990, Aspen.
33. Marshall E: Breast cancer: statement in the war on cancer, *Science* 254:1719, 1991.
34. Daly JM and others: Nutritional support in the cancer patients, *J Parenter Enteral Nutr* 14(suppl 5):244S, 1990.
35. Brody H, Noel MB: Dietitians' role in decisions to withhold nutrition and hydration, *J Am Diet Assoc* 91(5):580, 1991.

FURTHER READING

Ames BN and others: Ranking possible carcinogen hazards, *Science* 236:271, 1987.

Dr. Ames provides results from his Berkeley laboratory studies on a wide variety of environmental carcinogens, explains why animal cancer tests cannot be used to predict absolute human risks, and supplies a large table ranking hazards.

Burkitt D: An approach to the reduction of the most common Western cancers: the failure of therapy to reduce the disease, *Arch Surg* 126:345, 1991.

In his thought-provoking article, Dr. Burkitt discusses cancer and environment, dietary changes, and the future of cancer research. He makes a strong case for primary prevention, indicating that there is no evidence that the incidence of any disease was ever reduced by treatment alone.

Bloch AS, editor: *Nutrition management of the cancer patient,* Rockville, Md, 1990, Aspen.

This helpful reference by an experienced oncology dietitian and her contributors provides a comprehensive background for better understanding the complexities of caring for cancer patients.

CASE STUDY

Patient With Cancer

Catherine Schofield is a 35-year-old mother of three young children. She was admitted to Green Hills Hospital 3 weeks ago with multiple enterocutaneous fistulas. Her weight on admission was 52 kg (116 lb), height 165 cm (5 ft, 6 in). She had undergone a hysterectomy 4 months before admission, following a recurrence of cervical cancer. During the chemotherapy that followed for 7 months, she had regular bouts with nausea and anorexia. Surgery was performed again. Her fistulas continued to drain for 2 weeks postoperatively, during which time she tolerated clear liquids only. An intravenous drip of 10% glucose and 45% normal saline was ordered to supplement fluids and kcalories. This week Mrs. Schofield developed peritonitis and has had a fever of 39° C (102° F) for the past 24 hours. Her weight has dropped to 41 kg (90 lb); drainage from the fistulas has become odorous. She was placed in isolation today and was advised by her physician that he intended to start TPN and take some more tests to determine her progress.

Questions for Analysis

1. What types of nutritional assessment procedures would be used by the TPN team for planning Mrs. Schofield's nutritional therapy? Explain the purpose of each.
2. Calculate Mrs. Schofield's energy and protein needs, and account for increased needs.
3. Why did Mrs. Schofield develop nausea and anorexia during chemotherapy? What are the implications of this for recovery? Outline a plan for evaluating and controlling nausea and vomiting in patients undergoing chemotherapy.
4. What personal concerns would you expect Mrs. Schofield to have? What resources would you use to help her obtain the personal and physical support she probably needs?

When Does Feeding Become an Ethical Issue?

TO PROBE FURTHER

Plato believed that both the moral person and the physician should abide by the Hippocratic principle of medicine, "Above all, do no harm." In recent times others have returned to Plato's use of this medical model of ethics.

Current writers assert that an ethic of care rests on the "premise of nonviolence—that no one should be hurt." This outlook is unique in that it insists that women have made a valuable contribution to ethical theory by stressing values associated with caring. These implications are profound, especially for professions composed largely of women, such as dietetics and nursing.

Technology such as enteral and parenteral nutrition may sometimes support a caring intent and compassionate spirit, while at other times such modern technology becomes a value in and of itself with its own standard of efficiency. Enteral and parenteral feeding techniques may be used to maintain indefinitely patients who are unable to take food orally.

Concerned ethical thinkers use the following moral principles for decisions in regard to life-sustaining treatment that encompasses enteral or parenteral nutrition: benefit to patient, respect for patient autonomy or self-determination, maintenance of the moral integrity of health professionals, and justice in distributing scarce medical resources among eligible patients. They offer helpful views to guide clinicians in coming to a reasoned and defensible resolution of moral conflict.

- **Alternatives to artificial nutrition.** All options of nutritional support should be explored beyond simply considering whether or not to "Give food or fluids." Dietitians are particularly helpful in identifying alternative feeding strategies. It is wrong to assume that the question is "Let the patient die" versus "Keep the patient alive."
- **Patient prognosis for recovery of functions.** A widely held, ethically defensible view is that aggressive means of prolonging life becomes less morally desirable in proportion to the inability of the patient to regain what he or she considers useful function. The persistent vegetative state and permanent loss of consciousness are examples of extreme cases, in which recovery of function is not possible. In such cases, accurately determining the prognosis for recovery is critical.
- **Total management plans and goals of therapy.** The patient's prognosis and nature of the illness might determine whether the goal of medical care is to (1) at-

tempt cure, (2) manage a chronic illness that cannot be cured so as to maintain maximal patient function, or (3) allow a terminally ill patient to die with maximal comfort and symptom control. Nutritional treatment may make excellent sense within one plan of care, but no sense at all in another.

- **Wishes of the patient or patient surrogate.** It is legally and ethically acceptable that in almost all cases the voluntary choice of an informed patient should be overriding. When the patient cannot choose, a surrogate or other substitute decision maker who is familiar with the patient's values and wishes may be consulted.
- **Ability of the patient to choose.** It is important to assess the patient's ability to make the particular medical care choice relevant to the matter at hand. In some circumstances, expert psychiatric or psychologic evaluation is needed.
- **Benefits and burdens of artificial treatment.** The medical team often tends to overestimate the benefits and underestimate the burdens of the treatments they use routinely. When the means of administering nutrition becomes invasive and painful, the burdens may become substantial. Restraining the patient or drawing blood repeatedly to monitor the effects of total parenteral nutrition may be unacceptable burdens to the patient. Patients may feel that being kept alive by artificial means is an indignity and that life is no longer useful or meaningful. Spiritual and emotional burdens should be assessed equally with physical burdens in making accurate assessments of the moral obligations to patients.

Modern medical technology has produced circumstances that caregivers and patients have never faced before. Decisions regarding nutrition and hydration in terminally ill patients must be made more frequently. Ethical and moral questions do not always have black or white solutions; they are often grey. The ethics task for dietitians may be to achieve a balance between what works and those who care.

REFERENCES

Brody H, Noel MB: Dietitians' role in decisions to withhold nutrition and hydration, *J Am Diet Assoc* 91(5):580, 1991.

Dalton S: What are the sources and standards of ethical judgment in dietetics? *J Am Diet Assoc* 91(5):545, 1991.

Gilligan C: *In a different voice: psychological theory and women's development,* Cambridge, Mass, 1990, Harvard University Press.

The American Dietetic Association: Issues in feeding the terminally ill adult, *J Am Diet Assoc* 87:78, 1987.

Toward the Prevention of Cancer

Studies of geographic, socioeconomic, chronologic, and immigration patterns of cancer distribution indicate that the vast majority of cases are due primarily to environmental factors. The logical conclusion is that reduction of these causative factors may reduce or eliminate most forms of cancer.

The American Cancer Society suggests that two thirds of all cases of cancer in the United States are caused by only two factors: inhaled smoke and ingested food.

Tobacco, alone or in combination with alcohol, remains the most important cause of cancer, accounting for about one of every three cancer deaths in the United States. Cigarettes are the most important cause of tobacco-related cancer, but other forms of tobacco (chewing tobacco and snuff) are also established carcinogens. The cancer risk of former smokers remains elevated compared with life-long nonsmokers. However, quitting smoking, even late in life after heavy long-term abuse, greatly reduces cancer risk compared with the risk had smoking been continued. Despite the rhetoric of tobacco companies, even regular smokers of low-tar cigarettes still have a much higher cancer risk than nonsmokers.

Alcohol, in addition to its synergistic effects with tobacco, increases risk of cancers of the oral cavity, pharynx, liver, and esophagus. Alcohol use has also been consistently linked to colorectal cancer and female breast cancer. Liquor, wine, and beer seem to be equal in effect on cancer risk.

Major incriminating dietary factors that appear now to be carcinogenic are the food changes that contrast current Western diets with those of our paleolithic hunter-gatherer ancestors. We have reduced the amount of energy we obtain from starchy foods by half to two thirds. We have decreased our intake of dietary fiber by 75%. We have more than doubled the proportion of energy we derive from fat and changed from consuming mostly unsaturated fats to saturated fats. We have increased our salt intake fivefold. And sugar now accounts for one fifth of our total energy intake. The diet of our ancestors was energy-dilute, whereas our modern diet is energy-dense.

Many studies link what we eat and don't eat to the development of cancer. Direct relationships between pre-served or salty foods and nasopharynx and stomach cancer have been consistently observed in case-control and correlational studies. High consumption of fresh fruits and vegetables has consistently been found to decrease the risk of stomach cancer. Epidemiologic studies suggest a relation between high-animal-fat, low-fiber intakes and colorectal cancer. The basis for this relationship lies in the decreased transit time through the colon associated with high-fiber diets, and the increased water content in the intestinal lumen that dilutes other nutrients such as animal fat.

Considerable, though not yet conclusive, evidence indicates that ascorbic acid has a protective effect against cancer of the esophagus, larynx, and oral cavity. Nutrients such as vitamin A, beta-carotene, vitamin E, and ascorbic acid are thought to lower cancer risk in patients with elevated risk for cancers of the lung, esophagus, colon, and skin. Clinical and laboratory studies support findings that adequate intakes of vitamin D and calcium are associated with reduced incidence of colorectal cancer. These studies did not necessarily utilize supplemental amounts of these nutrients in addition to the RDAs, but were based more on low levels of intake of these nutrients, which would parallel the low levels of fresh fruit and vegetable intakes that are prevalent in our society.

Most causes of cancer (such as tobacco, alcohol, animal fat, obesity, and ultraviolet light) are associated with life-style, that is, personal choices and not environmental causes. This fact reinforces the basic truth that the best cure for cancer is prevention, and life-style changes are prevention.

REFERENCES

Burkitt D: An approach to the reduction of the most common Western cancers, *Arch Surg* 126:345, 1991.

Garland CF and others: Can colon cancer incidence and death rates be reduced with calcium and vitamin D? *Am J Clin Nutr* 54:193S, 1991.

Greenwald P, Sondik EJ: *Cancer control objectives,* Washington, DC, 1986, National Cancer Institute.

Henderson BE and others: Toward the primary prevention of cancer, *Science* 254:1131, 1991.

Prasad KN, Edwards-Prasad J: Expressions of some molecular cancer risk factors and their modification by vitamins, *J Am Coll Nutr* 9(1):28, 1990.

Wynder EL: Primary prevention of cancer: planning and policy considerations, *J Natl Cancer Inst* 83(7):475, 1991.

CHAPTER 26

Nutritional Support in Disabling Disease and Rehabilitation

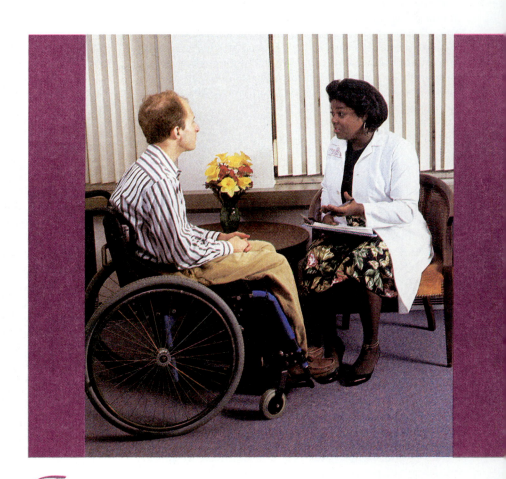

This chapter completes our clinical nutrition series. In addition to the primary care clinical problems we have reviewed in the preceding chapters of this section, we conclude with a focus on long-term disabling disease requiring rehabilitative care. Such situations often involve profound trauma and devastating effects that call for tremendous coping resources.

In this final chapter we examine the supportive role of nutrition in the rehabilitative process. We look at musculoskeletal disease, neuromuscular disease, and progressive neurologic disorders. In each case we see that personalized nutritional care plays a vital role in the healing and restoring process. Such care demands special knowledge and skills and much personal strength.

Nutritional Support and Rehabilitative Care

Goals of Supportive Care

Positive goals guide care for those with disabling disease or injury. Successful support is rooted in a positive philosophy based on the optimal potential of each person affected. This approach requires a specialized team working with the patient and family to meet individual needs. It is built on clearly defined *preventive* and *restorative* personal care objectives. To the greatest degree possible within each situation, two goals are fundamental in planning care: (1) to prevent further **disability,** and (2) to restore potential function. Health workers and clients alike have developed many creative techniques of care to meet these twin goals. Both of these key principles apply to nutritional support. Together with the other specialized therapists on the rehabilitation team, the registered dietitian functions as the nutrition specialist and carries numerous nutritional care responsibilities[1]:

1. *Nutritional assessment*—initial comprehensive evaluation and continuing reassessment at appropriate intervals
2. *Nutritional therapy*—to meet fundamental nutrient and energy requirements, as well as any specialized requirements
3. *Eating or feeding assessment*—needs for self-help eating devices of food marketing and preparation
4. *Coordination of community services*—referrals and communication to meet individual needs, home health care, rehabilitation, public health, vocational agencies, financial assistance, or other services
5. *Nutritional education and counseling*—with the individual client, the family, and other caregivers

Team Approach Method

How can these goals be met? How can the health care system draw on its various resources and levels of care to meet these tremendous needs? In some devastating cases, obstacles may seem almost insurmountable. In other cases, when the underlying disease may lack a cure, the prognosis is poor. Nonetheless, these support goals remain valid. Everyone involved persists in trying to achieve them. Often the patient's initial reaction is one of defeat and resignation or withdrawal. Certainly the patient and family cannot carry the overwhelming burden alone or accomplish the necessary care alone. Such a complex and complicated process requires a strong team approach. A number of sensitive and skilled specialists lend their particular expertise, bringing their unique training, insights and resources to identify specific personal needs.

At all times, however, these health care specialists remember that the most important member of the team is the patient. They always work *with,* not for, the patient and family to help develop solutions. Goal setting is always personal. These three partners—the professional specialist, the client, and the family—form a greater health team. It is always a shared, supportive undertaking, whatever the individual limitations or outcome (see To Probe Further, p. 504).

Socioeconomic and Psychologic Factors

Social Attitudes

The general attitudes of society toward disabled persons varies between extremes of overprotection and avoidance. These social attitudes result mainly from years of negative conditioning and are not easily changed. Some people are repelled by deformities or severe illness, perhaps because they sense their own vulnerability and mortality. Others completely ignore them. Neither extreme is helpful. But at the same time, overprotection robs persons of their selfhood and smothers the *will* to fight against surrounding odds and develop self-acceptance. However, disabled persons do have varying special needs, and social avoidance of these needs creates additional problems in everyday living. There are doorways not made for wheelchairs, unmanageable stairs and curbings, lack of access to public transportation, and many more daily barriers.

Economic Problems

Care for disabling injury or severe illness is a long and costly process. A major area of exploration for the health care team is one of financial resources and assistance needed. Also, continuing long-term economic problems may revolve around employment capabilities, earning capacities, or the means for providing care.

Living Situation

Disabled persons face many practical problems of everyday living. Whether an individual needs long-term hospital care or can maintain independent living, perhaps with an attendant, depends on a number of physical and situational factors. If with help the person can maintain a home, then the necessary special equipment

---

disability • A mental or physical impairment that prevents an individual from performing one or more gainful activities; not synonymous with *handicap,* which implies serious disadvantage.

TO PROBE FURTHER

Persons with obvious disabling conditions receive cues from others that help them adapt to their disabilities. Anyone with a disability undergoes some revision of self-concept, a disruption in familiar role patterns, and a period of adjustment to the limitations. This adjustment usually involves going through the stages of the classic medical model of the "sick role": (1) exemption from normal responsibility, (2) wanting to get well, and (3) cooperation with health professionals.

However, the person with an invisible disability—such as kidney failure, some types of cancer, cardiovascular disease, or diabetes—often does not receive these supportive cues and feedback in the difficult task of adjustment, and is often denied obtaining employment. These conditions are not apparent or easily observed by casual acquaintances. Often this reinforces the human desire to deny the actual limitations and creates more damage through poor self-care. The person with an invisible disability is tempted to avoid the adjustment process and

ignore the condition's limitations. Yet these persons need rehabilitative support and training as much as those with more obvious disabilities.

These psychologic aspects of invisible disability carry implications for all members of the health team. Because the loss is not tangible, the patient or client often lacks the support for living a normal life in the home or workplace, especially support for the initial grieving and adjustment needed for living with a chronic condition, which hinders adjustment. Health professionals must be aware of the psychodynamics of the adaptive process, anticipate needs, offer guidance, and assist the client in mourning outwardly. Then the healing process can begin.

REFERENCES

Cross EW: Implementing the Americans with Disabilities Act, *J Am Diet Assoc* 93(3):273, 1993.

Falvo DR, Allen H, Maki DR: Psychosocial aspects of invisible disability, *Rehabil Lit* 43:2, 1982.

for maximal self-care and added care by the attendant must be provided.

Psychologic Barriers

Positive resolution of many practical and emotional problems requires tremendous psychologic adjustment. Each person struggles with self-image and physical body trauma. It is small wonder that they often withdraw in defeat and exhaustion. Personality changes occur during rehabilitation processes that test both inner strength and physical stamina. Depending on personal resources and strengths, the person may or may not be able to function. Much of the health team's keen insight and concern are directed toward supporting each person's efforts to meet individual needs. That many disabled persons do reach self-care goals in some measure is evident in the remarkable achievements some of them attain, despite or perhaps because of their difficulties.

Special Needs of Older Disabled Persons

America is aging. Population projections indicate that by the year 2000, 13% of the population will be over 65; by 2030, 22%. Over the next decade the most rapid population increase will be among those over 85 years of age.[2] And with older age comes an increased number of disabled elderly persons. The U.S. Rehabilitation Services Administration, using a baseline of 1 disabled American in 10, estimates that the odds of being disabled increase to 1 in 3 after age 65. Increased services, including rehabilitation services, are needed. But reha-

bilitation needs of older persons differ from those of younger people. Three life-changing events of aging determine these needs: retirement, chronic illness, and general physical decline.

Vocational Rehabilitation

Without adequate planning, many older persons experience stressful disorientation with retirement. They have had a lifetime occupation of active involvement in a familiar working environment, and now that sense of stability and identity is no longer there. Supportive activities focus on vocational planning and effective use of leisure time. At this point, many persons have not been accustomed to viewing leisure activities in a positive manner and need help in making this adjustment. In addition, vocational programs can help persons find gainful employment after they retire from work. Or, they can help retired healthy Americans find ways of contributing their wisdom and skills to others now working in the same field. In turn, such activity can enhance the health and social assets of the older person.

Residual Disabilities from Illnesses

In the age period of 60 to 75 years (the young-old), rehabilitation must focus on problems remaining from chronic diseases of aging: heart disease, hypertension, stroke, or cancer. Chronic illnesses may also be related to damaging health behaviors such as alcoholism, smoking, excessive eating of foods high in fat and salt, and a sedentary life-style. Survival after a heart attack or stroke, which now occurs more frequently with modern medical care, may leave an older person with chronic disabilities. However, early efforts at rehabilitation help prevent disability, avoid complications, and restore reasonable function.

Physical Decline in Aging

In persons between 75 and 85 years of age and older (the old-old), disability increases sharply. Much of this increase comes from falls and resulting fractures, chronic brain failure, disorders in locomotion, impaired senses of perception, and increased problems with drug reactions and interactions. Older persons may have several different diseases and take a number of different drugs or receive a variety of medical treatments. In this age-group, minor disabilities often result in major handicaps. Mental and physical dependency may require supportive care in the home or long-term care facility. Common health problems in both the young-old and old-old groups involve nutritional care as well. These problems include arthritis, cardiorespiratory and cardiovascular insufficiency, depression, sensory deprivation, infections, skin and foot disorders, and nutritional deficiencies from poor dentition and fad diets.

In general, however, disease and disability do not affect only the young-old and old-old, nor are all members of these groups disabled. Many of the disabled are young people, and many older adults continue to be fit and healthy. But the increasing age of the general population inevitably brings with it an increasing number of older adults with chronic disease and various disabilities of aging. Even minor disabilities may cause major **handicaps** in everyday living, and minor injuries may bring major debilitating results. In any case, the twin goals of rehabilitation care continue to be prevention of further disability and restoration of the maximal function available.

Principles of Supportive Nutritional Care
Prevention of Malnutrition
Kilocalories

The rehabilitative process of physical therapy involves hard work. The patient tires easily, and the energy intake must be sufficient to meet the energy output demands. Excess kcalories must be avoided to prevent obesity, but sufficient energy for tissue metabolism is essential.

Protein

General protein needs are based on maintaining strength of tissue structure and function. Tissue and organ integrity protect against catabolism, infections, negative nitrogen balance, and **decubitus ulcers.**[3] Dietary protein in optimal quantity and quality ensures the necessary supply of all essential amino acids re-

quired for tissue synthesis. In addition to these general needs, severe trauma such as that involved in spinal cord injury brings special needs to meet the catabolic response.

Carbohydrate

General energy needs are great. They are met by optimal dietary carbohydrate as the body's major fuel source (see Chapters 2 and 14). Severe trauma requires maximal carbohydrate, especially in the early stages following injury. More breakdown of tissue protein and fat occurs to provide needed energy, but this only adds to the negative nitrogen balance. Thus, sufficient carbohydrate foods are important to provide the needed energy and spare protein for its essential tissue-rebuilding function.

Fat

At any point in rehabilitation care the diet must supply linoleic acid, the essential fatty acid, and a moderate amount of fat for the body's general metabolic activities and tissue integrity. The general dietary recommendation that fat supply about 30% of the total kilocalories is sufficient. Some fat for food palatability also enhances appetite, which tends to be poor in the course of long-term illness.

Vitamins and Minerals

Optimal intake of vitamins and minerals for metabolic activity and maintenance of tissue reserves is needed. The normal RDA standards for age and sex are adequate in most cases. However, a deficiency state such as anemia indicates need for supplementation. In some rehabilitation centers multivitamin preparations are given routinely to ensure adequate amounts.

Restoration of Eating Ability
Normal Development of the Eating Process

In the normal growth and development of a child, the feeding and eating process develops through an overlapping and interdependent series of physical and physiologic stages. The usual activities of eating—swallowing, chewing, hand and utensil use—gradually de-

---

decubitus ulcer • Pressure sores in long-term bed-bound or immobile patients at points of bony protuberances, where prolonged pressure of body weight in one position cuts off adequate blood circulation to that area, causing tissue death and ulceration.

handicap • A mental or physical defect that may or may not be congenital, which prevents the individual from participating in normal life activities; implies disadvantage.

velop with motor ability. The learning comes with much practice and patience. In a sense, the injured person must "start over" and relearn these basic skills.

Thus, with an understanding of these normal patterns, the disabled person works with the professional team of occupational and physical therapists, nutritionists, and nurses to find adaptive procedures to restore basic eating ability. For each client, four aspects of the eating process will require individual attention: (1) the nature and degree of motor control, (2) eating position, (3) use of adapted utensils, and (4) supportive individual needs. For example, blind persons will need a description of the food served, its placement on the plate (named generally in a clockwise direction to help remember), and a follow-up training course in preparing food with a number of assistive tools and techniques.

Nutritional Base

The personal food plan must fulfill basic nutritional needs, in increased amounts to meet additional metabolic demands. In addition, appetite and motivation must be supported to accomplish the task. Sensory stimuli such as variety in food texture, color, and flavor can enhance appetite and help motivate the learning of new adapted modes of eating. Also, "comfort foods" or familiar ethnic dishes and well-liked foods can encourage the client with the sometimes frustrating and difficult process of relearning how to eat.

Independence in Daily Living

With each disabled person, the goal is to achieve as much independence in daily living as possible (see Issues and Answers, p. 521). Maximal use is made of individual neuromotor resources and emotional reserves. These personal resources are aided by self-help devices as needed. A large number of these creative devices are available, many of them the product of the inventive mind of a concerned occupational therapist.[4]

A number of representative disabling conditions can illustrate various areas of need for supportive nutritional care. Here we briefly review examples of such conditions in three types of problems: musculoskeletal disease, neuromuscular disease, and progressive neurologic disorders.

Musculoskeletal Disease

Rheumatoid Arthritis

Clinical Characteristics

The general term arthritis comes from the Greek word *arthron,* meaning "joint." Its underlying chronic, systemic, inflammatory disease process usually occurs in the young adult years. It is a severe type of *autoimmune* disorder in which the body's immune system acts against its own tissues. It mainly attacks the joints of the

hands, arms, and feet, causing them to become extremely painful, stiff, and deformed. The precise triggering antigen is still unknown. However, a number of possible primary causes (a virus or several viruses) that stimulate the immune response in the genetically susceptible host are under study.[5] The joint damage involves tissue changes in the **synosheaths.** Progressive joint deformity and destruction usually progress rapidly.

This disability dramatically affects activities of daily living, especially the fundamental necessity of obtaining and eating food. There is hand and wrist involvement, including destruction of wrist ligaments and tendons, with weakened finger and hand grip strength, and limited finger movement (Fig. 26-1). All of these changes limit ability to self-feed, shop for food, or prepare it. Also, elbow and shoulder involvement hinder bringing food to the mouth. Further tissue damage of the *temporomandibular joint (TMJ)* of the jaws limits normal opening and closing of the mouth and alters chewing ability. Other nonjoint problems—such as anemia of chronic disease, decrease in salivary secretions, dysphagia, and bone disease—further complicate nutrition problems leading to overall malnutrition. In its juvenile form in children and adolescents, this resulting malnutrition can cause serious growth retardation.

Medical Management

Medical treatment may involve a number of drugs for control of the inflammatory process. Aspirin, as well as other nonsteroidal anti-inflammatory drugs (NSAIDs), is still a mainstay of medical therapy, with the use of enteric-coated preparations to avoid gastric irritation (see Chapter 19). Other drugs used to control the inflammatory process include gold salts, D-penicillamine, steroids, and immunosuppressive agents.[5] Weekly low-dose therapy with the anticancer drug methotrexate, which acts as as an antimetabolite to folic acid in DNA synthesis, is sometimes used but frequently causes the complicating viral condition **herpes zoster.**[7] When irreversible destruction of cartilage occurs in advanced stages of the disease, reconstructive joint surgery along with physical therapy and occupational therapy gives the best results.[5]

Nutritional Management

In all settings, planning nutritional support must begin with early assessment of individual patient status and needs, especially to detect any degree of malnutrition.[6] An initial history must thus assess potential drug-nutrition-food interactions and their nutritional effects (see Chapter 17). Also, the history should include any of the numerous unproven regimens for arthritis that the patient may be using.[6] In addition, attention may be given to dietary modifications under study that have shown therapeutic promise. Results indicate that

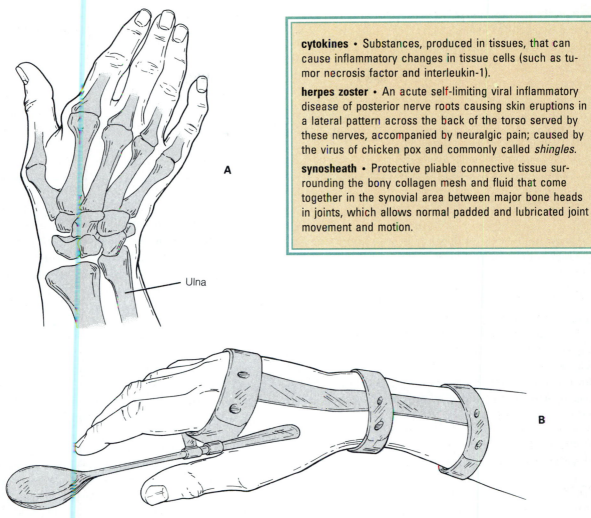

FIG. 26-1 **A,** Arthritic hand showing ulnar drift. **B,** Self-help device for stirring food during preparation and for eating assistance.

supplementation with the omega-3 fatty acids (see Chapter 3) suppresses synthesis of **cytokines** with potent inflammatory activities.[8]

Special functional assessment of eating ability is also needed, including any swallowing problem from lack of salivary secretions and dysphagia (see Clinical Application, p. 508).[9] Standard nutritional assessment is essential (see Chapter 16). On the basis of these data, nutritional needs can be determined and monitored.

1. **Energy.** Energy needs, especially for children, vary widely and must be determined on an individual basis. In general, needs will involve basal energy expenditure plus added multiples for increased metabolic activity factors, such as stress of disease activity, sepsis, fever, skeletal injury, or surgery (see Chapter 23). If the client is receiving physical therapy, an additional physical activity factor is used. Total kcalories are increased as needed to achieve desirable weight gain during growth,

or decreased if indicated for obese adults. Follow-up monitoring determines any needed adjustments in energy estimates.

2. **Protein.** Protein needs vary with protein status, surgical therapy, proteinuria, and nitrogen balance. A well-nourished adult patient needs about 0.5 to 1.0 g of protein/kg/day during quiet disease periods. An increase to 1.5 to 2.0 g/kg/day is needed during active inflammatory disease periods. The RDA standards for age and sex can guide protein needs for children to meet basic growth needs. States of malnutrition will require more.

3. **Vitamins and minerals.** Standard recommendations for vitamins and minerals are used. Specific supplementation may be used if needed, such as supplying calcium and vitamin D if bone disease is involved.

4. **Special enteral and parenteral feeding.** Tube

CLINICAL **A**PPLICATION   *Tilt and Swallow*

The swallowing reflex is frequently diminished or absent in disabled persons. The reflex may be enhanced, however, by the use of an ice collar or by brushing the neck with a small brush, such as a paint brush, just before eating. The liquid or semisolid food should be placed behind the front teeth, and the patient should slowly tilt the head back and swallow. This routine may be learned as the helper uses the repeated statement, "Tilt and swallow . . . tilt and swallow . . ."

REFERENCE
Price ME, Dilorio C: Swallowing: A practice guide, *Am J Nurs* 90(7):42, 1990. ◆

---

feeding may be used either to supplement oral intake or to supply total nutrition support (see Chapter 18). Parenteral nutrition support is seldom used, except for preoperative and postoperative needs or when bowel rest is indicated.

The course of rheumatoid arthritis is unpredictable. The disease is usually progressive, and some degree of permanent disability results. But many persons after years of disease are capable of self-care with rehabilitation training and are fully employable. Continuing optimal nutritional support is important maintenance therapy.

Osteoarthritis

This milder form of arthritis in older adults is more appropriately called *degenerative joint disease* because minimal inflammation is involved. Osteoarthritis affects approximately 44% of persons over age 40 in the United States. It is also chronic and may progress, limiting movement of affected joints, mainly the hands, knees, and hips. Marked disability is uncommon, but osteoarthritis may become a chronic disabling disease in the elderly.[10] There is no cure for the disease, which ultimately destroys cartilage between rubbing heads of bones in involved joints. However, damaged joints can be replaced by *arthroplasty*, surgical removal of the degenerated joint and replacement of a joint made with metal or plastic components. Hip replacements have been performed since the early 1960s, and the technique is now being refined and applied to other joints. In general, appropriate pain-controlling medication and nutritional support for general health promotion help relieve symptoms. Depending on degree of hand joint involvement, self-feeding devices may assist eating.

Osteoporosis

The metabolic bone disorder *osteoporosis* is the most common skeletal disorder in the United States, affecting about 24 million individuals. Approximately one third of postmenopausal women in the United States have osteoporosis and suffer from some 1.3 million associated fractures each year. Over age 70, osteoporosis affects both men and women after a slow, steady rate of bone loss and increasing fracture potential develop over many decades. When the porous bone mass finally falls below a fracture threshold, fractures occur spontaneously or with little trauma. These fractures in the elderly are a major cause of disabling illness and death. Bones of the vertebrae and the hip are most vulnerable, but hip fractures are more serious. The annual cost of treating patients with osteoporosis ranges from $7 to $12 billion.[11]

Medical treatment of postmenopausal osteoporosis in women is most effectively managed with estrogen replacement therapy. The slow, steadily developing form of osteoporosis in men and women responds more readily to nutritional therapy with a sound diet, including a calcium intake of 1200 to 1500 mg/day (see Chapters 8 and 13), increased physical activity, and weight control. Newer medical treatments under investigation include the cyclic use of bisphosphonate (etidronate), a structural analog of the naturally occurring pyrophosphate, a component of the hydroxyapatite crystals forming bone.[11,12] The best approach, of course, is prevention. This is achieved by ensuring that adolescents and young adults have sufficient dietary calcium for building bone mass, which peaks by age 30, stimulated by physical activity. Then a continuing sound diet and physical activity help sustain this normal bone mass.

Neuromuscular Disease

Growing Problem of Neurologic Injuries

In the United States, traumatic injury is the leading cause of death in the first four decades of life,[13,14] and the third leading cause of death for all ages. Some 150,000 persons per year are killed outright by automobile and industrial accidents, gunshot wounds and homicides, and sports injuries.[13,15] Increasingly, the strain on urban medical care centers comes into focus as special investigation reports in our local city newspapers remind us in bold front page Sunday headlines—"Trauma Care in Crisis."[16] Further realization of the problem of traumatic injury comes from the fact that more Americans die of highway trauma each year than have died of AIDS since that disease was first identified in 1981, and in both conditions the majority of the victims are young males between 16 and 30 years of age.[13]

Brain and Spinal Cord Injury

With current advances in emergency medicine, the number of persons surviving traumatic brain and spinal cord injury has increased dramatically. Here we review nutritional care of the injured patient in the acute care setting and follow-up nutritional management in rehabilitation.

Traumatic Brain Injury

Postinjury Metabolic Alterations

The brain is the control center of body functions and activities. Thus brain injury brings an immediate cascade of systemic metabolic responses that affect the entire body as the body mobilizes its resources to protect itself. The systemic inflammatory response is activated, and a sustained state of *hypermetabolism* develops. Ultimately, if the process continues unchecked, a sequence of organ failure follows. Any complication prolongs the hypermetabolic phase, and the increasing protein catabolism causes depletion of lean body mass.[17,18] Increased energy expenditure and urinary nitrogen excretion mark this increased metabolic demand in response to trauma.

Initial Nutrition Management

The immediate goals of the trauma team are control of the injury, maintenance of oxygen transport, and metabolic support.[17] Nutritional support as soon as possible is vital to meet the hypermetabolic drain on the body tissue resources for increased energy and protein demands.[18,19] Regular monitoring of energy needs is essential, often more than once a day. Most trauma centers now use indirect calorimetry at the bedside with a mobile calorimeter unit (see Chapter 6).

Early nutrition support may be delivered by either enteral or parenteral route (Chapter 18). Successful use has been reported of enteral feedings as early as 2 to 3 days after injury, achieving full caloric intake of 3020 kcal/24 hr by day 7 (Vital HN—Ross: 10% fat, 16% hydrolyzed protein, 74% carbohydrate, continuous infusion).[20] Parenteral nutrition is an alternate option because it can be started within the first 24 hours after injury and may be immediately adjusted to the nutritional requirements of each patient according to daily metabolic profile and urinary nitrogen analysis.[21] Some trauma centers prefer a combination of early total parenteral nutrition (TPN) through a central vein catheter (see Chapter 18) within 24 hours, starting enteral nutrition as soon as it can be tolerated, gradually tapering the TPN and discontinuing it when the enteral feeding is considered adequate.[17]

Rehabilitation Nutrition

Nutritional rehabilitation of the patient with traumatic brain injury presents a complex of individual problems that require skilled and sensitive nutrition management. To develop individual nutritional care plans, the rehabilitation dietitian works closely with other team members, especially the nurse, occupational therapist, speech pathologist, cognitive rehabilitation therapist, and physical therapist.[22] Together they assess the degree of *dysphagia,* difficulty with chewing and swallowing, level of language deficits and communication, and ability to perform basic daily living skills including food preparation and eating. Short- and long-range goals, as well as strategies to reach these goals, are developed along with many practical suggestions for adapting food forms and textures to meet eating problems.

Spinal Cord Injury

Postinjury Management

Each year catastrophic spinal cord injury in the United States affects some 10,000 trauma survivors between the ages of 16 and 30 years.[15] Over 200,000 quadriplegic and paraplegic patients now require lifetime care at an estimated annual cost of approximately $600,000.[23] Due to advanced medical care, the number of survivors is increasing each year. Most of these spinal cord injuries are due to automobile accidents (48%); other factors include falls (21%), sports injuries (14%), and physical assaults (15%).[23] Injury and loss of neurologic function in the upper cervical area of the spinal cord results in *quadriplegia,* paralysis from the neck down. Injuries and loss of neurologic function in the lower thoracic, lumbar, and sacral areas of the spine result in *paraplegia,* paralysis of the lower portion of the body. This spinal cord damage disrupts the nerve transmission of impulses from the brain to peripheral nerves and muscles, so that muscle function below the level of injury is lost. Immobilization brings complicating illnesses. Protein-energy malnutrition is common. About half of the hospitalized patients and two thirds of the patients admitted to a rehabilitation unit have clinical signs of malnutrition.

Nutrition Management

Enteral feeding tubes placed beyond the pylorus usually make it possible to start nutrition support within 3 to 5 days after the injury. The patients are usually well-nourished at the time of injury. Thus the goal of starting the feeding process as early as possible is to counteract the initial acute phase of spinal shock, and to prevent the onset of a malnutrition decline and secondary illnesses. There is wide variation in metabolic rates, hence energy needs, but they tend to be lower than those of other trauma patients due to decreased metabolic activity of denervated muscle.[23] The higher the injury to the spinal column, the greater the denervated muscle mass and the lower the measure of energy expenditure. Daily guidelines for energy needs are 23 kcal/kg for quadriplegics and 28 kcal/kg for paraplegics.[23]

Rehabilitation Nutrition

When the acute phase passes and the patient is stabilized, usually within 2 to 3 months after the injury, the extended rehabilitation training phase begins. This complex process of many parts is designed to restore the client to the best functional capacity possible to promote independent living.[24] The goal is to prevent and treat any complications associated with spinal cord injury. Combined therapies are used from the team of rehabilitation specialists: physiatrist, registered dietitian, registered nurse, physical therapist, occupational therapist, speech therapist, psychologist, social worker, and vocational counselor. Nutritional management involves individual assessment and care of (1) basic energy-nutrient needs and feeding capacities and (2) complications associated with the spinal cord injury.

Basic Nutritional Needs

Energy needs are based on sufficient kcalories to maintain an ideal body weight somewhat below that for a comparable person given in standard weight-height tables for healthy populations (see inside back book cover). For example, general weight goals for paraplegics have been recommended at 10 to 15 lb below standard body weight, and for quadriplegics, 15 to 20 lb below standard.[24,25] Excess weight gain is common in spinal cord injury clients due to the decreased metabolic rate that persists from the preceding acute postinjury phase and the continued relative immobilization.[23] Obesity contributes to medical problems, and adds physical problems in the frequent turning in bed necessary to prevent bed sores, and the transfers from bed to wheelchair. Adequate protein intake is essential for maintaining muscle mass and tissue integrity to prevent negative nitrogen balance, ulcer formation, and infection. Palatable high-protein supplements between meals may be needed to maintain an adequate intake. The client may be at risk for vitamin or mineral deficiencies if appetite and food intake are poor due to depression or fatigue. A standard multiple vitamin-mineral preparation is frequently recommended.

Associated Complications

Several nutrition-related complications in rehabilitation for spinal cord injury patients require special attention.

1. Pressure sores. Pressure sores, or decubitus ulcers, are caused by immobilization, loss of pressure sen-

sation around bony prominences, decreased blood circulation, skin breakdown, and ulcer formation open to infection and difficult to heal. Pressure sores occur in 60% of quadriplegic patients and 52% of paraplegics. Nutritional factors involved include anemia, which reduces oxygen supply to tissues; excessive weight loss, which reduces padding of bony prominences; and low levels of plasma proteins such as albumin, which lead to edema and loss of skin elasticity. The protein deficiency requires an increased protein intake. More severe ulcers require more intense nutritional intervention, with protein needs of 1.5 to 2.0 g/kg. Other nutrients important to the healing process include supplements of vitamin C and zinc.

2. Hypercalciuria. Immobility leads to an imbalance in calcium metabolism, with a loss of bone calcium and its increased excretion in the urine. In the long term, this loss of bone calcium leads to osteoporosis, which has been found to be present and progressive in 88% of patients with spinal cord injury, affecting the denervated musculoskeletal tissue below the level of injury.[23] A balance of calcium-vitamin D therapy and prudent control of excessive protein intake, which causes increased calcium withdrawal, is indicated. Bone fractures result in about 7% of these patients.

3. Kidney stones. Hypercalciuria also contributes to formation of kidney stones. The neurogenic effects following spinal cord injury cause loss of normal bladder control, resulting in problems of urinary reflux, retention, incontinence, infection, and stone formation.[24] Regular catheterization is necessary to prevent accumulation of bacteria and solutes such as calcium and other particles that can easily form stones. A high fluid intake of 2 to 3 L/day to dilute the urine and reduce the solute concentration must be a part of the overall nutrition care plan.

4. Neurogenic bowel. Gastrointestinal complications from loss of normal neuromuscular controls include decreased peristalsis and loss of bowel control. A regular schedule for emptying the bowel is necessary. About 12 hours before the scheduled time, 4 oz (120 ml) of prune juice with a little lemon juice is taken. About 20 to 30 minutes before the scheduled evacuation time, one or two glycerine suppositories are placed well above the anal sphincter, at least 2½ in. (6.5 cm) into the rectum, against the rectal mucosa. The patient is then placed on the toilet or bedside commode and provided with adequate support. This daily schedule and recording of results continues with no interruption by enemas. The patient is taught manual evacuation for continuing care at home. A vital part of this care is a high-fiber diet to provide added bulk and ample fluid intake to prevent impaction.

5. Depression. During the initial days of shock and survival, the patient does not yet realize full impact of the disability. When transfer to the rehabilitation unit occurs and the full extent of the disability is realized, a period of depression begins; this is a normal part of the personal grieving and healing process. The severity and duration of this period depends in large measure on the patient's personal strengths and resources. But the sensitive yet realistic support of the family and the rehabilitation team is also required if the serious and demanding work of rehabilitation is to be successful. The nutritionist must help ensure that adequate energy, protein, and fluid intake is maintained. Nutritional status is repleted with appetizing foods, especially when the patient's spirit is low. Even subtle improvements in muscle mass and function brought about by the nutritional care can be a source of strength to mind and body.

Cerebrovascular Accident (CVA)—Stroke

Brain injury due to a stroke also causes varying degrees of nerve damage and body paralysis (Chapter 20). Cerebrovascular disease from underlying atherosclerosis ranks third as a cause of death and second as a cause of disability in the United States.[26] In recent years the incidence of strokes has declined, largely because of improvement in control of hypertension and increased public education concerning hypertension. Nutrition management is detailed in Chapter 20. Rehabilitation care follows the same general goals and methods discussed in this chapter (see Case Study, p. 520).

Developmental Disabilities

During the developmental period of childhood, neuromuscular conditions such as cerebral palsy, epilepsy, spina bifida, and Down syndrome cause eating problems that can contribute to poor growth and delayed development.

Cerebral Palsy

Cerebral palsy is a general term for nonprogressive disorders of muscle control of movements and posture. It has many causes and results in brain damage that occurs largely before or at birth, probably due ultimately to hypoxia, poor oxygen supply to the brain.[27] Most affected children fall into one of two groups: *spastic*, in which muscles of one or more limbs are permanently contracted, making normal movements very difficult if at all possible; and *athetoid*, in which involuntary writhing movements are made. Mental retardation, with an IQ below 70, occurs in about 75% of persons with cerebral palsy, mostly in the spastic group. Exceptions, however, occurring mostly in the athetoid group, are important, and some of these individuals are highly intelligent. Some features of the condition during childhood change as the child grows older, often for the better, with patience and skillful treatment.

Early nutritional management focuses mainly on feeding problems. When the infant or young child cannot obtain sufficient nourishment due to oral motor dysfunction, or when satisfactory oral feeding is interrupted for a prolonged period due to illness or surgery, enteral nutrition support by nasoenteric or gastrostomy tube feeding (Chapter 18) may be necessary.[27] In such cases, transition to oral feeding is usually difficult. In any case, oral feeding poses numerous problems, both functional and behavioral. Feeding problems of oral motor dysfunction (such as difficulties in sucking, swallowing, or chewing), gross motor/self-feeding impairment, lack of appetite, and food aversions, as well as alternate feeding practices of prolonged assisted feeding and use of pureed foods significantly reduce energy and nutrient intake.[28] Early and ongoing nutrition assessment, intervention, and counseling are essential components of rehabilitation team care. When accurate height measures to assess growth are difficult due to joint contractures, spasticity, or inability to stand, reasonably accurate stature can be calculated from knee height measures (see Chapter 16), using the standard equations given in Table 26-1.[29] Growth retardation in children persists with age. Many adults still have feeding problems, but exercise helps promote better nutrition.[30]

Epilepsy

Epilepsy, literally "seizures," is a neuromuscular disorder in which abnormal electrical activity in the brain causes recurring transient seizures. Normally the brain regulates all human activities, thoughts, perceptions, and emotions through the regular orderly electrical excitation of its nerve cells. But in an epileptic state during a seizure, an unregulated chaotic electrical discharge occurs. Seizures often appear spontaneously, or, in some cases, they may be set off by some stimulus such as a flashing light. This brain dysfunction may develop for no obvious reason, or an individual may have an

---

TABLE 26-1

Equations for Estimating Stature from Knee Height

Age/Sex Group	Equation
White males	
6-18 years	stature = (knee height × 2.22) + 40.54
19-59 years	stature = (knee height × 1.88) + 71.85
White females	
6-18 years	stature = (knee height × 2.15) + 43.21
19-59 years	stature = (knee height × 1.86) − (age × 0.05) ± 70.25

Adapted from Estimating stature from knee height. In *Directions for the Ross Knee Height Caliper*, Columbus, Ohio, Ross Laboratories, 1990.

Equations are based on normal, healthy individuals. Stature and knee height are measured in centimeters.

inherited predisposition. In other cases it may result from a wide variety of disease or injury, such as birth trauma, metabolic imbalance in the body, head injury, brain infection (meningitis, encephalitis), stroke, brain tumor, drug intoxication, or alcohol or drug withdrawal states. Epilepsy occurs in about 1 person in 200; the number of epileptics in the United States is about 1 million. Usually the disorder starts in childhood or adolescence. About a third of these young people outgrow the condition and do not need medication. An-

other third find their seizures well controlled by drug treatment and require less medication over time. The remaining third find that their condition remains the same or becomes more resistant to drug therapy. Anticonvulsant drugs are the first line of treatment for epilepsy and in most cases decrease the frequency of seizures.

Nutritional management of epilepsy functions in several areas of care. First, it helps ensure an appropriate diet for normal growth during childhood and adolescence and for health maintenance in adulthood. Second, it seeks to ameliorate side effects of anticonvulsant drugs. Some of the most commonly used drugs and their relation to food and nutrients are shown in Table 26-2. Third, if a *ketogenic* diet is used, the clinical nutritionist is responsible for its calculations and for the education of staff, patient, and family in its use. This special high-fat diet was developed to control epilepsy before current anticonvulsant drugs became widely available in the 1940s. It is still successfully used for children with intractable myoclonic epilepsy that resists drug therapy.[31]

Spina Bifida

Spina bifida is a congenital defect in the formation of the spine. It develops during early embryonic life, when the neural tube, which forms the spinal cord, does not close completely, leaving part of one or more vertebrae of the spinal cord exposed at birth.[32] The vertebral canal usually closes within 4 weeks of conception. Thus, this congenital defect can often be diagnosed early in pregnancy by ultrasound scanning or by high levels of **alpha-fetoprotein** in the amniotic fluid or maternal blood, so that appropriate genetic counseling can be provided for the parents. The defect can occur anywhere along the spine but is more common in the lower back. The neurologic damage that occurs depends on the severity and level of the lesion on the spine.[33] The incidence is about 1 case per 1,000 babies born, but this number increases with either very young or old maternal age. A mother who has had one affected child is 10 times more likely than the average rate of having another affected child.

There are three main forms of spina bifida.

Spina bifida occulta. This is the least serious and most common form of spina bifida. The name indicates an "unseen cleft in the spine." It often goes unnoticed in otherwise healthy children save for a small dimple over the area of the underlying abnormality.

Myelomeningocele. Also known as myelocele, this is the most severe form of spina bifida, and the affected child is usually severely disabled. Here the spinal cord (mylo) and its enveloping membranes (meninges) protrude from the spine in a sac (cele).

TABLE 26-2

Anticonvulsant Drugs Used to Control Basic Types of Epilepsy and Their Nutrition-Related Side Effects

Most Commonly Used Drug	Drug Trade Name	Nutrition-Related Side Effects
Grand mal (tonic/clonic) seizures		
Phenytoin (adults)	Dilantin	Nausea, vomiting, and constipation; reduced taste sensation; vitamins D and K catabolism; reduced serum calcium, B_6, B_{12}, folate, and serum magnesium levels; overgrowth of gums
Phenobarbitol	Luminal	Increased appetite or anorexia, nausea, vomiting, vitamins D and K catabolism, reduced bone density
Primidone	Mysoline	Gastrointestinal upset, weight loss
Carbamazepine	Tegretol	Nausea, vomiting, diarrhea, abdominal pain, xerostomia (dry mouth), glossitis (sore tongue), stomatitis (sore mouth), increased blood urea nitrogen
Petit mal (absence) seizures		
Ethosuximide	Zarontin	Gastrointestinal upset, nausea, vomiting, anorexia, weight loss
Valproic acid	Depakane, Depakote	Nausea, vomiting, indigestion, diarrhea, abdominal pain, constipation, anorexia and weight loss, or increased appetite and weight gain
Clonazepam	Klonopin	Hyperactivity, short attention span, impulsive behavior, weight gain
Partial seizures		
Phenytoin (adults)	Dilantin	Nausea, vomiting, and constipation; reduced taste sensation; vitamins D and K catabolism; reduced levels of serum calcium, B_6, B_{12}, folate, and serum magnesium; overgrowth of gums
Phenobarbitol	Luminal	Increased appetite or anorexia, nausea, vomiting, vitamins D and K catabolism, reduced bone density
Carbamazepine	Tegretol	Nausea, vomiting, diarrhea, abdominal pain, xerostomia (dry mouth), glossitis (sore tongue), stomatitis (sore mouth), increased blood urea nitrogen

Meningocele. This form of spina bifida is less severe because the nerve tissue of the spinal cord is usually intact. Outer skin covers the bulging sac, and therefore there are usually no functional problems. Ideally, necessary surgical repairs are performed in the first few days of life.

Nutrition management of children with spina bifida focuses on growth pattern and individual degree of problems with growth retardation and short stature, low muscle mass and weakness, deformities or paralysis of lower extremities, and reduced ability to control bladder and bowels. Normal growth charts have been revised for use with nutrition assessment of these children.[32] Nutrition care plans give attention to the main problems of short statue and poor growth, increased weight, and constipation. Obesity is a particular problem due to several factors: (1) low basal metabolic rate related to lowered amount of lean body mass, (2) little physical activity related to the disabled condition and dependency on a wheelchair, and (3) use of food and overfeeding by parents or other caregivers to reward or show love or to counteract what is seen as frailty or weakness due to the disability. All of these factors become part of ongoing nutrition counseling.

Down Syndrome

A chromosomal abnormality accounts for the mental retardation and characteristic appearance of children with Down syndrome, a condition first described in the previous century by the English physician John L. H. Down (1828-1896). Its cause remained a mystery until 1959, when modern researchers discovered that persons with Down syndrome had one too many chromosomes in each of their cells (47 instead of the normal 46). Then, because the extra chromosome is usually number 21, they gave it the alternate name of *trisomy 21.* The two parent chromosomes numbered 21 fail to go into separate daughter cells during the first stage of sperm or egg cell formation, and some eggs or sperm are thus formed with an extra number 21 chromosome. If one of these takes part in fertilization, the resulting baby will have the extra chromosome and Down syndrome. This event is more likely if the mother is over age 35, indicating that defective egg formation, rather than sperm formation, is usually the cause. Down syndrome occurs in about 1 in 650 babies born. The rate rises steeply with increased maternal age to about 1 in 40 among mothers over age 40. The degree of mental retardation varies with an IQ between 30 and 80, but all children with Down syndrome are capable of limited learning. These children are usually affectionate, cheerful, and friendly, and they get along well with family and friends. They thrive and reach their full potential in a loving family.

Nutritional needs center on delayed learning of feeding skills; inappropriate, excessive, or inadequate intakes of food energy and nutrients; and poor eating habits. Studies indicate frequent obesity, possibly due to excessive fat, low physical activity, or both.[34] Diets need to be individualized because these children tend to gain excess weight if they are given the intakes recommended for most children. Plans for increasing physical activity are important.

Progressive Neurologic Disorders

Progressive neurologic disorders, especially during the middle and older years of adulthood, have disabling effects on the personal lives of many individuals. Examples reviewed here illustrate some of these effects and nutrition approaches to providing support.

Parkinson's Disease

Parkinson's disease is a long-known neurologic disease, first described by the English physician James Parkinson (1755-1824) nearly 2 centuries ago, but its underlying origin remains unknown. Current researchers speculate that the triggering cause may be related to some environmental factor such as a toxin.[35] Genetic factors are not the cause but may predispose persons in some families to the disease. It is a common disorder that has been reported in every race and region of the world, usually with onset of motor symptoms after age 40, rising in incidence with advancing age. In the United States, about 1 person in 200, mostly elderly, is affected by the disease, with some 50,000 new cases a year. Men are more likely to be affected than women.

The disorder affects the *basal ganglia* of the brain, a cluster of nerve cells at the central base of the brain. Signals from the brain's motor cortex pass via the brainstem *reticular formation* and the spinal cord to the muscles, which contract. Other signals pass through the basal ganglia, which provides a *damping effect* to help smooth and control the signal flow to reticular formation and spinal cord, thus preventing uncoordinated muscle contraction responses. This damping effect is produced by the balancing action of two neurotransmitters: *dopamine,* which is made in the basal ganglia, is necessary for the damping effect, and stimulates the signal flow, and *acetylcholine,* which is a widespread neu-

alpha-fetoprotein • A fetal antigen in amniotic fluid that provides an early pregnancy test for fetal malformations such as neural tube defect.

spina bifida • A congenital defect in the fetal closing of the neural tube to form a portion of the lower spine, leaving the spine unclosed and the spinal cord open in various degrees of exposure and damage.

rotransmitter in the body that inhibits the signal flow. In Parkinson's disease, degeneration of key parts of the basal ganglia causes a lack of dopamine within this part of the brain, thus preventing the basal ganglia from modifying nerve pathways that control muscle function.[36] The muscles become overly tense, causing joint rigidity and general body stiffness, a fine constant tremor even at rest, and slow movements.

Medical Management

Although there is no cure for Parkinson's disease, drug management has helped minimize symptoms for many patients. A dramatic change in treatment came in the 1960s with the advent of the drug levodopa, which the body can transform into the needed dopamine. Dopamine itself cannot be used since it does not cross the blood-brain barrier as does levodopa.[36] The major goals of present research are (1) to devise new methods of drug delivery to achieve a slow, steady release and (2) to find a means of slowing down the progression of Parkinson's disease.[37] Current surgical researchers are investigating transplants of dopamine-secreting adrenal medulla tissue and the brain grafting of fetal dopamine neurons.[37,38]

Nutritional Management

Nutritional care centers on nutrition-related drug effects, eating problems, and malnutrition. Common side effects of levodopa include severe nausea that affects food intake. Excessive intake of vitamin B_6 should be avoided because it interacts with levodopa and reduces the drug's beneficial effect. Hand tremors make it difficult to obtain and prepare food and to perform eating movements of carrying food from bowl or plate to the mouth. Thus, for example, soups should be avoided and more textured foods used. As the disease progresses, people with Parkinson's disease may have problems with chewing, swallowing, or aspiration of small food items such as peas or nuts, as well as discomfort from constipation, flatulence, or delayed gastric emptying. Small, frequent meals with increased carbohydrate and decreased fat content, chewing thoroughly and eating slowly with special utensils as needed, appropriate energy intake to maintain optimal weight, and adequate fiber and fluid to prevent constipation will all be helpful.

A recent study indicates that a special diet of daytime protein restriction to about 10 g provides a helpful adjunct therapy for patients experiencing unpredictable motor-response fluctuations from the drug levodopa.[39] Protein foods (such as meat and dairy products) to meet a day's total RDA intake (0.8 g/kg/day), are reserved for use in the evening meal and later snack. These beneficial effects of steady symptom control appear to result from a decrease during the day in the plasma concentration of dietary protein-derived large neutral amino acids that compete with L-dopa for transport into the brain.

Huntington's Chorea

First described by American physician George Huntington (1850-1916), Huntington's chorea is an uncommon genetic disease in which degeneration of the basal ganglia of the brain results in **chorea**—rapid, jerky, involuntary movements, and *dementia*—progressive mental impairment. Recently, after a decade-long search, a large group of scientists from six institutions finally discovered the defective gene that causes the disease, opening the way to future therapies and possibly to an eventual cure.[40] Symptoms do not usually appear until about age 35 to 50; cases of symptomatic effects beginning in childhood are rare. This genetic disease is inherited in an autosomal dominant pattern, with each child having a 50% chance of the condition developing. In the United States, the disease develops in about 5 persons per 100,000. Generally, the symptoms do not appear until middle adulthood, so affected persons may have children before learning that they have the disease.

Medical Management

As a result of recent advances in genetics, a test is now available for young adults whose parents have Huntington's chorea. The test allows these individuals to learn, with 95% accuracy, whether they carry the gene and thus have the disorder. The test can then help them decide whether or not to have children. Huntington's chorea has no known cure, but medical management helps lessen the characteristic chorea, which affects face, arms, and trunk with random grimaces, twitches, and general clumsiness. The drug chlorpromazine (Thorazine), the most widely used antipsychotic drug for its tranquilizing effect (it suppresses brain centers that control abnormal emotions and behaviors), has been found useful. The mental impairment causes behavior changes, difficulty making decisions, apathy, irritability, and memory loss.

Nutritional Management

The excessive muscular activity requires adequate energy and nutrient intake to prevent malnutrition and excess weight loss. As the disease progresses, patients become cachectic, and even with adequate food intake, a progressively catabolic state develops. Nutritional counseling involves help in planning diets dense in energy nutrients to combat malnutrition, and assistance with dysphagia or feeding problems and with the drug side effect of constipation.

Guillain-Barré Syndrome

This acute postinfectious polyneuritis was first described by two twentieth-century French neurologists,

Georges Guillain (1876-1961) and Jean Alexander Barré (1880-1965). Guillain-Barré syndrome is a rare form of damage to the peripheral nerves, in which the myelin sheaths covering nerve axons, and sometimes the axons themselves, deteriorate, causing loss of nerve conduction and partial or complete paralysis.[41] Nerve inflammation occurs particularly where the nerve roots leave the spine, impairing both movement and sensation. Muscular weakness in the legs, often accompanied by numbness and tingling, progresses upward to the trunk, arms, face, and head. A low-grade fever persists, and there may be urinary tract infection, respiratory failure requiring a ventilator, and personality changes. This acute syndrome is an autoimmune reaction, often following a viral infection and sometimes an immunization. In general, incidence in the United States is about 15 cases per million people per year.

Medical Management

Hospitalization for close monitoring of patients with an acute condition is essential, especially if a breathing difficulty occurs. Severe cases may require *plasmapheresis,* in which blood plasma is withdrawn from the patient, treated to remove antibodies, and replaced. Most people recover completely without specific treatment other than general supportive care, but some are left with permanent weakness in affected areas.

Nutritional Management

During early acute phases, enteral or parenteral nutrition support may be necessary, with attention to increased energy and protein needs in the formula solutions (see Chapter 18). Also, if respiratory distress requiring ventilator assistance occurs, increased fat for needed energy fuel rather than increased carbohydrate would be indicated, such as for patients with chronic obstructive pulmonary disease (see Chapter 20). Food consistency and texture may need to be adjusted in early oral feedings to accommodate any chewing and swallowing problems from weak facial and throat muscles. Continuing attention to energy and nutrient needs during convalescence is required to restore lost body weight and muscle mass.

Amyotrophic Lateral Sclerosis

Amyotrophic lateral sclerosis (ALS) is the most common of the motor neuron diseases.[42] It is also known as Lou Gehrig's disease, for the famous U.S. baseball player who was struck down by ALS at the height of his successful Major League career. In persons with these rare neuron disorders, nerves that control muscular activity degenerate within the brain and spinal cord. Researchers recently reported the discovery of the gene causing a hereditary form of the disease.[43,44] The gene controls the synthesis of an enzyme that helps cells get rid of highly toxic and destructive superoxide free radi-

cals, which are produced by a variety of oxidative cell reactions. If the enzyme were abnormal due to the defective ALS gene, free cell radicals might well build up, causing the death of the motor neurons affected in persons with ALS. As it is now, this relentless nerve degeneration of ALS progresses to involve the muscles of respiration and swallowing, usually killing its victims in about 3 years.[44] This giant step of identifying the responsible defective gene will lead to more knowledge of how the progressive destructive course of ALS may be slowed, controlled, or prevented.

Nutritional Management

Nutrition care planning and counseling focuses on increased energy intake and adjusted nutrient needs as the disease progresses.[45] Weakness of hands and arms, as well as problems with chewing, swallowing, delayed or absent response of gag reflex, and risk of aspiration require eating assistance and modification of food textures. Frequent small meals are better tolerated. In advanced stages, enteral and parenteral nutrition support can supply needed energy and nutrients in a variety of individualized formulas (see Chapter 18).

Multiple Sclerosis

Multiple sclerosis (MS) is a progressive disease of the central nervous system in which scattered patches of insulating myelin are destroyed. The myelin is the fatty covering of nerve fibers in the brain and spinal cord that protects the neurons and facilitates the passage of neuromuscular impulses. In these denuded patches, the myelin is replaced by nonfunctional plaques of scar tissue so that the nerve fiber can no longer conduct normal electrical impulses. The severity of the condition varies markedly among affected persons. The precise cause of MS is unknown, but it is an autoimmune disease in which the body's defense system begins to treat the myelin tissue in the central nervous system as a foreign substance and gradually sets out to destroy it, with subsequent scarring left. Ongoing studies are investigating triggering events for this mutiny in the immune system involving T cells and the protein antigens produced. Research is also investigating the possibili-

amyotrophic lateral sclerosis • A progressive neuromuscular disease characterized by the degeneration of the neurons of the spinal cord and the motor cells of the brain stem causing a deficit of upper and lower motor neurons; death usually occurs in 2 to 3 years.

chorea • A wide variety of ceaseless involuntary movements that are rapid, complex, and jerky, yet appear to be well coordinated; characteristic movements of Huntington's disease.

ties of using these autoimmune components as treatment strategies in a similar manner to that of vaccines.[46,47] A genetic factor, still unknown, is probably involved since relatives of affected persons are eight times more likely than others to develop the disease. Environment seems to play a role. MS is five times more common in temperate zones such as the United States and Europe than in the tropics. Perhaps the disease is induced by a virus picked up in the first 15 years of life in these temperate climates.[48] Approximately two thirds of persons with MS experience the beginning symptoms between ages 20 and 40. More women than men are affected (ratio, 2:1), and the disease is most common in white populations. In the relatively high-risk temperate areas, the incidence of MS is about 1 in every 1,000 people.

Depending on how extensive the tissue involvement and which parts of the brain and spinal cord are affected, the effects of MS vary widely from mild periodic feelings of tingling, numbness, constriction, or stiffness in any part of the body to more severe, disabling disease. The role of dietary factors remains uncertain, but considerable investigation has implicated a high-fat diet as an agent.[48]

Medical Management

Physicians have lacked specific means of treatment while the search for a cure goes on. Corticosteroid drugs have been used to alleviate symptoms of an acute attack. Currently, however, a more specifically effective drug is being made available. An advisory panel of the U.S. Food and Drug Administration has approved use of *beta-interferon (Betaseron)*, and this new drug will probably be on the market by 1994. It is the first drug shown in testing to be effective in reducing the number and severity of symptomatic episodes of MS, although hundreds have been tried over the past decades. Betaseron is a genetically engineered drug containing beta-interferon, a type of protein that helps regulate the immune system. Adjunct physical therapy helps maintain muscle strength and the ability to remain mobile and independent.

Nutritional Management

General nutritional care responds to basic nutritional needs for adequate energy and nutrient intake to maintain or restore optimal nutritional status. It also assists with symptomatic gastrointestinal problems in eating and elimination, as discussed with other neuromuscular diseases above. If steroid therapy is used, dietary sodium is reduced. Low-fat foods are wise in any case, in possible relation to disease control[48] and to healthy weight management. Nasoenteric or gastrostomy tube feeding may be needed for patients with advanced disease to provide enteral nutrition support.

Myasthenia Gravis

The neuromuscular disease **myasthenia gravis** occurs in about 1 of every 20,000 persons, causing the affected person to become paralyzed due to the inability of the neuromuscular junctions to transmit nerve fiber signals to the muscles.[36] It is an autoimmune disorder, in which, for unknown reasons, the body's immune system attacks and gradually destroys the receptors in muscles responsible for picking up nerve impulses. As a result, the affected muscles respond only weakly or not at all to nerve impulses. Only about two to five new cases of this rare disease per 100,000 people are diagnosed annually. Myasthenia gravis affects more women than men (ratio, 3:2). Although it can occur at any age, it usually occurs between ages 20 and 30 in women and 50 and 70 in men. Facial muscles are usually involved first, causing drooped eyelids, double vision, and sometimes a lack of facial animation, with an absent-stare appearance. Weak muscles of the face, throat, larynx, and neck cause difficulties in speaking and eating. As muscles in the arms and legs become involved, problems develop with other daily living activities, such as food shopping and preparation, dressing, combing the hair, and climbing stairs. In severe cases, respiratory muscles in the chest weaken and cause breathing difficulty.

Medical Management

Treatment may involve a thymectomy, removal of the thymus gland, a small gland in the upper chest thought to be partly responsible for the abnormal antibody activity, especially if a small tumor is found there. Temporary relief may be obtained by regular plasmapheresis, exchanges of the patient's antibody-containing blood for antibody-free blood. These antibodies produced by the disease attack the receptors on the muscle cells that bind the acetylcholine neurotransmitter necessary for muscle contraction, thus effectively reducing stimulation of muscle cells and weakening muscle action. Drugs used to treat myasthenia gravis, such as neostigmine (Prostigmin) or pyridostigmine (Mestinon, Regonol), increase the amount of the neurotransmitter acetylcholine at the nerve ending by blocking the action of the enzyme that normally breaks it down. The blocking action of these drugs increases levels of the acetylcholine transmitter by allowing more of it to accumulate in the synaptic cleft between nerve and muscle-fiber endings, thus permitting the remaining receptors to function more efficiently.

Nutritional Management

Nutritional care has three main goals: (1) to maintain optimal energy-nutrient intake for muscle strength and good nutritional status; (2) to solve any associated eating problems by adjusting meal patterns to a major meal at breakfast, when the patient is more rested, and frequent small meals through the day, and by modifying food texture and supplementing with enteral feedings as needed; and (3) to help counteract drug side effects of nausea and vomiting. The drugs described should be taken with liquid or food to lessen stomach irritation.

Alzheimer's Disease

Alzheimer's disease was named for the German neurologist Alois Alzheimer (1864-1915), who in 1907 first described the characteristic neurofibrillary tangles found in the postmortem brain of a 51-year-old demented woman.[49] The disease is a form of progressive dementia in which nerve cells degenerate in the brain, and the brain substance shrinks. The hallmark of the disease is the development of abnormal intracellular filaments in tangles of neurofibrils and extracellular deposits of amyloid-forming protein in senile plaques (**amyloid** plaques) and cerebral blood vessels, as first reported by Alzheimer. The density of these plaques has become the basis for the postmortem diagnosis of Alzheimer's disease; there is no absolute diagnostic test for the disease during life. Alzheimer's disease accounts for 60% to 80% of dementia in people over age 65; it afflicts 5% to 11% of the U.S. population over age 65 and about half of the population over age 85.[49]

In addition to its human cost to patient and family, Alzheimer's disease levies a tremendous social and financial burden. Currently, more than 4 million Americans have been diagnosed, many of whom require institutional care at a cost that exceeds $50 billion a year and is expected to increase to $80 billion in the next few years.[49] With the rapidly increasing population of persons over age 85, the health care problem of Alzheimer's disease is assuming enormous proportions. Research into causes and treatment has greatly expanded in recent years. However, the cause remains unknown, and there is still no means of stopping the progressive years of mental and personal decline until death. This declining progression of Alzheimer's disease has been divided into three broad stages: stage 1, the early period of increasing forgetfulness and anxious depression; stage 2, a middle period of severe memory loss for recent events, disorientation, and personality changes; and stage 3, the final period of severe confusion, psychosis, memory loss, personal neglect, confinement to bed, feeding problems, full-time nursing care, and finally death from an infection such as pneumonia.[50]

Medical Management

There is no treatment for the disease itself, except for suitable day-to-day nursing and social care for both the patient and the family. Keeping the patient well nourished, occupied, and exercised helps lessen anxiety and personal distress, especially in the earlier stages, when the patient is sufficiently aware of his or her condition. Some use of tranquilizing medication often helps improve difficult behavior and enables the patient to sleep. Research into drug therapy continues. Family counseling and respite care are essential.

Nutritional Management

Nutritional care in each stage of Alzheimer's disease becomes increasingly difficult and challenging. Adequate nutrition throughout the course of the disease is essential to improve physical well-being, help maximize the patient's functioning, and improve quality of life. Nutrition-related changes occur at each progressive stage of the illness (Table 26-3) and illustrate the major goals of maintaining adequate nutrition and preventing malnutrition, and devising practical ways of dealing with feeding problems.[50,51] Because these patients have lower body weight and require higher energy intakes than do normal elderly persons, they often require high-calorie supplemental beverages to help supply added nourishment.[52,53] Studies generally have identified four major factors that promote optimal intake in long-term care[54]:

- Using skilled individualized feeding techniques
- Selecting appropriate food consistency
- Providing adequate feeding time
- Focusing on the midday meal, when cognitive abilities are at peak level

To Sum Up

Individuals facing disabling illness and injury confront a myriad of interacting challenges, including social attitudes and financial, physical, and psychologic barriers. The team approach, involving family and friends in addition to health professionals, becomes an essential basis of care.

---

amyloid • A glycoprotein substance having a relation to starchlike structure but more a protein compound; an abnormal complex material forming characteristic brain deposits of fibrillary tangles always found in postmortem examinations of patients with Alzheimer's disease, the only means of definitive diagnosis; found in various body tissues which, when advanced, form lesions that destroy functional cells and injure the organ.

myasthenia gravis • A progressive neuromuscular disease caused by faulty nerve conduction due to presence of antibodies to acetylcholine receptors at the neuromuscular junction.

TABLE 26-3

Progression of Alzheimer's Disease

	General Symptoms	Nutrition-Related Effects
Stage 1 (early)	Loss of memory	Difficulty in shopping, cooking
	Decrease in social and vocational skills	Forgetting to eat
	Careless work, housekeeping, finances	Changes in taste and smell
	Easily lost	Unusual food choices
	Personality changes	Degeneration of appetite regulation
	Recognition of faces	
	Well-oriented to time	
Stage 2 (middle)	Inability to recall names	Increased energy requirement from agitation
	Disorientation to time	
	Delusions	Holding food in mouth
	Depression	Forgetting to swallow
	Agitation	Losing ability to use utensils
	Language problems	Using spoon only
		Eating with hands
Stage 3 (final)	Complete disorientation	No recognition of food
	Forgetting own name	Refusal to eat or open mouth for feeding
	Not recognizing family	Need for nasogastric feeding
	Loss of verbal skills	
	Loss of basic self-care skills	
	Urinary and fecal incontinence	
	Bedridden	

Adapted from Gra, GE: Nutrition and dementia, *J Am Diet Assoc* 89(12):1795, 1989.

The basic principles of nutrition care involve *prevention* of malnutrition and *restoration* of eating ability. To avoid malnutrition, the nutritionist must assess individual nutritional needs to meet basal energy expenditure needs, added metabolic activity factors due to any underlying disease process, and requirements of physical therapy and other activities. Nutrient intake must be sufficient to meet a variety of needs: protein and fat (linoleic acid) to promote tissue and organ integrity; carbohydrate to counteract impaired postinjury metabolism; and optimal intake of vitamins and minerals, which sometimes requires the use of supplements to guard against deficiencies. To restore eating ability, the occupational therapist and nurse play significant roles in promoting adequate swallowing, chewing, and skills in using hands and utensils. To meet individual nutritional needs, the nutritionist must assess eating skills, estimate eating desire (sensory stimuli, "comfort foods") and help the client develop new ways of eating with various self-help devices.

Special disabling conditions that require special nutrition support and modifications to treat underlying disease effects include (1) *musculoskeletal disease,* such as various forms of arthritis; (2) *neuromus-*

cular disease, caused by a sudden brain or spinal cord injury or a stroke, or by developmental disabilities due to cerebral palsy, epilepsy, or spina bifida; and (3) *progressive neurologic disorders,* such as Parkinson's and Huntington's diseases, ALS, MS, or dementia as seen in Alzheimer's disease.

QUESTIONS FOR REVIEW

1. What are the two major goals of rehabilitative therapy for persons with disabling conditions? How do the basic principles of nutritional care help meet these goals?

2. Describe the functions of major nutrients in preventing or retarding the catabolic process that often occurs in long-term disabling illness or injury.

3. Select six of the disease processes or injuries discussed that result in eating disabilities. Describe the nature of the disease or injury and relate it to the disability involved. Outline the medical and nutritional therapy used in each case, giving the rationale for the nutritional management.

REFERENCES

1. Gines DJ: Introduction to nutrition and rehabilitation. In Gines DJ, editor: *Nutrition management in rehabilitation,* Rockville, Md, 1990, Aspen.

2. Institute of Medicine: *The second fifty years: promoting health and preventing disability,* Washington, DC, 1991, National Academy Press.

3. Breslow RA and others: Malnutrition in tubefed nursing home patients with pressure sores, *J Parenter Enteral Nutr* 15(6):663, 1991.

4. Cassell JA: Interview: Fred Sammons, ORT, *Top Clin Nutr* 3(3):71, 1988.

5. Harris ED: Rheumatoid arthritis: pathophysiology and implications for therapy, *N Engl J Med* 322(18):1277, 1990.

6. Wolman PG: Arthritis. In Gines DJ, editor: *Nutrition management in rehabilitation,* Rockville, Md, 1990, Aspen.

7. Antonelli MAS and others: Herpes zoster in patients with rheumatoid arthritis treated with weekly, low-dose methotrexate, *Am J Med* 90:295, 1991.

8. Kremer JM and others: Dietary fish oil and olive oil supplementation in patients with rheumatoid arthritis: clinical and immunologic effects, *Arthritis Rheum* 33(6):810, 1990.

9. Price ME, Dilorio C: Swallowing: a practice guide, *Am J Nurs* 90(7):42, 1990.

10. White-O'Connor B and others: Dietary habits, weight history, and vitamin supplement use in elderly osteoarthritis patients, *J Am Diet Assoc* 89(3):378, 1989.

11. Tolstoi LG, Levin RM: Osteoporosis—the treatment controversy, *Nutr Today* 27(4):6, 1992.

12. Chesnut CH: Osteoporosis and its treatment, *N Engl J Med* 326:406, 1992.

13. US Department of Health and Human Services, Public Health Service: *Healthy people 2000: national health promotion and disease prevention objectives,* Pub No 91-50212, Washington, DC, 1990, US Government Printing Office.

14. Kearns P: Nutrition in neurological injury, *Nutr Clin Prac* 6(6):211, 1991.

15. National Center for Health Statistics: *Health, United States, 1989 and prevention profile,* Pub No 90-1232, Hyattsville, Md, 1990, US Department of Health and Human Services.

16. Hubert C: Trauma care crisis, *Sacramento Bee* 273:1, 1993.

17. Konvolinka CW, Morell VO: Nutrition in head trauma, *Nutr Clin Prac* 6(6):223, 1991.

18. Ott L, Young B: Nutrition in the neurologically injured patient, *Nutr Clin Prac* 6(6):223, 1991.

19. Varella L: Barbiturate therapy and nutrition support in head-injured patients, *Nutr Clin Prac* 6(6):239, 1991.

20. Kirby DF and others: Early enteral nutrition after brain injury by percutaneous endoscopic gastrojejunostomy, *J Parenter Enteral Nutr* 15(3):298, 1991.

21. Annis K and others: Nutritional support of the severe head-injured patient, *Nutr Clin Prac* 6(6):245, 1991.

22. Yankelson S: Traumatic brain injury. In Gines DJ, editor: *Nutrition management in rehabilitation,* Rockville, Md, 1990, Aspen.

23. Chin DE, Kearnes P: Nutrition in the spinal-injured patient, *Nutr Clin Prac* 6(6):213, 1991.

24. O'Brien RY: Spinal cord injury. In Gines DJ, editor: *Nutrition management in rehabilitation,* Rockville, Md, 1990, Aspen.

25. Peiffer SC and others: Nutritional assessment during rehabilitation of the spinal cord injury patient, *J Am Diet Assoc* 78:501, 1981.

26. Doolittle ND: Advances in the neurosciences and implications for nursing care, *J Neurosci Nurs* 23(4):207, 1991.

27. Kozlowski BW: Cerebral palsy. In Gines DJ, editor: *Nutrition management in rehabilitation,* Rockville, Md, 1990, Aspen.

28. Thommessen M and others: Energy and nutrient intakes of disabled children: Do feeding problems make a differences? *J Am Diet Assoc* 91(12):1522, 1991.

29. Johnson RK, Ferrara MS: Estimating stature from knee height for persons with cerebral palsy: an evaluation of estimating equations, *J Am Diet Assoc* 91(10):1283, 1991.

30. Ferrang TM and others: Dietary and anthromorphic assessment of adults with cerebral palsy, *J Am Diet Assoc* 92(9):1083, 1992.

31. Gasch AT: Use of the traditional ketogenic diet for treatment of intractable epilepsy, *J Am Diet Assoc* 90(10):1433, 1990.

32. Dustrude A, Prince A: Provision of optimal nutrition care in myelomeningocele, *Top Clin Nutr* 5(2):34, 1990.

33. Atencio PL and others: Effect of level of lesion and quality of ambulation on growth chart measurements in children with myelomeningocele, *J Am Diet Assoc* 92(7):858, 1992.

34. Unonu JN, Johnson AA: Feeding patterns, food energy, nutrient intakes, and anthropometric measurements of selected black preschool children with Down syndrome, *J Am Diet Assoc* 92(7):856, 1992.

35. Rajput AH: Frequency and cause of Parkinson's disease, *Can J Neurol Sci* 19:103, 1992.

36. Guyton AC: *Textbook of medical physiology,* ed 8, Philadelphia, 1991, WB Saunders.

37. Tsui JKC: Future treatment of Parkinson's disease, *Can J Neurol Sci* 19:160, 1992.

38. Lindvall O and others: Grafts of fetal dopamine neurons survive and improve motor function in Parkinson's disease, *Science* 247:574, 1990.

39. Paré S and others: Effect of daytime protein restriction on nutrient intakes of free-living Parkinson's disease patients, *Am J Clin Nutr* 55:701, 1992.

40. Gusella J and others: Discovery of Huntington's disease gene, *Cell,* Mar 22, 1993.

41. Honavar M and others: A clinicopathological study of the Guillain-Barré syndrome, *Brain* 114(3):1245, 1991.

42. McNamara JO, Fridovich I: Did radicals strike Lou Gehrig? *Nature* 362(6415):20, 1993.

43. Rosen DR and others: Mutations in Cu/Zn superoxide dismutase gene are associated with familial amyotrophic lateral sclerosis, *Nature* 362(6415):59, 1993.

44. Marx J: Gene linked to Lou Gehrig's disease, *Science* 259(5100):1393, 1993.

45. Miller CA: Nutritional needs and care in amytrophic lateral sclerosis, *Top Clin Nutr* 4(1):15, 1989.

46. Marx J: Testing of autoimmune therapy begins, *Science* 252(5002):27, 1991.

47. Hoffman M: On the trail of the errant T cells of multiple sclerosis, *Science* 254(5031):521, 1991.

48. Lowis GW: The social epidemiology of multiple sclerosis, *Sci Total Environ* 90:163, 1990.

49. Yankner BA, Mesulam M: β-Amyloid and the pathogenesis of Alzheimer's disease, *N Engl J Med* 325(26):1849, 1991.

50. Gray GE: Nutrition and dementia, *J Am Diet Assoc* 89(12):1795, 1989.

51. Claggett MS: Nutritional factors relevant to Alzheimer's disease, *J Am Diet Assoc* 89(3):392, 1989.

52. Renvall NJ and others: Body composition of patients with Alzheimer's disease, *JAMA* 93(1):47, 1993.

53. Riley ME, Volicer L: Evaluation of a new nutritional supplement for patients with Alzheimer's disease, *J Am Diet Assoc* 90(3):433, 1990.

54. Suski NS, Nielsen CC: Factors affecting food intake of women with Alzheimer's type dementia in long-term care, *J Am Diet Assoc* 89(12):1770, 1989.

FURTHER READING

Annis K and others: Nutritional support of the severe head-injured patient, *Nutr Clin Prac* 6(6):245, 1991.

Chin DE, Kearns P: Nutrition in the spinal-injured patient, *Nutr Clin Prac* 6(6):213, 1991.

These two articles in the same issue of this helpful journal provide a case study of a 17-year-old boy who suffered severe head injury when the car he was driving left the road and hit a tree, and a full review of care for persons with spinal injuries. Nutrition support plays an essential role in each case.

Breslow RA and others: Malnutrition in tubefed nursing home patients with pressure sores, *J Parenter Enteral Nutr* 15(6):663, 1991.

Price ME , Diloria C: Swallowing: a practice guide, *Am J Nurs* 90(7):42, 1990.

These two articles discuss two basic problems encountered with disabled persons: pressure sores in bedridden patients and swallowing problems in a variety of neuromuscular and progressive neurologic disorders, both of which often compromise nutritional status.

Gines DJ, editor: *Nutrition management in rehabilitation,* Rockville, Md, 1990, Aspen.

This small reference book provides a wealth of material for nutritional care of many conditions requiring patient rehabilitation following traumatic injury or chronic phases of disabling disease.

CASE STUDY

Patient with a Cerebrovascular Accident

James Braddock is a tall (182 cm, or 6 ft, 1 in.), 57-year-old black man who resided until 6 weeks ago at a rehabilitation center to recover from the results of a cerebrovascular accident (CVA), or stroke, that occurred 6 months ago. At that time he was brought to the local hospital emergency room, accompanied by his wife, who had found him unconscious on the bathroom floor after hearing a fall. He had flaccid paralysis on the right side. Pinprick response was normal on the left side but questionable on the right.

Within an hour Mr. Braddock began to regain consciousness but appeared to be confused, disoriented, and apprehensive. His personal physician examined him and found his weight to be 155 kg (345 lb), which was his usual weight. His pulse rate was 140 beats per minute; blood pressure, 190/100. The physician's impression was cerebral hemorrhage in the left-middle cerebral artery prefrontal area with massive extension, paralysis on the right side, and aphasia.

Laboratory tests were ordered for blood urea nitrogen, fasting blood glucose, serum cholesterol, hemoglobin, hematocrit, sodium, potassium, chloride, and carbon dioxide-combining power. The physician also ordered an intravenous infusion of 500 ml of 2.5% dextrose in 0.5% saline every 8 hours. The diet order was for clear liquids taken by mouth as tolerated. Later the laboratory reported these results: blood urea nitrogen, 16 mg/dl; blood glucose, 140 mg/dl; cholesterol, 290 mg/dl; hemoglobin, 14 gm/100 ml; hematocrit, 40 ml/100 ml; sodium, 135 mEq/L; potassium, 4.2 mEq/L; chloride, 98 mEq/L; and carbon dioxide, 60 vol/dl.

The diet was changed to full liquid the following day, and the intravenous infusion was discontinued. Mr. Braddock was advanced to a soft diet 4 days later. Nurses' notes indicated he was being fed by the staff. Two weeks later he was able to tolerate a full diet. The occupational therapist, together with the clinical nutritionist and the nurse, developed eating aids that would help him learn to feed himself.

After 4 weeks Mr. Braddock was transferred to the rehabilitation center for follow-up therapy. At that time he started on a vigorous physical and speech therapy program. Self-feeding skills helped him gain more independence, and a diet plan of 1500 kcalories (with cholesterol limited to 300 mg and sodium restricted to 1000 mg) was designed to promote weight loss and help control his hypertension and vascular disease.

Mr. Braddock's response to therapy was good. In 6 months he was able to walk with a cane and had regained much of his ability to speak. He was released to home care, following careful instructions regarding his home-care needs. Follow-up home visit reports indicate that Mr. Braddock has been losing weight gradually, has stopped smoking, and is practicing prescribed exercises daily. He is now inquiring about future job possibilities.

Questions for Analysis

1. What underlying conditions may have been responsible for the CVA? What factors indicate this possible association?

2. What was the purpose of each laboratory test ordered? Which values were elevated? Which values were inadequate?

3. Which members of the rehabilitative support team are identified? Was any member underused? How could this person's role have been expanded?

4. Outline the instructions you would give Mrs. Braddock to help her plan nutritional care for her husband at home.

ISSUES · AND · ANSWERS

Independent Living versus the Kindness of Strangers

"**I** have always relied on the kindness of strangers."
If Tennessee Williams' famous line in his play *A Streetcar Named Desire* for the lead character Blanche conjures up images of a blithe Southern belle, you're right—but think again. In today's reality, you may well think of a once-independent career woman now confined to her wheelchair, much of her financial resources gone to pay for lengthy and highly specialized care. Before 1978 she would have relied heavily on the "kindness of strangers" to meet most of her basic needs, including transportation to keep medical appointments and to purchase food, and to help in meal preparation and personal care.

In 1978 the Rehabilitation Act of 1973 was amended to allocate federal funds to establish independent living centers for disabled persons. The number of Americans who cannot perform even simple activities of daily living because of a major illness, disabling injury, or chronic health condition rose dramatically by 83.2% in the decade between 1966 and 1976, for example, and gradually rose during the 1980s and is still rising. In 1980 about 15% of the free-living population was disabled. This rise was caused primarily by new technologies that have virtually wiped out the infectious diseases that used to kill the disabled, as well as those that, together with nutrition, have extended the overall life span. The causes of disability also have changed, with rheumatoid arthritis and diabetes replacing heart disease and other causes.

Disabled persons traditionally have been barred from many activities because of limited mobility. Jobs, educa-tion, and recreational facilities have often been denied to them because of inadequate physical access or facilities, and even fear and prejudice. Promotion of physical access, independent living, and access to employment, have been strong civil rights issues in many parts of the United States, often with positive results.

The passage of legislation establishing independent living centers across the United States enabled disabled persons to meet their basic needs. It also promoted political awareness in local communities. Such legislation has opened the door to disabled persons who can and want to be self-reliant individuals capable of enriching their lives and contributing to their communities. Economic realities have caused federal authorities to be reluctant to issue costly new regulations regarding the needs of disabled persons, although employment access is now guaranteed under the Americans With Disabilities Act of 1990. But the recent record is mixed, since cutbacks have occurred in programs providing income support via the Social Security Administration. Public support for these programs is also lessening, since the proportion of the public being served is relatively small, with highly specialized needs.

Will the disabled person once again find it necessary to rely on "the kindness of strangers"? How will the loss of contributed income from working disabled persons affect the economy? And will the kind strangers be capable of filling the gap?

REFERENCES

Cross EW: Implementing the Americans with Disabilities Act, *J Am Diet Assoc* 93(3):273, 1993.

DeJong G, Lifchez R: Physical disability and public policy, *Sci Am* 248(6):40, 1983.

APPENDIX

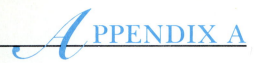

Nutritive Values of the Edible Part of Food

Key to Abbreviations

Kcal, Kcalories; *Prot,* protein; *Carb,* carbohydrate; *Fat,* fat; *Chol,* cholesterol; *Safa,* saturated fat; *Mufa,* monounsaturated fat; *Pufa,* polyunsaturated fat; *Sod,* sodium; *Pot,* potassium; *Mag,* magnesium; *Iron,* iron; *Zinc,* zinc; *VA,* vitamin A; *VC,* vitamin C; *Thia,* thiamin; *Ribo,* riboflavin; *Niac,* niacin; *VB_6,* vitamin B_6; *Fol,* folate; *VB_{12},* vitamin B_{12}; *Calc,* calcium; *Phos,* phosphorus; *Sel,* selenium; *Fibd,* dietary fiber; and *VE,* vitamin E.

Food name	Portion	Wt (g)	Kcal	Prot (g)	Carb (g)	Fat (g)	Chol (mg)	Safa (g)	Mufa (g)	Pufa (g)	Sod (mg)	Pot (mg)
Baby foods												
Apple Betty	oz	28.4	20	0.1	5.6	0	0	0	0	0	3	14
Apple blueberry	oz	28.4	17	0.1	4.6	0.1	0	—	—	—	0	20
Apple juice	Fl oz	31	14	0	3.6	0	0	0	0	0	1	28
Apple peach juice	Fl oz	31	13	0	3.2	0	0	0	0	0	—	30
Applesauce	oz	28.4	12	0.1	3.1	0	0	0	0	0	1	20
Beans-green	oz	28.4	7	0.4	1.7	0	0	0	0	0	1	45
Beans-green-buttered	oz	28.4	9	0.3	1.9	0.2	—	—	—	—	1	45
Beef	oz	28.4	30	3.9	0	1.5	—	0.73	0.62	0.06	23	62
Beef & egg noodles	oz	28.4	15	0.6	2	0.5	—	—	—	—	8	13
Beef lasagna	oz	28.4	22	1.2	2.8	0.6	—	—	—	—	129	35
Beef stew	oz	28.4	14	1.4	1.5	0.3	3.55	0.16	0.12	0.01	98	40
Beets	oz	28.4	10	0.4	2.2	0	0	0	0	0	24	52
Carrots	oz	28.4	8	0.2	1.7	0	0	0	0	0	11	56
Cereal & egg yolks	oz	28.4	15	0.5	2	0.5	18	0.17	0.22	0.04	9	11
Chicken	oz	28.4	37	3.9	0	2.2	—	0.58	1.01	0.54	13	40
Cookie-arrowroot	Item	6	24	0.4	4.3	0.9	0	0.2	0.52	0.02	22	9
Corn-creamed	oz	28.4	16	0.4	4	0.1	0	0	0	0	12	26
Egg yolks	Serving	28.4	58	2.8	0.3	4.9	223	1.47	1.8	0.54	11	22
Garden vegetables	oz	28.4	11	0.7	1.9	0.1	0	0	0	0	10	48
Ham	oz	28.4	32	3.9	0	1.6	—	0.55	0.78	0.22	12	58
Lamb	oz	28.4	29	4	0	1.3	0	0.66	0.53	0.06	18	58
Liver	oz	28.4	29	4.1	0.4	1.1	52	0.39	0.22	0.02	21	64
Mixed cereal/mix	oz	28.4	32	1.3	4.5	1	0	—	—	—	13	56
Mixed vegetables	oz	28.4	11	0.3	2.7	0	0	0	0	0	2	34
Oatmeal cereal/milk	oz	28.4	33	1.4	4.3	1.2	0	—	—	—	13	58
Orange juice	Fl oz	31	14	0.2	3.2	0.1	0	—	—	—	0	57
Peaches	oz	28.4	20	0.1	5.4	0	0	0	0	0	2	46
Pears	oz	28.4	12	0.1	3.1	0	0	0	0	0	1	37
Peas	oz	28.4	11	1	2.3	0.1	0	0	0	0	1	32
Peas-creamed	oz	28.4	15	0.6	2.5	0.5	0	—	—	—	4	25
Pork	oz	28.4	35	4	0	2	—	0.68	1.02	0.22	12	63
Pretzels	Item	6	24	0.7	4.9	0.1	—	0	0	0	16	8
Rice cereal/milk	oz	28.4	33	1.1	4.7	1	0	—	—	—	13	54
Spinach-creamed	oz	28.4	11	0.7	1.6	0.4	0	—	—	—	14	54
Squash	oz	28.4	7	0.2	1.6	0.1	0	0	0	0	1	51
Sweet potatoes	oz	28.4	16	0.3	3.7	0	0	0	0	0	6	75
Teething biscuits	Item	11	43	1.2	8.4	0.5	0	—	—	—	40	35
Turkey	oz	28.4	32	4	0	1.7	—	0.54	0.62	0.41	15	65
Turkey & rice	oz	28.4	14	0.5	2.1	0.4	2.84	0.12	0.15	0.04	5	12
Veal & vegetables	oz	28.4	20	1.7	1.7	0.8	—	—	—	—	7	43
Zwieback	Piece	7	30	0.7	5.2	0.7	1.46	0.28	0.24	0.05	16	21

Mag (mg)	Iron (mg)	Zinc (mg)	VA (RE)	VC (mg)	Thia (mg)	Ribo (mg)	Niac (mg)	VB$_6$ (mg)	Fol (µg)	VB$_{12}$ (µg)	Calc (mg)	Phos (mg)	Sel (mg)	Fibd (g)	VE (mg)
—	0.05	—	0	9.8	0.004	0.01	0.013	—	0.1	—	5	—	—	0	0.065
—	0.06	—	1	7.9	0.005	0.01	0.034	0.01	1	—	1	2	0	0.1	0.165
1	0.18	0.009	1	18	0.002	0.005	0.026	0.009	0	—	1	2	0	0.25	0.18
1	0.17	0.008	2	18.1	0.002	0.003	0.066	0.007	0.04	—	1	1	0	0.25	0.18
1	0.06	0.007	0	10.9	0.003	0.008	0.017	0.009	0.5	—	1	2	0	0.7	0.165
7	0.21	0.058	13	1.5	0.007	0.024	0.098	0.011	9.8	—	11	6	0	0.39	0.128
—	0.36	—	13	2.3	0.005	0.03	0.096	—	8.1	—	18	—	0.17	0.7	0.128
5	0.42	0.696	16	0.6	0.003	0.04	0.808	0.04	1.6	0.403	2	24	0.003	0	0.111
2	0.12	0.106	31	0.3	0.01	0.012	0.205	0.014	1.4	0.026	3	8	0.003	0.1	0.062
3	0.25	0.198	100	0.5	0.02	0.025	0.384	0.02	—	—	5	11	—	0.1	0.062
3	0.2	0.247	95	0.9	0.004	0.018	0.372	0.021	—	—	3	12	0.003	0.34	0.062
4	0.09	0.034	1	0.7	0.003	0.012	0.037	0.007	8.7	—	4	4	—	0.4	0.128
3	0.1	0.043	325	1.6	0.007	0.011	0.131	0.021	4.2	—	6	6	0	0.7	0.128
1	0.13	0.081	11	0.2	0.003	0.012	0.014	0.006	0.9	0.02	7	11	—	0	0.071
4	0.4	0.343	11	0.5	0.004	0.043	0.923	0.057	2.9	—	18	27	0.003	0	0.111
1	0.18	0.032	—	0.3	0.03	0.026	0.344	0.002	—	0.004	2	7	—	0	0.014
2	0.08	0.054	2	0.6	0.004	0.013	0.145	0.012	3.2	0.005	6	9	—	0.9	0.128
2	0.78	0.543	107	0.4	0.02	0.075	0.007	0.045	26.1	0.437	22	81	0.005	0	0.17
6	0.24	0.074	172	1.6	0.017	0.02	0.221	0.028	11.4	—	8	8	0	0.7	0.128
4	0.29	0.637	3	0.6	0.039	0.044	0.746	0.071	0.6	—	2	23	0.003	0	0.111
4	0.42	0.781	7	0.3	0.005	0.057	0.829	0.043	0.6	0.621	2	27	0.004	0	0.111
4	1.5	0.844	3247	5.5	0.014	0.514	2.36	0.097	95.7	0.612	1	58	0.007	0	0.111
8	2.96	0.202	6	0.3	0.122	0.165	1.64	0.019	3.2	—	62	40	—	0.25	0.045
—	0.09	—	77	0.8	0.004	0.009	0.142	—	2.3	—	6	—	0	0.25	0.128
10	3.44	0.262	6	0.4	0.143	0.16	1.7	0.017	2.8	—	62	45	0.001	0.7	0.054
3	0.05	0.017	2	19.4	0.014	0.009	0.074	0.017	8.2	—	4	3	0	0.25	0.18
2	0.07	0.024	5	8.9	0.003	0.009	0.173	0.004	1.1	—	2	3	0	0.7	0.165
2	0.07	0.021	1	7	0.004	0.008	0.054	0.002	1	—	2	3	0	0.25	0.165
4	0.27	0.099	16	1.9	0.023	0.017	0.289	0.02	7.4	—	6	12	0	0.7	0.128
—	0.16	0.11	2	0.5	0.025	0.016	0.23	0.013	6.4	0.023	4	9	—	0.7	0.128
3	0.28	0.644	3	0.5	0.041	0.058	0.643	0.058	0.5	0.281	1	27	0.004	0	0.111
2	0.23	0.047	0	0.2	0.028	0.021	0.214	0.005	—	—	1	7	—	0	0.009
13	3.46	0.182	6	0.3	0.132	0.142	1.48	0.032	2.3	—	68	50	0.001	0.25	0.074
16	0.18	0.088	118	2.5	0.004	0.029	0.061	0.021	17.2	—	25	15	—	1.12	0.128
3	0.08	0.04	57	2.2	0.003	0.016	0.1	0.018	4.4	—	7	4	0	0.7	0.128
4	0.1	0.058	183	2.8	0.008	0.009	0.101	0.026	2.8	—	4	7	0	0.7	0.128
4	0.39	0.102	1	1	0.026	0.059	0.476	0.012	—	0.008	29	18	—	0.1	—
4	0.34	0.519	48	0.6	0.005	0.059	1.04	0.051	3.2	0.284	7	36	0.003	0	0.111
—	0.07	—	27	0.3	0.001	0.006	0.087	0.009	0.9	—	6	6	—	0	0.062
2	0.17	0.284	21	0.5	0.006	0.021	0.457	0.024	—	0.128	3	15	—	0.1	0.062
1	0.04	0.038	0	0.4	0.015	0.017	0.092	0.006	—	—	1	4	—	0	—

Continued.

Key to Abbreviations

Kcal, Kcalories; *Prot*, protein; *Carb*, carbohydrate; *Fat*, fat; *Chol*, cholesterol; *Safa*, saturated fat; *Mufa*, monounsaturated fat; *Pufa*, polyunsaturated fat; *Sod*, sodium; *Pot*, potassium; *Mag*, magnesium; *Iron*, iron; *Zinc*, zinc; *VA*, vitamin A; *VC*, vitamin C; *Thia*, thiamin; *Ribo*, riboflavin; *Niac*, niacin; *VB₆*, vitamin B_6; *Fol*, folate; *VB₁₂*, vitamin B_{12}; *Calc*, calcium; *Phos*, phosphorus; *Sel*, selenium; *Fibd*, dietary fiber; and *VE*, vitamin E.

Food name	Portion	Wt (g)	Kcal	Prot (g)	Carb (g)	Fat (g)	Chol (mg)	Safa (g)	Mufa (g)	Pufa (g)	Sod (mg)	Pot (mg)
Beverages												
Beer-light	Fl oz	29.5	8	0.1	0.4	0	0	0	0	0	1	5
Beer-regular	Fl oz	29.7	12	0.1	1.1	C	0	0	0	0	2	7
Brandy/cognac-pony	Item	30	73	—	—	0	0	0	0	0	—	—
Carn inst break-choc(env)	Item	36	130	7	23	1	—	—	—	—	136	422
Champagne-domestic-glass	Item	120	84	0.2	3	0	0	0	0	0	—	—
Choc bev drink-no milk-dry	oz	28.4	97.7	0.924	25.3	0.868	0	0.513	0.283	0.025	58.8	165
Cider-fermeted	Fl oz	30	11.8	—	0.3	0	0	0+	0	0	0	—
Club soda	Fl oz	29.6	0	0	0	0	0	0	0	0	6	0
Coffee substitute-prep	Fl oz	30.3	1.52	0.03	0.192	0	0	0	0	0	1.21	7.27
Coffee-brewed	Fl oz	30	1	0	0.1	0	0	0	0	0	1	16
Coffee instant-prep	Fl oz	30.3	0.61	0	0.121	0	0	0	0	0	0.91	10.9
Cordials/liqueur-54-proof	Fl oz	34	97	—	11.5	0	0	0	0	0	1	1
Cream soda	Fl oz	30.9	16	0	4.1	0	0	0	0	0	4	0
Gatorade-thirst quencher	Fl oz	30.1	7	0	1.9	0	0	0	0	0	12	3
Grape drink-can	Cup	253	154	1.42	37.8	0.202	0	0.063	0.008	0.056	7.59	334
Hot cocoa-prep/milk-home	Cup	250	218	9.1	25.8	9.05	33	5.61	2.65	0.33	123	480
Lemon lime soda-7UP	Fl oz	30.7	12	0	3.2	0	0	0	0	0	3	0
Ovaltine-choc-prep/milk	Cup	265	227	9.53	29.2	8.79	—	—	—	—	228	600
Perrier-mineral water	Cup	237	0	0	0	0	0	0	0	0	3	0
Postum-inst grain bev-dry	oz	28.4	103	1.93	24.1	0.028	0	0	0	0	28.4	896
Soda-cola type-carbonated	Cup	246.4	100.8	0	25.6	0	0	0.016	0	0	9.84	2.464
Soda-diet cola-carbonated	Cup	236.8	2.368	0.24	0.24	0	0	0	0	0	14.24	0
Tang-inst drink-orange-dry	oz	28.4	104	0	26.1	0	0	0	0	0	12.8	80.9
Tea-brewed	Fl oz	29.6	0	0	0.1	0	0	0	0	0	1	11
Tea-herb-brewed	Fl oz	29.6	0.17	0.017	0.05	0	0	0	0	0	0	3
Tea-instant-prep-sweet	Cup	259	87	0.1	22.1	0.1	0	0.008	0.003	0.021	—	50
Tea-instant-prep unsweet	Cup	237	2	0.1	0.4	0	0	0	0	0	8	47
Tonic water-quinine soda	Fl oz	30.5	10	0	2.7	0	0	0	0	0	1	0
Water	Cup	237	0	0	0	0	0	0	0	0	7	1
Whis/gin/rum/vod-100 proof	Fl oz	27.8	82	0	0	0	0	0	0	0	0	0
Whis/gin/rum/vod-80 proof	Fl oz	27.8	64	0	0	0	0	0	0	0	0	1
Whis/gin/rum/vod-86 proof	Fl oz	27.8	69	0	0	0	0	0	0	0	0	1
Whis/gin/rum/vod-90 proof	Fl oz	27.7	73	0	0	0	0	0	0	0	1	0
Whis/gin/rum/vod-94 proof	Fl oz	27.8	76.5	0	0	0	0	0	0	0	0	0
Wine cooler-white wine/7UP	Serving	102	54.9	0.05	5.72	0	0	0	0	0	7.48	41
Wine-dessert	Fl oz	30	46	0.1	3.5	0	0	0	0	0	3	28
Wine-red table	Fl oz	29.5	21	0.1	0.5	0	0	0	0	0	19	40.7
Wine-rose table	Fl oz	29.5	21	0	0.4	0	0	0	0	0	1	29
Wine-vermouth-dry-glass	Item	100	105	0	1	0	0	0	0	0	4	75
Wine-vermouth-sweet-glass	Item	100	167	0	12	0	0	0	0	0	—	—
Wine-white table	Fl oz	29.5	20	0	0.2	0	0	0	0	0	18	33.3
Breads												
Bagel-egg	Item	55	163	6.02	30.9	1.41	8	—	—	—	198	40.7
Bagel-water	Item	55	163	6.02	30.9	1.41	0	0.2	0.4	0.6	198	40.7
Biscuits-prep/mix	Item	28.4	104	1.63	13	5.05	1.4	3.31	1.29	0.196	221	32.8
Bread stick-vienna type	Item	35	106	3.3	20.3	1.1	0	—	—	—	548	33
Corn-home rec	Slice	45	108	2.21	15.6	3.94	0	—	—	—	126	42.3
Cracked wheat	Slice	25	65.5	2.32	12.5	0.868	0	0.1	0.2	0.2	108	33.3
French-enr	Slice	35	98	3.33	17.7	1.36	0	0.2	0.4	0.4	193	30.1
Mixed grain	Slice	25	64.3	2.49	11.7	0.93	0	—	—	—	103	54.5
Pita	Item	38	105	3.95	20.6	0.57	0	—	—	—	215	44.8
Pumpernickel	Slice	32	81.6	2.93	15.4	1.1	0	—	—	—	173	139
Raisin-enr	Slice	25	69.5	2.05	13.2	0.99	0	0.2	0.3	0.2	94	60
Rye-american-light	Slice	25	65.5	2.12	12	0.913	0	—	—	—	174	51
Wheat-firm-toast	Slice	21	59	2.31	10.9	1.05	0	0.1	0.2	0.3	153	42.4
White-firm	Slice	23	61.4	1.9	11.2	0.902	0	0.2	0.3	0.3	118	25.8

Mag (mg)	Iron (mg)	Zinc (mg)	VA (RE)	VC (mg)	Thia (mg)	Ribo (mg)	Niac (mg)	VB$_6$ (mg)	Fol (µg)	VB$_{12}$ (µg)	Calc (mg)	Phos (mg)	Sel (mg)	Fibd (g)	VE (mg)
1	0.01	0.01	0	0	0.003	0.009	0.116	0.01	1.2	0	1	4	0	0	—
2	0.01	0	0	0	0.002	0.008	0.135	0.015	1.8	0.01	1	4	—	0.07	—
—	—	—	—	—	—	—	—	—	—	—	—	—	—	0	—
80	4.5	3	525	27	0.3	0.07	5	0.4	0	0.6	100	150	—	—	—
—	—	—	—	—	—	—	—	—	—	—	—	—	—	0	—
27.4	0.879	0.434	1.63	0.196	0.01	0.041	0.143	0.003	—	0	10.4	35.8	—	—	0.056
—	—	—	—	—	—	—	—	—	—	—	—	—	—	0	—
0	—	0.03	0	0	0	0	0	0	0	0	1	0	—	0	—
1.21	0.018	0.009	—	—	—	0	0.065	—	—	0	0.91	2.12	—	0	—
2	0.12	0	0	0	0	0	0.066	0	0	0	1	0	0	0	—
1.21	0.015	0.009	0	0	0	0	0.088	0	0	0	0.91	0.91	0	0	0
0	0.02	0.02	—	0	—	—	—	—	—	—	0	0	—	0	—
0	0.02	0.022	0	0	0	0	0	0	0	0	2	0	—	0	—
0	0.02	0.01	0	0	0.002	0	0	0	0	0	0	3	—	0	0
25.3	0.607	0.127	2.02	0.253	0.066	0.094	0.663	0.164	6.58	0	22.8	27.8	—	0	—
56	0.78	1.22	95.5	2.4	0.102	0.435	0.365	0.107	12	0.87	298	270	—	3	—
0	0.02	0.02	0	0	0	0	0.005	0	0	0	1	0	—	0	0
52	4.77	1.13	700	29	0.63	0.97	12.7	0.766	29	0.871	392	302	—	—	—
1	0	0	0	0	0	0	0	0	0	0	32	0	—	0	—
—	1.87	—	0	0	0.165	0.076	6.76	—	—	—	76.7	189	—	0	—
2.464	0.072	0.024	0	0	0	0	0	0	0	0	7.392	29.6	—	0	0
2.368	0.072	0.192	0	0	0.008	0.056	0	0	0	0	9.44	21.28	—	0	—
—	0.028	—	535	107	0	0	0	—	—	—	71	75.8	—	—	—
1	0.01	0.01	0	0	0	0.004	0	0	1.5	0	0	0	0	0	—
0	0.02	0.01	0	0	0.003	0.001	0	0	0.2	0	1	0	—	0	0
5	0.05	0.08	0	0	0	0.047	0.093	—	9.6	0	6	3	0	0	—
5	0.04	0.08	0	0	0	0.005	0.088	0.005	0.7	0	5	3	0	0	—
0	—	—	0	0	0	0	0	0	0	0	0	0	—	0	0
2	0.01	0.06	0	0	0	0	0	0	0	0	5	0	—	0	—
0	0.01	0.01	0	0	0.002	0.001	0.004	0	0	0	0	1	—	0	—
0	0.03	0.02	0	0	0.002	0	0	0	0	0	0	1	0	0	0
0	0.01	0.01	0	0	0.002	0	0.014	0	0	0	0	2	0	0	0
0	0	0	0	0	0	0	0	0	0	0	0	0	0	0	0
0	0.01	0.01	0	0	0.002	0.001	0.004	0	0	0	0	1	—	0	—
5	0.193	0.063	—	—	0.002	0.003	0.043	0.007	0.1	0	6.11	6.95	—	0	—
3	0.07	0.02	—	0	0.005	0.005	0.064	0	0.1	0	2	3	—	0	—
4	0.13	0.03	0	0	0.001	0.008	0.024	0.01	0.6	0	2	4	—	0	—
3	0.11	0.02	—	0	0.001	0.005	0.022	0.007	0.3	0	2	4	—	0	—
—	—	—	—	—	0.01	0.01	0.2	—	—	—	8	—	0.005	0	—
—	—	—	—	—	—	—	—	—	—	—	—	—	—	0	—
3	0.09	0.02	0	0	0.001	0.001	0.02	0.004	0.1	0	3	4	—	0	—
11	1.46	0.286	23.5	0	0.209	0.16	1.94	0.024	13.2	0.052	23.1	36.9	—	1.16	—
11	1.46	0.286	0	0	0.209	0.16	1.94	0.024	13.2	0	23.1	36.9	0.018	1.16	—
3.36	0.616	0.109	37	0	0.101	0.067	1.75	0.011	2.24	0.036	33.9	98.6	0.005	0.504	—
—	0.3	—	0	0	0.02	0.03	0.3	—	—	—	16	31	—	1.02	—
8.1	0.671	0.212	7.25	0	0.081	0.081	0.675	0.032	4.5	0.077	48.6	43.7	0.005	1.17	—
8.75	0.665	—	0	0	0.095	0.095	0.84	0.023	—	0	16.3	31.8	0.011	1.33	0.025
7	1.08	0.221	0	0	0.161	0.123	1.4	0.019	13	0	38.5	28.4	0.01	0.805	0.042
12.3	0.815	0.3	0	0	0.098	0.095	1.04	0.026	16.3	0	26	53	0.011	1.58	0.025
—	0.916	—	0	0	0.171	0.076	1.4	—	—	—	30.8	38	—	0.608	—
21.8	0.877	0.365	0	0	0.109	0.166	1.06	0.049	—	0	22.7	69.8	0.014	1.89	—
6.25	0.775	0.155	0	0	0.083	0.155	1.02	0.009	8.75	0	25.5	22.5	—	0.55	—
6	0.68	0.318	0	0	0.103	0.08	0.828	0.023	9.75	0	20	36.3	0.009	1.55	—
22.5	0.823	0.403	0	0	0.067	0.05	0.92	0.045	13.2	0	17.2	63	0.011	2.38	0.025
4.83	0.653	0.143	0	0	0.108	0.071	0.863	0.008	8.05	0	29	24.8	0.006	0.437	0.028

Continued.

Key to Abbreviations
Kcal, Kcalories; *Prot,* protein; *Carb,* carbohydrate; *Fat,* fat; *Chol,* cholesterol; *Safa,* saturated fat; *Mufa,* monounsaturated fat; *Pufa,* polyunsaturated fat; *Sod,* sodium; *Pot,* potassium; *Mag,* magnesium; *Iron,* iron; *Zinc,* zinc; *VA,* vitamin A; *VC,* vitamin C; *Thia,* thiamin; *Ribo,* riboflavin; *Niac,* niacin; *VB₆,* vitamin B₆; *Fol,* folate; *VB₁₂,* vitamin B₁₂; *Calc,* calcium; *Phos,* phosphorus; *Sel,* selenium; *Fibd,* dietary fiber; and *VE,* vitamin E.

Food name	Portion	Wt (g)	Kcal	Prot (g)	Carb (g)	Fat (g)	Chol (mg)	Safa (g)	Mufa (g)	Pufa (g)	Sod (mg)	Pot (mg)
Breads—cont'd												
White-firm-toast	Slice	20	65	2	12	1	0	0.2	0.3	0.3	117	28
Whole wheat-firm	Slice	25	61.3	2.41	11.3	1.09	0	0.1	0.2	0.3	159	44
Whole wheat-home rec	Slice	25	66.5	2.25	11.6	1.61	0	—	—	—	89	85
Breadcrumbs-dry-grated	Cup	100	390	13	73	5	0	1	1.6	1.4	736	152
Crackers												
Animal	Item	1.9	8.67	0.127	1.47	0.2	0	—	—	—	7.53	1.67
Cheddar snacks	Item	1.6	7.22	0.144	1.11	0.261	—	—	—	—	14.3	2.17
Cheese	Item	1	5.38	0.091	0.52	0.327	—	0.09	0.09	0.03	12	1.86
Graham-plain	Item	7	27.5	0.5	5	0.5	0	0.1	0.25	0.15	33	27.5
Graham-sug/honey	Item	7	30.1	0.519	5.4	0.732	0	0.1	0.4	0.1	32.9	11.7
Ritz	Item	3.33	18	0.233	2.13	0.967	0	—	—	—	32.3	2.67
Rye Krisp-natural	Item	2.1	7.5	0.25	1.67	0.033	0	0	0	0	18.5	10.2
Rye Wafers	Item	6.5	22.5	1	5	0	0	0	0	0	57	39
Saltines	Item	2.75	12.5	0.25	2	0.25	0.75	0.1	0.1	0.05	36.8	3.25
Triscuits	Item	4.5	21	0.4	3.1	0.75	0	—	—	—	—	—
Wheat Thins	Item	1.8	9	0.125	1.25	0.35	0	—	—	—	—	—
Croissant-roll-Sara Lee	Item	26	109	2.3	11.2	6.1	—	—	—	—	140	40
French toast-home rec	Slice	65	153	5.67	17.2	6.73	—	—	—	—	257	85.8
Muffins												
Blueberry-home rec	Item	40	110	3	17	4	21	1.1	1.4	0.7	252	46
Bran-home rec	Item	40	112	2.96	16.7	5.08	21	1.2	1.4	0.8	168	98.8
Corn-home rec	Item	40	125	3	19	4	21	1.2	1.6	0.9	192	54
English-plain	Item	56	133	4.43	25.7	1.09	0	—	—	—	358	314
English-plain-toast	Item	53	154	5.13	29.8	1.26	0	—	—	—	414	364
Plain-home rec	Item	40	120	3	17	4	21	1	1.7	1	176	50
Soy	Item	40	119	3.9	16.7	4.4	0	—	—	—	—	—
Others												
Pancakes-buckwheat-mix	Item	27	55	2	6	2	20	0.8	0.9	0.4	160	66
Pancakes-plain-home rec	Item	27	60	2	9	2	20	0.5	0.8	0.5	160	33
Pancakes-plain-mix	Item	27	58.9	1.85	7.87	2.17	20	0.7	0.7	0.3	160	43.2
Roll-Brown & Serve-enr	Item	26	85	2	14	2	0	0.4	0.7	0.5	144	25
Roll-hamburger/hotdog	Item	40	114	3.43	20.1	2.09	0	0.5	0.8	0.6	241	36.8
Roll-hard-enriched	Item	50	155	5	30	2	0	0.4	0.6	0.5	312	49
Roll-submarine/hoagie-enr	Item	135	390	12	75	4	0	0.9	1.4	1.4	761	122
Roll-whole wheat-homemade	Item	35	90	3.5	18.3	1	0	—	—	—	197	102
Waffles-enr-home rec	Item	75	245	6.93	25.7	12.6	45	2.3	2.8	1.4	445	129
Waffles-froz	Item	37	103	2.15	15.9	3.52	0	—	—	—	265	77.7
Breakfast cereals												
100% Bran	Cup	66	178	8.3	48.1	3.3	0	0.59	0.57	1.87	457	824
All Bran	Cup	85.2	212	12.2	63.4	1.53	0	—	—	—	961	1051
Alpha Bits	Cup	28.4	111	2.2	24.6	0.6	0	—	—	—	219	110
Bran Buds	Cup	85.2	220	11.8	64.8	2.04	0	—	—	—	523	1425
Bran Chex	Cup	49	156	5.1	39	1.4	0	—	—	—	455	394
Bran Flakes-Kellogg's	Cup	39	127	4.9	30.5	0.7	0	0	0	0	363	248
C.W. Post-plain	Cup	97	432	8.7	69.4	15.2	0	11.3	1.72	1.42	167	198
Cheerios	Cup	22.7	88.8	3.42	15.7	1.45	0	0.27	0.515	0.597	246	81
Corn Bran	Cup	36	124	2.5	30.4	1.3	0	—	—	—	310	70
Corn Chex	Cup	28.4	111	2	24.9	0.1	0	0	0	0	271	23
Corn Flakes-Kellogg's	Cup	22.7	88.3	1.84	19.5	0.068	0	0	0	0	281	20.9
Corn Grits-enr	Cup	242	146	3.5	31.4	0.5	0	0.06	0.11	0.2	0	54
Corn-shredded-sugar	Cup	25	95	2	22	0	0	0	0	0	247	—
Cracklin Bran	Cup	60	229	5.5	41.1	8.8	0	—	—	—	487	355
Cream/wheat-instant	Cup	241	53	4.4	31.6	0.6	0	0	0	0	6	48
Cream/wheat-packet	Item	150	132	2.5	28.9	0.4	0	0	0	0	241	55

Mag (mg)	Iron (mg)	Zinc (mg)	VA (RE)	VC (mg)	Thia (mg)	Ribo (mg)	Niac (mg)	VB6 (mg)	Fol (µg)	VB12 (µg)	Calc (mg)	Phos (mg)	Sel (mg)	Fibd (g)	VE (mg)
4.8	0.6	0.142	0	0	0.07	0.06	0.8	0.008	8	0	22	23	0.006	0.5	0.024
23.3	0.855	0.42	0	0	0.088	0.053	0.958	0.047	13.8	0	18	65	0.011	2.83	0.03
23.3	0.67	0.562	10.8	0	0.068	0.038	0.798	0.05	12.3	0.027	19.8	63.3	0.011	2.83	0.025
32	3.6	—	0	0	0.35	0.35	4.8	—	—	—	122	141	0.02	3.65	—
0.267	0.059	0.009	0	0	0.005	0.009	0.073	0	0.2	0.001	0.2	1.2	0	0.027	0.007
0.278	0.068	0.012	0.18	0	0.009	0.007	0.067	0.001	0.222	0.009	1.22	1.89	0.001	0.056	0.006
0.22	0.035	0.01	—	0	0.004	0.004	0.082	—	—	—	1.05	2.1	0	0.025	0.003
3.57	0.25	0.053	0	0	0.01	0.04	0.25	0.006	0.91	0	3	10.5	0.001	0.224	0.026
2.31	0.183	0.053	0	0	0.024	0.019	0.218	0.006	0.91	0	2.66	8.26	0.001	0.119	0.026
—	0.1	—	—	—	0.013	0.013	0.1	—	—	—	5	8	—	0.107	0.012
2.5	0.092	0.057	—	—	0.006	0.005	0.033	0.007	0.833	—	0.833	6.83	0.001	0.34	0.008
—	0.25	—	0	0	0.02	0.015	0.1	—	—	—	3.5	25	0.001	1.05	0.024
0.77	0.125	0.017	0	0	0.125	0.013	0.1	0.001	0.495	0	0.5	2.5	0.004	0.072	0.01
—	—	—	—	—	—	—	—	—	—	—	—	—	0.001	0.155	0.017
—	—	—	—	—	—	—	—	—	—	—	—	—	0	0.099	0.007
7	1.04	—	8.2	0	0.28	0.1	1.2	—	—	—	12	32	—	0.56	—
11.7	1.34	0.553	22.2	0	0.124	0.163	1.01	0.038	17.6	0.291	72.2	84.5	—	2.02	—
10	0.6	—	18	0	0.09	0.1	0.7	—	—	—	34	53	—	0.85	—
35.2	1.26	1.08	40	2.48	0.1	0.112	1.26	0.111	16.8	0.092	53.6	111	—	2.52	—
18.4	0.7	—	25	0	0.1	0.1	0.7	—	—	—	42	68	—	0.95	—
10.6	1.58	0.403	0	0	0.258	0.179	2.1	0.022	17.9	0	90.7	62.7	0.015	1.29	—
12.2	1.83	0.466	0	0	0.239	0.207	2.43	0.026	20.7	0	105	72.6	0.015	1.49	—
10.8	0.6	—	8	0	0.09	0.12	0.9	—	—	—	42	60	—	0.85	—
52	0.9	—	40	0	0.08	0.1	0.5	—	—	—	35	56	—	0.835	—
5.13	0.4	0.192	12	0	0.04	0.05	0.2	0.057	2.97	0.355	59	91	0.002	0.621	—
5.13	0.4	0.192	6	0	0.06	0.07	0.5	0.057	2.97	0.355	27	38	0.002	0.45	—
5.13	0.265	0.192	7.66	0	0.038	0.059	0.254	0.057	2.97	0.355	35.6	70.7	0.003	0.394	—
5.46	0.8	0.19	0	0	0.1	0.06	0.9	0.016	9.88	—	20	23	0.008	0.988	0.203
7.6	1.19	0.248	0	0	0.196	0.132	1.58	0.014	14.8	—	53.6	32.8	0.012	1.01	0.016
11.5	1.2	0.3	0	0	0.2	0.12	1.7	0.018	29.5	0	24	46	0.015	1.5	0.02
—	3	—	0	0	0.54	0.32	4.5	0.047	—	—	58	115	0.041	3.75	0.054
40	0.8	—	0	0	0.12	0.05	1.1	—	—	—	34	98	0.016	1.83	0.035
16.5	1.48	0.653	28	0	0.18	0.24	1.46	0.054	14.3	0.365	154	135	0.011	1.05	—
7.77	1.8	0.303	95	0	0.167	0.2	1.93	0.098	0.74	—	30	141	—	0.888	—
312	8.12	5.74	—	63	1.6	1.8	20.9	2.1	—	6.3	46	801	0.02	19.5	—
318	13.5	11.2	1125	45.2	1.11	1.28	15	1.53	301	—	69	794	0.025	25.5	1.27
17	1.8	1.5	375	—	0.4	0.4	5	0.5	100	1.5	8	51	0.01	0.3	—
271	13.5	11.2	1125	45.2	1.11	1.28	15	1.53	301	—	57.1	740	0.025	23.6	0.903
126	7.8	2.14	11	26	0.6	0.26	8.6	0.9	173	2.6	29	327	0.01	7.9	—
71	11.2	5.1	516	—	0.5	0.6	6.9	0.7	138	2.1	19	192	0.004	5.5	0.164
67	15.4	1.64	1284	—	1.3	1.5	17.1	1.7	342	5.1	47	224	—	2.2	—
31.3	3.61	0.629	300	12	0.295	0.341	4	0.409	4.99	1.2	38.8	107	0.01	0.863	—
18	12.2	4	—	—	0.38	0.7	10.9	0.858	232	1.39	41	52	0.002	6.84	—
4	1.8	0.1	14	15	0.4	0.07	5	0.5	100	1.5	3	11	0.002	0.5	—
2.72	1.43	0.064	300	12	0.295	0.341	4	0.409	80.1	—	0.681	14.3	0.001	0.454	0.023
11	1.55	0.17	—	—	0.24	0.15	1.96	0.058	1	—	1	29	0.024	0.6	0.29
3.5	0.6	0.088	0	13	0.33	0.05	4.4	0.45	88.3	1.33	1	10	0.002	1.54	0.09
116	3.8	3.2	794	32	0.8	0.9	10.6	1.1	212	—	40	241	0.01	9.1	—
14	12	0.41	—	—	0.2	0.1	1.8	—	11	—	59	43	—	2.21	—
9	8.1	0.23	1250	—	0.4	0.2	5	0.5	100	—	40	20	—	2.02	—

Continued.

Food name	Portion	Wt (g)	Kcal	Prot (g)	Carb (g)	Fat (g)	Chol (mg)	Safa (g)	Mufa (g)	Pufa (g)	Sod (mg)	Pot (mg)
Breakfast cereals—cont'd												
Cream/wheat-reg-hot	Cup	251	134	3.8	27.7	0.5	0	0	0	0	2	43
Crispy Rice	Cup	28.4	111	1.8	24.8	0.1	0	0	0	0	205	27
Farina-ckd-enr	Cup	233	116	3.4	24.6	0.2	0	0.02	0.02	0.07	1	30
Fortified Oat Flake	Cup	48	177	9	34.7	0.7	0	0	0	0	429	343
Frosted Flake-Kellogg's	Cup	35	133	1.8	31.7	0.1	0	0	0	0	284	22
Frosted Mini Wheats	Item	7.1	25.5	0.731	5.86	0.071	0	0	0	0	2.06	34.2
Granola-homemade	Cup	122	595	15	67.3	33.1	0	5.84	9.37	17.2	12	612
Granola-Nature Val	Cup	113	503	11.5	75.5	19.6	0	13	2.93	2.75	232	389
Grape Nuts	Cup	114	407	13.3	93.5	0.456	0	0	0	0	792	381
Grape Nuts Flakes	Cup	32.5	116	3.48	26.6	0.358	0	0	0	0	250	113
Heartland Natural	Cup	115	499	11.6	78.6	17.7	0	—	—	—	294	385
Honey Bran	Cup	35	119	3.1	28.6	0.7	0	0	0	0	202	151
Honey Nut Cheerios	Cup	33	125	3.6	26.5	0.8	0	0.13	0.31	0.3	299	115
Life-plain/cinnamon	Cup	44	162	8.1	31.5	0.8	0	0	0	0	229	197
Lucky Charms	Cup	32	125	2.9	26.1	1.2	0	0.22	0.43	0.49	227	66
Malt O Meal-ckd	Cup	240	122	3.5	25.8	0.3	0	0	0	0	2	—
Maypo-cook-hot	Cup	240	170	5.8	31.8	2.4	0	—	—	—	9	211
Nutri Grain-barley	Cup	41	153	4.5	33.9	0.3	0	0	0	0	277	108
Nutri Grain-corn	Cup	42	160	3.4	35.5	1	0	—	—	—	276	98
Nutri Grain-rye	Cup	40	144	3.5	33.9	0.3	0	0	0	0	272	72
Nutri Grain-wheat	Cup	44	158	3.8	37.2	0.5	0	0	0	0	299	120
Oatmeal-inst-packet	Item	177	104	4.4	18.1	1.7	0	0.289	0.597	0.697	286	100
Oatmeal-raw	Cup	81	311	13	54.2	5.1	0	0.94	1.8	2.08	3	284
Oats-puffed-sugar	Cup	25	100	3	19	1	0	0.185	0.075	0.465	294	—
Product 19	Cup	33	126	3.2	27.4	0.2	0	0	0	0	378	51
Raisin Bran-Kellogg's	Cup	49.2	154	5.3	37.1	0.984	0	—	—	—	359	256
Ralston-ckd	Cup	253	134	5.5	28.2	0.8	0	0	0	0	4	153
Rice Chex	Cup	25.2	99.5	1.34	22.5	0.101	0	0	0	0	211	29.2
Rice Krispies	Cup	28.4	112	1.9	24.8	0.2	0	0	0	0	340	30
Rice-puffed-plain	Cup	14	56	0.9	12.6	0.1	0	0	0	0	0	16
Rice-puffed-sugar	Cup	28.4	115	1	26	0	0	0	0	0	21	43
Roman meal-ckd	Cup	241	147	6.6	33	1	0	—	—	—	3	302
Special K	Cup	21.3	83.1	4.2	16	0.085	0	0	0	0	199	36.8
Sugar Corn Pops	Cup	28.4	108	1.4	25.6	0.1	0	0	0	0	103	17
Sugar Smacks	Cup	37.9	141	2.65	33	0.72	0	0	0	0	100	56.1
Team	Cup	42	164	2.7	36	0.7	0	0	0	0	259	71
Toasties	Cup	22.7	87.8	1.84	19.5	0.045	0	0	0	0	238	26.3
Total	Cup	33	116	3.3	26	0.7	0	0.1	0.07	0.34	409	123
Trix	Cup	28.4	108	1.5	24.9	0.4	0	0	0	0	179	26
Wheat Chex	Cup	46	169	4.5	37.8	1.1	0	—	—	—	308	174
Wheat Flakes-sugar	Cup	30	105	3	24	0	0	0	0	0	368	81
Wheat Germ-sugar	Cup	113	426	24.7	68.7	9.1	0	1.57	1.32	5.5	3	803
Wheat germ-toasted	Cup	113	431	32.9	56.1	12.1	0	2.07	1.7	7.48	4	1070
Wheat-puffed-plain	Cup	12	44	1.8	9.5	0.1	0	0	0	0	0.48	42
Wheat-puffed-sugar	Serving	38	138	5.59	30.2	0.456	0	—	0.122	0.141	1.52	132
Wheat-rolled-ckd	Cup	240	180	5	41	1	0	0.182	0.07	0.475	535	202
Wheat-shred-biscuit	Item	23.6	83	2.6	18.8	0.3	0	0	0	0	0.472	77
Wheat-whole meal	Cup	245	110	4	23	1	0	0.182	0.07	0.475	535	118
Wheatena-ckd	Cup	243	135	5	28.7	1.1	0	—	—	—	5	187
Wheaties	Cup	29	101	2.8	23.1	0.5	0	0.07	0.05	0.24	363	108
Whole Wheat Natural	Cup	242	151	4.9	33.2	0.9	0	—	—	—	1	171
Combination foods												
Beans/pork/frankfurter-can	Cup	257	366	17.3	39.6	16.9	15	6.05	7.27	2.15	1105	604
Beans/pork/sweet sauce-can	Cup	253	282	13.4	53.1	3.69	17	1.42	1.6	0.473	849	673
Beans/pork/tom sauce-can	Cup	253	247	13	49	2.6	17	1	1.12	0.331	1113	759
Beef & vegetable stew	Cup	245	220	16	15	11	72	4.9	4.5	0.5	1006	613

Mag (mg)	Iron (mg)	Zinc (mg)	VA (RE)	VC (mg)	Thia (mg)	Ribo (mg)	Niac (mg)	VB$_6$ (mg)	Fol (μg)	VB$_{12}$ (μg)	Calc (mg)	Phos (mg)	Sel (mg)	Fibd (g)	VE (mg)
10	10.3	0.33	—	—	0.2	0.1	1.5	—	9	—	51	42	—	1.94	—
12	0.7	0.46	—	1	0.1	0	2	0.044	3	0.082	5	31	0.004	1	—
4	1.16	0.16	—	—	0.19	0.12	1.28	0.023	6	—	4	28	—	3.26	—
58	13.7	1.5	636	—	0.6	0.7	8.4	0.9	169	2.5	68	176	0.01	1.2	—
3	2.2	0.05	463	19	0.5	0.5	6.2	0.6	124	—	1	26	—	0.77	—
55.8	0.447	0.376	94	3.76	0.092	0.107	1.25	0.128	25.1	—	2.34	18.5	—	0.54	0.026
141	4.84	4.47	10	1	0.73	0.31	2.14	0.428	99	—	76	494	0.023	12.8	—
116	3.78	2.19	—	—	0.39	0.19	0.83	—	85	—	71	354	0.037	4.2	—
76.3	4.95	2.51	1500	—	1.48	1.71	20.1	2.05	402	6.04	43.3	286	0.034	5.47	—
35.8	5.17	0.65	430	—	0.423	0.488	5.72	0.585	115	1.72	13	96.9	0.01	2.08	0.137
147	4.33	3.04	—	—	0.36	0.16	1.61	—	64	—	75	416	—	5.4	—
46	5.6	0.9	463	19	0.5	0.5	6.2	0.6	23	1.9	16	132	—	3.9	—
39	5.2	0.87	437	17	0.4	0.5	5.8	0.6	—	1.7	23	122	—	1.3	—
14	11.6	1.45	—	—	0.95	1	11.6	—	37	—	154	238	—	1.4	—
27	5.1	0.56	424	17	0.4	0.5	5.6	0.6	—	1.7	36	88	—	0.6	—
—	9.5	0.17	—	—	0.4	0.3	5.9	0.019	6	—	5	23	—	0.6	—
51	8.4	1.49	702	28	0.7	0.8	9.4	0.9	9	2.8	125	248	—	1.2	—
32	1.45	5.4	543	22	0.5	0.6	7.2	0.7	145	2.2	11	126	0.027	2.4	—
27	0.89	5.5	555	22	0.5	0.6	7.4	0.8	148	2.2	1	120	0.003	2.6	0.042
31	1.13	5.3	530	21	0.5	0.6	7	0.7	141	2.1	8	104	—	2.56	0.04
34	1.24	5.8	588	23	0.6	0.7	7.7	0.8	155	2.3	12	164	0.007	2.8	0.044
—	6.32	—	455	—	0.53	0.29	5.49	0.742	150	—	163	133	0.015	1.62	1.06
120	3.41	2.48	10	—	0.59	0.11	0.63	0.097	26	—	42	384	0.022	4.6	0.203
28	4	0.693	275	13	0.33	0.38	4.4	0.45	5.5	1.33	44	102	0.006	2.65	0.168
12	21	0.5	1748	70	1.7	2	23.3	2.3	466	7	4	47	—	0.4	—
63.5	6	5.02	500	—	0.492	0.59	6.69	0.689	133	2.02	17.2	183	0.005	5.31	—
59	1.64	1.42	—	—	0.2	0.18	2.05	0.114	18	0.109	14	148	—	4.2	—
6.3	1.59	0.348	1.85	13.4	0.328	—	4.44	0.454	89	1.34	3.53	24.7	0.004	0.151	0.01
10	1.8	0.48	375	15	0.4	0.4	5	0.5	100	—	4	34	0.004	0.1	0.011
3	0.15	0.14	0	0	0.02	0.01	0.42	0.011	3	—	1	14	0.001	0.1	0.094
7.56	0	1.48	300	15	0	0	0	0.504	98.8	1.48	3	14	0.002	0.2	0.188
109	2.12	1.78	—	—	0.24	0.12	3.08	0.113	24	—	30	215	—	2.31	—
11.7	3.39	2.81	28	11.3	0.277	0.32	3.75	0.383	75.2	—	6.18	41.3	0.013	0.17	—
2	1.8	1.5	375	15	0.4	0.4	5	0.5	100	—	1	28	—	0.2	0.026
18.2	2.39	0.379	500	20.1	0.493	0.569	6.67	0.682	134	—	4.17	41.3	—	0.531	—
19	2.57	0.58	555	22	0.5	0.6	7.4	0.8	—	2.2	6	65	0.007	0.4	—
3.41	0.597	0.066	300	—	0.295	0.341	4	0.409	80.1	1.2	0.908	10	—	0.386	—
37	21	0.78	1748	70	1.7	2	23.3	2.3	466	7	56	137	—	2.4	—
6	4.5	0.13	371	15	0.4	0.4	4.9	0.5	—	1.5	6	19	—	0.1	—
58	7.3	1.23	—	24	0.6	0.17	8.1	0.8	162	2.4	18	182	—	3.4	0.193
32.7	4.8	0.669	33	16	0.4	0.45	5.3	0.54	9	1.59	12	83	0.003	2.7	0.126
272	7.71	14.1	—	—	1.41	0.7	4.73	0.829	298	—	38	971	—	5.7	—
362	10.3	18.8	5	7	1.89	0.93	6.31	1.11	398	—	50	1294	—	14.6	15.9
17	0.57	0.28	0	0	0.02	0.03	1.3	0.02	4	—	3	43	—	0.4	0.08
55.1	1.8	0.897	0	0	0.076	0.087	4.1	0.065	12.2	0	10.6	135	—	2.11	—
52.8	1.7	1.15	0	0	0.17	0.07	2.2	—	26.4	—	19	182	—	2.87	2.54
40	0.74	0.59	0	0	0.07	0.06	1.08	0.06	12	—	10	86	—	2.2	0.085
53.9	1.2	1.18	0	0	0.15	0.05	1.5	—	27	—	17	127	—	1.61	2.6
49	1.36	1.68	—	—	0.02	0.05	1.34	0.046	17	—	11	146	0.058	2.6	—
32	4.6	0.65	384	15	0.4	0.4	5.1	0.5	9	1.5	44	100	0.003	2	0.122
54	1.5	1.16	—	—	0.17	0.12	2.15	—	26	—	17	167	0.058	2.7	2.57
71	4.45	4.79	80	5.9	0.149	0.144	2.32	0.118	77.1	0.87	123	267	—	12.8	0.561
87	4.2	3.8	35	7.7	0.119	0.154	0.888	0.215	94.5	0.06	155	266	—	14	0.561
88	8.3	14.8	62	7.8	0.132	0.116	1.26	0.175	56.8	0.03	141	297	—	13.8	0.561
—	2.9	—	480	17	0.15	0.17	4.7	—	—	0.002	29	184	—	3.19	0.515

Key to Abbreviations

Kcal, Kcalories; *Prot,* protein; *Carb,* carbohydrate; *Fat,* fat; *Chol,* cholesterol; *Safa,* saturated fat; *Mufa,* monounsaturated fat; *Pufa,* polyunsaturated fat; *Sod,* sodium; *Pot,* potassium; *Mag,* magnesium; *Iron,* iron; *Zinc,* zinc; *VA,* vitamin A; *VC,* vitamin C; *Thia,* thiamin; *Ribo,* riboflavin; *Niac,* niacin; *VB₆,* vitamin B₆; *Fol,* folate; *VB₁₂,* vitamin B₁₂; *Calc,* calcium; *Phos,* phosphorus; *Sel,* selenium; *Fibd,* dietary fiber; and *VE,* vitamin E.

Food name	Portion	Wt (g)	Kcal	Prot (g)	Carb (g)	Fat (g)	Chol (mg)	Safa (g)	Mufa (g)	Pufa (g)	Sod (mg)	Pot (mg)
Combination foods—cont'd												
Beef potpie-home rec	Slice	210	515	21	39	30	44	7.9	12.9	7.4	596	334
Beef raviolios-can	oz	28.4	27.5	1.14	4.26	0.568	—	0.11	0.16	0.254	131	45.7
Chicken A La King-home rec	Cup	245	470	27	12	34	186	12.9	13.4	6.2	759	404
Chicken Chow Mein-can	Cup	250	95	7	18	0	98	0	0	0	722	418
Chicken potpie-baked-home rec	Slice	232	545	23	42	31	72	11	13.5	5.5	593	343
Chili Con Carne/beans-can	Cup	255	340	19	31	16	38	7.5	7.2	1	1354	594
Chili with beans-can	Cup	255	286	14.6	30.4	14	43	6	5.95	0.923	1330	932
Macaroni & cheese-enr-can	Cup	240	230	9	26	10	42	4.2	3.1	1.4	729	139
Macronia & cheese-enr-hom	Cup	200	430	17	40	22	42	8.9	8.8	2.9	1086	240
Meat loaf-celery/onions	Serving	87.6	213	15.8	5.23	13.9	107	5.29	5.9	0.613	103	182
Pizza-cheese-baked	Slice	49	109	5.97	15.9	2.5	7	1.2	0.77	0.382	261	85
Pizza-pepperoni-baked	Slice	53	135	7.56	14.8	5.19	11	1.67	2.34	0.87	199	114
Salads												
Carrot raisin-home	Cup	268	306	3.8	55.8	11.6	—	—	—	—	—	—
Chef ham/cheese	Serving	200	196	13.4	7.42	12.7	46	6.98	4.09	0.739	567	415
Chicken	Cup	205	502	26	17.4	36.2	—	—	—	—	1395	521
Coleslaw	Tbsp	8	6	0.1	0.99	0.21	1	0.031	0.057	0.108	2	14
Fruit-can/juice	Cup	249	125	1.28	32.5	0.06	0	0.01	0.012	0.027	13	288
Green tossed	Serving	207	32	2.6	6.67	0.16	0	0.021	0.008	0.07	53	356
Macaroni	Serving	28.4	50.7	0.7	5.3	3	—	—	—	—	148	21
Mandarin orange gelatin	Serving	28.4	22.7	0.4	5.7	0	—	0	0	0	14	9
Potato	Cup	250	358	6.7	27.9	20.5	171	3.57	6.2	9.3	1323	635
Three bean-Del Monte	oz	28.4	22.4	0.71	5.06	0.056	0	0	0	0	101	38.3
Tuna	Cup	205	350	30	7	22	68	4.3	6.3	6.7	434	—
Others												
Sandwich-blt/mayo	Item	148	282	6.8	28.8	15.6	—	—	—	—	—	—
Sandwich-club	Item	315	590	35.6	41.7	20.8	—	—	—	—	—	—
Spaghetti/tom/cheese-can	Cup	250	190	6	39	2	4	0.5	0.3	0.4	955	303
Spaghetti/tom/che-home rec	Cup	250	260	9	37	9	4	2	5.4	0.7	955	408
Spaghetti/tom/meat-can	Cup	250	260	12	29	10	39	2.2	3.3	3.9	1220	245
Spaghetti/tom/meat-home rec	Cup	248	330	19	39	12	75	3.3	6.3	0.9	1009	665
Taco	Item	171	370	20.7	26.7	20.6	57	11.4	6.58	0.959	802	473
Dairy products												
Cheese food-American-proc	oz	28.4	93	5.56	2.07	6.97	18	4.38	2.04	0.2	337	79
Cheese spread-proc	oz	28.4	82	4.65	2.48	6.02	16	3.78	1.76	0.18	381	69
Cheeses												
American-proc	oz	28.4	106	6.28	0.45	8.86	27	5.58	2.54	0.28	406	46
Blue	oz	28.4	100	6.06	0.659	8.14	21	5.29	2.21	0.23	395	72.9
Camembert-wedge	Item	38	114	7.52	0.18	9.22	27	5.8	2.67	0.28	320	71
Cheddar-shred	Cup	113	455	28.1	1.45	37.5	119	23.8	10.6	1.06	701	111
Cottage, 4%-large curd	Cup	225	232	28.1	6.03	10.1	33.8	6.41	2.88	0.315	911	189
Cream	oz	28.4	100	2.17	0.759	10	31.4	6.31	2.82	0.365	85.1	34.4
Feta	oz	28.4	75	4.03	1.16	6.03	25	4.24	1.31	0.17	316	18
Gouda	oz	28.4	101	7.07	0.63	7.78	32	4.99	2.2	0.19	232	34
Limburger	oz	28.4	93	5.68	0.14	7.72	26	4.75	2.44	0.14	227	36
Monterey	oz	28.4	106	6.94	0.19	8.58	—	—	—	—	152	23
Mozzarella-skim milk	oz	28.4	72	6.88	0.78	4.51	16	2.87	1.28	0.13	132	24
Parmesan-grated	Cup	100	456	41.6	3.74	30	79	19.1	8.73	0.66	1862	107
Provolone	oz	28.4	100	7.25	0.61	7.55	20	4.84	2.1	0.22	248	39
Ricotta-skim milk	Cup	246	340	28	12.6	19.5	76	12.1	5.69	0.64	307	308
Romano	oz	28.4	110	9.02	1.03	7.64	29	—	—	—	340	—
Roquefort	oz	28.4	105	6.11	0.57	8.69	26	5.46	2.4	0.37	513	26
Swiss	oz	28.4	107	8.06	0.96	7.78	26	5.04	2.06	0.28	74	31
Swiss-proc	oz	28.4	95	7.01	0.6	7.09	24	4.55	2	0.18	388	61

Mag (mg)	Iron (mg)	Zinc (mg)	VA (RE)	VC (mg)	Thia (mg)	Ribo (mg)	Niac (mg)	VB$_6$ (mg)	Fol (µg)	VB$_{12}$ (µg)	Calc (mg)	Phos (mg)	Sel (mg)	Fibd (g)	VE (mg)
—	3.8	—	344	6	0.3	0.3	5.5	—	—	—	29	149	—	3.9	1.18
—	0.312	—	5	0.426	0.026	0.023	0.398	—	—	—	4.54	—	—	0.23	0.045
—	2.5	—	226	12	0.1	0.42	5.4	—	—	—	127	358	—	1.2	0.931
—	1.3	—	30	13	0.05	0.1	1	—	—	—	45	85	—	0.9	0
—	3	—	615	5	0.34	0.31	5.5	—	—	—	70	232	0.032	4.2	0.882
—	4.3	—	30	—	0.08	0.18	3.3	0.263	—	—	82	321	—	5	—
115	8.75	5.1	86	4.3	0.122	0.268	0.913	0.337	—	0.03	119	393	—	6.93	—
—	1	—	52	0	0.12	0.24	1	—	—	—	199	182	—	1.44	0.384
52	1.8	—	172	0	0.2	0.4	1.8	—	—	—	362	322	0.028	1.2	0.32
13.6	1.91	3.08	12.3	0.725	0.052	0.148	3.16	0.162	10.9	1.52	22.8	112	0.001	0.11	0.068
12	0.45	0.63	57	1	0.14	0.13	1.93	0.03	46	0.26	90	88	—	1.59	—
6	0.7	0.39	44	1.2	0.1	0.17	2.28	0.04	39	0.14	48	56	—	1.48	—
—	3	—	1100	12	0.16	0.16	1	—	—	—	96	130	—	16.7	—
28.4	1.17	1.73	740	24	0.337	0.24	2.21	0.206	46	0.474	227	251	0.019	2.39	0.719
1	0.05	0.02	7	2.6	0.005	0.005	0.022	0.01	2.1	0.002	4	3	—	0.297	—
21	0.62	0.36	143	8.3	0.027	0.035	0.886	—	—	0	28	36	0.001	1.64	—
22	1.3	0.43	235	48	0.06	0.1	1.15	0.16	77	0	26	80	0.001	2.11	0.483
—	—	—	—	—	—	—	—	—	—	—	—	—	—	0.29	—
—	—	—	—	—	—	—	—	—	—	—	—	—	—	0.57	—
39	1.63	0.78	82	24.9	0.193	0.15	2.23	0.353	16.8	0.385	48	130	—	5.26	—
6.25	0.284	0.093	3	0.852	0.014	0.014	0.085	—	—	—	9.66	16.2	—	1.52	—
—	2.7	—	113	2	0.08	0.23	10.3	—	—	—	41	291	—	1.03	0
—	1.5	—	174	13	0.16	0.14	1.6	—	—	—	53	89	—	2.88	—
—	4.3	—	350	27	0.38	0.41	10.2	—	—	—	103	394	—	4.17	—
28	2.8	—	185	10	0.35	0.28	4.5	—	—	—	40	88	0.025	2.5	—
—	2.3	—	215	13	0.25	0.18	2.3	—	—	—	80	135	—	2.5	—
28	3.3	—	200	5	0.15	0.18	2.3	—	—	—	53	113	—	2.75	—
—	3.7	—	—	22	0.25	0.3	4	—	—	—	124	236	0.022	2.73	—
71	2.42	3.93	147	2.2	0.15	0.45	3.22	0.24	23	1.04	221	203	—	2.67	—
9	0.24	0.85	77.8	0	0.008	0.125	0.04	—	—	0.317	163	130	0.006	0	0.179
8	0.09	0.73	67	0	0.014	0.122	0.037	0.033	2	0.113	159	202	0.006	0	0.179
6	0.11	0.85	103	0	0.008	0.1	0.02	0.02	2	0.197	174	211	0.003	0	0.179
6.99	0.09	0.749	61.2	0	0.008	0.108	0.287	0.047	9.98	0.344	150	110	0.006	0	0.179
8	0.12	0.9	105	0	0.011	0.185	0.239	0.086	24	0.492	147	132	0.008	0	0.243
31	0.77	3.51	359	0	0.031	0.424	0.09	0.084	21	0.935	815	579	0.018	0	0.723
11.3	0.315	0.833	110	0	0.047	0.367	0.284	0.151	27	1.4	135	297	0.052	0	1.44
2.03	0.344	0.152	122	0	0.005	0.057	0.029	0.013	4.05	0.122	23.3	30.4	0.001	0	0.181
5	0.18	0.82	—	0	—	—	—	—	—	—	140	96	—	0	0.179
8	0.07	1.11	55	0	0.009	0.095	0.018	0.023	6	—	198	155	0	0	0.179
6	0.04	0.6	109	0	0.023	0.143	0.045	0.024	16	0.295	141	111	—	0	0.179
8	0.2	0.85	80.8	0	—	0.111	—	—	—	—	212	126	0.013	0	0.179
7	0.06	0.78	49.8	0	0.005	0.086	0.03	0.02	2	0.232	183	131	0.003	0	0.179
51	0.95	3.19	211	0	0.045	0.386	0.315	0.105	8	—	1376	807	0.024	0	0.64
8	0.15	0.92	69.4	0	0.005	0.091	0.044	0.021	3	0.415	214	141	—	0	0.179
36	1.08	3.3	319	0	0.052	0.455	0.192	0.049	—	0.716	669	449	—	0	1.57
—	—	—	48.6	0	—	0.105	0.022	—	2	—	302	215	—	0	0.179
8	0.16	0.59	89.2	0	0.011	0.166	0.208	0.035	14	0.182	188	111	—	0	0.179
10.1	0.05	1.11	72.1	0	0.006	0.103	0.026	0.024	2	0.475	272	171	0.002	0	0.179
8	0.17	1.02	68.8	0	0.004	0.078	0.011	0.01	—	0.348	219	216	0.002	0	0.179

Continued.

Key to Abbreviations

Kcal, Kcalories; *Prot,* protein; *Carb,* carbohydrate; *Fat,* fat; *Chol,* cholesterol; *Safa,* saturated fat; *Mufa,* monounsaturated fat; *Pufa,* polyunsaturated fat; *Sod,* sodium; *Pot,* potassium; *Mag,* magnesium; *Iron,* iron; *Zinc,* zinc; *VA,* vitamin A; *VC,* vitamin C; *Thia,* thiamin; *Ribo,* riboflavin; *Niac,* niacin; *VB₆,* vitamin B₆; *Fol,* folate; *VB₁₂,* vitamin B₁₂; *Calc,* calcium; *Phos,* phosphorus; *Sel,* selenium; *Fibd,* dietary fiber; and *VE,* vitamin E.

Food name	Portion	Wt (g)	Kcal	Prot (g)	Carb (g)	Fat (g)	Chol (mg)	Safa (g)	Mufa (g)	Pufa (g)	Sod (mg)	Pot (mg)
Creams												
Coffee-table-light	Cup	240	469	6.48	8.78	46.3	159	28.9	13.4	1.72	95	292
Half & Half-fluid	Cup	242	315	7.16	10.4	27.8	89	17.3	8.04	1.03	98	314
Non dairy-powdered	Cup	94	514	4.5	51.6	33.4	0	30.6	0.91	0.01	170	763
Non dairy-coffeemate	Tbsp	15	16	0	2	1	0	0	—	0	5	20
Sour-cultured	Cup	230	493	7.27	9.82	48.2	102	30	13.9	1.79	123	331
Sour-Half & Half	Tbsp	15	20	0.44	0.64	1.8	6	1.12	0.52	0.07	6	19
Sour-imitation	oz	28.4	59	0.68	1.88	5.53	0	5.04	0.17	0.02	29	46
Whip-imit-froz	Cup	75	239	0.94	17.3	19	0	16.3	1.21	0.39	19	14
Whip-imit-pressurized	Cup	70	184	0.69	11.3	15.6	0	13.2	1.35	0.17	43	13
Whip-pressurized	Cup	60	154	1.92	7.49	13.3	46	8.3	3.85	0.5	78	88
Whipping-heavy	Cup	238	821	4.88	6.64	88.1	326	54.8	25.4	3.27	89	179
Milk												
1% Fat-lowfat-fluid	Cup	244	102	8.03	11.7	2.59	10	1.61	0.75	0.1	123	381
2% Fat-lowfat-fluid	Cup	244	121	8.12	11.7	4.68	18	2.92	1.35	0.17	122	377
2% Milk solids add	Cup	245	125	8.53	12.2	4.7	18	2.93	1.36	0.18	128	397
Buttermilk-fluid	Cup	245	99	8.11	11.7	2.16	9	1.34	0.62	0.08	257	371
Chocolate-whole	Cup	250	208	7.92	25.9	8.48	30	5.26	2.48	0.31	149	417
Condensed-sweet-can	Cup	306	982	24.2	166	26.6	104	16.8	7.43	1.03	389	1136
Eggnog-commercial	Cup	254	342	9.68	34.4	19	149	11.3	5.67	0.86	138	420
Evaporated-skim-can	Cup	255	199	19.3	28.9	0.51	10.2	0.309	0.158	0.015	293	847
Evaporated-whole-can	Cup	252	338	17.2	25.3	19.1	73.1	11.6	5.9	0.605	267	764
Human-whole-mature	Cup	246	171	2.53	17	10.8	34	4.94	4.08	1.22	42	126
Nonfat/skim-fluid	Cup	245	86	8.35	11.9	0.44	4	0.287	0.116	0.016	126	406
Whole-3.3% Fat-fluid	Cup	244	150	8.03	11.4	8.15	33	5.07	2.35	0.3	120	370
Whole-low sodium	Cup	244	149	7.56	10.9	8.44	33	5.26	2.44	0.31	6	617
Others												
Milkshake-choc-thick	Item	300	356	9.15	63.5	8.1	32	5.04	2.34	0.3	333	672
Milkshake-vanilla-thick	Item	313	350	12.1	55.6	9.48	37	5.9	2.74	0.35	299	572
Yogurt-fruit flavor-lowfat	Cup	227	231	9.92	43.2	2.45	10	1.58	0.67	0.07	133	442
Yogurt-plain-lowfat	Cup	227	144	11.9	16	3.52	14	2.27	0.97	0.1	159	531
Yogurt-plain-nonfat	Cup	227	127	13	17.4	0.41	4	0.264	0.112	0.012	174	579
Yogurt-plain-whole	Cup	227	139	7.88	10.6	7.38	29	4.76	2.03	0.21	105	351
Desserts												
Angelfood-mix/prep	Slice	53	142	4.2	31.5	0.122	0	—	—	—	142	51.9
Cheesecake-commercial	Slice	85	257	4.61	24.3	16.3	—	—	—	—	189	83.3
Fruit-dark-home rec	Slice	15	56.9	0.72	8.96	2.3	6.75	0.48	1.31	0.47	23.7	74.4
Gingerbread-mix/prep	Slice	63	175	2	32	4	1	1.1	1.8	1.1	90	173
Pound-home recipe	Slice	33	160	2	16	10	68	5.9	3	0.6	58	20
Sheet-no icing-home rec	Slice	86	315	4	48	12	1	3.3	4.9	2.6	382	68
Sponge-home recipe	Slice	66	188	4.82	35.7	3.14	162	1.1	1.3	0.5	164	59.4
Strawberry shortcake	Serving	175	344	4.8	61.2	8.9	—	—	—	—	—	—
Yellow/icing-home rec	Slice	69	268	2.9	40.3	11.4	36	3	3	1.4	191	72.5
Cookies												
Choc chip-home rec	Item	10	46.3	0.5	6.41	2.68	5.25	0.6	1.15	0.8	20.6	20.5
Choc chip-mix	Item	10.5	50	0.5	6.96	2.42	5.52	0.7	0.9	0.6	37.8	13.5
Macaroon	Item	19	90	1	12.5	4.5	0	—	—	—	6	88
Oatmeal/raisin-mix	Item	13	61.5	0.732	8.93	2.6	0	0.5	0.825	0.5	37.1	22.6
Peanut butter-mix	Item	10	50	0.8	5.87	2.64	—	—	—	—	56.6	19.4
Sandwich-choc/van	Item	10	50	0.5	7	2.25	0	0.55	0.975	0.55	63	3.75
Sugar-mix	Item	20	98.8	0.908	13.1	4.79	—	—	—	—	109	13.6
Vanilla wafer	Item	4	18.5	0.2	3	0.6	2.5	0.1	0.2	0.1	10	2.9

Mag (mg)	Iron (mg)	Zinc (mg)	VA (RE)	VC (mg)	Thia (mg)	Ribo (mg)	Niac (mg)	VB$_6$ (mg)	Fol (μg)	VB$_{12}$ (μg)	Calc (mg)	Phos (mg)	Sel (mg)	Fibd (g)	VE (mg)
21	0.1	0.65	519	1.82	0.077	0.355	0.137	0.077	6	0.528	231	192	0.001	0	—
25	0.17	1.23	315	2.08	0.085	0.361	0.189	0.094	6	0.796	254	230	0.001	0	—
4	1.08	0.48	57.4	0	0	0.155	0	0	0	0	21	397	—	0	—
—	—	—	—	—	—	—	—	—	—	—	—	18	—	—	—
26	0.14	0.62	546	1.98	0.081	0.343	0.154	0.037	25	0.69	268	195	—	0	—
2	0.01	0.08	20.4	0.13	0.005	0.022	0.01	0.002	2	0.045	16	14	—	0	—
—	—	—	0	0	0	0	0	0	0	0	1	13	—	0	—
1	0.09	0.02	194	0	0	0	0	0	0	0	5	6	—	0	—
1	0.01	0.01	99.4	0	0	0	0	0	0	0	4	13	—	0	—
6	0.03	0.22	165	0	0.022	0.039	0.042	0.025	—	0.175	61	54	—	0	—
17	0.07	0.55	1051	1.38	0.052	0.262	0.093	0.062	9	0.428	154	149	—	0	—
34	0.12	0.95	150	2.37	0.095	0.407	0.212	0.105	12	0.898	300	235	0.003	0	0.146
33	0.12	0.95	150	2.32	0.095	0.403	0.21	0.105	12	0.888	297	232	0.007	0	0.146
35	0.12	0.98	150	2.45	0.098	0.424	0.22	0.11	13	0.936	313	245	0.007	0	0.147
27	0.12	1.03	24.3	2.4	0.083	0.377	0.142	0.083	—	0.537	285	219	0.003	0	—
33	0.6	1.02	90.7	2.28	0.092	0.405	0.313	0.1	12	0.835	280	251	0.003	0.15	0.225
78	0.58	2.88	302	7.96	0.275	1.27	0.643	0.156	34	1.36	868	775	0.003	0	—
47	0.51	1.17	268	3.81	0.086	0.483	0.267	0.127	2	1.14	330	278	0.003	0	—
68.9	0.74	2.3	300	3.16	0.115	0.788	0.444	0.14	23	0.609	740	497	0.003	0	—
60.5	0.479	1.94	184	4.74	0.118	0.796	0.489	0.126	20.2	0.411	658	509	0.003	0	—
8	0.07	0.42	178	12.3	0.034	0.089	0.435	0.027	13	0.111	79	34	0.004	0	2.16
28	0.1	0.98	150	2.4	0.088	0.343	0.216	0.098	13	0.926	302	247	0.007	0	0.147
33	0.12	0.93	92.2	2.29	0.093	0.395	0.205	0.102	12	0.871	291	228	0.003	0	0.146
12	—	—	95.2	—	0.049	0.256	0.105	0.083	—	0.876	246	209	0.003	0	0.146
48	0.93	1.44	77.5	0	0.141	0.666	0.372	0.075	15	0.945	396	378	0.005	0.75	—
37	0.31	1.22	107	0	0.094	0.61	0.457	0.131	21	1.63	457	361	0.005	0.2	—
33	0.16	1.68	31.2	1.5	0.084	0.404	0.216	0.091	21	1.06	345	271	0.011	0.8	—
40	0.18	2.02	45	1.82	0.1	0.486	0.259	0.111	25	1.28	415	326	0.011	0	—
43	0.2	2.2	4.8	1.98	0.109	0.531	0.281	0.12	28	1.39	452	355	0.011	0	—
26	0.11	1.34	83.8	1.2	0.066	0.322	0.17	0.073	17	0.844	274	215	0.011	0	—
5.83	0.451	0.106	0	0	0.064	0.122	0.594	0.007	4.77	0.015	50	63	0.003	0.037	1.43
8.5	0.408	0.357	43	4.25	0.026	0.111	0.391	0.054	15.3	0.421	47.6	74.8	—	1.79	—
—	0.42	—	3.6	0.06	0.024	0.024	0.165	—	—	—	10.8	17	—	0.313	—
14	0.9	0.284	0	0	0.09	0.11	0.8	0.048	5	0.066	57	63	0.004	1.83	—
—	0.5	—	16	0	0.05	0.06	0.4	—	1.98	—	6	24	0.002	0.08	0.888
12	0.9	0.301	30	0	0.13	0.15	1.1	0.024	6.02	0.087	55	88	0.006	0.96	2.31
7.26	1.11	0.799	25	0	0.092	0.132	0.726	0.037	14.5	0.332	25.1	65.3	0.004	0	1.78
—	2	—	86	89	0.17	0.21	1.3	—	—	—	73	84	—	2.14	—
13.1	0.787	0.338	9.5	0	0.076	0.097	0.656	0.023	5.52	0.123	57.3	60.7	0.004	0.552	1.86
3.5	0.249	0.044	1	0	0.015	0.015	0.146	0.002	0.9	0.01	3.3	8.4	0.001	0.27	0.267
2.52	0.228	0.053	6.09	0	0.014	0.022	0.195	0.002	0.945	—	2.94	7.46	0.001	0.284	0.28
—	0.15	—	0	0	0.01	0.03	0.1	—	—	—	5	16	0.001	0.437	0.507
3.64	0.285	0.085	2.08	0	0.022	0.021	0.241	0.006	1.56	—	4.42	14.4	0.001	0.351	0.347
3.9	0.19	0.75	3.04	0	0.019	0.016	0.381	0.008	2.4	—	11.5	23.5	—	0.18	0.257
5.1	0.175	0.086	0	0	0.015	0.025	0.175	0.004	0.3	0	2.5	24	0.001	0.15	0.257
1.6	0.386	0.054	2.96	0	0.036	0.024	0.466	0.011	1.8	—	20.8	37.8	0.001	0.262	0.514
0.68	0.06	—	1	0	0.01	0.009	0.08	—	—	—	1.6	2.5	0	0.01	0.103

Continued.

Key to Abbreviations

Kcal, Kcalories; *Prot*, protein; *Carb*, carbohydrate; *Fat*, fat; *Chol*, cholesterol; *Safa*, saturated fat; *Mufa*, monounsaturated fat; *Pufa*, polyunsaturated fat; *Sod*, sodium; *Pot*, potassium; *Mag*, magnesium; *Iron*, iron; *Zinc*, zinc; *VA*, vitamin A; *VC*, vitamin C; *Thia*, thiamin; *Ribo*, riboflavin; *Niac*, niacin; *VB₆*, vitamin B6; *Fol*, folate; *VB₁₂*, vitamin B12; *Calc*, calcium; *Phos*, phosphorus; *Sel*, selenium; *Fibd*, dietary fiber; and *VE*, vitamin E.

Food name	Portion	Wt (g)	Kcal	Prot (g)	Carb (g)	Fat (g)	Chol (mg)	Safa (g)	Mufa (g)	Pufa (g)	Sod (mg)	Pot (mg)
Others												
Cupcake/choc icing	Item	36	130	2	21	5	15	2	1.7	0.7	120	42
Custard-baked	Cup	265	305	14	29	15	278	6.8	5.4	0.7	209	387
Danish pastry-plain	Item	65	250	4.06	29.1	13.6	0	4.7	6.1	3.2	249	60.5
Doughnuts-cake-plain	Item	25	104	1.28	12.2	5.77	10	1.2	1.2	2	139	27.3
Doughnuts-yeast-glazed	Item	50	205	3	22	11.2	13	3	5.8	3.3	117	34
Gel-D Zerta-low cal, prep	Cup	240	16	4	0	0	0	0	0	0	—	—
Frozen yogurt-choc	Cup	144	230	5.8	35.8	8.6	6	5.24	2.52	0.32	142	376
Frozen yogurt-fruit variety	Cup	226	216	7	41.8	2	—	—	—	—	—	—
Frozen yogurt-vanilla	Cup	144	28	5.6	34.8	8	4	4.92	2.28	0.3	126	304
Gelatin dessert-prep	Cup	240	140	4	34	0	0	0	0	0	0	—
Gelatin-dry-envelope	Item	7	25	6	0	0	0	0	0	0	8	180
Granola bar	Item	24	109	2.35	16	4.23	—	—	—	—	66.7	78.2
Ice cream-van-hard-10% fat	Cup	133	269	4.8	31.7	14.3	59	8.92	3.6	0.32	116	257
Ice cream-van-soft serve	Cup	173	377	7.04	38.3	22.5	153	13.5	5.85	0.65	153	338
Ice milk-van-soft-2.6% fat	Cup	175	223	8.03	38.4	4.62	13	2.88	1.16	0.1	163	412
Ice cream sundae-hot fudge	Item	165	297	5.89	49.8	9.01	21.5	5.25	2.43	0.843	190	413
Jello-gel-sugar free-prep	Cup	240	16	2	0	0	0	0	0	0	120	—
Pie												
Apple-home rec	Slice	135	323	2.75	49.1	13.6	0	3.9	6.4	3.6	207	115
Banana cream-home rec	Slice	130	285	6	40	12	40	3.8	4.7	2.3	252	264
Cherry-home rec	Slice	135	350	4	52	15	0	4	6.4	3.6	410	142
Crust-mix/prep-baked	Item	160	743	10	70.5	46.5	0	11.4	19.9	11.7	1300	89.5
Custard-home rec	Slice	130	285	8	30	14	—	4.8	5.5	2.5	373	178
Lemon meringue-home	Slice	120	300	3.86	47.3	11.2	0	3.7	4.8	2.3	223	52.8
Mince-home rec	Slice	135	365	3	56	16	0	4	6.6	3.6	604	240
Peach-home rec	Slice	135	345	3	52	14	0	3.5	6.2	3.6	361	21
Pecan-home rec	Slice	118	495	6	61	27	0	4	14.4	6.3	260	145
Pumpkin-home rec	Slice	130	275	5	32	15	0	5.4	5.4	2.4	278	208
Pudding												
Choc-ckd-mix/milk	Cup	260	320	9	59	8	32	4.3	2.6	2	335	354
Choc inst-mix/milk	Cup	260	325	8	63	7	28	3.6	2.2	0.3	322	335
Rice/raisins	Cup	265	387	9.5	70.8	8.2	—	—	—	—	188	469
Tapioca cream-home rec	Cup	165	220	8	28	8	80	4.1	2.5	0.5	257	223
Sherbet-orange-2% fat	Cup	193	270	2.16	58.7	3.82	14	2.38	0.96	0.09	88	198
Turnover-apple	oz	28.4	85.2	0.738	10.5	4.71	1.42	—	—	—	109	13.9
Twinkie-Hostess	Item	42	143	1.25	25.6	4.2	21	—	—	—	189	—
Eggs												
Hard-large-no shell	Item	50	75	6.25	0.61	5.01	213	1.55	1.91	0.682	63	60
Poached-whole-large	Item	50	75	6.25	0.61	5.01	213	1.55	1.91	0.682	63	60
Substitute-liquid	Cup	251	211	30.1	1.61	8.31	2.51	1.65	2.25	4.02	444	828
White-raw-large	Item	33.4	17	3.52	0.34	0	0	0	0	0	55	48
Whole-raw-large	Item	50	75	6.25	0.61	5.01	213	1.55	1.91	0.682	63	60
Yolk-raw-large	Item	16.6	59	2.78	0.3	5.12	213	1.59	1.95	0.698	7	16
Fast foods												
Arthur Treacher-chick sand	Item	156	413	16.2	44	19.2	—	—	—	6.7	708	279
Burger King-Whop hamburger	Item	261	630	26	50	36	104	16.5	13.8	2.22	990	520
Churchs Chick-white meat	Item	100	327	21	10	23	—	—	—	—	498	186
Dairy Queen-banana split	Item	383	540	10	91	15	30	—	—	—	—	—
Dairy Queen-cone, regular	Item	142	226	5.37	33.2	8.43	38.3	4.87	2.5	0.494	126	233
Dairy Queen-dip cone, reg	Item	156	300	7	40	13	20	—	—	—	—	—
Dairy Queen-float	Item	397	330	6	59	8	20	—	—	—	—	—
Dairy Queen-malt-regular	Item	418	600	15	89	20	50	—	—	—	—	—
Dairy Queen-sundae-regular	Item	177	319	6.31	53.4	9.66	23	5.63	2.61	0.904	204	443

Mag (mg)	Iron (mg)	Zinc (mg)	VA (RE)	VC (mg)	Thia (mg)	Ribo (mg)	Niac (mg)	VB$_6$ (mg)	Fol (µg)	VB$_{12}$ (µg)	Calc (mg)	Phos (mg)	Sel (mg)	Fibd (g)	VE (mg)
—	0.4	—	12	0	0.05	0.06	0.4	—	—	—	47	71	0.003	0.42	0.05
—	1.1	—	87	1	0.11	0.5	0.3	—	—	—	297	310	0.003	1.02	—
9.75	1.2	0.546	11	0	0.156	0.15	1.47	—	—	—	68.9	66.3	—	0.582	—
5.75	0.365	0.128	2.2	0	0.06	0.05	0.428	0.009	2	—	11	55	0.002	0.325	0.18
9.5	0.6	—	5	0	0.1	0.1	0.8	—	11	—	16	33	0.004	1.1	0.36
—	—	—	—	—	—	—	—	—	—	—	—	—	—	0	—
38	0.086	0.72	30.2	0.4	0.052	0.304	0.44	0.108	16	0.42	212	200	—	0	0.078
24	0	—	0	0	0.01	0.26	0	—	—	—	200	200	—	—	—
20	0.44	0.62	82	1.2	0.054	0.322	0.412	0.116	8	0.42	206	186	—	—	—
—	—	—	—	—	—	—	—	—	—	—	—	—	0.016	0	—
—	0.4	—	—	4	0	0	0	0	—	—	0	0	0.002	0	—
—	0.763	—	—	—	0.067	0.026	—	—	—	0	14.4	66.5	—	0.96	—
18	0.12	1.41	133	0.7	0.052	0.329	0.134	0.061	3	0.625	176	134	0.002	0	0.08
25	0.43	1.99	199	0.92	0.08	0.448	0.178	0.095	9	0.996	236	199	0.002	0	0.104
29	0.28	0.86	44	1.17	0.117	0.541	0.184	0.133	5	1.37	274	202	0.003	0	—
34.7	0.611	0.99	46.2	2.48	0.066	0.314	1.12	0.132	9.9	0.677	216	238	—	—	0.693
—	—	—	—	—	—	—	—	—	—	—	—	—	—	0	—
10.8	1.22	0.23	5.1	2	0.149	0.108	1.24	0.035	6.75	0	12.2	31.1	0.015	2.16	2.15
—	1	—	66	1	0.11	0.22	1	—	—	—	86	107	0.015	1.4	—
9.45	0.9	—	118	0	0.16	0.12	1.4	—	—	0	19	34	0.015	1.08	2.15
—	3.05	—	0	0	0.535	0.395	4.95	—	—	—	65.5	136	—	4.23	0.784
—	1.2	—	60	0	0.11	0.27	0.8	—	—	—	125	147	0.015	2.08	2.07
7.2	0.9	0.336	33.4	3.66	0.096	0.12	0.72	0.029	10.8	0.191	15.6	48	0.013	1.44	1.91
24.3	1.9	—	0	1	0.14	0.12	1.4	—	—	—	38	51	0.015	1.96	2.15
9.45	1.2	—	198	4	0.15	0.14	2	—	—	0	14	39	0.015	1.82	2.15
—	3.7	—	40	0	0.26	0.14	1	—	—	—	55	122	0.012	4.13	—
16.9	1	—	320	0	0.11	0.18	1	—	—	—	66	90	0.015	3.51	2.07
—	0.8	—	68	2	0.05	0.39	0.3	—	—	—	265	247	—	0	—
—	1.3	—	68	2	0.08	0.39	0.3	—	—	—	374	237	—	0	—
—	1.1	—	35	0	0.08	0.37	0.5	—	—	—	260	249	—	1.42	—
—	0.7	—	60	2	0.07	0.3	0.2	—	—	—	173	180	—	0.56	—
15	0.31	1.33	39	3.86	0.033	0.089	0.131	0.025	14	0.158	103	74	—	0	—
2.56	0.312	0.054	2.28	0.284	0.028	0.02	0.332	0.011	1.14	0.028	3.98	11.4	—	0.21	0.452
—	0.545	—	8.1	0	0.055	0.06	0.5	—	—	—	19	—	—	—	—
5	0.72	0.55	95.2	0	0.031	0.254	0.037	0.07	23	0.5	25	89	0.012	0	0.35
5	0.72	0.55	95.2	0	0.031	0.254	0.037	0.07	23	0.5	25	89	0.012	0	0.35
21.9	5.27	3.26	542	0	0.276	0.753	0.276	0.008	37.4	0.748	133	304	—	0	—
4	0.01	0	0	0	0.002	0.151	0.031	0.001	1	0.07	2	4	0.005	0	—
5	0.72	0.55	95.2	0	0.031	0.254	0.037	0.07	23	0.5	25	89	0.022	0	0.35
1	0.59	0.52	—	0	0.028	0.106	0.002	0.065	24	0.52	23	81	0.007	0	0.349
27	1.7	—	36.9	19	0.17	0.24	8.1	—	—	—	59	147	—	—	—
50	6	5.25	192	13	0.02	0.03	5.2	0.312	31.2	2.81	104	312	—	—	—
—	1	—	43	1	0.1	0.18	7.2	—	—	—	94	—	—	—	—
—	1.8	—	225	18	0.6	0.6	0.8	—	—	0.9	350	250	—	—	—
21.3	0.213	0.781	87.4	1.56	0.071	0.355	0.426	0.085	7.1	0.284	212	192	—	—	—
—	0.4	—	90.1	0	0.09	0.34	0	—	—	0.6	200	150	—	—	—
—	0	—	30	0	0.12	0.17	0	—	—	0.6	200	200	—	—	—
—	3.6	—	225	3.6	0.12	0.6	0.8	—	—	1.8	500	400	—	—	—
37.2	0.655	1.06	74.5	2.66	0.071	0.336	1.2	0.142	10.6	0.726	232	255	—	—	—

Continued.

Key to Abbreviations

Kcal, Kcalories; *Prot,* protein; *Carb,* carbohydrate; *Fat,* fat; *Chol,* cholesterol; *Safa,* saturated fat; *Mufa,* monounsaturated fat; *Pufa,* polyunsaturated fat; *Sod,* sodium; *Pot,* potassium; *Mag,* magnesium; *Iron,* iron; *Zinc,* zinc; *VA,* vitamin A; *VC,* vitamin C; *Thia,* thiamin; *Ribo,* riboflavin; *Niac,* niacin; *VB*$_6$, vitamin B$_6$; *Fol,* folate; *VB*$_{12}$, vitamin B$_{12}$; *Calc,* calcium; *Phos,* phosphorus; *Sel,* selenium; *Fibd,* dietary fiber; and *VE,* vitamin E.

Food name	Portion	Wt (g)	Kcal	Prot (g)	Carb (g)	Fat (g)	Chol (mg)	Safa (g)	Mufa (g)	Pufa (g)	Sod (mg)	Pot (mg)
Fast foods—cont'd												
Jack/Box-Break Jack sand	Item	121	301	18	28	13	182	—	—	—	1037	190
Jack/Box-Jumbo Jack hamburger	Item	246	551	28	45	29	80	11.4	12.6	2.42	1134	492
Jack/Box-Jumbo Jack/cheese	Item	272	628	32	45	35	110	15	12.6	2.03	1666	499
Jack/Box-Moby Jack	Item	141	455	17	38	26	56	—	—	—	837	246
Jack/Box-Onion rings-bag	Item	83	275	3.7	31.3	15.5	14	6.95	6.65	0.665	430	129
McDonald-Big Mac hamburger	Item	215	560	25.2	42.5	32.4	103	10.1	20.1	1.5	950	237
McDonald-QP hamburger w/ch	Item	194	520	28.5	35.1	29.2	118	11.2	16.5	1.51	1150	341
McDonalds-cheeseburger	Item	116	310	15	31.2	13.8	53	5.17	7.66	0.93	750	223
McDonalds-Egg McMuffin	Item	138	290	18.2	28.1	11.2	226	3.82	6.1	1.29	740	213
McDonalds-Filet O Fish	Item	142	440	13.8	37.9	26.1	50	5.16	10.2	10.8	1030	150
McDonalds-hamburger	Item	102	260	12.3	30.6	9.5	37	3.63	5.09	0.77	500	215
McDonalds-QP hamburger	Item	166	410	23.1	34	20.7	86	8.09	11.4	1.21	660	322
Taco Bell-Bean Burrito	Item	168	332	16.7	42.6	11.5	79	5.6	4.23	0.633	1030	405
Taco Bell-Beef Burrito	Item	110	262	13.3	29.3	10.4	32.5	5.23	3.7	0.427	746	370
Taco Bell-Beefy Tostada	Item	225	334	16.1	29.7	16.9	75	11.5	3.51	0.538	870	490
Taco Bell-Burrito Supreme	Item	225	457	21	43	22	126	7.7	7.35	1.65	367	350
Taco Bell-Taco-regular	Item	171	370	20.7	26.7	20.6	57	11.4	6.58	0.959	802	473
Taco Bell-Tostada-regular	Item	144	223	9.6	26.5	9.86	30	5.37	3.05	0.749	543	403
Wendys-Double hamburger	Item	226	540	34.3	40.3	26.6	122	10.5	10.3	2.8	791	569
Wendys-Single hamburger	Item	218	511	25.7	40.1	27.4	86	10.4	11.4	2.2	825	479
Wendys-Triple hamburger	Item	259	693	50	28.6	41.5	142	15.9	18.2	2.74	713	785
Fats and oils												
Animal fat-cooking-chicken	Tbsp	12.8	115	0	0	12.8	11	3.8	5.7	2.7	—	—
Butter-regular	Tbsp	14	100	0.119	0.008	11.4	30.7	7.07	3.28	0.421	116	3.64
Butter-whipped	Tbsp	9	64.5	0.077	0.005	7.3	19.7	4.54	2.11	0.271	74.3	2.34
Margarine-corn-reg-hard	Tsp	4.7	33.8	0	0	3.8	0	0.6	2.2	0.8	44.3	1.99
Margarine-corn-reg-soft	Tsp	4.7	33.7	0	0	3.8	0	0.7	1.5	1.5	50.7	1.77
Margarine-diet-mazola	Tbsp	14	50	0	0	5.7	0	1	2.1	2.6	130	—
Margarine-reg-hard-stick	Item	113	815	1	1	91.3	0	17.9	40.6	28.8	1070	48.1
Margarine-veg spray-Mazola	Serving	0.72	6	0	0	0.72	0	0.08	0.17	0.4	0	—
Mayonnaise-imitation-soy	Tbsp	15	34.7	0	2.4	2.9	4	0.5	0.7	1.6	74.6	—
Mayonnaise-light-low cal	Tbsp	14	40	0	1	4	5	—	—	—	—	—
Miracle Whip-light-low cal	Tbsp	14	45	0	2	4	5	—	—	—	95	—
Dressings												
Blue Cheese low cal	Tbsp	16	10	0	1	1	4	0.5	0.3	0	177	5
Blue Cheese	Tbsp	15.3	77.1	0.7	1.1	8	9	1.5	1.9	4.3	167	6.12
Caesar	Tbsp	15	70	0	1	7	—	—	—	—	—	—
French	Tbsp	15.6	67	0.1	2.7	6.4	1.95	1.5	1.2	3.4	214	12.3
French-low cal	Tbsp	16.3	21.9	0	3.5	0.9	1	0.1	0.2	0.5	128	13
Italian	Tbsp	14.7	68.7	0	1.5	7.1	0	1	1.7	4.1	116	2
Italian-low cal	Tbsp	15	15.8	0	0.7	1.5	1	0.2	0.3	0.9	118	2
Mayo-low cal	Tbsp	16	20	0	2	2	2	0.4	0.4	1	44	1
Mayonnaise type	Tbsp	14.7	57.3	0	3.5	4.9	4	0.7	1.3	2.6	104	1
Ranch style	Tbsp	15	54	0.4	0.6	5.7	—	—	—	—	97	—
Russian	Tbsp	15.3	76	0.2	1.6	7.8	0	1.1	1.8	4.5	133	24
Russian-low cal	Tbsp	16.3	23.1	0.1	4.5	0.7	1	0.1	0.2	0.4	141	26
Thou Isl-low cal	Tbsp	15.3	24.3	0.1	2.5	1.6	2	0.2	0.4	1	153	17
Thousand Island	Tbsp	15.6	58.9	0	2.4	5.6	4.9	0.9	1.3	3.1	109	18
Vinegar/oil-home	Tbsp	15.6	71.8	0	0.4	8	0	1.5	2.4	3.9	0.1	1.2
Others												
Sandwich spread-commercial	Tbsp	15.3	59.5	0.1	3.4	5.2	12	0.8	1.1	3.1	—	—
Shortening-vegetable-soy	Cup	205	1812	0	0	205	0	51.2	89	52.2	—	—
Vegetable oil-corn	Cup	218	1927	0	0	218	0	27.7	52.7	128	0	0
Vegetable oil-olive	Cup	216	1909	0	0	216	0	30.7	159	18.2	0.08	0

Mag (mg)	Iron (mg)	Zinc (mg)	VA (RE)	VC (mg)	Thia (mg)	Ribo (mg)	Niac (mg)	VB$_6$ (mg)	Fol (µg)	VB$_{12}$ (µg)	Calc (mg)	Phos (mg)	Sel (mg)	Fibd (g)	VE (mg)
24	2.5	1.8	133	3	0.41	0.47	5.1	0.14	—	1.1	177	310	—	—	—
44	4.5	4.2	73.9	3.7	0.47	0.34	11.6	0.3	—	2.68	134	261	—	—	—
49	4.6	4.8	220	4.9	0.52	0.38	11.3	0.31	—	3.05	273	411	—	—	—
30	1.7	1.1	72.1	1	0.3	0.21	4.5	0.12	—	1.1	167	263	—	—	—
15	0.85	0.35	2.4	0.6	0.09	0.1	0.92	0.06	11	0.12	73	86	—	—	0.587
38	4	4.7	106	1.68	0.48	0.41	6.81	0.27	21	1.8	256	314	—	—	—
41	3.72	5.7	211	3.24	0.37	0.39	6.73	0.23	23	2.15	295	382	—	—	—
21	2.3	2.09	118	2.15	0.29	0.21	3.86	0.12	18	0.94	199	177	—	—	0.53
33	2.77	1.8	150	1.38	0.47	0.33	3.71	0.16	44	0.8	256	319	—	—	—
27	1.83	0.9	43.8	0.06	0.3	0.15	2.68	0.1	20	0.82	165	229	—	1.11	—
23	2.29	2.05	45.6	2.15	0.28	0.16	3.84	0.12	17	0.84	122	110	—	—	0.428
37	3.68	5.1	67	3.24	0.36	0.29	6.7	0.27	23	1.88	142	249	—	—	—
0.407	3.84	3.04	240	3.3	0.275	0.6	3.86	0.205	73	0.995	144	143	—	—	—
40.5	3.05	2.37	41.7	0.55	0.115	0.46	3.23	0.16	19.5	0.985	42	87.5	—	—	—
68	2.45	3.18	383	3.9	0.09	0.5	2.85	0.26	0.26	1.13	190	173	—	—	—
51.8	3.8	5.85	216	8	0.45	0.923	6.17	0.27	42.8	1.53	146	245	—	—	—
71	2.42	3.93	257	2.2	0.15	0.45	3.22	0.24	23	1.04	221	203	—	—	—
59	1.88	1.9	187	1.3	0.1	0.33	1.33	0.17	75	0.68	211	116	—	—	—
49	5.95	5.68	30.6	1.2	0.36	0.39	7.57	0.54	27	4.07	102	314	—	—	—
43	4.92	4.87	93.4	2.5	0.42	0.38	7.28	0.33	36	2.38	96	233	—	—	—
55	8.33	10.8	47.4	1.4	0.31	0.56	11	0.62	31	4.92	65	393	—	—	—
—	—	—	—	—	—	—	—	—	—	—	—	—	—	0	—
0.28	0.022	0.007	105	0	0.001	0.005	0.006	0	0.42	—	3.36	3.22	0	0	0.221
0.18	0.014	0.005	67.9	0	0	0.003	0.004	0	0.27	—	2.16	2.07	0	0	0.142
0.12	—	—	47	0.008	0	0.002	0.001	0	0.06	0.004	1.41	1.08	0	0	0.606
0.11	—	—	47	0.007	0	0.002	0.001	0	0.05	0.004	1.25	0.95	0	0	0.5
—	0	—	130	0	0	0	0	—	—	—	0	—	0	0	0.112
2.95	0.07	—	338	0.181	0.011	0.042	0.026	0.01	1.34	0.108	33.9	26	0.002	0	13.2
—	0	—	0	0	0	0	0	—	—	—	0	0	—	0	—
—	—	0.02	—	—	—	—	—	—	—	—	—	—	—	0	3.11
—	—	—	—	—	—	—	—	—	—	—	—	—	—	0	2.9
—	—	—	—	—	—	—	—	—	—	—	—	—	—	0	—
—	0	—	9	0	0	0.001	0	—	—	—	10	8	—	0	—
—	0	—	9.5	0.3	0	0.02	0	—	—	—	12.4	11.3	—	0.05	—
—	—	—	—	—	—	—	—	—	—	—	—	—	—	0.04	—
—	0.1	0.01	—	—	—	—	—	—	—	—	1.7	2.2	—	0.1	—
—	0.1	0.03	—	—	—	—	—	—	—	—	2	2	—	0.09	—
—	0	0.02	—	—	0	0	0	—	—	—	1	1	—	0.05	—
—	0	—	—	—	0	0	0	—	—	—	0	1	—	0.09	—
—	0	—	12	—	0	0	0	—	—	—	3	4	—	0	—
0.29	0	—	9.6	—	0	0	0	—	—	—	2	4	—	0	—
—	—	—	—	—	—	—	—	—	—	—	—	—	—	0	—
—	0.1	0.07	31.8	1	0.01	0.01	0.1	—	—	—	3	6	—	0	—
—	0.1	—	—	—	—	—	—	—	—	—	3	6	—	0.2	—
—	0.1	—	14.8	0	0	0	0	—	—	—	2	3	—	0.3	—
—	0.1	0.02	15	0	0	0	0	—	—	—	2	3	—	0.6	—
—	—	—	—	—	—	—	—	—	—	—	—	—	—	0	—
—	—	—	—	—	—	—	—	—	—	—	—	—	—	0.02	—
—	—	—	—	—	—	—	—	—	—	—	—	—	—	0	27.9
0	0	0	—	0	0	0	0	0	0	0	0	0	—	0	31.1
0.02	0.83	0.13	—	0	0	0	0	0	0	0	0.38	2.63	—	0	25.7

Continued.

Food name	Portion	Wt (g)	Kcal	Prot (g)	Carb (g)	Fat (g)	Chol (mg)	Safa (g)	Mufa (g)	Pufa (g)	Sod (mg)	Pot (mg)
Fish
Anchovy-fillet-can	Item	4	8.4	1.16	0	0.388	3.4	0.088	0.151	0.102	147	21.8
Bluefish-baked/butter	Item	155	246	40.6	0	8.1	108	1.83	1.84	3.94	161	—
Carp-cooked-dry heat	Serving	85	138	19.4	0	6.1	72	1.18	2.54	1.56	54	363
Catfish-fried-breaded	Serving	85	194	15.4	6.83	11.3	69	2.8	4.77	2.83	238	289
Clam-can-solid/liquid	oz	28.4	12.8	2.33	0.667	0.333	17.7	0.067	0	0	14.7	39.7
Clams-breaded-fried	Serving	85	171	12.1	8.78	9.48	52	2.28	3.86	2.44	309	277
Clams-ckd-moist heat	Serving	85	126	21.7	4.36	1.65	57	0.16	0.146	0.469	95	534
Clams-raw-meat only	Serving	85	63	10.9	2.18	0.83	29	0.08	0.068	0.24	47	267
Cod-ckd-dry heat	Piece	180	189	41.1	0	1.55	99	0.302	0.223	0.526	141	440
Crab cake	Item	60	93	12.1	0.29	4.51	90	0.89	1.69	1.36	198	195
Crab meat-king-can	Cup	135	135	24	1	3.2	135	0.6	0.6	2	675	149
Crab-imitation-surimi	Serving	85	87	10.2	8.69	1.11	17	—	—	—	715	77
Crab-steamed-pieces	Cup	155	150	30	0	2.39	82.2	0.206	0.287	0.831	1662	406
Crayfish-ckd-moist	Serving	85	97	20.3	0	1.15	151	0.197	0.32	0.281	58	298
Flatfish-ckd-dry heat	Serving	85	99	20.5	0	1.3	58	0.309	0.263	0.35	89	292
Grouper-ckd-dry heat	Serving	85	100	21.1	0	1.11	40	0.254	0.228	0.343	45	403
Haddock-cook-dry heat	Serving	85	95	20.6	0	0.79	63	0.142	0.128	0.263	74	339
Halibut-broiled-dry	Serving	85	119	22.7	0	2.49	35	0.354	0.822	0.799	59	490
Lobster-ckd-moist	oz	28.4	27.8	5.82	0.364	0.168	20.4	0.03	0.045	0.026	108	100
Mackeral-Atlantic-can	Cup	190	296	44	0	12	150	3.39	5.16	0.165	720	369
Mackerel-ckd-dry heat	Serving	85	223	20.3	0	15.1	64	3.55	5.96	3.66	71	341
Mussel-blue-ckd-moist	Serving	85	147	20.2	6.28	3.81	48	0.723	0.862	1.03	313	228
Ocean perch-ckd-dry	Serving	85	103	20.3	0	1.78	46	0.266	0.681	0.465	82	298
Oyster-east-ckd-moist	Serving	85	117	12	6.65	4.21	93	1.07	0.425	1.26	190	389
Oyster-eastern-can	Cup	248	170	17.5	9.7	6.14	136	1.57	0.62	1.83	277	568
Oysters-Pacific-raw	Seving	85	69	8.03	4.21	1.96	—	0.434	0.304	0.76	90	143
Oysters-raw-meat only	Cup	248	171	17.5	9.7	6.14	136	1.57	0.62	1.83	277	568
Perch-breaded-fried	Piece	85	915	16	6	11	32	2.7	4.4	2.3	128	242
Perch-ckd-dry heat	Serving	85	99	21.1	0	1	98	0.201	0.166	0.401	67	293
Pollock-Atlantic-raw	Serving	85	78	16.5	0	0.83	60	0.115	0.095	0.411	73	302
Pollock-ckd-dry heat	Serving	85	96	20	0	0.95	82	0.196	0.148	0.445	98	329
Pompano-ckd-dry heat	Serving	85	179	20.1	0	10.3	54	3.82	2.82	1.24	65	541
Red snapper-ckd-dry	Serving	85	109	22.4	0	1.46	40	0.31	0.274	0.5	48	444
Rockfish-ckd-dry heat	Serving	100	121	24	0	2.01	44	0.474	0.447	0.594	77	520
Roe-raw-eggs	oz	28.4	39	6.25	0.42	1.8	105	0.408	0.465	0.744	—	—
Salmon-ckd-moist heat	Serving	85	157	23.3	0	6.4	42	1.19	2.22	1.87	50	454
Salmon-pink-can	Serving	85	118	16.8	0	5.14	—	1.31	1.54	1.74	471	277
Salmon-smoked	Serving	100	117	18.3	0	4.32	23	0.929	2.02	0.995	784	175
Sardine-can/oil	Item	12	25	2.96	0	1.38	17	0.184	0.465	0.618	60.5	47.5
Scallops-steamed	oz	28.4	31.8	6.59	0.511	0.398	15.1	—	—	—	75.2	135
Sea bass-ckd-dry heat	Serving	85	105	20.1	0	2.18	45	0.557	0.462	0.81	74	279
Shad-bake/marg/bacon	Serving	100	201	23.2	0	11.3	69.4	2.45	2.23	5.9	79	377
Shrimp-ckd-moist heat	Serving	85	84	17.8	0	0.92	166	0.246	0.167	0.374	190	154
Shrimp-French fried	Serving	85	206	18.2	9.75	10.4	150	1.77	3.19	3.83	292	191
Shrimp-meat-can	Cup	128	154	29.6	1.32	2.51	222	0.477	0.375	0.966	216	269
Smelt-ckd-dry heat	Serving	85	106	19.2	0	2.64	76	0.492	0.699	0.965	65	316
Sole/flounder-baked	Serving	127	148	30.7	0	1.94	86	0.461	0.392	0.523	133	436
Squid-ckd-fried	Serving	85	149	15.3	6.62	6.36	221	1.6	2.34	1.82	260	237
Stick-bread-froz-ckd	oz	28.4	76	4.38	6.65	3.42	31	0.882	1.42	0.886	163	73
Surimi	Serving	85	84	12.9	5.82	0.77	25.5	—	—	—	122	95
Swordfish-broil/marg	Serving	100	174	28	0	6	4	—	—	—	—	—
Swordfish-ckd-dry	Serving	85	132	21.6	0	4.37	43	1.2	1.68	1.01	98	314
Trout-brook-ckd	Serving	100	196	23.5	0.4	11.2	—	—	—	—	78.8	—
Trout-rainbow-ckd-dry	Serving	85	129	22.4	0	3.66	62	0.707	1.13	1.31	29	539
Tuna-can/oil-drained	Serving	85	169	24.8	0	6.98	15.3	1.3	2.51	2.45	301	176
Tuna-diet-low sodium	oz	28.4	35.5	7.67	0.011	0.54	9.94	0.09	0.163	0.199	11.4	73.8
Tuna-light-can/water	Serving	85	111	25.1	0	0.43	—	0.136	0.122	0.111	303	267

Mag (mg)	Iron (mg)	Zinc (mg)	VA (RE)	VC (mg)	Thia (mg)	Ribo (mg)	Niac (mg)	VB$_6$ (mg)	Fol (µg)	VB$_{12}$ (µg)	Calc (mg)	Phos (mg)	Sel (mg)	Fibd (g)	VE (mg)
2.8	0.186	0.098	—	—	0.003	0.015	0.796	0.008	—	0.035	9.2	10	0.002	0	0.012
43.3	1.1	—	24	—	0.17	0.16	2.9	—	—	1.64	44.6	445	0.047	0	—
32	1.35	1.62	8.11	1.4	—	—	—	0.186	—	1.25	44	451	0.026	0	—
23	1.22	0.73	7.21	0	0.062	0.113	1.94	—	—	—	37	183	—	0.8	—
—	1.17	0.347	—	—	0.003	0.03	0.3	—	—	5.4	15.7	38.7	0.046	0	0.629
12	11.8	1.24	77.2	—	—	0.207	1.75	—	—	34.2	54	160	—	0.32	—
16	23.8	2.32	145	—	—	0.362	2.85	—	—	84.1	78	287	—	0	—
8	11.9	1.16	76.6	—	—	0.181	1.5	—	—	42	39	144	0.016	0	0.209
76	0.88	1.04	24.9	1.8	0.158	0.142	4.52	0.509	—	1.89	25	248	0.081	0	—
20	0.65	2.46	—	—	—	—	—	—	—	3.56	63	128	0.013	0.03	—
29	1.1	5.83	—	—	0.11	0.11	2.6	—	—	13.5	61	246	0.03	0	1.65
—	0.33	—	—	—	0.027	0.023	0.153	—	—	—	11	—	0.019	0	—
52.7	1.18	11.8	13.5	—	0.082	0.085	2.08	—	—	—	91.5	434	0.034	0	—
27	2.67	1.42	—	2.8	—	0.065	2.5	—	—	2.94	26	280	—	0	—
50	0.28	0.53	9.61	—	0.068	0.097	1.85	0.204	—	2.13	16	246	—	0	—
32	0.96	0.43	—	—	0.069	0.005	0.324	—	—	0.558	18	121	—	0	—
43	1.14	0.41	16.2	—	0.034	0.038	3.94	0.294	—	1.18	36	205	0.025	0	0.51
91	0.91	0.45	45.6	—	0.059	0.077	6.06	0.337	—	1.16	51	242	0.051	0	—
9.94	0.111	0.829	7.42	—	0.002	0.019	0.304	0.022	3.15	0.883	17.3	52.5	0.023	0	—
70	3.88	1.94	248	1.7	0.076	0.403	11.7	0.399	10.2	13.2	458	572	0.089	0	—
82.5	1.33	0.8	45.9	0.3	0.135	0.35	5.82	0.391	—	16.2	13	236	0.03	0	—
32	5.71	2.27	—	—	—	—	—	—	—	—	28	242	—	0	—
33	1	0.52	11.7	—	—	0.114	2.07	—	—	0.981	117	235	0.03	0	—
92.7	11.4	155	—	—	—	0.282	2.12	0.081	15.2	32.5	76	236	0.051	0	—
135	16.6	226	—	—	—	0.412	3.09	0.236	22.1	47.5	111	344	0.149	0	—
19	4.34	14.1	—	—	0.057	0.198	1.71	—	—	—	7	138	0.056	0	0.723
135	16.6	226	222	—	0.34	0.412	3.25	0.124	24.6	47.5	111	344	0.141	0	2.04
—	1.1	—	—	—	0.1	0.1	1.6	—	—	0.85	28	192	0.02	0.05	1.06
33	0.98	1.21	—	—	—	—	—	—	—	—	87	218	0.03	0	—
57	0.39	0.4	9.01	—	0.04	0.157	2.78	0.244	—	2.71	51	188	—	0	—
—	0.24	0.51	19.5	—	0.063	0.065	1.4	0.059	3	3.57	5	—	—	0	—
27	0.57	0.59	—	—	—	—	—	—	—	—	36	290	—	0	—
31	0.2	0.37	—	—	0.045	0.003	0.294	—	—	—	34	171	—	0	—
34	0.53	0.53	65.8	0.87	0.044	0.084	3.92	—	—	—	12	228	0.039	0	—
—	0.17	—	—	3.98	0.028	0.216	0.398	—	—	—	4.25	98.1	0.014	0	—
—	0.76	0.44	—	0.9	—	—	—	—	—	—	—	—	0.026	0	—
29	0.72	0.78	14.1	0	0.02	0.158	5.56	0.255	13.1	5.85	—	279	0.045	0	1.15
18	0.85	0.31	26.4	—	0.023	0.101	4.72	0.278	1.9	3.26	11	164	0.061	0	—
4.5	0.35	0.155	8.11	—	0.01	0.027	0.63	0.02	1.4	1.07	45.8	58.8	0.006	0	—
—	0.852	—	—	—	—	—	—	—	—	—	32.7	96	0.015	0	—
45	0.32	0.44	54.4	—	—	—	—	—	—	—	11	211	—	0	—
—	0.6	—	9.01	—	0.13	0.26	8.6	—	—	—	24	313	—	0	2
29	2.62	1.33	—	—	0.026	0.027	2.2	0.108	2.9	1.27	33	116	0.054	0	—
34	1.07	1.17	—	—	0.11	0.116	2.61	0.083	6.9	1.59	57	185	0.027	0.48	0.807
53	3.5	1.61	22.6	—	0.035	0.047	3.53	0.142	2.3	1.44	75	299	0.041	0	3.64
33	0.98	1.8	—	—	—	0.124	1.5	—	—	3.37	65	251	0.105	0	—
74	0.43	0.8	14.4	—	0.102	0.145	2.77	0.305	—	3.19	23	368	0.16	0	—
33	0.86	1.48	—	3.5	0.048	0.389	2.21	0.049	—	1.04	33	213	—	0.3	—
7	0.21	0.19	9.01	—	0.036	0.05	0.596	0.017	5.1	0.503	6	51	0.003	0.665	—
—	0.22	—	—	—	0.017	0.018	0.187	—	—	—	7	—	—	0	—
—	1.3	—	616	—	0.04	0.05	10.9	—	—	—	—	275	0.047	0	—
29	0.88	1.25	35.1	0.9	0.037	0.099	10	0.324	—	1.72	5	287	—	0	—
35	1.1	—	95.8	1	0.12	0.06	2.5	—	—	—	218	272	—	0	—
33	2.07	1.18	18.9	3.1	0.072	0.191	—	—	—	—	73	272	—	0	—
26	1.18	0.77	19.8	—	0.032	—	—	0.094	4.5	—	11	265	0.061	0	1.42
9.09	0.341	0.142	6.91	—	0.009	0.014	3.52	0.105	0	0.398	1.42	62.5	0.033	0	—
25	2.72	0.37	—	—	—	—	—	0.321	4	—	10	158	0.061	0	—

Continued.

Key to Abbreviations

Kcal, Kcalories; *Prot*, protein; *Carb*, carbohydrate; *Fat*, fat; *Chol*, cholesterol; *Safa*, saturated fat; *Mufa*, monounsaturated fat; *Pufa*, polyunsaturated fat; *Sod*, sodium; *Pot*, potassium; *Mag*, magnesium; *Iron*, iron; *Zinc*, zinc; *VA*, vitamin A; *VC*, vitamin C; *Thia*, thiamin; *Ribo*, riboflavin; *Niac*, niacin; *VB₆*, vitamin B₆; *Fol*, folate; *VB₁₂*, vitamin B₁₂; *Calc*, calcium; *Phos*, phosphorus; *Sel*, selenium; *Fibd*, dietary fiber; and *VE*, vitamin E.

Food name	Portion	Wt (g)	Kcal	Prot (g)	Carb (g)	Fat (g)	Chol (mg)	Safa (g)	Mufa (g)	Pufa (g)	Sod (mg)	Pot (mg)
Fish—cont'd												
Tuna-white-can/water	Serving	85	116	22.7	0	2.09	35	0.556	0.551	0.78	333	241
Tuna-yellowfin-raw	Serving	85	92	19.9	0	0.81	38	0.2	0.131	0.241	31	—
White perch-fried filet	Item	65	108	12.5	0	5.3	—	—	—	—	—	—
Whitefish-bake/stuff	Serving	100	215	15.2	5.8	14	—	—	—	—	195	291
Whiting-ckd-dry heat	Serving	85	98	20	0	1.43	71	0.269	0.309	0.456	113	369
Frozen dinners												
Beef dinner-Swanson	Item	326	320	25	34	9	—	—	—	—	1085	—
Beef sirloin tips-Le Menu	Item	326	400	29	27	19	—	—	—	—	1100	—
Beef/green peppers-Stouffer	Item	220	225	10	18	11	—	—	—	—	960	420
Cabbage roll/tom sauc-Horm	oz	28.4	23	1.1	3.2	0.7	3	0.281	0.226	0.043	127	87
Chicken cacciatore-Stouffer	Item	319	310	25	29	11	—	—	—	—	1135	300
Chicken dinner-Swanson	Item	326	660	26	64	33	—	—	—	—	1610	—
Chicken Kiev-Le Menu	Item	234	500	21	35	30	—	—	—	—	745	—
Chicken parmigiana-Le Menu	Item	333	390	26	28	19	—	—	—	—	900	—
Egg roll-beef/shrimp-froz	Item	12	27	0.9	3.5	1	—	—	—	—	80.5	—
Fettucini Alfredo-Stouffer	Item	142	270	8	19	18	—	—	—	—	1195	240
Fish & chips-Van De Kamps	Item	224	500	16	45	30	—	—	—	—	551	—
Fish Divan-Lean Cuisine	Item	351	270	31	16	10	85	—	—	—	780	850
Ham-froz din-Banquet	Item	284	369	16.8	47.7	12.2	—	—	—	—	1590	125
Lasagna-Stouf	Item	298	385	28	36	14	—	—	—	—	1200	580
Manicotti-cheese-Le Menu	Item	241	310	18	29	13	—	—	—	—	840	—
Meatballs/noodles-Stouffer	Item	312	475	25	33	27	—	—	—	—	1620	395
Meatloaf-froz din-Banquet	Item	312	412	20.9	29	23.7	—	—	—	—	1991	468
Mexican dinner-Swanson	Item	454	590	20	64	29	—	—	—	—	1865	—
Salisbury steak din-Banq	Item	312	390	18.1	24	24.6	—	—	—	—	2059	387
Sole-light-Van De Kamp's	Item	142	293	16	17	18	—	—	—	—	412	—
Turkey dinner-Swanson	Item	326	340	20	42	10	—	—	—	—	1295	—
Turkey pie-Stouffer	Item	284	460	20	35	26	—	—	—	—	1735	270
Veal parmigiana-froz din	Item	213	296	24	17	14	—	—	—	—	973	466
Vegetable lasagna-Le Menu	Item	312	400	15	30	24	—	—	—	—	1135	—
Fruits												
Apple juice-can/bottled	Cup	248	116	0.15	29	0.28	0	0.047	0.012	0.082	7	296
Apple juice-froz-diluted	Cup	239	111	0.34	27.6	0.25	0	0.043	0.005	0.074	17	301
Apples-raw-peeled-boiled	Cup	171	91	0.45	23.3	0.61	0	0.099	0.024	0.178	1	150
Apples-raw-unpeeled	Item	138	81	0.27	21.1	0.49	0	0.08	0.021	0.145	1	159
Applesauce-can-sweet	Cup	255	194	0.47	50.8	0.47	0	0.077	0.018	0.138	8	156
Applesauce-can-unsweet	Cup	244	106	0.4	27.6	0.12	0	0.02	0.005	0.034	5	183
Apricot-raw-without pit	Item	35.3	16.9	0.494	3.93	0.138	0	0.01	0.06	0.027	0.353	104
Apricots-can/juice	Cup	248	119	1.56	30.6	0.09	0	0.007	0.042	0.017	9	409
Apricots-dried-ckd-unsweet	Cup	250	211	3.24	54.8	0.41	0	0.028	0.178	0.08	9	1222
Apricots-dried-unckd	Cup	130	310	4.75	80.3	0.6	0	0.042	0.26	0.117	13	1791
Bananas-raw-peeled	Item	114	105	1.18	26.7	0.55	0	0.211	0.047	0.101	1	451
Blackberries-froz-unsweet	Cup	151	97	1.78	23.7	0.65	0	—	—	—	2	211
Blackberries-raw	Cup	144	74	1.04	18.4	0.56	0	0.07	0.17	0.299	0	282
Blueberries-froz-unsweet	Cup	155	78	0.65	18.9	0.99	0	—	—	—	1	83
Blueberries-raw	Cup	145	82	0.97	20.5	0.55	0	0.07	0.16	0.292	9	129
Boysenberries-froz-unsweet	Cup	132	66	1.46	16.1	0.35	0	—	—	—	2	183
Cherries-sweet-raw	Item	6.8	4.9	0.082	1.13	0.065	0	0.015	0.018	0.02	0	15.2
Cranapple juice-can	Cup	253	170	0.253	43.2	0	0	0	0	0	5.06	68.3
Cranberry sauce-can-sweet	Cup	277	419	0.55	108	0.42	0	0.06	0.14	0.22	80	71
Dates-natural-dried-chop	Cup	178	489	3.5	131	0.8	0	0.05	0.31	0.42	5	1161
Figs-dried-unckd	Cup	199	508	6.06	130	2.32	0	0.466	0.513	1.11	22	1418
Fruit cocktail-can/juice	Cup	248	113	1.13	29.4	0.03	0	0.005	0.007	0.015	9	235
Fruit punch drink-can	Fl oz	31	14	0	3.7	0	0	0	0	0	7	8

Mag (mg)	Iron (mg)	Zinc (mg)	VA (RE)	VC (mg)	Thia (mg)	Ribo (mg)	Niac (mg)	VB$_6$ (mg)	Fol (µg)	VB$_{12}$ (µg)	Calc (mg)	Phos (mg)	Sel (mg)	Fibd (g)	VE (mg)
—	0.51	—	—	—	0.003	0.039	4.93	—	3.5	—	—	—	0.061	0	—
—	0.62	0.45	15	—	0.369	0.04	8.33	—	—	—	14	163	0.085	0	—
—	0.7	—	0	0	0.04	0.05	2.7	—	—	—	9	113	0.016	0	0.813
—	0.5	—	601	0	0.11	0.11	2.3	—	—	—	—	246	—	0.58	—
23	0.36	0.45	29.1	—	0.058	0.051	1.42	0.153	12.8	2.21	53	242	—	0	—
—	—	—	—	—	—	—	—	—	—	—	—	—	—	—	—
—	—	—	—	—	—	—	—	—	—	—	—	—	—	—	—
—	2.33	—	136	0	0.078	0.155	3.88	—	—	—	0	—	—	—	—
4	0.25	0.19	—	0.18	0.76	0.02	0.29	0.03	2.9	0.1	5.9	15.7	—	—	—
—	—	—	—	—	—	—	—	—	—	—	—	—	—	—	—
—	—	—	—	—	—	—	—	—	—	—	—	—	—	—	—
—	—	—	—	—	—	—	—	—	—	—	—	—	—	0.12	—
—	—	—	—	—	—	—	—	—	—	—	—	—	—	—	—
—	—	—	—	—	—	—	—	—	—	—	—	—	—	—	—
—	2.5	—	1311	57	0.57	0.23	3.4	—	—	—	151	278	—	—	—
—	3.15	—	248	0	0.21	0.42	4.2	—	—	—	410	—	—	—	—
—	—	—	—	—	—	—	—	—	—	—	—	—	—	—	—
—	4.3	—	427	8	0.16	0.22	4.2	—	—	—	84	243	—	—	—
—	—	—	—	—	—	—	—	—	—	—	—	—	—	—	—
—	3.5	—	791	7	0.16	0.19	3.6	—	—	—	90	206	—	—	—
—	—	—	—	—	—	—	—	—	—	—	—	—	—	—	—
—	—	—	—	—	—	—	—	—	—	—	—	—	—	—	—
—	—	—	—	—	—	—	—	—	—	—	—	—	—	—	—
—	2.3	—	123	6.4	0.3	0.38	6.8	—	—	—	97	—	—	—	—
—	—	—	—	—	—	—	—	—	—	—	—	—	—	—	—
8	0.92	0.07	0.2	2.3	0.052	0.042	0.248	0.074	0.2	0	16	18	0.002	0.52	0.025
12	0.61	0.09	—	1.4	0.007	0.036	0.091	0.079	0.7	0	14	16	0.002	0	0.024
5	0.32	0.07	7.5	0.3	0.027	0.021	0.162	0.075	1	0	8	13	0.001	4.1	0.086
6	0.25	0.05	7.4	7.8	0.023	0.019	0.106	0.066	3.9	0	10	10	0.001	3.04	0.814
7	0.89	0.1	2.8	4.4	0.033	0.071	0.479	0.066	1.5	0	9	17	0.001	3.06	0.23
7	0.29	0.06	7	2.9	0.032	0.061	0.459	0.063	1.4	0	7	18	0.001	3.66	0.22
2.82	0.191	0.092	92.2	3.53	0.011	0.014	0.212	0.019	3.04	0	4.94	6.71	0	0.67	0.314
24	0.74	0.27	420	12.2	0.045	0.047	0.853	—	—	0	30	50	0.001	2.81	2.21
42	4.17	0.66	591	3.9	0.015	0.075	2.36	0.285	0	—	40	104	—	19.5	—
61	6.11	0.97	941	3.1	0.01	0.196	3.9	0.203	13.4	0	59	152	—	10.1	—
33	0.35	0.19	9.2	10.3	0.051	0.114	0.616	0.659	21.8	0	7	22	0.001	1.82	0.308
33	1.21	0.37	17.2	4.7	0.044	0.069	1.82	0.092	51.3	0	44	46	0.001	7.55	—
29	0.83	0.39	23.7	30.2	0.043	0.058	0.576	0.084	18	0	46	30	0.001	8.93	5.04
8	0.28	0.11	12.6	3.8	0.05	0.057	0.806	0.091	10.4	0	12	18	0.001	4.94	—
7	0.24	0.16	14.5	18.9	0.07	0.073	0.521	0.052	9.3	0	9	15	0.001	3.34	—
21	1.12	0.29	8.9	4.1	0.07	0.049	1.01	0.074	83.6	0	36	36	0.001	5.15	—
0.8	0.026	0.004	1.46	0.48	0.003	0.004	0.027	0.002	0.28	0	1	1.3	0	0.1	0.009
5.06	0.152	0.101	—	81	0.013	0.051	0.152	—	0.5	0	17.7	7.59	0.001	0	—
8	0.61	0.14	5.5	5.5	0.042	0.058	0.277	0.039	—	0	10	16	0.001	3.2	—
63	2.05	0.52	8.9	0	0.16	0.178	3.92	0.342	22.4	0	58	70	—	15.5	—
118	4.45	1	26.4	1.7	0.141	0.175	1.38	0.446	15	0	286	136	—	18.5	—
17	0.53	0.21	75.7	6.8	0.03	0.04	0.999	—	—	0	20	34	0.001	1.51	—
1	0.06	0.04	1.2	9.2	0.007	0.007	0.007	0	0.4	0	2	0	0	0	—

Continued.

Key to Abbreviations

Kcal, Kcalories; *Prot*, protein; *Carb*, carbohydrate; *Fat*, fat; *Chol*, cholesterol; *Safa*, saturated fat; *Mufa*, monounsaturated fat; *Pufa*, polyunsaturated fat; *Sod*, sodium; *Pot*, potassium; *Mag*, magnesium; *Iron*, iron; *Zinc*, zinc; *VA*, vitamin A; *VC*, vitamin C; *Thia*, thiamin; *Ribo*, riboflavin; *Niac*, niacin; *VB₆*, vitamin B₆; *Fol*, folate; *VB₁₂*, vitamin B₁₂; *Calc*, calcium; *Phos*, phosphorus; *Sel*, selenium; *Fibd*, dietary fiber; and *VE*, vitamin E.

Food name	Portion	Wt (g)	Kcal	Prot (g)	Carb (g)	Fat (g)	Chol (mg)	Safa (g)	Mufa (g)	Pufa (g)	Sod (mg)	Pot (mg)
Fruits—cont'd												
Fruit roll up-cherry	Item	14.4	50	0	12	1	0	—	—	—	5	45
Grape juice-can/bottle	Cup	253	155	1.41	37.9	0.19	0	0.063	0.008	0.056	7	334
Grape juice-froz-diluted	Cup	250	128	0.47	31.9	0.23	0	0.073	0.01	0.065	5	53
Grapefruit juice-can-sweet	Cup	250	116	1.45	27.8	0.23	0	0.03	0.03	0.053	4	405
Grapefruit juice-can-unsweet	Cup	247	93	1.29	22.1	0.24	0	0.032	0.032	0.057	3	378
Grapefruit juice-froz-diluted	Cup	247	102	1.37	24	0.33	0	0.047	0.044	0.079	2	337
Grapefruit juice-raw	Cup	247	96	1.24	22.7	0.25	0	0.035	0.032	0.059	2	400
Grapefruit-raw-pink/red	Item	246	74	1.36	18.5	0.246	0	0.034	0.032	0.06	0	312
Grapefruit-raw-white	Item	236	78	1.63	19.8	0.24	0	0.034	0.03	0.057	0	350
Kiwifruit-raw	Item	76	46	0.75	11.3	0.34	0	0	0	0	4	252
Lemonade-froz-diluted	Cup	248	105	0	28	0	0	0	0	0	0	40
Lemon juice-can/bottle	Cup	244	52	0.98	15.8	0.7	0	0.093	0.027	0.207	50	248
Lemon juice-raw	Cup	244	60	0.92	21.1	0	0	0	0	0	2	303
Lemons-raw-peeled	Item	58	17	0.64	5.41	0.17	0	0.023	0.006	0.052	1	80
Lime juice-can/bottle	Cup	246	51	0.61	16.5	0.57	0	0.064	0.054	0.157	39	185
Lime juice-raw	Cup	246	66	1.08	22.2	0.25	0	0.027	0.025	0.066	2	268
Limes-raw	Item	67	20	0.47	7.06	0.13	0	0.015	0.013	0.037	1	68
Melons-cantaloupe-raw	Cup	160	57	1.4	13.4	0.44	0	0	0	0	14	494
Melons-casaba-raw	Cup	170	45	1.53	10.5	0.17	0	0	0	0	20	357
Melons-honeydew-raw	Cup	170	60	0.77	15.6	0.17	0	0	0	0	17	461
Nectarines-raw	Item	136	67	1.28	16	0.62	0	—	—	—	0	288
Orange juice-can	Cup	249	104	1.46	24.5	0.36	0	0.045	0.062	0.085	6	436
Orange juice-froz-diluted	Cup	249	112	1.68	26.8	0.14	0	0.017	0.025	0.03	2	474
Orange juice-raw	Cup	248	111	1.74	25.8	0.5	0	0.06	0.089	0.099	2	496
Oranges-raw-all varieties	Item	131	62	1.23	15.4	0.16	0	0.02	0.03	0.033	0	237
Papaya nectar-can	Cup	250	142	0.43	36.3	0.38	0	0.118	0.103	0.088	14	78
Papayas-raw	Cup	140	54	0.86	13.7	0.2	0	0.06	0.053	0.043	4	359
Peaches-can/water pack	Cup	244	58	1.07	14.9	0.14	0	0.015	0.051	0.068	8	241
Peaches-dried-ckd-unsweet	Cup	258	198	2.99	50.8	0.63	0	0.067	0.23	0.304	6	825
Peaches-dried-unckd	Cup	160	383	5.77	98.1	1.22	0	0.131	0.445	0.587	12	1594
Peaches-froz-sliced-sweet	Cup	250	235	1.56	59.9	0.33	0	0.035	0.12	0.16	16	325
Peaches-raw-sliced	Cup	170	73	1.19	18.9	0.16	0	0.017	0.058	0.077	1	334
Peaches-raw-whole	Item	87	37	0.61	9.65	0.08	0	0.009	0.03	0.039	0	171
Pears-can/juice	Cup	248	123	0.85	32.1	0.16	0	0.01	0.035	0.037	10	238
Pears-raw-bartlet-unpeeled	Item	166	98	0.65	25.1	0.66	0	0.037	0.139	0.156	1	208
Pineapple-can/juice	Cup	250	150	1.04	39.2	0.21	0	0.015	0.025	0.073	4	304
Pineapple juice-can	Cup	250	139	0.8	34.4	0.2	0	0.013	0.023	0.07	2	334
Pineapple juice-froz-diluted	Cup	250	129	1	31.9	0.08	0	0.005	0.008	0.025	3	340
Pineapple-raw-diced	Cup	155	77	0.6	19.2	0.66	0	0.05	0.074	0.226	1	175
Plums-raw-prune type	Item	28.4	20	0	6	0	0	0	0	0	0	48
Pomegranates-raw	Item	154	104	1.47	26.4	0.46	0	—	—	—	5	399
Prune juice-can/bottle	Cup	256	181	1.55	44.7	0.08	0	0.008	0.054	0.018	11	706
Prunes-dried-unckd	Cup	161	385	4.2	101	0.83	0	0.066	0.547	0.18	6	1200
Raisins-seedless	Cup	145	434	4.67	115	0.67	0	0.218	0.026	0.196	17	1089
Raisins-seedless-packet	Item	14	42	0.451	11.1	0.064	0	0.021	0.003	0.019	1.68	105
Raspberries-raw	Cup	123	61	1.11	14.2	0.68	0	0.023	0.065	0.385	0	187
Rhubarb-raw-ckd-sugar	Cup	270	380	1	97	0	0	0	0	0	5	548
Strawberries-froz-unsweet	Cup	149	52	0.63	13.6	0.16	0	0.009	0.022	0.08	3	220
Strawberries-raw-whole	Cup	149	45	0.91	10.5	0.55	0	0.03	0.077	0.277	2	247
Tangerines-raw-peeled	Item	84	37	0.53	9.4	0.16	0	0.018	0.029	0.031	1	132
Watermelon-raw	Cup	160	50	0.99	11.5	0.68	0	—	—	—	3	186
Grains												
Bisquick mix-dry	Cup	112	480	8	76	16	—	—	—	—	1400	—
Corn chips	oz	28.4	155	1.7	16.9	9.14	0	1.5	3.39	4.25	164	43.3
Cornmeal-degerm-enr-ckd	Cup	240	125	2.88	26.4	0.56	0	0.076	0.14	0.241	1	55
Croutons-herb seasoned	Cup	30	100	4.29	20	0	0	0	0	0	372	38.6

Mag (mg)	Iron (mg)	Zinc (mg)	VA (RE)	VC (mg)	Thia (mg)	Ribo (mg)	Niac (mg)	VB$_6$ (mg)	Fol (µg)	VB$_{12}$ (µg)	Calc (mg)	Phos (mg)	Sel (mg)	Fibd (g)	VE (mg)
—	—	—	—	—	—	—	—	—	—	—	—	—	—	—	—
24	0.6	0.13	2	0.2	0.066	0.094	0.663	0.164	6.5	0	22	27	0.001	0	—
11	0.26	0.1	1.9	59.7	0.038	0.065	0.31	0.105	3.1	0	9	11	0.001	0	—
24	0.89	0.15	0	67.3	0.1	0.058	0.798	0.05	25.9	0	20	27	0.001	0	0.1
24	0.5	0.21	1.8	72	0.104	0.049	0.571	0.049	25.6	0	18	27	0.001	0.442	0.099
26	0.34	0.13	2.2	83.4	0.101	0.054	0.536	0.109	8.9	0	19	34	0.001	0	0.099
30	0.49	0.13	2.47	93.9	0.099	0.049	0.494	—	51.2	0	22	37	0.001	0.5	0.098
20	0.3	0.18	63.7	91	0.098	0.05	0.492	0.104	23.1	0	36	22	0.001	3.2	0.615
21.2	0.142	0.165	2.4	78.6	0.088	0.048	0.634	0.102	23.6	0	28	18	0.001	2.5	0.59
23	0.31	—	13.3	74.5	0.015	0.038	0.38	—	—	0	20	31	—	2.58	—
—	0.1	—	1	17	0.01	0.02	0.2	—	12	—	2	3	0.001	0.56	—
20	0.31	0.15	3.7	60.4	0.1	0.022	0.481	0.105	24.6	0	26	21	0.001	0.732	—
16	0.08	0.12	4.9	112	0.073	0.024	0.244	0.124	31.5	0	18	14	0.001	0.732	—
—	0.35	0.04	1.7	30.7	0.023	0.012	0.058	0.046	6.2	0	15	9	0.001	0.58	—
16	0.56	0.15	4	15.7	0.081	0.007	0.401	0.066	19.5	0	30	24	0.001	0	—
14	0.08	0.15	2.5	72.1	0.049	0.025	0.246	0.106	—	0	22	18	—	0	—
—	0.4	0.07	0.7	19.5	0.02	0.013	0.134	—	5.5	0	22	12	0.001	0.353	—
17	0.34	0.25	516	67.5	0.058	0.034	0.918	0.184	27.3	0	17	27	0.001	1.28	0.224
14	0.68	—	5.1	27.2	0.102	0.034	0.68	—	—	0	9	12	0.001	2	0.238
12	0.12	—	6.8	42.1	0.131	0.031	1.02	0.1	—	0	10	17	0.001	1.53	0.238
11	0.21	0.12	100	7.3	0.023	0.056	1.35	0.034	5.1	0	6	22	0.001	2.18	—
27	1.1	0.17	43.7	85.7	0.149	0.07	0.782	0.219	136	0	21	36	0.001	0.26	0.1
24	0.24	0.13	19.4	96.9	0.197	0.045	0.503	0.11	109	0	22	40	0.001	0.498	0.1
27	0.5	0.13	49.6	124	0.223	0.074	0.992	0.099	136	0	27	42	0.001	1.98	0.099
13	0.13	0.09	25.9	69.7	0.114	0.052	0.369	0.079	39.7	0	52	18	0.002	3.14	0.314
8	0.86	0.38	27.7	7.5	0.015	0.01	0.375	0.023	5.2	0	24	1	0.001	0.125	—
14	0.14	0.1	282	86.5	0.038	0.045	0.473	0.027	—	0	33	7	0.001	1.27	—
12	0.77	0.22	130	7	0.022	0.046	1.27	0.046	8.2	0	6	25	0.001	1.08	—
35	3.37	0.47	50.8	9.5	0.013	0.054	3.92	0.098	0.2	0	23	99	0.001	6.7	—
67	6.5	0.92	346	7.7	0.003	0.339	7	0.107	10.6	0	45	191	0.001	14	—
12	0.93	0.13	70.9	235	0.033	0.088	1.63	0.045	—	0	6	28	0.001	5.99	—
11	0.19	0.23	91	11.2	0.029	0.07	1.68	0.031	5.8	0	9	21	0.001	2.72	0.17
6	0.1	0.12	46.5	5.7	0.015	0.036	0.861	0.016	3	0	5	11	0.001	1.39	0.087
17	0.71	0.22	1.4	4	0.027	0.027	0.496	—	—	0	21	29	0.001	4.71	—
9	0.41	0.2	3.3	6.6	0.033	0.066	0.166	0.03	12.1	0	19	18	0.001	4.32	0.82
35	0.7	0.24	9.5	23.8	0.238	0.048	0.71	—	—	0	34	16	0.002	1.88	0.25
34	0.65	0.29	1.2	26.7	0.138	0.055	0.643	0.24	57.7	0	42	20	0.002	0.25	—
23	0.75	0.29	2.5	30	0.175	0.05	0.5	0.185	—	0	28	20	0.002	0.3	—
21	0.57	0.12	3.5	23.9	0.143	0.056	0.651	0.135	16.4	0	11	11	0.001	1.86	0.155
1.96	0.1	0.028	8	1	0.01	0.01	0.1	0.023	0.616	0	3	5	0	0.588	0.196
—	0.46	—	—	9.4	0.046	0.046	0.462	0.162	—	0	5	12	0.001	1.1	—
36	3.03	0.52	0.9	10.6	0.041	0.179	2.01	—	1	0	30	64	0.001	2.56	—
73	3.99	0.85	320	5.4	0.13	0.261	3.16	0.425	5.9	0	82	127	0.001	11	—
48	3.02	0.38	1.1	4.8	0.226	0.128	1.19	0.361	4.8	0	71	140	0.001	7.69	1.02
4.62	0.291	0.039	0.112	0.462	0.022	0.012	0.115	0.035	0.462	0	6.86	13.6	0	0.742	0.098
22	0.7	0.57	16	30.8	0.037	0.111	1.11	0.07	6	0	27	15	0.001	5.5	0.369
32.4	1.6	0.216	22	16	0.05	0.14	0.8	0.054	14.3	0	211	41	0.001	5.4	0.54
16	1.12	0.19	6.6	61.4	0.033	0.055	0.688	0.042	25	0	23	20	0.001	3.9	0.313
16	0.57	0.19	4.1	84.5	0.03	0.098	0.343	0.088	26.4	0	21	28	0.001	3.87	0.179
10	0.09	—	77.3	25.9	0.088	0.018	0.134	0.056	17.1	0	12	8	0.001	1.68	—
17	0.28	0.11	58.5	15.4	0.128	0.032	0.32	0.23	3.4	0	13	14	0.001	0.64	—
—	—	—			—	—	—	—	—		—	—	—	3.02	0.302
21.9	0.376	0.435	—	—	0.048	0.026	0.554	0.054	—	0	37.1	54.6	0.002	1.66	—
14	1.4	0.24	14	0	0.243	0.138	1.71	0.087	16	0	2	29	0.006	0.7	0.192
11.4	1.54	0.3	0	—	0.129	0.2	1.72	0	0	—	—	—	—	1.41	—

Continued.

Key to Abbreviations
Kcal, Kcalories; *Prot,* protein; *Carb,* carbohydrate; *Fat,* fat; *Chol,* cholesterol; *Safa,* saturated fat; *Mufa,* monounsaturated fat; *Pufa,* polyunsaturated fat; *Sod,* sodium; *Pot,* potassium; *Mag,* magnesium; *Iron,* iron; *Zinc,* zinc; *VA,* vitamin A; *VC,* vitamin C; *Thia,* thiamin; *Ribo,* riboflavin; *Niac,* niacin; *VB₆,* vitamin B₆; *Fol,* folate; *VB₁₂,* vitamin B₁₂; *Calc,* calcium; *Phos,* phosphorus; *Sel,* selenium; *Fibd,* dietary fiber; and *VE,* vitamin E.

Food name	Portion	Wt (g)	Kcal	Prot (g)	Carb (g)	Fat (g)	Chol (mg)	Safa (g)	Mufa (g)	Pufa (g)	Sod (mg)	Pot (mg)
Grains—cont'd												
Flour-wheat-enr-sifted	Cup	115	419	11.9	87.7	1.12	0	0.178	0.1	0.475	1.84	123
Macaroni-ckd-firm-hot	Cup	130	183	6.2	36.9	0.865	0	0.124	0.102	0.355	0.93	40.9
Noodles-egg-enr-ckd	Cup	160	200	7	37	2	50	—	—	—	3	70
Noodles-ramen-oriental	Cup	227	207	5.9	30.7	8.6	—	—	—	—	829	—
Popcorn-popped-plain	Cup	6	25	1	5	0	0	0	0	0	0	—
Popcorn-popped-sugar coat	Cup	35	135	2	30	1	0	0.5	0.2	0.4	0	—
Potato pancakes-home rec	Item	76	495	4.63	26.4	12.6	93	3.42	5.35	2.54	388	538
Pretzel-thin-stick	Item	0.3	1.19	0.028	0.242	0.011	0	0	0	0	4.83	0.303
Rice cake-regular	Item	9.31	35	0.7	7.6	0.28	0	—	—	—	10.8	27.2
Rice-brown-Uncle Ben's	Cup	146	220	5	46.4	1.82	0	0.462	0.425	0.616	2.4	172
Rice-Spanish-home rec	Cup	245	213	4.4	40.7	4.2	0	—	—	—	774	566
Rice-white-instant-hot	Cup	165	161	3.4	35.1	0.27	0	0.073	0.084	0.072	4	7
Rice-white-long grain-ckd	Cup	205	264	5.51	57.2	0.58	0	0.158	0.181	0.155	4	80
Rice-white-parboil-ckd	Cup	175	199	4.01	43.3	0.47	0	0.128	0.147	0.126	6	66
Shake n Bake	oz	28.4	116	2.44	17.7	4.26	—	—	—	—	984	56.8
Spaghetti-cdk-tender-hot	Cup	140	155	5	32	1	0	—	—	—	1	85
Stuffing-mix-dry form	Cup	30	111	3.9	21.7	1.1	—	—	—	—	399	52
Stuffing-mix-prep	Cup	140	501	9.1	49.8	30.5	—	—	—	—	1254	126
Taco shells	Item	11	49.8	0.967	7.24	2.15	0	—	—	—	—	—
Tortilla chips-Doritos	oz	28.4	139	2	18.6	6.6	0	1.43	3.19	1.77	180	51
Tortilla-corn	Item	30	67.2	2.15	12.8	1.14	0	—	—	—	53.4	52.2
Tortilla-flour	Item	30	95	2.5	17.3	1.8	0	—	—	—	—	—
Meats												
Bacon bits	Tbsp	6	26.6	1.92	1.72	1.55	0	—	—	—	165	—
Bacon-pork-broiled/fried	Slice	6.3	36.3	1.93	0.036	3.12	5.33	1.1	1.5	0.367	101	30.7
Beef-liver-fried/marg	Slice	85	184	22.7	6.68	6.8	410	2.4	1.46	1.53	90	309
Bologna-pork	Slice	23	57	3.52	0.17	4.57	14	1.58	2.25	0.49	272	65
Braunschweiger-saus-pork	Slice	18	65	2.43	0.56	5.78	28	1.96	2.68	0.67	206	36
Canadian bacon-pork-grill	Slice	23.3	43	5.64	0.315	1.96	13.5	0.66	0.94	0.185	360	90.5
Corned beef hash-can	Cup	220	400	19	24	25	50	11.9	10.9	0.5	1188	440
Deviled ham-can	Tbsp	13	45	2	0	4	10	1.5	1.8	0.4	160	—
Frankfurter-hot dog-no bun	Item	57	183	6.43	1.46	16.6	29	6.13	7.79	1.56	639	95
Ham-reg-lunch meat-11% fat	Slice	28.4	52	4.98	0.88	3	16	0.96	1.4	0.34	373	94
Ham-reg-roasted-pork	Cup	140	249	31.7	0	12.6	83	4.36	6.22	1.98	2100	573
Hamburger-ground-reg-baked	Serving	85	244	19.6	0	17.8	74	6.99	7.79	0.66	51	188
Hamburger-ground-reg-fried	Serving	85	260	20.3	0	19.2	75	7.53	8.39	0.71	71	255
Italian sausage-pork-link	Item	67	217	13.4	1.01	17.2	52	6.05	8.01	2.2	618	204
Kielbasa-pork/beef	Slice	26	81	3.45	0.56	7.06	17	2.58	3.36	0.8	280	70
Knockwurst-pork/beef-link	Item	68	209	8.08	1.2	18.9	39	6.94	8.71	1.98	687	136
Lamb-chop-lean/fat-broiled	Item	85	307	18.8	0	25.2	84	10.8	10.3	2.02	64	230
Lamb-chop/rib-lean-broiled	Item	57	134	15.8	0	7.38	51.9	2.65	2.97	0.673	48.5	178
Lamb-leg-lean/fat-roast	Slice	85	219	21.7	0	14	79	5.85	5.92	1.01	56	266
Liverwurst/liver saus-pork	Slice	18	59	2.54	0.4	5.14	28	1.91	2.4	0.47	215	—
Mortadella-pork/beef	Slice	15	47	2.46	0.46	3.81	8	1.43	1.71	0.47	187	24
Polish sausage-pork	Item	227	740	32	3.7	65.2	159	23.4	30.6	6.99	1989	538
Pork-chop-lean-broiled	Item	66	169	18.4	0	10.1	63	3.48	4.53	1.23	49	276
Pork-chop-lean/fat-broiled	Item	82	284	19.3	0	22.3	77	8.06	10.2	2.53	54	287
Pork-loin-lean-roast	Slice	72	180	21.4	0	9.81	68	3.38	4.41	1.19	52	271
Pork-loin-lean/fat-roast	Item	88	268	22.4	0	19.1	80	6.92	8.76	2.18	56	284
Pork-tenderloin-lean-roast	oz	28.4	47	8.16	0	1.36	26.3	0.47	0.613	0.163	19	152
Pot roast-arm-beef-ckd	Slice	100	231	33	0	9.98	101	3.79	4.35	0.4	66	289
Roast beef-rib-lean	Slice	51	122	13.9	0	7.03	41.3	2.96	3.06	0.209	37.7	192
Roast beef-rib-lean/fat	Slice	85	308	18.3	0	25.5	73	10.8	11.4	0.9	52	257
Salami-ckd-beef	Slice	23	58	3.38	0.57	4.62	14	1.94	2.14	0.2	266	52
Salami-dry or hard-pork	Slice	10	41	2.26	0.16	3.37	8	1.19	1.6	0.37	226	—
Sausage-link-pork-ckd	Item	13	48	2.55	0.13	4.05	11	1.4	1.81	0.5	168	47

Mag (mg)	Iron (mg)	Zinc (mg)	VA (RE)	VC (mg)	Thia (mg)	Ribo (mg)	Niac (mg)	VB$_6$ (mg)	Fol (μg)	VB$_{12}$ (μg)	Calc (mg)	Phos (mg)	Sel (mg)	Fibd (g)	VE (mg)
24.8	5.34	0.81	—	0	0.903	0.569	6.79	0.051	30.4	0	16.6	124	0.005	3.11	0.046
23.3	1.82	0.688	—	0	0.266	0.127	2.18	0.046	0.93	0	0.93	70.7	0.032	2.08	0.026
43.2	1.4	—	11	0	0.22	0.13	1.9	0.141	19.2	0	16	94	0.094	3.52	—
—	—	—	—	—	—	—	—	—	—	—	—	—	—	2.04	—
—	0.2	0.5	—	0	—	0.01	0.1	0.012	—	0	1	17	0.001	0.4	—
—	0.5	—	—	0	—	0.02	0.4	—	—	—	2	47	0.007	1.35	—
24	1.21	0.68	8.9	0.4	0.104	0.095	1.61	0.29	21.5	0.217	21	78	—	—	—
0.072	0.006	0.003	0	0	0.001	0.001	0.013	0	0.048	0	0.078	0.273	—	—	0
—	—	—	—	—	—	—	—	—	—	—	—	—	—	0.158	—
—	0.9	—	0	0	0.18	0.04	4.2	—	—	—	16	222	0.057	2.48	0.993
—	1.5	—	162	37	0.1	0.07	1.7	—	—	—	34	96	—	1.83	—
9	1.04	0.4	—	0	0.124	0.076	1.45	0.016	6	0	13	23	0.033	1.32	0.182
26	2.25	0.94	—	0	0.334	0.027	3.03	0.191	7	0	23	95	0.041	2.13	0.226
20	1.97	0.53	—	0	0.437	0.031	2.45	0.033	6	0	33	73	0.035	0.875	0.193
—	0.71	—	62	0.284	0.162	0.184	2.19	—	—	—	13.9	43.5	—	—	—
23.8	1.3	0.7	0	0	0.2	0.11	1.5	0.09	16.8	0	11	70	0.085	2.24	0.084
—	1	—	0	0	0.07	0.08	1	—	—	—	37	57	—	—	—
—	22	—	91	0	0.13	0.17	2.1	—	—	—	92	136	—	—	—
11.4	0.286	0.142	—	—	0.032	0.017	0.189	—	—	0	15.6	25.4	—	0.88	—
21	0.5	0.24	5.2	0	0.03	0.03	0.04	0.1	4	—	30	59	—	1.85	—
19.5	0.57	0.426	—	0	0.048	0.03	0.384	0.091	5.7	0	42	54.9	0.002	1.56	—
7	1.1	—	0.2	0	0.01	0.08	1	—	—	—	46	25	0.005	0.778	—
—	0.3	—	0	0.18	0.025	0.018	0.138	—	—	—	8.4	18.1	—	—	—
1.67	0.103	0.206	0	2.13	0.044	0.018	0.464	0.017	0.333	0.11	0.667	21.3	0.001	0	0.033
20	5.34	4.63	9216	19.4	0.179	3.52	12.3	1.22	187	95	9	392	0.048	0	0.536
3	0.18	0.47	—	8.1	0.12	0.036	0.897	0.06	1	0.21	3	32	0.004	0	0.014
2	1.68	0.51	759	2	0.045	0.275	1.51	0.06	—	3.62	2	30	0.002	0	0.063
5	0.19	0.395	0	5	0.192	0.046	1.61	0.105	1	0.18	2.5	69	0.003	0	—
—	4.4	—	—	—	0.02	0.2	4.6	—	—	—	29	147	—	—	0.066
1.69	0.3	0.238	0	—	0.2	0.01	0.2	0.042	—	0.091	1	12	0.002	0	—
6	0.66	1.05	—	15	0.113	0.068	1.5	0.08	2	0.74	6	49	0.005	0	0.08
5	0.28	0.61	0	8	0.244	0.071	1.49	0.1	1	0.24	2	70	0.013	0	—
30	1.88	3.46	0	31.7	1.02	0.462	8.61	0.43	—	0.98	12	393	0.066	0	0.392
13	2.05	4.16	—	0	0.026	0.136	4.04	0.2	7	1.99	8	117	—	0	0.315
17	2.08	4.31	—	0	0.026	0.17	4.96	0.2	8	2.3	10	145	—	0	0.315
12	1.01	1.59	—	1.3	0.417	0.156	2.79	0.22	—	0.87	16	114	0.022	0	0.107
4	0.38	0.52	—	6	0.059	0.056	0.749	0.05	—	0.42	11	38	0.004	0	0.042
8	0.62	1.13	—	18	0.233	0.095	1.86	0.11	—	0.8	7	67	0.01	0	—
20	1.6	3.4	—	—	0.08	0.19	5.95	0.09	12	2.16	16	151	0.014	0	0.142
16.5	1.26	3	—	—	0.057	0.143	3.73	0.086	12	1.5	9.12	121	0.01	0	0.091
20	1.69	3.74	—	—	0.09	0.23	5.6	0.13	17	2.2	9	162	0.014	0	0.043
—	1.15	—	—	—	0.049	0.185	—	0.03	5	2.42	5	41	0.003	0	0.063
2	0.21	0.32	—	4	0.018	0.023	0.401	0.019	—	0.22	3	15	0.002	0	0.024
31.8	3.27	4.38	—	2.27	1.14	0.336	7.82	0.431	—	2.22	27.2	309	0.066	0	0.363
19	0.61	1.93	1.5	0.2	0.641	0.278	3.93	0.3	4	0.71	5	184	0.011	0	0.106
20	0.66	2.01	2.1	0.2	0.69	0.294	4.32	0.31	4	0.81	5	193	0.014	0	0.131
16	0.82	1.71	1.8	0.3	0.681	0.196	4.09	0.34	0.72	0.45	4	164	0.023	0	0.114
17	0.87	1.8	2.1	0.3	0.727	0.21	4.44	0.35	1	0.53	5	173	0.028	0	0.139
7	0.437	0.85	0.601	0.1	0.266	0.111	1.33	0.12	1.67	0.157	2.33	81.7	0.009	0	0.113
24	3.79	8.66	0	0	0.081	0.289	3.72	0.33	11	3.4	9	268	0.006	0	0.14
12.8	1.33	3.54	0	0	0.042	0.107	2.1	0.153	4.08	1.49	5.1	109	0.012	0	0.092
17	1.77	4.27	0	0	0.065	0.146	2.65	0.25	5	2.37	10	140	0.02	0	0.119
3	0.46	0.49	—	3	0.029	0.059	0.785	0.05	0.46	1.11	2	23	0.004	0	0.025
2	0.13	0.42	—	—	0.093	0.033	0.56	0.06	—	0.28	1	23	0.002	0	0.011
2	0.16	0.33	—	0	0.096	0.033	0.587	0.04	—	0.22	4	24	0.004	0	0.021

Continued.

Key to Abbreviations

Kcal, Kcalories; *Prot,* protein; *Carb,* carbohydrate; *Fat,* fat; *Chol,* cholesterol; *Safa,* saturated fat; *Mufa,* monounsaturated fat; *Pufa,* polyunsaturated fat; *Sod,* sodium; *Pot,* potassium; *Mag,* magnesium; *Iron,* iron; *Zinc,* zinc; *VA,* vitamin A; *VC,* vitamin C; *Thia,* thiamin; *Ribo,* riboflavin; *Niac,* niacin; *VB6,* vitamin B6; *Fol,* folate; *VB12,* vitamin B12; *Calc,* calcium; *Phos,* phosphorus; *Sel,* selenium; *Fibd,* dietary fiber; and *VE,* vitamin E.

Food name	Portion	Wt (g)	Kcal	Prot (g)	Carb (g)	Fat (g)	Chol (mg)	Safa (g)	Mufa (g)	Pufa (g)	Sod (mg)	Pot (mg)
Meats—cont'd												
Sausage-patty-pork-ckd	Item	27	100	5.31	0.28	8.41	22	2.92	3.75	1.03	349	97
Spareribs-pork-braised	oz	28.4	113	8.23	0	8.58	34.3	3.33	4.01	0.997	26.3	90.7
Steak-chicken fried	Item	100	389	17.9	12.3	30	—	—	—	—	815	126
Steak-rib-ckd	Item	100	225	28	0	11.6	80	4.93	5.1	0.35	69	394
Steak-round-lean/fat	Slice	85	179	26.2	0	7.49	72	2.8	3.08	0.33	51	365
Steak-sirloin-lean-broiled	Item	56	133	17	0	6.63	50	2.71	2.92	0.28	37	226
Steak-sirloin-lean/fat	Item	85	271	22.7	0	19.4	77	8.07	8.67	0.77	52	297
Miscellaneous												
Baking powder-home use	Tsp	3	3.87	0.003	0.936	0	0	0	0	0	329	4.5
Baking powder-low sodium	Tsp	4.3	7.4	0.004	1.79	0	0	0	—	—	0.258	471
Baking soda	Tsp	3	0	0	0	0	0	0	0	0	821	—
Chewing gum-candy coated	Item	1.7	5	—	1.6	—	0	0	0	0	—	—
Chewing gum-Wrigleys	Item	3	10	0	2.3	—	0	0	0	0	0	0
Pickle relish-sweet	Tbsp	15	20	0	5	0	0	0	0	0	124	—
Pickle/hamburger relish	oz	28.4	30	0	7	0	0	0	0	0	325	—
Pickle/hot dog relish	oz	28.4	35	0	8	0	0	0	0	0	200	—
Vinegar-cider	Tbsp	15	0	0	1	0	0	0	0	0	0.125	15
Vinegar-distilled	Cup	240	29	0	12	0	0	0	0	0	2	36
Yeast-baker-dry-act-packet	Serving	7	20	3	3	0	0	0	0	0	1	140
Yeast-brewers-dry	Tbsp	8	25	3	3	0	0	0	0	0	9	152
Nuts and seeds												
Nut-filbert/hazel-dri-chop	Cup	115	727	15	17.6	72	0	5.3	56.5	6.9	3	512
Nut-walnut-Persian/English	Cup	120	770	17.2	22	74.2	0	6.7	17	47	12	602
Nuts-almond-shelled-sliver	Cup	115	677	22.9	23.5	60	0	5.69	39	12.6	12.7	842
Nuts-brazil-dried-shelled	Cup	140	919	20.1	17.9	92.7	0	22.6	32.2	33.8	2	840
Nuts-cashews-dry roast	Cup	137	787	21	44.8	63.5	0	12.5	37.4	10.7	21	774
Nuts-chestnuts-roast	oz	28.4	68	1.27	14.9	0.34	0	0.05	0.176	0.087	1	135
Nuts-coconut cream-raw	Cup	240	792	8.7	16	83.2	0	73.8	3.54	0.91	10	781
Nuts-coconut-dri-flake-can	Cup	77	341	2.58	31.5	24.4	0	21.6	1.04	0.267	15	249
Nuts-coconut-dried-shred	Cup	93	466	2.68	44.3	33	0	29.3	1.4	0.361	244	313
Nuts-macadamia-dried	Cup	134	940	11.1	18.4	98.8	0	14.8	77.9	1.7	6	493
Nuts-mixed-dry roast	Cup	137	814	23.7	34.7	70.5	0	9.45	43	14.8	16	817
Nuts-mixed-oil roast	Cup	142	876	23.8	30.4	80	0	12.4	45	18.9	16	825
Nuts-peanuts-oil roast	Cup	145	840	38.8	26.7	71.3	0	9.9	35.5	22.6	22	1020
Nuts-peanuts-oil-salted	Cup	145	841	38.8	26.8	71.3	0	9.93	35.5	22.6	626	1020
Nuts-peanuts-Spanish-dried	Cup	146	827	37.5	23.6	71.8	0	9.96	35.6	22.7	23	1047
Nuts-Pecans-dried-halves	Cup	108	721	8.37	19.7	73.1	0	5.85	45.5	18.1	1	423
Nuts-pecans-oil roast	Cup	110	754	7.65	17.7	78.3	0	6.27	48.8	19.4	1	395
Nuts-pistachio-dri	Cup	128	739	26.3	31.8	61.9	0	7.84	41.8	9.36	7	1399
Nuts-pistachio-dry roast	Cup	128	776	19.1	35.2	67.6	0	8.56	45.6	10.2	8	1242
Nuts-walnut-black-dried-chop	Cup	125	759	30.4	15.1	70.7	0	4.54	15.9	46.9	2	655
Peanut butter-chunk style	Tbsp	16.1	95	3.88	3.48	8.07	0	1.54	3.8	2.31	78.5	121
Peanut butter-low sodium	Tbsp	16	95	5	2.5	8.5	0	1.36	3.95	2.46	5	110
Peanut butter-old fashion	Tbsp	16	95	4.2	2.7	8.1	0	1.5	—	2.7	75	110
Peanut butter-smooth type	Tbsp	16	95	4.56	2.53	8.18	0	1.36	3.95	2.46	75	110
Seeds-pumpkin/squash-roast	Cup	64	285	11.9	34.4	12.4	0	2.35	3.86	5.66	12	588
Seeds-sesame-roast-whole	oz	28.4	161	4.82	7.31	13.6	0	1.91	5.15	5.98	3	135
Seeds-sunflower-oil roast	Cup	135	830	28.8	19.9	77.6	0	8.13	14.8	51.2	4	652
Poultry												
Chicken-breast-no skin-roast	Item	172	284	53.4	0	6.14	146	1.74	2.14	1.32	126	440
Chicken-thigh-no skin-roast	Item	52	109	13.5	0	5.66	49	1.57	2.16	1.29	46	124
Chicken roll-light	Slice	28.4	45	5.54	0.695	2.09	14	0.575	0.84	0.455	166	64.5
Chicken spread-can	Tbsp	13	25	2	0.7	1.52	—	—	—	—	—	—
Breast-fried/batter	Item	280	728	69.6	25.2	36.9	238	9.86	15.3	8.62	770	564

Mag (mg)	Iron (mg)	Zinc (mg)	VA (RE)	VC (mg)	Thia (mg)	Ribo (mg)	Niac (mg)	VB6 (mg)	Fol (µg)	VB12 (µg)	Calc (mg)	Phos (mg)	Sel (mg)	Fibd (g)	VE (mg)
5	0.34	0.68	—	0	0.2	0.069	1.22	0.09	—	0.47	9	50	0.003	0	0.043
7	0.527	1.3	0.901	—	0.116	0.108	1.55	0.1	1.33	0.307	13.3	74	0.005	0	0.045
—	2.3	—	781	—	0.11	0.14	2.7	—	—	—	11	110	—	0	0.13
27	2.57	6.99	0	0	0.105	0.216	4.8	0.4	8	3.32	13	208	0.006	0	0.092
26	2.39	4.59	0	0	0.097	0.221	4.98	0.46	10	2.08	5	203	0.029	0	0.111
17.9	1.88	3.65	3	0	0.071	0.165	2.4	0.252	5.6	1.6	6.16	137	0.019	0	0.073
23	2.49	4.73	15	0	0.092	0.218	3.21	0.33	7	2.22	9	180	0.029	0	0.111
—	0	—	0	0	0	0	0	—	—	—	58	87.1	—	—	—
—	0	—	0	0	0	0	0	—	—	—	207	314	—	—	—
—	—	—	—	0	0	0	0	0	0	0	—	—	—	0	—
—	—	—	—	0	0	0	0	—	—	—	—	—	—	—	—
0	0	0	0	0	0	0	0	0	0	0	3	0	—	—	—
—	0.1	0.01	—	—	—	—	—	—	—	—	3	2	0	—	—
—	0.189	—	—	—	—	—	—	—	—	—	5.67	3.78	0	—	—
—	0.189	—	—	—	—	—	—	—	—	—	5.6	3.7	0	—	—
—	0.1	0.02	—	—	—	—	—	0	—	—	1	1	0.013	0	—
0	—	—	—	—	—	—	—	—	—	—	—	—	0.074	0	—
3.78	1.1	—	0	0	0.16	0.38	2.6	0.14	286	0	3	90	0	2.21	0.006
18.4	1.4	—	0	0	1.25	0.34	3	0.2	313	0	17	140	0	—	—
328	3.76	2.76	7.7	1.2	0.575	0.127	1.3	0.704	82.6	0	216	359	0.002	9.77	27.3
203	2.93	3.28	14.3	3.9	0.458	0.178	1.25	0.67	79.2	0	113	380	0.023	5.76	3.14
340	4.21	3.36	0	0.69	0.243	0.896	3.87	0.13	67.5	0	306	598	0.005	10.7	27.6
315	4.76	6.42	—	1	1.4	0.171	2.27	0.351	5.6	0	246	840	2.26	10.8	8.97
356	8.22	7.67	0	0	0.274	0.274	1.92	0.351	94.8	0	62	671	0.007	10	0.781
26	0.43	0.26	0.1	—	0.043	0.026	0.426	—	—	0	5	29	0.002	2.19	0.142
—	5.47	2.3	0	6.7	0.072	0	2.14	—	—	0	26	293	—	1.6	—
38	1.42	1.23	0	0	0.023	0.015	0.235	—	—	0	11	79	—	4.4	0.539
47	1.78	1.69	0	0.6	0.029	0.019	0.441	—	—	0	14	99	0.016	3.9	0.651
155	3.23	2.29	0	—	0.469	0.147	2.87	—	—	0	94	183	0.007	12.4	—
308	5.07	5.21	2.1	0.6	0.274	0.274	6.44	0.406	69	0	96	596	0.007	11.6	—
333	4.56	7.22	2.3	0.7	0.707	0.315	7.19	0.341	118	0	153	659	0.007	12.8	—
273	2.78	9.6	0	0	0.425	0.146	21.5	0.576	153	0	125	733	0.055	12.8	9.99
273	2.78	9.6	0	0	0.425	0.146	21.5	0.577	153	0	125	733	0.055	12.8	10.1
262	4.71	4.78	0	0	0.969	0.191	20.7	0.432	147	0	85	560	0.007	11.7	11.4
138	2.3	5.91	13.3	2.1	0.916	0.138	0.958	0.203	42.3	0	39	314	0.003	8.3	3.35
142	2.33	6.05	—	—	—	—	—	—	—	0	37	324	0.006	8.47	1.36
203	8.67	1.71	29.3	—	1.05	0.223	1.38	—	74.2	0	173	644	0.007	13.8	6.67
166	4.06	1.74	—	—	0.541	0.315	1.8	—	—	0	90	609	0.007	13.8	6.67
252	3.84	4.28	37	—	0.271	0.136	0.863	—	—	—	72	580	0.024	8.08	1.05
25.6	0.306	0.448	0	0	0.02	0.018	2.21	0.073	14.8	0	6.56	51.1	0.001	1.06	0.969
28	0.29	0.47	—	0	0.024	0.017	2.15	0.062	13.1	0	5	60	0.002	1.7	1.12
30	0.3	0.5	—	—	0.01	0.01	2.3	—	—	—	5	60	0.002	1.06	0.96
28	0.29	0.47	—	0	0.024	0.017	2.15	0.062	13.1	0	5	60	0.002	0.96	1.12
168	2.12	6.59	—	—	—	—	—	—	—	0	35	59	—	29.4	—
101	4.19	2.03	—	—	—	—	—	—	—	0	281	181	—	5.32	—
171	9.05	7.04	—	1.9	0.432	0.378	5.58	—	316	0	76	1538	0.104	9.18	66.8
50	1.78	1.72	10.8	0	0.12	0.196	23.6	1.02	6	0.58	26	392	0.046	0	0.602
12	0.68	1.34	10.2	0	0.038	0.12	3.39	0.18	4	0.16	6	95	0.021	0	0.182
5	0.275	0.205	—	—	0.019	0.037	1.5	—	—	—	12	44.5	—	0	—
—	0.3	—	—	—	0.001	0.015	0.357	—	—	—	16	—	—	—	0.036
68	3.5	2.66	56.5	0	0.322	0.408	29.5	1.2	16	0.82	56	516	0.03	—	0.98

Continued.

Key to Abbreviations

Kcal, Kcalories; *Prot,* protein; *Carb,* carbohydrate; *Fat,* fat; *Chol,* cholesterol; *Safa,* saturated fat; *Mufa,* monounsaturated fat; *Pufa,* polyunsaturated fat; *Sod,* sodium; *Pot,* potassium; *Mag,* magnesium; *Iron,* iron; *Zinc,* zinc; *VA,* vitamin A; *VC,* vitamin C; *Thia,* thiamin; *Ribo,* riboflavin; *Niac,* niacin; *VB$_6$,* vitamin B$_6$; *Fol,* folate; *VB$_{12}$,* vitamin B$_{12}$; *Calc,* calcium; *Phos,* phosphorus; *Sel,* selenium; *Fibd,* dietary fiber; and *VE,* vitamin E.

Food name	Portion	Wt (g)	Kcal	Prot (g)	Carb (g)	Fat (g)	Chol (mg)	Safa (g)	Mufa (g)	Pufa (g)	Sod (mg)	Pot (mg)
Poultry—cont'd												
Breast-fried/flour	Item	196	436	62.4	3.22	17.4	176	4.8	6.86	3.84	150	506
Breast-no skin-fried	Item	172	322	57.5	0.88	8.1	156	2.22	2.96	1.84	136	474
Breast-roast	Item	196	386	58.4	0	15.3	166	4.3	5.94	3.26	138	480
Breast-stewed	Item	220	404	60.3	0	16.3	166	4.58	6.38	3.48	136	390
Drumstick-fried	Item	49	120	13.2	0.8	6.72	44	1.79	2.66	1.58	44	112
Frankfurter	Item	45	116	5.82	3.06	8.76	45	2.49	3.81	1.82	617	—
Giblets-fried/flour	Cup	145	402	47.2	6.31	19.5	647	5.5	6.41	4.9	164	478
Giblets-simmered	Cup	145	228	37.5	1.37	6.92	570	2.16	1.73	1.56	85	229
Leg-no skin-roast	Item	95	182	25.7	0	8.01	89	2.18	2.9	1.87	87	230
Leg-no skin-stewed	Item	101	187	26.5	0	8.14	90	2.22	2.95	1.9	78	192
Leg-roast	Item	114	265	29.6	0	15.4	105	4.24	5.97	3.42	99	256
Liver pate-can	Tbsp	13	26	1.75	0.85	1.7	—	—	—	—	—	—
Liver-simmered	Cup	140	219	34.1	1.23	7.63	883	2.58	1.88	1.25	71	196
Thigh-fried/flour	Item	62	162	16.6	1.97	9.29	60	2.54	3.64	2.11	55	147
Wing-fried/flour	Item	32	103	8.36	0.76	7.09	26	1.94	2.84	1.58	25	57
Wing-roast	Item	34	99	9.13	0	6.62	29	1.85	2.6	1.41	28	62
Wing-stewed	Item	40	100	9.11	0	6.73	28	1.88	2.64	1.43	27	56
Duck												
Flesh & skin-roast	Item	764	2574	145	0	217	640	73.9	98.6	27.9	454	1560
No skin-roast	Item	442	890	104	0	49.5	396	18.4	16.4	6.3	286	1114
Turkey												
Ham-cured thigh meat	Slice	28.4	36.5	5.37	0.105	1.44	—	0.485	0.325	0.43	283	92
Breast-no skin-roast	Item	612	826	184	0	4.5	510	1.44	0.78	1.2	318	1784
Loaf-breast	Serving	28.4	31.2	6.38	0	0.447	11.5	0.137	0.127	0.078	406	78.8
Pastrami	Slice	28.4	40	5.21	0.47	2.06	—	1.03	0.58	0.45	297	73.5
Roll-light	oz	28.4	42	5.3	0.15	2.05	12	0.57	0.71	0.49	139	71
Dark meat-no skin	Cup	140	262	40	0	10.1	119	3.4	2.29	3.03	110	406
Light-no skin-roast	Cup	140	219	41.9	0	4.5	97	1.44	0.79	1.2	89	426
Light/dark-no skin	Cup	140	238	41	0	6.95	107	2.29	1.45	2	99	418
Sauces and dips												
Dip-French onion-Kraft	Tbsp	15	30	0.5	1.5	2	0	—	—	—	120	—
Dip-guacamole-Kraft	Tbsp	15	25	0.5	1.5	2	0	—	—	—	108	—
Gravy-beef-can	Cup	233	124	8.73	11.2	5.49	7	2.75	2.3	0.21	117	189
Gravy-chicken-can	Cup	238	189	4.59	12.9	13.6	5	3.36	6.08	3.58	1375	260
Gravy-turkey-can	Cup	238	122	6.2	12.2	5.01	5	1.48	2.15	1.17	—	—
Horseradish-prep	Tbsp	15	6	0.2	1.4	0	0	0	0	0	165	44
Mustard-brown-prep	Cup	250	228	14.8	13.3	15.8	0	—	—	—	3268	325
Mustard-yellow-prep	Tsp	5	5	0.1	0.1	0.1	0	0	0	0	65	7
Sauces												
Barbecue	Cup	250	188	4.5	32	4.5	0	0.67	1.94	1.71	2032	435
Bearnaise-mix/milk	Cup	255	701	8.32	17.5	68.2	189	41.8	19.9	3.03	1265	—
Cheese-mix/milk	Cup	279	307	16	23.2	17.1	53	9.32	5.31	1.58	1566	554
Chili-bottled	Tbsp	15	16	0.4	3.7	0	0	0	0	0	201	56
Curry-mix/milk	Cup	272	270	10.7	25.7	14.7	35	6.05	5.16	2.76	1276	—
Heinz 57	Tbsp	15	15	0.4	2.7	0.2	0	0	0	0	265	—
Marinara-can	Cup	250	171	4	25.5	8.38	0	1.2	4.28	2.3	1572	1061
Mushroom-mix/milk	Cup	267	228	11.3	23.8	10.3	34	5.4	3.27	1.1	1533	—
Picante-can	Fl oz	16	9	0.3	1.9	0.5	0	0	0	0	218	77
Salsa/chilies-can	Fl oz	16	10	0.4	2	0.7	0	0	0	0	111	87
Sour cream-mix/milk	Cup	314	509	19.1	45.4	30.3	91	16.1	9.88	2.76	1007	733
Soy	Tbsp	18	11	1.56	1.5	0	0	0	0	0	1029	64
Spaghetti-can	Cup	249	272	4.53	39.7	11.9	0	1.7	6.07	3.25	1236	957
Sweet/sour-mix/prep	Cup	313	294	0.76	72.7	0.08	0	0.01	0.02	0.04	779	66
Tabasco	Tsp	5	0	0.1	0.1	0	0	0	0	0	22	3

Mag (mg)	Iron (mg)	Zinc (mg)	VA (RE)	VC (mg)	Thia (mg)	Ribo (mg)	Niac (mg)	VB6 (mg)	Fol (µg)	VB12 (µg)	Calc (mg)	Phos (mg)	Sel (mg)	Fibd (g)	VE (mg)
58	2.34	2.14	29.4	0	0.16	0.256	26.9	1.14	8	0.68	32	456	0.021	0.07	0.686
54	1.96	1.86	12	0	0.136	0.216	25.4	1.1	8	0.62	28	424	0.031	0	0.602
54	2.08	2	54.7	0	0.13	0.234	24.9	1.08	6	0.64	28	420	0.053	0	0.686
48	2.02	2.12	54.1	0	0.09	0.254	17.2	0.64	6	0.46	28	344	0.053	0	0.77
11	0.66	1.42	12.3	0	0.04	0.11	2.96	0.17	4	0.16	6	86	0.005	0	0.172
—	0.9	—	—	—	0.03	0.052	1.39	—	—	—	43	—	0.01	0	—
37	15	9.09	5195	12.7	0.141	2.21	15.9	0.88	550	19.3	26	414	0.025	—	—
30	9.34	6.63	3234	11.6	0.126	1.38	5.95	0.49	545	14.7	18	331	0.025	0	—
23	1.24	2.71	13	0	0.071	0.22	6	0.35	8	0.31	12	174	0.013	0	0.333
21	1.41	2.81	13	0	0.06	0.218	4.85	0.22	8	0.23	11	151	0.013	0	0.354
26	1.52	2.96	46.2	0	0.078	0.243	7.06	0.37	8	0.35	14	199	0.016	0	0.399
—	1.19	—	28.2	1.3	0.007	0.182	0.977	—	—	—	1	—	—	0	0.036
29	11.9	6.07	6886	22.2	0.214	2.45	6.23	0.82	1077	27.1	20	437	0.099	0	—
15	0.93	1.56	18.3	0	0.058	0.151	4.31	0.21	5	0.19	8	116	0.011	0.04	0.217
6	0.4	0.56	12	0	0.019	0.044	2.14	0.13	1	0.09	5	48	0.006	0	0.112
7	0.43	0.62	16.2	0	0.014	0.044	2.26	0.14	1	0.1	5	51	0.006	0	0.119
6	0.45	0.65	15.9	0	0.016	0.041	1.85	0.09	1	0.07	5	48	0.006	0	0.14
124	20.6	14.2	483	0	1.33	2.06	36.9	1.4	50	2.26	86	1190	—	0	—
88	11.9	11.5	103	0	1.15	2.08	22.5	1.1	44	1.76	52	898	—	0	—
—	0.785	—	—	—	0.015	0.07	1	—	—	—	2.5	54	—	0	—
178	9.36	10.6	0	0	0.264	0.802	45.9	3.42	38	2.36	76	1370	0.049	0	0.551
5.67	0.113	0.318	0	0	0.011	0.03	2.36	0.1	—	0.572	2	64.8	—	0	—
4	0.47	0.61	—	—	0.016	0.071	1	—	—	—	2.5	56.5	—	0	—
5	0.36	0.44	—	—	0.025	0.064	1.99	—	—	—	11	52	—	0	—
34	3.27	6.25	0	0	0.088	0.347	5.11	0.5	13	0.52	45	286	0.035	0	0.896
39	1.88	2.85	0	0	0.085	0.181	9.57	0.75	8	0.52	27	307	—	0	0.126
37	2.49	4.34	0	0	0.087	0.255	7.62	0.64	10	0.52	35	298	0.035	0	0.896
—	—	—	—	—	—	—	—	—	—	—	—	—	—	—	—
—	1.63	2.33	0	0	0.074	0.084	1.54	0.023	—	0.23	14	70	—	0.093	—
—	1.12	1.91	264	0	0.041	0.103	1.06	0.024	—	—	48	69	—	—	—
—	1.67	—	0	0	0.048	0.191	3.1	—	—	0	10	—	—	—	—
—	0.1	—	—	—	—	—	—	—	—	—	9	5	—	—	—
—	4.5	—	—	—	—	—	—	—	—	—	310	335	—	—	4.38
2	0.1	—	—	—	—	—	—	—	—	—	4	4	0	0.06	0.088
—	2.25	—	218	17.5	0.075	0.05	2.25	0.188	—	0	48	50	—	2.3	—
47	0.27	0.972	—	2.3	0.148	0.564	0.318	—	—	—	570	437	—	0.1	—
—	0.1	—	21	2	0.01	0.01	0.2	—	—	—	3	8	0	—	—
—	—	—	—	—	—	—	—	—	—	—	485	280	—	0.9	—
—	—	—	—	—	—	—	—	—	—	—	—	—	0	—	—
59	2	0.67	240	31.9	0.113	0.148	3.98	—	—	0	44	88	—	—	—
—	—	—	—	—	—	—	—	—	—	—	—	—	—	0.5	—
—	0.25	—	23	8.8	0.02	0.01	0.22	—	—	—	3.8	8	—	—	—
—	0.28	—	39	9.1	0.02	0.01	0.29	—	—	—	4.2	9.3	—	—	—
—	0.61	1.37	—	—	—	0.704	0.556	—	—	—	546	—	—	—	—
8	0.49	0.036	0	0	0.009	0.023	0.605	0.031	1.9	0	3	38	—	—	—
60	1.62	0.53	306	27.9	0.137	0.147	3.75	—	—	0	70	90	—	—	—
—	1.62	0.091	—	—	—	0.097	—	—	—	0	41	—	—	—	—
—	—	—	—	—	0	0.01	0	—	—	—	—	—	—	—	—

Continued.

Key to Abbreviations
Kcal, Kcalories; *Prot*, protein; *Carb*, carbohydrate; *Fat*, fat; *Chol*, cholesterol; *Safa*, saturated fat; *Mufa*, monounsaturated fat; *Pufa*, polyunsaturated fat; *Sod*, sodium; *Pot*, potassium; *Mag*, magnesium; *Iron*, iron; *Zinc*, zinc; *VA*, vitamin A; *VC*, vitamin C; *Thia*, thiamin; *Ribo*, riboflavin; *Niac*, niacin; *VB₆*, vitamin B₆; *Fol*, folate; *VB₁₂*, vitamin B₁₂; *Calc*, calcium; *Phos*, phosphorus; *Sel*, selenium; *Fibd*, dietary fiber; and *VE*, vitamin E.

Food name	Portion	Wt (g)	Kcal	Prot (g)	Carb (g)	Fat (g)	Chol (mg)	Safa (g)	Mufa (g)	Pufa (g)	Sod (mg)	Pot (mg)
Sauces—cont'd												
Taco-can	Fl oz	16	11	0.4	2.2	0.7	0	—	—	—	128	88
Tartar-regular	Tbsp	14	75	0	1	8	9	1.5	1.8	4.1	98	11
Teriyaki-bottled	Tbsp	18	15	1.07	2.87	0	0	0	0	0	690	41
Tomato-can-low sod	Cup	226	90	4	18	0	—	0	0	0	65	—
Tomato-can-salt add	Cup	245	74	3.25	17.6	0.41	0	0.059	0.061	0.164	1481	908
Tomato-Spanish-can	Cup	244	80	3.52	17.7	0.64	0	0.092	0.098	0.264	1152	—
Worcestershire	Tbsp	15	12	0.3	2.7	0	0	0	0	0	147	120
Tomato catsup	Tbsp	15	15	0	4	0	0	0	0	0	156	54
Soups												
Bean/bacon-can-water	Cup	253	173	7.89	22.8	5.94	3	1.53	2.18	1.82	952	403
Beef broth-can-ready	Cup	240	16	2.74	0.1	0.53	0.605	0.26	0.22	0.02	782	130
Beef broth-dehy-cubed	Item	3.6	6	0.62	0.58	0.14	0.144	0.07	0.06	0.01	864	15
Beef-chunky-can	Cup	240	171	11.7	19.6	5.14	14	2.55	2.14	0.2	867	336
Black bean-can-water	Cup	247	116	5.64	19.8	1.51	0	0.4	0.54	0.47	1198	273
Cheese-can-milk	Cup	251	230	9.45	16.2	14.6	48	9.12	4.1	0.44	1020	340
Chick broth-can/water	Cup	244	39	4.93	0.93	1.39	1	0.41	0.63	0.29	776	210
Chicken noodle-can	Cup	241	75	4.04	9.35	2.45	7	0.65	1.11	0.55	1107	55
Chicken-chunky-can	Cup	251	178	12.7	17.3	6.63	30	1.98	2.97	1.39	887	176
Chicken/rice-can	Cup	240	127	12.3	13	3.19	12	0.95	1.43	0.67	888	—
Clam-Manhattan-water	Cup	244	78	4.18	12.2	2.31	2	0.44	0.41	1.32	1808	262
Clam-New England-milk	Cup	248	163	9.46	16.6	6.6	22	2.95	2.26	1.08	992	300
Cream/celery-can-milk	Cup	248	165	5.69	14.5	9.68	32	3.95	2.47	2.65	1010	309
Cream/chick-can-milk	Cup	248	191	7.46	15	11.5	27	4.63	4.45	1.64	1046	273
Cream/mushroom-milk	Cup	248	203	6.05	15	13.6	20	5.12	2.98	4.61	1076	270
Cream/potato-can-milk	Cup	248	148	5.78	17.2	6.45	22	3.76	1.73	0.56	1060	323
Minestrone-can-water	Cup	241	83	4.26	11.2	2.51	2	0.54	0.69	1.11	911	312
Onion-can-water	Cup	241	57	3.75	8.18	1.74	0	0.26	0.75	0.65	1053	69
Onion-dehy-packet	Serving	39	115	4.52	20.9	2.33	2	0.54	1.36	0.27	3493	260
Pea-green-can-water	Cup	250	164	8.59	26.5	2.94	0	1.41	1	0.38	987	190
Pea-split-can-water	Cup	253	189	10.3	28	4.4	8	1.76	1.8	0.63	1008	399
Tomato rice-can-water	Cup	247	120	2.11	21.9	2.72	2	0.52	0.6	1.35	815	330
Tomato-can-milk	Cup	248	160	6.09	22.3	6.01	17	2.91	1.6	1.11	932	450
Tomato-can-water	Cup	244	86	2.06	16.6	1.92	0	0.36	0.43	0.96	872	263
Turkey noodle-can	Cup	244	69	3.9	8.63	1.99	5	0.56	0.81	0.49	815	75
Turkey vegetable-can	Cup	241	74	3.09	8.64	3.02	2	0.9	1.33	0.67	905	175
Turkey-chunky-can	Cup	236	136	10.2	14.1	4.41	9	1.22	1.78	1.08	923	361
Vegetable beef-can	Cup	245	79	5.58	10.2	1.9	5	0.85	0.8	0.11	957	173
Vegetarian-can-water	Cup	241	72	2.1	12	1.93	0	0.29	0.83	0.73	823	209
Spices and herbs												
Chili powder	Tsp	2.6	8	0.32	1.42	0.44	0	—	—	—	26	50
Cinnamon-ground	Tsp	2.3	6	0.09	1.84	0.07	0	0.01	0.01	0.01	0.598	11
Oregano-ground	Tsp	1.5	5	0.17	0.97	0.15	0	0.04	0.01	0.08	0.225	25
Paprika	Tsp	2.1	6	0.31	1.17	0.27	0	0.04	0.03	0.17	0.714	49
Parsley-dried	Tsp	0.3	1	0.07	0.15	0.01	0	0	0	0	1.36	11
Pepper-black	Tsp	2.1	5	0.23	1.36	0.07	0	0.02	0.02	0.02	0.924	26
Salt-table	Tsp	5.5	0	0	0	0	0	0	0	0	2132	0
Sugars and sweets												
Almond Joy	oz	28.4	151	1.7	18.5	7.8	—	1.74	2.47	1.72	—	—
Bit O Honey	oz	28.4	121	0.9	21.2	3.6	—	1.65	1.63	0.188	—	—
Caramels-plain/choc	oz	28.4	115	1	22	3	0	1.6	1.1	0.1	74	54
Choc coated peanuts	oz	28.4	160	5	11	12	0	4	4.7	2.1	16	143
Chocolate-semisweet	Cup	170	860	7	97	61	0	36.2	19.8	1.7	3	553
Fondant-uncoated	oz	28.4	105	0	25	1	0	0.1	0.3	0.1	60	1
Fudge-choc-plain	oz	28.4	115	1	21	3	0	1.3	1.4	0.6	54	42

Mag (mg)	Iron (mg)	Zinc (mg)	VA (RE)	VC (mg)	Thia (mg)	Ribo (mg)	Niac (mg)	VB$_6$ (mg)	Fol (µg)	VB$_{12}$ (µg)	Calc (mg)	Phos (mg)	Sel (mg)	Fibd (g)	VE (mg)
—	0.3	—	4.4	6.2	0.02	0.01	0.27	—	—	—	5.9	9.8	—	—	—
—	0.1	—	3	0	0	0	0	—	—	—	3	4	—	—	—
11	0.31	0.018	0	0	0.005	0.013	0.229	0.018	3.6	0	4	28	—	—	—
—	—	—	—	—	—	—	—	—	—	—	—	—	0.002	3.39	—
46	1.88	0.6	240	32.1	0.162	0.142	2.82	—	—	0	34	78	—	3.68	—
—	8.5	—	240	21	0.18	0.152	3.15	—	—	0	40	—	—	3.66	—
—	0.9	—	5.1	27	0	0.03	0	—	—	—	15	9	—	—	—
3.6	0.1	0.034	21	2	0.01	0.01	0.2	0.016	0.75	0	3	8	0	—	—
44	2.05	1.03	89	1.6	0.089	0.033	0.567	0.04	31.9	—	81	132	0.008	3.2	—
—	0.41	—	0	0	0.005	0.05	1.87	—	—	—	15	31	0.008	0	—
2	0.08	0.008	—	—	0.007	0.009	0.119	—	—	—	8	—	0	—	—
—	2.32	2.64	261	7	0.058	0.151	2.71	0.132	13.4	0.61	31	120	0.008	—	—
42	2.16	1.41	49	0.8	0.077	0.054	0.534	0.094	24.7	0.02	45	107	0.008	—	—
20	0.81	0.688	147	1.2	0.063	0.334	0.502	0.078	—	0.44	288	250	0.008	—	—
2	0.51	0.249	0	0	0.01	0.071	3.35	0.024	—	0.24	9	73	0.008	0	—
5	0.78	0.395	72	0.2	0.053	0.06	1.39	0.027	2.2	—	17	36	0.008	1.45	—
—	1.73	1	130	1.3	0.085	0.173	4.42	0.05	4.6	0.25	24	113	0.008	—	—
—	1.87	—	586	3.8	0.024	0.098	4.1	—	3.8	—	35	—	0.008	1.44	—
10	1.89	0.927	93	3.2	0.063	0.049	1.34	0.083	9.5	2.19	34	57	0.008	—	—
23	1.48	0.799	40	3.5	0.067	0.236	1.03	0.126	9.7	10.3	187	157	0.008	—	—
22	0.69	0.196	68	1.4	0.074	0.248	0.436	0.064	8.5	—	186	151	0.008	0.77	—
18	0.67	0.675	94	1.3	0.074	0.258	0.923	0.067	7.7	—	180	152	0.008	0.5	—
20	0.59	0.64	38	2.3	0.077	0.28	0.913	0.064	—	—	178	156	0.008	—	—
17	0.54	0.675	67	1.1	0.082	0.236	0.642	0.089	9.2	—	166	160	0.008	—	—
7	0.92	0.735	234	1.1	0.053	0.043	0.942	0.099	16.1	0	34	56	0.008	1.9	—
2	0.67	0.612	0	1.2	0.034	0.024	0.6	0.048	15.2	0	26	11	0.008	—	—
25	0.58	0.231	1	0.9	0.111	0.238	1.99	—	6.3	—	55	126	0	2.2	—
39	1.95	1.71	20	1.7	0.108	0.068	1.24	0.053	1.8	0	27	124	0.008	—	—
48	2.28	1.32	44	1.4	0.147	0.076	1.48	0.068	2.5	0	22	213	0.008	—	—
5	0.79	0.514	76	14.8	0.062	0.049	1.06	0.077	—	0	23	33	0.008	1.7	—
23	1.82	0.29	108	67.7	0.134	0.248	1.52	0.164	20.9	0.44	159	148	0.008	0.8	—
8	1.76	0.244	69	66.5	0.088	0.051	1.42	0.112	14.7	0	13	34	0.008	0.9	—
5	0.94	0.583	29	0.2	0.073	0.063	1.4	0.037	—	—	12	48	0.008	0.7	—
4	0.76	0.612	244	0	0.029	0.039	1.01	0.048	—	0.17	17	40	0.008	0.964	—
—	1.91	2.12	716	6.4	0.035	0.106	3.59	0.307	11.1	2.12	50	104	0.008	2.5	—
6	1.11	1.55	189	2.4	0.037	0.049	1.03	0.076	10.6	0.31	17	40	0.008	0.98	—
7	1.08	0.46	300	1.4	0.053	0.046	0.916	0.055	10.6	0	21	35	0.008	1.21	—
4	0.37	0.07	908	1.67	0.009	0.021	0.205	—	—	0	7	8	0.001	0.889	—
1	0.88	0.05	6	0.65	0.002	0.003	0.03	—	—	0	28	1	0.001	—	—
4	0.66	0.07	104	—	0.005	—	0.093	—	—	0	24	3	—	—	—
4	0.5	0.08	127	1.49	0.014	0.037	0.322	—	—	0	4	7	0	—	—
1	0.29	0.01	7	0.37	0.001	0.004	0.024	0.003	—	0	4	1	—	—	—
4	0.61	0.03	0	—	0.002	0.005	0.024	—	—	0	9	4	0	0.525	—
0	0	—	0	0	0	0	0	0	0	0	14	—	—	0	0
—	—	—	—	—	—	—	—	—	—	—	—	—	0.001	—	0.308
—	0.25	—	—	—	0	0.13	1.4	—	—	—	13	—	0.001	—	0.048
1	0.4	—	0	0	0.01	0.05	0.1	—	—	—	42	35	0.001	0.784	0.048
—	0.4	—	0	0	0.1	0.05	2.1	—	—	—	33	84	0.001	—	0.196
—	4.4	—	9	0	0.02	0.14	0.9	—	—	—	51	255	0.006	—	1.19
—	0.3	—	0	0	0	0	0	—	—	—	4	2	0.001	0	—
12.6	0.3	—	0	0	0.01	0.03	0.1	—	—	—	22	24	0.001	—	0.196

Continued.

Key to Abbreviations
Kcal, Kcalories; *Prot*, protein; *Carb*, carbohydrate; *Fat*, fat; *Chol*, cholesterol; *Safa*, saturated fat; *Mufa*, monounsaturated fat; *Pufa*, polyunsaturated fat; *Sod*, sodium; *Pot*, potassium; *Mag*, magnesium; *Iron*, iron; *Zinc*, zinc; *VA*, vitamin A; *VC*, vitamin C; *Thia*, thiamin; *Ribo*, riboflavin; *Niac*, niacin; *VB6*, vitamin B6; *Fol*, folate; *VB12*, vitamin B12; *Calc*, calcium; *Phos*, phosphorus; *Sel*, selenium; *Fibd*, dietary fiber; and *VE*, vitamin E.

Food name	Portion	Wt (g)	Kcal	Prot (g)	Carb (g)	Fat (g)	Chol (mg)	Safa (g)	Mufa (g)	Pufa (g)	Sod (mg)	Pot (mg)
Sugars and sweets—cont'd												
Gum Drops	oz	28.4	100	0	25	0	0	0	0	0	10	1
Hard	oz	28.4	110	0	28	0	0	0	0	0	9	1
Jelly Beans	Item	2.8	6.6	0	2.64	0	—	0	0	0	0.3	0
Kit Kat bar	Item	43	210	3	25	11	—	5.6	3.77	0.448	38	129
Life Savers	Item	2	7.8	0	1.94	0.02	0	0	0	0	0.6	0
Lollipop	Item	28.4	108	0	28	0	0	0	0	0	—	—
M & M's-package	Item	45	220	3	31	10	—	—	—	—	—	—
Milk choc/almonds	oz	28.4	151	2.6	14.5	10.1	—	4.06	3.92	1.38	23	125
Milk choc/peanuts	oz	28.4	154	4	12.6	10.8	—	5.22	5.04	1.78	19	138
Milk choc-plain	oz	28.4	145	2	16	9	0	5.5	3	0.3	28	109
Milky Way bar	Item	60	260	3	43	9	—	5.05	3.61	0.336	—	—
Peanut Brittle	oz	28.4	123	2.4	20.4	4.4	—	1.85	1.79	0.632	9	43
Peanut Butter Cup	Piece	17	92	2.2	8.7	5.35	2.5	2.8	1.83	0.751	54.5	68
Snickers bar	Item	57	270	6	33	13	—	4.73	5.03	2.04	—	—
Honey-strained/extracted	Tbsp	21	65	0	17	0	0	0	0	0	1	11
Icing-cake-choc-mix/prep	Cup	275	1035	9	185	38	0	23.4	11.7	1	882	536
Icing-cake-fudge-mix/water	Cup	245	830	7	183	16	0	5.1	6.7	3.1	568	238
Icing-cake-white-boiled	Cup	94	295	1	75	0	0	0	0	0	134	17
Icing-cake-white-unckd	Cup	319	1200	2	260	21	0	12.7	5.1	0.5	156	57
Icing-cake-white/coco-boil	Cup	166	605	3	124	13	0	11	0.9	0	195	277
Jams/preserves-regular	Tbsp	20	55	0	14	0	0	0	0	0	2	18
Marshmallows	oz	28.4	90	1	23	0	0	0	0	0	11	2
Molasses-cane-blackstrap	Tbsp	20	45	0	11	—	0	—	—	—	18	585
Molasses-cane-light	Tbsp	20	50	0	13	—	0	—	—	—	3	183
Popsicle	Item	95	70	0	18	0	0	0	0	0	0	—
Sugar-brown-pressed down	Cup	220	820	0	212	0	0	0	0	0	66	757
Sugar-Equal-packet	Item	1	4	0	1	0	0	0	0	0	0	0
Sugar-Sweet & Low-packet	Item	1	4	—	0.9	—	0	—	—	—	4	3
Sugar-white-granulated	Tbsp	12	45	0	12	0	0	0	0	0	0.12	0
Sugar-white-powder-sifted	Cup	100	385	0	100	0	0	0	0	0	0.83	3
Vegetables												
Alfalfa seeds-sprouted-raw	Cup	33	10	1.32	1.25	0.23	0	0.023	0.018	0.135	2	26
Artichokes-boil-drain	Item	120	53	2.76	12.4	0.2	0	0.048	0.006	0.086	79	316
Asparagus-froz-boil-spears	Cup	180	50.4	5.31	8.77	0.756	0	0.171	0.023	0.331	7.2	392
Avocado-raw-California	Item	173	306	3.64	12	30	0	4.48	19.4	3.53	21	1097
Beans-baked beans-can	Cup	254	235	12.2	52.1	1.14	0	0.295	0.099	0.493	1008	752
Beans-garbanzo-can	Serving	28.4	27.8	1.31	4.66	0.511	0	0.07	0.17	0.26	113	54.8
Beans-green-froz-French	Cup	135	36	1.84	8.26	0.18	0	0.041	0.007	0.093	17	151
Beans-lima-can	Cup	248	186	11.3	34.4	0.74	0	0.168	0.043	0.358	618	668
Beans-lima-froz-boil-drain	Cup	170	170	10.3	32	0.58	0	0.13	0.034	0.278	90	694
Beans-mung-sprouted-boil	Cup	125	26	2.52	5.2	0.11	0	0.031	0.015	0.04	12	125
Beans-navy pea-dry-ckd	Cup	190	225	15	40	1	0	—	—	—	13	790
Beans-pinto-froz-boil	oz	28.4	46	2.64	8.77	0.135	0	0.017	0.01	0.078	—	—
Beans-red kidney-can	Cup	255	230	15	42	1	0	—	—	—	833	673
Beans-refried beans	Cup	253	270	15.8	46.8	2.7	—	1.04	—	—	1071	994
Beans-shellie-can	Cup	245	75	4.3	15.2	0.47	0	0.056	0.034	0.27	819	268
Beans-snap-green-can-cuts	Cup	135	27	1.55	6	0.135	0	0.03	0.006	0.07	339	147
Beans-snap-green-raw-boil	Cup	125	44	2.36	9.86	0.36	0	0.08	0.014	0.181	4	373
Beans-snap-wax-raw-boil	Cup	125	44	2.36	9.86	0.36	0	0.08	0.014	0.181	4	373
Beans-snap-yellow/wax-can	Cup	136	26	1.56	6.12	0.14	0	0.03	0.006	0.07	340	148
Beets-can-sliced-drain	Cup	170	54	1.56	12.2	0.24	0	0.04	0.048	0.086	479	284
Broccoli-froz-boil-drain	Cup	185	51	5.71	9.85	0.21	0	0.03	0.015	0.101	44	332
Broccoli-raw	Cup	88	24	2.62	4.62	0.3	0	0.048	0.022	0.148	24	286
Broccoli-raw-boil-drain	Cup	155	46	4.64	8.68	0.44	0	0.068	0.032	0.21	16	254
Cabbage-celery-raw	Cup	76	12	0.91	2.46	0.15	0	0.033	0.017	0.055	7	181
Cabbage-common-boil-drain	Cup	145	30.5	1.39	6.92	0.363	0	0.046	0.026	0.173	27.6	297

Mag (mg)	Iron (mg)	Zinc (mg)	VA (RE)	VC (mg)	Thia (mg)	Ribo (mg)	Niac (mg)	VB$_6$ (mg)	Fol (µg)	VB$_{12}$ (µg)	Calc (mg)	Phos (mg)	Sel (mg)	Fibd (g)	VE (mg)
—	0.1	—	0	0	0	0	0	—	—	—	2	0	0.001	0	—
—	0.5	—	0	0	0	0	0	—	—	—	6	2	0.001	0	0.048
—	0.03	—	0	0	0	—	—	—	—	—	0.3	0.1	0	0	—
19	0.56	0.43	9	—	0.03	0.11	0.1	—	—	—	65	78	0.002	—	0.301
—	0.04	—	0	0	0	0	0	—	—	—	0.4	0.2	0	0	—
—	0	—	0	0	0	0	0	—	—	—	0	0	0.001	0	—
—	—	—	—	—	—	—	—	—	—	—	—	—	0.002	—	0.495
—	0.5	—	21	0	0.02	0.12	0.2	—	—	—	65	77	0.001	—	0.308
—	0.4	—	15	0	0.07	0.07	1.4	—	—	—	49	83	0.001	—	0.308
16	0.3	—	24	0	0.02	0.1	0.1	—	1.96	—	65	65	0.001	—	0.196
—	—	—	—	—	—	—	—	—	—	—	—	—	0.002	—	0.66
—	0.56	—	24	0	0.02	0.01	1.3	—	—	—	11	35	0.001	—	—
14.5	0.24	0.24	1	—	0.05	0.03	0.8	—	—	—	14.5	41	0.001	—	0.187
—	—	—	—	—	—	—	—	—	—	—	—	—	0.002	—	0.627
0.63	0.1	0.02	0	0	0	0.01	0.1	0.004	—	0	1	1	0.001	0.06	—
—	3.3	—	174	1	0.06	0.28	0.6	—	—	—	165	305	0.003	—	—
—	2.7	—	0	0	0.05	0.2	0.7	—	—	—	96	218	0.003	—	—
—	0	—	0	0	0	0.03	0	—	—	—	2	2	0.001	0	—
—	0	—	258	0	0	0.06	0	—	—	—	48	38	0.003	0	—
—	0.8	—	0	0	0.02	0.07	0.3	—	—	—	10	50	0.002	—	—
—	0.2	—	0	0	0	0.01	0	0.004	1.6	0	4	2	0	0.2	0.018
—	0.5	0.01	0	0	0	0	0	—	—	—	5	2	0	0	—
—	3.2	—	—	—	0.02	0.04	0.4	0.04	—	0	137	17	0.013	0	0.082
—	0.9	—	—	—	0.01	0.01	0	0.04	—	0	33	9	0.013	0	0.082
—	0	—	0	0	0	0	0	—	—	—	0	—	—	—	—
—	7.5	—	0	0	0.02	0.07	0.4	—	—	—	187	42	0.003	0	—
0	0	0	0	0	0	0	0	0	0	0	0	0	0	—	—
—	—	—	—	—	—	—	—	—	—	—	—	—	0	—	—
—	0	0.006	0	0	0	0	0	—	—	—	0	0	0	0	—
—	0.1	—	0	0	0	0	0	—	—	—	0	0	0.001	0	—
9	0.32	0.3	5.1	2.7	0.025	0.042	0.159	0.011	12.2	0	10	23	—	0.726	—
47	1.62	0.43	17.2	8.9	0.068	0.059	0.709	0.104	53.4	0	47	72	—	4	0.228
23.4	1.15	1	147	43.9	0.117	0.185	1.87	0.036	242	0	41.4	99	0.007	2.16	2.52
70	2.04	0.73	106	13.7	0.187	0.211	3.32	0.484	113	0	19	73	—	6.13	3.66
82	0.74	3.55	43.4	—	0.389	0.152	1.09	0.34	60.7	0	128	264	—	19.6	—
9.37	0.71	0.264	0.568	1.42	0.003	0.011	0.085	—	—	—	11.1	30.1	—	1.4	—
29	1.11	0.84	71.3	11.1	0.065	0.1	0.563	0.076	44.2	0	61	33	0.001	2.16	0.176
84	3.94	1.58	42.3	21.6	0.072	0.106	1.32	0.154	—	0	70	176	0.004	10.4	—
58	2.32	0.74	32.4	21.8	0.12	0.104	1.8	0.208	111	0	38	153	0.001	8.33	0
18	0.81	0.58	1.7	14.1	0.062	0.126	1.01	—	166	0	15	34	—	2.7	—
—	5.1	1.8	0	0	0.27	0.13	1.3	1.06	66.5	0	95	281	0.021	9.31	0.646
—	0.77	—	0	0.19	0.078	0.031	0.18	—	—	0	14.9	—	—	1.39	—
9.94	4.6	1.91	1	7.65	0.13	0.1	1.5	1.12	35.7	0	74	278	0.009	12.5	—
99	4.47	3.45	—	15.2	0.124	0.139	1.23	—	—	—	118	214	—	11.6	—
—	2.43	—	55.9	7.5	0.078	0.132	0.502	—	—	0	72	—	—	12	—
17.5	1.2	0.39	47.1	6.5	0.02	0.075	0.27	0.054	43	0	35	34	0.001	1.76	0.041
32	1.6	0.45	83.3	12.1	0.093	0.121	0.768	0.07	41.6	0	58	46	0.001	2.25	0.025
32	1.6	0.45	83.3	12.1	0.093	0.121	0.768	0.07	41.6	0	58	48	0.001	2.25	0.363
18	1.22	0.4	47.4	6.4	0.02	0.076	0.274	0.057	43	0	36	26	0.001	1.77	0.394
22.1	3.1	0.36	3	5	0.02	0.05	0.2	0.085	40.8	0	32	31	0.001	3.2	0.051
37	1.13	0.56	348	73.7	0.101	0.15	0.843	0.239	104	0	94	101	0.003	7.3	0.851
22	0.78	0.36	136	82	0.058	0.104	0.562	0.14	62.4	0	42	58	0.001	2.46	0.405
94	1.78	0.24	220	98	0.128	0.322	1.18	0.308	107	0	178	74	0.003	4.03	0.713
10	0.23	0.17	91.2	20.5	0.03	0.038	0.304	0.176	59.8	0	58	22	0.002	1.63	0.09
21.8	0.566	0.232	12.5	35.2	0.083	0.08	0.33	0.093	29.4	0	47.9	36.3	0.003	4	2.42

Continued.

Key to Abbreviations

Kcal, Kcalories; *Prot,* protein; *Carb,* carbohydrate; *Fat,* fat; *Chol,* cholesterol; *Safa,* saturated fat; *Mufa,* monounsaturated fat; *Pufa,* polyunsaturated fat; *Sod,* sodium; *Pot,* potassium; *Mag,* magnesium; *Iron,* iron; *Zinc,* zinc; *VA,* vitamin A; *VC,* vitamin C; *Thia,* thiamin; *Ribo,* riboflavin; *Niac,* niacin; *VB₆,* vitamin B₆; *Fol,* folate; *VB₁₂,* vitamin B₁₂; *Calc,* calcium; *Phos,* phosphorus; *Sel,* selenium; *Fibd,* dietary fiber; and *VE,* vitamin E.

Food name	Portion	Wt (g)	Kcal	Prot (g)	Carb (g)	Fat (g)	Chol (mg)	Safa (g)	Mufa (g)	Pufa (g)	Sod (mg)	Pot (mg)
Vegetables—cont'd												
Cabbage-common-raw-shred	Cup	90	21.6	1.09	4.83	0.162	0	0.021	0.012	0.078	16.2	221
Cabbage-red-raw-shred	Cup	70	19	0.97	4.29	0.18	0	0.024	0.013	0.088	7	144
Cabbage-white mustard-boil	Cup	170	20	2.65	3.03	0.27	0	0.036	0.02	0.131	57	630
Cabbage-white mustard-raw	Cup	70	9	1.05	1.53	0.14	0	0.018	0.011	0.067	45	176
Carrot-raw-shred-scraped	Cup	110	48	1.12	11.2	0.2	0	0.034	0.008	0.084	38	356
Carrot-raw-whole-scraped	Item	72	31	0.74	7.3	0.14	0	0.022	0.006	0.055	25	233
Carrots-boil-drain-sliced	Cup	156	70	1.7	16.3	0.28	0	0.054	0.014	0.138	104	354
Carrots-can-sliced-drain	Cup	146	34	0.94	8.08	0.28	0	0.052	0.014	0.134	352	262
Carrots-froz-boil-drain	Cup	146	52	1.73	12	0.16	0	0.031	0.007	0.077	86	230
Cauliflower-froz-boil	Cup	180	34	2.9	6.76	0.39	0	0.06	0.028	0.186	32	250
Cauliflower-raw-boil-drain	Cup	124	30	2.32	5.74	0.22	0	0.046	0.022	0.144	8	400
Cauliflower-raw-chop	Cup	100	24	1.99	4.92	0.18	0	0	0	0	15	355
Celery-Pascal-raw-diced	Cup	120	18	0.8	4.36	0.14	0	0.038	0.028	0.072	106	340
Celery-Pascal-raw-stalk	Item	40	6	0.26	1.45	0.05	0	0.013	0.01	0.024	35	114
Chives-raw-chop	Tbsp	3	1	0.08	0.11	0.02	0	0.003	0.003	0.007	0	8
Collards-froz-boil-drain	Cup	170	61	5.04	12.1	0.69	0	—	—	—	85	427
Collards-raw-boil-drain	Cup	190	27	2.1	5.02	0.29	0	—	—	—	36	177
Corn-froz-boil-kernels	Cup	165	134	4.94	33.7	0.12	0	0.018	0.034	0.056	8	228
Corn-kernels	1 Ear	77	83	2.56	19.3	0.98	0	0.152	0.288	0.464	13	192
Corn-kernels & cob-froz-boil	Item	126	118	3.92	28.1	0.92	0	0.144	0.272	0.438	6	316
Corn-sweet-can-drain	Cup	165	132	4.3	30.5	1.64	0	0.254	0.478	0.772	470	160
Corn-sweet-cream style-can	Cup	256	186	4.46	46.4	1.08	0	0.166	0.314	0.506	730	344
Cowpeas-blackeye-froz-boil	Cup	170	224	14.4	40.4	1.13	0	0.298	0.102	0.476	9	638
Cowpeas-blackeye-raw-boil	Cup	165	179	13.4	29.9	1.32	0	0.345	0.117	0.558	7	693
Cucumber-raw-sliced	Cup	104	14	0.56	3.02	0.14	0	0.034	0.004	0.054	2	156
Eggplant-boil-drain	Cup	96	27	0.8	6.37	0.22	0	0.042	0.019	0.089	3	238
Endive-raw-chop	Cup	50	8	0.62	1.68	0.1	0	0.024	0.002	0.044	12	158
Garlic-raw-clove	Item	3	4	0.19	0.99	0.02	0	0.003	0	0.007	1	12
Leeks-boil-drain	Item	124	38	1.01	9.45	0.25	0	0.033	0.004	0.138	13	108
Lettuce-butterhead-leaves	Slice	15	2	0.19	0.35	0.03	0	0.004	0.001	0.018	1	39
Lettuce-iceberg-raw-chop	Cup	55	7.15	0.556	1.15	0.105	0	0.014	0.003	0.055	4.95	86.9
Lettuce-iceberg-raw-leaves	Piece	20	2.61	0.201	0.418	0.038	0	0.005	0.001	0.02	1.81	31.6
Lettuce-looseleaf-raw	Cup	55	10	0.72	1.96	0.16	0	0.022	0.006	0.09	6	148
Lettuce-Romaine-raw-shred	Cup	56	8	0.9	1.32	0.12	0	0.014	0.004	0.06	4	162
Miso-fermented soybeans	Cup	275	565	32.5	76.9	16.7	0	2.42	3.69	9.43	10030	451
Mushrooms-boil-drain	Item	12	3	0.26	0.62	0.06	0	0.007	0.001	0.022	0	43
Mushrooms-can-drain	Item	12	3	0.22	0.6	0.04	0	0.005	0.001	0.014	—	—
Mushrooms-raw-chop	Cup	70	18	1.46	3.26	0.3	0	0.04	0.004	0.12	2	260
Olives-green-pickled-can	Item	4	3.75	0.1	0.1	0.5	0	0.05	0.35	0.035	80.8	1.75
Olives-mission-rip-can	Item	3	5	0.1	0.1	0.667	0	0.067	0.41	0.034	19.2	0.667
Onions-mature-boil-drain	Cup	210	58	1.9	13.2	0.34	0	0.056	0.048	0.132	16	318
Onions-mature-raw-chop	Cup	160	54	1.88	11.7	0.42	0	0.07	0.06	0.164	4	248
Onion rings-froz-prep-heat	Item	10	40.7	0.534	3.82	2.67	0	0.858	1.09	0.511	37.5	12.9
Onions-young-green	Item	5	1.25	0.087	0.278	0.007	0	0.001	0	0	0.2	12.8
Parsley-raw-chop	Tbsp	4	1.2	0.088	0.276	0.012	0	0	0	0	1.6	21.6
Peas-green-can-drain	Cup	170	118	7.52	21.4	0.58	0	0.106	0.052	0.278	372	294
Peas-green-froz-boil-drain	Cup	160	126	8.24	22.8	0.44	0	0.078	0.038	0.206	140	268
Peas-split-dry-ckd	Cup	200	230	16	42	1	0	—	—	—	8	592
Peppers-hot chili-raw	Cup	150	60	3	14.2	0.3	0	0.032	0.016	0.164	10	510
Peppers-hot-red-dried	Tsp	2	5	0	1	0	0	0	0	0	20	20
Peppers-sweet-green-raw	Cup	226	61.1	2.01	14.6	0.43	0	0.063	0.029	0.231	4.53	401
Peppers-jalapeno-can-chop	Cup	136	33	1.09	6.66	0.82	0	0.084	0.046	0.445	1990	185
Pickle-dill-cucumber-med	Item	65	5	0	1	0	0	0	0	0	928	130
Pickle-fresh pack-cucumber	Item	7.5	5	0	1.5	0	0	0	0	0	50	—
Pickle-sweet/gherkin-small	Item	15	20	0	5	0	0	0	0	0	128	—
Potato chips-salt add	Item	2	10.5	0.128	1.04	0.708	0	0.181	0.125	0.36	9.4	26
Potato skin-baked	Item	58	115	2.49	26.7	0.06	0	0.015	0.001	0.025	12	332

Mag (mg)	Iron (mg)	Zinc (mg)	VA (RE)	VC (mg)	Thia (mg)	Ribo (mg)	Niac (mg)	VB$_6$ (mg)	Fol (µg)	VB$_{12}$ (µg)	Calc (mg)	Phos (mg)	Sel (mg)	Fibd (g)	VE (mg)
13.5	0.504	0.162	113	42.6	0.045	0.027	0.27	0.086	51	0	42.3	20.7	0.002	1.8	1.5
11	0.35	0.15	28	39.9	0.035	0.021	0.21	0.147	14.5	0	36	29	0.002	1.7	0.14
18	1.77	—	437	44.2	0.054	0.107	0.728	—	—	0	158	49	0.004	2.1	1.19
13	0.56	—	210	31.5	0.028	0.049	0.35	—	—	0	74	26	0.002	1.3	0.084
16	0.54	0.22	3094	10.2	0.106	0.064	1.02	0.162	15.4	0	30	48	0.002	3.52	0.484
11	0.36	0.14	2025	6.7	0.07	0.042	0.668	0.106	10.1	0	19	32	0.002	2.3	0.317
20	0.96	0.46	3830	3.6	0.054	0.088	0.79	0.384	21.6	0	48	48	0.002	5.77	0.651
12	0.94	0.38	2011	4	0.026	0.044	0.806	0.164	13.4	0	38	34	0.002	2.19	0.613
14	0.69	0.35	2585	4.1	0.039	0.054	0.639	0.188	15.8	0	41	39	0.003	5.4	0.613
16	0.74	0.24	4	56.4	0.066	0.096	0.558	0.158	73.8	0	30	44	0.001	3.24	0.054
14	0.52	0.3	18	68.6	0.078	0.064	0.684	0.25	63.4	0	34	44	0.001	2.73	0.038
14	0.58	0.18	16	71.5	0.076	0.057	0.633	0.231	66.1	0	29	46	0.001	2.4	0.03
14	0.58	0.2	152	7.6	0.036	0.036	0.36	0.036	10.6	0	44	32	0	1.92	0.432
5	0.19	0.07	51	2.5	0.012	0.012	0.12	0.012	3.6	0	14	10	0	0.64	0.144
2	0.05	—	192	2.4	0.003	0.005	0.021	0.005	—	0	2	2	—	0.096	—
52	1.9	0.46	1017	44.9	0.08	0.196	1.08	0.194	129	0	357	46	0.001	5.2	—
21	0.78	1.22	422	18.6	0.032	0.082	0.448	0.08	12.4	0	148	19	0.001	2.1	—
30	0.5	0.56	408	4.2	0.114	0.12	2.1	0.164	33.4	0	4	78	0.001	3.47	0.05
24	0.47	0.37	167	4.8	0.166	0.055	1.24	0.046	35.7	0	2	79	0.001	6.6	0.056
36	0.78	0.8	266	6	0.22	0.086	1.91	0.282	38.4	0	4	94	0.001	2.65	0.069
28	1.4	0.64	256	7	0.05	0.08	1.5	0.33	59.4	0	8	81	0.001	2.15	0.066
44	0.98	1.36	248	11.8	0.064	0.136	2.46	0.162	115	0	8	130	0.001	3.07	0.102
85	3.6	2.42	128	4.5	0.442	0.109	1.24	0.162	240	0	40	208	—	9.8	0.204
83	2.36	1.3	105	2.6	0.112	0.177	1.77	0.083	173	0	46	197	—	11	0.215
12	0.28	0.24	46	4.8	0.032	0.02	0.312	0.054	14.4	0	14	18	0.001	1.04	0.156
13	0.34	0.14	61	1.3	0.073	0.019	0.576	0.083	13.8	0	5	22	—	2.69	0.029
8	0.42	0.4	103	3.2	0.04	0.038	0.2	0.01	71	0	26	14	—	—	—
1	0.05	—	0	0.9	0.006	0.003	0.021	—	0.1	0	5	5	0	—	0
18	1.36	—	57	5.2	0.032	0.025	0.248	—	30.1	0	37	21	0	3.97	1.14
1.65	0.04	0.03	146	1.2	0.01	0.01	0.045	0.008	11	0	5	4	0	0.15	0.06
4.95	0.275	0.121	182	2.15	0.025	0.017	0.103	0.022	30.8	0	10.5	11	0	0.55	0.22
1.81	0.1	0.044	6.61	0.781	0.009	0.006	0.037	0.008	11.2	0	3.81	4	0	0.2	0.08
6	0.78	0.121	106	10	0.028	0.044	0.224	0.03	76	0	38	14	0	0.76	0.22
4	0.62	—	146	13.4	0.056	0.056	0.28	—	76	0	20	26	0	0.952	0.224
116	7.52	9.13	24	0	0.267	0.688	2.37	0.591	90.8	0.57	183	420	—	9.9	—
1	0.21	0.1	0	0.5	0.009	0.036	0.535	0.011	2.2	0	1	10	0.001	0.264	0.01
—	0.1	0.09	0	—	—	—	—	—	1.5	0	—	—	0.005	0.216	0.01
8	0.86	0.344	0	2.4	0.072	0.314	2.88	0.068	14.8	0	4	72	0.009	0.91	0.056
—	0.05	—	1	—	—	—	—	—	0.04	0	2	0.5	0	0.104	—
—	0.033	0.01	1	—	0	0	—	0	0.033	0	3	0.333	0	0.09	—
22	0.42	0.38	0	12	0.088	0.016	0.168	0.378	26.6	0	58	48	0.007	1.68	0.252
16	0.58	0.28	0	13.4	0.096	0.016	0.16	0.252	31.8	0	40	46	0.003	2.64	0.496
1.9	0.169	0.042	2.25	0.14	0.028	0.014	0.361	0.008	1.3	0	3.1	8.1	—	0.382	0.069
1	0.095	0.022	25	2.25	0.004	0.007	0.001	—	0.685	0	3	1.65	0	0.12	0.006
1.6	0.248	0.028	208	3.6	0.003	0.004	0.028	0.006	7.32	0	5.2	1.6	0	0.176	0.07
30	1.62	1.2	131	16.2	0.206	0.132	1.24	0.108	75.4	0	34	114	0.001	6.97	0.034
46	2.52	1.5	107	15.8	0.452	0.16	2.37	0.18	93.8	0	38	144	0.001	6.08	0.192
—	3.4	2.1	8	—	0.3	0.18	1.8	—	—	—	22	178	0.003	10.5	0.18
38	1.8	0.46	116	364	0.136	0.136	1.43	0.418	35	0	26	68	—	3.55	1.03
3.4	0.3	0.054	130	0	0	0.02	0.2	—	—	0	5	4	0	0.685	—
22.6	1.04	0.272	143	202	0.149	0.068	1.15	0.561	49.8	0	20.4	43	—	4.19	1.56
16	3.81	0.26	231	17.7	0.041	0.068	0.68	—	—	0	35	23	0	—	—
7.8	0.7	0.176	7	4	0	0.01	0	0.005	0.65	0	17	14	0	0.78	—
—	0.15	0.02	1	0.5	0	0	0	0.001	0.075	0	2.5	2	0	0.09	—
0.15	0.2	0.02	1	1	0	0	0	0.001	0.15	0	2	2	0	0.165	—
1.2	0.024	0.021	0	0.83	0.003	0	0.084	0.01	0.9	0	0.5	3.1	0	0.029	0.085
25	4.08	0.28	—	7.8	0.071	0.061	1.78	0.356	12.5	0	20	59	—	3.02	—

Continued.

Key to Abbreviations
Kcal, Kcalories; *Prot,* protein; *Carb,* carbohydrate; *Fat,* fat; *Chol,* cholesterol; *Safa,* saturated fat; *Mufa,* monounsaturated fat; *Pufa,* polyunsaturated fat; *Sod,* sodium; *Pot,* potassium; *Mag,* magnesium; *Iron,* iron; *Zinc,* zinc; *VA,* vitamin A; *VC,* vitamin C; *Thia,* thiamin; *Ribo,* riboflavin; *Niac,* niacin; *VB₆,* vitamin B₆; *Fol,* folate; *VB₁₂,* vitamin B₁₂; *Calc,* calcium; *Phos,* phosphorus; *Sel,* selenium; *Fibd,* dietary fiber; and *VE,* vitamin E.

Food name	Portion	Wt (g)	Kcal	Prot (g)	Carb (g)	Fat (g)	Chol (mg)	Safa (g)	Mufa (g)	Pufa (g)	Sod (mg)	Pot (mg)
Vegetables—cont'd												
Potato-Au Gratin-home rec	Cup	245	322	12.4	27.6	18.6	58	11.6	5.27	0.676	1060	970
Potato-french fried-froz	Item	5	11.1	0.173	1.7	0.438	0	0.208	0.178	0.033	1.5	22.9
Potato-french fried-raw	Item	5	13.5	0.2	1.8	0.7	0	0.17	0.178	0.033	11.1	42.7
Potato-hash brown-prep-raw	Cup	156	326	3.77	33.3	21.7	—	8.48	9.69	2.5	38	501
Potato-hash brown-froz	Cup	156	340	4.92	43.8	17.9	0	7.01	8.01	2.07	54	680
Potato-mashed-dehy-prep	Cup	210	166	4.2	27.5	4.62	4	1.43	1.35	1.33	491	704
Potato-mashed-milk/butter	Cup	210	222	3.95	35.1	8.87	4	2.17	3.72	2.54	619	607
Potato-scallop-home rec	Cup	245	210	7.03	26.4	9.02	29	5.53	2.55	0.407	821	925
Potato-scallop-mix-prep	oz	28.4	26.4	0.602	3.63	1.22	—	0.748	0.344	0.055	96.8	57.7
Pumpkin pie mix-can	Cup	270	282	2.93	71.3	0.34	0	0.176	0.043	0.019	561	372
Radishes-raw	Item	4.5	0.7	0.027	0.161	0.024	0	0.001	0.001	0.002	1.1	10.4
Rutabagas-boil-drain	Cup	170	58	1.88	13.2	0.32	0	0.042	0.04	0.142	30	488
Sauerkraut-can	Cup	236	44	2.15	10.1	0.33	0	0.083	0.031	0.144	1561	401
Seaweed-wakame-raw	oz	28.4	12.8	0.86	2.6	0.182	0	0.037	0.016	0.062	248	14.2
Soybean-dry-ckd	Cup	180	234	19.8	19.4	10.3	0	—	—	—	4	972
Spinach-can-solids/liquids	Cup	234	44	4.93	6.84	0.87	0	0.14	0.023	0.363	747	539
Spinach-froz-boil-chop	Cup	205	57.4	6.44	10.9	0.431	0	0.068	0.012	0.176	176	611
Spinach-raw-boil-drain	Cup	180	41	5.35	6.75	0.47	0	0.076	0.013	0.194	126	838
Spinach-raw-chop	Cup	56	12	1.6	1.96	0.2	0	0.032	0.006	0.082	44	312
Squash-acorn-baked	Cup	205	115	2.29	29.9	0.29	0	0.059	0.021	0.121	9	896
Squash-butternut-baked	Cup	205	83	1.84	21.5	0.18	0	0.039	0.014	0.078	7	583
Squash-hubbard-boil-mash	Cup	236	70	3.5	15.2	0.88	0	0.179	0.066	0.368	12	504
Squash-summer-boil-sliced	Cup	180	36	1.63	7.76	0.56	0	0.115	0.041	0.236	2	346
Squash-winter-bake-mashed	Cup	205	79	1.81	17.9	1.29	0	0.267	0.096	0.543	3	895
Squash-zucchini-froz-boil	Cup	223	37	2.56	7.94	0.29	0	0.06	0.022	0.123	5	434
Squash-zucchini-italia-can	Cup	227	65	2.33	15.6	0.25	0	0.052	0.018	0.107	850	622
Squash-zucchini-raw-boil	Cup	180	28	1.14	7.08	0.1	0	0.018	0.008	0.038	4	456
Squash-zucchini-raw-sliced	Cup	130	19	1.5	3.78	0.18	0	0.038	0.014	0.078	3	322
Succotash-boil-drain	Cup	192	222	9.73	46.8	1.53	0	0.284	0.298	0.732	32	787
Sweet potato-bake-peel	Item	114	118	1.96	27.7	0.13	0	0.027	0.005	0.056	12	397
Sweet potato-boil-mashed	Cup	328	344	5.4	79.6	0.97	0	0.21	0.036	0.433	42	602
Sweet potato-can-mashed	Cup	255	258	5.05	59.2	0.51	0	0.11	0.02	0.227	191	536
Sweet potato-candied	Piece	105	144	0.91	29.3	3.41	0	1.42	0.658	0.154	73	198
Tofu-soybean curd	Piece	120	86	9.4	2.9	5	0	—	—	—	8	50
Tomato juice-can	Cup	244	42	1.86	10.3	0.14	0	0.02	0.022	0.058	882	536
Tomato juice-low sodium	Cup	244	42	1.86	10.3	0.14	0	0.01	0.022	0.058	24.4	536
Tomato paste-can-low sodium	Cup	262	220	9.9	49.3	2.33	0	0.332	0.351	0.948	172	2442
Tomato paste-can-salt add	Cup	262	220	9.9	49.3	2.33	0	0.332	0.351	0.948	2070	2442
Tomato powder	oz	28.4	85.8	3.67	21.2	0.125	0	0.018	0.019	0.05	38.1	547
Tomato puree-can-low sodium	Cup	250	102	4.18	25.1	0.29	0	0.04	0.043	0.118	49	1051
Tomato puree-can-salt add	Cup	250	102	4.18	25.1	0.29	0	0.04	0.043	0.118	998	1051
Tomato-can-low sodium-diet	Cup	240	47	2.24	10.3	0.59	0	0.084	0.089	0.238	31.2	529
Tomato-raw-red-rip	Item	123	24	1.09	5.34	0.26	0	0.037	0.039	0.107	10	254
Tomato-red-can-stewed	Cup	255	68	2.37	16.5	0.36	58	0.051	0.054	0.148	647	611
Tomato-red-can-whole	Cup	240	47	2.24	10.3	0.59	0	0.084	0.089	0.238	390	529
Tomato-red-raw-boil	Cup	240	60	2.68	13.5	0.65	0	0.091	0.096	0.262	25	624
Tomato-stew-cook-home rec	Cup	101	59	1.77	10.4	2.21	0	0.4	0.701	0.447	374	170
V-8 veg juice-low sodium	Cup	243	51	0	9.72	0	0	0	0	0	58.3	571
Vegetable juice-can	Cup	242	44	1.52	11	0.22	0	0.032	0.034	0.092	884	468
Vegetables-mixed-froz-boil	Cup	182	108	5.22	23.8	0.28	0	0.056	0.018	0.132	64	308

Mag (mg)	Iron (mg)	Zinc (mg)	VA (RE)	VC (mg)	Thia (mg)	Ribo (mg)	Niac (mg)	VB$_6$ (mg)	Fol (µg)	VB$_{12}$ (µg)	Calc (mg)	Phos (mg)	Sel (mg)	Fibd (g)	VE (mg)
48	1.56	1.69	64.6	24.3	0.157	0.284	2.43	0.426	19.9	0.492	292	278	—	4.41	—
1.1	0.067	0.021	0	0.55	0.006	0.002	0.115	0.012	0.83	0	0.4	4.3	0	0.16	0.01
—	0.07	—	0	1.1	0.007	0.004	0.16	0.009	1.1	0	0.8	5.6	0	0.16	0.01
32	1.27	0.46	—	8.9	0.115	0.031	3.12	0.434	12	0	13	65	—	3.12	—
26	2.34	0.5	—	9.8	0.174	0.032	3.78	0.196	38.8	0	24	112	0.001	1.5	0.295
—	1.26	—	18.9	6.3	0.063	0.105	1.68	—	—	—	65	92	0.001	1.2	—
37	0.55	0.58	35.5	12.9	0.176	0.084	2.27	0.47	16.7	0	54	97	0.001	3.15	0.084
46	1.41	0.98	33.2	26.1	0.169	0.225	2.58	0.436	21.3	0.348	140	154	—	4.41	—
3.98	0.108	0.071	—	0.937	0.005	0.016	0.292	0.012	0.312	—	10.2	15.9	—	0.54	—
43	2.87	0.72	2241	9.5	0.043	0.319	1.01	—	—	0	99	120	—	—	—
0.4	0.013	0.013	0.03	1.03	0	0.002	0.014	0.003	1.22	0	0.9	0.8	0	0.1	—
36	0.8	0.52	0	37.2	0.122	0.062	1.07	0.154	26.4	0	72	84	—	2.5	0.255
31	3.47	0.44	4.2	34.8	0.05	0.052	0.337	0.307	7.05	0	72	46	0.024	6.06	—
30.4	0.619	0.108	10.2	0.852	0.017	0.065	0.454	—	—	0	42.6	22.7	0.001	1.2	—
—	4.9	—	5	0	0.38	0.16	1.1	—	—	—	131	322	—	—	—
132	3.7	0.99	1505	31.6	0.042	0.248	0.634	0.187	136	0	195	74	0.003	5.08	0.047
141	3.12	1.44	1596	25.2	0.123	0.344	0.859	0.299	220	0	299	98.4	0.002	4.51	3.85
157	6.42	1.37	1474	17.7	0.171	0.425	0.882	0.436	262	0	244	100	0.002	3.96	3.38
44	1.52	0.3	376	15.8	0.044	0.106	0.406	0.11	108	0	56	28	0.001	1.46	1.03
87	1.91	0.35	87.3	22.1	0.342	0.027	1.81	0.398	38.4	0	90	93	0.002	4.3	0.246
59	1.22	0.27	1435	30.9	0.148	0.035	1.99	0.254	39.3	0	84	55	0.002	3.5	0.246
32	0.67	0.22	945	15.4	0.099	0.066	0.788	0.243	23	0	23	33	0.002	4.2	0.283
44	0.64	0.71	51.7	10	0.079	0.074	0.923	0.117	36.2	0	48	69	0.006	2.52	0.216
16	0.67	0.54	729	19.7	0.174	0.049	1.44	0.148	57.4	0	28	41	0.006	5.74	0.246
28	1.08	0.44	96.2	8.2	0.091	0.089	0.861	0.1	17.5	0	38	55	0.007	3.23	0.268
31	1.55	0.58	123	5.2	0.095	0.091	1.2	—	—	0	38	66	—	7.02	—
38	0.64	0.32	43.2	8.4	0.074	0.074	0.77	0.14	30.2	0	24	72	0.006	2.3	0.216
28	0.55	0.26	44.2	11.7	0.091	0.039	0.52	0.116	28.8	0	20	42	0.004	2	0.156
102	2.93	1.22	56.4	15.7	0.323	0.184	2.55	0.223	—	0	32	224	—	14	—
23	0.52	0.33	2488	28	0.083	0.145	0.689	0.275	25.7	0	32	62	0.001	3.42	5.2
32	1.83	0.87	5594	55.9	0.174	0.459	2.1	0.8	36.3	0	70	88	0.022	9.84	15
61	3.39	0.54	3857	13.3	0.069	0.23	2.44	0.168	—	0	76	133	0.002	4.59	—
12	1.19	0.16	440	7	0.019	0.044	0.414	0.043	12	0.032	27	27	0.001	1.1	—
—	2.3	—	0	0	0.07	0.04	0.1	—	—	—	154	151	0.002	1.44	—
28	1.42	0.36	136	44.6	0.114	0.076	1.64	0.27	48.4	0	20	46	0.001	2.9	0.535
28	1.42	0.36	136	44.6	0.114	0.076	1.64	0.27	48.4	0	20	46	0.001	2.8	0.537
134	7.83	2.1	647	111	0.406	0.498	8.44	0.996	—	0	91.7	207	0.003	11.3	—
134	7.83	2.1	647	111	0.406	0.498	8.44	0.996	—	0	91.7	207	0.003	11.3	—
50.6	1.3	0.486	490	33.1	0.259	0.216	2.59	0.13	34.1	0	47.1	83.8	—	—	—
60	2.32	0.54	340	88.2	0.178	0.135	4.29	0.38	—	0	37	99	0.003	5.75	0.55
60	2.32	0.54	340	88.2	0.178	0.135	4.29	0.38	—	0	37	99	0.003	5.75	0.55
29	1.45	0.38	145	36.3	0.108	0.074	1.76	0.216	—	0	63	46	0.002	1.69	0.528
14	0.59	0.13	139	21.6	0.074	0.062	0.738	0.059	11.5	0	8	29	0.001	1.6	0.418
29	1.86	0.42	142	33.8	0.117	0.089	1.82	—	7.4	0	84	51	0.002	2.04	0.561
29	1.45	0.38	145	36.3	0.108	0.074	1.76	0.216	7	0	63	46	0.002	1.93	0.53
33	1.44	0.32	325	50.3	0.17	0.144	1.72	0.086	22.6	0	20	70	0.001	1.92	0.816
13	0.78	0.17	102	14.8	0.067	0.064	0.75	0.031	9.9	0	19	32	0.001	1.04	0.343
—	1.46	—	437	53	0.049	0.073	1.94	—	—	—	38.9	—	0.001	2.7	—
26	1.02	0.48	283	67	0.104	0.068	1.76	0.339	—	0	26	40	0.001	2.7	—
40	1.5	0.9	1360	5.8	0.13	0.218	1.55	0.134	34.6	0	44	92	0.001	4.19	—

Continued.

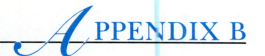

APPENDIX B

Cholesterol Content of Foods

	Amount of cholesterol		
Item	100 g edible portion* (mg)	Edible portion of 450 g (1 lb) as purchased (mg)	Refuse from item as purchased (%)
Beef, raw			
With bone†	70	270	15
Without bone†	70	320	0
Brains, raw	>2000	>9000	0
Butter	250	1135	0
Caviar or fish roe	>300	>1300	0
Cheese			
Cheddar	100	455	0
Cottage, creamed	15	70	0
Cream	120	545	0
Other (25%-30% fat)	85	385	0
Cheese spread	65	295	0
Chicken, flesh only, raw	60	—	0
Crab			
In shell†	125	270	52
Meat only†	125	565	0
Egg, whole	550	2200	12
Egg white	0	0	0
Egg yolk			
Fresh	1500	6800	0
Frozen	1280	5800	0
Dried	2950	13,380	0
Fish			
Steak†	70	265	16
Fillet†	70	320	0
Heart, raw	150	680	0
Ice cream	45	205	0
Kidney, raw	375	1700	0
Lamb, raw			
With bone†	70	265	16
Without bone†	70	320	0
Lard and other animal fat	95	430	0
Liver, raw	300	1360	0
Lobster			
Whole†	200	235	74
Meat only†	200	900	0
Margarine			
All vegetable fat	0	0	0
Two-thirds animal fat, one-third vegetable fat	65	295	0

From Watt, BK, Merrill, AL: *Composition of foods—raw, processed, prepared,* U.S. Department of Agriculture, Agriculture Handbook No 8, Dec 1963.   *Continued.*

*Data apply to 100 g of edible portion of the item, although it may be purchased with the refuse indicated and described or implied in the first column.
†Items that have the same chemical composition for the edible portion but differ in the amount of refuse.

Item	Amount of cholesterol		Refuse from item as purchased (%)
	100 g edible portion* (mg)	Edible portion of 450 g (1 lb) as purchased (mg)	
Milk			
Fluid, whole	11	50	0
Dried, whole	85	385	0
Fluid, skim	3	15	0
Mutton			
With bone†	65	250	16
Without bone†	65	295	0
Oysters			
In shell†	>200	>90	90
Meat only†	>200	>900	0
Pork			
With bone†	70	260	18
Without bone†	70	320	0
Shrimp			
In shell†	125	390	31
Flesh only†	125	565	0
Sweetbreads (thymus)	250	1135	0
Veal			
With bone†	90	320	21
Without bone†	90	410	0

*A*PPENDIX C

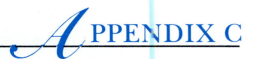

Dietary Fiber in Selected Plant Foods

Food	Amount	Weight (g)	Total dietary fiber (g)	Noncellulose polysaccharides (g)	Cellulose (g)	Lignin
Apple	1 med					
Flesh		138	1.96	1.29	0.66	0.01
Skin		100	3.71	2.21	1.01	0.49
Banana	1 small	119	2.08	1.33	0.44	0.31
Beans						
Baked	1 cup	255	18.53	14.45	3.59	0.48
Green, cooked	1 cup	125	4.19	2.31	1.61	0.26
Bread						
White	1 slice	25	0.68	0.50	0.18	Trace
Whole meal	1 slice	25	2.13	1.49	0.33	0.31
Broccoli, cooked	1 cup	155	6.36	4.53	1.78	0.05
Brussels sprouts, cooked	1 cup	155	4.43	3.08	1.24	0.11
Cabbage, cooked	1 cup	145	4.10	2.55	1.00	0.55
Carrots, cooked	1 cup	155	5.74	3.44	2.29	Trace
Cauliflower, cooked	1 cup	125	2.25	0.84	1.41	Trace
Cereals						
All-Bran	1 oz	30	8.01	5.35	1.80	0.86
Corn Flakes	1 cup	25	2.75	1.82	0.61	0.33
Grapenuts	¼ cup	30	2.10	1.54	0.38	0.17
Puffed Wheat	1 cup	15	2.31	1.55	0.39	0.37
Rice Krispies	1 cup	30	1.34	1.04	0.23	0.07
Shredded Wheat	1 biscuit	25	3.07	2.20	0.66	0.21
Special K	1 cup	30	1.64	1.10	0.22	0.32
Cherries	10 cherries	68	0.84	0.63	0.17	0.05
Cookies						
Ginger	4 snaps	28	0.56	0.41	0.08	0.07
Oatmeal	4 cookies	52	2.08	1.64	0.21	0.22
Plain	4 cookies	48	0.80	0.68	0.05	0.06
Corn	1 cup	165	7.82	7.11	0.51	0.20
Canned	1 cup	165	9.39	8.20	1.06	0.13
Flour						
Bran	1 cup	100	44.00	32.70	8.05	3.23
White	1 cup	115	3.62	2.90	0.69	0.03
Whole meal	1 cup	120	11.41	7.50	2.95	0.96
Grapefruit	½ cup	100	0.44	0.34	0.04	0.06
Jam, strawberry	1 tbsp	20	0.22	0.17	0.02	0.03
Lettuce	¼ head	100	1.53	0.47	1.06	Trace
Marmalade, orange	1 tbsp	20	0.14	0.13	0.01	Trace
Onions, raw, sliced	1 cup	100	2.10	1.55	0.55	Trace
Orange	1 cup	200	0.58	0.44	0.08	0.06
Parsnips, raw, diced	1 cup	100	4.90	3.77	1.13	Trace
Peach, flesh and skin	1 med	100	2.28	1.46	0.20	0.62
Peanuts	1 oz	30	2.79	1.92	0.51	0.36
Peanut butter	1 tbsp	16	1.21	0.90	0.31	Trace

Adapted from Southgate, DAT, et al: A guide to calculating intakes of dietary fiber, *J Hum Nutr* 30:303, 1976.

Continued.

Food	Amount	Weight (g)	Total dietary fiber (g)	Noncellulose polysaccharides (g)	Cellulose (g)	Lignin
Pear	1 med					
Flesh		164	4.00	2.16	1.10	0.74
Skin		100	8.59	3.72	2.18	2.67
Peas, canned	1 cup	170	13.35	8.84	3.91	0.60
Peas, raw or frozen	1 cup	100	7.75	5.48	2.09	0.18
Plums	1 plum	66	1.00	0.65	0.15	0.20
Potato, raw	1 med	135	4.73	3.36	1.38	Trace
Raisins	1 oz	30	1.32	0.72	0.25	0.35
Strawberries	1 cup •	149	2.65	1.39	1.04	0.22
Tomato						
Raw	1 med	135	1.89	0.88	0.61	0.41
Canned, drained	1 cup	240	2.04	1.08	0.89	0.07
Turnips, raw	1 med	100	2.20	1.50	0.70	Trace

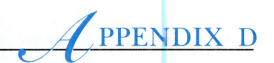

APPENDIX D

Sodium and Potassium Content of Foods, 100 g, Edible Portion

Food and description	Sodium (mg)	Potassium (mg)
Almonds		
Dried	4	773
Roasted and salted	198	773
Apple brown betty	153	100
Apple butter	2	252
Apple juice, canned or bottled	1	101
Apples		
Raw, pared	1	110
Frozen, sliced, sweetened	14	68
Applesauce, canned, sweetened	2	65
Apricot nectar, canned (approx. 40% fruit)	Trace	151
Apricots		
Raw	1	281
Canned, syrup pack, light	1	239
Dried, sulfured, cooked, fruit, and liquid	8	318
Asparagus		
Cooked spears, boiled, drained	1	183
Canned spears, green		
Regular pack, solids and liquid	236[1]	166
Special dietary pack (low sodium), solids and liquid	3	166
Frozen		
Cuts and tips, cooked, boiled, drained	1	220
Spears, cooked, boiled, drained	1	238
Avocados, raw, all commercial varieties	4	604
Bacon, cured, cooked, broiled or fried, drained	1021	236
Bacon, Canadian, cooked, broiled or fried, drained	2555	432
Baking powders		
Home use		
Straight phosphate	8220	170
Special low-sodium preparations	6	10,948
Bananas, raw, common	1	370
Barbecue sauce	815	174
Bass, black sea, raw	68	256
Beans, common, mature seeds, dry		
White		
Cooked	7	416
Canned, solids and liquid, with pork and tomato sauce	463	210
Red, cooked	3	340
Beans, lima		
Immature seeds		
Cooked, boiled, drained	1	422
Canned		
Regular pack, solids and liquid	236[1]	222

Numbers in parentheses denote values imputed, usually from another form of the food or from a similar food. Dashes denote lack of reliable data for a constituent believed to be present in measurable amount. Values are selected from Watt, BK, Merrill, AL: *Composition of foods—raw, processed, prepared,* U.S. Department of Agriculture, Agriculture Handbook No 8, Dec 1963.

For notes see p. A-53. *Continued.*

Food and description	Sodium (mg)	Potassium (mg)
Special dietary pack (low sodium), solids and liquid	4	222
Frozen, thin-seeded types, commonly called baby limas, cooked, boiled, drained	129	394
Mature seeds, dry, cooked	2	612
Beans, mung, sprouted seeds, cooked, boiled, drained	4	156
Beans, snap		
Green		
Cooked, boiled, drained	4	151
Canned		
Regular pack, solids and liquid	236[1]	95
Special dietary pack (low sodium), solids and liquid	2	95
Frozen, cut, cooked, boiled, drained	1	152
Yellow or wax		
Cooked, boiled, drained	3	151
Canned		
Regular pack, solids and liquid	236[1]	95
Special dietary pack (low sodium), solids and liquid	2	95
Frozen, cut, cooked, boiled, drained	1	164
Beans and frankfurters, canned	539	262
Beef		
Retail cuts, trimmed to retail level		
Round	60	370
Rump	60	370
Hamburger, regular ground, cooked	47	450
Beef and vegetable stew, canned	411	174
Beef, corned, boneless		
Cooked, medium fat	1740	150
Canned corned-beef hash (with potato)	540	200
Beef, dried, cooked, creamed	716	153
Beef potpie, commercial, frozen, unheated	366	93
Beet greens, common, cooked, boiled, drained	76	332
Beets, common, red		
Canned		
Regular pack, solids and liquid	236[1]	167
Special dietary pack (low sodium), solids and liquid	46	167
Beverages, alcoholic		
Beer, alcohol 4.5% by volume (3.6% by weight)	7	25
Gin, rum, vodka, whisky		
80 proof (33.4% alcohol by weight)	1	2
86 proof (36.0% alcohol by weight)	1	2
90 proof (37.9% alcohol by weight)	1	2
94 proof (39.7% alcohol by weight)	1	2
100 proof (42.5% alcohol by weight)	1	2
Wines		
Dessert, alcohol 18.8% by volume (15.3% by weight)	4	75
Table, alcohol 12.2% by volume (9.9% by weight)	5	92
Biscuit dough, commercial, frozen	910	86
Biscuit mix, with enriched flour, and biscuits baked from mix		
Dry form	1300	80
Made with milk	973	116
Biscuits, baking powder, made with enriched flour	626	117
Blackberries, including dewberries, boysenberries, and youngberries, raw	1	170
Blackberries, canned, solids and liquid		
Water pack, with or without artificial sweetener	1	115
Syrup pack, heavy	1	109
Blueberries		
Raw	1	81
Frozen, not thawed, sweetened	1	66
Bluefish, cooked		
Baked or broiled	104	—
Fried	146	—
Boston brown bread	251	292
Bouillon cubes or powder	24,000	100
Boysenberries, frozen, not thawed, sweetened	1	105
Bran, added sugar and malt extract	1060	1070
Bran flakes (40% bran), added thiamine	925	—

For notes see p. A-53.

Food and description	Sodium (mg)	Potassium (mg)
Bran flakes with raisins, added thiamine	800	—
Brazil nuts	1	715
Bread crumbs, dry, grated	736	152
Bread stuffing mix and stuffings prepared from mix, dry form	1331	172
Breads		
Cracked wheat	529	134
French or Vienna, enriched	580	90
Italian, enriched	585	74
Raisin	365	233
Rye, American (⅓ rye, ⅔ clear flour)	557	145
White enriched, made with 3%-4% nonfat dry milk	507	105
Whole wheat, made with 2% nonfat dry milk	527	273
Broccoli		
Cooked spears, boiled, drained	10	267
Frozen, spears, cooked, boiled, drained	12	220
Brussels sprouts, frozen, cooked, boiled, drained	14	295
Buffalo fish, raw	52	293
Bulgur (parboiled wheat), canned, made from hard red winter wheat		
Unseasoned[2]	599	87
Seasoned[3]	460	112
Butter[4]	987	23
Buttermilk, fluid, cultured (made from skim milk)	130	140
Cabbage		
Common varieties (Danish, domestic, and pointed types)		
Raw	20	233
Cooked, boiled until tender, drained, shredded, cooked in small amount of water	14	163
Red, raw	26	268
Cabbage, Chinese (also called celery cabbage or petsai)	23	253
Cakes		
Baked from home recipes		
Angle food	283	88
Fruit cake, made with enriched flour, dark	158	496
Gingerbread, made with enriched flour	237	454
Plain cake or cupcake, without icing	300	79
Pound, modified	178	78
Frozen, commercial, devil's food, with chocolate icing	420	119
Candy		
Caramels, plain or chocolate	226	192
Chocolate, sweet	33	269
Chocolate coated, chocolate fudge	228	193
Gum drops, starch jelly pieces	35	5
Hard	32	4
Marshmallows	39	6
Peanut bars	10	448
Carp, raw	50	286
Carrots		
Raw	47	341
Canned		
Regular pack, solids and liquid	236[1]	120
Special dietary pack (low sodium), solids and liquid	39	120
Cashew nuts	15[5]	464
Catfish, freshwater, raw	60	330
Cauliflower		
Cooked, boiled, drained	9	206
Frozen, cooked, boiled, drained	10	207
Caviar, sturgeon, granular	2200	180
Celery, all, including green and yellow varieties		
Raw	126	341
Cooked, boiled, drained	88	239
Chard, Swiss, cooked, boiled, drained	86	321
Cheese straws	721	63
Cheeses		
Natural cheeses		
Cheddar (domestic type, commonly called American)	700	82

Food and description	Sodium (mg)	Potassium (mg)
Cottage (large or small curd)		
Creamed	229	85
Uncreamed	290	72
Cream	250	74
Parmesan	734	149
Swiss (domestic)	710	104
Pasteurized process cheese, American	1136[6]	80
Pasteurized process cheese spread, American	1625[6]	240
Cherries		
Raw, sweet	2	191
Canned		
Sour, red, solids and liquid, water pack	2	130
Sweet, solids and liquid, syrup pack, light	1	128
Frozen, not thawed, sweetened	2	130
Chicken, all classes		
Light meat without skin, cooked, roasted	64	411
Dark meat without skin, cooked, roasted	86	321
Chicken potpie, commercial, frozen, unheated	411	153
Chicory, Witloof (also called French or Belgian endive), bleached head (forced), raw	7	182
Chili con carne, canned, with beans	531	233
Chocolate, bitter or baking	4	830
Chocolate syrup, fudge type	89	284
Chop suey, with meat, canned	551	138
Chow mein, chicken (without noodles), canned	290	167
Citron, candied	290	120
Clams, raw		
Soft, meat only	36	235
Hard or round, meat only	205	311
Clams, canned, including hard, soft, razor, and unspecified solids and liquid	—	140
Cocoa and chocolate-flavored beverage powders		
Cocoa powder with nonfat dry milk	525	800
Mix for hot chocolate	382	605
Cocoa, dry powder, high-fat or breakfast		
Plain	6	1522
Processed with alkali	717	651
Coconut cream (liquid expressed from grated coconut meat)	4	324
Coconut meat, fresh	23	256
Cod		
Cooked, broiled	110	407
Dehydrated, lightly salted	8100	160
Coffee, instant, water-soluble solids		
Dry powder	72	3256
Beverage	1	36
Coleslaw, made with French dressing (commercial)	268	205
Collards, cooked, boiled, drained, leaves, including stems, cooked in small amount of water	25	234
Cookie dough, plain, chilled in roll, baked	548	48
Cookies		
Assorted, packaged, commercial	365	67
Butter, thin, rich	418	60
Gingersnaps	571	462
Molasses	386	138
Oatmeal with raisins	162	370
Sandwich type	483	38
Vanilla wafer	252	72
Corn, sweet		
Cooked, boiled, drained, white and yellow, kernels, cut off cob before cooking	Trace	165
Canned		
Regular pack, cream style, white and yellow, solids and liquid	236[1]	(97)
Special dietary pack (low sodium), cream style, white and yellow, solids and liquid	2	(97)
Frozen, kernels cut off cob, cooked, boiled, drained	1	184
Corn fritters	477	133
Corn grits, degermed, enriched, dry form	1	80

For notes see p. A-53.

Food and description	Sodium (mg)	Potassium (mg)
Corn products used mainly as ready-to-eat breakfast cereals		
Corn flakes, added nutrients	1005	120
Corn, puffed, added nutrients	1060	—
Corn, rice, and wheat flakes, mixed, added nutrients	950	—
Cornbread, baked from home recipes, southern style, made with degermed corn-meal, enriched	591	157
Cornbread mix and cornbread baked from mix, cornbread, made with egg, milk	744	127
Cornmeal, white or yellow, degermed, enriched, dry form	1	120
Cornstarch	Trace	Trace
Cowpeas, including blackeye peas		
Immature seeds, canned, solids and liquid	236[1]	352
Young pods, with seeds, cooked, boiled, drained	3	196
Crab, canned	1000	110
Crackers		
Butter	1092	113
Graham, plain	670	384
Saltines	(1100)	(120)
Sandwich type, peanut-cheese	992	226
Soda	1100	120
Cranberries, raw	2	82
Cranberry juice cocktail, bottled (approx. 33% cranberry juice)	1	10
Cranberry sauce, sweetened, canned, strained	1	30
Cream, fluid, light, coffee, or table, 20% fat	43	122
Cream substitutes, dried, containing cream, skim milk (calcium reduced), and lac-tose	575	—
Cream puffs with custard filling	83	121
Cress, garden, raw	14	606
Croaker, Atlantic, cooked, baked	120	323
Cucumbers, raw, pared	6	160
Custard, baked	79	146
Dates, domestic, natural and dry	1	648
Doughnuts, cake type	501	90
Duck, domesticated, raw, flesh only	74	285
Eggplant, cooked, boiled, drained	1	150
Eggs, chicken		
Raw		
Whole, fresh and frozen	122	129
Whites, fresh and frozen	146	139
Yolks, fresh	52	98
Endive (curly endive and escarole), raw	14	294
Farina		
Enriched		
Regular		
Dry form	2	83
Cooked	144	9
Quick-cooking, cooked	165	10
Instant-cooking, cooked	188	13
Nonenriched, regular, dry form	2	83
Figs, canned, solids and liquid, syrup pack, light	2	152
Flatfishes (flounders, soles, sand dabs), raw	78	342
Fruit cocktail, canned, solids and liquid, water pack, with or without artificial sweet-ener	5	168
Garlic, cloves, raw	19	529
Ginger root, fresh	6	264
Gizzard, chicken, all classes, cooked, simmered	57	211
Goose, domesticated, flesh only, cooked, roasted	124	605
Gooseberries, canned, solids and liquid, syrup pack, heavy	1	98
Grapefruit		
Raw, pulp, pink, red, white, all varieties	1	135
Canned, juice, sweetened	1	162
Grapefruit juice and orange juice blended, canned, sweetened	1	184
Grapes, raw, American type (slip skin), such as Concord, Delaware, Niagara, Ca-tawba, and Scuppernong	3	158
Grapejuice, canned or bottled	2	116

Continued.

Food and description	Sodium (mg)	Potassium (mg)
Guavas, whole, raw, common	4	289
Haddock, cooked, fried	177	348
Hake, including Pacific hake, squirrel hake, and silver hake or whiting; raw	74	363
Halibut, Atlantic and Pacific, cooked, broiled	134	525
Ham croquette	342	83
Heart, beef, lean, cooked, braised	104	232
Herring		
Raw, Pacific	74	420
Smoked, hard	6231	157
Honey, strained or extracted	5	51
Horseradish, prepared	96	290
Ice cream and frozen custard, regular, approximately 17% fat	63[7]	181
Ice cream cones	232	244
Ice milk	68[7]	195
Jams and preserves	12	88
Kale, cooked, boiled, drained, leaves including stems	43	221
Kingfish; southern, gulf, and northern (whiting); raw	83	250
Lake herring (cisco), raw	47	319
Lamb, retail cuts	70	290
Lemon juice, canned or bottled, unsweetened	1	141
Lettuce, raw crisphead varieties such as Iceberg, New York, and Great Lakes strains	9	175
Lime juice, canned or bottled, unsweetened	1	104
Liver, beef, cooked, fried	184	380
Lobster, northern, canned or cooked	210	180
Loganberries, canned, solids and liquid, syrup pack, light	1	111
Macadamia nuts	—	164
Macaroni, unenriched, dry form	2	197
Macaroni and cheese, canned	304	58
Margarine[8]	987	23
Marmalade, citrus	14	33
Milk, cow		
Fluid (pasteurized and raw)		
Whole, 3.7% fat	50	144
Skim	52	145
Canned, evaporated (unsweetened)	118	303
Dry, skim (nonfat solids), regular	532	1745
Malted		
Dry powder	440	720
Beverage	91	200
Chocolate drink, fluid, commercial		
Made with skim milk	46	142
Made with whole (3.5% fat) milk	47	146
Molasses, cane		
First extraction or light	15	917
Third extraction or blackstrap	96	2927
Muffin mixes, corn, and muffins baked from mixes		
Made with egg, milk	479	110
Made with egg, water	346	104
Mushrooms		
Raw	15	414
Canned, solids and liquid	400	197
Muskmelons, raw, cantaloupes, other netted varieties	12	251
Mussels, Atlantic and Pacific, raw, meat only	289	315
Mustard greens, cooked, boiled, drained	18	220
Mustard, prepared		
Brown	1307	130
Yellow	1252	130
Nectarines, raw	6	294
New Zealand spinach, cooked, boiled, drained	92	463
Noodles, egg noodles, enriched, cooked	2	44
Oat products used mainly as hot breakfast cereals, oatmeal or rolled oats		
Dry form	2	352
Cooked	218	61

For notes see p. A-53.

Food and description	Sodium (mg)	Potassium (mg)
Oat products used mainly as ready-to-eat breakfast cereals, with or without corn, puffed, added nutrients	1267	—
Ocean perch, Atlantic (redfish)		
Raw	79	269
Cooked, fried	153	284
Ocean perch, Pacific, raw	63	390
Oils, salad or cooking	0	0
Okra		
Raw	3	249
Cooked, boiled, drained	2	174
Olives, pickled; canned or bottled		
Green	2400	55
Ripe, Ascolano (extra large, mammoth, giant jumbo)	813	34
Ripe, salt-cured, oil-coated, Greek style	3288	—
Onions, mature (dry), raw	10	157
Onions, young green (bunching varieties), raw, bulb and entire top	5	231
Oranges, raw, peeled fruit, all commercial varieties	1	200
Orange juice		
Raw, all commercial varieties	1	200
Canned, unsweetened	1	199
Frozen concentrate, unsweetened, diluted with 3 parts water, by volume	1	186
Oysters		
Raw, meat only, Eastern	73	121
Cooked, fried	206	203
Frozen, solids and liquid	380	210
Oyster stew, commercial frozen, prepared with equal volume of milk	366	176
Pancake and waffle mixes and pancakes baked from mixes, plain and buttermilk, made with egg, milk	564	154
Parsnips, cooked, boiled, drained	8	379
Peaches		
Raw	1	202
Canned, solids and liquid, water pack, with or without artificial sweetener	2	137
Frozen, sliced, sweetened, not thawed	2	124
Peanut butters made with small amounts of added fat, salt	607	670
Peanuts		
Roasted with skins	5	701
Roasted and salted	418	674
Pears		
Raw, including skin	2	130
Canned, solids and liquid, syrup pack, light	1	85
Peas, green, immature		
Cooked, boiled, drained	1	196
Canned, Alaska (early or June peas)		
Regular pack, solids and liquid	236[1]	96
Special dietary pack (low sodium), solids and liquid	3	96
Frozen, cooked, boiled, drained	115	135
Peas, mature seeds, dry, whole, raw	35	1005
Peas and carrots, frozen, cooked, boiled, drained	84	157
Pecans	Trace	603
Peppers, hot, chili, mature, red, raw, pods excluding seeds	25	564
Peppers, sweet, garden varieties, immature, green, raw	13	213
Perch, yellow, raw	68	230
Pickles, cucumber, dill	1428	200
Piecrust or plain pastry, made with enriched flour, baked	611	50
Pies, baked, piecrust made with unenriched flour		
Apple	301	80
Cherry	304	105
Mince	448	178
Pumpkin	214	160
Pike, walleye, raw	51	319
Pineapple		
Raw	1	146
Frozen chunks, sweetened, not thawed	2	100

For notes see p. A-53.

Continued.

Food and description	Sodium (mg)	Potassium (mg)
Pizza, with cheese, from home recipe, baked		
With cheese topping	702	130
With sausage topping	729	168
Plate dinners, frozen, commercial, unheated		
Beef pot roast, whole oven-browned potatoes, peas, corn	259	244
Chicken, fried; mashed potatoes; mixed vegetables (carrots, peas, corn, beans)	344	112
Meat loaf with tomato sauce, mashed potatoes, peas	393	115
Turkey, sliced; mashed potatoes; peas	400	176
Plums		
Raw, Damson	2	299
Canned, solids and liquid, purple (Italian prunes), syrup pack, light	1	145
Popcorn, popped		
Plain	(3)	—
Oil and salt added	1940	—
Pork, fresh, retail cuts, trimmed to retail level, loin	65	390
Pork, lightly cured, commercial, ham, medium-fat class, separable, lean, cooked, roasted	930	326
Pork, cured, canned ham, contents of can	(1100)	(340)
Potatoes		
Cooked, boiled in skin	3[9]	407
Dehydrated mashed, flakes without milk		
Dry form	89	1600
Prepared, water, milk, table fat added	231	286
Pretzels	1680[10]	130
Prunes, dried, "softenized," cooked (fruit and liquid), with added sugar	3	262
Pudding mixes and puddings made from mixes, with starch base		
With milk, cooked	129	136
With milk, without cooking	124	129
Pumpkin, canned	2	240
Radishes, raw, common	18	322
Raisins, natural (unbleached), cooked, fruit and liquid, added sugar	13	355
Raspberries		
Canned, solids and liquid, water pack, with or without artificial sweetener, red	1	114
Frozen, red, sweetened, not thawed	1	100
Rennin products		
Tablet (salts, starch, rennin enzyme)	22,300	—
Dessert mixes and desserts prepared from mixes		
Chocolate, dessert made with milk	52	125
Other flavors (vanilla, caramel, fruit flavorings)		
Mix, dry form	6	—
Dessert, made with milk	46	128
Rhubarb, cooked, added sugar	2	203
Rice		
Brown		
Raw	9	214
Cooked	282	70
White (fully milled or polished), enriched, common commercial varieties, all types		
Raw	5	92
Cooked	374	28
Rice products used mainly as ready-to-eat breakfast cereals		
Rice flakes, added nutrients	987	180
Rice, puffed; added nutrients, without salt	2	100
Rice, puffed or open-popped, presweetened, honey and added nutrients	706	—
Rockfish, including black, canary, yellowtail, rasphead, and bocaccio, cooked, oven-steamed	68	446
Roe, cooked, baked or broiled, cod and shad[11]	73	132
Rolls and buns, commercial, ready-to-serve		
Danish pastry	366	112
Hard rolls, enriched	625	97
Plain (pan rolls), enriched	506	95
Sweet rolls	389	124
Rusk	246	161
Rutabagas, cooked, boiled, drained	4	167
Rye, flour, medium	(1)	203

For notes see p. A-53.

Food and description	Sodium (mg)	Potassium (mg)
Rye wafers, whole grain	882	600
Salad dressings, commercial[12]		
Blue and Roquefort cheese		
Regular	1094	37
Special dietary (low calorie), low fat (approx. 5 kcal/tsp)	1108	34
French		
Regular	1370	79
Special dietary (low calorie), low fat (approx. 5 kcal/tsp)	787	79
Mayonnaise	597	34
Thousand Island		
Regular	700	113
Special dietary (low calorie, approx. 10 kcal/tsp)	700	113
Salmon, coho (silver)		
Raw	48[13]	421
Canned, solids and liquid	351[14]	339
Salt pork, raw	1212	42
Salt sticks, regular type	1674	92
Sandwich spread (with chopped pickle)		
Regular	626	92
Special dietary (low calorie, approx. 5 kcal/tsp)	626	92
Sardines, Atlantic, canned in oil, drained solids	823	590
Sardines, Pacific, in tomato sauce, solids and liquid	400	320
Sauerkraut, canned, solids and liquid	747[15]	140
Sausage, cold cuts, and luncheon meats		
Bologna, all samples	1300	230
Frankfurters, raw, all samples	1100	220
Luncheon meat, pork, cured ham or shoulder, chopped, spiced or unspiced, canned	1234	222
Pork sausage, links or bulk, cooked	958	269
Scallops, bay and sea, cooked, steamed	265	476
Soups, commercial, canned		
Beef broth, bouillon, and consomme, prepared with equal volume of water	326	54
Chicken noodle, prepared with equal volume of water	408	23
Tomato		
Prepared with equal volume of water	396	94
Prepared with equal volume of milk	422	167
Vegetable beef, prepared with equal volume of water	427	66
Soy sauce	7325	366
Spaghetti, enriched, cooked, tender stage	1	61
Spaghetti, in tomato sauce with cheese, canned	382	121
Spinach		
Cooked, boiled, drained	50	324
Canned		
Regular pack, drained solids	236[1]	250
Special dietary pack (low sodium), solids and liquid	34	250
Frozen, chopped, cooked, boiled, drained	52	333
Squash, summer, all varieties, cooked, boiled, drained	1	141
Squash, frozen		
Summer, yellow crookneck, cooked, boiled, drained	3	167
Winter, heated	1	207
Strawberries		
Raw	1	164
Frozen, sweetened, not thawed, sliced	1	112
Sturgeon, cooked, steamed	108	235
Succotash (corn and lima beans), frozen, cooked, boiled, drained	38	246
Sugars, beet or cane, brown	30	344
Sweet potatoes		
Cooked, all, baked in skin	12	300
Canned, liquid pack, solids and liquid, regular pack in syrup	48	(120)
Dehydrated flakes, prepared with water	45	140
Tangerines, raw (Dancy variety)	2	126
Tapioca, dry	3	18
Tapioca desserts, tapioca cream pudding	156	135
Tartar sauce, regular	707	78

For notes see p. A-53.   *Continued.*

Food and description	Sodium (mg)	Potassium (mg)
Tea, instant (water-soluble solids), carbohydrate added		
Dry powder	—	4530
Beverage	—	25
Tomato catsup, bottled	1042[16]	363
Tomato juice, canned or bottled		
Regular pack	200	227
Special dietary pack (low sodium)	3	227
Tomato juice cocktail, canned or bottled	200	221
Tomato puree, canned		
Regular pack	399	426
Special dietary pack (low sodium)	6	426
Tomatoes, ripe		
Raw	3	244
Canned, solids and liquid, regular pack	130	217
Tongue, beef, medium fat, cooked, braised	61	164
Tuna, canned		
In oil, solids and liquid	800	301
In water, solids and liquid	41[17]	279[17]
Turkey, all classes		
Light meat, cooked, roasted	82	411
Dark meat, cooked, roasted	99	398
Turkey potpie, commercial, frozen, unheated	369	114
Turnips, cooked, boiled, drained	34	188
Turnip greens, leaves, including stems		
Canned, solids and liquid	236[1]	243
Frozen, cooked, boiled, drained	17	149
Veal, retail cuts, untrimmed	80	500
Vinegar, cider	1	100
Waffles, frozen, made with enriched flour	644	158
Walnuts		
Black	3	460
Persian or English	2	450
Watercress leaves including stems, raw	52	282
Watermelon, raw	1	100

For notes, see p. A-53.

Food and description	Sodium (mg)	Potassium (mg)
Wheat flours		
Whole (from hard wheats)	3	370
Patent		
All-purpose or family flour, enriched	2	95
Self-rising flour, enriched (anhydrous monocalcium phosphate used as a baking acid)[18]	1079	—[19]
Wild rice, raw	7	220
Yeast		
Baker's, compressed	16	610
Brewer's, debittered	121	1894
Yogurt, made from whole milk	47	132
Zweiback	250	150

[1]Estimated average based on addition of salt in the amount of 0.6% of the finished product.

[2]Processed, partially debranned, whole-kernel wheat with salt added.

[3]Processed, partially debranned, whole-kernel wheat with chicken fat, chicken stock base, dehydrated onion flakes, salt, monosodium glutamate, and herbs.

[4]Values apply to salted butter. Unsalted butter contains less than 10 mg of either sodium or potassium per 100 g. Value for vitamin A is the year-round average.

[5]Applies to unsalted nuts. For salted nuts, value is approximately 200 mg per 100 g.

[6]Values for phosphorus and sodium are based on use of 1.5% anhydrous disodium phosphate as the emulsifying agent. If emulsifying agent does not contain either phosphorus (P) or sodium (Na), the content of these two nutrients in milligrams per 100 g is as follows:

	Na	P
American process cheese	650	444
Swiss process cheese	681	540
American cheese food	—	427
American cheese spread	1139	548

[7]Value for product without added salt.

[8]Values apply to salted margarine. Unsalted margarine contains less than 10 mg/100 g of either sodium or potassium. Vitamin A value based on the minimum required to meet federal specifications for margarine with vitamin A added, 15,000 IUA/lb.

[9]Applies to product without added salt. If salt is added, an estimated average value for sodium is 236 mg/100 g.

[10]Sodium content is variable. For example, very thin pretzel sticks contain about twice the average amount listed.

[11]Prepared with butter or margarine, lemon juice or vinegar.

[12]Values apply to products containing salt. For those without salt, sodium content is low, ranging from less than 10 to 50 mg/100 g; the amount usually is indicated on the label.

[13]Sample dipped in brine contained 215 mg sodium/100 g.

[14]For product canned without added salt, value is approximately the same as for raw salmon.

[15]Values for sauerkraut and sauerkraut juice are based on salt content of 1.9% and 2.0%, respectively, in the finished products. The amounts in some samples may vary significantly from this estimate.

[16]Applies to regular pack. For special dietary pack (low sodium), values range from 5-35 mg/100 g.

[17]One sample with salt added contained 375 mg of sodium/100 g and 275 mg of potassium.

[18]The acid ingredient most commonly used in self-rising flour. When sodium acid pyrophosphate in combination with either anhydrous monocalcium phosphate or calcium carbonate is used, the value for calcium is approximately 120 mg/100 g; for phosphorus, 540 mg; for sodium, 1360 mg.

[19]90 mg of potassium/100 g contributed by flour. Small quantities of additional potassium may be provided by other ingredients.

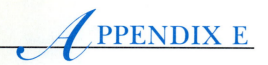

Sodium Levels in Mineral Waters and Soft Drinks

Sodium Levels in Mineral Waters

Sodium levels	Beverage (8 fl oz)
Low (less than 5 mg)	Black Mountain spring water
	Bel-Air mineral water
	Perrier
	Poland Springs sparkling water
	Sheffield's O_2 sparkling spring water
Moderate-low (30-60 mg)	Calistoga mineral water
	Canada Dry club soda
	Napa Valley springs mineral water
	Schweppes club soda
Moderate-high (100-110 mg)	Calso water
High (more than 400 mg)	Lady Lee club soda

Adapted from *Sodium in mineral waters—8 fluid ounce servings*, American Heart Association, Alameda County Chapter. Oakland, Calif, Feb 1981.

Sodium Levels in Soft Drinks

Regular beverage	Sugar-free beverage
Less than 20 mg/12 fl oz	
Aspen, Bubble-Up, Canada Dry ginger ale, Canada Dry tonic water, Orange Crush, Pepsi, Schweppes ginger ale, Schweppes tonic water, Shasta cola, Squirt	
20-40 mg/12 fl oz	
Canada Dry collins mix, Coca-Cola, Dr. Pepper, Fanta (orange, grape, root beer), Mountain Dew, Mr. Pibb, Seven-Up, Shasta (all flavors except cola, strawberry, lemon-lime), Sunkist, Teem	Sugar-free Dr. Pepper, Diet Shasta grape, Diet Squirt
40-60 mg/12 fl oz	
Fanta ginger ale, Schweppes bitter lemon, Shasta (lemon-lime, strawberry), Sprite	Fresca, Sugar-free Mr. Pibb, Pepsi Light, Diet Seven-Up, Diet Shasta (all flavors except grape), Tab, Tab-Strawberry
60-80 mg/12 fl oz	
	Diet-Rite Cola, Diet Pepsi, Sugar-free Sprite, Tab (black cherry, ginger ale, grape, lemon-lime, orange, root beer)
80-100 mg/12 fl oz	
	Sugar-free Bubble-Up, Diet Mug Root Beer, Diet Sunkist

Adapted from *Sodium in soft drinks—12 fl oz servings*, American Heart Association, Alameda County Chapter, Oakland, Calif, Feb 1981.

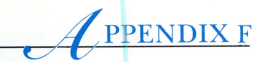

Salt-Free Seasoning Guide

Fish

Breaded, battered fillets
  Dry mustard, onion;
    oregano, basil,
    garlic; thyme
Broiled steaks or fillets
  Chili or curry powder;
    tarragon
Fillets in butter sauce
  Thyme, chervil; dill;
    fennel
Fish soup
  Italian seasoning; bay
    leaf, thyme, tarra-
    gon
Fish cakes
  Tarragon, savory; dry
    mustard, white
    pepper; red pep-
    per, oregano

Beef

Swiss steak
  Rosemary, black pep-
    per; bay leaf,
    thyme; clove
Roast beef
  Basil, oregano; bay
    leaf; nutmeg; tarra-
    gon, marjoram
Beef stew
  Chili powder; bay leaf,
    tarragon; caraway;
    marjoram
Meatballs
  Garlic, thyme; basil,
    oregano, onion;
    thyme, garlic; black
    pepper, dry mus-
    tard
Beef stroganoff
  Red pepper, onion,
    garlic; nutmeg, on-
    ion; curry powder

Poultry and veal

Fried chicken
  Basil, oregano,
    garlic; onion, dill;
    sesame seed, nut-
    meg
Roast chicken or turkey
  Ginger, garlic; onion,
    thyme, tarragon
Chicken croquettes
  Dill; curry; chili,
    cumin; tarragon,
    oregano
Veal patties
  Italian seasoning;
    tarragon; dill, on-
    ion, sesame seed
Barbecue chicken
  Garlic, dry mustard;
    clove, allspice, dry
    mustard; basil,
    garlic, and ore-
    gano

Gravies and sauces

Barbecue
  Bay leaf, thyme, red pep-
    per; cinnamon, ginger,
    allspice, dry mustard,
    red pepper; chili powder
Brown
  Chervil, onion; onion, bay
    leaf, thyme; onion, nut-
    meg; tarragon
Chicken
  Dry mustard; ginger, garlic;
    marjoram, thyme, bay
    leaf
Cream
  White pepper, dry mustard;
    curry powder; dill, on-
    ion, paprika; tarragon,
    thyme

Soups

Chicken
  Thyme, savory; gin-
    ger; clove, white
    pepper, allspice
Clam chowder
  Basil, oregano; nut-
    meg, white pep-
    per; thyme, garlic
    powder
Mushroom
  Ginger; oregano;
    thyme, tarragon;
    bay leaf, black pep-
    per; chili powder
Onion
  Curry, caraway; mar-
    joram, garlic;
    cloves
Tomato
  Bay leaf, thyme; Ital-
    ian seasoning; ore-
    gano, onion; nut-
    meg
Vegetable
  Italian seasoning; pa-
    prika, caraway;
    rosemary, thyme;
    fennel, thyme

Salads

Chicken
  Curry or chili powder;
    Italian seasoning;
    thyme, tarragon
Coleslaw
  Dill; caraway; poppy;
    dry mustard, ginger
Fish or seafood
  Dill; tarragon, ginger,
    dry mustard, red
    pepper; ginger, on-
    ion, garlic
Macaroni
  Dill; basil, thyme, ore-
    gano; dry mustard,
    garlic
Potato
  Chili powder; curry;
    dry mustard, onion

Pasta, beans, and rice

Baked beans
  Dry mustard; chili
    powder; clove, on-
    ion; ginger, dry
    mustard
Rice and vegetables
  Curry; thyme, onion,
    paprika; rosemary,
    garlic; ginger, on-
    ion, garlic
Spanish rice
  Cumin, oregano,
    basil; Italian sea-
    soning
Spaghetti
  Italian seasoning,
    nutmeg; oregano,
    basil, nutmeg; red
    pepper, tarragon
Rice pilaf
  Dill; thyme; savory,
    black pepper

Vegetables

Asparagus
  Ginger; sesame seed;
    basil, onion
Broccoli
  Italian seasoning; mar-
    joram, basil; nutmeg,
    onion; sesame seed
Cabbage
  Caraway; onion, nutmeg;
    allspice, clove
Carrots
  Ginger; nutmeg; onion, dill
Cauliflower
  Dry mustard; basil; pa-
    prika, onion
Tomatoes
  Oregano; chili powder; dill,
    onion
Spinach
  Savory, thyme; nutmeg;
    garlic, onion

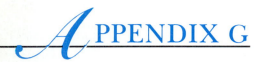

Nutritional Analysis of Fast Foods

Food Name	Portion	WT. Gm	KCAL Kc	PROT Gm	CARB Gm	FAT Gm	CHOL Mg	SAFA Gm	MUFA Gm	PUFA Gm	SOD Mg	POT Mg
ARBY'S-BEEF AND CHEESE SAND-WICH	ITEM	176	402	32.2	27.1	18	77	9.03	3.66	3.51	1634	345
ARBY'S-CHICKEN BREAST SAND-WICH	ITEM	184	493	23	47.9	25	91	5.1	9.6	10.3	1019	330
ARBY'S-CLUB SANDWICH	ITEM	252	560	30	43	30	100	11.6	9.28	8.4	1610	466
ARBY'S-HAM AND CHEESE SAND-WICH	ITEM	146	353	20.7	33.4	15.5	58	6.44	6.74	1.38	772	290
ARBY'S-ROAST BEEF SANDWICH	ITEM	139	346	21.5	33.5	13.8	52	3.61	6.8	1.71	792	316
ARBY'S-SUPER ROAST BEEF SAND-WICH	ITEM	234	501	25.1	50.4	22.1	40	8.5	8.2	5.4	798	503
ARBY'S-TURKEY DELUXE	ITEM	236	510	28	46	24	70	—	—	—	1220	—
ARBYS-SOUP-BOSTON CLAM CHOWDER	SERVING	227	207	10	18	11	28	4	5	2	1157	319
ARBYS-SOUP-CREAM OF BROC-COLI	SERVING	227	180	9	19	8	3	5	2	1	1113	455
ARBYS-SOUP-FRENCH ONION	SERVING	227	67	2	7	3	0	1	2	1	1248	106
ARBYS-SOUP-LUMBERJACK MIXED VEGETABLE	SERVING	227	89	2	13	4	4	2	1	1	1075	268
ARBYS-SOUP-OLD FASHIONED CHICKEN NOODLE	SERVING	227	99	6	15	2	25	1	1	1	929	78
ARBYS-SOUP-PILGRIM CLAM CHOWDER	SERVING	227	193	10	18	11	28	4	5	2	1157	379
ARBYS-SOUP-ROAST BEEF AND VEGETABLE	SERVING	227	96	5	14	3	10	1	1	1	996	211
ARBYS-SOUP-SPLIT PEA AND HAM	SERVING	227	200	8	21	10	30	5	1	1	1029	272
ARBYS-SOUP-TOMATO FLOR-ENTINE	SERVING	227	84	3	15	2	2	1	1	1	910	221
ARBYS-SOUP-WISCONSIN CHEESE	SERVING	227	287	9	19	19	31	8	8	3	1129	441
BEEF BURGER-FAST FOOD	OUNCE	28.3	72.3	4.99	7.26	2.58	—	—	—	—	54.7	45.9
BUN-HAMBURGER/HOTDOG-FAST FOOD	OUNCE	28.3	97.8	2.66	16.3	2.41	—	—	—	—	22.1	31.2
BURGER KING-BACON DOUBLE CHEESE-DELUXE	SERVING	195	592	33	28	39	111	16	14	6	804	463
BURGER KING-BARBECUE BACON DOUBLE CHEESE	ITEM	174	536	32	31	31	105	14	13	2	795	429
BURGER KING-BK BROILER	ITEM	168	379	24	31	18	53	3	7.96	3.84	764	324
BURGER KING-BK BROILER SAUCE	SERVING	14	90	0	0	10	7	1	2	5	95	—
BURGER KING-CHICKEN TENDERS	PIECE	90	39.3	2.67	2.33	2.17	7.67	0.5	0.833	0.5	90.2	249
BURGER KING-CROISSANT-EGG AND CHEESE	ITEM	127	369	12.8	24.3	24.7	216	14.1	7.54	1.37	551	174
BURGER KING-CROISSANT-EGG/CHEESE/HAM	ITEM	152	475	18.9	24.2	33.6	213	17.5	11.4	2.36	1080	272
BURGER KING-DOUBLE CHEESE-BURGER	ITEM	172	483	30	29	27	100	13	11	2	851	344
BURGER KING-FISH TENDERS	SERVING	99	267	12	18	16	28	3	7	4	870	176
BURGER KING-MUSHROOM SWISS DOUBLE CHEESE	ITEM	176	473	31	27	27	95	12	11	2	746	—
BURGER KING-RANCH DIP SAUCE	SERVING	28	171	0	2	18	0	3	4	10	208	—
BURGER KING-SWEET & SOUR SAUCE	SERVING	28	45	0	11	0	0	0	0	0	52	9.14
BURGER KING-TARTAR DIP SAUCE	SERVING	28	174	0	3	18	16	3	4	11	302	13.8
BURGER KING-TATER TENDERS	SERVING	71	213	2	25	12	3	3	6	3	318	—

MAG Mg	IRON Mg	ZINC Mg	V-A RE	V-C Mg	THIA Mg	RIBO Mg	NIAC Mg	V-B6 Mg	FOL Ug	VB12 Ug	CALC Mg	PHOS Mg	SEL Mg	FIBD Gm	V-E Mg
40	5.05	5.37	58	0	0.38	0.46	5.9	0.34	41	2.05	183	401	—	1.06	0.484
45.8	3.45	1.66	15.3	0	0.447	0.388	14.8	0.65	32.3	0.339	111	290	—	1.56	3.1
46.2	3.6	3.13	127	28.3	0.68	0.43	7	0.396	43.6	0.937	200	433	—	2.27	3.92
16	3.25	1.38	95.8	2.7	0.31	0.49	2.69	0.2	71	0.54	130	152	—	1.04	1.36
31	4.23	3.39	63.1	2.1	0.38	0.31	5.86	0.27	40	1.22	54	239	—	0.974	0.257
58.3	6.38	10.7	0	0	0.526	0.601	9.44	0.484	41.1	4.29	115	402	—	1.64	0.432
—	2.7	—	—	—	0.45	0.34	8	—	—	—	80	—	—	—	—
20.4	1.36	0.731	100	3.6	0.061	0.216	0.944	0.116	8.85	9.38	170	143	—	1.36	0.163
54.8	0.792	0.738	50	9	0.113	0.422	0.751	0.175	45.5	0.588	237	193	—	1.75	1.7
2.27	0.636	0.577	10	2.4	0.032	0.023	0.565	0.045	14.3	0	25	11.4	—	0.908	0.326
5.68	1.87	2.72	250	9	0.061	0.102	1.85	0.152	14.2	0.295	40.9	90.8	—	1.25	0.436
4.54	0.726	0.372	200	1.2	0.05	0.057	1.31	0.025	2.04	0.136	15.9	34	—	0.681	0.079
19.2	1.95	1.06	350	3.6	0.061	0.163	1.34	0.148	9.36	9.67	134	126	—	1.92	0.275
4.54	1.04	1.44	300	4.8	0.034	0.045	0.96	0.07	9.76	0.295	15.9	38.6	—	0.454	0.354
36.3	2.02	2.95	300	1.2	0.109	0.089	2.38	0.204	4.31	0.227	31.8	168	—	3.86	0.163
10.2	1.64	0.236	100	12	0.091	0.093	1.34	0.116	15	0.102	44.8	57.9	—	0.454	2.8
6.81	1.32	1.13	90.1	2.4	0.03	0.238	0.704	0.045	6.81	0	252	241	—	1.82	0.436
—	0.255	—	8.22	0.17	0.017	0.037	0.822	—	—	—	3.4	24.9	—	0.028	—
—	0.227	—	0	0.142	0.071	0.023	0.397	—	—	—	9.36	13	—	0	—
37.5	3.95	6.36	71.4	7.59	0.298	0.392	8.12	0.365	31.4	3.24	156	373	—	1.06	1.78
36.1	3.96	6.52	48.7	4.42	0.294	0.393	8.25	0.348	27.1	3.34	158	379	—	0.799	0.758
29.1	3.23	3.17	43.7	6.22	0.274	0.262	5.21	0.242	37.5	1.52	73.7	153	—	1.8	3.1
—	—	—	—	—	—	—	—	—	—	—	—	—	—	0	
21.6	1.03	0.738	25.2	0	0.135	0.117	6.21	0.315	9	0.297	9	234	—	0.27	0.362
22	2.2	1.76	300	0.2	0.19	0.38	1.51	0.1	36	0.78	244	349	—	2.05	0.83
26	2.13	2.17	135	11.4	0.52	0.3	3.19	0.23	36	1.01	144	336	—	—	—
30.6	2.95	3.95	100	5.84	0.215	0.308	4.94	0.237	31.4	1.81	189	305	—	1.44	2.12
33.1	1.7	0.589	19.6	0.005	0.232	0.167	2.29	0.055	22.7	1.05	60	191	—	1.12	1.55
—	4.14	—	—	—	—	—	—	—	—	—	—	—	—	—	—
—	—	—	—	—	—	—	—	—	—	—	—	—	—	—	—
2.09	0.1	0.013	0	0	0.001	0.003	0.059	0.003	0.301	0	1.02	2.65	—	0.014	—
1.01	0.255	0.053	25.5	0.248	0.002	0.005	0.013	0.076	2.17	0.059	6.99	7.81	—	0.042	4.67
—															

Continued.

Food Name	Portion	WT. Gm	KCAL Kc	PROT Gm	CARB Gm	FAT Gm	CHOL Mg	SAFA Gm	MUFA Gm	PUFA Gm	SOD Mg	POT Mg
CHEESE BURGER-FAST FOOD	OUNCE	28.3	78	5.61	6.55	3.26	12.3	1.73	1.65	0.241	198	68
CHICKEN-BREAST AND WING-BREADED-FRIED	SERVING	163	494	35.7	19.6	29.5	149	7.84	12.2	6.79	975	566
CHICKEN-BREAST-FAST FOOD	OUNCE	28.3	73.1	7.65	2.61	3.57	23.6	0.616	0.852	0.467	142	85
CHICKEN-DRUMSTICK & THIGH-BREADED-FRIED	SERVING	148	430	30.1	15.7	26.7	165	7.05	10.9	6.32	756	446
CHICKEN-DRUMSTICK-FAST FOOD	OUNCE	28.3	59	7.03	4.2	1.56	25.6	0.858	1.2	0.703	133	73.7
CHICKEN-FRIED-FAST FOOD-VARIOUS PORTIONS	OUNCE	28.3	82.2	4.71	5.67	4.51	25.4	1.14	1.66	0.958	153	70.9
CHICKEN-MEAT-SHAPED-FRIED-FAST FOOD	OUNCE	28.3	81.6	4.85	4.65	4.85	—	—	—	—	141	39.7
CHICKEN-SHOULDER-FAST FOOD	OUNCE	28.3	92.4	5.33	3.18	6.49	—	—	—	—	150	73.7
CHICKEN-THIGH-FAST FOOD	OUNCE	28.3	104	7.26	2.75	7.14	26.2	1.22	1.73	0.962	139	68
CHICKEN-WING-FAST FOOD	OUNCE	28.3	91.9	7.85	2.78	5.47	—	—	—	—	198	53.9
COLESLAW-FAST FOOD	OUNCE	28.3	23.8	0.68	2.75	1.13	1.07	0.206	0.374	0.759	76.5	45.4
DOUBLE CHEESE BURGER-FAST FOOD	OUNCE	28.3	66.3	4.2	6.63	2.55	16.6	2.2	1.94	0.238	49.9	85.3
FAST FOOD-PIZZA WITH CHEESE	OUNCE	28.4	63.2	3.46	9.23	1.45	4.25	0.693	0.445	0.221	151	49.3
FAST FOOD-PIZZA WITH PEPPERONI	OUNCE	28.4	72.3	4.04	7.93	2.78	5.67	0.893	1.25	0.465	107	61
FISH CAKE-FRIED-WITH BUN-FAST FOOD	OUNCE	28.3	84.5	2.72	7.63	4.79	19.7	0.388	0.761	0.455	167	51.6
FRANKFURTER-CONEY DOG-FAST FOOD	OUNCE	28.3	69.2	3.12	6.95	3.2	14.7	3.09	3.99	0.81	242	48.8
FRANKFURTER-HOT DOG-FAST FOOD	OUNCE	28.3	77.7	3.12	7.37	3.97	14.7	3.09	3.99	0.81	219	48.2
HAMBURGER-DOUBLE PATTY-EVERYTHING ON IT	OUNCE	28.4	67.8	4.3	5.05	3.33	15.3	1.32	1.3	0.351	99.2	71.4
HARDEE-BACON AND EGG BISCUIT	SERVING	124	410	15	35	24	155	5	14	5	990	180
HARDEE-BACON EGG AND CHEESE BISCUIT	SERVING	137	460	17	35	28	165	8	15	5	1220	200
HARDEE-BIG COUNTRY BREAKFAST-COUNTRY HAM	SERVING	254	670	29	52	38	345	9	21	8	2870	710
HARDEE-BIG COUNTRY BREAKFAST-SAUSAGE	SERVING	274	850	33	51	57	340	16	31	11	1980	670
HARDEE-BIG COUNTRY BREAKFAST-WITH BACON	SERVING	217	660	24	51	40	305	10	22	8	1540	530
HARDEE-BIG COUNTRY BREAKFAST-WITH HAM	SERVING	251	620	28	51	33	325	7	19	8	1780	620
HARDEE-BIG ROAST BEEF SANDWICH	SERVING	134	300	18	32	11	45	5	5	2	880	320
HARDEE-BIG TWIN HAMBURGER	SERVING	173	450	23	34	25	55	11	9	5	580	280
HARDEE-BISCUIT N GRAVY	SERVING	221	440	9	45	24	15	6	14	5	1250	210
HARDEE-CHICKEN N PASTA SALAD	SERVING	414	230	27	23	3	55	1	1	1	380	620
HARDEE-CRISPY CURLS	SERVING	85	300	4	36	16	0	3	8	5	840	370
HARDEE-GRILLED CHICKEN SANDWICH	SERVING	192	310	24	34	9	60	1	3	5	890	410
HARDEE-HAM & EGG BISCUIT	SERVING	138	370	15	35	19	160	4	12	4	1050	210
HARDEE-HAM EGG & CHEESE BISCUIT	SERVING	151	420	18	35	23	170	6	13	4	1270	230
HARDEE-MUSHROOM N SWISS HAMBURGER	SERVING	186	490	30	33	27	70	13	12	2	940	370
HARDEE-REGULAR ROAST BEEF SANDWICH	SERVING	114	260	15	31	9	35	4	4	2	730	260
HARDEE-THE LEAN ONE SANDWICH	ITEM	220	420	27	37	18	85	8	8	2	760	510
HARDEE-THREE PANCAKES	SERVING	137	280	8	56	2	15	1	1	1	890	240
KFC-CHICKEN HOT WINGS	PIECE	119	62.6	3.66	2.99	3.99	24.6	0.832	10.3	0.666	113	218
KFC-CHICKEN SANDWICH	SERVING	166	482	21	39	27	47	6	3.91	9	1060	297
KFC-CRISPY CHICKEN-BREAST	PIECE	135	342	33	12	20	114	5	4.7	2	790	347
KFC-CRISPY CHICKEN-DRUMSTICK	PIECE	69	204	14	6	14	71	3	3.72	2	324	157
KFC-CRISPY CHICKEN-THIGH	PIECE	119	406	20	14	30	129	8	6.95	4	688	280
KFC-CRISPY CHICKEN-WING	PIECE	65	254	12	9	19	67	4	5.74	3	422	115
LONG JOHN SILVER-BATTERED SHRIMP-9 PIECE	PIECE	357	95.4	2.66	9.76	4.99	13.9	1.11	3.22	0.555	163	94.3

MAG Mg	IRON Mg	ZINC Mg	V-A RE	V-C Mg	THIA Mg	RIBO Mg	NIAC Mg	V-B6 Mg	FOL Ug	VB12 Ug	CALC Mg	PHOS Mg	SEL Mg	FIBD Gm	V-E Mg
5.88	0.567	0.722	9.36	0.283	0.023	0.048	0.624	0.038	6.79	0.311	25.2	33.2	—	0.057	0.142
38	1.49	1.55	57.7	0	0.14	0.3	12	0.57	9	0.67	60	307	—	0.261	1.18
7.6	0.17	0.287	9.36	0.68	0.02	0.048	1.98	0.158	1.13	0.09	3.97	51.9	—	0	0.089
37	1.6	3.24	66.7	0	0.14	0.43	7.21	0.33	10	0.83	36	240	—	0.237	1.58
6.47	0.312	0.807	6.52	0.425	0.02	0.062	1.42	0.096	2.25	0.09	4.25	41.1	—	0	0.089
7.05	0.283	0.575	6.52	0.454	0.02	0.051	1.62	0.116	1.76	0.087	4.25	38.6	—	0	0.212
—	0.312		5.95	0.425	0.009	0.006	0.794	—	—	—	3.97	33.5	—	0	—
—	0.142	—	4.25	0.34	0.02	0.037	1.87	—	—	—	3.69	31.8	—	0	—
6.19	0.085	0.664	6.24	0.283	0.023	0.068	1.42	0.087	1.97	0.082	4.25	36.9	—	0	0.089
—	0.227	—	6.52	0.624	0.017	0.043	1.47	—	—	—	5.1	31.2	—	0	—
3.81	0.51	0.045	7.65	0.425	0.009	0.003	0.028	0.022	8.87	0.008	9.92	9.07	—	0	0.498
5.86	0.624	0.906	7.94	0.057	0.02	0.04	0.765	0.045	5.39	0.422	3.4	30.9	—	0.142	0.139
7.09	0.261	0.366	33.2	0.567	0.082	0.074	1.12	0.02	26.4	0.15	52.4	50.7	—	0.576	0.386
3.4	0.374	0.207	21.8	0.652	0.054	0.094	1.22	0.023	21	0.074	25.8	30.1	—	0.576	—
7.98	0.482	0.682	5.67	0.113	0.017	0.043	1.39	0.033	11.8	0.845	13.9	34.3	—	0	0.389
2.86	0.964	0.554	7.37	0.51	0.065	0.068	1.08	0.031	1.02	0.333	12.2	30.3	—	0	0.08
2.86	0.567	0.554	4.54	0.454	0.011	0.006	0.567	0.031	1.02	0.333	5.67	33.2	—	0	0.08
6.24	0.734	0.712	1.42	0.142	0.045	0.048	0.95	0.068	5.84	0.51	12.8	39.4	—	0.285	0.172
24.8	2.18	1.37	116	2.92	0.331	0.445	3.01	0.136	13.9	0.467	253	358	—	0.625	1.45
27.4	2.41	1.52	129	3.23	0.366	0.492	3.32	0.151	15.4	0.516	279	396	—	0.69	1.61
—	—	—	—	—	—	—	—	—	—	—	—	—	—	—	—
—	—	—	—	—	—	—	—	—	—	—	—	—	—	—	—
23.4	2.46	2.54	333	0	0.312	0.796	1.84	0.343	52.8	1.5	77.5	347	—	0	5.69
—	—	—	—	—	—	—	—	—	—	—	—	—	—	—	—
33.4	3.65	6.14	0	0	0.301	0.344	5.41	0.277	23.5	2.45	66	230	—	0.939	0.247
34.9	4	4.57	16.7	3.26	0.277	0.306	6.72	0.27	33.9	2.27	79.6	197	—	1.74	1.05
—	9	—	—	—	—	—	—	—	—	—	—	—	—	—	—
—	—	—	—	—	—	—	—	—	—	—	—	—	—	—	—
44.1	3	2.66	413	0.033	0.43	0.593	4.17	0.1	31	0.472	542	611	—	2.21	4.09
25.5	2.75	1.62	127	8.73	0.56	0.535	3.87	0.207	39.3	0.73	94.9	234	—	1.06	2.33
30.2	2.65	1.67	142	3.56	0.403	0.542	3.66	0.166	16.9	0.569	308	436	—	0.761	1.78
—	—	—	—	—	—	—	—	—	—	—	—	—	—	—	—
28.4	3.11	5.22	0	0	0.257	0.293	4.6	0.236	20	2.09	56.1	196	—	0.799	0.211
—	—	—	—	—	—	—	—	—	—	—	—	—	—	—	—
25.4	1.86	0.914	63.2	0.719	0.215	0.388	1.39	0.099	13.5	0.415	341	411	—	1.35	1.86
22.3	1.48	2.1	63.4	0.206	0.05	0.149	7.65	0.491	3.69	0.333	17.9	175	—	0.061	1.05
41.4	3.11	1.5	13.8	0	0.403	0.35	13.4	0.586	29.1	0.305	99.9	261	—	1.41	2.8
40.2	1.61	1.47	20	0	0.113	0.171	18.4	0.771	5.38	0.459	21.4	312	—	0.08	0.742
16	0.92	1.98	17.4	0	0.057	0.155	4.14	0.238	5.54	0.217	8.42	120	—	0.041	0.637
28.8	1.77	2.97	35.2	0	0.108	0.293	8.22	0.395	9.75	0.362	16	221	—	0.136	0.668
12.4	0.81	1.14	24.5	0	0.038	0.089	4.33	0.265	2.33	0.18	9.87	97.2	—	0.056	0.72
132	10.3	4.23	242	4.89	0.3	0.496	9.86	0.364	33.5	3.4	214	764	—	1.77	16.9

Continued.

Food Name	Portion	WT. Gm	KCAL Kc	PROT Gm	CARB Gm	FAT Gm	CHOL Mg	SAFA Gm	MUFA Gm	PUFA Gm	SOD Mg	POT Mg
LONG JOHN SILVER-BREADED SHRIMP	PIECE	420	51	1.19	6.19	2.43	5.95	0.524	1.57	0.286	85.2	41
LONG JOHN SILVER-CATFISH FILLET	SERVING	373	860	28	90	42	65	10	26	6	990	1180
LONG JOHN SILVER-CHICKEN PLANK-4 PIECE	SERVING	415	940	39	94	44	70	10	29	5	1660	1320
LONG JOHN SILVER-CHICKEN-LIGHT HERB	SERVING	498	630	35	85	17	85	3	5	7	2170	790
LONG JOHN SILVER-CLAM CHOWDER WITH COD	SERVING	198	140	11	10	6	20	2	3	2	590	380
LONG JOHN SILVER-CLAM DINNER	SERVING	363	980	21	122	45	15	10	30	6	1200	870
LONG JOHN SILVER-COLE SLAW	SERVING	98	140	1	20	6	15	1	2	4	260	190
LONG JOHN SILVER-FISH & CHICKEN ENTREE	SERVING	398	870	35	91	40	70	9	26	5	1520	1290
LONG JOHN SILVER-FISH & MORE ENTREE	SERVING	381	800	31	88	37	70	8	23	5	1390	1260
LONG JOHN SILVER-FISH AND FRYES-3 PIECE	SERVING	358	810	42	77	38	85	9	27	2	1630	1340
LONG JOHN SILVER-FISH SAND-WICH PLATTER	SERVING	379	870	26	108	38	55	8	22	7	1110	1050
LONG JOHN SILVER-FRIES	SERVING	85	220	3	30	10	5	3	7	1	60	390
LONG JOHN SILVER-GARDEN SALAD	SERVING	246	170	9	13	9	5	0.846	1	0.777	380	20
LONG JOHN SILVER-GUMBO-COD & SHRIMP BOBS	SERVING	198	120	9	4	8	25	2	3	3	740	310
LONG JOHN SILVER-HOMESTYLE FISH SANDWICH	SERVING	196	510	22	58	22	45	5	13	3	780	470
LONG JOHN SILVER-HOMESTYLE FISH-3 PIECE	SERVING	456	960	43	97	44	100	10	29	5	1890	1540
LONG JOHN SILVER-HOMESTYLE FISH-6 PIECE	SERVING	513	1260	49	124	64	130	14	43	6	1590	1660
LONG JOHN SILVER-HUSH-PUPPIES	PIECE	24	70	2	10	2	5	1	1	1	25	65
LONG JOHN SILVER-LIGHT FISH-LEMON	SERVING	291	320	24	49	4	75	1	1	1	900	470
LONG JOHN SILVER-LIGHT FISH-PAPRIKA	SERVING	284	300	24	45	2	70	1	1	1	650	460
LONG JOHN SILVER-MIXED VEGE-TABLES	SERVING	113	60	2	9	2	0	1	1	1	330	120
LONG JOHN SILVER-OCEAN CHEF SALAD	SERVING	321	250	24	19	9	80	2	2	2	1340	160
LONG JOHN SILVER-RICE PILAF	SERVING	142	210	5	43	2	0	1	1	1	570	140
LONG JOHN SILVER-SEAFOOD PLATTER	SERVING	400	970	30	109	46	70	10	30	6	1540	1100
LONG JOHN SILVER-SEAFOOD SALAD	SERVING	337	270	16	36	7	90	1	2	3	670	100
LONG JOHN SILVER-SEAFOOD SALAD-SCOOP	SERVING	142	210	14	26	5	90	1	2	3	570	100
LONG JOHN SILVER-SHRIMP & FISH DINNER	SERVING	348	770	25	85	37	80	8	23	5	1250	1030
LONG JOHN SILVER-SHRIMP FISH & CHICKEN	SERVING	380	840	31	89	40	80	9	26	5	1450	1170
LONG JOHN SILVER-SHRIMP SCAMPI	SERVING	529	610	25	87	18	220	3	6	7	2120	560
MCDONALDS-APPLE BRAN MUFFIN	SERVING	85	190	5	46	0	0	0	0	0	230	202
MCDONALDS-APPLE DANISH	SLICE	115	390	5.8	51.2	17.9	25.7	3.49	10.8	1.96	370	68.6
MCDONALDS-APPLE PIE	SERVING	83	260	2.2	30	14.8	0	4.83	9.11	0.87	240	49.5
MCDONALDS-BACON AND EGG BISCUIT	SERVING	156	440	17.5	33.3	26.4	253	8.22	16.1	2.01	1230	237
MCDONALDS-BACON BITS	SERVING	3	16	1.3	0.1	1.19	0	0	1.19	0	95	4.35
MCDONALDS-BARBEQUE (BARBE-CUE) SAUCE	SERVING	32	50	0.3	12.1	0.5	0	0.06	0.19	0.22	340	55.7
MCDONALDS-BISCUIT WITH SPREAD	SERVING	75	260	4.6	31.9	12.7	1	3.39	8.64	0.64	730	99.5
MCDONALDS-CHEF SALAD	SERVING	283	230	20.5	7.5	13.3	128	5.91	6.52	0.91	490	—
MCDONALDS-CHICKEN MCNUG-GETS-6 PIECE	SERVING	113	290	19	16.5	16.3	65	4.1	10.4	1.78	520	—

MAG Mg	IRON Mg	ZINC Mg	V-A RE	V-C Mg	THIA Mg	RIBO Mg	NIAC Mg	V-B6 Mg	FOL Ug	VB12 Ug	CALC Mg	PHOS Mg	SEL Mg	FIBD Gm	V-E Mg
156	12.1	4.97	285	5.75	0.353	0.584	11.6	0.428	39.4	3.99	252	899	—	2.08	19.9
121	4.63	3.43	317	11	0.201	0.489	9.69	0.869	67.4	9.41	200	1017	—	0.071	6.85
—															
94.6	4.83	3.59	120	0	0.324	0.647	26.3	1.05	9.96	0.747	214	782	—	0	1.58
16.7	1.7	0.923	73.9	4.21	0.053	0.143	1.17	0.129	8.17	8.44	117	110	—	1.67	0.24
40.6	56.7	6.18	365	46.9	0.341	0.911	7.17	0.258	54.1	201	209	572	—	0	5.41
13.1	0.5	0.149	225	29.8	0.039	0.026	0.256	0.127	36.8	0.032	36.1	23.1	—	2.33	5.28
—	—														
131	3.25	2.14	71.2	5	0.392	0.495	12.3	0.724	46.4	5.17	133	769	—	1.69	9.28
93.7	6.39	2.25	64.6	2.14	0.872	0.648	11.1	0.421	89.1	2.29	238	488	—	4.06	6.82
28.9	0.646	0.323	0	8.76	0.15	0.024	2.76	0.201	24.6	0	16.1	79.1	—	2.93	0.209
40	1.73	1.1	239	25.6	0.14	0.15	11.4	0.561	65.7	0.268	42	217	—	2.07	1.12
41.1	2.28	0.776	300	21.4	0.117	0.079	1.98	0.168	46.5	0.24	100	105	—	3.02	2.09
48.4	18	1.16	33.4	1.11	0.451	0.335	5.73	0.218	46.1	1.19	123	252	—	2.1	3.53
157	3.89	2.56	85.3	5.99	0.47	0.593	14.7	0.866	55.5	6.19	159	920	—	2.02	11.1
177	4.38	2.88	95.9	6.74	0.528	0.667	16.6	0.975	62.4	6.97	179	1035	—	2.27	12.5
—															—
56.1	2.29	1.39	79.7	10.2	0.291	0.146	3.38	0.335	46.1	0.576	40.4	238	—	2.43	3.66
97.7	2.43	1.6	53.1	3.73	0.293	0.369	9.18	0.54	34.6	3.86	99	573	—	1.26	6.91
24.1	0.899	0.536	75	3.5	0.078	0.132	0.931	0.081	20.8	0.003	28.5	56.4	—	5.9	0.935
—	—	—	—	—	—	—	—	—	—	—	—	—	—	—	—
16.6	1.77	0.618	59.5	0.565	0.148	0.016	1.51	0.082	5.32	0.006	16.9	44.6	—	0.778	0.936
114	4.13	2.2	59	13.4	0.42	0.368	8.22	0.876	36.9	1.68	109	484	—	5.33	5.2
86	3.22	5.2	129	19.9	0.128	0.158	3.72	0.27	46.7	2.89	148	444	—	1.33	8.9
36.2	1.36	2.19	250	8.38	0.054	0.067	1.57	0.114	19.7	1.22	62.5	187	—	0.562	3.76
81.7	3.45	1.55	27.5	16.5	0.372	0.212	6.64	0.64	35	1.06	54.1	422	—	7.33	5.29
—	—	—	—	—	—	—	—	—	—	—	—	—	—	—	—
203	13.6	6.22	364	11.3	0.132	0.196	13.6	0.55	9.89	5.57	299	1156	—	0	15.5
54.8	0.6	1.23	1	0.7	0.02	0.08	0.4	0.374	76.8	0.784	31	178	—	4.47	0.454
8.09	1.37	0.232	34.5	16.1	0.28	0.2	2.2	0.026	3.42	0	14	30.7	—	1.57	4.51
5.84	0.71	0.168	0	11.4	0.06	0.02	0.32	0.019	2.47	0	10.7	22.1	—	1.13	3.25
31.2	2.56	1.73	160	0	0.36	0.33	2.47	0.172	17.5	0.588	185	451	—	0.786	1.82
2.85	0	0.056	0	0	0	0	0	0.002	3.81	0.036	0	6.51	—	0	0.248
5.76	0.31	0.064	30	2.34	0.01	0.01	0.17	0.024	1.28	0	12.8	6.4	—	1.89	2.1
14.1	1.31	0.704	0	0	0.23	0.11	1.65	0.028	5.95	0.102	75	168	—	0.977	2.14
—	1.51	—	411	13.6	0.31	0.29	3.6	—	—	—	256	—	—	—	—
	1		0	0	0.11	0.12	8.97				12.8				

Continued.

Food Name	Portion	WT. Gm	KCAL Kc	PROT Gm	CARB Gm	FAT Gm	CHOL Mg	SAFA Gm	MUFA Gm	PUFA Gm	SOD Mg	POT Mg
MCDONALDS-CHOCOLATE MILK-SHAKE-LOWFAT	SERVING	293	320	11.6	66	1.7	10	0.76	0.92	0.05	240	—
MCDONALDS-CHUNKY CHICKEN SALAD	SERVING	250	140	23.1	5.3	3.4	78	0.94	1.99	0.52	230	436
MCDONALDS-CINNAMON AND RAISIN DANISH	ITEM	110	440	6.4	57.5	21	34.7	4.2	13	1.6	430	—
MCDONALDS-COOKIE-CHOCOLATY	SERVING	56	330	4.2	41.9	15.6	4	5.04	10.2	0.39	280	71.7
MCDONALDS-COOKIE-MCDONALD-LAND	SERVING	56	290	4.2	47.1	9.2	0	1.85	6.8	0.52	300	37.5
MCDONALDS-CROUTONS	SERVING	11	50	1.39	6.8	2.17	0	0.45	1.32	0.11	140	19.9
MCDONALDS-ENGLISH MUFFIN	SERVING	59	170	5.4	26.7	4.6	9	2.38	1.68	0.5	270	74.3
MCDONALDS-FRENCH FRIES-LARGE	SERVING	122	400	5.61	45.9	21.6	16	9.06	11.6	0.89	200	866
MCDONALDS-FRENCH FRIES-MEDIUM	SERVING	97	320	4.44	36.3	17.1	12	7.17	9.21	0.7	150	692
MCDONALDS-FRENCH FRIES-REGULAR ORDER	SERVING	68	220	3.13	25.6	12	9	5.05	6.49	0.5	110	484
MCDONALDS-GARDEN SALAD	SERVING	213	110	7.1	6.2	6.6	83	2.9	3.16	0.53	160	450
MCDONALDS-HASHBROWN POTATO	SERVING	55	130	1.4	14.9	7.3	9	3.24	3.66	0.37	330	238
MCDONALDS-HONEY SAUCE	SERVING	14	45	0	11.5	0	0	0	0	0	0	—
MCDONALDS-HOT CAKES WITH SYRUP	SERVING	176	410	8.2	74.4	9.2	21	3.66	3.09	2.46	640	187
MCDONALDS-HOT CARAMEL SUNDAE	SERVING	174	270	6.6	59.3	2.8	13	1.51	1.22	0.09	180	414
MCDONALDS-HOT FUDGE SUNDAE	SERVING	169	240	7.3	50.5	3.2	6	2.35	0.76	0.05	170	274
MCDONALDS-HOT MUSTARD SAUCE	SERVING	30	70	0.5	8.2	3.6	5	0.51	1.23	1.86	250	25.6
MCDONALDS-ICED CHEESE DANISH	SERVING	110	390	7.4	42.3	21.8	47	5.95	12.1	1.77	420	—
MCDONALDS-McCHICKEN SAND-WICH	SERVING	190	490	19.2	39.8	28.6	42.6	5.4	11.5	11.6	780	340
MCDONALDS-McDLT HAMBURGER	ITEM	234	580	26.3	36	36.8	109	11.5	16.7	8.5	990	—
MCDONALDS-MCLEAN DELUXE HAMBURGER	SERVING	206	320	22	35	10	60	4	5	1	670	290
MCDONALDS-MILKSHAKE-CHOCO-LATE-LOWFAT	SERVING	293	320	12	66	2	10	1	1	0	240	—
MCDONALDS-MILKSHAKE-STRAW-BERRY-LOWFAT	SERVING	293	320	11	67	1	10	1	1	0	170	—
MCDONALDS-MILKSHAKE-VA-NILLA-LOWFAT	SERVING	293	290	11	60	1	10	1	1	0	170	643
MCDONALDS-PORK SAUSAGE	SERVING	48	180	8.4	0	16.3	48	5.88	8.51	1.9	350	—
MCDONALDS-RASPBERRY DANISH	ITEM	117	410	6.1	61.5	15.9	26	3.11	10.2	1.1	310	—
MCDONALDS-SALAD DRESSING-PEPPERCORN	OUNCE	28.4	160	0	2	18	14	2	4	10	170	22.4
MCDONALDS-SALAD DRESSING-RED FRENCH	OUNCE	28.4	80	0	10	4	0	0	2	2	220	22.4
MCDONALDS-SAUSAGE AND EGG BISCUIT	ITEM	180	520	19.9	32.6	34.5	275	11.2	20	2.54	1250	319
MCDONALDS-SAUSAGE BISCUIT	ITEM	123	440	13	31.9	29	49	9.27	17.2	2.54	1080	196
MCDONALDS-SAUSAGE MCMUFFIN	ITEM	117	370	16.5	27.3	21.9	64	7.79	11.7	2.43	830	179
MCDONALDS-SAUSAGE MCMUFFIN WITH EGG	ITEM	167	440	22.6	27.9	26.8	263	9.45	14.2	3.15	980	255
MCDONALDS-SCRAMBLED EGGS	SERVING	98	140	12.4	1.2	9.8	399	3.33	5.03	1.44	290	102
MCDONALDS-SIDE SALAD	SERVING	115	60	3.7	3.3	3.3	41	1.45	1.59	0.27	85	219
MCDONALDS-STRAWBERRY MILK-SHAKE-LOWFAT	SERVING	293	320	10.7	67	1.3	10	0.63	0.64	0.05	170	—
MCDONALDS-STRAWBERRY SUNDAE	SERVING	171	210	5.7	49.2	1.1	5	0.63	0.39	0.04	95	263
MCDONALDS-SWEET AND SOUR SAUCE	SERVING	32	60	0.2	13.8	0.2	0	0.03	0.1	0.1	190	10.4
MCDONALDS-VANILLA MILK-SHAKE-LOWFAT	SERVING	293	290	10.8	60	1.3	10	0.63	0.67	0.05	170	—
MCDONALDS-VANILLA-FROZEN YOGURT	SERVING	80	100	4	22	0.75	3	0.41	0.28	0.06	80	—
PIZZA-BEEF/CHICKEN/ONION	OUNCE	28.3	72.6	5.53	7.23	2.38	—	—	—	—	267	49
PIZZA-BEEF/ONION	OUNCE	28.3	72.9	4.34	7.88	2.66	—	—	—	—	132	49.9
PIZZA-CHICKEN CURRY/PEAS	OUNCE	28.3	81.6	3.74	9.41	3.23	—	—	—	—	146	44.5
PIZZA-CHICKEN/MUSHROOM/TOMATO	OUNCE	28.3	60.7	4.9	7.31	1.3	—	—	—	—	167	44.2

MAG Mg	IRON Mg	ZINC Mg	V-A RE	V-C Mg	THIA Mg	RIBO Mg	NIAC Mg	V-B6 Mg	FOL Ug	VB12 Ug	CALC Mg	PHOS Mg	SEL Mg	FIBD Gm	V-E Mg
—	0.84	—	91.9	0	0.13	0.5	0.4	—	—	—	332	—	—	—	—
36.6	1.02	2.94	366	19.9	0.22	0.17	8.5	0.6	26.6	0.63	33.8	257	—	0.955	13
—	1.81	—	33	3.2	0.32	0.24	2.8	—	—	—	35.1	—	—	—	—
20.2	2.18	0.515	0	0	0.18	0.21	2.47	0.028	5.04	0.073	23.9	71.1	—	1.12	1.73
12.9	2.07	0.325	0	0	0.25	0.18	2.54	0.028	3.92	0.067	8.91	91.3	—	0.56	1.73
4.62	0.35	0.103	0	0.14	0.05	0.03	0.42	0.007	3.41	0	6.48	15.4	—	0.517	0.114
12.2	1.61	0.396	36.6	0	0.33	0.14	2.47	0.097	51.1	0.001	151	59.8	—	1.56	0.16
40.1	0.93	0.633	0	14.6	0.24	0	3.29	0.317	40.1	0.147	17.8	162	—	4.21	0.3
32	0.73	0.506	0	11.6	0.19	0	2.6	0.253	32	0.117	14.1	129	—	3.35	0.239
22.4	0.52	0.354	0	8.16	0.14	0	1.84	0.177	22.4	0.082	9.93	90.4	—	—	—
34.7	1.26	0.956	391	13.5	0.1	0.16	0.59	0.486	56.9	0.232	149	188	—	1.8	0.974
9.3	0.27	0.175	0	1.59	0.06	0.02	0.85	0.069	3.55	0	5.58	39.4	—	1.09	0.125
—	0.07	—	0	0.14	0	0.01	0.04	—	—	—	—	—	—	—	—
25	2.08	0.6	52	4.71	0.32	0.33	2.82	0.12	9	0.19	114	501	—	—	—
50.5	0.08	1.1	87.4	0	0.08	0.35	0.26	0.383	19.1	0.661	222	198	—	1.04	1.38
32	0.48	1.29	64.3	0	0.08	0.35	0.3	0.074	7.23	0.597	235	178	—	1.25	1.36
5.47	0.22	0.094	1.6	0.45	0.01	0.01	0.15	0.01	1.27	0	15	7.3	—	0.252	1.45
—	1.42	—	37.6	1.1	0.29	0.23	2.1	—	—	—	32.9	—	—	—	—
47.3	2.61	1.72	31.2	2.42	0.96	0.21	8.92	0.671	33.3	0.35	143	299	—	1.61	3.19
—	3.91	—	226	7.38	0.39	0.36	6.87	—	—	—	225	—	—	—	—
34.8	3.78	3.24	66.6	9.74	0.354	0.311	5.81	0.257	47.7	1.48	92.5	170	—	2.4	3.2
—	—	—	—	—	—	—	—	—	—	—	332	—	—	—	—
—	—	—	—	—	—	—	—	—	—	—	327	—	—	—	—
48.1	0.205	2.43	38.1	2.2	0.123	0.589	0.314	0.132	30.8	1.54	327	394	—	0	0.12
—	0.67	—	0	0	0.27	0.1	2.31	—	—	—	8.24	—	—	0	—
—	1.47	—	35.1	3.2	0.33	0.21	2.1	—	—	—	14.2	—	—	—	—
0	0.114	0.023	5.68	0	0.002	0.005	0.001	0.003	1.19	0.039	3.12	3.98	—	0	2.87
0	0.114	0.023	5.68	0	0.002	0.005	0.001	0.003	1.19	0.039	3.12	3.98	—	0	2.87
25	3.16	2.16	88.3	0.1	0.53	0.35	3.99	0.2	40	1.37	116	490	—	—	—
19.8	1.98	1.54	0	0	0.49	0.21	3.96	0.114	8.73	0.504	83.2	443	—	1.35	3.66
20	2.3	1.67	72.1	1.27	0.6	0.29	4.8	0.133	47.7	0.503	235	273	—	1.1	1.94
28.6	3.34	2.39	150	0	0.64	0.42	4.82	0.19	68.1	0.718	263	390	—	1.56	2.77
10.2	2.08	1.09	156	1.18	0.07	0.26	0.05	0.075	27.2	1.68	57	136	—	0	3.44
12.4	0.67	0.252	217	7.4	0.05	0.08	0.32	0.059	40.3	0	763	25.5	—	1.23	0.469
—	0.09	—	91.9	0	0.13	0.48	0.31	—	—	—	327	—	—	—	—
19	0.16	1.17	54.3	1.3	0.07	0.29	0.25	0.067	8.77	0.54	190	127	—	0.687	0.754
2.38	0.17	0.014	54.8	0.64	0	0.01	0.08	0.004	0.344	0	10.9	3.03	—	0.016	—
—	0.1	—	91.9	0	0.13	0.48	0.31	—	—	—	327	—	—	—	—
—	0.23	—	88.4	0	0.04	0.18	0.37	—	—	—	112	—	—	—	—
—	0.709	—	23.2	1.25	0.026	0.023	1.25	—	—	—	72.9	53	—	0.028	—
—	0.17	—	23.2	0.227	0.011	0.017	0.879	—	—	—	21.3	35.7	—	0.113	—
—	0.17	—	29.8	0.198	0.02	0.026	1.73	—	—	—	19.3	36.6	—	0.198	—
—	0.198	—	22.7	0.312	0.009	0.011	0.765	—	—	—	24.1	36.6	—	0.085	—

Continued.

Food Name	Portion	WT. Gm	KCAL Kc	PROT Gm	CARB Gm	FAT Gm	CHOL Mg	SAFA Gm	MUFA Gm	PUFA Gm	SOD Mg	POT Mg
PIZZA-CHICKEN/PINEAPPLE	OUNCE	28.3	80.5	4.22	6.32	4.25	—	—	—	—	267	37.4
PIZZA-COMBINATION SUPREME	OUNCE	28.3	50.5	4.14	7.09	0.624	5.66	1.33	1.47	0.408	165	45.1
PIZZA-CURRY BEEF/PEAS	OUNCE	28.3	70.6	4.51	7.31	2.58	8.33	0.856	1.62	1.01	130	47.3
PIZZA-ONION/TOMATO/GREEN PEPPER/MUSHROOM	OUNCE	28.3	45.4	3.49	6.58	0.567	—	—	—	—	136	42.8
PIZZA-PEPPERONI/BEEF/SALAMI/ MUSHROOM/ETC	OUNCE	28.3	83.3	5.07	4.56	4.96	—	—	—	—	367	61.2
PIZZA-SHRIMP/CUCUMBER	OUNCE	28.3	68.6	4.45	6.83	2.61	—	—	—	—	143	46.2
PIZZA-SHRIMP/SQUID/MUSH-ROOM	OUNCE	28.3	70.3	4.96	7.43	2.3	—	—	—	—	160	33.2
POTATOES-FRENCH FRIED-FAST FOOD	OUNCE	28.3	91.3	1.08	10.3	5.07	2.76	1.8	1.93	0.755	17	130
POTATOES-MASHED-FAST FOOD	OUNCE	28.3	26.4	0.624	5.44	0.227	0.544	0.284	0.481	0.328	82.2	48.2
RAX-GRILLED CHICKEN SAND-WICH	ITEM	190	440	24	36	19	87.9	2.92	4.48	5.37	1050	340
SALAD-FAST FOOD	OUNCE	28.3	33.5	0.454	3.29	2.04	—	—	—	—	128	39.7
SPAGHETTI-VEGETABLES/ SAUCE/CHEESE	OUNCE	28.3	28.3	3.8	3.01	0.113	—	—	—	—	83.6	52.4
SUBWAY SANDWICH-HAM AND CHEESE-ON WHEAT	ITEM	194	673	39	86	22	73	7	8	4	2508	918
SUBWAY-BMT SANDWICH-ON HONEY WHEAT ROLL	ITEM	220	1011	45	88	57	133	20	25	7	3199	1002
SUBWAY-BMT SANDWICH-ON ITALIAN ROLL	ITEM	213	982	44	83	55	133	20	24	7	3139	917
SUBWAY-CLUB SANDWICH-ON HONEY WHEAT	ITEM	220	722	47	89	23	84	7	9	4	2777	1055
SUBWAY-CLUB SANDWICH-ON ITALIAN ROLL	ITEM	213	693	46	83	22	84	7	8	4	2717	971
SUBWAY-COLD CUT COMBO SAND-WICH-ITALIAN	ITEM	184	853	46	83	40	166	12	15	10	2218	876
SUBWAY-COLD CUT COMBO SAND-WICH-ON WHEAT	ITEM	191	883	48	88	41	166	12	15	10	2278	1010
SUBWAY-HAM & CHEESE SAND-WICH-ON ITALIAN	ITEM	184	643	38	81	18	73	7	8	4	1710	834
SUBWAY-MEATBALL SANDWICH-ON ITALIAN ROLL	ITEM	215	918	42	96	44	88	17	17	4	2022	1210
SUBWAY-MEATBALL-ON HONEY WHEAT ROLL	ITEM	224	947	44	101	45	88	17	18	4	2082	1498
SUBWAY-ROAST BEEF SANDWICH-ITALIAN ROLL	ITEM	184	689	42	84	23	83.3	8	9	4	2288	910
SUBWAY-ROAST BEEF SANDWICH-ON WHEAT ROLL	ITEM	189	717	41	89	24	75	8	9	4	2348	994
SUBWAY-SALAD DRESSING-BUTTERMILK RANCH	SERVING	56.7	348	1	2	37	6	5	7	24	492	17
SUBWAY-SALAD DRESSING-LITE ITALIAN	SERVING	56.7	23	1	4	1	0	3.97	6.35	15.9	952	13
SUBWAY-SEAFOOD/CRAB SAND-WICH-ON ITALIAN	ITEM	210	986	29	94	57	56	11	15	28	1967	557
SUBWAY-SEAFOOD/CRAB SAND-WICH-ON WHEAT	ITEM	219	1015	31	100	58	56	11	16	28	2027	641
SUBWAY-SPICY ITALIAN SAND-WICH-ON ITALIAN	ITEM	213	1043	42	83	63	137	23	28	7	2282	880
SUBWAY-STEAK & CHEESE SAND-WICH-ITALIAN	ITEM	213	765	43	83	32	82	12	12	4	1556	909
SUBWAY-TURKEY BREAST SAND-WICH-WHEAT ROLL	ITEM	192	674	42	88	20	67	6	7	7	2520	605
TACO BELL-DOUBLE BEEF BURRITO SUPREME	ITEM	255	457	23.6	41.7	21.8	56.8	10.1	15.4	2.09	1053	431
TACO BELL-ENCHIRITO	ITEM	213	382	19.8	30.9	19.7	54.2	9.32	—	1.51	1243	—
TACO BELL-MEXICAN PIZZA	SERVING	223	575	21.3	39.7	36.8	52	11.4	8.16	9.74	1031	408
TACO BELL-NACHOS	SERVING	106	346	7.49	37.5	18.5	8.82	5.74	9.96	1.55	399	159
TACO BELL-NACHOS BELL-GRANDE	SERVING	287	649	21.6	60.6	35.3	36.3	12.3	—	2.61	997	674
TACO BELL-PINTOS & CHEESE	SERVING	128	190	8.97	19	8.72	16.2	3.6	4.92	0.814	642	399
TACO BELL-SOFT TACO	ITEM	92.1	228	11.8	17.9	11.8	31.8	5.37	3.71	1.21	516	178
TACO BELL-TACO BELLGRANDE	ITEM	163	355	18.3	17.7	23.1	55.9	10.9	6.57	1.32	472	334
TACO BELL-TACO LIGHT	ITEM	170	410	19	18.1	28.8	55.6	11.6	—	5.36	594	316
TACO BELL-TACO SALAD WITH SALSA/NO SHELL	SERVING	530	520	30.6	30	31.4	79.8	14.4	19.2	1.7	1431	1151

MAG Mg	IRON Mg	ZINC Mg	V-A RE	V-C Mg	THIA Mg	RIBO Mg	NIAC Mg	V-B6 Mg	FOL Ug	VB12 Ug	CALC Mg	PHOS Mg	SEL Mg	FIBD Gm	V-E Mg
—	0.397	—	25.2	0.879	0.026	0.026	2.13	—	—	0.084	85.9	114	—	0.057	—
6.45	0.227	0.343	9.64	0.624	0.017	0.017	1.81	0.038	6.9	0.084	26.6	39.4	—	0.17	0.348
7.03	0.17	0.725	28.6	0.879	0.02	0.023	3.57	0.058	2.45	0.366	23.8	37.7	—	0.17	0.784
—	0.227	—	9.07	0.425	0.014	0.023	1.64	—	—	—	24.7	32.9	—	0.227	—
—	0.227	—	21.5	0.198	0.02	0.003	3.06	—	—	—	76.3	58.7	—	0.085	—
—	0.198	—	11.9	0.397	0.009	0.011	2.32	—	—	—	24.7	48.2	—	0.142	—
—	0.17	—	13	0.369	0.009	0.014	0.936	—	—	—	22.4	37.7	—	0.142	—
9.62	0.595	0.108	6.24	0.312	0.023	0.011	0.369	0.067	8.21	0	2.27	20.1	—	0	0.07
5.15	0.765	0.077	14.7	0.227	0.017	0.011	0.198	0.063	2.25	0.016	3.12	14.2	—	0	0.208
47.3	3.56	1.72	15.8	0	0.462	0.401	15.3	0.671	33.3	0.35	114	299	—	1.61	3.19
—	0.652	—	4.25	0.85	0.017	0.006	0.028	—	—	—	5.39	14.2	—	0	—
—	0.312	—	3.97	0.085	0.011	0.011	0.227	—	—	—	3.97	9.64	—	0.34	—
—	—	—	—	—	—	—	—	—	—	—	—	—	—	6	—
—	—	—	—	—	—	—	—	—	—	—	—	—	—	6	—
66.1	4.26	6.08	66.5	5.4	0.271	0.341	5.06	0.481	62.6	2.33	63.6	308	—	5	6.1
39.7	3.18	1.39	83	15.1	0.486	0.348	9.3	0.455	43.1	0.44	96.3	247	—	6	5.04
65.6	3.09	2.5	74	20.2	0.477	0.334	12.5	0.581	47	0.946	57.5	384	—	5	1.61
27.5	2.86	2.73	87	17.3	0.359	0.333	3.8	0.201	39	1.23	227	315	—	5	1.08
28.5	2.97	2.83	90.3	18	0.372	0.346	3.94	0.208	40.5	1.28	23.5	327	—	6	1.13
49.6	2.17	2.8	174	16.8	0.528	0.388	3.56	0.335	45.1	0.756	304	527	—	5	4.6
47.1	4.97	6.2	71.9	18.7	0.333	0.391	9.36	0.4	34.9	3.21	77.6	263	—	3.02	1.18
—	—	—	—	—	—	—	—	—	—	—	—	—	—	—	—
57.1	3.68	5.26	57.5	4.67	0.234	0.294	4.37	0.416	54.1	2.01	54.9	266	—	5	5.26
58.6	3.78	5.4	59	4.79	0.24	0.302	4.49	0.427	55.6	2.07	56.4	273	—	6	5.4
1.13	0.113	0.102	47.6	0	0.007	0.014	0.002	0.01	3.56	0.118	7.94	14.7	—	0	2.72
0.363	0.113	0.062	13.6	0	0.006	0.011	0.002	0.007	2.77	0.092	5.67	2.84	—	0	5.86
—	—	—	—	—	—	—	—	—	—	—	—	—	—	—	—
61.7	4.41	5.28	107	5.49	0.51	0.383	6.95	0.258	91.3	6.54	230	336	—	2.49	3.01
—	—	—	—	—	—	—	—	—	—	—	—	—	—	5	—
43.1	4.22	6.78	119	5.82	0.33	0.464	5.06	0.381	36.4	2.54	231	456	—	6	1.01
—	—	—	—	—	—	—	—	—	—	—	—	—	—	7	—
87.2	3.95	5.93	286	8.68	0.427	2.19	3.68	0.354	132	2.18	145	548	—	5.68	2.78
—	2.84	—	290	28.1	0.256	0.418	2.32	—	—	—	269	—	—	—	—
62.9	3.74	2.32	295	30.9	0.319	0.326	2.96	0.274	113	0.198	257	360	—	5.75	3.02
42.8	0.934	2.58	169	1.88	0.006	0.163	0.679	0.122	15.7	0.615	191	439	—	1.39	3.36
—	3.48	—	341	57.8	0.104	0.339	2.17	—	—	—	297	—	—	—	—
49.8	1.42	1.08	132	51.4	0.05	0.146	0.396	0.192	98.1	0.076	156	175	—	4.87	1.68
30.6	2.27	1.36	64	1.22	0.387	0.224	2.74	0.159	40.3	0.31	116	132	—	2.56	1.1
54.1	1.92	2.4	254	5.48	0.107	0.291	2.02	0.282	71.3	0.549	182	234	—	4.54	1.94
—	2.44	—	199	4.7	0.199	0.325	2.51	—	—	—	155	—	—	—	—
111	5.14	9.14	908	76.1	0.264	0.64	3.17	0.779	98.8	4.29	367	567	—	7.04	7.25

Continued.

Food Name	Portion	WT. Gm	KCAL Kc	PROT Gm	CARB Gm	FAT Gm	CHOL Mg	SAFA Gm	MUFA Gm	PUFA Gm	SOD Mg	POT Mg
TACO BELL-TACO SALAD WITH SALSA/SHELL	SERVING	595	941	36	63.1	61.3	80.4	18.7	21.6	12.1	1662	1212
TACO BELL-TACO SALAD-NO SALSA-NO SHELL	SERVING	530	502	29.5	26.3	31.3	79.8	14.4	19.2	1.7	1056	988
WENDYS-BACON AND CHEESE POTATO	SERVING	347	450	15	57	18	10	37.1	38.2	14.1	1125	1580
WENDYS-BIG CLASSIC-QUARTER POUND BURGER	SERVING	277	570	27	46	33	85	15.9	14.8	4.26	1075	590
WENDYS-BROCCOLI AND CHEESE POTATO	SERVING	377	400	9	59	16	0	—	—	—	470	1555
WENDYS-CHEESE POTATO	SERVING	348	470	13	57	21	0	12.1	9.26	4	580	1435
WENDYS-CHEESE SAUCE	SERVING	56	40	1	5	2	0	1.87	1.06	0.319	300	70
WENDYS-CHEESE TORTELLINI/ SPAGHETTI SAUCE	SERVING	112	120	4	24	1	5	2.8	2.15	0.888	280	110
WENDYS-CHICKEN CLUB SAND- WICH	SERVING	231	500	30	42	24	75	5.45	8.46	8.02	950	515
WENDYS-CHICKEN SALAD	SERVING	56	120	7	4	8	0	3	2.81	3	215	60
WENDYS-CHILI	SERVING	255	220	21	23	7	45	3	5.66	1.05	750	495
WENDYS-FRENCH FRIES-REGULAR SIZE	SERVING	134	440	5	53	23	25	8.51	9.13	3.58	265	855
WENDYS-KIDS MEAL HAMBURGER	SERVING	104	260	14	30	9	35	3.5	4.75	0.768	545	205
WENDYS-REFRIED BEANS	SERVING	56	70	4	10	3	0	1	2.21	1	215	210
WENDYS-SEAFOOD SALAD	SERVING	56	110	4	7	7	0	1	4.46	4	455	40
WENDYS-SINGLE CHEESEBURGER/ EVERYTHING	SERVING	252	490	29	35	27	90	10.8	11.2	4.58	1155	495
WENDYS-SINGLE HAMBURGER/ EVERYTHING	SERVING	234	420	25	35	21	70	6.72	9.4	4.43	865	495
WENDYS-SPANISH RICE	SERVING	56	70	2	13	1	0	0.121	0.298	1	440	130
WENDYS-TACO SALAD WITH TACO CHIPS	SERVING	791	660	40	46	37	35	28.8	28.7	15.4	1110	1330
WENDYS-TUNA SALAD	SERVING	56	100	8	4	6	0	1	0.796	3	290	90

MAG Mg	IRON Mg	ZINC Mg	V-A RE	V-C Mg	THIA Mg	RIBO Mg	NIAC Mg	V-B6 Mg	FOL Ug	VB12 Ug	CALC Mg	PHOS Mg	SEL Mg	FIBD Gm	V-E Mg
125	7.1	10.3	888	77	0.508	0.753	4.78	0.875	111	4.82	398	637	—	7.91	8.14
111	4.54	9.14	572	74.3	0.246	0.498	3.17	0.779	98.8	4.29	331	567	—	7.04	7.25
167	15.3	6.99	266	76.5	1.04	0.805	14.5	1.94	75.4	2.26	713	1015	—	9.85	5.83
49.2	4.75	6.36	162	9.41	0.346	0.496	7.95	0.382	50.5	2.92	304	491	—	2.32	3.42
—	—	—	—	—	—	—	—	—	—	—	—	—	—	—	—
71.9	2.25	2.43	288	33.9	0.223	0.425	3.47	0.574	30.6	0.299	417	398	—	3.59	2.75
9.52	0.056	0.195	23.5	0.448	0.03	0.113	0.064	0.028	2.52	0.224	114	87.9	—	0.168	0.08
14.3	1.34	0.643	110	4.24	0.12	0.175	1.21	0.085	12.2	0.17	74.5	92.3	—	1.01	1.14
41.7	14.4	1.46	87.1	15.8	0.511	0.365	16	0.478	45.3	0.462	101	259	—	2.3	5.29
8.2	0.5	0.659	21.5	1.08	0.022	0.077	1.79	0.134	5.96	0.141	12.8	57.5	—	0.214	2.89
53.2	6.3	4.12	146	18.9	0.158	0.258	4.81	0.232	41.3	1.46	55.2	228	—	6	2.11
45.6	1.02	0.509	0	13.8	0.237	0.038	4.36	0.316	38.9	0	25.5	125	—	4.62	0.33
21.6	2.47	2.22	7.3	1.43	0.226	0.198	3.82	0.135	24.9	0.998	62.6	110	—	1.32	0.641
24.7	1.16	0.493	0	1.68	0.082	0.039	0.177	0.087	71.1	0	24.6	72.3	—	3	0.566
14.3	0.535	0.865	21.4	3.3	0.021	0.026	0.619	0.045	7.76	0.481	24.7	73.7	—	0.222	1.48
43.7	4.31	4.27	136	10.9	0.403	0.423	6.52	0.302	55.1	1.8	234	348	—	2.69	3.8
39.5	4.29	3.69	75.6	11.1	0.402	0.353	6.6	0.292	54.2	1.68	105	193	—	2.73	3.64
8.92	0.692	0.196	23.9	9.2	0.046	0.017	0.586	0.057	3.6	0	15.3	17.4	—	0.744	0.36
166	9.23	13.6	1478	67.4	0.396	0.925	15.2	1.16	147	6.41	532	847	—	10.5	10.8
10.3	0.557	0.176	14.9	1.23	0.018	0.041	3.75	0.045	3.9	0.679	9.25	61.9	—	0.312	0.638

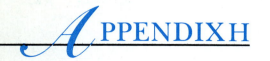

APPENDIX H

Physical Growth NCHS Percentiles

GIRLS: BIRTH TO 36 MONTHS
PHYSICAL GROWTH
NCHS PERCENTILES*

NAME _____   RECORD # _____

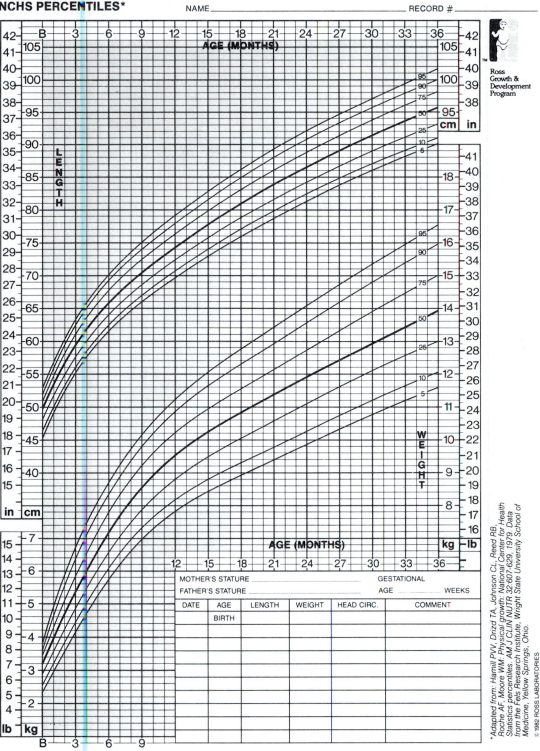

Ross
Growth &
Development
Program

MOTHER'S STATURE _____   GESTATIONAL

FATHER'S STATURE _____   AGE _____ WEEKS

DATE	AGE	LENGTH	WEIGHT	HEAD CIRC.	COMMENT
	BIRTH				

*Adapted from: Hamill PVV, Drizd TA, Johnson CL, Reed RB, Roche AF, Moore WM. Physical growth: National Center for Health Statistics percentiles. AM J CLIN NUTR 32:607-629, 1979. Data from the Fels Research Institute, Wright State University School of Medicine, Yellow Springs, Ohio.

© 1982 ROSS LABORATORIES

BOYS: BIRTH TO 36 MONTHS
PHYSICAL GROWTH
NCHS PERCENTILES*

NAME _____   RECORD # _____

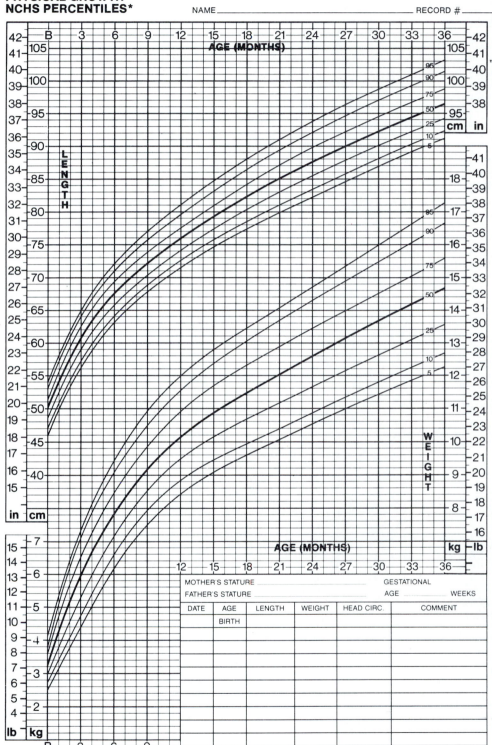

*Adapted from: Hamill PVV, Drizd TA, Johnson CL, Reed RB, Roche AF, Moore WM: Physical growth: National Center for Health Statistics percentiles. AM J CLIN NUTR 32:607-629, 1979. Data from the Fels Research Institute, Wright State University School of Medicine, Yellow Springs, Ohio.

© 1982 ROSS LABORATORIES

Ross
Growth &
Development
Program

**GIRLS: BIRTH TO 36 MONTHS
PHYSICAL GROWTH
NCHS PERCENTILES***

NAME_____   RECORD #_____

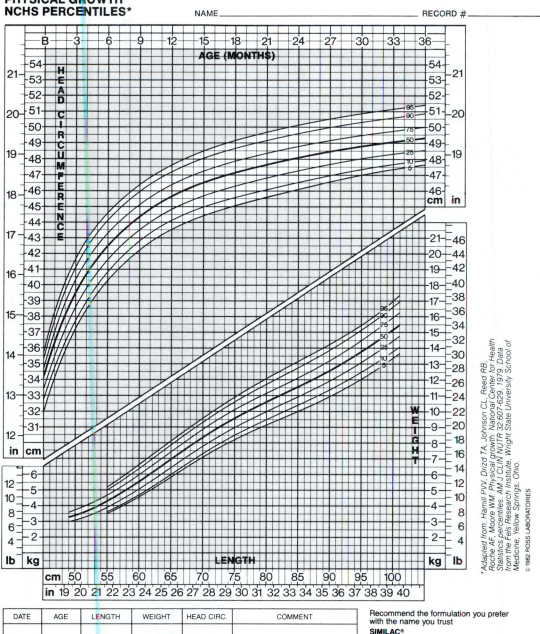

*Adapted from: Hamill PVV, Drizd TA, Johnson CL, Reed RB, Roche AF, Moore WM: Physical growth: National Center for Health Statistics percentiles. AM J CLIN NUTR 32:607-629, 1979. Data from the Fels Research Institute, Wright State University School of Medicine, Yellow Springs, Ohio.
© 1982 ROSS LABORATORIES

DATE	AGE	LENGTH	WEIGHT	HEAD CIRC.	COMMENT

Recommend the formulation you prefer
with the name you trust

**SIMILAC®
SIMILAC® WITH IRON
SIMILAC® WITH WHEY
Infant Formulas**

**The ISOMIL® System of
Soy Protein Formulas**

**ADVANCE®
Nutritional Beverage**

ROSS LABORATORIES
COLUMBUS, OHIO 43216
Division of Abbott Laboratories, USA

G106/JUNE 1983   LITHO IN USA

BOYS: BIRTH TO 36 MONTHS
PHYSICAL GROWTH
NCHS PERCENTILES*

NAME _____   RECORD # _____

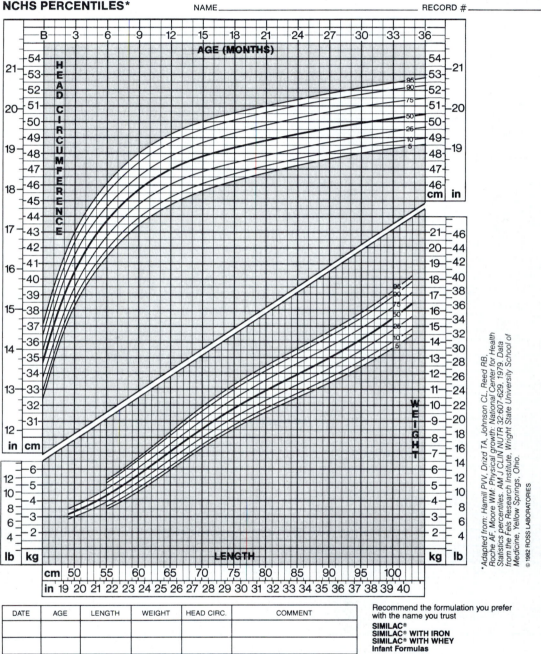

*Adapted from: Hamill PVV, Drizd TA, Johnson CL, Reed RB, Roche AF, Moore WM: Physical growth: National Center for Health Statistics percentiles. AM J CLIN NUTR 32:607-629, 1979. Data from the Fels Research Institute, Wright State University School of Medicine, Yellow Springs, Ohio.

© 1982 ROSS LABORATORIES

DATE	AGE	LENGTH	WEIGHT	HEAD CIRC.	COMMENT

Recommend the formulation you prefer
with the name you trust

SIMILAC®
SIMILAC® WITH IRON
SIMILAC® WITH WHEY
Infant Formulas

The **ISOMIL®** System of
Soy Protein Formulas

ADVANCE®
Nutritional Beverage

ROSS LABORATORIES
COLUMBUS, OHIO 43216
Division of Abbott Laboratories, USA

G105/JUNE 1983   LITHO IN USA

GIRLS: 2 TO 18 YEARS
PHYSICAL GROWTH
NCHS PERCENTILES*

NAME _____ RECORD # _____

DATE	AGE	STATURE	WEIGHT	COMMENT

MOTHER'S STATURE _____ FATHER'S STATURE _____

AGE (YEARS)

STATURE

WEIGHT

Ross
Growth &
Development
Program

*Adapted from: Hamill PVV, Drizd TA, Johnson CL, Reed RB,
Roche AF, Moore WM: Physical growth: National Center for Health
Statistics percentiles. AM J CLIN NUTR 32:607-629, 1979. Data
from the National Center for Health Statistics (NCHS) Hyattsville,
Maryland.

BOYS: 2 TO 18 YEARS
PHYSICAL GROWTH
NCHS PERCENTILES*

NAME _____   RECORD # _____

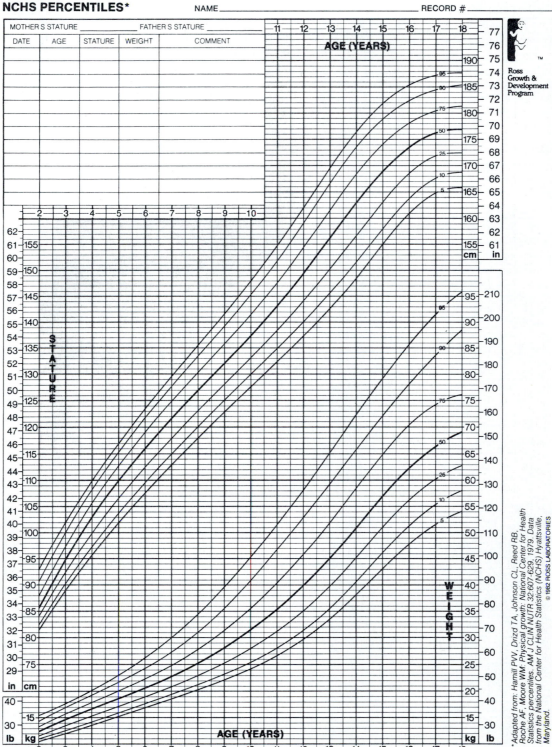

* Adapted from: Hamill PVV, Drizd TA, Johnson CL, Reed RB, Roche AF, Moore WM: Physical growth: National Center for Health Statistics percentiles. AM J CLIN NUTR 32:607-629, 1979. Data from the National Center for Health Statistics (NCHS) Hyattsville, Maryland.

Ross Growth & Development Program

© 1982 ROSS LABORATORIES

GIRLS: PREPUBESCENT
PHYSICAL GROWTH
NCHS PERCENTILES*

NAME _____   RECORD # _____

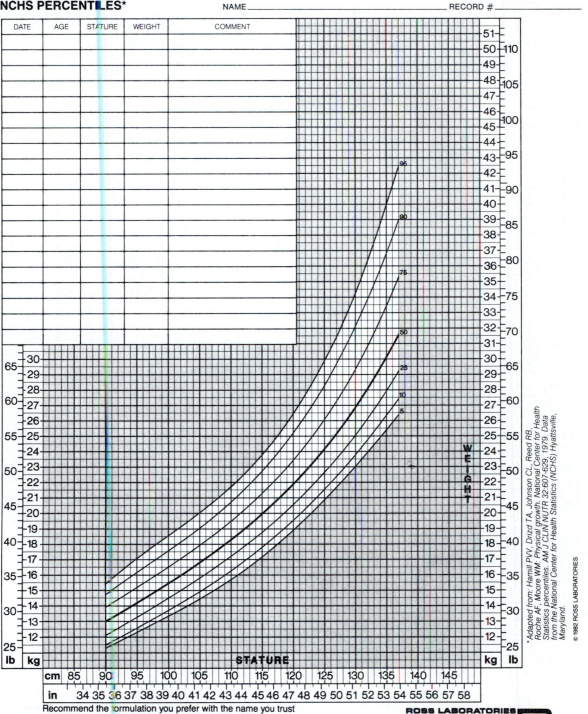

DATE	AGE	STATURE	WEIGHT	COMMENT

STATURE

WEIGHT

cm 85 90 95 100 105 110 115 120 125 130 135 140 145

in 34 35 36 37 38 39 40 41 42 43 44 45 46 47 48 49 50 51 52 53 54 55 56 57 58

Recommend the formulation you prefer with the name you trust

SIMILAC®
SIMILAC® WITH IRON
SIMILAC® WITH WHEY
Infant Formulas

The **ISOMIL®** System of
Soy Protein Formulas

ADVANCE®
Nutritional Beverage

ROSS LABORATORIES
COLUMBUS, OHIO 43216
Division of Abbott Laboratories, USA

G108/JUNE 1983   LITHO IN USA

BOYS: PREPUBESCENT
PHYSICAL GROWTH
NCHS PERCENTILES*

NAME_____ RECORD #_____

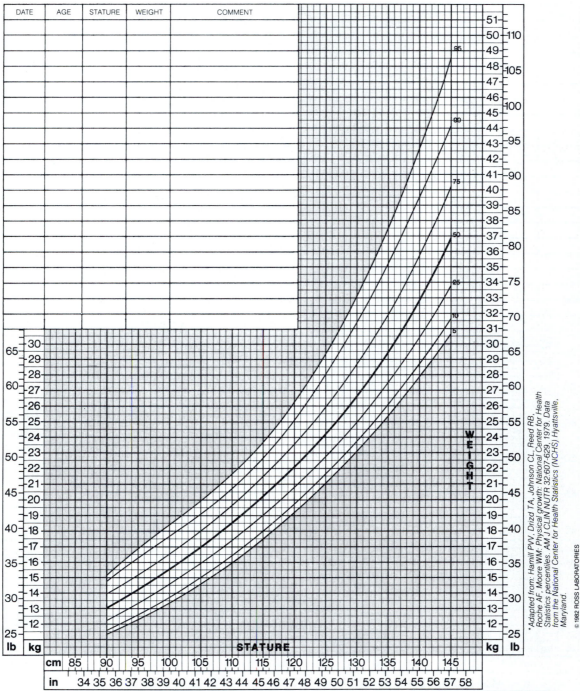

DATE	AGE	STATURE	WEIGHT	COMMENT

STATURE

WEIGHT

cm 85 90 95 100 105 110 115 120 125 130 135 140 145

in 34 35 36 37 38 39 40 41 42 43 44 45 46 47 48 49 50 51 52 53 54 55 56 57 58

*Adapted from: Hamill PVV, Drizd TA, Johnson CL, Reed RB, Roche AF, Moore WM: Physical growth: National Center for Health Statistics percentiles. AM J CLIN NUTR 32:607-629, 1979. Data from the National Center for Health Statistics (NCHS) Hyattsville, Maryland.

© 1982 ROSS LABORATORIES

Recommend the formulation you prefer with the name you trust

SIMILAC®
SIMILAC® WITH IRON
SIMILAC® WITH WHEY
Infant Formulas

The ISOMIL® System of
Soy Protein Formulas

ADVANCE®
Nutritional Beverage

ROSS LABORATORIES
COLUMBUS, OHIO 43216
Division of Abbott Laboratories, USA

G107/JUNE 1983   LITHO IN USA

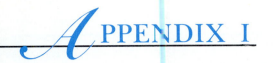

APPENDIX I

Assessment of Nutritional Status: Percentiles

Mid–Upper-Arm Circumference Percentiles (cm)

Age (yr)	Female percentiles					Male percentiles				
	5th	25th	50th	75th	95th	5th	25th	50th	75th	95th
1	13.8	14.8	15.6	16.4	17.7	14.2	15.0	15.9	17.0	18.3
2	14.2	15.2	16.0	16.7	18.4	14.1	15.3	16.2	17.0	18.5
3	14.3	15.8	16.7	17.5	18.9	15.0	16.0	16.7	17.5	19.0
4	14.9	16.0	16.9	17.7	19.1	14.9	16.2	17.1	18.0	19.2
5	15.3	16.5	17.5	18.5	21.1	15.3	16.7	17.5	18.5	20.4
6	15.6	17.0	17.6	18.7	21.1	15.5	16.7	17.9	18.8	22.8
7	16.4	17.4	18.3	19.9	23.1	16.2	17.7	18.7	20.1	23.0
8	16.8	18.3	19.5	21.4	26.1	16.2	17.7	19.0	20.2	24.5
9	17.8	19.4	21.1	22.4	26.0	17.5	18.7	20.0	21.7	25.7
10	17.4	19.3	21.0	22.8	26.5	18.1	19.6	21.0	23.1	27.4
11	18.5	20.8	22.4	24.8	30.3	18.6	20.2	22.3	24.4	28.0
12	19.4	21.6	23.7	25.6	29.4	19.3	21.4	23.2	25.4	30.3
13	20.2	22.3	24.3	27.1	33.8	19.4	22.8	24.7	26.3	30.1
14	21.4	23.7	25.2	27.2	32.2	22.0	23.7	25.3	28.3	32.3
15	20.8	23.9	25.4	27.9	32.2	22.2	24.4	26.4	28.4	32.0
16	21.8	24.1	25.8	28.3	33.4	24.4	26.2	27.8	30.3	34.3
17	22.0	24.1	26.4	29.5	35.0	24.6	26.7	28.5	30.8	34.7
18	22.2	24.1	25.8	28.1	32.5	24.5	27.6	29.7	32.1	37.9
19-25	21.1	24.7	26.5	29.0	34.5	26.2	28.8	30.8	33.1	37.2
25-35	23.3	25.5	27.7	30.4	36.8	27.1	30.0	31.9	34.2	37.5
35-45	24.1	26.7	29.0	31.7	37.8	27.8	30.5	32.6	34.5	37.4
45-55	24.2	27.4	29.9	32.8	38.4	26.7	30.1	32.2	34.2	37.6
55-65	24.3	28.0	30.3	33.5	38.5	25.8	29.6	31.7	33.6	36.9
65-75	24.0	27.4	29.9	32.6	37.3	24.8	28.5	30.7	32.5	35.5

Data derived from the Health and Nutrition Examination Survey data of 1971-1974, using same population samples as those of the National Center for Health Statistics (NCHS) growth percentiles for children. Adapted from Frisancho, AR: New norms of upper limb fat and muscle areas for assessment of nutritional status, *Am J Clin Nutr* 34:2540, 1981.

Mid–Upper-Arm Muscle Circumference Percentiles (cm)

Age (yr)	Female percentiles					Male percentiles				
	5th	25th	50th	75th	95th	5th	25th	50th	75th	95th
1	10.5	11.7	12.4	13.9	14.3	11.0	11.9	12.7	13.5	14.7
2	11.1	11.9	12.6	13.3	14.7	11.1	12.2	13.0	14.0	15.0
3	11.3	12.4	13.2	14.0	15.2	11.7	13.1	13.7	14.3	15.3
4	11.5	12.8	13.8	14.4	15.7	12.3	13.3	14.1	14.8	15.9
5	12.5	13.4	14.2	15.1	16.5	12.8	14.0	14.7	15.4	16.9
6	13.0	13.8	14.5	15.4	17.1	13.1	14.2	15.1	16.1	17.7
7	12.9	14.2	15.1	16.0	17.6	13.7	15.1	16.0	16.8	19.0
8	13.8	15.1	16.0	17.1	19.4	14.0	15.4	16.2	17.0	18.7
9	14.7	15.8	16.7	18.0	19.8	15.1	16.1	17.0	18.3	20.2
10	14.8	15.9	17.0	18.0	19.7	15.6	16.6	18.0	19.1	22.1
11	15.0	17.1	18.1	19.6	22.3	15.9	17.3	18.3	19.5	23.0
12	16.2	18.0	19.1	20.1	22.0	16.7	18.2	19.5	21.0	24.1
13	16.9	18.3	19.8	21.1	24.0	17.2	19.6	21.1	22.6	24.5
14	17.4	19.0	20.1	21.6	24.7	18.9	21.2	22.3	24.0	26.4
15	17.5	18.9	20.2	21.5	24.4	19.9	21.8	23.7	25.4	27.2
16	17.0	19.0	20.2	21.6	24.9	21.3	23.4	24.9	26.9	29.6
17	17.5	19.4	20.5	22.1	25.7	22.4	24.5	25.8	27.3	31.2
18	17.4	19.1	20.2	21.5	24.5	22.6	25.2	26.4	28.3	32.4
19-25	17.9	19.5	20.7	22.1	24.9	23.8	25.7	27.3	28.9	32.1
25-35	18.3	19.9	21.2	22.8	26.4	24.3	26.4	27.9	29.8	32.6
35-45	18.6	20.5	21.8	23.6	27.2	24 7	26.9	28.6	30.2	32.7
45-55	18.7	20.6	22.0	23.8	27.4	23.9	26.5	28.1	30.0	32.6
55-65	18.7	20.9	22.5	24.4	28.0	23.6	26.0	27.8	29.5	32.0
65-75	18.5	20.8	22.5	24.4	27.9	22.3	25.1	26.8	28.4	30.6

Data derived from the Health and Nutrition Examination Survey data of 1971-1974, using same population samples as those of the National Center for Health Statistics (NCHS) growth percentiles for children. Adapted from Frisancho, AR: New norms of upper limb fat and muscle areas for assessment of nutritional status, *Am J Clin Nutr* 34:2540, 1981.

Triceps Skinfold Percentiles (mm)

Age (yr)	Female percentiles					Male percentiles				
	5th	25th	50th	75th	95th	5th	25th	50th	75th	95th
1	6	8	10	12	16	6	8	10	12	16
2	6	9	10	12	16	6	8	10	12	15
3	7	9	11	12	15	6	8	10	11	15
4	7	8	10	12	16	6	8	9	11	14
5	6	8	10	12	18	6	8	9	11	15
6	6	8	10	12	16	5	7	8	10	16
7	6	9	11	13	18	5	7	9	12	17
8	6	9	12	15	24	5	7	8	10	16
9	8	10	13	16	22	6	7	10	13	18
10	7	10	12	17	27	6	8	10	14	21
11	7	10	13	18	28	6	8	11	16	24
12	8	11	14	18	27	6	8	11	14	28
13	8	12	15	21	30	5	7	10	14	26
14	9	13	16	21	28	4	7	9	14	24
15	8	12	17	21	32	4	6	8	11	24
16	10	15	18	22	31	4	6	8	12	22
17	10	13	19	24	37	5	6	8	12	19
18	10	15	18	22	30	4	6	9	13	24
19-25	10	14	18	24	34	4	7	10	15	22
25-35	10	16	21	27	37	5	8	12	16	24
35-45	12	18	23	29	38	5	8	12	16	23
45-55	12	20	25	30	40	6	8	12	15	25
55-65	12	20	25	31	38	5	8	11	14	22
65-75	12	18	24	29	36	4	8	11	15	22

Data derived from the Health and Nutrition Examination Survey data of 1971-1974, using same population samples as those of the National Center for Health Statistics (NCHS) growth percentiles for children. Adapted from Frisancho, AR: New norms of upper limb fat and muscle areas for assessment of nutritional status, *Am J Clin Nutr* 34:2540, 1981.

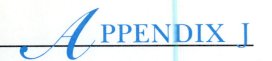

APPENDIX I

Normal Blood and Urine Valves

Normal Constituents of the Blood in the Adult

Physical measurements

Specific gravity		1.025-1.029
Viscosity (water as unity)		4.5
Bleeding time (capillary)	Minutes	1-3
Prothrombin time (plasma) (Quick)	Seconds	10-20
Sedimentation rate (Wintrobe method)		
Men	mm/hr	0-9
Women	mm/hr	0-20

Hemologic studies

Cell volume	%	39-50
Red blood cells	Million per mm³	4.25-5.25
White blood cells	Per mm³	5000-9000
Lymphocytes	%	25-30
Neutrophils	%	60-65
Monocytes	%	4-8
Eosinophils	%	0.5-4
Basophils	%	0-1.5
Platelets	Per mm³	125,000-300,000

Proteins

Total protein (serum)	g/dl	6.5-7.5
Albumin (serum)	g/dl	4.5-5.5
Globulin (serum)	g/dl	1.5-2.5
Albumin: globulin ratio		1.8-2.5
Fibrinogen (plasma)	g/dl	0.2-0.5
Hemoglobin		
Males	g/dl	14-17
Females	g/dl	13-16

Nitrogen constituents

Nonprotein N (serum)	mg/dl	20-36
(whole blood)	mg/dl	25-40
Urea (whole blood)	mg/dl	18-38
Urea N (whole blood)	mg/dl	8-18
Creatinine (whole blood)	mg/dl	1-2
Uric acid (whole blood)	mg/dl	2.5-5.0
Amino acid N (whole blood)	mg/dl	3-6

Carbohydrates and lipids

Glucose (whole blood)	mg/dl	70-90
Ketones—as acetone (whole blood)	mg/dl	1.5-2
Fats (total lipids) (serum)	mg/dl	570-820
Cholesterol (serum)	mg/dl	100-230
Bilirubin (serum)	mg/dl	0.1-0.25
Icteric index (serum)	units	4-6

Blood gases

CO_2 content (serum)	vol %	55-75
	mmol/L	(24.5-33.5)
CO_2 content (whole blood)	vol %	40-60
	mmol/L	(18.0-27.0)
Oxygen capacity (whole blood)		
Males	vol %	18.7-22.7
Females	vol %	17.0-21.0
Oxygen saturation		
Arterial blood	%	94-96
Venous blood	%	60-85

Acid-base constituents

Base, total fixed (serum)	mEq/L	142-150
Sodium (serum)	mg/dl	320-335
	mEq/L	(139-146)
Potassium (serum)	mg/dl	16-22
	mEq/L	(4.1-5.6)
Calcium (serum)	mg/dl	9.0-11.5
	mEq/L	(4.5-5.8)
Magnesium (serum)	mg/dl	1.0-3.0
	mEq/L	(1.0-2.5)
Phosphorus, inorganic (serum)	mg/dl	3.0-5.0
	mEq/L	(1.0-1.6)
Chlorides, expressed as Cl (serum)	mg/dl	352-383
	mEq/L	(99-108)
As NaCl (serum)	mg/dl	580-630
	mEq/L	(99-108)
Sulfates, inorganic as SO_4 (serum)	mg/dl	2.5-5.0
	mEq/L	(0.5-1.0)
Lactic acid (venous blood)	mg/dl	10-20
	mEq/L	(1.1-2.2)

Abbreviations and conversion factors:
 dl = deciliter
 ml = milliliter
 µg = microgram

$$mEq/L = \frac{mg/L}{\text{Equivalent weight}}$$

$$\text{Equivalent weight} = \frac{\text{Atomic weight}}{\text{Valence of element}}$$

g = gram
mm³ = cubic millimeter
mEq = milliequivalent

$$mmol \text{ (millimole)}/L = \frac{mg/L}{\text{Molecular weight}}$$

vol % (volumes percent) = mmol/L × 2.24

Normal Constituents of the Blood in the Adult—cont'd

Acid-base constituents—cont'd

Serum protein base binding power	mEq/L	(15.5-18.0)
Base bicarbonate HCO$_3$ (serum)	mEq/L	(19-30)
pH (blood or plasma at 38° C)		7.3-7.45

Miscellaneous

Phosphatase (serum)	Bodansky units per deciliter	5
Iron (whole blood)	mg/dl	46-55
Ascorbic acid (whole blood)	mg/dl	0.75-1.50
Carotene (serum)	µg/dl	75-125

Normal Constituents of the Urine in the Adult

Urine constituents	g/24 hr
Total solids	55-70
Nitrogenous constituents	
Total nitrogen	10-17
Ammonia	0.5-1.0
Amino acid N	0.4-1
Creatine	None
Creatinine	1-1.5
Protein	None
Purine bases	0.016-0.060
Urea	20-35
Uric acid	0.5-0.7
Acetone bodies	0.003-0.015
Bile	None
Calcium	0.2-0.4
Chloride (as NaCl)	10-15
Glucose	None
Indican	0-0.030
Iron	0.001-0.005
Magnesium (as MgO)	0.15-0.30
Phosphate, total (as phosphoric acid)	2.5-3.5
Potassium (as K$_2$O)	2.0-3.0
Sodium (as Na$_2$O)	4.0-5.0
Sulfates, total (as sulfuric acid)	1.5-3.0

Physical measurements

Specific gravity	1.010-1.025
Reaction (pH)	5.5-8.0
Volume (ml/24 hr)	800-1600

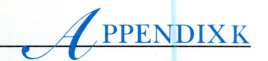

APPENDIX K

Exchange Lists for Meal Planning

Milk Exchange List

Skim milk (12 g carbohydrate, 8 g protein, 0 g fat, 90 kcal)

1 cup	Skin or nonfat milk (½% and 1%)
⅓ cup	Powdered (nonfat dry, before adding liquid)
½ cup	Canned, evaporated skim milk
1 cup	Buttermilk made from skim milk
1 cup	Yogurt made from skim milk (plain, unflavored)

Low-fat milk (12 g carbohydrate, 8 g protein, 5 g fat, 120 kcal)

1 cup	2% fat milk
1 cup	Plain nonfat yogurt (added milk solids)

Whole milk (12 g carbohydrate, 8 g protein, 8 g fat, 150 kcal)

1 cup	Whole milk
1 cup	Custard-style yogurt made from whole milk (plain, unflavored)

Vegetable Exchange List

(5 g carbohydrate, 2 g protein, 0 g fat, 25 kcal). 1 exchange equals ½ cup cooked vegetables or vegetable juice and 1 cup raw vegetables

Artichoke (½ medium)	Mushrooms (cooked)
Asparagus	Onions
Beans (green, wax, Italian)	Pea pods
Bean sprouts	Sauerkraut
Beets	Spinach (cooked)
Broccoli	Squash, summer, zucchini
Brussels sprouts	String beans (green, yellow)
Cabbage, cooked	Tomato
Carrots	Tomato juice
Cauliflower	Turnips
Eggplant	Vegetable juice
Green pepper	Zucchini (cooked)
Greens	

Fruit Exchange List

(15 g carbohydrate, 0 g protein, 0 g fat, 60 kcal). 1 fruit exchange equals:

1	Apple (2 in diameter)
4 rings	Dried apple
½ cup	Apple juice
½ cup	Applesauce (unsweetened)
½ cup	Apricots, canned
7 halves	Apricots, dried
4	Apricots, fresh
½	Banana, 9 in
¾ cup	Blackberries
¾ cup	Blueberries
1 cup	Raspberries
1¼ cup	Strawberries
⅓ melon	Cantaloupe (5 in diameter)
½ cup	Cherries, canned
12	Cherries (large, raw)
½ cup	Cider
⅓ cup	Cranberry juice cocktail
2½ medium	Dates
1½	Figs, dried
2	Figs, fresh (2 in diameter)
⅓ cup	Grape juice
½	Grapefruit
½ cup	Grapefruit juice
15	Grapes
⅛ melon	Honeydew melon (7 in diameter; cubes = 1 cup)
1	Kiwi (large)
¾ cup	Mandarin oranges
½ small	Mango
1 small	Nectarine (1½ in diameter)
1 small	Orange (2½ in diameter)
½ cup	Orange juice
½ cup or 2 halves	Peach, canned
1 medium or ¾ cup	Peach, fresh (2¾ in diameter)
½ cup or 2 halves	Pear, canned
1 small or ½ large	Pear, fresh
⅓ cup	Pineapple, canned
¾ cup	Pineapple, raw
½ cup	Pineapple juice
2	Plums (2 in diameter)
⅓ cup	Prune juice
3	Prunes, dried
2 tbsp	Raisins
2	Tangerine (2½ in diameter)
1¼ cups	Watermelon (cubes)

Starch/Bread Exchange List

(15 g carbohydrate, 3 g protein, 0 g fat, 80 kcal) 1 starch/bread exchange equals:

Bread

½ (1 oz)	Bagel, small
2 (⅔ oz)	Bread sticks (crisp, 4 in long, ½ in wide)
3 tbsp	Dried bread crumbs
½	English muffin
½ (1 oz)	Frankfurter bun
½ (1 oz)	Hamburger bun
½	Pita (6 in diameter)
1 (small)	Plain roll
1 slice	Raisin (unfrosted)
1 slice	Rye or pumpernickel
1	Tortilla (6 in diameter)
1 slice	White (including French and Italian)
1 slice	Whole wheat

Cereal/Grains/Pasta

½ cup	Bran flakes
½ cup	Cereal (cooked)
2½ tbsp	Cornmeal (dry)
2½ tbsp	Flour (dry)
3 tbsp	Grapenuts
¾ cup	Other ready-to-eat unsweetened cereal
½ cup	Pasta (cooked spaghetti, noodles, macaroni)
1½ cups	Puffed cereal (unfrosted)
⅓ cup	Rice or barley (cooked)
½ cup	Shredded wheat
3 tbsp	Wheat germ

Crackers/Snacks

8	Animal
3	Graham (2½-in square)
¾ oz	Matzoh (4 × 6 in)
5 slices	Melba toast
24	Oyster
3 cups	Popcorn (popped with no added fat)
¾ oz	Pretzels
4	Rye crisp (2 × 3½ in)
6	Saltines

Dried Beans/Peas/Lentils

¼ cup	Baked beans
⅓ cup	Dried beans, such as kidney, white, split, blackeye (cooked)
⅓ cup	Lentils (cooked)

Starchy Vegetables

½ cup	Corn
1	Corn on the cob (6 inches)
½ cup	Lima beans
½ cup	Peas, green (canned or frozen)
½ cup	Potato, mashed
1 small	Potato, white (3 ounces baked)
1 cup	Winter squash, acorn or butternut
⅓ cup	Yam or sweet potato

Starch Group (with Fat)

1 starch/bread exchange
1 fat exchange

1	Biscuit (2½ in across)
1 (2 oz)	Corn bread (2-in cube)
6	Cracker, round butter type
10 (1½ oz)	French fries (2-3½ in)
1	Muffin, plain, small
2	Pancake (4 in diameter)
¼ cup	Stuffing, bread (prepared)
2	Taco shell (6 in across)
1	Waffle (4½ in square)
4-6 (1 oz)	Whole-wheat crackers (such as Triscuits)

Meat Exchange List

Lean (0 g carbohydrate, 7 g protein, 3 g fat, 55 kcal)

Beef	1 oz	Baby beef (lean), chipped beef, chuck, flank steak, tenderloin, plate ribs, round (bottom, top), all cuts rump, spare ribs, tripe
Cheese	1 oz	Cottage, farmer's, or pot (low-fat), grated parmesan
Fish	2 oz	Fresh or frozen, any type canned salmon, tuna, mackerel, crab, or lobster
Pork	1 oz	Leg (whole rump, center shank), ham (center slices), USDA good or choice grades such as round, sirloin, flank, and tenderloin
Poultry	1 oz	Chicken, turkey, cornish hen (without skin)
Veal	1 oz	Leg, loin, rib, shank, shoulder, chops, roasts, all cuts except cutlets (ground or cubed)

Medium Fat (0 g carbohydrate, 7 g protein, 5 g fat, 75 kcal)

Beef	1 oz	All ground beef, roast (rib, chuck, rump), steak (cubed, porterhouse, T-bone), meat loaf
Cheese	¼ cup or 1 oz	Cottage (creamed), mozzarella (made with skim milk), ricotta, Neufchatel
Egg	1	Egg
Fish	¼ cup	Tuna (canned in oil); salmon (canned)
Lamb	1 oz	Leg, rib, sirloin, loin (roast and chops), shank, shoulder
Organ meat	1 oz	All types
Other	4 oz	Tofu
Pork	1 oz	Loin (all cuts tenderloin), chops, roast, Boston butt, cutlets

Poultry	1 oz	Capon, duck (domestic), goose, ground turkey, chicken with skin
Veal	1 oz	Cutlets

High Fat (0 g carbohydrate, 7 g protein, 8 g fat, 100 kcal)

Beef	1 oz	Brisket, corned beef (commercial), chuck (ground commercial), roasts (rib), steaks (club and rib); most USDA prime cuts of beef
Cheese	1 oz	All regular cheeses (American, blue, brick, Camembert, cheddar, Gouda, Limburger, Muenster, Swiss, Monterey), all processed cheeses
Cold cuts	1 oz	Bologna, salami, pimento loaf
Frankfurter	1 oz	Turkey, chicken
Lamb	1 oz	Patties (ground lamb)
Peanut butter	1 tbsp	
Pork	1 oz	Spare ribs, loin (back ribs), pork (ground), country-style ham, deviled ham, pork sausage
Sausage	1 oz	Polish, Italian

Fat Exchange List

(0 g carbohydrate, 0 g protein, 5 g fat, 45 kcal)

⅛ medium	Avocado
1 strip	Bacon, crisp
1 tsp	Butter, margarine
1 tbsp	Cream, heavy
2 tbsp	Cream, light
2 tbsp	Cream, sour
1 tbsp	Cream cheese
Dressing	
2 tsp	All varieties
	Mayonnaise type
1 tbsp	Gravy, meat
1 tbsp	Reduced kcalorie
Olives	10 small or 5 large
Nuts	
6	Almonds, whole, dry roasted
1 tbsp	Cashews, dry roasted
1 tbsp	Other
20 small or 10 large	Peanuts, Spanish, whole
10	Peanuts, Virginia, whole
2 large	Pecans, whole
2 tsp	Pumpkin seeds
1 tbsp	Seeds (pine, sunflower)
2 whole	Walnuts
Oil	
1 tsp	Corn, cottonseed, safflower, soy, sunflower, olive, peanut, canola

Free Foods

A free food is any food or drink that contains less than 20 kcal per serving. You can eat as much as you want of those items that have no serving size specified. You may eat two or three servings per day of those items that have a specific serving size. Be sure to spread them out through the day.

Drinks

Bouillon or broth without fat
Bouillon, low-sodium
Carbonated drinks, sugar-free
Carbonated water
Club soda
Cocoa powder, unsweetened (1 tbsp)
Coffee/tea
Drink mixes, sugar-free
Tonic water, sugar-free

Nonstick pan spray

Fruit

Cranberries, unsweetened (½ cup)
Rhubarb, unsweetened (½ cup)

Vegetables

(raw, 1 cup)
Cabbage
Celery
Chinese cabbage
Cucumber
Green onion
Hot peppers
Mushrooms (fresh)
Radishes
Zucchini

Seasonings

Basil (fresh)
Celery seeds
Cinnamon
Chili powder
Chives
Curry
Dill
Flavoring extracts (vanilla, almond, walnut, peppermint, butter, lemon, etc.)
Garlic
Garlic powder
Herbs
Hot pepper sauce

Salad greens

Endive
Escarole
Lettuce
Romaine
Spinach

Sweet substitutes

Candy, hard, sugar-free
Gelatin, sugar-free
Gum, sugar-free
Jam/jelly, sugar-free (2 tsp)
Pancake syrup, sugar-free (1-2 tbsp)
Sugar substitutes (saccharin, aspartame)
Whipped topping (2 tbsp)

Condiments

Catsup (1 tbsp)
Horseradish
Mustard
Pickles, dill, unsweetened
Salad dressing, low-kcalorie (2 tbsp)
Taco sauce (3 tbsp)
Vinegar

Lemon
Lemon juice
Lemon pepper
Lime
Lime juice
Mint
Onion powder
Oregano
Paprika
Pepper
Pimento
Soy sauce
Soy sauce, low-sodium (lite)
Spices
Wine, used in cooking (¼ cup)
Worcestershire sauce

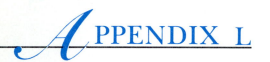

*A*PPENDIX L

Recommended Nutrient Intakes for Canadians

Summary Examples of Recommended Nutrient Intake Based on Age and Body Weight Expressed as Daily Rates										
Age	Sex	Energy (kcal)	Thiamin (mg)	Riboflavin (mg)	Niacin NE	n-3 PUFA (g)	n-6 PUFA (g)	Weight (kg)	Protein (g)	Vitamin A RE
0-4 months	Both	600	0.3	0.3	4	0.5	3	6.0	12*	400
5-12 months	Both	900	0.4	0.5	7	0.5	3	9.0	12	400
1 year	Both	1100	0.5	0.6	8	0.6	4	11	13	400
2-3 years	Both	1300	0.6	0.7	9	0.7	4	14	16	400
4-6 years	Both	1800	0.7	0.9	13	1.0	6	18	19	500
7-9 years	M	2200	0.9	1.1	16	1.2	7	25	26	700
	F	1900	0.8	1.0	14	1.0	6	25	26	700
10-12 years	M	2500	1.0	1.3	18	1.4	8	34	34	800
	F	2200	0.9	1.1	16	1.2	7	36	36	800
13-15 years	M	2800	1.1	1.4	20	1.5	9	50	49	900
	F	2200	0.9	1.1	16	1.2	7	48	46	800
16-18 years	M	3200	1.3	1.6	23	1.8	11	62	58	1000
	F	2100	0.8	1.1	15	1.2	7	53	47	800
19-24 years	M	3000	1.2	1.5	22	1.6	10	71	61	1000
	F	2100	0.8	1.1	15	1.2	7	58	50	800
25-49 years	M	2700	1.1	1.4	19	1.5	9	74	64	1000
	F	1900	0.8	1.0	14	1.1	7	59	51	800
50-74 years	M	2300	0.9	1.2	16	1.3	8	73	63	1000
	F	1800	0.8§	1.0§	14§	1.1§	7§	63	54	800
75 + years	M	2000	0.8	1.0	14	1.1	7	69	59	1000
	F‖	1700	0.8§	1.0§	14§	1.1§	7§	64	55	800
Pregnancy (additional)										
1st Trimester		100	0.1	0.1	0.11	0.05	0.3		5	0
2nd Trimester		300	0.1	0.3	0.22	0.16	0.9		20	0
3rd Trimester		300	0.1	0.3	0.22	0.16	0.9		24	0
Lactation (additional)		450	0.2	0.4	0.33	0.25	1.5		20	400

From Scientific Review Committee: Nutrition recommendations, *Health and Welfare,* Ottawa, 1990.

NE, Niacin equivalents; PUFA, polyunsaturated fatty acids; RE, retinol equivalents.

*Protein is assumed to be from breast milk and must be adjusted for infant formula.

†Infant formula with high phosphorus should contain 375 mg of calcium.

‡Breast milk is assumed to be the source of the mineral.

¶Smokers should increase vitamin C by 50%.

§Level below which intake should not fall.

‖Assumes moderate physical activity.

Vitamin D (µg)	Vitamin E (mg)	Vitamin C (mg)	Folate (µg)	Vitamin B12 (µg)	Calcium (mg)	Phosphorus (mg)	Magnesium (mg)	Iron (mg)	Iodine (µg)	Zinc (mg)
10	3	20	25	0.3	250†	150	20	0.3‡	30	2‡
10	3	20	40	0.4	400	200	32	7	40	3
10	3	20	40	0.5	500	300	40	6	55	4
5	4	20	50	0.6	550	350	50	6	65	4
5	5	25	70	0.8	600	400	65	8	85	5
2.5	7	25	90	1.0	700	500	100	8	110	7
2.5	6	25	90	1.0	700	500	100	8	95	7
2.5	8	25	120	1.0	900	700	130	8	125	9
2.5	7	25	130	1.0	1100	800	135	8	110	9
2.5	9	30	175	1.0	1100	900	185	10	160	12
2.5	7	30	170	1.0	1000	850	180	13	160	9
2.5	10	40¶	220	1.0	900	1000	230	10	160	12
2.5	7	30¶	190	1.0	700	850	200	12	160	9
2.5	10	40¶	220	1.0	800	1000	240	9	160	12
2.5	7	30¶	180	1.0	700	850	200	13	160	9
2.5	9	40¶	230	1.0	800	1000	250	9	160	12
2.5	6	30¶	185	1.0	700	850	200	13	160	9
5	7	40¶	230	1.0	800	1000	250	9	160	12
5	6	30¶	195	1.0	800	850	210	8	160	9
5	6	40¶	215	1.0	800	1000	230	9	160	12
5	5	30¶	200	1.0	800	850	210	8	160	9
2.5	2	0	200	1.2	500	200	15	0	25	6
2.5	2	10	200	1.2	500	200	45	5	25	6
2.5	2	10	200	1.2	500	200	45	10	25	6
2.5	3	25	100	0.2	500	200	65	0	50	6

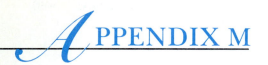

Guidelines for Nutritional Assessment and Care of Cystic Fibrosis

Step One: Calculation of Basal Metabolic Rate (BMR)

In cystic fibrosis care, if a patient fails to grow adequately while receiving kcalorie intake based on RDAs, use this table to calculate Basal Metabolic Rate (BMR) daily energy requirement.

World Health Organization Equations for Calculating Basal Metabolic Rate (kcal) from Body Weight (kg)

Age (years)	BMR (kcal)	
	Females	Males
0-3	$61.0 \times$ (wt kg) $- 51$	$60.9 \times$ (wt kg) $- 54$
3-10	$22.5 \times$ (wt kg) $+ 499$	$22.7 \times$ (wt kg) $+ 495$
10-18	$12.2 \times$ (wt kg) $+ 746$	$17.5 \times$ (wt kg) $+ 651$
18-30	$14.7 \times$ (wt kg) $+ 496$	$15.3 \times$ (wt kg) $+ 679$
30-60	$8.7 \times$ (wt kg) $+ 829$	$11.6 \times$ (wt kg) $+ 879$

Adapted from World Health Organization: Energy and protein requirements, WHO Technical Report Series, Volume 924, No 724, 1985, Ramsey, BW et al: Nutritional assessment and management in cystic fibrosis, *Am J Clin Nutr* 55:108, 1992, and Cystic Fibrosis Foundation guidelines.

Step Two: Calculation of Daily Energy Expenditure (DEE) in Therapy

$$DEE = BMR \times (AC + DC)$$

Abbreviations

DEE = daily energy expenditure (kcal)
BMR = basal metabolic rate (kcal)
AC = activity coefficient
DC = disease coefficient

Guidelines for AC and DC Values

Use the following tables to establish the appropriate activity coefficient and disease coefficient values.

Activity Coefficients (AC)

Activity level of patient	AC value
Confined to bed	1.3
Sedentary	1.5
Active	1.7

Disease Coefficients (DC)

Lung functioning level in cystic fibrosis	Forced air expiration volume in 1 second ($FEV_{1.0}$) (100% = normal FEV)	DC value
Close to normal lung function	>80%	0.0
Moderate lung disease	40%-79%	0.2
Severe lung disease	<40%	0.3
Very severe lung disease	<40%	0.5

Adapted from Ramsey BW et al: Nutritional assessment and management in cystic fibrosis, *Am J Clin Nutr* 55:108, 1992, and Cystic Fibrosis Foundation guidelines.

DEE Calculation

Determine the DEE for a school-age child with cystic fibrosis who is attending school, is relatively sedentary, and has a measured $FEV_{1.0}$ of 50% of predicted normal value.

$$
\begin{aligned}
DEE &= BMR \times (AC + DC) \\
&= BMR \times (1.5 + 0.2) \\
&= BMR \times 1.7
\end{aligned}
$$

Step Three: Calculation of Daily Energy Requirement (DER) from Daily Energy Expenditure (DEE)

Calculation Method

1. Calculate the coefficient of fat absorption (CFA):

$$CFA = \frac{\text{Fat absorption (FA)}}{\text{Fat intake (FI)}} = \text{Fat absorption \%*}$$

2. Use one of the following guideline formulas for DER:

$$\text{If CFA} > 0.93, \text{ then DER} = \text{DEE}$$

or

$$\text{If CFA} = 0.93, \text{ then DER} = \text{DEE} \times \frac{0.93}{\text{CFA}}$$

Abbreviations

CFA = coefficient of fat absorption
FA = fat absorption (kcal)
FI = fat intake (kcal)
DEE = daily energy expenditure (kcal)
DER = daily energy requirement (kcal)

---

*NOTE 1: The fat absorption % (CFA) is usually calculated in a clinical setting by medical laboratory analysis from a patient stool sample.
NOTE 2: If no laboratory analysis report is available, then use CFA = 0.85 as an approximation value in the DER calculation.
Adapted from Ramsey BW et al: Nutritional assessment and management in cystic fibrosis, *Am J Clin Nutr* 55:108, 1992, and Cystic Fibrosis Foundation guidelines.

DER Calculation Example

The fat absorption of a cystic fibrosis patient on enzyme therapy has been determined by laboratory analysis to be 78% of normal. Therefore, the CFA for this patient is 0.78. The DEE for this same patient is calculated to be 2000 kcal. Therefore, the DER for this patient is:

$$DER = DEE \times \frac{0.93}{CFA}$$

$$DER = 2000 \text{ kcal} \times \frac{0.93}{0.78}$$

$$DER = 2384 \text{ kcal/day}$$

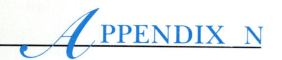

APPENDIX N

Diets for Nutritional Management of Kidney Stone Disease

TABLE W–1		
Low-Calcium Diet (approximately 400 mg calcium)		
	Foods allowed	**Foods not allowed**
Beverage*	Carbonated beverage, coffee, tea	Chocolate-flavored drinks, milk, milk drinks
Bread	White, light rye bread, crackers	
Cereals	Refined cereals	Oatmeal, whole-grain cereals
Desserts	Cake, cookies, gelatin desserts, pastries, pudding, sherbets, all made without chocolate, milk or nuts; if egg yolk is used, it must be from one egg allowance	
Fat	Butter, cream, 2 tbsp/day; French dressing, margarine, salad oil, shortening	Cream (except in amount allowed), mayonnaise
Fruits	Canned, cooked, or fresh fruits or juice except rhubarb	Dried fruit, rhubarb
Meat, eggs	224 g (8 oz) daily of any meat, fowl, fish except clams, oysters, shrimp; not more than one egg daily, including those used in cooking	Clams, oysters, shrimp, cheese
Potato or substitute	Potato, hominy, macaroni, noodles, refined rice, spaghetti	Whole-grain rice
Soup	Broth, vegetable soup made from vegetables allowed	Bean or pea soup, cream or milk soup
Sweets	Honey, jam, jelly, sugar	
Vegetables	Any canned, cooked, fresh vegetables or juice except those listed	Dried beans, broccoli, green cabbage, celery, chard, collards, endive, greens, lettuce, lentils, okra, parsley, parsnips, dried peas, rutabagas
Miscellaneous	Herbs, pickles, popcorn, relishes, salt, spices, vinegar	Chocolate, cocoa, milk gravy, nuts, olives, white sauce

*Depending on calcium content of local water supply. In instances of high calcium content, distilled water may be indicated.

TABLE W–2

Low-Phosphorus Diet (approximately 1 g phosphorus and 40 g protein)

	Foods allowed	Foods not allowed
Milk	Not more than 1 cup daily; whole, skim, buttermilk or 3 tbsp powdered, including the amount used in cooking	
Beverages	Fruit juices, tea, coffee, carbonated drinks, Postum	Milk and milk drinks except as allowed
Bread	White only; enriched commercial, French, hard rolls, soda crackers, rusk	Rye and whole-grain breads, cornbread, biscuits, muffins, waffles
Cereals	Refined cereals, such as Cream of Wheat, Cream of Rice, rice, cornmeal, dry cereals, cornflakes, spaghetti, noodles	All whole-grain cereals
Desserts	Berry or fruit pies, cookies, cakes in average amounts; Jell-O, gelatin, angel food cake, sherbet, meringues made with egg whites, puddings if made with one egg or milk allowance	Desserts with milk and eggs, unless made with the daily allowance
Eggs	Not more than one egg daily, including those used in cooking; extra egg whites may be used	
Fats	Butter, margarine, oils, shortening	
Fruits	Fresh, frozen, canned, as desired	Dried fruits such as raisins, prunes, dates, figs, apricots
Meat	One large serving or two small servings daily of beef, lamb, veal, pork, rabbit, chicken, turkey	Fish, shellfish (crab, oyster, shrimp, lobster), dried and cured meats (bacon, ham, chipped beef), liver, kidney, sweetbreads, brains
Cheese	None	Avoid all cheese and cheese spreads
Vegetables	Potatoes as desired; at least two servings per day of any of the following: asparagus, carrots, beets, green beans, squash, lettuce, rutabagas, tomatoes, celery, peas, onions, cucumber, corn; no more than 1 serving daily of either cabbage, spinach, broccoli, cauliflower, brussels sprouts, artichokes	Dried vegetables such as peas, mushrooms, lima beans
Miscellaneous	Sugar, jams, jellies, syrups, salt, spices, seasonings; condiments in moderation	Chocolate, nuts, nut products such as peanut butter, cream sauces

Sample menu pattern

Breakfast	Lunch	Dinner
Fruit juice	Meat, 56 g (2 oz)	Meat, 56 g
Refined cereal	Potato	Potato
Egg	Vegetable	Vegetable
White toast	Salad	Salad
Butter	Bread, white	Bread, white
½ cup milk	Butter	Butter
Coffee or tea	½ cup milk	Dessert
	Dessert	Coffee or tea
	Coffee or tea	

TABLE W–3

Low-Calcium Test Diet (200 mg Calcium)

	Grams	Calcium (mg)
Breakfast		
Orange juice, fresh	100	19.00
Bread (toast), white	25	19.57
Butter	15	3.00
Rice Krispies	15	3.70
Cream, 20% butterfat	35	33.95
Sugar	7	0.00
Jam	20	2.00
Distilled water, coffee, or tea*		0.00
TOTAL		81.22
Lunch		
Beef steak, cooked	100	10.00
Potato	100	11.00
Tomatoes	100	11.00
Bread	25	19.57
Butter	15	3.00
Honey	20	1.00
Applesauce	20	1.00
Distilled water, coffee, or tea		0.00
TOTAL		56.57
Dinner		
Lamb chop, cooked	90	10.00
Potato	100	11.00
Frozen green peas	80	10.32
Bread	25	19.57
Butter	15	3.00
Jam	20	2.00
Peach sauce	100	5.00
Distilled water, coffee, or tea		0.00
TOTAL		60.89
TOTAL MILLIGRAMS CALCIUM		198.68

*Use distilled water only for cooking and for beverages.

TABLE W–4

Acid Ash Diet

The purpose of this diet is to furnish a well-balanced diet in which the total acid ash is greater than the total alkaline ash each day. It lists (1) unrestricted foods, (2) restricted foods, (3) foods not allowed, and (4) sample of a day's diet.

Unrestricted foods: Eat as much as desired of the following foods.

- Bread: any, preferably whole grain; crackers, rolls
- Cereals: any, preferably whole grain
- Desserts: angel food or sunshine cake; cookies made without baking powder or baking soda; cornstarch pudding, cranberry desserts, custards, gelatin desserts, ice cream, sherbet, plum or prune desserts; rice or tapioca pudding
- Fats: any, as butter, margarine, salad dressings, shortening, lard, salad oils, olive oil
- Fruits: cranberries, plums, prunes
- Meat, eggs, cheese; any meat, fish, or fowl, two servings daily; at least one egg daily
- Potato substitutes: corn, hominy, lentils, macaroni, noodles, rice, spaghetti, vermicelli
- Soup: broth as desired; other soups from foods allowed
- Sweets: cranberry or plum jelly; sugar, plain sugar candy
- Miscellaneous: cream sauce, gravy, peanut butter, peanuts, popcorn, salt, spices, vinegar, walnuts

Restricted foods: Do not eat any more than the amount allowed each day.

- Milk: 2 cups daily (may be used in other ways than as beverage)
- Cream: ⅓ cup or less daily
- Fruits: one serving of fruit daily (in addition to prunes, plums, cranberries); certain fruits listed under "Sample menu" are not allowed at any time
- Vegetables including potato: two servings daily; certain vegetables listed under "Foods not allowed" are not allowed at any time

Foods not allowed

- Carbonated beverages, such as ginger ale, cola, root beer
- Cakes or cookies made with baking powder or soda
- Fruits: dried apricots, bananas, dates, figs, raisins, rhubarb
- Vegetables: dried beans, beet greens, dandelion greens, carrots, chard, lima beans
- Sweets: chocolate or candies other than those under "Unrestricted foods"; syrups
- Miscellaneous: other nuts, olives, pickles

Sample menu

Breakfast	Lunch	Dinner
Grapefruit	Creamed chicken	Broth
Wheatena	Steamed rice	Roast beef, gravy
Scrambled eggs	Green beans	Buttered noodles
Toast, butter, plum jam	Stewed prunes	Sliced tomato
Coffee, cream, sugar	Bread, butter	Mayonnaise
	Milk	Vanilla ice cream
		Bread, butter

TABLE W–5

Low-Purine Diet (approximately 125 mg purine)

General directions

- During acute stages use only list 1.
- After acute stage subsides and for chronic conditions, use the following schedule:
  Two days a week, not consecutive, use list 1 entirely.
  The remaining days add foods from list 2 and 3, as indicated.
  Avoid list 4 entirely.
- Keep diet moderately low in fat.

Typical meal pattern

Breakfast	Lunch	Dinner
Fruit	Egg or cheese dish	Egg or cheese dish
Refined cereal and/or egg	Vegetables, as allowed (cooked or salad)	Cream of vegetable soup, if desired
White toast	Potato or substitute	Starch (potato or substitute)
Butter, 1 tsp	White bread	Colored vegetable, as allowed
Sugar	Butter, 1 tsp	White bread, butter, 1 tsp, if desired
Coffee	Fruit or simple dessert	Salad, as allowed
Milk, if desired	Milk	Fruit or simple dessert
		Milk

Food list 1: may be used as desired; foods that contain an insignificant amount of purine bodies

Beverages	Cheese of all kinds*	Celery
Carbonated	Eggs	Corn
Chocolate	Fats of all kinds* (moderation)	Cucumber
Cocoa	Fruits of all kinds	Eggplant
Coffee	Gelatin, Jell-O	Endive
Fruit juices	Milk: buttermilk, evaporated, malted, sweet	Kohlrabi
Postum	Nuts of all kinds,* peanut butter*	Lettuce
Tea	Pies* (except mincemeat)	Okra
Butter*	Sugar and sweets	Parsnips
Bread: white and crackers, cornbread	Vegetables	Potato, white and sweet
Cereals and cereal products	Artichokes	Pumpkin
Corn	Beets	Rutabagas
Rice	Beet greens	Sauerkraut
Tapioca	Broccoli	String beans
Refined wheat	Brussels sprouts	Summer squash
Macaroni	Cabbage	Swiss chard
Noodles	Carrots	Tomato
		Turnips

*High in fat.

TABLE W–5

Low-Purine Diet (approximately 125 mg purine)—cont'd

Food list 2: one item four times a week; foods that contain a moderate amount (up to 75 mg) of purine bodies in 100 g serving

Asparagus	Finnan haddie	Mushrooms	Salmon
Bluefish	Ham	Mutton	Shad
Bouillon	Herring	Navy beans	Spinach
Cauliflower	Kidney beans	Oatmeal	Tripe
Chicken	Lima beans	Oysters	Tuna fish
Crab	Lobster	Peas	Whitefish

Food list 3: one item once a week; foods that contain a large amount (75-150 mg) of purine bodies in 100 g serving

Bacon	Duck	Perch	Sheep
Beef	Goose	Pheasant	Shellfish
Calf tongue	Halibut	Pigeon	Squab
Carp	Lentils	Pike	Trout
Chicken soup	Liver sausage	Pork	Turkey
Codfish	Meat soups	Quail	Veal
	Partridge	Rabbit	Venison

Food list 4: avoid entirely; foods that contain large amounts (150-1000 mg) of purine bodies in 100 g serving

Sweetbreads	825 mg	Liver (calf, beef)	233 mg	Meat extracts	160-400 mg
Anchovies	363 mg	Kidneys (beef)	200 mg	Gravies	Variable
Sardines (in oil)	295 mg	Brains	195 mg		

TABLE W–6

Low-Methionine Diet

	Foods allowed	Foods not allowed
Soup	Any soup made without meat stock or addition of milk	Rich meat soups, broths, canned soups made with meat broth
Meat or meat substitute	Peanut butter sandwich; spaghetti, or macaroni dish made without addition of meat, cheese, or milk; one serving per day: chicken, lamb, veal, beef, pork, crab, or bacon (3)	Fish and those not listed above
Beverages	Soy milk, tea, coffee	Milk in any form
Vegetables	Asparagus, artichoke, beans, beets, carrots, chicory, cucumber, eggplant, escarole, lettuce, onions, parsnips, potatoes, pumpkin, rhubarb, tomatoes, turnips	Those not listed as allowed
Fruits	Apples, apricots, bananas, berries, cherries, fruit cocktail, grapefruit, grapes, lemon juice, nectarines, oranges, peaches, pears, pineapple, plums, tangerines, watermelon, cantaloupe	Those not listed as allowed
Salads	Raw or cooked vegetable or fruit salad	
Cereals	Macaroni, spaghetti, noodles	
Bread	Whole wheat, rye, white	
Nuts	Peanuts	
Desserts	Fresh or cooked fruit, ices, fruit pies	
Eggs		In any form
Cheese		All varieties
Concentrated sweets	Sugar, jams, jellies, syrup, honey, hard candy	
Concentrated fats	Butter, margarine, cream	
Miscellaneous	Pepper, mustard, vinegar, garlic, oil, herbs, spices	

Meal pattern

Breakfast	Lunch	Dinner
1 cup fruit juice	1 serving soup	56 g (2 oz) meat
½ cup fruit	1 serving sandwich	1 med starch
1 slice toast	1 cup fruit	½ cup vegetable
1½ pats butter	240 ml (8 oz) soy milk*	1 serving salad
2 tsp jelly	3 tsp sugar	1 tbsp dressing
1 tbsp sugar	1 tbsp cream	1 slice bread
Beverage	Beverage	1 serving dessert
1 tbsp cream		1 tbsp sugar
		1 tbsp cream
		1½ pats butter
		Beverage

Sample menu

Breakfast	Lunch	Dinner
Orange juice	Vegetable soup, vegetarian	Chicken, roast
Applesauce	Peanut butter sandwich	Baked potato
Whole-wheat toast	Canned peaches	Artichoke
Butter	Soy milk*	Sliced tomatoes
Jelly	Sugar	French dressing
Sugar	Cream	Whole-wheat bread
Coffee	Coffee or tea	Fruit ice
Cream		Sugar
		Cream
		Butter
		Coffee or tea

Adapted from Smith DR, Kolb FO, and Harper HA: The management of cystinuria and cystine-stone disease, J Urol 81:61, 1959.
*Optional: use in children to include protein intake. Omit if urine calcium is elevated in adults.

Calculation Aids and Conversion Tables

More than 185 years ago a group of French scientists set up the metric system of weights and measures. Today, with refinements over years of use, it is called the "Systeme International" (SI). In 1975 our American Congress passed the Metric Conversion Act, which provides for conversion of our customary British/American system to the simpler metric system used by the rest of the world. We are now in the midst of this conversion, as evidenced by distance signs along highways and labels on many packaged foods in supermarkets. Here are a few conversion factors to help you make these transitions in your necessary calculations.

Metric System of Measurement

Like our money system, this is a simple decimal system based on units of 10. It is uniform and used internationally.

Weight units: 1 kilogram (kg) = 1000 grams (gm or g)
1 g = 1000 milligrams (mg)
1 mg = 1000 micrograms (mcg or μg)
Length units: 1 meter (m) = 100 centimeters (cm)
1000 meters = 1 kilometer (km)
Volume units: 1 liter (L) = 1000 milliliters (ml)
1 milliliter = 1 cubic centimeter (cc)
Temperature units: Celcius (C) scale, based on 100 equal units between 0° C (freezing point of water) and 100° C (boiling point of water); this scale is used entirely in all scientific work.
Energy units: Kilocalorie (kcal) = Amount of energy required to raise 1 kg water 1° C
Kilojoule (kJ) = Amount of energy required to move 1 kg mass 1 m by a force of 1 newton
1 kcal = 4.184 kJ

In 1970 the American Institute of Nutrition's Committee on Nomenclature recommended that the term *kilojoule* (kJ) replace the kilocalorie (kcal). This change is gradually coming about.

British/American System of Measurement

Our customary system is a confusion of units with no uniform relationships. It is not a decimal system, but rather a jumbled collection of different units collected in usage and language over time. It is used mainly in America.

Weight units: 1 pound (lb) = 16 ounces (oz)
Length units: 1 foot (ft) = 12 inches (in)
1 yard (yd) = 3 feet (ft)
Volume units: 3 teaspoons (tsp) = 1 tablespoon (tbsp)
16 tbsp = 1 cup
1 cup = 8 fluid ounces (fl oz)
4 cups = 1 quart (qt)
5 cups = 1 imperial quart (qt), Canada
Temperature units: Fahrenheit (F) scale, based on 180 equals units between 32° F (freezing point of water) and 212° F (boiling point of water) at standard atmospheric pressure

Conversions Between Measurement Systems

Weight: 1 oz = 28.35 g (usually used as 28 or 30 g)
2.2 lb = 1 kg
Length: 1 in = 2.54 cm
1 ft = 30.48 cm
39.37 in = 1 m
Volume: 1.06 qt = 1 L
0.85 imperial qt = 1 L (Canada)

Temperature:

Boiling point of water	100° C	212° F
Body temperature	37° C	98.6° F
Freezing point of water	0° C	32° F

Interconversion formulas:

$$\text{Fahrenheit temperature (°F)} = \tfrac{9}{5}\,(\text{°C}) + 32$$
$$\text{Celsius temperature (°C)} = \tfrac{5}{9}\,(\text{°F} - 32)$$

Retinol Equivalents

The following definitions and equivalences that are internationally agreed on provide a basis for calculating retinol equivalent conversions.

Definitions: International units (IU) and retinol equivalents (RE) are defined as follows:

1 IU = 0.3 µg retinol (0.0003 mg)
1 IU = 0.6 µg beta-carotene (0.0006 mg)
1 RE = 6 µg retinol
1 RE = 6 µg beta-carotene
1 RE = 12 µg other provitamin A carotenoids
1 RE = 3.33 IU retinol
1 RE = 10 IU beta-carotene

Conversion formulas: On the basis of weight beta-carotene is ½ as active as retinol; on the basis of structure the other provitamin carotenoids are ¼ as active as retinol. In addition, retinol is more completely absorbed in the intestine, whereas the provitamin carotenoids are much less well utilized, with an average absorption of about ⅓. Therefore in overall activity beta-carotene is ⅙ as active as retinol, and the other carotenoids are 1/12 as active. These differences in utilization provide the basis for the 1:6:12 relationship shown in the equivalences given and in the following formulas for calculating retinol equivalents from values of vitamin A, beta-carotene, and other active carotenoids, expressed either as international units or micrograms:

If retinol and beta-carotene are given in micrograms:
Micrograms of retinol + (Micrograms of beta-carotene ÷ 6) = RE

If both are given as IU:
International units of retinol ÷ 3.33) + (International units of beta-carotene ÷ 10) = RE

If beta-carotene and other carotenoids are given in micrograms:
(Micrograms of beta-carotene ÷ 6) + (Micrograms of other carotenoids ÷ 12) = RE

Approximate Metric Conversions

When you know	Multiply by	To find
Weight		
Ounces	28	Grams
Pounds	0.45	Kilograms
Length		
Inches	2.5	Centimeters
Feet	30	Centimeters
Yards	0.9	Meters
Miles	1.6	Kilometers
Volume		
Teaspoons	5	Millimeters
Tablespoons	15	Millimeters
Fluid ounces	30	Millimeters
Cups	0.24	Liters
Pints	0.47	Liters
Quarts	0.95	Liters
Temperature		
Fahrenheit temperature	⅝ (after subtracting 32)	Celsius temperature

GLOSSARY

achlasia (Gr *a-*, negative, without; *cholasis*, relaxation) Failure to relax the smooth muscle fibers of the gastrointestinal tract at any point of juncture of its parts; especially failure of the esophagogastric sphincter to relax when swallowing, caused by degeneration of ganglion cells in the wall of the organ. The lower esophagus also loses its normal peristaltic activity. Also called cardiospasm.

actin (Gr *aktis*, a radiating activating substance) Myofibril protein whose synchronized meshing action in conjunction with **myosin** causes muscles to contract and relax.

adenosine triphosphate (ATP) The high-energy compound formed in the cell, called the "energy currency " of the cell because of the binding of energy in its high-energy phosphate bonds for release for cell work as these bonds are split. A compound of adenosine (a nucleotide containing adenine and ribose) that has three phosphoric acid groups, ATP is a high-energy phosphate compound important in energy exchange for cellular activity. The splitting off of the terminal phosphate bond (PO_4) of ATP to produce adenosine diphosphate (ADP) releases bound energy and transfers it to free energy available for body work. The reforming of ATP in cell oxidation again stores energy in high-energy phosphate bonds for use as needed. They may be charged and discharged according to conditions in the cell.

adipocyte (L *adipis*, fat; Gr *kytos*, hollow vessel) A fat cell. All cell names end in the suffix *-cyte*, with the type of cell indicated by the root word to which it is added.

adipose (L *adeps*, fat; *adiposus*, fatty) Fat present in cells of adipose (fatty) tissue.

admixture (L *admixtus*, admixture) A mixture resulting from adding or mingling another ingredient; a combination of two or more substances that are not chemically united or that exist in no fixed proportion to each other.

aerobic capacity (Gr *aer*, air or gas) Milliliters of oxygen consumed per kilogram of body weight per minute; influenced by body composition.

aldosterone Potent hormone of the cortex of the adrenal glands, which acts on the distal renal tubule to cause reabsorption of sodium in an ion exchange with potassium. The aldosterone mechanism is essentially a sodium-conserving mechanism but indirectly also conserves water, since water absorption follows the sodium reabsorption.

alpha-fetoprotein A fetal antigen in amniotic fluid that provides an early pregnancy test for fetal malformations such as neural tube defect.

amine An organic compound containing nitrogen. Many different amine organic compounds are found.

amino acid (*amino*, the monovalent chemical group —NH_2) An acid containing the essential element nitrogen (in the chemical group —NH_2). Amino acids are the structural units of protein and the basic building blocks of the body.

aminopeptidase (Chemistry: *amino*, nitrogen-containing; Gr *pepsis*, digestion) Protein-splitting enzyme that cuts the peptide bond (linkage) at the amino end of amino acids, splitting off the amino group —NH_2.

amnionic fluid (Gr *amnion*, bowl) The watery fluid within the membrane enveloping the fetus, in which the fetus is suspended.

amphoteric (Gr *amphoteros*, both) Having opposite characteristics; capable of acting either as an acid or a base, combining with both acids and bases.

ampullae (L *ampulla*, a jug) A general term for flasklike wider portions of a tubular structure; spaces under the nipple of the breast for storing milk.

amyloid (Gr *amylon*, starch; *-oid, eidos*, form, shape) A glycoprotein substance having a relation to starchlike structure but more a protein compound; an abnormal complex material forming characteristic brain deposits of fibrillary tangles always found in postmortem examinations of patients with Alzheimer's disease, the only means of definitive diagnosis; found in various body tissues that can form lesions that destroy functional cells and injure the organ.

amyotrophic lateral sclerosis (Gr *a-*, negative; *mys*, muscle; *trophē*, nourishment; L *lateralis*, to the side; *sklerōsis*, hardness) A progressive neuromuscular disease characterized by the degeneration of the neurons of the spinal cord and the motor cells of the brain stem, causing a deficit of upper and lower motor neurons; death usually occurs in 2 to 3 years.

anabolism (Gr *anabole*, a building up) Metabolic process by which body tissues are built.

anemia (Gr *an-*, negative prefix; *haima*, blood) Blood condition characterized by decreased number of circulating red blood cells, hemoglobin, or both.

anergy (Gr *an-*, negative prefix, *ergon*, work) Diminished immunologic reactivity to specific antigens.

anorexia nervosa (Gr "want of appetite") Extreme psychophysiologic aversion to food, resulting in life-threatening weight loss; a psychiatric eating disorder caused by a morbid fear of fatness, in which the person's distorted body image is reflected as fat when the body is actually malnourished and extremely thin from self-starvation.

anthropometry (Gr *anthropos,* man; *metron,* measure) The science of measuring the size, weight, and proportions of the human body.

antibody Any of numerous protein molecules produced by B cells as a primary immune defense for attaching to specific related **antigens;** animal protein made up of a specific sequence of amino acids that is designed to interact with its specific antigen during an allergic response or to prevent infection.

antigen (antibody + Gr *gennan,* to produce) Any foreign or "non-self" substances, such as toxins, viruses, bacteria, and foreign proteins, that stimulate the production of **antibodies** specifically designed to interact with them.

antimetabolite A substance bearing a close structural resemblance to one required for normal physiologic functioning and exerting its effect by interfering with the utilization of the essential metabolite.

antioxidant (Gr *anti,* against; *oxys* keen) A substance that inhibits oxidation of polyunsaturated fatty acids and formation of free radicals in the cells.

apoprotein (Gr *apo,* from, separation or derivation from; *prōtos,* first, protein compound) A separate protein compound that attaches to its specific receptor site on a particular lipoprotein and activates certain functions, such as synthesis of a related enzyme. An example is apoprotein C II, an apoprotein of HDL and VLDL that functions to activate the enzyme lipoprotein lipase.

areola (L *areola,* area, space) A defined space; a circular area of different color surrounding a central point, such as the darkened pigmented ring surrounding the nipple of the breast.

ariboflavinosis Group of clinical manifestations of riboflavin deficiency.

arteriosclerosis (Gr *arteria,* from *aēr,* air, and *tērein,* to keep, because of the ancient belief that the arteries contained vital air; *sklēros,* hard) Blood vessel disease characterized by thickening and hardening of artery walls, with loss of functional elasticity, mainly affecting the intima (inner lining) of the arteries.

arthroplasty (Gr *arthron,* joint; *plassein,* to form) Surgical procedure for replacing degenerated joints such as the hip with a mechanical joint of metal or special plastic; formation of movable joint replacement, developed by team of biomedical engineers and orthopedists.

asterixis (Gr *a,* negative prefix; *sterixis,* a fixed position) Neuromotor disturbance marked by an inability to hold outstretched hands in a steady position, resulting in an intermittent flapping of the hands, characteristic of hepatic coma.

atheroma (Gr *athērē,* gruel; *-oma,* a mass or body of tissue) A mass of fatty plaque formed in inner arterial walls in atherosclerosis.

atherosclerosis (Gr *athere,* gruel; *skleros,* hard) Common form of arteriosclerosis, characterized by the gradual formation,—beginning in childhood in genetically predisposed individuals,—of yellow cheese like streaks of cholesterol and fatty material that develop into hardened plaques in the intima or inner lining of major blood vessels, such as coronary arteries, eventually in adulthood cutting off blood supply to the tissue served by the vessels; the underlying pathology of coronary heart disease.

atrium (L *atrion,* hall) An anatomical chamber; usually used alone to designate one of the pair of smaller upper chambers of the heart, with thin muscular walls, which receives blood from the body's inflowing circulation via the superior and inferior vena cava and delivers it to the thicker walled ventricles.

autonomy (Gr *autos,* self; *nomos,* law) The state of functioning independently, without extraneous influence.

azotemia (Gr *a,* negative; *zoe,* life; *azote,* nitrogen; haima, blood) An excess of urea or other nitrogenous substances in the blood.

basal metabolic rate (BMR) Amount of energy required to maintain the resting body's internal activities after an overnight fast. See also **resting metabolic rate (RMR).**

benign (L *benignus,* kind, generous) Not malignant or recurrent; favorable for recovery.

beriberi (Singhalese "I cannot, I cannot") A disease of the peripheral nerves caused by a deficiency of thiamin (vitamin B_1). It is characterized by pain (neuritis) and paralysis of the extremities, cardiovascular changes, and edema. Beriberi is common in the Orient, where diets consist largely of milled rice with little protein.

bile (L *bilis,* bile) A fluid secreted by the liver and transported to the gallbladder for concentration and storage. It is released into the duodenum upon entry of fat to facilitate enzymatic fat digestion by acting as an emulsifying agent.

bilirubin (L *bilis,* bile; *ruber,* red) A reddish bile pigment resulting from the degradation of heme by reticuloedothelial cells in the liver; a high level in the blood produces the yellow skin symptomatic of jaundice.

bioavailability Amount of a nutrient ingested in food that is absorbed and thus available to the body for metabolic use.

blood urea nitrogen (BUN) The nitrogen component of urea in the blood; a measure of kidney function; elevated levels of BUN indicate a disorder of kidney function.

body composition The relative sizes of the four basic body compartments that make up the total body: lean body mass (muscle mass), fat, water, and bone.

bolus (Gr *bolos,* lump) Rounded mass of food formed in the mouth and ready to be swallowed.

buffer Mixture of acidic and alkaline components that, when added to a solution, is able to protect the solution against wide variations in its pH, even when strong acids and bases are added to it. If an acid is added, the alkaline partner reacts to counteract the acidic effect. If a base is added, the acid partner reacts to counteract the alkalizing effect. A solution to which a buffer has been added is called a buffered solution.

bulimia nervosa (L *bous,* ox; *limos,* hunger) A psychiatric eating disorder related to the person's fear of fatness, in which cycles of gorging on large quantities of food are followed by self-induced vomiting and use of diuretics and laxatives to maintain a "normal" body weight.

cachexia (Gr *kakos*, bad; *hexis*, habit) A specific profound effect caused by malnutrition and a disturbance in glucose metabolism usually seen in patients with terminal cancer or heart failure; general poor health and malnutrition indicated by an emaciated appearance.

calcitonin (L *calx*, lime, calcium; *tonus*, balance) A polypeptide hormone secreted by the thyroid gland in response to hypercalcemia, which acts to lower both calcium and phosphate in the blood.

calcitriol Activated hormone form of vitamin D $(1,25[OH]_2D_3)$-1,25-dihydroxycholecalciferol.

callus (L *callositis*, callus, bone) Unorganized meshwork of newly grown, woven bone developed on pattern of original fibrin clot (formed after fracture or surgery) and normally replaced in the healing process by hard adult bone.

calorie (L *calor*, heat) A unit of heat energy. The calorie used in the study of metabolism is the large calorie, or *kilocalorie*, defined as the amount of heat required to raise the temperature of 1 kg of water 1° Celsius (centigrade).

calorimetry (L *calor*, heat; Gr *metron*, measure) Measurement of amounts of heat absorbed or given out. *Direct method:* measurement of amount of heat produced by a subject enclosed in a small chamber. *Indirect method:* measurement of amount of heat produced by a subject by the quantity of nitrogen and carbon dioxide eliminated.

cancer (L *cancer*, crab) A malignant cellular tumor with properties of tissue invasion and spread to other parts of the body.

candidiasis (L *candidus*, glowing white) Infection with the fungus of the genus *Candida*, generally caused by *C. albicans*, so-named for the whitish appearance of its small lesions; usually a superficial infection in moist areas of the skin or inner mucous membranes.

capillary fluid shift mechanism Process that controls the movement of water and small molecules in solution (electrolytes, nutrients) between the blood in the capillary and the surrounding interstitial area. Filtration of water and solutes out of the capillary at the arteriole end and reabsorption at the venule end are accomplished by shifts in balance between the intracapillary hydrostatic blood pressure and the colloidal osmotic pressure exerted by the plasma proteins.

carbohydrate Compound of carbon, hydrogen, and oxygen; starches, sugars, cellulose, and gums made and stored in plants; major energy source in the human diet.

carboxyl (COOH) The monovalent radical, —COOH occurring in those organic acids termed carboxylic acids.

carboxypeptidase (L *carbo-*, carbon; *oxy*, oxygen) A protein enzyme that splits off the chemical group *carboxyl* (—COOH) at the end of peptide chains, acting on the peptide bond of the terminal amino acid having a free-end carboxyl group.

carcinoma (Gr *karkinos*, crab; *onkoma*, a swelling) A malignant new growth made up of epithelial cells, infiltrating the surrounding tissue and spreading to other parts of the body.

cardiac output (Gr *kardia*, heart) Total volume of blood propelled from the heart with each contraction; equal to the stroke output multiplied by the number of beats per the time unit used in the calculation.

carnitine A naturally occurring amino acid $(C_{17}H_{15}NO_3)$ formed from methionine and lysine, required for transport of long-chain fatty acids across the mitochondrial membrane, where they are oxidized as fuel substrate for metabolic energy.

casein hydrolysate formula (L *caseus*, cheese) Infant formula with base of hydrolyzed casein, major milk protein, produced by partially breaking down the casein into smaller peptide fragments, making a product that is more easily digested.

catabolism (Gr *katabole*, a throwing down) The breaking-down phase of metabolism, the opposite of anabolism. Catabolism includes all the processes in which complex substances are progressively broken down into simpler ones. Catabolism usually involves the release of energy. Together, anabolism and catabolism constitute metabolism, which is the coordinated operation of anabolic and catabolic processes into a dynamic balance of energy and substance.

chemical bonding Process of linking the radicals, chemical elements, or groups of a chemical compound.

cholecalciferol Chemical name for vitamin D in its inactive dietary form (D_3). When the inactive cholecalciferol is consumed or its counterpart cholesterol compound is developed in the skin, its first stage of activation occurs in the liver and then is completed in the kidney to the active vitamin D hormone form *calcitriol* (1,25-dihydroxycholecalciferol, or shorter form $1,25[OH]_2D_3$).

cholecystectomy (Gr *cholē*, bile; *kystis*, bladder; *ektomē*, a cutting out) Surgical removal of the gallbladder.

cholecystokinin (CCK) (Gr *chole*, bile or gall; *kystis*, bladder, *kinein*, to move) A peptide hormone secreted by the duodenal mucosa in the presence of fat. The cholecystokinin causes the gallbladder to contract. This contraction propels bile into the duodenum, where it is needed to emulsify the fat. The fat is thus prepared for digestion and absorption.

cholesterol A fat-related compound, a sterol $(C_{27}H_{45}OH)$. It is a normal constituent of bile and a principal constituent of gallstones. In body metabolism cholesterol is important as a precursor of various steroid hormones, such as sex hormones and adrenal corticoids. Cholesterol is synthesized by the liver. It is widely distributed in nature, especially in animal tissue such as glandular meats and egg yolk.

chorea (L *choreia*, dance) A wide variety of ceaseless involuntary movements that are rapid, complex, and jerky, yet appear to be well coordinated; characteristic movements of Huntington's disease.

chronic dieting syndrome (Gr *chronos*, time, persisting over a long period of time; *diaita*, way of living, customary allowance of food and drink; *syndrome*, concurrence, a set of symptoms that occur together) A compulsive eating disorder, commonly referred to as **compulsive over-eating.** It includes binge eating episodes, but without the purging behavior of persons with bulimia nervosa. This is an emotional, reactive eating pattern occurring in response to stress or anxiety and used to soothe painful feelings.

chylomicrons (L *chylus,* juice, milky fluid taken up by lacteals of the intestinal villi; Gr *mikros,* small) Initial lipoproteins, carrying a large fat load, formed in the intestinal wall after a meal for absorption of the food fats into circulation.

chyme (Gr *chymos,* juice) Semifluid food mass in gastrointestinal tract following gastric digestion.

chymotrypsin (Gr *chymos,* chyme, creamy gruel-like material produced by gastric digestion of food) One of the protein-splitting and milk-curdling pancreatic enzymes, activated in the intestine from precursor chymotrypsinogen. It breaks peptide linkages of the amino acids phenylalanine and tyrosine.

cirrhosis (Gr *kirrhos,* orange-yellow) Chronic liver disease, characterized by loss of functional cells, with fibrous and nodular regeneration.

cisterni chyli Cistern or receptacle of the chyle is a dilated sac at the origin of the thoracic duct, which is the common truck that receives all the lymphatic vessels. The cisterna chyli lies in the abdomen between the second lumbar vertebra and the aorta. It receives the lymph from the intestinal trunk, the right and left lumbar lymphatic trunks, and two descending lymphatic trunks. The chyle, after passing through the cisterna chyli, is carried upward into the chest through the thoracic duct and empties into the venous blood at the point where the left subclavian vein joins the left internal jugular vein.

clinical nutrition specialist Specialty practice of a registered dietitian with an advanced degree in nutritional science and training in clinical nutrition.

coenzyme factors A major metabolic role of the micronutrients, vitamins and minerals, as essential partners with cell enzymes in a variety of reactions in both energy and protein metabolism.

cognitive (L *cognoscere,* to know) Pertaining to the mental processes of perceptions, memory, judgment, and reasoning, as contrasted with emotional and volitional processes.

collagen (Gr *kolla,* glue; *gennan,* to produce) The protein substance of the white fibers (collagenous fibers) of skin, tendon, bone, cartilage, and all other connective tissue; it is converted into gelatin by boiling.

collagen disease (Gr *kolla,* glue; *gennan,* to produce) Diseases attacking collagen tissues, the protein substance of the white fibers (collagenous fibers) of skin, tendon, bone, cartilage, and other connective tissue; any of a group of diseases that are clinically distinct but have in common widespread pathologic changes in the connective tissue, such as rheumatoid arthritis, lupus erythematosus, scleroderma, and rheumatic fever.

colloid (Gr *kollōdēs,* glutinous) Glutinous, gluelike; a dispersion of matter throughout a liquid.

colloidal osmotic pressure (COP) Pressure produced by the protein molecules in the plasma and in the cell. Because proteins are large molecules, they do not pass through the separating membranes of the capillary cells. Thus they remain in their respective compartments, exerting a constant osmotic pull that protects vital plasma and cell fluid volumes in these compartments.

colon (Gr *kolon,* colon) The part of the large intestine extending from the cecum to the rectum.

colostrum (L *colostrum,* premilk) Thin yellow fluid first secreted by the mammary gland a few days before and after childbirth, preceding the mature breast milk. It contains up to 20% protein including a large amount of lactalbumin, more minerals and less lactose and fat than does milk, and immunoglobulins representing the antibodies found in maternal blood.

compartment The collective quantity of material of a given type in the body. The four body compartments are lean body mass (muscle), bone, fat, and water.

complement (L *complere,* to fill) A complex series of enzymatic proteins occurring in normal serum that interact to combine with and augment (fill out, complete) the antigen-antibody complex of the body's immune system, producing lysis when the antigen is an intact cell; composed of 11 discrete proteins or functioning components, activated by the immunoglobulin factors IgG and IgM.

corticotropin-releasing factor (CRF) (L *cortex,* shell or rind, external layer; Gr *tropikos,* turning, *-tropic,* suffix indicating turning toward or changing) Hypothalamus factor stimulating release of anterior pituitary hormone ACTH (adrenocorticotropic hormone).

creatinine (Gr *kreas,* flesh) End product of the breakdown of body tissue; found in muscles and blood and excreted in urine. High levels indicate abnormally high catabolism of body proteins and possibly inadequate intake of carbohydrate and fat, which have a protein-sparing effect.

cretinism (F *cretinisine*) A congenital disease resulting from absence or deficiency of normal thyroid secretion, characterized by physical deformity, dwarfism, & mental retardation, and often goiters.

cruciferous (L *cruces,* cross; *forma,* form) Bearing a cross; botanical term for plants belonging to the botanical family *Cruciferae* or *Brassicaceae,* the mustard family, so called because of crosslike, four-petaled flowers; name given to certain vegetables of this family, such as broccoli, cabbage, brussels sprouts, and cauliflower.

cyclosporine An immunosuppressant drug widely used following organ transplants to control the immune system and prevent rejection of the new tissue.

cytokines (Gr *kytos,* hollow vessel, cell; *kinētos,* movable, changing) Substances produced in tissues that can cause inflammatory changes in tissue cells, e.g., tumor necrosis factor and interleukin-1.

deamination Removal of amino group (NH_2) from amino acid.

decubitus ulcer (L *decubitus,* lying down; *ulcus,* ulcer) Pressure sores in long-term bed-bound or immobile patients at points of bony protuberances, where prolonged pressure of body weight in one position cuts off adequate blood circulation to that area, causing tissue death and ulceration.

dehiscence (L *dehiscere,* to gape) A splitting open; the separation of the layers of a surgical wound, either (1) partial or superficial or (2) complete, with total disruption requiring resuturing.

dehydrocholesterol A precursor cholesterol compound in the skin that is irratiated by sunlight to produce an initial stage in the process of forming activated vitamin D hormone.

demographic (Gr *demos,* people; *graphein,* to write) The statistical data of a population, especially those showing average age, income, education, births, deaths, and so on.

diabetes insipidus (Gr *dia,* through; *bainein,* to go; *diabetes,* siphon; L *insipidus,* tasteless, not sweet, as compared to diabetes *mellitus,* L honey) A condition of the pituitary gland and insufficiency of one of its hormones, vasopressin or antidiuretic hormone; characterized by a copious output of a nonsweet urine, great thirst, and sometimes a large appetite. In diabetes insipidus these symptoms result from a specific injury to the pituitary gland, not a collection of metabolic disorders as in diabetes mellitus. The injured pituitary gland produces less vasopressin, a hormone that normally helps the kidneys reabsorb adequate water.

dialysis (Gr *dia,* through; *lysis,* dissolution) Process of separating crystalloids and colloids in solution by the difference in their rates of diffusion through a semipermeable membrane; crystalloids pass through readily and colloids very slowly or not at all.

dideoxynucleosides (chemistry *di-,* two; *de-,* removal; *oxy-,* oxygen; *nucleoside,* basic type of chemical compound involved) A class of drugs used treat HIV-infected persons; a nucleoside is a combination of a sugar (a pentose) with a purine or pyrimidine (two types of compounds that provide the cross-linking "ladders" of the double strands of DNA) base.

dietary fiber Nondigestible form of carbohydrate that is of nutritional importance in gastrointestinal disease such as diverticulosis and in reducing serum lipid and glucose levels related to chronic conditions such as heart disease and diabetes.

dietetics Management of diet and the use of food; the science concerned with the nutritional planning and preparation of foods.

disability Mental or physical impairment that prevents an individual from performing one or more gainful activities; not synonymous with **handicap,** which implies serious disadvantage.

disaccharides (Gr *di,* two; *saccharide,* sugar) Class of compound sugars composed of two molecules of monosaccharide. The three most common are sucrose, lactose, and maltose.

disulfiram White to off-white crystalline antioxidant; inhibits oxidation of the acetaldehyde metabolized from alcohol. It is used in the treatment of alcoholism, producing extremely uncomfortable symptoms when alcohol is ingested following oral administration of the drug.

diverticulitis (L *divertere,* to turn aside) Inflammation of pockets of tissue (diverticuli) in the lining of the mucous membrane of the colon.

dysentery (Gr *dys,* painful, bad; *enteron,* intestine) A general term given to a number of disorders marked by inflammation of the intestines, especially of the colon, and attended by abdominal pain and frequent stools containing blood and mucus. The causative agent may be chemical irritants, bacteria, protozoa, or parasites.

dyspnea (Gr *dysnoia,* difficulty of breathing) Labored, difficult breathing.

eclampsia (Gr *eklampein,* to shine forth) Advanced pregnancy-induced hypertension (PIH), manifested by convulsions.

ecology (Gr *oikos,* house) Relations between organisms and their environments.

eicosanoids (Gr *eikosa,* twenty) Long chain fatty acids composed of 20 carbon atoms.

electrolytes (Gr *electron,* amber [which emits electricity when rubbed]; *lytos,* soluble) A chemical element or compound that in solution dissociates as ions carrying a positive or negative charge (for example, H^+, Na^+, K^+, Ca^{++}, Mg^{++}, and Cl^-, HCO_3^-, HPO_4^-, SO_4^-. Electrolytes constitute a major force controlling fluid balances within the body through their concentrations and shifts from one place to another to restore and maintain balance—**homeostasis.**

elemental formula A nutrition support formula composed of simple elemental nutrient components that require no further digestive breakdown and are thus readily absorbed; infant formula produced with elemental ready-to-be-absorbed components of free amino acids and carbohydrate as simple sugars.

emulsifier An agent that breaks down large fat globules to smaller, uniformly distributed particles. This action is accomplished in the intestine chiefly by the bile acids, which lower surface tension of the fat particles. Emulsification greatly increases the surface area of fat, facilitating contact with fat-digesting enzymes.

encephalopathy (Gr *enkephalos,* brain; *pathos,* disease) Any degenerative disease of the brain.

endemic (Gr *endemos,* dwelling in a place) Characterizing a disease of low morbidity that remains constantly in a human community but is clinically recognizable in only a few.

endocarditis (Gr *endon,* within; *kardia,* heart) Inflammation of the endocardium, the serous membrane that lines the cavities of the heart.

endothelium (Gr *endo-,* within; *thēlē,* nipple) Layer of epithelial cells that line the cavities of the heart, the blood and lymph vessels, and the serous cavities of the body, originating from the mesoderm.

energy (Gr *en,* in, with; *ergon,* work) The capacity of a system for doing work; available power. Energy is manifest in various forms—motion, position, light, heat, and sound. Energy is interchangeable among these various forms and is constantly being transformed and transferred among them.

enteral (Gr *enteron,* intestine) A mode of feeding that uses the gastrointestinal tract, oral or tube feeding.

enterogastrone (Gr *enteron,* intestine; *gaster,* stomach; *-one,* suffix for hormones) A duodenal peptide hormone that inhibits gastric hydrochloric acid secretion and motility.

enzyme (Gr *en,* in; *zyme,* leaven) Various complex proteins produced by living cells that act independently of these cells. Enzymes are capable of producing certain chemical changes in other substances without themselves being changed in the process. Their action is therefore that of a catalyst. Digestive enzymes of the gastrointestinal secretions act on food substances to break them down into simpler compounds and greatly accelerate the speed of these chemical reactions. An enzyme is usually named according to the substance (substrate) on which it acts, with the common suffix -ase; for example, sucrase is the specific enzyme for sucrose and breaks it down to glucose and fructose.

epidemiology (Gr *epidemois*, prevalent; *-ology*, study) The study of factors determining the frequency, distribution, and strength of diseases in population groups.

ergogenic (Gr *ergo*, work; *gennan*, to produce) Tendency to increase work output; various substances that increase work or exercise capacity and output.

erythema (Gr *erythros*, red; *erythema*, flush upon the skin) Redness of the skin produced by coagulation of the capillaries; results from a variety of causes, e.g., radiant heat or burns.

essential amino acid Any one of nine amino acids that the body cannot synthesize at all or in sufficient amounts to meet body needs, so it must be supplied by the diet, and is hence a *dietary* essential. These nine specific amino acids are histidine, isoleucine, leucine, lysine, methionine, phenylalanine, threonine, tryptophan, and valine.

essential fatty acid (L *essentialis*, necessary or inherent) A fatty acid required in the diet because the body cannot synthesize it.

essential hypertension An inherent form of hypertension with no specific discoverable cause and considered to be familial; also called primary hypertension.

ester A compound produced by the reaction between an acid and an alcohol with elimination of a molecule of water. This process is called *esterification*. For example, a triglyceride is a glycerol ester. Cholesterol esters are formed in the mucosal cells by combination with fatty acids, largely linoleic acid.

exudate (L *exsudare*, to sweat out) Various materials such as cells, cellular debris, and fluids, usually resulting from inflammation, that have escaped from blood vessels and are deposited in or on surface tissues; has a high protein content.

fasciculi (L *fascis*, bundle) A general term for a small bundle or cluster of muscle, tendon, or nerve fibers.

fatty acid The structural components of fats.

ferritin Protein-iron compound in which iron is stored in tissues; the storage form of iron in the body.

fetor hepaticus (L *fetor*, stench, offensive odor; *hepaticus*, liver) The peculiar odor of the breath that is characteristic of advanced liver disease.

fetus (L *fetus*, unborn offspring) The unborn offspring in the postembryonic period, after major structures have been outlined; in humans the growing offspring from 7 to 8 weeks after fertilization until birth.

filtration (L *filtrum*, felt used to strain liquids) Passage of a fluid through a semipermeable membrane (a membrane that permits passage of water and small solutes but not large molecules) as a result of a difference in pressures on the two sides of the membrane. For example, the net filtration pressure in the capillaries is the difference between the outward-pushing hydrostatic force of the blood pressure and the opposing inward-pulling force of the colloidal osmotic pressure exerted by the plasma proteins retained in capillary.

fistula (L *fistula*, pipe) Abnormal passageway, usually between two internal organs, or leading from an internal organ to the surface of the body.

flushing reaction Short-term reaction resulting in redness of neck and face.

fuel factor The kilocalorie value (energy potential) of food nutrients; that is, the number of kilocalories that 1 g of the nutrient yields when oxidized. The kilocalorie fuel factor for carbohydrate is 4; for protein, 4; and for fat, 9. The basic figures are used in computing diets and energy values of foods. (For example, 10 g of fat yields 90 kcal.)

fulminant (L *fulminare*, to flare up) Sudden, severe; occurring suddenly with great intensity.

gastrectomy (Gr *gaster*, stomach; *ektomē*, excision) Surgical removal of the whole (total gastrectomy) or part (partial gastrectomy) of the stomach.

gastrin Hormone secreted by mucosal cells in the antrum of the stomach that stimulates the parietal cells to produce hydrochloric acid. Gastrin is released in response to stimulants, especially coffee, alcohol, and meat extractives, into the stomach. When the gastric pH reaches 2.0 to 3.0, a feedback mechanism cuts off gastrin secretion and prevents excess acid formation.

gastritis (Gr *gaster*, stomach) Inflammation of the stomach.

geriatrics (Gr *geras*, old age; *iatrike*, surgery, medicine) Branch of medicine specializing in medical problems associated with old age.

gerontology (Gr *geronto*, old man; *logy*, work, reason, study) Study of the aging process and its remarkable progressive events.

gestation (L *gestatio*, from; *gestare*, to bear) The period of embryonic and fetal development from fertilization to birth; pregnancy.

glomerulosclerosis (L *glomus*, ball, cluster; *sklērōsis*, hardness) Intercapillary degeneration of the nephron glomerulus, a cluster of capillary loops cupped at the head of each nephron, resulting in the degeneration of the entire nephron; a diabetic complication, with symptoms of albuminuria, nephrotic edema, hypertension, and renal insufficiency.

glossitis (Gr *glossa*, tongue + *itis*) Swollen, reddened tongue; riboflavin deficiency symptom.

glucagon (Gr *glykys*, sweet; *gonē*, seed) A polypeptide hormone secreted by the A cells of the pancreatic islets of Langerhans in response to hypoglycemia; has an opposite balancing effect to that of insulin, raising the blood sugar, thus is used as a quick-acting antidote for the hypoglycemic reaction of insulin. It stimulates the breakdown of glycogen (glycogenolysis) in the liver by activating the liver enzyme phosphorylase and thus raises blood sugar levels during fasting states to ensure adequate levels for normal nerve and brain function.

gluconeogenesis (Gr *gleukos*, sweetness; *neos*, new; *genesis*, production, generation) Production of glucose from keto-acid carbon skeleton from deaminated amino acids and the glycerol portion of fatty acids.

glucose tolerance factor (GTF) A biologically active complex of chromium and nicotinic acid that facilitates the reaction of insulin with receptor sites on tissues.

glyceride Group name for fats; any of a group of esters obtained from glycerol by the replacement of one, two, or three hydroxyl (OH) groups with a fatty acid. Monoglycerides contain one fatty acid; diglycerides contain two fatty acids; triglycerides contain three fatty acids. Glycerides are the principal constituent of adipose tissue and are found in animal and vegetable fats and oils.

glycerol A colorless, odorless, syrupy, sweet liquid; a constituent of fats usually obtained by the hydrolysis of fats. Chemically glycerol is an alcohol; it is esterified with fatty acids to produce fats.

glycogen (Gr *glykys,* sweet; *genes,* born, produced) A polysaccharide, that is, a large compound of many saccharide (i.e., sugar) units. It is the main body storage form of carbohydrate, largely stored (with relatively rapid turnover) in the liver, with lesser amounts stored in muscle tissue.

glycogenolysis (*glycogen* + Gr *lysis,* dissolution) Specific term for conversion of glycogen into glucose in the liver; chemical process of enzymatic hydrolysis or breakdown by which this conversion is accomplished.

glycolysis Initial energy production enzyme pathway outside the mitochondria, by which 6-carbon glucose is changed to active 3-carbon fragments of acetyl CoA, the fuel ready for final energy production in the mitochondria to the high-energy phosphate bond compound adenosine triphosphate (ATP).

goiter (L *guttur,* throat) Enlargement of the thyroid gland caused by lack of sufficient available iodine to produce the thyroid hormone, thyroxine.

gravida (L *gravida,* heavy, loaded) A pregnant woman.

growth acceleration (L *celerare,* to quicken) Period of increased speed of growth at different points of childhood development.

growth channel The progressive regular growth pattern of children, guided along individual genetically controlled channels, influenced by nutritional and health status.

growth chart grids Grids comparing stature (length), weight, and age of children by percentile; used for nutritional assessment to determine how their growth is progressing. The most commonly used grids are those of the National Center for Health Statistics (NCHS), by the Fels Research Institute.

growth deceleration (L *de,* from; *celerare,* to quicken) Period of decreased speed of growth at different points of childhood development.

growth velocity (L *velocitas,* speed) Rapidity of motion or movement; rate of childhood growth over normal periods of development, as compared with a population standard.

handicap Mental or physical defect that may or may not be congenital that prevents the individual from participating in normal life activities; implies disadvantage.

Heimlich maneuver A first-aid maneuver to relieve a person who is choking from blockage of the breathing passageway by a swallowed foreign object or food particle. Standing behind the person, clasp the victim around the waist, placing one fist just under the sternum (breastbone) and grasping the fist with the other hand. Then make a quick, hard, thrusting movement inward and upward to dislodge the object.

hematuria (Gr *haima,* blood; *ouron,* urine) The abnormal presence of blood in the urine.

heme iron Dietary iron from animal sources, from the heme portion of hemoglobin in red blood cells. Heme iron is more easily absorbed and transported in the body than nonheme iron from plant sources, but it supplies the smaller portion of the body's total dietary iron intake.

hemodialysis (Gr *haima,* blood; *dia,* through; *lysis,* dissolution) Removal of certain elements from the blood according to their rates of diffusion through a semipermeable membrane, e.g., by a hemodialysis machine.

hemoglobin (Gr *haima, blood;* L *globus,* a ball) Oxygen-carrying pigment in red blood cells; a conjugated protein containing four heme groups combined with iron and four long polypeptide chains forming the protein globin, named for its ball-like form; made by the developing red blood cells in bone marrow. Hemoglobin carries oxygen in the blood to body cells.

hemolytic anemia (Gr *haima,* blood; *lysis,* dissolution) An anemia (reduced number of red blood cells) caused by breakdown of red blood cells and loss of their hemoglobin.

hemophilia (Gr *hemo-,* blood; *philein,* to love) A heredity hemorrhagic disease caused by deficiency of blood coagulation factor VIII; characterized by spontaneous or traumatic bleeding; transmitted as an X-linked (maternal) recessive trait to male children. This X chromosome–linked deficiency of factor VIII has played a major role in the history of royal families of Europe.

hemosiderin (Gr *haima,* blood; *sideros,* iron) Insoluble iron oxide–protein compound in which iron is stored in the liver if the amount of iron in the blood exceeds the storage capacity of ferritin, for example, during rapid destruction of red blood cells (malaria, hemolytic anemia).

herpes zoster (Gr *herpēs,* herpes; *zoster,* a girdle or encircling structure or pattern) An acute self-limiting viral inflammatory disease of posterior nerve roots causing skin eruptions in a lateral pattern across the back of the torso served by these nerves, accompanied by neuralgic pain; caused by the virus of chickenpox and commonly called *shingles.*

homeostasis (Gr *homoios,* like, unchanging; *stasis,* standing, stable) State of relative dynamic equilibrium within the body's internal environment; a balance achieved through the operation of various interrelated physiologic mechanisms.

hormones Various internally secreted substances from the endocrine organs, which are conveyed by the blood to another organ or tissue on which they act to stimulate increased functional activity or secretion. This tissue or substance is called its target organ or substance.

hydrogenation Process of hardening liquid vegetable oils by injecting hydrogen gas to produce margarines and shortenings.

hydrolysis (Gr *hydro,* water; *lysis,* dissolution) Process by which a chemical compound is split into other simpler compounds by taking up the elements of water, as in the manufacture of infant formulas to produce easier-to-digest derivatives of the main protein casein in the cow's milk base. This process occurs naturally in digestion.

25-hydroxycholecalciferol (25, [OH]D$_3$) Initial product formed in the liver in the process of developing the active vitamin D hormone.

hygroscopic (Gr *hygros,* moist) Taking up and retaining moisture readily.

hypercapnia (Gr *hyper,* above; *kapnos,* smoke) Excess carbon dioxide in the blood.

hyperemesis gravidarum (Gr *hyper,* above, excessive; *emesis,* vomiting; L *gravida,* heavy loaded) Severe vomiting during pregnancy that is potentially fatal.

hyperlipoproteinemia (Gr *hyper,* above; *lipoprotein,* fat-protein compound; *-emia,* suffix referring to *haima,* blood) Elevated level of lipoproteins in the blood.

hypernatremia (Gr *hyper,* above; L *natron,* sodium; *haima,* blood) Excessive levels of sodium in the blood.

hyperparathyroidism (Gr *hyper,* above; *para,* along side; *thyroidism,* thyroid gland function and, by extension, parathyroid gland function) Abnormally increased activity of the parathyroid gland, resulting in excessive secretion of parathyroid hormone, which normally helps regulate serum calcium levels in balance with vitamin D hormone; excess secretion occurs when the serum calcium level falls below normal, as in chronic renal disease or in vitamin D deficiency.

hypovolemia (Gr *hypo,* under; *haima,* blood) Abnormally decreased volume of circulating blood in the body.

hypoxemia (Gr *hypo,* under; *-ox-,* oxygen; *emia (haima),* blood) Deficient oxygenation of the blood, resulting in *hypoxia,* reduced oxygen supply to tissue.

iatrogenic (Gr *iatros,* healer; *genesis,* origin or source) Describing a medical disorder caused by physician diagnosis, manner, or treatment.

icterus (Gr *ikteros,* jaundice) Alternate term for jaundice: **nonicteric** indicates absence of jaundice; **preicteric** indicates a state prior to development of icterus, or jaundice.

immunocompetence (L *immunis,* free, exempt) The ability or capacity to develop an immune response—that is, antibody production and/or cell-mediated immunity—following exposure to antigen.

incomplete protein food A protein food having a ratio of amino acids different from that of the average body protein and therefore less valuable for nutrition than complete protein food.

indole A compound produced in the intestines by the decomposition of tryptophan; also found in the oil of jasmine and clove.

infarct (L *infarcire,* to stuff in) An area of tissue necrosis caused by local ischemia, resulting from obstruction of blood circulation to that area.

insulin (L *insula,* island) Hormone formed in the B cells of the islets of Langerhans in the pancreas. Insulin is secreted when blood glucose and amino acid levels rise and assists their entry into body cells. It also promotes glycogenesis and conversion of glucose into fat and inhibits lipolysis and gluconeogenesis (protein breakdown). Commercial insulin is manufactured from pigs and cows; new "artificial" human insulin products have recently been made available.

interferon (L *inter,* between; *ferire,* to strike) One of a class of small soluble proteins produced and released by cells invaded by a virus, which induces in noninfected cells the formation of an antiviral protein that interferes with viral multiplication.

intermittent claudication (L *claudicatio,* limping or lameness) A symptomatic pattern of peripheral vascular disease, characterized by absence of pain or discomfort in a limb, usually the legs, when at rest, which is followed by pain and weakness when walking, intensifying until walking becomes impossible, and then disappearing again after a rest period; seen in occlusive arterial disease.

interstitial fluid (L *inter,* between; *sistere,* to set) The fluid situated between parts or in the interspaces of a tissue.

intima (L *intima,* inner area) General term indicating an innermost part of a structure or vessel; inner layer of the blood vessel wall.

intramural nerve plexus (L *intra,* within; *murus,* wall; plexus, plait or network) Network of nerves in the walls of the intestine that make up the enteric nervous system controlling muscle action and secretions for digestion and absorption.

ischemia (Gr *ischein,* to suppress; *haima,* blood) Deficiency of blood to a particular tissue, caused by functional blood vessel constriction or actual obstruction.

jaundice (Fr *jaune,* yellow) A syndrome characterized by hyperbilirubinemia and deposits of bile pigment in the skin, mucous membranes, and sclera, giving a yellow appearance to the patient.

joule (James Prescott Joule, 1818-1889, English physicist) The international (SI) unit of energy and heat, defined as the work done by the force of 1 newton acting over the distance of 1 meter. A newton (named for Sir Isaac Newton, 1643-1727, English mathematician, physicist, and astronomer) is the international unit of force, defined as the amount of force that, when applied in a vacuum to a body having a mass of 1 kg, accelerates it at the rate of 1 meter per second. These are examples of the exactness with which terms and values used by the world's scientific community must be defined, as illustrated in the *Système International d'Unités (SI).*

keratinization The process of creating the protein *keratin,* which is the principal constituent of skin, hair, nails, horny tissues, and the organizing matrix of the enamel of the teeth. It is a very insoluble protein.

keto acid Amino acid residue after deamination. The glycogenic keto acids are used to form carbohydrates. The ketogenic keto acids are used to form fats.

kilocalorie (Fr *chilioi,* thousand; L *calor,* heat) The general term **calorie** refers to a unit of heat measure and is used alone to designate the *small calorie.* The calorie used in nutritional science and the study of metabolism is the *large calorie,* 1000 calories, or kilocalori (kcalorie), to be more accurate and avoid use of very large numbers in calculations.

kinetic (Gr *kinetikos,* moving) Energy released from body fuels by cell metabolism and now active in moving muscles and energizing all body activities.

kyphosis (Gr *hyphos,* a hump) Increased, abnormal convexity of the upper part of the spine; hunchback.

lactase Enzyme that splits the disaccharide lactose into its two monosaccharides, glucose and galactose.

lactated Ringer's solution Sterile solution of calcium chloride, potassium chloride, sodium chloride, and sodium lactate in water given to replenish fluid and electrolytes; developed by English physiologist Sydney Ringer (1835-1910).

lactiferous ducts (L *lac,* milk; *ferre,* to bear) Branching channels in the mammary gland that carry breast milk to holding spaces near the nipple, ready for the infant's feeding.

limiting amino acid The amino acid in foods occurring in the smallest amount, thus limiting its availability for tissue structure.

linoleic acid The ultimate essential fatty acid for humans.

lipase (Gr *lipos,* fat; *-ase,* enzyme) Group of fat enzymes that cut the ester linkages between the fatty acids and glycerol of triglycerides (fats).

lipids (Gr *lipos,* fat) Chemical group name for fats and fat-related compounds such as cholesterol, lipoproteins, and phospholipids; general group name for organic substances of a fatty nature, including fats, oils, waxes, and related compounds.

lipoprotein Noncovalent complexes of fat with protein. The lipoproteins function as major carriers of lipids in the plasma, since most of the plasma fat is associated with them. Such a combination makes possible the transport of fatty substances in a water medium such as plasma.

lumen (L *lumen,* light) The cavity or channel within a tube or tubular organ, such as the intestines.

lymphocytes (L *lympho-,* water; Gr *kytos,* hollow vessel, suffix for a cell type of the root to which it is designated or attached) Special white cells from lymphoid tissue that participate in humeral and cell-mediated immunity.

lymphoma (L *lympha,* water; Gr *sōma,* body) General term applied to any neoplastic disorder (cancer) of the lymphoid tissue.

macrocytic anemia (Gr *makros,* large; *cyte,* hollow vessel, cell) An anemia (deficiency of normal red cells) characterized by abnormally large red cells.

macronutrients (Gr *makros,* large; L *nutriens,* nourishment) The three large energy-yielding nutrients: carbohydrates, fats, and proteins.

malignant (L *malignare,* to act suspiciously) An abnormal condition such as a tumor that tends to become progressively worse and results in death.

malignant melanoma (L *malignans,* acting maliciously; Gr *melos,* black) A tumor tending to become progressively worse, composed of melanin, the dark pigment of the skin and other body tissues, usually arising from the skin and aggravated by excessive sun exposure.

maltase Enzyme that breaks down the disaccharide maltose into two units of glucose, a monosaccharide.

median (L *medianus,* middle, midpoint) In statistics, the middle number in a sequence of numbers.

medical foods Specially formulated nutrient mixtures for use under medical supervision to treat various metabolic diseases.

medulla (L *medulla,* marrow, center) General term for the inner or central portion of an organ or structure. The renal medulla is the inner part of the kidney, holding the lower parts (loop of Henle and collecting tubule) of the nephron, which are organized grossly into pyramids with glomerular heads of the nephrons in the outer portion (cortex) of the kidney.

megaloblastic anemia (Gr *mega,* great size; *blastos,* embryo, germ) Anemia resulting from faulty production of abnormally large immature red blood cells, caused by a deficiency of vitamin B_{12} and folate.

menadione The parent compound of vitamin K in the body; called also *vitamin* K_3.

menaquinone Form of vitamin K synthesized by intestinal bacteria; called also *vitamin* K_2.

menarche (Gr *men,* month; *arche,* beginning) The beginning of first menstruation with the onset of puberty.

meningitis (Gr *meninx,* membrane) Inflammation of the *meninges,* the three membranes that envelop the brain and spinal cord, caused by a bacterial or viral infection and characterized by high fever, severe headache, and stiff neck or back muscles.

metabolism (Gr *metaballein,* to change, alter) Sum of all the various biochemical and physiologic processes by which the body grows and maintains itself **(anabolism)** and breaks down and reshapes tissue **(catabolism),** transforming energy to do its work. Products of these various reactions are called **metabolites.**

metabolite Any substance produced by metabolism or by a metabolic process.

micellar bile-fat complex (L *mica,* crumb, particle) A combination of bile and fat in which the bile emulsifies fat into very minute globules or particles that can be absorbed easily into the small intestine wall in preparation for the final stage of absorption into circulation to the cells.

microaneurysm (Gr *mikros,* small; *aneurysma,* a widening) A small sac formed by the widening of the wall of small blood vessels; diabetic aneurysms may form in the basement membrane of capillaries throughout vascular beds, as in the eye.

micronutrients (Gr *mikros,* small; L *nutriens,* nourishment) The two classes of small non-energy-yielding elements and compounds—minerals and vitamins—essential in very small amounts for regulation and control functions in cell metabolism and building certain body structures.

microvilli (Gr *mikros,* small; L *villus,* tuft of hair) Minute vascular structures protruding from the surface of villi covering the inner surface of the small intestine, forming a "brush border" that facilitates absorption of nutrients.

monosaccharide (Gr *mono,* single; *sakcharon,* sugar) Simple single sugar; a carbohydrate containing a single saccharide (sugar) unit.

motivation Forces that affect individual goal-directed behavior toward satisfying needs or achieving personal goals.

mucosa (L *mucus*) The mucous membrane comprising the inner surface layer of gastrointestinal tract tissues, providing extensive nutrient absorption and transport functions.

mucus Viscid fluid secreted by mucous membranes and glands, consisting mainly of mucin (a glycoprotein), inorganic salts, and water. Mucus serves to lubricate and protect the gastrointestinal mucosa and to help move the food mass along the digestive tract.

myasthenia gravis (Gr *mys*, muscle; *asthenia*, weakness; L *gravis*, heavy, weighty, grave) A progressive neuromuscular disease caused by faulty nerve conduction resulting from the presence of antibodies to acetylcholine receptors at the neuromuscular junction.

myelin (Gr *myelos*, marrow) High lipid-to-protein substance forming a fatty sheath to insulate and protect neuron axons and facilitate their neuromuscular impulses.

myelin sheath (Gr *myelos*, marrow; *thēkē*, sheath) Covering of myelin, a lipid-protein substance with a high fat proportion to protein, surrounding nerve axons; serves as electrical insulator and speeds the conduction of nerve impulses; interrupted at intervals along the length of the axon by gaps known as Ranvier's nodes.

myofibril (Gr mys, muscle; L *fibrilla*, very small fiber) Slender thread of muscle; runs parallel to the muscle fiber's long axis.

myofilaments (Gr *mys*, muscle; L *filare*, to wind thread, spin) Threadlike filaments of actin or myosin, which are components of myofibrils.

myosin (Gr *mys*, muscle) Myofibril protein whose synchronized meshing action in conjunction with **actin** causes muscles to contract and relax.

necrosis (Gr *nekrosis*, deadness) Cell death caused by progressive enzyme breakdown.

neoplasm (Gr *neos*, new; *plasma*, formation) Any new or abnormal cellular growth, specifically one that is uncontrolled and progressive.

nephron (Gr *nephros*, kidney) Microscopic anatomic and functional unit of the kidney that selectively filters and reabsorbs essential blood factors, secretes hydrogen ions as needed for maintaining acid-base balance, then reabsorbs water to protect body fluids, and forms and excretes a concentrated urine for elimination of wastes. The nephron includes the renal corpuscle (glomerulus), the proximal convoluted tubule, the loop of Henle, the distal convoluted tubule, and the collecting tubule, which empties the urine into the renal medulla. The urine passes into the papilla and then to the pelvis of the kidney. Urine is formed by filtration of blood in the glomerulus and by the selective reabsorption and secretion of solutes by cells that comprise the walls of the renal tubules. There are approximately 1 million nephrons in each kidney.

nephropathy (Gr *nephros*, kidney; *pathos*, disease) Disease of the kidneys; in diabetes, renal damage associated with functional and pathologic changes in the nephrons, which can lead to glomerulosclerosis and chronic renal failure.

nephrosis (Gr *nephros*, kidney) Nephrotic syndrome caused by degenerative epithelial lesions of the renal tubules of the nephrons, especially the *mesangium*, the thin basement membrane that helps support the capillary loops in a renal glomerulus; marked by edema, albuminuria, and decreased serum albumin.

neuropathy (Gr *neuron*, nerve; *pathos*, disease) General term for functional and pathologic changes in the peripheral nervous system; in diabetes, a chronic sensory condition affecting mainly the nerves of the legs, marked by numbness from sensory impairment, loss of tendon reflexes, severe pain, weakness, and wasting of muscles involved.

niacin equivalent (NE) A measure of the total dietary sources of niacin equivalent to 1 mg of niacin. Thus an NE is 1 mg of niacin or 60 mg of tryptophan.

night blindness Inability to see well at night in diminished light, resulting from lack of required vitamin A.

nitrogen balance The metabolic balance between nitrogen intake in dietary protein and output in urinary nitrogen compounds such as urea and creatinine. For every 6.25 g dietary protein consumed, 1 g nitrogen is excreted.

nonheme iron The larger portion of dietary iron, including all the plant food sources and 60% of the animal food sources, which lacks the more easily absorbed and bioavailable heme iron in the remaining 40% of the animal food sources that contain hemoglobin residues of iron-containing heme.

norepinephrine (*nor-*, prefix, normal or parent form of a compound; Gr *epi-*, on, upon, or over; *nephros*, kidney) One of the catecholamines; a neurohormone, principal neurotransmitter of adrenergic nerves; secreted by inner part of the adrenal glands, which lie on top of the kidneys.

nulligravida (L *nullus*, none; *gravida*, pregnant) A woman who has never been pregnant.

nutrients (L *nutriens*, nourishment) Substances in food that are essential for energy, growth, normal functioning of the body, and maintenance of life.

nutrition (L *nutritio*, nourishment) The sum of the processes involved in taking in food nutrients, assimilating and using them to maintain body tissue and provide energy; a foundation for life and health.

nutritional science The body of scientific knowledge, developed through controlled research, that relates to the processes involved in nutrition—national, international, community, and clinical.

obesity (L *obesus*, excessively fat) Fatness; an excessive accumulation of fat in the body.

occult bleeding (L *occultus*, concealed) Obscure, difficult to detect, concealed from observation; such a small blood loss that it can be detected only by a microscope or chemical test.

oligosaccharides (Gr *oligos*, little; *saccharide*, sugar) Intermediate products of polysaccharide carbohydrate breakdown that contain a small number (from 4 to 10) of single sugar units of the monosaccharide glucose.

oliguria (Gr *oligos*, little; *ouron*, urine) Secretion of a very small amount of urine in relation to fluid intake.

oncogene (Gr *onkos*, mass; *genesis*, generation, production) Any of various genes that, when activated as by radiation or a virus, may cause a normal cell to become cancerous; viral genetic material carrying the potential of cancer and passed from parent to offspring.

organic (Gr *organikos*, organ) Carbon-based chemical compounds.

orthotopic (Gr *ortho*, straight, normal, correct; *topos*, place) Occurring at the normal place in the body; placement of a transplanted organ in the position formerly occupied by tissue of the same kind.

osmolality (Gr *osmos*, impulse, osmotic force) Property of a solution that depends on the concentration of the solute per unit of the solvent.

osteodystrophy (Gr *osteon*, bone) Defective bone formation.

osteoporosis (Gr *osteon*, bone; *poros*, passage, pore) Abnormal thinning of bone, producing a porous, fragile, latticelike bone tissue of enlarged spaces that is prone to fracture or deformity.

palliative (L *palliatus*, cloaked) Care affording relief but not cure; useful for comfort when cure is still unknown or obscured.

palmar grasp (L *palma*, palm) Early grasp of the young infant, clasping an object in the palm and wrapping the whole hand around it.

pancreatic enzyme preparations Commercial preparations of pancreatic enzymes—protease, lipase, and amylase—that have the same action as do the human enzymes from the pancreas; used in the treatment of pancreatic insufficiency.

pandemic (Gr *pan*, all; *dēmos*, people) A widespread epidemic, distributed through a region, continent, or the world.

pantothenic acid (Gr *pantothen*, "from all sides" or "in every corner") A B vitamin found widely distributed in nature and occurring throughout the body tissues. Pantothenic acid is an essential constituent of coenzyme A, which has extensive metabolic responsibility as an activating agent of a number of compounds in many tissues.

paradigm (Gr *para*, side-by-side; *deiknynai*, to show) A pattern or model serving as an example; a standard or ideal for practice or behavior based on a fundamental value or theme.

parasite (Gr *para*, along side; *sitos*, food, grain; *parasitos*, one who eats at another's table; in ancient Greece, a term for a person who received free meals in return for amusing or flattering conversation) An organism that lives on or in an organism of another species, known as the host, from whom all life-cycle nourishment is obtained.

parenchymal cells (Gr *parenchyma*, "anything poured in beside") Functional cells of an organ, as distinguished from the cells comprising its structure or framework.

parenteral (Gr *para*, along side, beyond, accessory; *enteron*, intestine) A mode of feeding that does not use the gastrointestinal tract but instead provides nutrition by intravenous delivery of nutrient solutions.

paresthesia (Gr *para*, beyond; *aisthesis*, perception) Abnormal sensations such as prickling, burning, and "crawling" of skin.

parity (L *parere*, to bring forth, produce) The condition of a woman with respect to having borne viable offspring.

pepsin The main gastric enzyme specific for proteins. Pepsin begins breaking large protein molecules into shorter chain polypeptides, proteoses, and peptones. Gastric hydrochloric acid is necessary to activate pepsin.

peptide bond The characteristic joining of amino acids to form proteins. Such a chain of amino acids is termed a peptide. Depending on its size, it may be a dipeptide fragment of protein digestion or a large polypeptide.

percentile (L *per*, throughout, in space or time; *centrum*, a hundred) One of 100 equal parts of a measured series of values; rate or proportion per hundred.

peristalsis (Gr *peri*, around; *stalsis*, contraction) A wavelike progression of alternate contraction and relaxation of the muscle fibers of the gastrointestinal tract.

peritoneal dialysis Dialysis through the peritoneum into and out of the peritoneal cavity.

peritoneum (Gr *per*, around; *teinein*, to stretch) A strong smooth surface, a serous membrane, lining the abdominal/pelvic walls and the undersurface of the diaphragm, forming a sac enclosing the body's vital visceral organs within the peritoneal cavity.

pernicious anemia A chronic macrocytic anemia occurring most commonly after age 40. It is caused by absence of the intrinsic factor normally present in the gastric juices and necessary for the absorption of cobalamin vitamin B_{12} and controlled by intramuscular injections of vitamin B_{12}.

phagocytes (Gr *phagein*, to eat; *kytos*, hollow vessel, cell) Cells that ingest microorganisms, other cells, or foreign particles; macrophages.

phospholipid Any of a class of fat-related substances that contain phosphorus, fatty acids, and a nitrogenous base. The phospholipids are essential elements in every cell.

photosynthesis (Gr *photos*, light; *synthesis*, putting together) Process by which plants containing chlorophyll are able to manufacture carbohydrate by combining CO_2 from air and water from soil. Sunlight is used as energy; chlorophyll is a catalyst. $6 CO_2 + 6 H_2O + Energy \rightarrow$ Chlorophyll $\rightarrow C_6H_{12}O_6 + 6 O_2$

phylloquinone A fat-soluble vitamin of the K group, $C_3H_{46}O_2$, found in green plants or prepared synthetically.

physiologic age (Gr *physis*, nature; *logikos*, or speech or reason) Rate of biologic maturation in individual adolescents that varies widely and accounts more for wide and changing differences in their metabolic rates, nutritional needs, and food requirements than does chronologic age.

pincer grasp Later digital grasp of the older infant, usually picking up smaller objects with a precise grip between thumb and forefinger.

placenta (L *placenta*, a flat cake) Special organ developed in early pregnancy that provides nutrients to the fetus and removes metabolic waste.

plaque (Fr *plaque*, patch or flat area) Thickened deposits of fatty material, largely cholesterol, within the arterial wall that eventually may fill the lumen and cut off blood supply to the tissue served by the damaged vessel.

polysaccharides (Gr *poly*, many; *saccharide*, sugar) Class of complex carbohydrates composed of many monosaccharide units. Common members are starch, dextrins, dietary fiber, and glycogen.

portal An entryway, usually referring to the portal circulation of blood through the liver. Blood is brought into the liver by the portal vein and out by the hepatic vein.

postprandial (L *post* after; *prandium*, breakfast, a meal) Occurring after a meal.

potential (L *potentia*, power) Energy existing in stored fuels and ready for action, but not yet released and active.

prealbumin (PAB) Plasma protein with short life used as a biochemical measure for assessing current nutritional status.

precursor (L *praecursor*, a forerunner) Something that precedes; in biology, a substance from which another substance is derived.

primigravida (L *prima*, first; *gravida*, pregnant) A woman pregnant for the first time.

proctocolectomy (Gr *prŏktos*, anus; *-col-*, colon; *ektomē*, excision) Surgical removal of the rectum and colon.

proenzyme An inactive precursor converted to the active enzyme by the action of an acid, another enzyme, or other means; also called zymogen.

prostaglandins (Gr *prostates*, standing before; L *glans*, acorn; hence, male prostate gland) Group of naturally occurring substances, first discovered in semen, derived from long-chain fatty acids that have multiple local hormonelike actions, including regulation of gastric acid secretion, platelet aggregation, body temperature, and tissue inflammation.

protein balance (Gr *protos*, first) Body tissue protein balance between building up tissue (**anabolism**) and breaking down tissue (**catabolism**) to maintain healthy body growth and maintenance.

proteinuria (Gr *protos*, first, protein; *ouron*, urine) The presence of an excess of serum proteins, such as albumin in the urine.

prothrombin (Gr *pro*, before; *thrombos*, clot) Blood-clotting factor (number II) synthesized in the liver from glutamic acid and carbon dioxide, catalyzed by vitamin K.

P/S ratio Ratio of polyunsaturated to saturated fats in the diet.

public health nutritionist A professional nutritionist, accredited by academic degree course of university and special graduate study (MPH, DrPH) in schools of public health accredited by the American Association of Public Health, responsible for nutrition components of public health programs in varied community settings—county, state, national, international.

pulmonary edema Accumulation of fluid in tissues of the lung.

pyrosis (Gr *pyro*, fire, burning) Heartburn.

raffinose (Fr *raffin*, to refine) A colorless crystalline trisaccharide component of legumes, composed of galactose and sucrose connected by bonds that human enzymes cannot break, thus it remains whole in the intestines and produces gas as bacteria attack it.

receptor (L *receptor*, receiver) Any one of various specific protein molecules in surface membranes of cells and cell organelles, to which complementary molecules (such as hormones, neurotransmitters, drugs, viruses, or other antigens or antibodies) may become bound.

Recommended Dietary Allowances (RDAs) Recommended daily allowances of nutrients and energy intake for population groups according to age and sex, with defined weight and height. The RDAs are established and reviewed periodically by a representative group of nutritional scientists in response to current research. These standards vary very little among the developed countries.

Registered Dietitian (RD) A professional dietitian, accredited by academic degree course of university and graduate study (MS, PhD), clinical and administration training, and passing required registration examinations administered by the American Dietetic Association.

renal solute load (L *ren*, kidney) Collective number and concentration of solute particles in a solution, carried by the blood to the kidney nephrons for excretion in the urine. These particles are usually nitrogenous products from protein metabolism and the electrolytes Na^+, K^+, Cl-, and $HPO_4=$.

renin-angiotensin-aldosterone mechanism Three-stage system of sodium conservation, hence control of water loss, in response to diminished filtration pressure in the kidney nephrons: (1) pressure loss causes kidney to secrete the enzyme renin, which combines with and activates angiotensinogen from the liver; (2) active angiotensin stimulates of the adjacent adrenal gland to release the hormone aldosterone; (3) the hormone causes reabsorption of sodium from the kidney nephrons and water follows.

replicate (L *replicare*, to fold back) To make an exact copy; to repeat, duplicate, or reproduce. In genetics, replication is the process by which double-stranded DNA makes copies of itself, each separating strand synthesizing a complementary strand. Cell replication is the process by which living cells, under gene control, make exact copies of themselves a programmed number of times during the life span of the organism. The process can be reproduced in the laboratory with cultured cell lines for special studies in cell biology.

resting metabolic rate (RMR) Amount of energy required to maintain the resting body's internal activities when in a normal environment temperature. Because of small differences in measuring techniques, RMR may be slightly different from the same person's **basal metabolic rate (BMR).** In practice, however, RMR and BMR measurments may be used interchangeably.

retinal Organic compound that is the aldehyde form of **retinol,** derived by the enzymatic splitting of absorbed carotene. It performs vitamin A activity. In the retina of the eye, retinal combines with opsins to form visual pigments. In the rods it combines with scotopsin to form rhodopsin (visual purple). In the cones it combines with photopsin to form the three pigments responsible for color vision.

retinol Chemical name for vitamin A, derived from its function relating to the retina of the eye and light-dark adaptation. Daily RDA standards are stated in retinol equivalents (RE) to account for sources of the preformed vitamin A and its precursor provitamin A, beta-carotene.

retinol Equivalent (RE) Unit of measure for dietary sources of vitamin A, both preformed vitamin, retinol, and the precursor provitamin, beta-carotene. 1 RE = 1 μg retinol or 6 μg beta-carotene.

retinopathy (L *rete*, net, network; *retina*, innermost layer covering the eyeball; *pathos*, disease) Noninflammatory disease of the retina, visual tissue of the eye, characterized by microaneurysms, intraretinal hemorrhages, waxy yellow exudates, "cotton wool" patches, and macular edema; a complication of diabetes that may lead to proliferation of fibrous tissue, retinal detachment, and blindness.

retrovirus (L *retro-*, backward) Any of a family of single-strand RNA viruses having an envelope and containing a reverse coding enzyme that allows for a reversal of genetic transcription from RNA to DNA rather than the usual DNA to RNA, the newly transcribed viral DNA then being incorporated into the host cell's DNA strand for the production of new RNA retroviruses.

rooting reflex A reflex in a newborn in which stimulation of the side of the cheek or the upper or lower lip causes the infant to turn its mouth and face to the stimulus.

sarcoma (Gr *sarkos*, flesh; *onkoma*, a swelling) Tumors, usually malignant, arising from connective tissue.

saturated (L *saturare*, to fill) To cause to unite with the greatest possible amount of another substance through solution, chemical combination, or the like. A saturated fat, for example, is one in which the component fatty acids are filled with hydrogen atoms. A fatty acid is said to be saturated if all available chemical bonds of its carbon chain are filled with hydrogen. If one bond remains unfilled, it is a monounsaturated fatty acid. If two or more bonds remain unfilled, it is a polyunsaturated fatty acid. Fats of animal sources are more saturated. Fats of plant sources are unsaturated.

scurvy A hemorrhagic disease caused by lack of vitamin C. Diffuse tissue bleeding occurs, limbs and joints are painful and swollen, bones thicken as a result of subperiosteal hemorrhage, ecchymoses (large irregular discolored skin areas caused by tissue hemorrhages) form, bones fracture easily, wounds do not heal well, gums are swollen and bleeding, and teeth loosen.

sebaceous (L *sebum*, suet) Secreting the fatty lubricating substance *sebum*.

secretin Hormone produced in the mucous membrane of the duodenum in response to the entrance of the acid contents of the stomach into the duodenum. Secretin in turn stimulates the flow of pancreatic juice, providing needed enzymes and the proper alkalinity for their action.

senescence (L *senescere*, to grow old) The process of growing old; a consequence of advancing age or of premature aging process from disease.

sepsis (Gr *sēpsis*, decay) Presence in the blood or other tissues of pathogenic microorganisms or their toxins; conditions associated with such pathogens.

serosa Outer surface layer of the intestines interfacing with the blood vessels of the portal system going to the liver.

serotonin A neurotransmitter in the brain that effectively suppresses appetite and heavy eating.

solutes (Gr *solvere*, to solve) Particles of a substance in solution; a solution consists of solutes and a dissolving medium (solvent), usually a liquid.

somatostatin (Gr *soma*, body; *stasis*, standing still, maintaining a constant level) A hormone formed in the D cells of the pancreatic islets of Langerhans and the hypothalamus. It is a balancing factor in maintaining normal blood glucose levels by inhibiting insulin and glucagon production in the pancreas as needed.

spina bifida (L *spina*, spine; *bifidus*, cleft into two parts or branches) Congenital defect in the fetal closing of the neural tube to form a portion of the lower spine, leaving the spine unclosed and the spinal cord open in various degrees of exposure and damage.

sprue Alternate term for adult celiac disease, a malabsorption syndrome.

steroids (Gr *stereos*, solid; L *-ol, oleum*, oil) Group name for lipid-based sterols, including hormones, bile acids, and cholesterol.

stoma (Gr *stoma*, mouth, opening) The opening established in the abdominal wall, connecting with the ileum or colon, for elimination of intestinal wastes after surgical removal of diseased portions of the intestinal tract.

stomatitis (Gr *stoma*, mouth; *-itis*, inflammation) Inflammation of the oral mucosa, especially the buccal tissue lining the inside of the cheeks, but also possibly the tongue, palate, floor of the mouth, and gums.

stroke volume (Gr *streich*, to strike or stretch) The amount of blood pumped from a ventricle (chamber of the heart releasing blood to body circulations) with each beat of the heart.

substrate (L *sub*, under; *stratum*, layer) The specific organic substance on which a particular enzyme acts to produce new metabolic products.

sucrase Enzyme splitting the disaccharide sucrose into its two monosaccharides of glucose and fructose.

synergism (Gr *syn*, with or together; *ergon*, work) The joint action of separate agents in which the total effect of their combined action is greater than the sum of their separate actions. (Adjective: **synergistic.**)

synosheath (Gr *syno-*, with, together; *thēkē*, sheath) Protective pliable connective tissue surrounding the bony-collagen meshwork and fluid that come together in the synovial area between major bone heads in joints, allows normal padded and lubricated joint movement and motion.

tachycardia (Gr *tachys*, swift; *kardia*, heart) Excessively rapid action of the heart; usually applied to a heart rate above 100 beats per minute.

tactile (L *tactus*, touch) Pertaining to the sense of touch.

taurine A sulfur-containing amino acid, $NH_2(CH_2)_2 SO_2OH$, formed from the essential amino acid methionine. It is found in various body tissues, such as lungs and muscles, and in bile and breast milk.

thermic effect of food (Gr *therme*, heat, of or pertaining to heat) Body heat produced by food; amount of energy required to digest and absorb food and transport nutrients to the cells. This basic preparatory work accounts for about 10% of the day's total energy (kcalories) requirement.

thiamin pyrophosphate (TPP) Activating coenzyme form of thiamin that plays a key role in carbohydrate metabolism.

tocopherol (Gr *tokos*, childbirth; *pherein*, to carry) Chemical name for vitamin E. It was so named by early investigators because their initial work with rats indicated a reproductive function, which did not turn out to be the case with humans. In humans it functions as a strong antioxidant to preserve structural membranes, such as cell walls.

transmural (L *trans-*, through; *murrus*, wall) Through the wall of an organ; extending through or affecting the entire thickness of the wall of an organ or cavity.

triglyceride (Gr *tri*, three) Chemical name for fat, indicating structure: attachment of three fatty acids to a glycerol base; a neutral fat, synthesized from carbohydrate and stored in adipose tissue. It releases free fatty acids into the blood when hydrolyzed by enzymes.

trypsin (Gr *trypein*, to rub; *pepsis*, digestion) A protein-splitting enzyme formed in the intestine by action of enterokinase on the inactive precursor trypsinogen.

vagotomy (L *vagus*, wandering; Gr *tomē*, a cutting) A cutting of the vagus nerve (tenth cranial nerve), which regulates muscular and secretory actions of the stomach.

valence (L *valens*, powerful) Power of an element or a radical to combine with or to replace other elements or radicals. Atoms of various elements combine in definite proportions. The valence number of an element is the number of atoms of hydrogen with which one atom of the element can combine.

varices (plural form) (L *varix* [singular], enlarged vein) Varicose veins; enlarged and tortuous veins, full of twists, turns, curves, or windings.

vasoactive (L *vas*, vessel) Having an effect on the diameter of blood vessels.

ventricle (L *venter*, belly, abdomen; *ventriculus*, diminutive form indicating relation to front aspect of the body) A small cavity; one of the pair of lower chambers of the heart, with thick muscular walls, that make up the bulk of the heart. The ventricles receive blood from the atria and in turn force blood out into body circulation to the lungs for oxygenation and then into systemic body circulation to service the cells.

villi (L *villus*, "tuft of hair") Small protrusions from the surface of a membrane; fingerlike projections covering the mucosal surfaces of the small intestine.

virus (L *virus*, poison; *virion*, individual virus particle) Minute infectious agent characterized by lack of independent metabolism and by the ability to reproduce with genetic continuity only within living host cells. Viruses range in decreasing size from about 200 nanometers (nm) down to only 15 nanometers (nm). (A nanometer is a linear measure equal to one-billionth of a meter; it is also called a millimicron.) Each particle (virion) consists basically of nucleic acids (genetic material) and a protein shell that protects and contains the genetic material and any enzymes present.

viscous (viscid) (L *viscidus*, glutinous or sticky) Physical property of a substance dependent on the friction of its component molecules as they slide by one another; viscosity.

VO$_2$max Maximum uptake volume of oxygen during exercise; used to measure the intensity and duration of exercise a person can perform.

xanthoma (Gr *xanthos*, yellow; *-oma*, mass or body of material) A plaque of yellow lipid deposits in the skin; fatty streaks or nodules.

Zollinger-Ellison syndrome An intractable, sometimes fulminating atypical peptic ulcer disease, characterized by extreme gastric hyperacidity.

$\mathcal{I}$NDEX